DORLAND'S
MEDICAL
SPELLER

DORLAND'S MEDICAL SPELLER

Second Edition

Consultant
ELLEN DRAKE, CMT, FAAMT

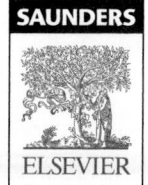

SAUNDERS

ELSEVIER

SAUNDERS
ELSEVIER

11830 Westline Industrial Drive
St. Louis, Missouri 63146

DORLAND'S MEDICAL SPELLER   ISBN: 978-1-4160-4573-1

Library of Congress Cataloging-in-Publication Data
Dorland's medical speller / Ellen Drake [consultant]. -- 2nd ed.
     p. ; cm.
     ISBN 978-1-4160-4573-1 (pbk. : alk. paper) 1. Medicine--Terminology.
I. Drake, Ellen, 1948- II. Dorland, W. A. Newman (William Alexander
Newman), 1864-1956. III. Title: Medical speller.
     [DNLM: 1. Medicine--Terminology--English. W 15 D711 2008]
     R123.D67 2008
     610.1'4--dc22
                               2008025101

Publishing Director: Andrew Allen
Acquisitions Editor: Jennifer Allen
Developmental Editor: Kelly Brinkman
Publishing Services Manager: Patricia Tannian
Design Direction: Renee Duenow

Working together to grow
libraries in developing countries

www.elsevier.com | www.bookaid.org | www.sabre.org

ELSEVIER   BOOK AID International   Sabre Foundation

Printed in United States of America

Last digit is the print number: 9   8   7   6   5   4   3   2   1

To all the medical transcriptionists
who over the years have asked for a revision
and to all those who have just wished silently for one

Preface

No book can attempt to present more than a small fraction of the large and growing body of medical terminology. The aim of this edition of the *Dorland's Medical Speller* is to present as many medical terms as possible within the confines of a book of reasonable size. Although this book was written primarily for medical transcriptionists, others who need a quick, accurate, and fairly comprehensive medical spelling reference may find it useful. Health information managers, abstractors, coders, nurses, ward clerks, court reporters, legal secretaries, medical assistants, allied health students, physicians, pharmacists, and even medical editors may appreciate a quick, easy-to-use alphabetical reference that provides correct spellings and capitalization for so many medical terms.

Although it is impossible to include the entire biomedical vocabulary, we have attempted to make this book as complete as possible. Our consultant, Ellen Drake, CMT, FAAMT, has added a large number of entries and expanded the cross-referencing, making it even easier to find a term. Outdated terms, obscure chemical terms, and terms relating to the plant and animal kingdoms have been culled to make room for the extensive new material. Except for anesthetics, imaging agents, and a few drugs that may appear in laboratory reports, drugs have not been included in this reference, primarily because it is impossible to keep them up to date in a reference that is not revised yearly. *Saunders Pharmaceutical Word Book and CD* is an excellent resource for up-to-date information on drugs.

Although we have exhaustively researched and documented the terms in this book, no book is ever perfect. We hope that you, our readers, will let us know if you find an error or note a glaring omission. To do so, please call Elsevier Customer Service toll-free at 1-800-545-2522.

Acknowledgments

Many thanks and hugs to my faithful friends, Georgia and Susan. I owe a huge debt of gratitude to my employer, Sally Pitman of Health Professions Institute, who graciously allowed me to take off huge amounts of time to work on this project. You three have encouraged me and lifted me up, and I love that you love me no matter what. To Peg Nelson, my dear friend and assistant, I am so appreciative of your attention to detail, alertness, and critical thinking. You went beyond what I asked of you, and that has made a difference in the book. Jennifer Weidley also provided some helpful research, and I appreciate her efforts.

I am grateful beyond words to have been blessed with a wonderful editor, Loren Wilson, and development editor, Lynda Huenefeld. You believed in the project and believed in me, you tolerated my occasional vents and whining with grace and tact, and you cut me some slack when I needed it. To Jennifer Allen and Kelly Brinkman, who replaced Loren and Lynda when we *thought* we were near the end of the project but were really in the thick of it: you've shown patience and understanding, but you must have been tearing your hair out at times. Thanks also go to Doug Anderson, Chief Lexicographer for the *Dorland's Illustrated Medical Dictionary*, and the entire Elsevier development team, especially Patricia (Trish) Tannian, whose work made this a better book. All those mentioned above did their jobs with professionalism and skill.

Finally, to my husband Randy, your name really deserves to be next to mine. Without you, this book would not have been possible, nor indeed would any of my projects. You work tirelessly to make things easy for me. I love the database and elegant Web interface—truly a work of art—that you designed for me. You put in many hours and long nights to help me complete this book, without so much as a hint of irritation or complaint. Your patience and determination amaze me, even after all these years. My love to you.

ELLEN DRAKE

How This Book Is Arranged

Order of Entries

Dorland's Medical Speller follows the same scheme of arrangement as *Dorland's Illustrated Medical Dictionary*. Main entries follow one another in letter-by-letter alphabetical order regardless of spaces or hyphens that occur within them (see below for special rules for eponyms and chemical names); compound entries consisting of one or more adjectives and a noun can be found as subentries under the noun. There is much more cross-referencing in this book than in the previous edition, with common adjectives appearing as main entries and the phrases in which they are used as subentries. For common (nonproper) main entries, a placeholder is used to designate the main entry; the placeholder may appear at the beginning, at the end, or within a subentry.

Chemical Prefixes

Italicized chemical prefixes such as the letters *p-* and *o-* and *cis-* and *trans-*, together with numbers, Greek letters, and the small capitals L- and D-, do not count for alphabetization. When prefixes are written out in full, however, for example as *para-* instead of *p-*, they are counted for alphabetical order.

Subentries

Each subentry appears on a new line following the main entry and is indented. Subentries may incorporate the main entry at any point in a phrase. Except for eponyms and a few trademarked terms, the main entry word in a subentry is represented only by the initial letter (for example, *blast c.* under *cell*) or letters if the main entry is compound. Regular English plurals are represented by the initial letter followed by 's (for example, *b's* for *bones*), and irregular or Greek or Latin plurals by the entire plural form written out (for example, *teeth* under *tooth* and *ligamenta* under *ligamentum*).

The main entry placeholder may appear at the beginning, end, or anywhere within a subentry phrase. In subentries the main entry placeholder is ignored for alphabetization, as are prepositions, conjunctions, and articles.

Eponymic Terms

The use of the possessive in eponyms is controversial. However, in keeping with widely accepted style for medical reporting and with the recommendations in *The Book of Style for Medical Transcription* (Association for Healthcare Documentation Integrity, Modesto, California), the possessive form of most eponyms has not been used. Exceptions in this reference include *law, theory, principle,* and *rule.* Owing to the present lack of consistency and consensus, no prescription can be given. Therefore, whether or not to use the possessive form is a matter left to the individual;. There are some terms in which the possessive is never used, such as *Christmas disease* and *Down syndrome.*

Terms containing a proper name are listed twice, once after the thing named and once under the eponym; thus *Down syndrome* is listed at both *Down* and *syndrome.* For such terms, only the proper name is counted for alphabetical order. For the example just given, the term is alphabetized as if it were only the name *Down* both at the main entry at D and as a subentry under *syndrome.* Everything following the name is ignored (including 's if it occurs) unless there are a number of terms containing the same name, in which case the words after the name are treated as subentries without a placeholder. Thus the following terms occur in this order:

McKee line
McKee-Farrar
    acetabular cup
    arthroplasty
    prosthesis

If more than one proper name occurs in a term, only the first one determines alphabetical order, unless the first name in consecutive terms is the same. In that case the second name and, if necessary, subsequent names are counted for alphabetization. This is illustrated by the following list:

McCarthy
    cystoscope
    electrode
    evacuator
    forceps

McCarthy-Alcock forceps
McCarthy-Campbell cystoscope

Umlauts are ignored for alphabetization:

Löwe ring
Lowe syndrome
Löwenberg canal
Löwenthal tract
Lower rings

Abbreviations and Acronyms

A number of abbreviations and acronyms are given, together with the words or phrases they stand for. The selection is only a small fraction of the abbreviations and acronyms in actual use. If more than one word or phrase is listed with an abbreviation, the terms are given in alphabetical order and each additional term is placed on a new line and indented.

Alternative Spellings

A number of words have alternative spellings, ranging from the difference of a single letter to the use of variant forms of Greek and Latin stems. Although every effort has been made to ensure that the spellings included in this book are valid, no indications of preference are given; in some cases a spelling that is favored by one specialty is not the same as the spelling preferred by another specialty.

Plurals

Plurals for foreign words, nearly all of them Greek and Latin, are given with the appropriate entries. In addition, they are given again as separate entries if they do not occur within a few lines of the singular form.

Diacritical Marks and Special Characters

Diacritical marks or accent marks, umlauts, and other special characters appear in many foreign expressions and eponyms. Superscripts and subscripts are common in chemical and mathematical expressions. They have been included in this book for the sake of accuracy and because this book has a wide audience, including editors of medical journals. Such marks often cause problems for the medical transcriptionist because they are not always correctly transferred electronically. Accents can generally be ignored, umlauts may or may not be replaced by diphthongs, and institutions have designated how subscripts and superscripts should be handled. Where possible, alternative renderings have been provided.

Brackets and Parentheses

In a few cases alternative spellings are enclosed by parentheses; these are mainly proper names, particularly proper names that have been transliterated from another alphabet. Some entries require a bit of explanation; these explanations are enclosed in brackets. Brackets are sometimes used as a part of Latin anatomical nomenclature to enclose an eponym in the genitive case; in this book such eponyms generally appear all lower case (as in *Dorland's Illustrated Medical Dictionary*), but an initial capital for the name is acceptable.

Brackets also are used in this book at the ends of entries for chemical names containing the symbols *o-, p-,* and *m-*; in these cases the brackets are not part of the term but enclose the full form of the prefix that may be used instead of the symbol, for example, *p*-aminobenzoic acid [para-] to indicate that it may also be written *para*-aminobenzoic acid.

DORLAND'S
MEDICAL
SPELLER

ā—L. ante (before)

α—
   alpha (Greek letter)
   heavy chain of IgA

α-1,4-glucan: α-1,4-glucan
6-glucosyl-transferase deficiency

a—[as a subscript] symbol for
arterial blood

α₁-antitrypsin

A—
   accommodation
   adenine
   adenosine
   [as a subscript] symbol for
      alveolar gas
   ampere
   anode
   atropine
   start of anesthesia

Å—Angström (law, unit)

A₁c (A1C)—hemoglobin A₁c
(glycosylated hemoglobin)

A₂ (A2)—aortic second sound

A-a, (A-a)O₂, P(A-a)O₂—alveolar-
arterial (oxygen gradient)

AA—
   achievement age
   Alcoholics Anonymous
   ascending aorta

AAA—
   abdominal aortic aneurysm
   acquired aplastic anemia
   acute anxiety attack

AABB—American Association of
Blood Banks

AAC—antibiotic-associated colitis

AACAP—American Academy of
Child and Adolescent Psychiatry

AACN—
   American Association of
      Colleges of Nursing
   American Association of
      Critical-Care Nurses

AAD—
   American Academy of
      Dermatology
   antibiotic-associated diarrhea

AAE—active assistive exercise

AAFP—
   American Academy of Family
      Practice
   American Association of
      Family Physicians

AAGP—American Academy of
General Practice

AAI—
   acute adrenal insufficiency
   American Association of
      Immunologists
   arm-ankle index

AAL—anterior axillary line

AAMA—American Association of
Medical Assistants

AAMD—age-associated memory
disorder

AAMT—American Association for
Medical Transcription
(now: Association for Healthcare
Documentation Integrity
[AHDI])

AAN—American Academy of
Neurology

AANA—American Association of
Nurse Anesthetists

AAO—
   American Academy of
      Ophthalmology
   American Academy of
      Otolaryngology

AAO3, AAOx3—awake, alert, and
oriented times three

AAOP—American Academy of Oral
Pathology

AAOS—American Academy of
Orthopaedic Surgeons

AAP—
   American Academy of
      Pediatrics
   American Association of
      Pathologists

AAPB—American Association of
Pathologists and Bacteriologists

AAPMC—antibiotic-associated
pseudomembranous colitis

AAPMR—American Academy
of Physical Medicine and
Rehabilitation

AARC—American Association for
Respiratory Care

Aaron sign

Aarskog syndrome

Aarskog-Scott syndrome

AAS—
   acute abdominal series
   aortic arch syndrome

Aase syndrome

AAT—auditory apperception test

AAV—adeno-associated virus

Ab—antibody

Ab, ab—abortion

AB—
- Ace bandage
- apex beat
- asthmatic bronchitis
- axiobuccal

A/B—apnea-bradycardia

A&B—apnea and bradycardia

ABA—allergic bronchopulmonary aspergillosis

abacterial

Abadie sign

abandonment

abaptiston

abarticular

abarticulation

abasia
- a.-astasia
- a. atactica
- choreic a.
- paralytic a.
- paroxysmal trepidant a.
- spastic a.
- trembling a.
- a. trepidans

abasic

abate

abatement

abaxial

Abbé (Abbe) condenser

Abbe
- cheiloplasty (stage I, stage II)
- flap
- intestinal anastomosis
- lip flap
- neurectomy
- operation
- repair
- rings
- small-bowel operation

Abbe-Estlander
- cheiloplasty
- operation

Abbé-Zeiss (Abbe-Zeiss)
- apparatus
- counting cell, counting chamber

Abbott
- method
- operation

Abbott-Luca operation

Abbott-Miller tube

Abbott-Rawson tube

ABC—
- Adriamycin, bleomycin, cisplatin

ABC— (continued)
- airway-breathing-circulation (protocol)
- antigen-binding capacity
- apnea, bradycardia, cyanosis
- applesauce, bananas, cereal (diet)
- aspiration biopsy cytology
- axiobuccocervical

ABCD—Adriamycin (doxorubicin), bleomycin, CCNU (lomustine), and dacarbazine

ABD, Abd, abd—abdomen, abdominal

abdomen
- acute a.
- boat-shaped a.
- carinate a.
- gridiron a.
- navicular a.
- pendulous a.
- scaphoid a.
- surgical a.

abdominal
- a. abscess
- a. aortic aneurysm
- a. aortography
- a. cavity
- a. crisis
- a. decompression
- a. gestation
- a. hysterectomy
- a. hysterotomy
- a. incision
- a. inguinal ring
- a. myomectomy
- a. nephrectomy
- a. nephrotomy
- a. ovariotomy
- a. reflexes
- a. retractor
- a. splenectomy
- total a. hysterectomy (TAH)

abdominalgia
- periodic a.

abdominocardiac reflex

abdominocentesis

abdominogenital

abdominohysterectomy

abdominohysterotomy

abdominoperineal resection (APR)

abdominoplasty
- Mladick a.

abdominoposterior

abdominoscopy

abdominoscrotal
abdominothoracic
    a. arch
    a. incision
abdominouterotomy
abdominovaginal hysterectomy
abdominovesical pouch
abducens
    a. nerve
    nervus a.
    a. palsy
abducent
    a. muscle
    a. nerve
abduct
abduction
abductor
ABE—acute bacterial endocarditis
Abegg rule
Abell operation
Abelson
    adenotome
    cannula
    murine leukemia virus
abenteric
ABEP—auditory brain stem evoked
  potential
Abercrombie
    degeneration
    syndrome
Aberdeen knot
Abernethy
    fascia
    operation
    sarcoma
aberrancy
aberrant
    a. cementosis
    a. cementum
    a. conduction
    a. regeneration
aberratio
    a. lactis
    a. testis
aberration
    chromatic a., lateral
    chromatic a., longitudinal
    chromatic-type a.
    chromosome a.
    dioptric a.
    distantial a.
    heterosomal a.
    intrachromosomal a.
    lateral a.
    longitudinal a.

aberration *(continued)*
    mental a.
    meridional a.
    monochromatic a.
    newtonian a.
    optical a.
    penta-X chromosomal a.
    spherical a., negative
    spherical a., positive
    tetra-X chromosomal a.
    triple-X chromosomal a.
    zonal a.
aberrometer
abetalipoproteinemia
ab externo incision
abeyance
ABF—aortobifemoral
ABG—axiobuccogingival
ABG, ABGs—arterial blood gas(es)
ABI—ankle-brachial index
abient
abietic acid
ability
    general a.
    impaired urinary
      concentrating a.
    primary mental a.
    verbal a.
abiotrophic
abiotrophy
    retinal a.
abirritation
abiuret
abiuretic
ABL—axiobuccolingual
ablactation
ablate
ablatio
    a. placentae
    a. retinae
ablation
    alcohol a.
    androgen a.
    catheter a.
    chemical a.
    electrical a.
    endometrial a.
    photochemical a.
    photomechanical a.
    photothermal a.
    radiofrequency a.
    radiofrequency catheter a.
    rotational a.
    transurethral needle a.
      (TUNA)

ABLB—alternate binaural loudness balance (test)
abluent
abluminal
ablution
ablutomania
ABMT—autologous bone marrow transplantation
ABN, Abn, abn—abnormal, abnormality
abnerval
abnormal
abnormality
abnormity
ABO
    antibodies
    antigens
    blood groups
    compatibility
    incompatibility
    typing
aborad
aboral
abort
aborticide
abortient
abortifacient
abortigenic
abortion
    accidental a.
    afebrile a.
    ampullar a.
    artificial a.
    cervical a.
    complete a.
    contagious a.
    elective a.
    epizootic a.
    habitual a.
    idiopathic a.
    imminent a.
    incomplete a.
    induced a.
    inevitable a.
    infected a.
    infectious a.
    justifiable a.
    late a.
    missed a.
    natural a.
    nontherapeutic a.
    partial a.
    partial birth a.
    recurrent a.
    saline a.

abortion *(continued)*
    septic a.
    spontaneous a.
    therapeutic a.
    threatened a.
    tubal a.
    vibrio a.
abortive
abortus
abouchement
ABP—arterial blood pressure
ABR—
    absolute bed rest
    American Board of Radiology
    auditory brain stem response
abrachia
abrachiatism
abrachius
abradant
abrade
abrader
    Howard a.
    Abraham cannula
Abrahams sign
Abrami disease
Abrams
    heart reflex
    needle
    test
Abramson catheter
abrasio
    a. corneae
    a. dentinum
abrasion
    acid a.
    bobby pin a.
    cervical a.
    dental a., denture a.
    dentifrice a.
    dicing a's
    gingival a.
    a. of gingiva
    marginal a.
    occupational a.
    tooth a.
abrasive
    aluminum oxide a.
    diatomaceous silicon dioxide a.
    a. disk
    FF a., FFF a. [degree of fineness]
    flint a.
    garnet a.
    iron oxide a.

abrasive *(continued)*
- a. point
- polishing a.
- quartz a.
- silicon carbide a.
- silicon dioxide a.
- a. strip
- zirconium silicate a.

abrasor

abreaction
- motor a.

Abrikosov (Abrikossoff) tumor

abruptio
- a. placentae
- a. placentae marginalis

abruption of placenta

ABS—acute brain syndrome

abscess
- acute a.
- acute dentoalveolar a.
- alveolar a.
- amebic a.
- anorectal a.
- apical a., acute
- apical a., chronic
- appendiceal a.
- appendicular a.
- atheromatous a.
- axillary a.
- Bartholin a.
- bartholinian a.
- Bezold (von Bezold) a.
- bicameral a.
- bile duct a.
- bilharziasis a.
- biliary a.
- blind a.
- bone a.
- brain a.
- breast a.
- broad ligament a.
- Brodie a.
- buccal space a.
- bursal a.
- canalicular a.
- caseocavernous a.
- caseous a.
- central mammary a.
- cerebellar a.
- cerebral a.
- cheesy a.
- cholangitic a.
- chronic a.
- circumscribed a.
- circumtonsillar a.

abscess *(continued)*
- cold a.
- collar button a.
- crypt a.
- deep a.
- dental a.
- dentoalveolar a.
- diaphragmatic a.
- diffuse a.
- diverticular a.
- Douglas a.
- dry a.
- Dubois a.
- dural a.
- embolic a.
- emphysematous a.
- encapsulated a.
- encysted a.
- entamebic a.
- eosinophilic a.
- epidural a.
- epiploic a.
- extradural a.
- fecal a.
- filarial a.
- follicular a.
- frontal a.
- fungal a.
- gangrenous a.
- gas a.
- gingival a.
- glandular a.
- gravitation a.
- gravity a.
- gummatous a.
- helminthic a.
- hematogenous a.
- hemorrhagic a.
- hepatic a.
- hot a.
- hypostatic a.
- idiopathic a.
- infraorbital space a.
- interlobular a.
- interlobular mammary a.
- interradicular a.
- intersphincteric a.
- intra-abdominal a.
- intracranial a.
- intradural a.
- intramastoid a.
- intramedullary a.
- ischiorectal a.
- kidney a.
- lacrimal a.

abscess *(continued)*

lacunar a.
lateral alveolar a.
lateral root a.
liver a.
lumbar a.
lung a.
lymphatic a.
mammary a.
marginal a.
masticator a.
mastoid a.
mediastinal a.
metastatic a.
metastatic tuberculous a.
midabdominal a.
migrating a.
miliary a.
milk a.
mother a.
Munro a.
mural a.
myocardial a.
nocardial a.
orbital a.
ossifluent a.
otic cerebral a.
otogenic a.
Paget a.
palatal a.
pancreatic a.
parafrenal a.
parametrial a.
parametric a.
parametritic a.
paranephric a.
parapancreatic a.
parapharyngeal space a.
parietal a.
parotid a.
Pautrier a.
pelvic a.
pelvirectal a.
perianal a.
periapical a.
periarticular a.
pericemental a.
pericholecystic a.
pericoronal a.
peridental a.
periductal mammary a.
perinephric a.
periodontal infrabony a.
peripleuritic a.
perirectal a.

abscess *(continued)*

perirenal a.
peritoneal a.
peritonsillar a.
periureteral a.
periurethral a.
perivesical a.
phlegmonous a.
phoenix a.
pilonidal a.
pneumococcic a.
postcecal a.
Pott a.
prelacrimal a.
premammary a.
preperitoneal a.
primary a.
prostatic a.
protozoal a.
psoas a.
pulmonary a.
pulp a.
pulpal a.
pyemic a.
pyogenic a.
radicular a.
recrudescent a.
renal a.
residual a.
retrocecal a.
retroesophageal a.
retromammary a.
retroperitoneal a.
retropharyngeal a.
retrotonsillar a.
retrovesical a.
ring a.
root a.
sacrococcygeal a.
satellite a.
scrofulous a.
secondary a.
septal a.
septicemic a.
serous a.
shirt-stud a.
spermatic a.
spirillar a.
splenic a.
stellate a.
stercoraceous a.
stercoral a.
sterile a.
stitch a.
streptococcal a.

abscess *(continued)*
    strumous a.
    subacute a.
    subaponeurotic a.
    subarachnoid a.
    subareolar a.
    subcutaneous a.
    subdiaphragmatic a.
    subdural a.
    subepidermal a.
    subfascial a.
    subgaleal a.
    subhepatic a.
    sublingual space a.
    submammary a.
    submandibular space a.
    submasseteric space a.
    submental space a.
    subpectoral a.
    subperiosteal a.
    subperitoneal a.
    subphrenic a.
    subscapular a.
    subungual a.
    sudoriparous a.
    superficial a.
    suprahepatic a.
    supralevator a.
    sympathetic a.
    syphilitic a.
    temporal lobe a.
    thecal a.
    thymic a.
    tonsillar a.
    tooth a.
    Tornwaldt (Thornwaldt) a.
    traumatic a.
    tropical a.
    tuberculous a.
    tubo-ovarian a.
    tympanitic a.
    tympanocervical a.
    tympanomastoid a.
    urethral a.
    urinary a.
    urinous a.
    verminous a.
    vestibular a.
    vitreous a.
    von Bezold a.
    walled-off a.
    wandering a.
    warm a.
    Welch a.
    worm a.

abscessogram
abscise
abscission
    corneal a.
absconsio (absconsiones)
absence
    atypical a. seizure
    complex a. seizure
    congenital ossicular a.
    enuretic a.
    a. epilepsy
    myoclonic a.
    a. seizure
    subclinical a. seizure
absentia epileptica
Absidia
    A. corymbifera
    A. ramosa
absinthe
absinthism
absinthium
absolute
    a. glaucoma
    a. hyperopia
    a. scotoma
absorb
absorbable
    a. dressing
    a. surgical suture
absorbed fraction
absorbefacient
absorbency
absorbent
absorber
absorptiometer
absorptiometry
    dual photon a.
    photon a.
absorption
    agglutinin a.
    bone a.
    broad-beam a.
    a. coefficient
    cutaneous a.
    enteral a.
    external a.
    fat a.
    internal a.
    interstitial a.
    intestinal a.
    iron a.
    net a.
    parenteral a.
    pathologic a., pathological a.
    percutaneous a.

absorption *(continued)*
    protein a.
    x-ray a.
absorptive
absorptive lenses
absorptivity
    molar a.
    specific a.
abstinence
    alimentary a.
abstract
abstraction
absurdity (absurdities)
abterminal
abtorsion
abulia
    cyclic a.
abulic
abundance
Aburel operation
abuse
    alcohol a.
    chemical a.
    child a.
    drug a.
    elder a.
    ethanol a.
    inhalant a.
    laxative a.
    mixed drug a.
    physical a.
    polydrug a.
    polypharmacy a.
    polysubstance a.
    psychoactive substance a.
    sexual a.
    spousal a.
    spouse a.
    substance a.
    tobacco a.
abut
abutment
    anterior a.
    auxiliary a.
    bombed a.
    bridge a.
    a. groove
    implant a.
    intermediate a.
    isolated a.
    multiple a.
    multirooted a.
    a. post
    primary a.

abutment *(continued)*
    screw-type a.
    secondary a.
    splinted a.
    terminal a.
ABV—Adriamycin, bleomycin, vinblastine
ABVD—Adriamycin (doxorubicin), bleomycin, vinblastine, and dacarbazine
AC—
    acromioclavicular
    adrenal cortex
    air conduction
    anterior chamber
    anterior colporrhaphy
    anticoagulant
    aortic closure
    axiocervical
ACA—
    adenocarcinoma
    anterior cerebral artery
acacia, gum
acalculia
acampsia
acantha
acanthamebiasis
Acanthamoeba
    A. astronyxis
    A. castellanii
    A. culbertsoni
    A. hatchetti
    A. polyphaga
    A. rhisodes
acanthesthesia
acanthion
acanthocyte
acanthocytosis
acanthoid
acantholysis
acantholytic
acanthoma
    a. adenoides cysticum
    basal cell a.
    clear cell a.
    Degos a.
    a. inguinale
    pilar sheath a.
    a. tropicum
acanthopelvis
acanthosis
    congenital a.
    malignant a. nigricans
    a. nigricans

acanthosis *(continued)*
    a. papulosa nigra
    a. verrucosa
acanthotic
a capite ad calcem
acapnial
acapnic
acarbia
acardia
acardiac
acardius
acari (plural of acarus)
acarian
acariasis
acaricide
acarid
acarine
acarodermatitis urticarioides
acaroid
acarophobia
acarotoxic
Acarus
    A. folliculorum
    A. hordei
    A. rhyzoglypticus hyacinthi
    A. siro
ACAT—automated computerized axial tomography
acatalasia
acathectic
acathexia
acathexis
acaudate
ACBE—air contrast barium enema
ACBG—aortocoronary bypass graft
ACBGS—aortocoronary bypass graft surgery
ACBS—aortocoronary bypass surgery
Acc.—
    accommodation
ACC—
    adenoid cystic carcinoma
    alveolar cell carcinoma
    ambulatory care center
    American College of Cardiology
accede
accelerant
accelerated idioventricular rhythm
acceleration
    angular a.
    central a.
    centripetal a.

acceleration *(continued)*
    developmental a.
    linear a.
    negative a.
    positive a.
    standard a. of free fall
accelerator
    C3b inactivator a.
    linear a.
    serum prothrombin conversion a. (SPCA)
    serum thrombotic a.
    thromboplastin generation a.
    a. urinae
accelerin
accentuation
    presystolic a.
acceptor
    hydrogen a.
    oxygen a.
access
    arteriovenous a.
    hemodialysis a.
    hemodialysis vascular a.
    vascular a.
    venovenous a.
accessiflexor
accessorius
accessory
    a. muscles of respiration
    a. nerve
    a. sign
accident
    cardiovascular a.
    car versus pedestrian a.
    cerebrovascular a. (CVA)
    motor vehicle a. (MVA)
accident prone
acclimate, acclimated
acclimation
acclimatization
acclimatize
Accolate
accolé
accommodate
accommodation
    absolute a.
    amplitude of a.
    binocular a.
    excessive a.
    histologic a.
    negative a.
    nerve a.
    obstetric a.

accommodation *(continued)*
   positive a.
   range of a.
   reflex a.
   a. reflex
   relative a.
   subnormal a.
accommodative
   a. convergence
   a. effort syndrome
   a. equipment
   a. esotropia
   a. iridoplegia
   a. palsy
   a. spasm
   a. target
accommodometer
accomplice
accordion drain
accouchement forcé
accoucheur
accoucheuse
accrementition
accretio
   a. cordis
   a. pericardii
accretion
accrochage ventilatoire
acculturation
accuracy
ACD—
   absolute cardiac dullness
   acid citrate dextrose
   adult celiac disease
   allergic contact dermatitis
   anterior chest discomfort
   anticonvulsant drug
ACDF—
   adult child of dysfunctional
     family
   anterior cervical diskectomy
     and fusion
ACE—
   adrenocortical extract
   angiotensin-converting enzyme
Ace-Fischer external fixator
acellular
acenesthesia
acentric
ACEP—American College of
  Emergency Physicians
acephalia
acephalic
acephalobrachia
acephalobrachius

acephalocardia
acephalocardius
acephalochiria
acephalochirus
acephalogaster
acephalogastria
acephalopodia
acephalopodius
acephalorhachia
acephalostomia
acephalostomus
acephalothoracia
acephalothorus
acephalous
acephalus
   a. dibrachius
   a. dipus
   a. monobrachius
   a. monopus
   a. paracephalus
   a. sympus
acephaly
acerate
acerbity
acerola
acervuline
acetabula (plural of acetabulum)
acetabular
   a. cup
   a. rim
acetabulectomy
acetabuloplasty
acetabulum (acetabula)
   sunken a.
acetaldehyde
acetamidine
acetaminophen poisoning
acetanilid poisoning
acetate
   cellulose a.
Acetest
acetic aldehyde
acetic acid
   glacial a.
acetic anhydride
acetify
acetimeter
acetin
acetoacetate
acetoacetic acid
acetoacetyl-CoA (coenzyme A)
acetoacetyl-CoA (coenzyme A)
   reductase
acetoacetyl-CoA (coenzyme A)
   thiolase

Acetobacter aceti
acetoin
acetolysis
acetonation
acetonemia
acetonemic
acetonitrile
acetonumerator
acetosoluble
acetous
acetowhite
acetowhitening
acetrizoate
acetrizoate sodium
acetum
acetyl
    a. chloride
    a. peroxide
acetylase
acetylated
acetylation
acetylator
acetylcholine (ACh)
    a. chloride
    a. receptor antibody (AChRab)
acetyl-CoA acetyltransferase
acetyl-CoA acyltransferase
acetyl-CoA: α-glucosaminide-
    N-acetyltransferase
acetyl-CoA carboxylase
acetyl-CoA: heparan-
    α-D-glucosaminide
    N-acetyltransferase
acetyl-CoA synthetase
N-acetylgalactosamine
N-acetylgalactosamine-4-sulfatase
N-acetylgalactosamine-4-sulfatase
    deficiency
N-acetylgalactosamine-6-sulfatase
    deficiency
α-*N*-acetylgalactosaminidase
    [alpha-]
β-*N*-acetylgalactosaminidase
    [beta-]
N-acetylglucosamine-6-sulfatase
N-acetylglucosamine-6-sulfatase
    deficiency
α-*N*-acetylglucosaminidase [alpha-]
N-acetylglucosaminylphospho-
    transferase
N-acetyl-β-hexosaminidase
acetylization
acetylsalicylic acid poisoning
acetylsulfadiazine
acetylsulfaguanidine

acetylsulfathiazole
acetyltransferase
acetyltributyl citrate
acetyltriethyl citrate
ACF—acute care facility
ACG—
    angiocardiogram
    angiocardiography
    angle closure glaucoma
    apexcardiogram
ACG, A.C.G.—American College of
    Gastroenterology
ACh—acetylcholine
achalasia
    cricopharyngeal a.
    pelvirectal a.
    sphincteral a.
Achard syndrome
Achard-Thiers syndrome
ache
AChE—acetylcholinesterase
acheilia
acheilous
acheiria
acheiropodia
acheirus
achievement scores
Achilles
    bursa
    bursitis
    jerk
    reflex
    tendon
achillobursitis
achillodynia
achillorrhaphy
achillotenotomy
    plastic a.
achillotomy
achlorhydria
achlorhydric
Acholeplasma laidlawii
acholia
acholic
acholuria
acholuric
achondrogenesis
achondroplasia
achondroplastic
achondroplasty
AChoR—acetylcholine receptor
AChRab—acetylcholine receptor
    antibody
achrestic
achromasia

achromatic
   a. lens
   a. perimetry
achromatin
achromatinic
achromatism
achromatize
achromatolysis
achromatophil
achromatophilia
achromatopsia
achromatosis
achromatous
achromaturia
achromia
   central a.
   congenital a.
   consecutive a.
   cortical a.
   a. parasitica
achromic nevus
achromocyte
achromoderma
achromophilous
achromotrichia
achrooamyloid
achroodextrin
Achúcarro stain
achylia
achymia
acicular
aciculate
aciculum
acid
   acetic a.
   acetoacetic a.
   acetylsalicylic a. (ASA)
   alpha-lipoic a. (ALA)
   amino a.
   aminoacetic a.
   aminobenzoic a.
   aminocaproic a.
   aminoglutaric a.
   aminolevulinic a. (ALA)
   6-aminopenicillanic a. (6-APA)
   aminosalicylic a.
   aminosuccinic a.
   arachidonic a.
   argininosuccinic a.
   aurintricarboxylic a.
   ascorbic a.
   bile a's
   binary a.
   boric a.
   Brønsted (Bronsted) a.

acid *(continued)*
   cahincic a.
   carbonic a.
   carboxylic a.
   chloroacetic a.
   chlorogenic a.
   choleic a's
   chromic a.
   13-*cis*-retinoic a.
   a. citrate dextrose (ACD)
   citric a.
   conjugate a.
   deoxyribonucleic a. (DNA)
   diacetic a.
   dichloroacetic a.
   dihydrolipoic a.
   ethacrynic a.
   ethylenediaminetetraacetic a.
   fatty a.
   folic a.
   formic a.
   gallic a.
   γ-aminobutyric a. (GABA) [gamma-]
   γ-carboxyglutamic a. [gamma-]
   glucuronic a.
   glutamic a.
   glyceric a.
   glycolic a.
   haloid a.
   hexadecanoic a.
   hippuric a.
   homogentisic a.
   homovanillic a.
   hydrochloric a.
   5-hydroxyindoleacetic a.
   inorganic a.
   lactic a.
   linoleic a.
   lysergic a.
   monobasic a.
   muriatic a.
   nalidixic a.
   nicotinic a.
   nitric a.
   nucleic a.
   oleic a.
   organic a.
   oxalic a.
   oxygen a.
   p-aminobenzoic a. (PABA)
   p-aminohippuric a. (PAHA)
   p-aminosalicylic a.
   pantothenic a.
   pentanoic a.

acid *(continued)*
    perchloric a.
    phenylpyruvic a.
    phosphoric a.
    polybasic a.
    polyene a's
    pyruvic a.
    ribonucleic a. (RNA)
    salicylic a.
    saturated fatty a's (SFAs)
    sodium *p*-aminohippuric
        (PAH) a. [p-, para-]
    stearic a.
    succinic a.
    sulfosalicylic a.
    sulfuric a.
    tannic a.
    teichoic a.
    thymidine diphosphoric a.
    thymidine triphosphoric a.
    titratable a.
    tribasic a.
    tricarboxylic a.
    trichloroacetic a.
    unsaturated fatty a's (UFAs)
    uric a.
    valproic a.
    vanillylmandelic a.
    xanthurenic a.
acidemia
    argininosuccinic a.
    free fatty a.
    glutaric a.
    isovaleric a.
    methylmalonic a.
    propionic a.
acid-fast
acid-fast bacillus (AFB)
acid-forming
acidic
acidifiable
acidification
acidifier
acidify
acidimeter
acidimetry
acidism
acidity
acid-maltase deficiency
acidogenic
acidophil
    alpha a.
    epsilon a.
acidophilia
acidophilic

acidophilus milk
acidosis
    bicarbonate wastage renal
        tubular a.
    carbon dioxide a.
    compensated metabolic a.
    compensated respiratory a.
    diabetic a.
    hypercapnic a.
    hyperchloremic renal a.
    lactic a.
    metabolic a.
    non-anion gap a.
    nonrespiratory a.
    renal hyperchloremia a.
    renal tubular a. (RTA), types
        1, 2, 4
    respiratory a.
    starvation a.
    uremic a.
acidosteophyte
acidotic
acid-proof
acid rain
acidulated
acidulous
aciduria
    acetoacetic a.
    argininosuccinic a.
    β-aminoisobutyric a.
    ethylmalonic-adipic a.
    glutamic a.
    glutaric a. (GA)
    L-glyceric a.
    glycolic a.
    methylmalonic a.
    orotic a.
    paradoxical a.
    pyroglutamic a.
    xanthurenic a.
aciduric
acinar
acinar-like
Acinetobacter
    A. calcoaceticus
    A. lwoffii
acini (plural of acinus)
acinic
aciniform
acinitis
acinose
acinotubular
acinous
acinus (acini)
    liver a.

acinus (acini) *(continued)*
    pancreatic a.
    pulmonary a.
    thyroid acini
acipenserin
ackee, akee
ACL—anterior cruciate ligament
Acland clip
aclasis
    diaphyseal a.
    metaphyseal a.
    tarsoepiphyseal a.
aclastic
ACLF—adult congregate living
  facility
ACLS—advanced cardiac life
  support
aclusion
acme
    a. of contraction
    a. of disease
ACMI
    bronchoscope
    gastroscope
    laparoscope
    Martin endoscopy forceps
    proctoscope
    telescope
    valve
ACMI-stat catheter
ACMI-Valentine tube
acne
    adolescent a.
    a. albida
    apocrine a.
    a. artificialis
    a. atrophica
    a. bacillus
    bromide a.
    a. cachecticorum
    a. cheloidalis
    chlorine a.
    a. ciliaris
    colloid a.
    comedo a.
    common a.
    a. conglobata
    conglobate a.
    contact a.
    a. cosmetica
    cystic a.
    a. cystica
    a. decalvans
    a. detergicans
    a. disseminata

acne *(continued)*
    a. dorsalis
    epidemic a.
    a. erythematosa
    a. estivalis
    excoriated a.
    a. excoriée des filles
    a. excoriée des jeunes filles
    a. frontalis
    a. fulminans
    a. generalis
    halogen a.
    a. hypertrophica
    a. indurata
    infantile a.
    a. inversa
    iodide a.
    a. keloid
    a. keloidalis nuchae
    a. keratosa
    lupoid a.
    Mallorca a.
    a. mechanica
    mechanical a.
    a. medicamentosa
    menstrual a.
    a. mentagra
    a. miliaris
    miliary a.
    a. necrotica miliaris
    a. necroticans et exulcerans
      serpiginosa nasi
    neonatal a.
    a. neonatarum
    nodulocystic a.
    a. nodulocystica
    occupational a.
    oil a.
    papular a.
    papulopustular a.
    a. papulopustulosa
    a. papulosa
    petroleum a.
    pickers' a.
    pomade a.
    premenstrual a.
    a. punctata
    pustular a.
    a. pustulosa
    a. rosacea
    a. scorbutica
    a. scrofulosorum
    a. seborrheica
    a. simplex
    steroid a.

acne *(continued)*
    summer a.
    a. syphilitica
    systemic a.
    tar a.
    a. tarsi
    a. telangiectodes
    tropical a.
    a. tropicalis
    a. urticata
    a. varioliformis
    a. venenata
    a. vulgaris
acnegen
acnegenic
acneiform
acnemia
acnitis
ACNM—American College of
  Nurse-Midwives
ACOG—American College of
  Obstetricians and Gynecologists
acolous
aconative
aconite
aconitine
acoprosis
acoprous
acorea
acoria
acorn-tip catheter
Acosta disease
acousma (acousmata)
acousmatamnesia
acoustic
    a. neuroma
    a. reflex
acousticophobia
acoustics
acoustogram
ACP—acid phosphatase
ACPS—acrocephalopolysyndactyly
acquisition time
ACR—American College of Radiology
acral
acrania
acranial
acranius
Acrel ganglion
acremoniosis
acrid
acridine orange
acrids
acrimony
acritical

ACRM—American College of
  Rehabilitation Medicine
acroagnosis
acroanesthesia
acroarthritis
acroblast
acrobrachycephaly
acrocentric
acrocephalopolysyndactyly (ACPS)
acrocephalosyndactyly of Apert
acrocephalous
acrochordon
acrocinesis
acrocinetic
acrocontracture
acrocyanosis
acrodermatitis
    a. chronica atrophicans
    a. continua
    a. enteropathica
    Hallopeau a.
    infantile a.
    papular a. of childhood
    a. perstans
acrodermatosis (acrodermatoses)
acrodolichomelia
acrodynia
acrodysesthesia
acroesthesia
acrogenous
acrognosis
acrohypothermy
acrokeratoelastoidosis
acrokeratosis
    paraneoplastic a.
    a. verruciformis
acrolein
acromastitis
acromegalic
acromegalogigantism
acromegaloidism
acromegaly
acromelia
acromelic
acrometagenesis
acromial
acromicria
acromioclavicular
acromiocoracoid
acromiohumeral
acromion
acromionectomy
acromionizer
acromioplasty
acromioscapular

acromiothoracic
acromphalus
acromyotonia
acromyotonus
acronarcotic
acroneuropathy
acroneurosis
acro-osteolysis
acropachyderma with
    pachyperiostitis
acroparalysis
acroparesthesia
    Nothnagel-type a.
    Schultze-type a.
acropathology
acropathy
    amyotrophic a.
    ulcerative mutilating a.
acrophobia
acropigmentatio reticularis
acropustulosis
acrosclerosis
acrosome
acrospiroma
    eccrine a.
acrostealgia
acrosyndactyly
acroteric
acrotic
acrotism
acrotrophodynia
acrotrophoneurosis
acrylate
acrylic acid
acrylonitrile
ACS—
    American Cancer Society
    American College of Surgeons
    antireticular cytotoxic serum
ACSM—American College of
    Sports Medicine
ACT—activated coagulation time
act
    compulsive a.
    Controlled Substances Act
    forced a.
    imperious a.
    impulsive a.
    reflex a.
ACTH—adrenocorticotropic
    hormone
ACTH-RF—adrenocorticotropic
    hormone–releasing factor
ACTH stimulation test
actin

acting out
actinic
    a. elastosis
    a. keratosis
    a. porokeratosis
    a. reticuloid
    a. telangiectasis
actiniform
actinism
actinium (Ac)
actinobacillosis
actinodermatitis
actinolyte
Actinomadura pelletieri
actinometer
actinometry
actinomycelial
Actinomyces
    A. israelii
    A. naeslundii
    A. odontolyticus
actinomycete
    nocardioform a.
actinomycetic
actinomycetin
actinomycetoma
actinomycin
actinomycoma
actinomycosis
    cervicofacial a.
    pulmonary a.
actinomycotic
actinophage
actinophytosis
actinotoxin
action
    adipokinetic a.
    antagonistic a.
    automatic a.
    bacteriocidal a.
    bacteriostatic a.
    ball-valve a.
    buffer a.
    capillary a.
    compulsive a.
    contact a.
    cumulative a.
    diastatic a.
    disordered a. of heart
    electrocapillary a.
    nicotinic a.
    a. potential
    protein-sparing a.
    reflex a.
    specific dynamic a. (SDA)

action *(continued)*
    a. spectrum
    synergistic a.
    tampon a.
    trigger a.
activated charcoal
activated coagulation time (ACT)
activated partial thromboplastin
    time (APTT, aPTT)
activation
    epileptic a.
    lymphocyte a.
activator
    bow a.
    functional a.
    monoblock a.
    plasminogen a.
    polyclonal a.
    Schwarz a.
    single-chain urokinase-type
      plasminogen (scu-PA) a.
      (prourokinase)
    tissue plasminogen a. (t-PA,
      tPA, TPA)
    urinary plasminogen a.,
      u-plasminogen a.
      (urokinase)
active
    a. motion
    optically a.
    a. range of motion
activity
    alpha wave a.
    asynchronous a.
    background a.
    bactericidal a.
    beta wave a.
    blocking a.
    continuous muscle fiber a.
    a's of daily living (ADL, ADLs)
    delta wave a.
    discrete a.
    electrical a.
    end-plate a.
    enzyme a.
    epileptiform a.
    insertional a.
    instrumental a's of daily living
      (IADL)
    intermittent rhythmic delta a.
    intrinsic sympathomimetic a.
      (ISA)
    involuntary a.
    leukemia-associated inhibitory
      a. (LIA)

activity *(continued)*
    nonsuppressible insulinlike a.
      (NSILA)
    optical a.
    partial agonist a.
    plasma renin a.
    polymorphic delta a.
    pseudomotor a.
    pulseless electrical a. (PEA)
    salaam a.
    serum bactericidal a.
    slow a.
    specific a.
    spike and wave a.
    spontaneous a.
    synchronous a.
    theta wave a.
    triggered a.
    voluntary a.
actomyosin
Acufex
    forceps
    instrument
    punch
acuity
    auditory a.
    Vernier a.
    visual a.
acuminatum (acuminata, acuminatae)
    condyloma acuminatum,
      condylomata acuminata
    verruca acuminata, verrucae
      acuminatae
acupoint
acupressure
acupuncture
acus
acute
    a. angle closure glaucoma
    a. demyelinating disease
acute on chronic
    a.o.c. fracture
    a.o.c. illness
    a.o.c. symptoms
Acutrol suture
ACVD—
    acute cardiovascular disease
    arteriosclerotic cardiovascular
      disease
    autoimmune collagen vascular
      disease
acyanotic
acyclic
acycloguanosine
acyl-CoA (coenzyme A)

acyl-CoA dehydrogenase
acyl-CoA desaturase
acyl-CoA synthetase
acyltransferase
acystia
AD—
    admitting diagnosis
    advance directive
    alcohol dehydrogenase
    axiodistal
    right ear (L. auris dextra)
ADA—
    adenosine deaminase
    American Dental Association
    American Diabetes
        Association
    anterior descending artery
ADAA—American Dental
    Assistants Association
adactylous
adactyly
Adair
    forceps
    tenaculum
Adair-Dighton syndrome
Adamantiades-Behçet syndrome
adamantine
adamantinoma
    a. of long bones
    pituitary a.
    tibial a.
adamantoblast
adamantoblastoma
Adam's apple
adamas dentis
Adamkiewicz
    artery
    test
Adams
    clasp
    disease
    forceps
    operation
    position
    saw
Adams-DeWeese device
Adams-Stokes
    disease
    syncope
    syndrome
A/D (analog-to-digital) converter
adaptability
adaptation
    auditory a.
    chromatic a.

adaptation (continued)
    color a.
    dark a.
    enzymatic a.
    genetic a.
    light a.
    phenotypic a.
    photopic a.
    physiologic a.
    retinal a.
    scotopic a.
    sensory a.
    social a.
adapter, adaptor
    House a.
    McReynolds a.
    Ralks a.
    social a.
Adaptic gauze dressing
adaxial
ADC—axiodistocervical
ADCC—antibody-dependent cell-
    mediated cytotoxicity
ADD—attention deficit disorder
ADDH—attention deficit disorder
    with hyperactivity
addict
addiction
    alcohol a.
    drug a.
    polysurgical a.
addictologist
addictology
Addis
    count
    method
    test
Addison
    anemia
    crisis
    disease
    keloid
    morphea
    pigmentation
    planes
    point
Addison-Biermer anemia
Addison-Gull disease
addisonian
    a. anemia
    a. crisis
    a. syndrome
addisonism
additive
addressin

ADDU—alcohol and drug
dependency unit
adducent
adducin
adduct
adduction
adductor
ADE—acute disseminated
encephalitis
Adelmann operation
adelomorphous
ADEM—acute disseminated
encephalomyelitis
adenalgia
adendritic
adenectomy
adenectopia
adenia
adenic
adeniform
adenine
    a. arabinoside
    a. deaminase
    a. nucleotide
    a. phosphoribosyl transferase
    (APRT) deficiency
adenitis
    acute epidemic infectious a.
    acute infectious a.
    acute salivary a.
    Bartholin a.
    cervical a.
    mesenteric a.
    phlegmonous a.
    syphilitic inguinal a.
    tuberculous a.
    vestibular a.
adenoacanthoma
adenoameloblastoma
adenoblast
adenocarcinoma
    acinar a.
    acinic cell a.
    acinous a.
    alveolar a.
    bronchioalveolar a.
    bronchiolar a.
    bronchioloalveolar a.
    bronchoalveolar a.
    bronchogenic a.
    clear cell a.
    ductal a. of prostate
    follicular a.
    gastric a.
    a. of infantile testis

adenocarcinoma *(continued)*
    a. of kidney
    a. of lung
    mammary a.
    mucinous a.
    mucoid a.
    papillary a.
    polymorphous low-grade a.
    polypoid a.
    renal a.
    scirrhous a.
    sebaceous a.
    terminal duct a.
    testicular a. of infancy
    urachal a.
adenocellulitis
adenocyte
adenodynia
adenoepithelioma
adenofibroma
    a. edematodes
    a. of ovary
    pseudomucinous a.
    serous a.
adenofibrosis
adenogenous
adenographic
adenography
adenohypophysectomy
adenohypophysial,
    adenohypophyseal
adenohypophysis
adenoid
    a. curet
    a. forceps
    a. hypertrophy
adenoidectomy
    tonsillectomy and a. (T&A)
adenoidism
adenoiditis
adenolipoma
adenolipomatosis
adenologaditis
adenolymphitis
adenolymphocele
adenolymphoma
adenoma
    acinar a.
    adamantinum a.
    adnexal a.
    adrenocortical a.
    a. alveolare
    apocrine a.
    basophilic a.
    bronchial a.

adenoma *(continued)*
    carcinoid a. of bronchus
    ceruminous a.
    chief cell a.
    chondromatous a.
    chromophobic a.
    clear cell a.
    colloid a.
    cortical a
    cystic a.
    duct a.
    embryonal a.
    endometrioid a.
    feminizing a.
    fetal a.
    fibroid a.
    a. fibrosum
    a. gelatinosum
    hepatocellular a.
    a. hidradenoides
    islet cell a.
    langerhansian a.
    liver cell a.
    macrofollicular a.
    malignant a.
    mesonephric a.
    microfollicular a.
    mucinous a.
    mucoid cell a.
    multiple endocrine a's
    oncocytic a.
    a. ovarii testiculare
    oxyphil a.
    papillary a.
    Pick testicular a.
    Pick tubular a.
    pituitary a.
    pleomorphic a.
    pseudomucinous a.
    racemose a.
    renal cortical a.
    sebaceous a.
    a. sebaceum
    serous cell a.
    a. simplex
    a. substantiae corticalis
        suprarenalis
    a. sudoriparum
    testicular a.
    toxic thyroid a.
    trabecular a.
    tubular a. of Pick
    a. tubulare testiculare ovarii
    tubulovillous a.
    villous a.

adenoma *(continued)*
    water-clear cell a.
    wolffian a.
adenomalacia
adenomatoid
adenomatome
adenomatosis
    erosive a. of nipple
    fibrosing a.
    multiple endocrine a. (MEA)
    a. oris
    pancreatic-islet a.
    pluriglandular a.
    polyendocrine a.
    pulmonary a.
adenomatous polyposis
adenomegaly
adenomyoepithelioma
adenomyofibroma
adenomyoma psammopapillare
adenomyomatosis
adenomyomatous
adenomyometritis
adenomyosarcoma
    embryonal a.
adenomyosis
    a. externa
    stromal a.
    a. tubae
    a. uteri
adenoneural
adenopathy
    axillary a.
    cervical a.
    hilar a.
    inguinal a.
    tracheobronchial a.
adenopharyngitis
adenophlegmon
adenophthalmia
adenopituicyte
adenosarcoma
    embryonal a.
adenosclerosis
adenosine
    cyclic a. monophosphate
        (cAMP; cyclic AMP; 3´,
        5´-AMP)
    a. deaminase
    a. diphosphate (ADP)
    a. kinase
    a. monophosphate (AMP)
    a. phosphate
    a. triphosphatase (ATPase)
    a. triphosphate (ATP)

adenosis
    blunt duct a.
    florid a.
    mammary sclerosing a.
    sclerosing a. of breast
    a. vaginae
    vaginal a.
adenosquamous
adenosyl
adenosylcobalamin
S-adenosylhomocysteine
S-adenosylmethionine
adenosyltransferase
    methionine a.
adenotome
    Abelson a.
    Kelly a.
    LaForce a.
    LaForce-Grieshaber a.
    Shambaugh a.
    Sluder a.
adenotomy
adenotonsillectomy
adenoviral
adenovirus
adenylate
    a. cyclase
    a. deaminase
    a. kinase
adenyl cyclase
adenylic acid
adenylosuccinase
adenylosuccinate lyase
adenylyl
adenylyltransferase
adequacy
    velopharyngeal a.
adermia
adermogenesis
ADG—
    atrial diastolic gallop
    axiodistogingival
ADH—
    alcohol dehydrogenase
    antidiuretic hormone
ADHA—American Dental
  Hygienists Association
ADHD—attention deficit
  hyperactivity disorder
adhere
adherence
    bacterial a.
    graft a.
    immune a.
    a. syndrome

adherent
adhesiectomy
adhesio (adhesiones)
    a. interthalamica
adhesiolysis
adhesion
    amniotic a.
    anomalous mesenteric a's
    attic a.
    banjo-string a.
    fibrinous a's
    fibromembranous a's
    filamentous a's
    filmy a's
    interthalamic a.
    periadnexal a.
    a. of pleura
    preputial a.
    primary a.
    secondary a.
    serologic a.
    sublabial a.
    traumatic uterine a.
adhesiotomy
adhesive
    Biobrane a.
    cyanoacrylate a.
    dental a.
    denture a.
    a. dressing
    methylmethacrylate a.
    a. syndrome
adhesiveness
    platelet a.
ADI—
    acceptable daily intake
    axiodistoincisal
adiabatic fast passage
adiadochokinesia, adiadochokinesis
adiaphoria
adiaspiromycosis
adiaspore
adiasporosis
adiastole
adiathermancy
Adie
    pupil
    syndrome
adiemorrhysis
adient
adipectomy
adipocele
adipocellular
adipoceratous
adipocere

adipocyte
adipofibroma
adipogenic
adipogenous
adipohepatic
adipoid
adipokinesis
adipokinetic
adipokinin
adipometer
adiponecrosis subcutanea
   neonatorum
adiponectin
adipopectic
adipopexis
adiposalgia
adipose
adiposis
   a. cerebralis
   a. dolorosa
   a. hepatica
   a. tuberosa simplex
   a. universalis
adipositas
   a. cerebralis
   a. cordis
   a. ex vacuo
adipositis
adiposity
   cerebral a.
   pituitary a.
adiposogenital dystrophy
adiposuria
adipsia
aditus
   a. ad antrum
     mastoideum
   a. ad pelvem
   a. laryngis
   a. orbitae
   a. orbitalis
   a. vaginae
adjacent
adjunct
adjunctive
adjuster
   Negus ligature a.
adjustment
   a. disorder
   occlusal a.
adjuvant
   a. chemotherapy
   double-emulsion a.
   Freund a.
   immunologic a.

adjuvant *(continued)*
   mycobacterial a.
   oil emulsion a.
   pertussis a.
   solubilized water-in-oil a.
   a. therapy
   water-in-oil-in-water
     emulsion a.
adjuvanticity
ADL, ADLs—activities of daily
  living
Adler
   punch
   test
   theory
adlerian psychoanalysis
adlerian psychology
ad lib.—as desired, at pleasure
  (L. ad libitum)
adm., admit—admission
admaxillary
admedial
admedian
adminiculum (adminicula)
   a. lineae albae
admittance
   acoustic a.
admixture
ad nauseam
adnerval
adneural
adnexa
   a. mastoidea
   a. oculi
   a. uteri
adnexal
adnexectomy
adnexitis
adnexopexy
adnexorganogenic
ADO—axiodisto-occlusal
adolescence
adolescent
adoral
ADP—adenosine diphosphate
ADP glucose
ADR—
   absence of deep reflexes
   adverse drug reaction
adrenal
   a. adenoma
   a. cortex
   a. crisis
   a. gland
   a. hyperplasia

adrenal *(continued)*
    a. hypoplasia
    a. insufficiency
    Marchand a.
    a. medulla
    a. steroids
    a. virilism
adrenalectomize
adrenalectomy
adrenaline acid tartrate
adrenalinemia
adrenalinuria
adrenalism
adrenalitis
adrenalopathy
adrenalotropic
adrenarche
adrenergic
    a. agonists
    a. antagonist
    a. nervous system
    a. stimulant
adrenoceptive
adrenoceptor
adrenochrome
adrenocortical
adrenocorticohyperplasia
adrenocorticoid
adrenocorticomimetic
adrenocorticosteroid
adrenocorticotrophic
adrenocorticotropic hormone
  (ACTH)
adrenocorticotropin
adrenodoxin
adrenogenous
adrenoglomerulotropin
adrenogram
adrenokinetic
adrenoleukodystrophy
adrenolutin
adrenolytic
adrenomedullary
adrenomedullotropic
adrenomegaly
adrenomimetic
adrenopathy
adrenoprival
adrenoreceptor
adrenostatic
adrenosterone
adrenosympathetic
adrenotoxin
adrenotropic
adrenotropin

adrenotropism
Adrian-Crooks–type cassette
adromia
ADS—
    anonymous donor sperm
    antibody-deficient syndrome
    antidiuretic substance
Adson
    bur
    cannula
    chisel
    clip
    conductor
    drill
    elevator
    forceps
    hook
    knife
    maneuver
    needle
    procedure
    retractor
    rongeur
    scissors
    suction tube
    syndrome
    test
    tube
adsorb
adsorbate
adsorbent
adsorption
    agglutinin a.
    immune a.
adsorption-hemagglutination
adsternal
adterminal
ADTP—alcohol dependency
  treatment program
adult
adulterant
adulteration
adumbration
AdV—adenovirus
advance
advancement
    capsular a.
    a. flap
    maxillary a.
    tendon a.
adventitia
adventitia dermis
adventitious sounds
adverse effects
adversive

advocate
    patient a.
adynamia episodica hereditaria
adynamic ileus
AE—
    above-elbow
    air entry
AEA—
    above-elbow amputation
    allergic extrinsic alveolitis
Aebli scissors
Aeby
    muscle
    plane
AED—
    antiepileptic drug
    automatic external
        defibrillator
Aedes aegypti
aedoeocephalus
Ae-H interval
AEP—auditory evoked potential
AEq—age equivalent
aequorin
AER—
    albumin excretion rate
    auditory evoked response
aerate, aerated
aeration
aeremia
aerial haze
aeriferous
aeriform
aeroallergen
aerobe
    facultative a.
    obligate a.
aerobic
aerobic capacity
aerocele
    epidural a.
    intracranial a.
Aerococcus viridans
aerocolpos
aerocystography
aerodermectasia
aerodigestive
aerodontalgia
aeroembolism
aerogastria
    blocked a.
aerogel
aerogen
aerogenesis
aerogenic

aerogenous
aeromedicine
aeromonad
Aeromonas
    A. caviae
    A. hydrophila
    A. sobria
aeroneurosis
aeropathy
aerophagia
aerophilic
aerophobia
Aeroplast dressing
aerosis
aerosol
aerosolization
aerotonometer
Af—
    atrial flutter
AF—
    acid-fast
    amniotic fluid
    Asian female
    atrial fibrillation
AFB—acid-fast bacillus, acid-fast
    bacilli
AFBG—aortofemoral bypass
    graft
AFC—acid-fast culture
afebrile
afetal
affect
    apathetic a.
    bland a.
    blunted a.
    congruent a.
    constricted a.
    depressed a.
    depressive a.
    euphoric a.
    flat a.
    impaired a.
    inappropriate a.
    labile a.
    restricted a.
affection
affective
affectivity
affectomotor
afferent
    a. defect
    flexor reflex a's
    a. nerve
    pressoreceptor a.
    primary a.

afferent *(continued)*
    somatic a.
    tendon organ a.
    visceral a.
afferentia
    tendon organ a.
    visceral a.
afferentiation
affiliation
affinity
    antibody a. chromatography
    chemical a.
    a. chromatography
    elective a.
    functional a.
    genetic a.
    a. labeling
    selective a.
affinous
afflux
affricate
affricative
A Fib—atrial fibrillation
afibrinogenemia
    congenital a.
AFl—atrial flutter
α-fluorocortisol [alpha-]
AFO—ankle-foot orthosis
aforementioned
AFP—
    alpha-fetoprotein
    atrial filling pressure
AFRD—acute febrile respiratory
   disease
AFS—
    acid-fast smear
    Alzheimer fugue state
    American Fertility Society
afterbirth
aftercare
aftercataract
after-coming head (of infant)
aftercontraction
aftercurrent
afterdamp
afterdepolarization
    delayed a. (DAD)
    early a. (EAD)
    late a.
afterdischarge
aftereffect
aftergilding
afterglow
afterhearing
afterhyperpolarization

afterimage
    negative a.
    positive a.
    Purkinje a.
afterimpression
    ventricular a.
afterload
    a. matching
    a. mismatching
    a.-reducing agent
    a. reduction
    ventricular a.
aftermath
aftermovement
afterpains
afterperception
afterpotential
    negative a.
    positive a.
    a. wave
afterpressure
aftersensation
aftertaste
α-L-fucosidase
afunction
AFV—amniotic fluid volume
Ag—
    antigen
    silver
AG—
    anion gap
    antiglobulin
    atrial gallop
    axiogingival
AGA—
    acute gonococcal arthritis
    American Gastroenterological
      Association
    appropriate for gestational
      age
against medical advice
   (AMA)
agalactia
α-D-galactosidase [alpha-]
agalactous
agalorrhea
agamete
agammaglobulinemia
    Bruton a.
    common variable a.
    lymphopenic a.
    Swiss-type a.
    X-linked infantile a.
aganglionic
aganglionosis

agar
  bacteriostasis a.
  bile-esculin a.
  bird seed a.
  bismuth sulfite a.
  blood a.
  Bordet-Gengou a.
  brain-heart infusion a.
  Brucella a.
  Campylobacter selective a.
  cetrimide a.
  charcoal yeast extract a.
  chocolate a.
  clostrisel a.
  Columbia blood a.
  corn meal a.
  Czapek-Dox a.
  deoxycholate-citrate a.
  deoxyribonuclease a.
  dextrose a.
  DNase a.
  egg-yolk a.
  Endo a.
  eosin–methylene blue
    (EMB) a.
  GC a.
  gelatin a.
  heart infusion a.
  Hektoen a.
  inhibitory mold a.
  Kligler iron a.
  Krumwiede triple sugar a.
  Levine EMB a.
  Löffler serum a.
  Löwenstein-Jensen
    (Lowenstein-Jensen,
    Loewenstein-Jensen) a.
  lysine iron a.
  MacConkey a.
  Middlebrook a.
  Mueller-Hinton a.
  mycobiotic a.
  Mycoplasma a.
  neomycin assay a.
  nitrate a.
  nutrient a.
  nystatin assay a.
  phenylalanine a.
  phenylethyl alcohol a.
  polymyxin test a's
  potato-blood a.
  potato dextrose a.
  Pseudomonas-selective a.
  rabbit blood a.
  Russell double-sugar a.

agar *(continued)*
  Sabhi a.
  Sabouraud dextrose a.
  saccharose-mannitol a.
  Salmonella-Shigella a.
  Schaedler blood a.
  seed a.
  Simmons citrate a.
  standard methods a.
  streptomycin assay a. with
    yeast extract
  sulfite a.
  tellurite a.
  tellurite glycine a.
  Thayer-Martin (TM) a.
  thistle seed a.
  Trichophyton a.
  triple sugar iron a.
  tryptic soy a.
  urea a.
  Wilkins-Chalgren a.
  xylose-lysine-deoxycholate a.
  Zein a.
agastria
agastric
AGC—absolute granulocyte count
AGE—
  acute gastroenteritis
  angle of greatest extension
age
  achievement a.
  anatomical a.
  Binet a.
  bone a.
  childbearing a.
  chronologic a., chronological a.
  coital a.
  a. of consent
  developmental a.
  emotional a.
  fertilization a.
  fetal a.
  functional a.
  gestational a.
  a. of menarche
  menarcheal a.
  menstrual a.
  mental a.
  ovulational a.
  physical a.
  physiologic a., physiological a.
  postovulatory a.
  reproductive a.
  skeletal a.
agenesia corticalis

agenesis
    anorectal a.
    callosal a.
    gonadal a.
    müllerian a.
    nuclear a.
    ovarian a.
    renal a.
    sacral a.
    vaginal a.
agenitalism
agenosomia
agenosomus
agent
    activating a.
    adrenergic blocking a.
    adrenergic neuron
        blocking a.
    afterload reducing a.
    alkylating a.
    alpha-adrenergic blocking a.
    antibacterial a.
    antifoaming a.
    beta-adrenergic blocking a.
    Bittner a.
    caudalizing a.
    chelating a.
    chemotherapeutic a.
    cholinergic blocking a.
    clearing a.
    complexing a.
    contrast a.
    desensitizing a.
    disclosing a.
    dorsalizing a.
    Eaton a.
    embedding a.
    fixing a's
    ganglionic blocking a.
    inducing a.
    luting a.
    mouse mammary tumor a.
    myoneural blocking a.
    neuromuscular blocking a.
    oncotic a.
    oxidizing a.
    progestational a.
    reducing a.
    sequestering a.
    transforming a.
    uncoupling a.
    virus-inactivating a.
    wetting a.
Agent Orange
agerasia

ageusia
    central a.
    conduction a.
    peripheral a.
ageusic
AGF—angle of greatest flexion
AGG—agammaglobulinemia
agger (aggeres)
    a. nasi
    a. perpendicularis
    a. valvae venae
agglomerated
agglutinable
agglutinant
agglutination
    acid a.
    alpha a.
    bacteriogenic a.
    beta a.
    cold a.
    cross a.
    flagellar a.
    group a.
    H a.
    heterophil a.
    immune a.
    intravascular a.
    latex a.
    macroscopic a.
    mediate a.
    microscopic a.
    O a.
    passive a.
    platelet a.
    Rh a.
    salt a.
    spontaneous a.
    T a.
    Vi a.
    warm a.
agglutinative
agglutinator
agglutinin
    alpha a.
    anti-A a.
    anti-B a.
    anti-M a.
    anti-N a.
    anti-P a.
    anti-Rh a.
    anti-S a.
    beta a.
    chief a.
    cold a.
    complete a.

agglutinin *(continued)*
    cross a.
    cross-reacting a.
    febrile a.
    flagellar a.
    group a.
    H a.
    immune a.
    incomplete a.
    latex a.
    leukocyte a.
    major a.
    Mg a.
    minor a.
    natural a.
    O a.
    partial a.
    platelet a.
    Rh a.
    saline a.
    serum a.
    somatic a.
    T a.
    warm a.
agglutinogen
agglutinogenic
agglutinophilic
agglutogenic
aggregate
    tubular a.
aggregated human IgG (AHuG)
aggregation
    cell a.
    familial a.
    platelet a.
aggregometry
aggression
    covert a.
    displaced a.
    healthy a.
aggressive
    a. behavior
    a. manner
    a. treatment
AGH—amenorrhea-galactorrhea
  hypothyroidism
aged, aging
agitated
agitation
agitographia
AGL—acute granulocytic leukemia
aglandular
aglomerular
aglossia
aglossostomia

α-glucan glycosyl 4:6-transferase
aglucon
α-glucosaminide-*N*-
    acetyltransferase
α-glucosidase
    lysosomal α.
aglycemia
aglycon
aglycosuric
agminated follicles
agmination
AGN—acute glomerulonephritis
agnathia
agnathous
agnathus
agnea
Agnew
    keratome
    operation
    splint
Agnew-Verhoeff incision
agnosia
    acoustic a.
    apraxic a.
    auditory a.
    body-image a.
    chromatic a.
    developmental a.
    digital a.
    facial a.
    finger a.
    geometrical a.
    gustatory a.
    ideational a.
    localization a.
    nonsymbolic visual a.
    position a.
    spatial a.
    symbolic visual a.
    tactile a.
    time a.
    topographical a.
    visual a.
    visual-spatial a.
    visuospatial a.
agnosic
agonad
agonadal
agonadism
agonal
agonist
    beta-2 a.
    beta-adrenergic a.
    cholinergic a's
    muscarinic a's

agonist *(continued)*
    narcotic a's
    prostaglandin a's
agonistic
agony
agoraphobia
agrammatism
agranular
agranulocyte
agranulocytic
agranulocytosis
    infantile genetic a.
    infantile lethal a.
agranuloplastic
agraphesthesia
agraphia
    absolute a.
    acoustic a.
    a. amnemonica
    a. atactica
    cerebral a.
    jargon a.
    literal a.
    mental a.
    motor a.
    musical a.
    optic a.
    sensory a.
    verbal a.
agraphic
Agrikola retractor
agrypnotic
AGS—
    adrenogenital syndrome
    American Geriatrics Society
AGT—antiglobulin test
AGV—aniline gentian violet
agyria
agyric
Ah—hypermetropic astigmatism
AH—abdominal hysterectomy
A&H—amenorrhea and hirsutism
AHA—
    acquired hemolytic anemia
    American Heart Association
    autoimmune hemolytic anemia
ahaptoglobinemia
AHC—acute hemorrhagic cystitis
AHD—
    arteriosclerotic heart disease
    atherosclerotic heart disease
    autoimmune hemolytic
      disease
AHDI—Association for Healthcare
  Documentation Integrity

AHF—antihemophilic factor
AHG—antihemophilic globulin
Ahlfeld sign
AHuG—aggregated human IgG
Ahumada-del Castillo
  syndrome
17α-hydrolase [17-alpha-]
17α-hydroxyprogesterone
  [17-alpha-]
17α-hydroxyprogesterone aldolase
  [17-alpha-]
$15-\alpha$-hydroxy prostaglandin
  dehydrogenase [-alpha-]
AI—
    anaphylatoxin inactivator
    anaphylatoxin inhibitor
    aortic incompetence
    aortic insufficiency
    apical impulse
    artificial insemination
    axioincisal
Aicardi syndrome
AICD—automatic implantable
  cardioverter-defibrillator
aichmophobia
AID—
    acute infectious disease
    artificial insemination by
      donor
aid
    air-conduction hearing a.
    binaural hearing a.
    body-worn hearing a.
    bone-conduction hearing a.
    contralateral routing of
      signals (CROS) a.
    electric hearing a.
    first a.
    in-the-ear (ITE) hearing a.
    mechanical hearing a.
    pharmaceutic a.,
      pharmaceutical a.
    prosthetic speech a.
    ultrasonic mobility a.
aide
    nurse's a.
AIDS—acquired immunodeficiency
  syndrome
α-L-iduronidase deficiency
AIH—
    American Institute of
      Homeopathy
    artificial insemination by
      husband
AII (atrial inhibited) pacing

AILD—angioimmunoblastic
lymphadenopathy with
dysproteinemia
ailment
ailurophobia
Ainsworth punch
AIP—acute intermittent porphyria
air
    alveolar a.
    ambient a.
    a. arthrography
    a. bed
    a. bronchogram
    a. bronchogram sign
    complementary a.
    a. conduction
    a. crescent sign
    a. curtain
    a. cushion
    a. cushion sign
    dead space a.
    a. embolism
    a. encephalography
    functional residual a.
    a. gap
    a. hunger
    a. insufflation
    laminar a. flow
    liquid a.
    a. monitor
    a. myelography
    a. pyelography
    reserve a.
    residual a.
    a. splint
    stationary a.
    supplemental a.
    a. swallowing
    tidal a.
    a. tube
    venous alveolar a.
    vitiated a.
air-bone gap
airborne
air-cuff plethysmography
airflow obstruction disease (AOD)
air-fluid level
AirGEL
airplane splint
airsickness
air space disease
airway
    anatomical a.
    artificial a.
    Brain [eponym] a.
    a. closure

airway *(continued)*
    a. conductance
    conducting a.
    endotracheal a.
    a. epithelium
    esophageal obturator a.
    a. heat loss
    a. hyperactivity
    laryngeal mask a.
    lower a.
    a. narrowing
    nasopharyngeal a.
    oropharyngeal a.
    a. osmolarity
    a. permeability
    a. reactivity
    a. receptors
    a. resistance
    respiratory a.
    a. tone
    upper a.
AIU—absolute iodine uptake
AIUM—American Institute of
    Ultrasound in Medicine
AK—above-knee, above-the-knee
AKA—above-knee amputation
akathisia
    psychic a.
akee, ackee
Åkerlund (Akerlund)
    deformity
    diaphragm
α-ketoglutarate glyoxylate
    carboligase
α-ketoglutaric acid
Akin
    bunionectomy
    operation
akinesia
    a. algera
    a. amnestica
    cerebral a.
    Nadbath a.
    O'Brien a.
    reflex a.
    spinal a.
    van Lint a.
akinesis
akinesthesia
akinetic
AL—axiolingual
ala (alae)
    alae lingulae cerebelli
    a. auris
    a. cerebelli
    a. cinerea

ala (alae) *(continued)*
    a. cristae galli
    a. ilii
    a. lobuli centralis
    a. major ossis sphenoidalis
    a. minor ossis sphenoidalis
    a. nasi
    a. ossis ilii
    a. ossis ilium
    a. sacri
    a. vomeris
Ala—alanine
ALA—
    α-aminolevulinic acid
    alpha-lipoic acid
    aminolevulinic acid
alacrima
alactasia
Alajouanine
    disease
    syndrome
alanine (Ala, A)
    a. aminotransferase (ALAT)
    a. racemase
    a. transaminase
Al-Anon
Alanson amputation
alar incision
ALARA—as low as reasonably
  achievable
Albarran
    disease
    gland
    test
    tubules
albedo
    a. retinae
    a. unguium
Albee
    fracture table
    operation
    osteotome
    saw
Albee-Delbet operation
Albers-Schönberg (Albers-Schoenberg)
    bone
    disease
    syndrome
Albert
    bronchoscope
    diphtheria stain
    disease
    operation
    position
    suture
Albert-Andrews laryngoscope

albicans
albiduria
albidus
Albini nodules
albinism
    a. I, a. II
    acquired a.
    Amish a.
    autosomal dominant
      oculocutaneous a.
    autosomal recessive ocular a.
      (AROA)
    brown a.
    complete imperfect a.
    complete perfect a.
    cutaneous a.
    Forsius-Eriksson ocular a.
    Forsius-Eriksson–type ocular a.
    localized a.
    Nettleship-Falls–type ocular a.
    ocular a. (OA)
    oculocutaneous a. (OCA)
    partial a.
    piebald a.
    red a.
    rufous a.
    tyrosinase-negative (ty-neg)
      oculocutaneous a.
    tyrosinase-positive (ty-pos)
      oculocutaneous a.
    xanthous a.
    X-linked ocular a. (Nettleship-
      Falls) (XOAN)
    yellow mutant (ym)
      oculocutaneous a.
albinismus
    a. circumscriptus
    a. totalis
    a. universalis
albino
albinoidism
    oculocutaneous a.
    punctate oculocutaneous a.
albinotic
Albinus muscle
Albrecht
    bone
    suture
Albright
    disease
    dystrophy
    hereditary osteodystrophy
    solution
    syndrome
albuginea
    a. oculi

albuginea *(continued)*
    a. ovarii
    a. penis
    a. testis
albugineotomy
albugineous
albuginitis
albumin
    a. A
    acetosoluble a.
    acid a.
    alkali a.
    a. of Bence Jones
    blood a.
    coagulated a.
    derived a.
    egg a.
    hematin a.
    human a.
    iodinated I 125 serum a.
    iodinated I 131 serum a.
    macroaggregated a. (MAA)
    native a.
    normal human serum a.
    radioiodinated (^{125}I) serum a.
      (human)
    radioiodinated (^{131}I) serum a.
      (human)
    tannate a.
    technetium Tc 99m aggregated a.
    triphenyl a.
    vegetable a.
albuminate
albuminaturia
albuminemia
albuminimetry
albuminocholia
albuminocytological
albuminoid
albuminolysis
albuminoptysis
albuminoreaction
albuminorrhea
albuminous
albuminuria
    adventitious a.
    Bamberger hematogenic a.
    globular a.
    nephrogenous a.
    postrenal a.
    renal a.
    residual a.
albuminuric retinitis
Alcaligenes
    A. denitrificans
    A. faecalis

Alcian blue
Alcock
    canal
    catheter
    lithotrite
Alcock-Hendrickson lithotrite
Alcock-Timberlake obturator
alcohol
    absolute a.
    acid a.
    amyl a., tertiary
    anisyl a.
    aromatic a.
    azeotropic isopropyl a.
    benzyl a.
    camphyl a.
    ceryl a.
    cinnamyl a.
    a. dehydrogenase
    denatured a.
    dihydric a.
    diluted a.
    fatty a.
    fetal a. syndrome
    grain a.
    a. intoxication
    isoamyl a.
    isobutyl a.
    isopropyl rubbing a.
    ketone a.
    methyl a.
    monohydric a.
    nicotinyl a.
    palmityl a.
    pantothenyl a.
    polyglucosic a.
    polyvinyl a.
    rubbing a.
    secondary a.
    stearyl a.
    sugar a's
    tertiary a.
    tribromoethyl a.
    trihydric a.
    unsaturated a.
    wood a.
alcoholemia
alcoholic psychosis
Alcoholics Anonymous (AA)
alcoholism
    epsilon a.
    paroxysmal a.
alcoholization
alcoholize
alcoholometer
alcoholysis

Alcon suture
Alco-Sensor
aldehyde
    cinnamic a.
    a. dehydrogenase (NAD+)
    a. fuchsin
    glycolic a.
    keto a.
    a.-lyase
    a. oxidase
    salicylic a.
    a.-tanned
Alder anomaly
Alder-Reilly bodies
aldohexose
aldolase
aldosterone
    a. adenoma
    a. suppression test
aldosteronism
    idiopathic a.
    juvenile a.
    primary a.
    pseudoprimary a.
    secondary a.
aldosteronogenesis
aldosteronoma
Aldrich syndrome
Aldrich-Mees lines
Aldridge operation
aldrin
aleurone
aleuronoid
Alexander
    chisel
    deafness
    disease
    gouge
    hearing loss
    incision
    operation
    osteotome
    periosteotome
Alexander-Adams operation
Alexander-Farabeuf
    elevator
    periosteotome
alexanderism
alexandrine
alexia
    a. with agraphia
    a. without aphasia
    aphasic a.
    cortical a.
    Dejerine a.

alexia *(continued)*
    developmental a.
    geometric a.
    isolated a.
    motor a.
    musical a.
    occipital a.
    optical a.
    parietal a.
    pure a.
    semantic a.
    sensory a.
    subcortical a.
    symbolic a.
    tactile a.
    verbal a.
alexic
aleydigism
Alezzandrini syndrome
ALG—antilymphocyte globulin
algedonic
algefacient
Alger brush
algesia
algesic
algesimetry
algesthesia
algicide
algid
alginate
algiomotor
algiovascular
algogenesia
algogenic
algolagnia
algophilia
algophobia
algor mortis
algorithm
algospasm
Alibert
    disease
    keloid
    mentagra
alible
Alice in Wonderland syndrome
alienation
aliflurane
aliform
align
alignment
    anatomical a.
    Cooley-Tukey a.
    optimal a.
alimentary

alimentation
    artificial a.
    forced a.
    parenteral a.
    rectal a.
    total parenteral a. (TPA)
alinasal
alipogenic
alipoidic
alipotropic
alisphenoid
alkalemia
alkalescence
alkalescent
alkali
alkaligenous
alkalimetry
    Engel a.
alkaline phosphatase (ALP)
alkalinity
alkalinuria
alkalization
alkalizer
alkalogenic
alkaloid
    vinca a's
alkalosis
    acapnial a.
    altitude a.
    carbon dioxide a.
    compensated a.
    congenital gastrointestinal a.
    hypochloremic a.
    hypokalemic a.
    metabolic a., compensated
    respiratory a., compensated
alkalotic
alkaluria
alkane
alkannin
alkaptonuria
    spontaneous a.
alkaptonuric
alkatriene
alkene
alkyl
alkylamine
alkylate
alkylation
ALL—
    acute lymphoblastic leukemia
    acute lymphocytic leukemia
allantiasis
allantochorion
allantogenesis

allantoic
allantoid
allantoin
allantoinuria
allantois
Allarton operation
allele
    multiple a's
    silent a.
allelic exclusion
allelism
Allemann syndrome
Allen
    clamp
    cyclodialysis
    implant
    law
    maneuver
    operation
    orbital implant
    paradoxical law
    root pliers
    test
    treatment
    trocar
Allen-Masters syndrome
allergen
allergenic extracts
allergic
    a. bronchopulmonary
      aspergillosis
    a. contact dermatitis (ACD)
    a. granulomatosis
    a. orchitis
    a. purpura
    a. rhinitis
    a. salute
    a. shiner
    a. urticaria
allergist
allergization
allergize
allergoid
allergologic, allergological
allergologist
allergology
allergosis
allergy
    atopic a.
    bacterial a.
    bronchial a.
    cold a.
    contact a.
    delayed a.
    drug a.

allergy *(continued)*
    food a.
    gastrointestinal a.
    hereditary a.
    humoral a.
    immediate a.
    intrinsic a.
    latent a.
    nasal a.
    physical a.
    pollen a.
    polyvalent a.
    seasonal a.
    spontaneous a.
allesthesia
    alleviant a.
    visual a.
allethrin
All-Flex diaphragm
alliance
    therapeutic a.
    working a.
allicin
Allingham
    colotomy
    fissure
    operation
    rectal speculum
    rectum excision
    ulcer
Allis
    clamp
    forceps
    inhaler
    sign
Allis-Ochsner forceps
Allison
    retractor
    suture
alliteration
alloalbumin
alloantigen
allodynia
alloeroticism
allogeneic
allograft
    cadaveric a.
    living related a.
    living unrelated a.
    nerve a.
alloimmune
alloimmunization
allokeratoplasty
allokinesis
allokinetic

allopathic
allopathist
allopathy
alloplast
alloplastic
alloplasty
allopregnanediol
allopsychic
alloreactive
allorhythmia
allorhythmic
all or none
allosensitization
allotoxin
allotransplantation
allotriodontia
allotriogeustia
allotropic
allotropy
allotypy
allowance
    recommended dietary a. (RDA)
alloy
    amalgam a.
    chrome-cobalt a.
    dental a.
    Newton silver-tin a.
    solid solution a.
Allport
    operation
    retractor
    searcher
allude, alluded
allusion
allyl isothiocyanate
allylamines
Alm retractor
Almeida disease
Almén test
almond
    bitter a.
Almoor operation
α-lobeline [alpha-]
alochia
Aloe, aloe
aloetic
alopecia
    a. acquisita
    androgenetic a.
    a. areata
    a. capitis totalis
    cicatricial a.
    a. cicatrisata
    a. circumscripta
    a. congenitalis

alopecia *(continued)*
    congenital sutural a.
    congenital triangular a.
    a. disseminata
    drug-induced a.
    favid a.
    female pattern a.
    follicular a.
    a. follicularis
    a. hereditaria
    hereditary a.
    a. leprotica
    a. liminaris
    male pattern a.
    marginal a.
    a. marginalis
    mechanical a.
    a. medicamentosa
    moth-eaten a.
    a. mucinosa
    physiologic a.
    pityriasic a.
    postpartum a.
    a. prematura
    premature a.
    a. presenilis
    pressure a.
    psychogenic a.
    radiation-induced a.
    senile a.
    a. senilis
    stress a.
    a. symptomatica
    a. syphilitica
    a. totalis
    a. toxica
    traction a.
    a. traumatica
    traumatic marginal a.
    a. triangularis congenitalis
    a. universalis
    x-ray a.
alopecic
Alouette
    amputation
    operation
ALP—alkaline phosphatase
Alpar implant
Alpers
    disease
    polioencephalopathy
alpha
    Greek letter
      (α; alphabetized as a)
    a.-*N*-acetylgalactosaminidase

alpha *(continued)*
    a.-*N*-acetylglucosaminidase
    a. chamber
    a. acid glycoprotein
    a.-adrenergic receptor
    a. amino acids
    a. amino nitrogen
    a.-amylose
    a. antichymotrypsin
    a. antiplasmin
    a.$_1$-antitrypsin
    a. band
    a.-beta variation
    a. cells
    a. chain
    a.-chymotrypsin
    a. decay
    a.-dextrinase
    a.-difluoromethylornithine
    a.-dinitrophenol
    a.-estradiol [now: estradiol
      17α (17-alpha)]
    a.-fetoprotein (AFP)
    a.-L-fucosidase
    a.-galactosidase A
    a. globulin
    a. globulin antibodies
    a.$_2$ globulins
    1,4-a.-glucan branching
      enzyme
    a. 1,4-glucosidase
    a.-helix
    a.-hemolytic streptococci
    17-a.-hydroxyprogesterone
      aldolase
    a.-hypophamine
    a.-L-iduronidase
    a.-interferon
    a.-keto acid dehydrogenase
    a.-ketoglutarate
    a.-ketoglutaric acid
    a.-lipoprotein
    a.-lobeline
    a.$_2$-macroglobulin
    a.-mannosidase
    a. melanocytic-stimulating
      hormone
    a.-methylacetoacetic acid
    a.-methylacetaceticaciduria
    a.-methylacetoacetyl CoA
      thiolase
    a.-methyldopa
    a.-naphthol thiourea
    a.-naphthyl acetate esterase
      reaction

alpha *(continued)*
    a. nerve fibers
    a. particles
    a. protease inhibitor
    a. radiation
    a. ray
    a. receptors
    a. seromucoid
    a.-streptococci
    a.-thalassemia
    a. threshold
    a.$_1$-thymosin
    a.-tocopherol
    a.-trypsin
alpha heavy chain disease
alphalytic
alphamimetic
alphanumeric
alphavirus
Alport syndrome
ALS—
    advanced life support
    amyotrophic lateral sclerosis
    antilymphocyte serum
Alsberg
    angle
    triangle
Alström (Alstrom)
    disease
    syndrome
Alström-Olsen syndrome (Alstrom-Olsen)
Alsus-Knapp operation
alterative
alteregoism
alternans
    auditory a.
    auscultatory a.
    electrical a.
    a. of the heart
    mechanical a.
alternating
    a. esotropia
    a. strabismus
    a. sursumduction
    a. suture
alternation
    cardiac a.
Altmann
    aniline-acid fuchsin stain
    fixative
    fluid
    granule
    liquid
    theory

Altmann-Gersh method
alum
    ammonium a.
    burnt a.
    chrome a.
    dried a.
    a. hematoxylin
    iron a.
aluminated
aluminosis
aluminum (Al)
    a. acetate
    a. aminoacetate
    a. ammonium sulfate
    basic a. carbonate
    a. chlorhydrex
    colloidal a. hydroxide
    a. glycinate
    a. hydrate
    a. hydroxide
    a. monostearate
    a. nicotinate
    a. oxide
    a. penicillin
    a. phosphate
    a. potassium sulfate
    a. sulfate
alveobronchiolitis
alveolabial
alveolalgia
alveolar
    a. arch
    a. capillary membrane
    a. hypoventilation
    a. proteinosis
    a. ridge
    segmental a. osteotomy
alveolate
alveolectomy
    transseptal a.
alveoli (genitive and plural of alveolus)
alveolitis
    allergic a.
    cryptogenic fibrosing a.
    diffuse sclerosing a.
    extrinsic allergic a.
    fibrosing a.
    a. sicca dolorosa
    a. with honeycombing
alveolocapillary
alveoloclasia
alveolodental
alveololabial
alveololingual

alveolomerotomy
alveolonasal
alveolopalatal
alveoloplasty
    interradicular a.
    intraseptal a.
alveolotomy
alveolus (alveoli)
    dental a.
    alveoli dentales mandibulae
    alveoli dentales maxillae
    alveoli dentis
    pulmonary a.
    alveoli pulmonis
    alveoli pulmonum
alveolysis
alveus (alvei)
    a. hippocampi
Alvis operation
Alyea clamp
alymphia
alymphocytosis
alymphoplasia
    thymic a.
Alzheimer
    cell
    dementia
    disease
    fibril
    primary degenerative
      dementia
    sclerosis
    stain
    syndrome
am—
    meterangle ametropia
    myopic astigmatism
a.m.—before noon
    (L. ante meridiem)
AM—Asian male
ama [ayurvedic]
AMA—
    Aerospace Medical Association
    against medical advice
    American Medical
      Association
    antimitochondrial antibody
amacrinal
amacrine cells
Amadori
    product
    rearrangement
amalgam
    copper a.
    dental a.

amalgam *(continued)*
    retrograde a.
    silver a.
amalgamate
amalgamation
Amanita
    A. muscaria
    A. pantherina
    A. phalloides
    A. verna
    A. virosa
amanitine
amanitotoxin
amaranth
amarine
amaroid
amaroidal
amasesis
amastia
amathophobia
amatol
amaurosis
    albuminuric a.
    Burns a.
    cat-eye s., cat's eye a.
    central a.
    a. centralis
    cerebral a.
    compression a.
    congenital a.
    a. congenita of Leber
    diabetic a.
    a. fugax
    hysterical a.
    intoxication a.
    Leber congenital a.
    a. partialis fugax
    reflex a.
    saburral a.
    toxic a.
    uremic a.
amaurotic
    a. nystagmus
    a. pupil
Amberg lateral sinus line
Amberlite
AMBI
    hip screw
    nail
ambidexterity
ambidextrous
ambient
ambiguity
    lexical a.
    ribosomal a.

ambiguity *(continued)*
    role a.
    sexual identity a.
    structural a.
ambiguous
ambilateral
ambilevosity
ambilevous
ambivalence
ambivalent
ambiversion
ambivert
AMBL—acute myeloblastic
  leukemia
amblychromasia
amblychromatic
amblyope
amblyopia
    a. alcoholica
    ametropic a.
    arsenic a.
    astigmatic a.
    color a.
    crossed a.
    a. cruciata
    deprivation a.
    eclipse a.
    a. ex anopsia
    nocturnal a.
    nutritional a.
    quinine a.
    receptor a.
    reflex a.
    strabismic a.
    suppression a.
    tobacco a.
    toxic a.
    traumatic a.
    uremic a.
amblyoscope
ambon
Ambu bag
ambulance
ambulant
ambulation
ambulatory
ameba
amebiasis
    a. of bladder
    a. cutis
    hepatic a.
    intestinal a.
    pulmonary a.
amebic
amebicidal

amebicides
amebiform
ameboid
ameboma
ameburia
amelanosis
amelanotic
amelia
    brachial a.
    complete a.
    unilateral a.
ameliorate, ameliorated
amelioration
ameloblastoma
    acanthomatous a.
    basal cell a.
    cystic a.
    extraosseous a.
    follicular a.
    granular cell a.
    malignant a.
    melanotic a.
    multicystic a.
    peripheral a.
    pigmented a.
    pituitary a.
    plexiform unicystic a.
    solid a.
    spindle cell a.
    unicystic a.
amelodentinal
amelogenesis imperfecta
amelogenic
amelogenin
amelus
amenable
amenorrhea
    absolute a.
    dietary a.
    dysponderal a.
    functional a.
    hypothalamic a.
    lactation a.
    nutritional a.
    ovarian a.
    pathologic a.
    physiologic a.
    pituitary a.
    post-pill a.
    premenopausal a.
    primary a.
    relative a.
    secondary a.
    traumatic a.
amenorrheal

American Academy of Orthopaedic
   Surgeons (AAOS)
American Board of Radiology (ABR)
American College of Radiology (ACR)
American College of Sports
   Medicine (ACSM)
American Institute of Ultrasound
   in Medicine (AIUM)
American Physical Therapy
   Association (APTA)
American Psychiatric Association
   (APA)
American Registry of Diagnostic
   Medical Sonographers (ARDMS)
American Thoracic Society (ATS)
American Type Culture Collection
   (ATCC)
americium (Am)
Ames test
α-methylacetoacetyl CoA-
   β-ketothiolase
ametria
ametropia
      axial a.
      curvature a.
      index a.
      position a.
      refractive a.
ametropic
Amh—mixed astigmatism with
   myopia predominating
AMH—automated medical history
AMI—acute myocardial
   infarction
amianthoid
Amici
      disk
      line
      striae
Amico
      drill
      extractor
      nail nipper
      skin lifter
amiculum (amicula)
      a. olivare
      a. of olive
amidine
amidine-lyase
amidinotransferase
amidobenzene
amidogen
amidohydrolase
amido-ligase
amidoxime

amimia
      amnesic a.
      ataxic a.
amine
      adrenergic a.
      vasoactive a's
amino acid
      α-a.a.
      D-a.a. oxidase
      aromatic a.a.
      basic a.a's
      essential a.a's
      ketogenic a.a.
      nonessential a.a's
      a.a. residue
      a.a. sequence
      sulfur-containing a.a's
      uncoded a.a.
aminoacidemia
aminoacidopathy
aminoaciduria
      imidazole a.
      overflow a.
      renal a.
      transport a.
aminoacyl
      a. adenylate
      a. histidine dipeptidase
      a.-tRNA synthetase
aminoacyltransferase
aminoacylase
o-aminoazotoluene [o-, ortho-]
aminobenzene
p-aminobenzoate (PAB) [p-, para-]
p-aminobenzoic acid (PABA)
      [p-, para-]
γ-aminobutyrate [gamma-]
γ-aminobutyric acid (GABA)
      [gamma-]
aminoglycoside
p-aminohippuric acid (PAH, PAHA)
      [p-, para-]
β-aminoisobutyricaciduria [beta-]
aminolevulinate dehydratase
5-aminolevulinate synthase
aminolevulinic acid (ALA)
aminolysis
aminopeptidase
      leucine a.
aminopurine
aminosalicylate
aminosis
aminosuria
aminuria
AML—acute myeloblastic leukemia

Ammon
- blepharoplasty
- canthoplasty
- dacryocystotomy
- filaments
- fissure
- horn
- operation

ammonia hemate
ammoniacal
ammonia-lyase
ammoniate
ammonification
ammonium
- a. bromide
- a. chloride
- ferric a. citrate
- ferric a. sulfate
- a. mandelate
- a. muriate
- a. oxalate
- a. purpurate
- a. sulfate
- a. tungstate

ammoniuria
ammonolysis
amnesia
- affective a.
- anterograde a.
- auditory a.
- Broca a.
- circumscribed a.
- concussion a.
- continuous a.
- elective a.
- emotional a.
- episodic a.
- generalized a.
- graphokinetic a.
- hysterical a.
- immunologic a.
- incomplete a.
- infantile a.
- Korsakoff a.
- lacunar a.
- localized a.
- mimokinetic a.
- olfactory a.
- organic a.
- patchy a.
- postconcussional a.
- posthypnotic a.
- posttraumatic a.
- psychogenic a.
- retroactive a.

amnesia *(continued)*
- retrograde a.
- selective a.
- systematic a.
- tactile a.
- transient global a.
- traumatic a.
- verbal a.
- visual a.

amnesiac
amnesic
amnestic
amniocele
amniocentesis
amniochorial
amniocyte
amniogenesis
amniogram
amnioma
amnion
- anterior cul-de-sac a.
- caudal cul-de-sac a.
- ectoplacental a.
- a. nodosum

amnionic
amnionitis
amniorrhea
amniorrhexis
amnioscope
amnioscopy
Amniostat-FLM
  (fetal lung maturity) test
amniotic fluid
amniotome
- Baylor a.
- Beacham a.

amniotomy
A-mode ultrasonography
Amoils
- cryoextractor
- cryoprobe
- retractor

amok, amuck
AMOL—acute monoblastic leukemia
amoral
amorphagnosia
amorphia
amorphous
amorphus
Amoss sign
amotio retinae
AMP—
- adenosine monophosphate
- average mean pressure

AMP deaminase

3′,5′-AMP, cyclic AMP—cyclic
  adenosine monophosphate
ampere (A)
ampere-second (A-s)
amphetamine
amphibious
amphibolic
amphicentric
amphichroic
amphicreatinine
amphidiarthrosis
amphigastrula
amphigenetic
amphigonadism
amphigony
amphileukemic
amphimorula
amphinucleus
amphipathic
amphipyrenin
amphitheater
amphitypy
amphogenic
ampholyte
amphophilic
    a.-basophil
    gram-a.
    a.-oxyphil
amphoric
amphoricity
amphoriloquy
amphorophony
amphoteric
amphoterism
amphotony
AMP kinase
Amplatz
    cardiac catheter
    coronary catheter
amplification
    compression a.
    gas a.
    gene a.
    image a.
amplifier
    buffer a.
    linear a.
    nuclear pulse a.
    pulse a.
    voltage a.
amplitude
    a. of accommodation
    a. of convergence
    a. image
    a. modulation

amplitude *(continued)*
    peak a.
    peak-to-peak a.
AMPPE—acute multifocal placoid
  pigment epitheliopathy
ampule
ampulla (ampullae)
    ampullae lactiferae
    anterior membranaceous a.
    a. canaliculi lacrimalis
    a. ductus deferentis
    a. ductus lacrimalis
    duodenal a.
    a. duodeni
    a. of gallbladder
    Henle a.
    a. hepatopancreatica
    a. of lacrimal canaliculus
    lateral membranaceous a.
    a. of Mascagni
    a. membranacea anterior
    a. membranacea lateralis
    a. membranacea posterior
    a. ossea anterior
    a. ossea lateralis
    a. ossea posterior
    phrenic a.
    posterior membranaceous a.
    rectal a.
    a. recti
    a. of Thoma
    a. of thoracic duct
    a. tubae uterinae
    a. of uterine tube
    a. of vas deferens
    a. of Vater
ampullar
ampullary
ampullate
ampullitis
ampullula
amputate
amputation
    AK (above-knee) a.
    Alanson a.
    Alouette a.
    Anderson a.
    aperiosteal a.
    Béclard a.
    Berger a.
    Bier a.
    BK (below-knee) a.
    bloodless a.
    Bunge a.
    a. by transfixion

amputation *(continued)*
   Callander a.
   Carden a.
   central a.
   cervix a.
   chop a.
   Chopart a.
   cinematic a.
   cineplastic a.
   circular a.
   closed a.
   coat-sleeve a.
   cutaneous a.
   definitive a.
   Dieffenbach a.
   double-flap a.
   Dupuytren a.
   eccentric a.
   elliptical a.
   end-bearing a.
   Farabeuf a.
   flap a.
   flapless a.
   Forbes a.
   forequarter a.
   Gritti a.
   Gritti-Stokes a.
   guillotine a.
   Guyon a.
   Hancock a.
   Hey a.
   hindquarter a.
   interilioabdominal a.
   interinnominoabdominal a.
   intermediary a.
   interpelviabdominal a.
   interscapulothoracic a.
   Jaboulay a.
   kineplastic a.
   Kirk a.
   Langenbeck
     (von Langenbeck) a.
   Larrey a.
   Le Fort a.
   linear a.
   Lisfranc a.
   Mackenzie a.
   Maisonneuve a.
   major a.
   Malgaigne a.
   mediotarsal a.
   metacarpal a.
   minor a.
   mixed a.
   musculocutaneous a.

amputation *(continued)*
   oblique a.
   open a.
   osteoplastic a.
   oval a.
   pathologic a.
   periosteoplastic a.
   phalangophalangeal a.
   Pirogoff a.
   primary a.
   provisional a.
   pulp a.
   racket a.
   ray a.
   rectangular a.
   Ricard a.
   root a.
   secondary a.
   semicircular flap a.
   spontaneous a.
   Stokes a.
   subastragalar a.
   submalleolar a.
   subperiosteal a.
   supracondylar a.
   Syme a.
   Teale a.
   tertiary a.
   through-the-knee a.
   transfixation a.
   transmetatarsal a.
   traumatic a.
   traverse a.
   Tripier a.
   Vladimiroff-Mikulicz a.
amputee
Amsler
   chart
   corneal graft operation
   grid
   marker
   needle
   test
amuck, amok
amusia
   instrumental a.
   sensory a.
   vocal motor a.
Amussat
   operation
   valve
   valvula
amychophobia
amyctic
amyelencephalia

amyelencephalus
amyelia
amyelic
amyelonic
amyelus
amygdala
    a. amara
    a. of cerebellum
    a. dulcis
amygdalin
amygdaline
amygdalohippocampectomy
amygdaloid
amylaceous
amylase
    pancreatic a.
    salivary a.
    serum a.
    urinary a.
amylasuria
amylemia
amylic
amylin
amylism
amylodextrin
amylodyspepsia
amylogenesis
amylogenic
amylo-1,6-glucosidase deficiency
amyloid
amyloidosis
    AA a.
    a. of aging
    AL a.
    Andrade-type a.
    cutaneous a.
    a. cutis
    familial a.
    hereditary a.
    heredofamilial a.
    idiopathic a.
    immunocyte-derived a.
    immunocytic a.
    Indiana-type a.
    Iowa-type a.
    kidney a.
    a. of larynx
    lichen a.
    light chain–related a.
    macular a.
    a. of multiple myeloma
    nodular a.
    Portuguese-type a.
    primary a.
    reactive systemic a.

amyloidosis *(continued)*
    renal a.
    secondary a.
    senile a.
amylolysis
amylolytic
amylopectin
amylopectinosis
amylophagia
amyloplastic
amylorrhea
amylose
amyluria
amyoplasia congenita
amyostasia
amyostatic
amyotonia
    a. congenita
    Oppenheim a.
amyotrophia
    neuralgic a.
    a. spinalis progressiva
amyotrophic
amyotrophy
    Aran-Duchenne a.
    diabetic a.
    neuralgic a.
    neuritic a.
    primary progressive a.
    progressive nuclear a.
    syphilitic a.
amyous
amyxia
amyxorrhea
ANA—antinuclear
    antibody
anabolic
anabolism
anachronism
anacidity
    gastric a.
anaclisis
anaclitic
anacobra
anacrotic, anadicrotic
anacrotism, anadicrotism
anadidymus
anadrenalism
anaerobic
anagen
Anagnostakis operation
anagogic
anagogy
anagotoxic
anakatadidymus

anakmesis
anal
  a. canal
  a. manometry
  a. speculum
  a. sphincter
analbuminemia
analeptic
analgesia
  a. algera
  audio a.
  conduction a.
  congenital a.
  continuous epidural a.
  a. dolorosa
  electrical a.
  epidural a.
  hysterical a.
  infiltration a.
  obstetric a.
  paretic a.
  perineural a.
  relative a.
  serial caudal a.
  spinal a.
analgesic
anallergic
analog
analogous
analog-to-digital (A/D) converter
analogue
  folic acid a.
  homologous a.
  metabolic a.
  purine a.
  pyrimidine a.
  substrate a.
analogy
analphalipoproteinemia
analysis
  acoustic a. of speech
  basic volume image a.
  bite a.
  blood gas a.
  bradykinetic a.
  cephalometric a.
  character a.
  chemical a.
  densimetric a.
  displacement a.
  Downs a.
  ego a.
  fluctuation a.
  Fourier a.
  gastric a.

analysis *(continued)*
  gravimetric a.
  group a.
  isotope dilution a.
  occlusal a.
  organic a.
  pentagastrin stimulated a.
  radiochemical a.
  saturation a.
  Simkin
  spectroscopic a.
  stop-flow a.
  structural a.
  tetrad a.
  transactional a.
  tubeless gastric a.
  vector a.
  volumetric a.
analysor
analyst
analyte
analytic, analytical
analyzer
  amino acid a.
  auditory a.
  blood gas a.
  breath a.
  centrifugal fast a.
  frequency a.
  image a.
  kinetic a.
  multichannel a's
  oxygen gas a.
  pulse-height a.
  sensory a.
  sequential multiple a. (SMA)
  visual a.
  voice a.
  wave a.
anamnesis
  associative a.
anamnestic response
anancastic
anangioid
anapepsia
anaphase
anaphia
anaphoresis
anaphoretic
anaphoria
anaphrodisiac
anaphylactic
anaphylactin
anaphylactogen
anaphylactogenesis

anaphylactogenic
anaphylactoid
anaphylactotoxin
anaphylatoxin inactivator
anaphylaxis
    active a.
    aggregate a.
    antiserum a.
    generalized a.
    heterocytotropic a.
    homocytotropic a.
    inverse a.
    local a.
    passive a.
    passive cutaneous a.
    reverse a.
    systemic a.
anaplasia
    monophasic a.
    polyphasic a.
anaplastic
anaplasty
anapophysis
anaptic
anarrhexis
anarthria
anasarca
anasarcous
anascitic
anastalsis
anastaltic
anastigmatic
anastomose
anastomosis (anastomoses)
    antiperistaltic a.
    aorticopulmonary a.
    a. arteriolovenularis simplex
    a. arteriovenosa glomeriformis
    a. arteriovenosa simplex
    arteriovenous a.
    Baffe a.
    Billroth a., Billroth I a.,
        Billroth II a.
    Braun a.
    Clado a.
    a. clamp
    Coffey a.
    crucial a.
    end-to-end a.
    end-to-side a.
    enteric a.
    esophagojejunal a.
    faciohypoglossal a.
    Furniss a.
    Galen a.
    genicular a.

anastomosis (anastomoses)
    (continued)
        glomeriform arteriolovenular a.
        glomeriform arteriovenous a.
        Haight a.
        heterocladic a.
        homocladic a.
        hypoglossal-facial nerve a.
        Hyrtl a.
        ileorectal a.
        intermesenteric arterial a.
        intestinal a.
        isoperistaltic a.
        Jacobson a.
        meningeal arterial a's
        nerve a.
        peristaltic a.
        portacaval a.
        portosystemic a.
        postcostal a.
        precapillary a.
        precostal a.
        pyeloileocutaneous a.
        rectosigmoid a.
        a. of Riolan
        Roux a.
        Roux-en-Y a.
        side-to-end a.
        side-to-side a.
        simple arteriolovenular a.
        simple arteriovenous a.
        splenorenal a.
        stirrup a.
        Sucquet-Hoyer a.
        sutureless a.
        terminoterminal a.
        transureteroureteral a.
        triple a.
        ureteroileocutaneous a.
        ureterotubal a.
        ureteroureteral a.
        ventriculocisternal a.
anastomotic operation
anatomical
anatomical snuffbox
anatomic equator
anatomist
anatomy
    applied a.
    comparative a.
    cross-sectional a.
    dental a.
    descriptive a.
    developmental a.
    general a.
    gross a.

anatomy *(continued)*
    histologic a.
    macroscopic a.
    medical a.
    microscopic a.
    pathological a.
    physiological a.
    radiological a.
    regional a.
    surface a.
    surgical a.
    systematic a.
    x-ray a.
anatricrotic
anatrophic nephrotomy
anatropia
anatropic
anavenin
ANC—absolute neutrophil
    count
ANCA—antineutrophil cytoplasmic
    autoantibody
anchor
    endosteal implant a.
anchorage
    cervical a.
    compound a.
    extramaxillary a.
    extraoral a.
    intermaxillary a.
    intraoral a.
    maxillomandibular a.
    multiple a.
    occipital a.
    reciprocal a.
    reinforced a.
    simple a.
    stationary a.
anchoring suture
ancillary
    a. measures
    a. therapy
ancipital
anconad
anconagra
anconal
anconeal
anconeus
anconitis
anconoid
Ancylostoma braziliense
ancylostomiasis
    cutaneous a.
    a. cutis
    a. dermatitis
ancyroid

Andernach ossicles
Anders disease
Andersch
    ganglion
    nerve
Andersen
    disease
    syndrome
    triad
Anderson
    amputation
    appliance
    operation
    pin fixation
    splint
    tibial lengthening
Anderson and Goldberger test
Andogsky syndrome
Andrade
    indicator
    syndrome
Andral
    decubitus
    sign
Andresen
    appliance
    diet
André Thomas sign
Andrews
    applicator
    disease
    gouge
    operation
    retractor
Andrews-Hartmann forceps
Andrews-Pynchon suction tube
androblastoma
androdedotoxin
androgalactozemia
androgen
    a. ablation
    adrenal a.
    a. deprivation
    a. precursors
    a. suppression
androgenic
androgenicity
androgenized
androgenous
androgyne
androgynous
androgyny
android
andromimetic
andropathy
androstane

androstanediol glucuronide
androstanolone
androstene
androstenediol
androstenedione
androsterone
anecdotal
anechoic
anectasis
Anel
    lacrimal duct dilation
    method
    operation
    probe
    syringe
anelectrotonic
anelectrotonus
anemia
    achlorhydric a.
    achrestic a.
    achylic a.
    a. achylica
    acquired hemolytic a.
    acquired sideroblastic a.
    acute hemolytic a.
    acute posthemorrhagic a.
    Addison a.
    Addison-Biermer a.
    addisonian a.
    ancylostome a.
    aplastic a.
    Arctic a.
    asiderotic a.
    atrophic a.
    autoimmune hemolytic a.
    Biermer-Ehrlich a.
    Blackfan-Diamond a.
    breast a.
    cameloid a.
    chronic congenital
      aregenerative a.
    a. of chronic disease
    Chvostek a.
    congenital a. of newborn
    congenital dyserythropoietic a.
    congenital hemolytic a.
    congenital hypoplastic a.
    congenital nonspherocytic
      hemolytic a.
    constitutional aplastic a.
    Cooley a.
    Coombs-negative immune
      hemolytic a.
    cow's milk a.
    crescent cell a.

anemia *(continued)*
    cytogenic a.
    Czerny a.
    deficiency a.
    Diamond-Blackfan a.
    dilution a.
    dimorphic a.
    Dresbach a.
    drug-induced immune
      hemolytic a.
    Edelmann a.
    elliptocytary a.
    elliptocytotic a.
    enzyme deficiency hemolytic a.
    erythroblastic a. of childhood
    essential a.
    Faber a.
    familial erythroblastic a.
    familial megaloblastic a.
    Fanconi a.
    febrile pleiochromic a.
    folic acid deficiency a.
    fragmentation hemolytic a.
    globe cell a.
    glucose-6-phosphate
      dehydrogenase deficiency a.
    goat's milk a.
    ground itch a.
    Heinz body a's
    hemolytic a.
    hemorrhagic a.
    hereditary nonspherocytic
      hemolytic a.
    Herrick a.
    hookworm a.
    hyperchromic a.
    hypochromic a.
    a. hypochromica
      sideroachrestica hereditaria
    hypochromic microcytic a.
    hypoplastic a.
    enterohemolytic a.
    idiopathic hypochromic a.
    immune hemolytic a.
    infectious hemolytic a.
    iron deficiency a.
    Israels-Wilkinson a.
    Jaksch a.
    juvenile pernicious a.
    Larzel a.
    lead a.
    Lederer a.
    Leishman a.
    leukoerythroblastic a.
    lysolecithin hemolytic a.

anemia *(continued)*
- macrocytic a.
- malignant a.
- Mediterranean a.
- megaloblastic a.
- megalocytic a.
- meniscocytic a.
- microangiopathic hemolytic a.
- microcytic a.
- milk a.
- miners' a.
- mountain a.
- myelopathic a.
- myelosclerotic a.
- a. neonatorum
- normochromic a.
- normocytic a.
- nutritional a.
- nutritional macrocytic a.
- osteosclerotic a.
- ovalocytary a.
- pernicious a.
- physiologic a.
- polar a.
- posthemorrhagic a. of newborn
- primaquine-sensitive a.
- primary a.
- pure red cell a.
- pyridoxine-responsive a.
- pyruvate-kinase deficiency a.
- radiation a.
- Rietti-Greppi-Micheli a.
- Rundles-Falls a.
- Runeberg a.
- scorbutic a.
- secondary a.
- sex-linked hypochromatic a. of Rundles and Falls
- sickle cell a.
- sideremic a.
- sideroachrestic a.
- sideroblastic a.
- sideropenic a.
- spherocytic a.
- a. splenetica
- splenic a.
- spur cell a.
- target cell a.
- thrombopenic a.
- thrombotic microangiopathic hemolytic a.
- toxic hemolytic a.
- traumatic a.
- triose-phosphate isomerase deficiency a.

anemia *(continued)*
- tunnel a.
- unstable hemoglobin hemolytic a.
- von Jaksch a.
- Wills a.
- Witts a.
- x-ray a.

anemic

anemonin

anemonism

anemonol

anencephalic

anencephalus

anencephaly

anenterous

anephric

anephrogenesis

anepiploic

anergic

anergy
- cutaneous a.
- negative a.
- positive a.

aneroid

anerythropoiesis

anerythroregenerative

anesthecinesia, anesthekinesia

anesthesia
- absorption a.
- angiospastic a.
- axillary a.
- balanced a.
- basal a.
- Bier local a.
- block a.
- brachial a.
- bulbar a.
- carbon dioxide absorption a.
- caudal a.
- central a.
- cerebral a.
- chloroform a.
- closed-circuit a.
- colonic a.
- compression a.
- conduction a.
- continuous epidural a.
- Corning a.
- crossed a.
- doll's head a.
- a. dolorosa
- electric a.
- endobronchial a.
- endotracheal a.

anesthesia *(continued)*
> epidural a.
> extradural a.
> facial a.
> field block a.
> fractional a.
> gas-oxygen-ether a.
> gauntlet a.
> general a.
> girdle a.
> glove a.
> glove and stocking a.
> gustatory a.
> Gwathmey oil-ether a.
> high-pressure a.
> hyperbaric spinal a.
> hypnosis a.
> hypobaric spinal a.
> hypotensive a.
> hypothermic a.
> hysterical a.
> infiltration a.
> inhalation a.
> insufflation a.
> intercostal a.
> intramedullary a.
> intranasal a.
> intraoral a.
> intraosseous a.
> intrapulpal a.
> intraspinal a.
> intratracheal a.
> intravenous a.
> intubation a.
> isobaric spinal a.
> Kulenkampff a.
> local a.
> lumbar epidural a.
> Meltzer a.
> mental a.
> mixed a.
> muscular a.
> nasoendotracheal a.
> nasotracheal intubation a.
> nausea a.
> nerve-blocking a.
> olfactory a.
> one-lung a.
> open a.
> orotracheal a.
> paracervical block a.
> paraneural a.
> parasacral a.
> paravertebral a.
> partial a.

anesthesia *(continued)*
> peridural a.
> perineural a.
> periodontal a.
> peripheral a.
> permeation a.
> plexus a.
> presacral a.
> pressure a.
> pudendal block a.
> rectal a.
> refrigeration a.
> regional a.
> retrobulbar a.
> sacral a.
> saddle block a.
> segmental a.
> semiclosed a.
> semiopen a.
> sexual a.
> spinal a.
> splanchnic a.
> stellate block a.
> stocking a.
> subarachnoid a.
> surface a.
> surgical a.
> sympathetic block a.
> tactile a.
> thalamic hyperesthetic a.
> topical a.
> total a.
> transsacral a.
> transtracheal a.
> traumatic a.
> twilight a.
> unilateral a.
> visceral a.

anesthesiologist
anesthesiology
anesthetic
> general a.
> local a.
> topical a.
> volatile a.

anesthetist
anesthetization
anesthetize
anetoderma
> Jadassohn a.
> Jadassohn-Pellizari a.
> perifollicular a.
> postinflammatory a.
> Schweninger-Buzzi a.

aneugamy

aneuploid
aneuploidy
Aneuroform
aneurogenic
aneurysm
    abdominal aortic a. (AAA)
    ampullary a.
    aortic arch a.
    aortic sinusal a.
    arterial a.
    arteriovenous a.
    atherosclerotic a.
    axial a.
    axillary a.
    bacterial a.
    Bérard a.
    berry a.
    brain a.
    cardiac a.
    caroticocavernous a.
    cerebral a.
    Charcot-Bouchard a.
    cirsoid a.
    compound a.
    congenital cerebral a.
    cylindroid a.
    cystogenic a.
    dissecting a.
    ectatic a.
    embolic a.
    embolomycotic a.
    endogenous a.
    erosive a.
    exogenous a.
    false a.
    hernial a.
    infected a.
    innominate a.
    intracavernous a.
    intracranial a.
    intrathoracic a.
    lateral a.
    luetic a.
    miliary a.
    mycotic a.
    orbital a.
    Park a.
    pelvic a.
    peripheral a.
    phantom a.
    popliteal a.
    posterior inferior
      communicating artery
      (PICA) a.
    Pott a.

aneurysm *(continued)*
    racemose a.
    Rasmussen a.
    renal a.
    Richet a.
    Rodrigues a.
    saccular a.
    serpentine a.
    Shekelton a.
    silent a.
    a. of sinus of Valsalva
    suprasellar a.
    syphilitic a.
    thoracic a.
    thoracoabdominal aortic a.
    traumatic a.
    true a.
    tubular a.
    varicose a.
    venous a.
    ventricular a.
    verminous a.
    worm a.
aneurysmal
aneurysmatic
aneurysmectomy
aneurysmoplasty
aneurysmorrhaphy
aneurysmotomy
ANF—antinuclear factor
Angelchik antireflux prosthesis
Angelucci
    operation
    syndrome
Anger camera
Anghelescu sign
angialgia
angiasthenia
angiectasis
angiectatic
angiectomy
angiectopia
angiitis
    allergic granulomatous a.
    leukocytoclastic a.
    necrotizing a.
    visceral a.
angina
    abdominal a.
    a. abdominalis
    a. abdominis
    a. acuta
    agranulocytic a.
    Bretonneau a.
    a. catarrhalis

angina *(continued)*
   a. cordis
   a. cruris
   a. decubitus
   a. diphtheritica
   a. dyspeptica
   a. epiglottidea
   a. equivalent
   exertional a.
   exudative a.
   a. follicularis
   a. gangrenosa
   hippocratic a.
   hypercyanotic a.
   hysterical a.
   intestinal a.
   a. inversa
   lacunar a.
   a. laryngea
   Ludwig a.
   malignant a.
   a. membranacea
   monocytic a.
   a. nervosa
   neutropenic a.
   a. pectoris
   a. pectoris vasomotoria
   Plaut a.
   Plaut-Vincent a.
   preinfarction a.
   Prinzmetal a.
   pseudomembranous a.
   a. rheumatica
   a. scarlatinosa
   Schultz a.
   a. simplex
   a. sine dolore
   a. tonsillaris
   a. trachealis
   ulceromembranous a.
   a. ulcerosa
   unstable a.
   variant a. pectoris
   vasomotor a.
   Vincent a.
anginal
anginiform
anginoid
anginophobia
angioaccess
angioarchitecture
angiocardiography (ACG)
   gas a.
   intravenous a.
   radionuclide a.

angiocardiography (ACG)
   (continued)
   rapid biplane a.
   retrograde a.
   right-sided a.
   selective a.
   venous a.
angiocardiokinetic
angiocarditis
angiocatheter
angiocholitis
Angio-Conray contrast medium
angiocrine
angiocrinosis
angiodermatitis
   disseminated pruritic a.
angiodiascopy
angiodynia
angiodysplasia
angiodystrophy
angioedema
   hereditary a.
   vibratory a.
angioedematous
angioelephantiasis
angioendotheliomatosis
   systemic proliferating a.
angiofibroma
   juvenile nasopharyngeal a.
angiofollicular
angiogenesis
   tumor a.
angiogenic
angioglioma
angiogram
   fluorescein a.
   renal a.
angiogranuloma
angiography
   aortic arch a.
   biliary a.
   carotid a.
   cerebral a.
   coronary a. (CA)
   digital subtraction a. (DSA)
   emission a.
   fluorescein a.
   four-vessel a.
   intravenous digital
     subtraction a.
   intravenous renal a.
   magnetic resonance a. (MRA)
   multigated a.
   orbital a.
   peripheral a.

angiography *(continued)*
  pulmonary a.
  radionuclide a.
  renal a.
  spinal cord a.
  subtraction a.
  vertebral a.
  visceral a.
angiohyalinosis
angioid
angioimmunoblastic
  lymphadenopathy with
  dysproteinemia (AILD)
angioinvasive
angiokeratoma
  a. circumscriptum
  a. corporis diffusum universale
  diffuse a.
  a. of Fordyce
  a. of Mibelli
  scrotal a.
  solitary a.
  vulvar a.
angioleiomyoma
angiolipoleiomyoma
angiology
angiolupoid
angiolymphangioma
angiolysis
angioma (angiomata)
  a. arteriale racemosum
  arteriovenous a. of brain
  capillary a.
  a. cavernosum
  cavernous a.
  cerebral a.
  cherry a.
  a. cutis
  encephalic a.
  fissural a.
  hereditary hemorrhagic a.
  infectious a.
  a. lymphaticum
  a. pigmentosum
  plane a.
  plexiform a.
  sclerosing a.
  senile a.
  a. serpiginosum
  simple a.
  spider a.
  spinal a.
  stellate a.
  strawberry a.
  telangiectatic a.

angioma (angiomata) *(continued)*
  tuberous a.
  a. venosum racemosum
  venous a. of brain
angiomatoid
angiomatosis
  cephalotrigeminal a.
  cerebroretinal a.
  congenital dysplastic a.
  diffuse corticomeningeal a.
  encephalofacial a.
  encephalotrigeminal a.
  hemorrhagic familial a.
  hepatic a.
  oculoencephalic a.
  a. retinae
  retinocerebral a.
  Sturge-Weber a.
angiomatous
angiomegaly
angiomyolipoma
angiomyosarcoma
angiomyxoma
angionecrosis
angioneoplasm
angioneuralgia
angioneurectomy
angioneuropathic
angioneuropathy
angioneurosis
angioneurotic edema
angioneurotomy
angiopathology
angiopathy
angioplasty
  balloon a.
  coronary a.
  laser a.
  patch a.
  percutaneous transluminal a.
    (PTA)
  percutaneous transluminal
    coronary a. (PTCA)
  percutaneous transluminal
    renal a. (PTRA)
angiopoiesis
angiopoietic
angiopressure
angiorrhaphy
  arteriovenous a.
angiosclerosis
angiosclerotic
angioscopy
  fiberoptic a.
angioscotoma

angiostenosis
angiosteosis
angiostomy
angiotelectasis
angiotensin
    a. I through II
    a.-converting enzyme (ACE)
    a.-converting enzyme
        inhibitors (ACEIs)
angiotome
angiotomy
Angle [eponym]
    classification
    splint
angle
    a. of aberration
    acromial a. of scapula
    a.-former
    alpha a.
    Alsberg a.
    alveolar a.
    a. of anomaly
    antegonial a.
    anterior a. of petrous portion
        of temporal bone
    a. of anterior chamber of eye
    anterior inferior a. of parietal
        bone
    a. of aperture
    auriculo-occipital a.
    axial line a.
    basal a.
    Baumann a.
    Bennett a.
    beta a.
    biorbital a.
    a. board
    Böhler a.
    Boogaard a.
    Broca a.
    buccal a's
    Bull a.
    cardiodiaphragmatic a.
    cardiohepatic a.
    cardiophrenic a.
    carrying a.
    cavity a's
    cavosurface a.
    cephalic a's
    cephalometric a.
    cerebellopontine a.
    chi a.
    a. closure glaucoma
    collodiaphyseal a.
    conchal mastoid a.

angle *(continued)*
    condylar a.
    a. of convergence
    a. of convexity
    coronary a.
    costophrenic a.
    costosternal a.
    costovertebral a.
    craniofacial a.
    critical a.
    cusp plane a.
    Daubenton a.
    a. of declination
    a. of deviation
    a. of direction
    distal a's
    duodenojejunal a.
    Ebstein a.
    elevation a.
    epigastric a.
    ethmocranial a.
    ethmoid a.
    external a. of border of tibia
    external a. of scapula
    facial a.
    a. of femoral torsion
    filtration a.
    Frankfort-mandibular plane a.
    frontal a. of parietal bone
    gamma a.
    gonial a.
    horizontal a.
    ileocolic a.
    a. of incidence
    incisal guide a.
    incisal mandibular plane a.
    a. of inclination
    inferior a. of duodenum
    inferior a. of parietal bone,
        anterior
    inferior a. of parietal bone,
        posterior
    inferior a. of scapula
    infrasternal a. of thorax
    inner a. of eye
    inner a. of humerus
    internal a. of tibia
    iridial a.
    iridocorneal a.
    a. of iris
    Jacquart a.
    a. of jaw
    kappa a.
    kyphotic a.
    labial a's

angle *(continued)*
- lambda a.
- limiting a.
- line a.
- lingual a's
- Louis a.
- Ludwig a.
- lumbosacral a.
- mandibular a.
- manubriosternal a.
- mastoid a. of parietal bone
- maxillary a.
- mesial a's
- metafacial a.
- meter a.
- Mikulicz a.
- a. of minimum deviation
- minimum separable a.
- minimum visible a.
- minimum visual a.
- a. of mouth
- a. of Mulder
- nasal a. of eye
- neck shaft a.
- occipital a. of parietal bone
- ocular a's
- olfactive a.
- olfactory a.
- ophryospinal a.
- optic a.
- orificial a.
- orofacial a.
- outer a. of eye
- parietal a. of sphenoid bone
- a. of pelvis
- pelvivertebral a.
- phrenopericardial a.
- Pirogoff a.
- point a.
- a. of polarization
- posterior inferior a. of parietal bone
- principal a.
- prism a.
- a. of pubis
- QRST a.
- Quatrefages a.
- Ranke a.
- a. of reflection
- refracting a.
- a. of refraction
- a. of rib
- rolandic a.
- a. of Rolando
- sacrovertebral a.

angle *(continued)*
- scaphoconchal a.
- scattering a.
- Serres a.
- sigma a.
- sinodural a.
- solid a.
- somatosplanchnic a.
- sphenoidal a.
- sphenoidal a. of parietal bone
- squint a.
- sternal a.
- sternoclavicular a.
- subcarinal a.
- subcostal a.
- subpubic a.
- subscapular a.
- substernal a.
- a. of supination
- a. suture
- a. of Sylvius
- temporal a.
- tentorial a.
- tooth a's
- Topinard a.
- a. of torsion
- tuber a.
- uterine a.
- venous a.
- vertical a.
- vesicourethral a., anterior
- vesicourethral a., posterior
- a. of Virchow
- visual a.
- Vogt a.
- Weisbach a.
- Welcker a.
- xiphoid a's
- Y a.

angle-former
angor
- a. animi
- a. ocularis

Angström unit
angular
- a. blepharitis
- a. frequency
- a. incision
- a. momentum

angulated
angulation osteotomy
angulus (anguli)
- a. costae
- a. inferior scapulae
- a. infrasternalis

angulus (anguli) *(continued)*
    a. iridis
    a. iridocornealis
    a. lateralis scapulae
    a. mandibulae
    a. mastoideus ossis parietalis
    a. oculi lateralis
    a. oculi medialis
    a. oris
    a. sterni
    a. subpubicus
    a. superior scapulae
anhedonia
anhidrosis
    postmiliarial a.
    thermogenic a.
anhidrotic
anhydrase
anhydride
    acetic a.
    arsenous a.
    chromic a.
    perosmic a.
    silicic a.
    sorbitol a.
    sulfurous a.
    trimellitic a.
anhydrous
aniacinamidosis
Anichkov
    cell
    myocyte
anicteric
anile
anilide
aniline
    a. fuchsin
    a. gentian violet
    a. red
anilingus
anilinism
anility
animation
    suspended a.
anion gap
anionic
aniridia
anisakiasis
Anisakis marina
anise
    star a.
aniseikonia
anisoaccommodation
anisochromasia
anisochromatic

anisocoria
anisocytosis
anisodactylous
anisodactyly
anisodiametric
anisodont
anisokaryosis
anisomastia
anisomelia
anisometrope
anisometropia
anisometropic
anisophoria
anisopia
anisopiesis
anisopoikilocytosis
anisosmotic
anisospore
anisosthenic
anisotonic
anisotropic
anisotropy
anisuria
Anitschkow (Anichkov)
    cell
    myocyte
ankle
    cocked a.
    deck a's
    a. mortise
    tailor's a.
ankyloblepharon filiforme adnatum
ankylocheilia
ankylocolpos
ankylodactyly
ankyloglossia
    complete a.
    partial a.
    a. superior
ankylopoietic
ankyloproctia
ankylosed
ankylosing
    a. hyperostosis
    a. spondylitis
ankylosis (ankyloses)
    artificial a.
    bony a.
    capsular a.
    cricoarytenoid joint a.
    dental a.
    extra-articular a.
    extracapsular a.
    false a.
    fibrous a.

ankylosis (ankyloses) *(continued)*
 intracapsular a.
 ligamentous a.
 operative a.
 partial a.
 spurious a.
 stapedial a.
 a. of stapes
 true a.
 unsound a.
ankylotic
ankylotome
ankylotomy
ANLL—acute nonlymphocytic
 leukemia
Annandale operation
annectent
annihilation
 a. photons
 a. radiation
annular
 a. plexus
 a. scotoma
annulate
annulet
annuloplasty
 DeVega a.
 Kay a.
annulorrhaphy
annulus (annuli)
 annuli tracheae
 a. ciliaris
 a. ovalis
 a. tracheae
 tympanic a.
 a. tympanicus
 a. urethralis
 Vieussens a.
 a. of Zinn
anochromasia
anociassociation
anociated
anococcygeal
anocutaneous fistula
anodal
anoderm
anodontia
 partial a.
 total a.
 true a.
 a. vera
anodyne
anogenital
anomaloscope
anomalotrophy

anomalous
 a. retinal correspondence
 a. trichromatism
anomaly
 Alder constitutional
  granulation a.
 Alder-Reilly a.
 Alius-Grignaschi a.
 Aristotle a.
 Axenfeld a.
 Chédiak-Higashi a.
 Chédiak-Steinbrinck-
  Higashi a.
 Chiari a.
 chromosomal a.
 congenital a.
 cor triatriatum a.
 craniovertebral a's
 developmental a.
 Ebstein a.
 fetal a.
 Freund a.
 Hegglin a.
 Huët-Pelger nuclear a.
 Jordan a.
 May-Hegglin a.
 morning glory a.
 Pelger-Huët nuclear a.
 Pelger nuclear a.
 Peters a.
 Pierre Robin a.
 Poland a.
 Rieger a.
 Shone a.
 Steinbrinck a.
 Taussig-Bing a.
 Uhl a.
 Undritz a.
anomia
anonychia
anonymous
anoperineal
Anopheles maculipennis
anophthalmia
anophthalmus
anoplasty
anorchia
anorchid
anorchism
anorectal
anorectic
anorectitis
anorectocolonic
anorectoplasty
 Laird-McMahon a.

anorexia
  hysterical a.
  a. nervosa
anorexigenic
anorgasmy
anorthopia
anorthoscope
anoscope
  Bacon a.
  Bodenheimer a.
  Boehm a.
  Brinkerhoff a.
  Buie-Hirschman a.
  Fansler a.
  Goldbacher a.
  Hirschman a.
  Ives a.
  Muer a.
  Otis a.
  Pratt a.
  Pruitt a.
  rotating a.
  Sims a.
  speculum a.
  Welch-Allyn a.
anoscopy
anosigmoidoscopic
anosigmoidoscopy
anosmia
  a. gustatoria
  preferential a.
  a. respiratoria
anosmic
anosognosia
anospinal
anosteoplasia
anostosis
anotia
anotropia
anotus
anovaginal
anovarism
anovesical
anovular
anovulation
anovulatory
anovulomenorrhea
anoxemia
anoxemic
anoxia
  altitude a.
  anemic a.
  anoxic a.
  diffuse cerebral a.
  fetal a.

anoxia *(continued)*
  fulminating a.
  histotoxic a.
  myocardial a.
  a. neonatorum
  stagnant a.
anoxiate
anoxic
ANP—atrial natriuretic peptide
ANS—
  acute nephritic syndrome
  anterior nasal spine
  autonomic nervous system
ansa (ansae)
  a. cervicalis
  a. of Galen
  a. of Haller
  Henle a.
  a. hypoglossi
  a. lenticularis
  a. of lenticular nucleus
  a. nephroni
  ansae nervorum spinalium
  a. peduncularis
  a. sacralis
  a. subclavia
  a. of Vieussens
  a. vitellina
  a. of Wrisberg
ansate
anserine
Anson-McVay operation
ansotomy
antacid
antagonism
  bacterial a.
  metabolic a.
antagonist
  adrenergic a.
  aldosterone a.
  alpha-adrenergic a.
  associated a's
  beta-adrenergic a.
  calcium a.
  competitive a.
  contralateral a.
  direct a's
  enzyme a.
  folic acid a.
  insulin a's
  ipsilateral a.
  metabolic a.
  narcotic a.
  sulfonamide a.
antalgesia

antalgic
antalkaline
antaphrodisiac
antapoplectic
antatrophic
ante—before
antebrachial
antebrachium
antecedent
    plasma thromboplastin a. (PTA)
antecolic gastrectomy
antecubital
antecurvature
anteflect
anteflexed
anteflexion
antegonial
    a. angle
    a. notch
antegrade
    percutaneous a. pyelography
    percutaneous a. urography
antelocation
ante mortem, antemortem
antenatal
antenna
antepartal
antepartum
antephialtic
anteposition
anteprostate
antepyretic
anteriad
anterior
    a. cervical diskectomy and
      fusion (ACDF)
    a. chamber
    a. chamber angle
    a. chamber cleavage
    a. ciliary arteries
    a. corneal staphyloma
    a. focal point
    a. hyaloid membrane
    a. megalophthalmos
    a. nephrectomy
    a. palatine suture
    a. pharyngotomy
    a. pole
    a. rhinoscopy
    a. rhizotomy
    a. sclerotomy
    a. segment
    a. synechia
    a. thalamotomy
    a. uveitis

anteriorly
anterograde
anteroinferior
anterointernal
anterolateral
anteromedial
anteromedian
anteroparietal
anteroposteriorly
anteroposterior (AP) view
anteroseptal
anterosuperior
anterosuperiorly
anteroventral
anteversion
anteverted
anthelix
anthelmintic
anthelotic
antherpetic
Anthony
    compressor
    tube
anthracene
anthracic
anthracoid
anthraconecrosis
anthracosilicosis
anthracosis linguae
anthrax
    agricultural a.
    a. bacillus
    cerebral a.
    cutaneous a.
    gastrointestinal a.
    industrial a.
    inhalational a.
    intestinal a.
    malignant a.
    meningeal a.
    pulmonary a.
    symptomatic a.
anthrone
anthropogenic
anthropoid
anthropometry
    forensic a.
anthropomorphic
anthropomorphism
anthroponosis
anthropopathy
anthropophobia
anthroposcopy
antiabortifacient
Antia-Buch chondrocutaneous flap

antiadrenergic
antiagglutinin
antialbumin
antiamebic
antianaphylaxis
antiandrogen
antianemic
antianginal
antianopheline
antiantibody
antiantitoxin
antianxiety
antiarin
antiarrhythmic
antiarthritic
antiasthmatic
antiatherogenic
antiautolysin
antibacterial
antibiotic
antibody (antibodies)
    ABO a.
    acetylcholine receptor a's
    a. affinity chromatography
    anaphylactic a.
    anti–acetylcholine receptor
      (anti-AChR) a's
    anti–glomerular basement
      membrane a's
    anti-A a.
    anti-B a.
    anti-basement membrane a.
    anticardiolipin a.
    anticentromere a.
    anticytoplasmic a.
    anti-D a.
    anti-DNA a.
    antifibrin a.
    anti–glomerular basement
      membrane (anti-GBM) a.
    anti-idiotype a.
    anti-La a.
    anti-M a.
    antimicrosomal a.
    antimitochondrial a.
    antinuclear a. (ANA)
    anti-P a.
    antipeptide a.
    antireceptor a.
    anti-Rh (Rhesus) a.
    anti-Ro a.
    anti-S a.
    anti-Sm a.
    anti-smooth muscle a.
    anti-T-cell a.
    antithyroglobulin a's

antibody (antibodies) *(continued)*
    antithyroid a's
    autoimmune a.
    autologous a.
    basement membrane a.
    B-cell a.
    bispecific a.
    bivalent a.
    blocking a.
    cell-bound a.
    cell-fixed a.
    cold a.
    cold-reactive a.
    combining-site a.
    complement-fixing a.
    complete a.
    cross-reacting a.
    cryptosporidiosis a.
    cytophilic a.
    cytotoxic a.
    cytotropic a.
    a. deficiency syndrome
    a.-dependent cell–mediated
      cytotoxicity
    Donath-Landsteiner a.
    duck virus hepatitis yolk a.
    enhancing a.
    a. excess
    fluorescein-labeled a.
    Forssman a.
    H a.
    hepatitis B core a. (HBcAb)
    hepatitis B e a. (HBeAb)
    hepatitis B surface a. (HBsAb)
    heteroclitic a.
    heterocytotropic a.
    heterogenetic a.
    heterophil a., heterophile a.
    homocytotropic a.
    humoral a.
    hybrid a.
    hybridoma a.
    immune a.
    immunosorbent a.
    incomplete a.
    inhibiting a.
    isophil a.
    maternal a.
    mitochondrial a's
    monoclonal a.
    natural a's
    neutralizing a.
    nuclear a.
    O a.
    opsonizing a.
    polyclonal a.

antibody (antibodies) *(continued)*
    protective a.
    reaginic a.
    Rh a's
    saline a.
    sensitizing a.
    skin-sensitizing a.
    T a.
    thyroglobulin a.
    thyroid microsomal a's
    TSH-displacing a. (TDA)
    Vi a.
    warm a.
    warm-reactive a.
antibromic
anticalculous
anticarcinogen
anticarcinogenic
anticariogenic
anticatalyst
anticephalalgic
anticholelithogenic
anticholesteremic
anticholinergic
anticholinesterase
anticipation
anticlinal
anticnemion
anticoagulant
    circulating a.
    lupus a.
anticoagulated
anticomplement
anticonvulsant
anticrotin
anticurare
anticytolysin
anticytotoxin
antidepressant
    atypical a.
    tetracyclic a.
    tricyclic a.
antidiabetic
antidiabetogenic
antidiarrheal
antidiuresis
antidiuretic hormone
antidotal
antidote
    chemical a.
    Hall a.
    mechanical a.
    physiologic a.
    universal a.
antidromic
antidysenteric

antiedemic
antiemetic
antienzyme
antiepileptic
antiestrogen
antiestrogenic
antifibrillatory
antifibrinolysin
antifibrinolytic
antifilarial
antiflatulent
antifolate
antifungal
antigalactic
antigen (Ag)
    A a.
    ABO a.
    accessible a.
    allogeneic a.
    alpha a. of adenovirus
    alum-precipitated a.
    Am a's
    a.-antibody complex
    autologous a.
    B a.
    bacterial a.
    a.-binding capacity
    blood group a's
    C a.
    capsular a.
    carbohydrate a's
    carcinoembryonic a. (CEA)
    class I, II, and III a's
    common acute lymphoblastic
      leukemia a.
    common enterobacterial a.
    common leukocyte a's
    complement-fixing a.
    complete a.
    conjugated a.
    cross-reacting a.
    cryptic T a.
    cryptococcal a.
    D a.
    delta a.
    differentiation a.
    Duffy a.
    E a.
    endogenous a.
    epsilon a.
    erythrocyte a.
    a. excess
    exogenous a.
    extractable nuclear a's
    F a.
    factor VIII a.

antigen (Ag) *(continued)*
    febrile a's
    fetal a's
    Forssman a.
    Frei a.
    gamma a.
    Gm a's
    group-specific a.
    H a.
    H-2 a's
    hepatitis B e a. (HBeAg)
    hepatitis B core a. (HBcAg)
    hepatitis B surface a. (HBsAg)
    heterologous a.
    heterophil a.
    heterophile a.
    histocompatibility a's, major
    histocompatibility a's, minor
    homologous a.
    human leukocyte a. (HLA)
    human thymus lymphocyte a.
    H-Y a.
    I a.
    Ia a.
    idiotypic a.
    incomplete a.
    inhalant a.
    Inv group a.
    K a.
    Kell a.
    Kidd a.
    Km a's
    Kveim a.
    LD a's
    lens a's
    leukocyte common a.
    Ly a.
    Lyb a's
    lymphocyte-defined a's (LD a's)
    lymphocyte function–associated a. 1 (LFA-1)
    lymphocyte function–associated a. 2 (LFA-2)
    lymphocyte function–associated a. 3 (LFA-3)
    lymphogranuloma venereum a.
    Lyt a's
    M a.
    mumps skin test a.
    NP a.
    nuclear a's
    O a.
    oncofetal a.
    organ-specific a.
    Oz a.

antigen (Ag) *(continued)*
    P54 a.
    pancreatic oncofetal a.
    partial a.
    PHA (phytohemagglutinin) a.
    plasma cell a.
    pollen a.
    Pr a.
    a. presentation
    a.-presenting cell
    private a's
    proliferating cell nuclear a.
    prostate specific a.
    protective a.
    public a's
    QA a.
    R a.
    recall a.
    Rh (Rhesus) factor a.
    S a.
    SD a.
    self-a.
    sequestered a's
    sero-defined a's (SD a's)
    serologically defined a's (SD a's)
    serum hepatitis a. (SH a.)
    SH a.
    shock a.
    skin-specific histocompatibility a.
    Sm a.
    somatic a's
    species-specific a's
    surface a.
    SV 40 T a.
    synthetic a.
    T a.
    Tac a.
    T-cell a.
    T-dependent a.
    theta a. (τ a.)
    Thy 1 a.
    thymus-dependent a.
    thymus-independent a.
    thymus leukemia a. (TL a.)
    T-independent a.
    tissue-specific a.
    TL a.
    transplantation a.
    tumor-associated a.
    tumor-specific a. (TSA)
    tumor-specific transplantation a. (TSTA)
    VDRL a.
    Vi a.

antigen (Ag) *(continued)*
    viral capsid a.
    xenogeneic a.
antigenemia
antigenemic
antigenic
antigenicity
antiglobulin
anti–glomerular basement
  membrane (anti-GBM)
antigoitrogenic
antigonadotropic
antigravity suit
antihallucinatory
anti-HBc
anti-HBs
antihelix
antihemagglutinin
antihemolysin
antihemolytic
antihemophilic
antihemorrhagic
antiheterolysin
antihidrotic
antihistamine
antihistaminic
antihormone
antihypercholesterolemic
antihyperglycemic
antihyperlipoproteinemic
antihypertensive
antihypnotic
antihypotensive
antihysteric
antiicteric
anti-idiotype
antiinfective
antiinflammatory
anti-insulin
anti-isolysin
antiketogenic
antileishmanial
antileprotic
antileukocidin
antileukocytic
antilewisite
    British a. (BAL)
antilipotropic
antilipotropism
antilithic
antilysin
antilysis
antilytic
antimalarial
antimephitic

antimesenteric
antimetabolite
antimicrobial
antimineralocorticoid
antimony (Sb)
    a. potassium tartrate
    a. sodium dimercaptosuccinate
    tartrated a.
antimuscarinic
antimutagen
antimyasthenic
antimycobacterial
antimycotic
antinarcotic
antinatriuresis
antinauseant
antineoplastic
antinephritic
antineuralgic
antineuritic
antineurotoxin
antiniad
antinial
antinion
antinociceptive
antinuclear
antiodontalgic
antioncogene
antiopsonin
antiovulatory
antioxidant
antioxidation
antiparallel
antiparalytic
antiparasitic
antiparasympathomimetic
antiparkinsonian
antipedicular
antipediculotic
antiperiodic
antiperistalsis
antiperistaltic
antiperspirant
antiphagocytic
antiphlogistic
antiplasmin
    α_2-a. [alpha2-]
antiplasmodial
antiplastic
antiplatelet
antipneumococcal
antipodagric
antipodal
antipolycythemic
antiprecipitin

antiprothrombin
antiprotozoal
antipruritic
antipsoriatic
antipsychomotor
antipsychotic
antipyretic
antipyrotic
antiradiation
antireflective coating
antirheumatic
anti-Rho-D titer
antiricin
antirickettsial
antischistosomal
antiscorbutic
antiseborrheic
antisecretory
antisepsis
    physiologic a.
antiseptic
antiserum
    rabies a.
    Rh (Rhesus) a.
    therapeutic a.
antisialagogue
antisialic
antisocial
antispasmodic
    biliary a.
    bronchial a.
antispastic
antistaphylococcal
antisterility
antisternum
antistreptococcal
antistreptolysin O titer
antisudorific
antisyphilitic
antitetanic
antithenar
antithrombin
    a. I
    a. III
antithromboplastin
antithrombotic
antithymocyte
antithyroid
antithyrotoxic
antithyrotropic
antitonic
antitoxic
antitoxin
    botulism a.
    bovine a.

antitoxin *(continued)*
    Clostridium perfringens types
      C and D a.
    Crotalus a.
    diphtheria a.
    gas gangrene a.
    perfringens a.
    scarlet fever a.
    Staphylococcus a.
    Streptococcus a.
    tetanus and gas gangrene a's
    tetanus perfringens a.
antitragicus muscle
antitragus
antitreponemal
antitrichomonal
antitrismus
antitropin
antitrypanosomal
α_1-antitrypsin [alpha-1-]
antituberculin
antituberculotic
antituberculous
antitumorigenic
antitussive
antityphoid
antiulcerative
antivenereal
antivenin
    black widow spider a.
    Latrodectus mactans a.
    polyvalent crotaline a.
antivenomous
antiviral
antixenic
antixerophthalmic
antixerotic
Anton
    symptom
    syndrome
Anton-Babinski syndrome
Antoni neurilemoma, type A, type B
antophthalmic
antra (plural of antrum)
antral resection
antrectomy
antritis
antrobuccal
antrocele
antroduodenectomy
antrodynia
antronasal
antropyloric
antroscope
antroscopy

antrostomy
    intranasal a.
    radical maxillary a.
antrotomy
    sublabial a.
antrotympanic
antrotympanitis
antrum (antra)
    a. auris
    cardiac a.
    ethmoid a.
    a. ethmoidale
    a. folliculare
    frontal a.
    gastric a.
    a. of Highmore
    a. highmori
    mastoid a.
    a. mastoideum
    a. maxillare
    maxillary a.
    pyloric a.
    a. pyloricum
    a. of stomach
    tympanic a.
    a. tympanicum
    a. of Willis
anuclear
anucleated
anucleolar
ANUG—acute necrotizing
  ulcerative gingivitis
anuloplasty
anulus (anuli)
    atrioventricular valve anuli
    a. of conjunctiva, a.
      conjunctivae
    a. femoralis
    a. fibrocartilagineus
      membranae tympani
    a. fibrosus disci
      intervertebralis
    a. inguinalis profundus
    a. inguinalis superficialis
    a. iridis major
    a. iridis minor
    a. lymphaticus cardiae
    mitral valve a.
    a. of spermatozoon
    a. tendineus communis
    tricuspid valve a.
    a. tympanicus
    a. umbilicalis
    a. urethralis
    a. of Zinn

anuresis
anuretic
anuria
    angioneurotic a.
    calculous a.
    compression a.
    obstructive a.
    postrenal a.
    prerenal a.
    renal a.
    suppressive a.
anuric
anus
    artificial a.
    ectopic a.
    imperforate a.
    a. of Rusconi
    a. vesicalis
    a. vestibularis
    vulvovaginal a.
anusitis
anvil
    Bunnell a.
anxiety
    castration a.
    existential a.
    free-floating a.
    neurotic a.
    separation a.
    signal a.
anxiolytic
AO—opening of the
  atrioventricular valves
AOA—American Optometric
  Association
AOA splint
AOB—alcohol on breath
aorta (aortas, aortae)
    abdominal a.
    a. abdominalis
    a. ascendens
    ascending a.
    bicuspal a.
    buckled a.
    a. chlorotica
    a. descendens
    descending a.
    descending thoracic a.
    dextropositioned a.
    dorsal embryonic a.
    double a.
    dynamic a.
    kinked a.
    overriding a.
    palpable a.

aorta (aortas, aortae) *(continued)*
    pericardial a.
    primitive a.
    retroesophageal a.
    root of a.
    a. sacrococcygea
    straddling a.
    a. thoracalis
    thoracic a.
    throbbing a.
    ventral a.
aortalgia
aortectomy
aortic
    a. aneurysm
    a. arch
    a. arch angiography
    a. arteritis
    a. cross-clamp
    a. dissection
    a. embolism
    a. flush pigtail catheter
    a. impedance
    a. insufficiency
    a. knob
    a. prosthesis
    a. regurgitation
    a. root
    a. septal defect
    a. sinus
    a. stenosis
    a. thrombosis
    trileaflet a. prosthesis
    a. valve
    a. valvulitis
    a. valvuloplasty
aorticopulmonary
aorticorenal
aortitis
    Döhle-Heller a.
    luetic a.
    nummular a.
    rheumatic a.
    a. syphilitica
    a. syphilitica obliterans
    ulcerative a.
aortoarteritis
aortobifemoral
aortocaval
aortocoronary
aortoduodenal
aortoenteric
aortoesophageal
aortofemoral
aortogastric

aortogram
    flush a.
    transbrachial arch a.
    translumbar a.
aortography
    abdominal a.
    catheter a.
    intravenous a.
    lumbar a.
    retrograde a.
    selective visceral a.
    thoracic a.
    translumbar a.
    venous a.
    visceral a.
aortoiliac
aortopathy
aortoplasty
aortopulmonary
aortorrhaphy
aortosclerosis
aortotomy incision
AO soft lens
AP—
    alkaline phosphatase
    angina pectoris
    antepartum
    anterior pituitary
    anteroposterior
    aortic pressure
    apical pulse
    arterial pressure
A&P—
    anterior and posterior
    auscultation and percussion
APA—
    American Psychiatric Association
    American Psychological
        Association
6-APA—6-aminopenicillanic acid
APACHE—acute physiology and
   chronic health evaluation
apaconitine
apancreatic
aparalytic
aparathyrosis
aparthrosis
apathetic
apathy
apatite
A pattern
APB—atrial premature beat
APC—
    adenomatous polyposis coli
    atrial premature contraction

APD—
- action potential duration
- ambulatory peritoneal dialysis
- anteroposterior diameter
- atrial premature depolarization

APE—
- acute psychotic episode
- acute pulmonary edema
- anterior pituitary extract

apeidosis

apellous

apepsia
- achlorhydria a.

aperiodic

aperistalsis

Apert
- acrocephalosyndactyly
- disease
- hirsutism
- syndrome

Apert-Crouzon disease

apertognathia
- Le Fort a. repair (I)

apertura (aperturae)
- a. chordae tympani
- a. externa aqueductus vestibuli
- a. nasalis posterior
- a. pelvis inferior
- a. pelvis superior
- a. piriformis
- a. sinus frontalis
- a. sinus sphenoidalis
- a. thoracis inferior
- a. thoracis superior
- a. tympanica canaliculi
- a. tympanica canaliculi chordae tympani

aperture
- angle of a.
- angular a.
- bony anterior nasal a.
- cloacal a.
- coded-image a.
- a. of frontal sinus
- inferior a. of thorax
- laryngeal a.
- a. of larynx
- lateral a. of fourth ventricle
- a. of lens
- median a. of fourth ventricle
- nasal a., anterior
- nasal a., posterior
- numerical a.
- orbital a.

aperture (continued)
- pharyngeal a.
- piriform a.
- posterior nasal a.
- a. of sphenoid sinus
- superior a. of axillary fossa
- superior a. of minor pelvis
- superior a. of thorax
- thoracic a., inferior
- thoracic a., superior
- tympanic a. of canaliculus of chorda tympani

apex (apices, apexes)
- a. of arytenoid cartilage
- a. auriculae
- a. auriculare
- a. of bladder
- a. capitis fibulae
- a. cartilaginis arytenoideae
- a. cordis
- a. cuspidis dentis
- darwinian a.
- flaring a.
- a. of head of fibula
- a. of heart
- a. linguae, a. lingualis
- a. of lung
- a. nasi
- a. ossis sacralis
- a. ossis sacri
- a. of patella, a. patellae
- a. prostatae, a. of prostate gland
- a. pulmonalis
- a. pulmonis
- a. radicis dentis
- radiographic a.
- root a.
- a. of sacrum
- a. of tongue
- a. vesicae
- a. vesicalis

Apgar
- rating
- scale
- score
- test

APGAR—adaptability, partnership, growth, affection, resolve (questionnaire)

APH—
- adenohypophysial hormone
- antepartum hemorrhage

aphagia algera

aphake

aphakia

aphakic
aphalangia
aphasia
    acoustic a.
    ageusic a.
    amnesic a., amnestic a.
    anosmic a.
    apractic a.
    associative a.
    ataxic a.
    Broca a.
    central a.
    color name a.
    combined a.
    cortical a.
    crossed a.
    efferent motor a.
    expressive a.
    expressive-receptive a.
    finger a.
    fluent a.
    frontocortical a.
    frontolenticular a.
    functional a.
    gestural a.
    gibberish a.
    global a.
    intellectual a.
    kinetic motor a.
    mixed a.
    motor a.
    paroxysmal a.
    pictorial a.
    psychosensory a.
    puerperal a.
    pure motor a.
    receptive a.
    semantic a.
    sensory a.
    subcortical a.
    tactile a.
    total a.
    true a.
    verbal a.
    visual a.
    Wernicke a.
aphasiac
aphasic
aphemic
apheresis
aphonia
    hysterical a.
    a. paralytica
    spastic a.
aphonic

aphonogelia
aphosphagenic
aphosphorosis
aphotesthesia
aphotic
aphrasia
aphrodisiac
aphtha (aphthae)
    Bednar a.
    Behçet a.
    cachectic a.
    epizootic a.
    a. febriles
    Mikulicz a.
    recurring scarring a.
    a. tropicae
aphthoid
aphthongia
aphthosis
    Touraine a.
aphthous
aphylactic
aphylaxis
apical
    a. clearance
    a. impulse
    a. radius
    a. zone
apicectomy
apices (plural of apex)
apicitis
    orbital a.
apicoectomy
apicolysis
apicostomy
apicotomy
apiotherapy
apiphobia
apitoxin
apituitarism
APKD—adult polycystic kidney
    disease
aplacental
aplanatic
aplanatism
aplasia
    a. axialis extracorticalis
      congenita
    a. cutis congenita
    germinal cell a.
    gonadal a.
    hereditary retinal a.
    Leydig cell a.
    lobular a.
    nuclear a.

aplasia *(continued)*
    pure red cell a.
    retinal a.
    thymic-parathyroid a.
aplastic
    a. anemia
    a. crisis
    a. pancytopenia
apleuria
Apley
    grinding test
    knee test
    maneuver
    sign
    traction
APN—acute pyelonephritis
apnea
    chemoreceptor a.
    deglutition a.
    hypersomnia sleep a.
    induced a.
    initial a.
    late a.
    a. neonatorum
    obstructive sleep a.
    postanesthesia a.
    sleep a.
    traumatic a.
apneic
apneumatosis
apneusis
apneustic
apo—apolipoprotein
apochromatic
apocrine
    a. chromhidrosis
    a. cystadenoma
    a. gland(s)
    a. metaplasia
apodal
apodia
apoenzyme
apoferritin
apogamia, apogamy
apokamnosis
apolar
apolipoprotein
    a. A-I
    a. B
    a. C-II
    a. C-II deficiency, familial
    a. D
    a. E (apo-E)
apomorphine
aponeurectomy

aponeurorrhaphy
aponeurosis (aponeuroses)
    abdominal a.
    bicipital a.
    a. bicipitalis
    clavicoracoaxillary a.
    crural a.
    Denonvilliers a.
    epicranial a.
    extensor a.
    a. of external oblique muscle
    femoral a.
    a. of insertion
    intercostal aponeuroses
    ischiorectal a.
    a. linguae
    lingual a.
    a. musculi bicipitis brachii
    a. of origin
    a. palatina, palatine a.
    palmar a., a. palmaris
    perineal a.
    pharyngeal a.
    pharyngobasilar a.
    plantar a., a. plantaris
    Sibson a.
    subscapular a.
    superficial perineal a.
    supraspinous a.
    temporal a.
    vertebral a.
    a. of Zinn
aponeurositis
aponeurotic
aponeurotomy
apophlegmatic
apophyseal
apophyseopathy
apophysis (apophyses)
    basilar a.
    calcaneal a.
    cerebral a.
    a. cerebri
    genial a.
    a. helicis
    odontoid a.
    a. ossium
    pterygoid a.
apophysitis tibialis adolescentium
apoprotein
apoptosis
apoptotic
apostasis
aposthia
apothecary

apparatus
- Abbe-Zeiss a.
- absorption a.
- acoustic a.
- attachment a.
- auditory a.
- Barcroft a.
- Beckmann a.
- Benedict-Knipping a.
- Benedict-Roth a.
- biliary a.
- Calandruccio compression a.
- cerebellovestibular a.
- Charnley a.
- chromatic a.
- ciliary a.
- cytopharyngeal a.
- a. derivatorius
- Desault a.
- digestive a.
- a. digestorius
- electro-oculogram a.
- Fell-O'Dwyer a.
- Finsen a.
- genital a. of the female
- Golgi a.
- a. of Goormaghtigh
- Hodgen a.
- Horsley-Clarke a.
- Howard-Dolman a.
- hyoid a.
- ICLH (Imperial College, London Hospital) a.
- inhalation anesthesia a.
- inhalation therapy a.
- Jaquet a.
- Junker a.
- juxtaglomerular a.
- Kirschner a.
- lacrimal a.
- a. lacrimalis
- locomotor a.
- masticatory a.
- mytotic a.
- parabasal a.
- a. of Perroncito
- pilosebaceous a.
- reproductive a.
- a. respiratorius
- respiratory a.
- rocking a.
- Sayre a.
- Scholander a.
- sound-conducting a.
- Soxhlet a.
- spindle a.

apparatus *(continued)*
- spine a.
- steadiness a.
- stereotaxic a.
- suspensory a. of pleura
- Taylor a.
- a. of Timofeew
- Tiselius a.
- urogenital a.
- a. urogenitalis
- vasomotor a.
- vestibular a.
- vocal a.
- Waldenberg a.
- Wangensteen a.
- Warburg a.

appearance
- angry a.
- applecore-like a.
- ball-in-hand a.
- beaded a.
- beaked a.
- beaten-brass a.
- beaten-silver a.
- beavertail a. of balloon profile
- bone-within-bone a.
- bubble-like a.
- bullneck a.
- candle drippings a.
- cluster-of-grapes a.
- coarse a.
- cobblestone a.
- cobblestone-like a.
- cobra-head a.
- coiled-spring a.
- cotton ball a.
- cotton-wool a.
- cushingoid a.
- cystlike a.
- double-bubble a.
- drumstick a.
- eggshell a.
- enamel paint spot a.
- fine-speckled a.
- finger-in-glove a.
- fish-flesh a.
- Florence flask a.
- frayed-string a.
- frondlike a.
- ground-glass a.
- hair-on-end a., hair-standing-on-end a.
- hammered-brass a.
- heterogeneous a.
- homogeneous a.
- honeycomb a.

appearance *(continued)*
  hot-cross-bun a.
  inverse comma a.
  jail bars a.
  kernel-of-corn a., kernel-of-popcorn a.
  lacelike a.
  lamina dura–like a.
  leafless-tree a.
  light bulb a.
  lobulated saccular a.
  moth-eaten a.
  onion peel a.
  onion skin a.
  pancake a.
  panda a.
  picket fence a.
  picture frame a.
  pigtail a.
  plucked-chicken a.
  popcorn-like a.
  pruned-tree a.
  punched-out a.
  railroad track a.
  reticulogranular a.
  rugger jersey a.
  saber-shin a.
  sandwich a.
  scottie dog a.
  shell-of-bone a.
  shocklike a.
  shocky a.
  slapped-cheek a.
  slapped-face a.
  soap-bubble a.
  spadelike a.
  stack-of-coins a.
  string-of-beads a.
  stuck-on a.
  sunburst a.
  sun-ray a., sunray a.
  Swiss Alps a.
  tadpole-like a.
  toxic a.
  trefoil a.
  trilayer a.
  weblike a.
  whorled a.
  wineglass a.
  worm-eaten a.
  wormy a.
appendage
  atrial a.
  caudal a.
  cecal a.
  cutaneous a's

appendage *(continued)*
  drumstick a.
  a. of epididymis
  epiploic a's
  a's of eye
  fibrous a. of liver
  preauricular a.
  testicular a.
  a's of the fetus
  a's of the skin
  a. of the testis
  uterine a's
  a. of ventricle of larynx
  vermicular a.
appendagitis
  epiploic a.
appendectomy
  auricular a.
appendiceal
appendices (plural of appendix)
appendicitis
  actinomycotic a.
  acute a.
  amebic a.
  a. by contiguity
  chronic a.
  foreign-body a.
  fulminating a.
  gangrenous a.
  a. granulosa
  helminthic a.
  left-sided a.
  lumbar a.
  myxoglobulosis a.
  nonobstructive a.
  a. obliterans
  obstructive a.
  perforating a.
  perforative a.
  protective a.
  purulent a.
  recurrent a.
  relapsing a.
  segmental a.
  skip a.
  stercoral a.
  subperitoneal a.
  suppurative a.
  traumatic a.
  verminous a.
appendicocecostomy
appendicocele
appendicoenterostomy
appendicolith
appendicolithiasis
appendicolysis

appendicopathy
appendicostomy
appendicular ataxia
appendix (appendices)
 auricular a.
 cecal a.
 a. cerebri
 ensiform a.
 a. epididymidis
 a. of epididymis
 epiploic a's
 a. epiploicae
 a. fibrosa hepatis
 fibrous a. of liver
 Morgagni a.
 omental a's
 a. omentales
 pelvic a.
 a. testis
 a. of ventricle of larynx
 a. vermicularis
 vermiform a.
 a. vermiformis
 a. vesiculosae epöophori
 xiphoid a.
apperception
apperceptive
appersonification
appestat
appetite
 perverted a.
appetizers
applanate
applanation tonometry
apple
 Adam's a.
 bitter a.
 May a.
 thorn a.
applecore-like appearance
appliance
 Andresen a.
 Begg a.
 Bimler a.
 craniofacial a.
 crown of thorns a.
 Crozat a.
 Denholz a.
 edgewise a.
 expansion plate a.
 extraoral a.
 fixed a.
 Fränkel a.
 functional a.
 habit-breaking a.

appliance *(continued)*
 Hawley a.
 Jackson a.
 Johnston twin wire a.
 jumping-the-bite a.
 Kesling a.
 Kingsley a.
 labiolingual a.
 light round-wire a.
 monoblock a.
 multibanded a.
 occlusal overlay a.
 orthodontic a.
 permanent a.
 pin and tube a.
 prosthetic a.
 regulating a.
 removable a.
 retaining a.
 ribbon arch a.
 Roger Anderson pin fixation a.
 Schwarz a.
 speech a.
 split plate a.
 twin wire a.
 universal a.
 Walker a.
application
applicator
 Andrews a.
 beam-therapy a.
 Brown a.
 cotton-tipped a. test
 Dean a.
 Ernst a.
 Fletcher-Suit a.
 Gifford a.
 Holinger a.
 Lejeune a.
 Plummer-Vinson
  radium a.
 Pynchon a.
 Roberts a.
 sandwich-mold a.
 sonic a.
 surface a.
applique
Appolito
 operation
 suture
appose
apposition suture
appraisal
 health risk a.
apprehension test

approach
  idiographic a.
  Kocher-McFarland a.
  nomothetic a.
  Risdon a.
  transcranial a.
  transnasal a.
  transseptal a.
  transthoracic a.
approximate
approximation
  successive a.
  a. suture
approximator
  rib a.
  skin-edge a.
APR—abdominoperineal resection
apractic
apraxia
  agnosic a.
  akinetic a.
  amnestic a.
  classic a.
  congenital a.
  constructional a.
  cortical a.
  developmental a.
  geometric a.
  ideational a.
  ideokinetic a.
  ideomotor a.
  innervatory a.
  limb-kinetic a.
  motor a.
  oculomotor a.
  optic a.
  sensory a.
  tongue a.
  transcortical a.
  trunk a.
  visual a.
A&P repair—anterior and posterior
  repair
aproctia
apron
  abdominal a.
  lead-rubber a.
aprosody
aprosopia
aprotinin
APTA—American Physical
  Therapy Association
aptitude
APTT, aPTT—activated partial
  thromboplastin time

aptyalia
aptyalism
APUD—amine precursor uptake
  and decarboxylation
apudoma
apyetous
apyknomorphous
apyogenous
apyous
apyrene
apyretic
apyrexia
apyrexial
apyrogenic
AQ—achievement quotient
AQS—additional qualifying
  symptoms
aqua (aquae)
Aquaflex lens
aquaphobia
aquapuncture
aquatic
aqueduct
  cerebral a.
  a. of cochlea
  a. of Cotunnius
  fallopian a.
  a. of Fallopius
  a. of mesencephalon
  a. of midbrain
  a. of Sylvius
  ventricular a.
  a. of the vestibule
aqueductal
aqueductus (gen. and pl.
  aqueductus)
  a. cerebri
  a. cochleae
  a. endolymphaticus
  a. mesencephali
  a. vestibuli
aqueous
  a. flare
  a. humor
  a. outflow
aquiparous
AR—
  alarm reaction
  aortic regurgitation
  artificial respiration
arabin
arabinose
arabinosis
arabinosuria
arabitol

arachidate
arachidic acid
arachidonate 5-lipoxygenase
arachidonate 12-lipoxygenase
arachidonic acid
Arachnia propionica
arachnid
arachnidism
arachnodactyly
    congenital contractural a.
      (CCA)
    contractural a.
arachnogastria
arachnoid
    a. of brain
    cranial a.
    spinal a.
arachnoidal
arachnoidea (arachnoideae)
    a. mater encephali
    a. mater spinalis
arachnoiditis
    basal a.
    a. of cerebral hemispheres
    cisternal a.
    opticochiasmatic a.
    a. of posterior cerebral fossa
    spinal a.
arachnophobia
Aran-Duchenne
    amyotrophy
    disease
    muscular atrophy
    muscular dystrophy
araneous
Aran's law
Arantius
    body
    canal
    duct
    ligament
    nodules
    ventricle
arbor (arbores)
    a. bronchialis
    a. medullaris vermis
    a. vitae cerebelli
    a. vitae uteri
arboreal
arborescent
arborization
    cervical mucus a.
Arbuckle probe
arc.—abnormal retinal
  correspondence

arc
    auricular a.
    autonomic reflex a.
    binauricular a.
    bregmatolambdoid a.
    carbon a.
    dorsal venous a.
    epiploic a. of Haller and Barkow
    external marginal a. of
      Zuckerkandl
    mercury a.
    nasobregmatic a.
    naso-occipital a.
    neural a.
    nuclear a.
    retruded a. of closure
    Riolan a.
    sensorimotor a.
ARC—AIDS-related complex
arcade
    anomalous mitral a.
    arterial a's
    Flint a.
    Riolan a.
    temporal a.
    vascular a.
Arcelin views
arch
    abdominothoracic a.
    alveolar a.
    anastomotic a.
    anterior a. of atlas
    a. of aorta, aortic a.
    arterial a's of colon
    arterial a's of ileum
    arterial a's of jejunum
    auricular a.
    axillary a.
    a. of azygos vein
    basal a.
    branchial a's
    carpal a's
    cervical a.
    cervical aortic a.
    a. of Corti
    cortical a's of kidney
    costal a.
    a. of cricoid cartilage
    crural a.
    dental a.
    diaphragmatic a.
    dorsal a. of wrist
    dorsal venous a. of hand
    double aortic a.
    epiphyseal a.

arch *(continued)*
    fallen a's
    fibrous a. of soleus muscle
    a's of foot
    glossopalatine a.
    Haller a's
    hyoid a.
    hyothyroid a.
    iliopectineal a.
    inferior palpebral a.
    inguinal a.
    intermesenteric arterial a.
    ischiopubic a.
    jugular venous a.
    Langer axillary a.
    lingual a.
    longitudinal a. of foot
    lumbocostal a.
    malar a.
    mandibular a.
    marginal a. of eyelid
    maxillary a.
    nasal a.
    neural a.
    open pubic a.
    oral a.
    palatal a.
    palatine a., anterior
    palatine a., posterior
    palatoglossal a.
    palatomaxillary a.
    palatopharyngeal a.
    palmar arterial a.
    palmar carpal a.
    palmar venous a.
    palpebral a.
    paraphysial a.
    parieto-occipital a.
    a. of pelvis
    persistent right aortic a.
    pharyngeal a's
    pharyngoepiglottic a.
    pharyngopalatine a.
    plantar a.
    plantar venous a.
    popliteal a.
    postaural a's
    posterior a. of atlas
    prepancreatic a.
    primitive costal a's
    pubic a., a. of pubis
    pulmonary a's
    Reichert a.
    residual a.
    residual dental a.

arch *(continued)*
    rhinencephalic a.
    ribbon a.
    right aortic a.
    Riolan a.
    saddle a.
    Salus a.
    Shenton a.
    superciliary a.
    superficial femoral a.
    supraorbital a. of frontal bone
    systemic a.
    tarsal a's
    tendinous a.
    a. of thoracic duct
    thyrohyoid a.
    transverse a. of foot
    trapezoidal a.
    Treitz a.
    U-shaped a.
    venous a's of kidney
    vertebral a.
    visceral a's
    volar venous a.
    V-shaped a.
    Zimmermann a.
    zygomatic a.
archaic
arch bar
    Erich a.b.
    Jelanko a.b.
    Winter a.b.
archetype
archiblast
archiblastic
archicerebellum
archistriatum
architectonic
arciform
Arco pacemaker
arctation
arcual
arcuate
    a. incision
    a. scotoma
    a. suture
arcuation
arcus
    a. adiposus
    a. alveolaris mandibulae
    a. alveolaris maxillae
    a. anterior atlantis
    a. aortae
    a. aorticus
    a. cartilaginis cricoideae

arcus *(continued)*
  a. corneae
  corneal a.
  a. cornealis
  a. costalis
  a. costarum
  a. dentalis mandibularis
  a. dentalis maxillaris
  a. dorsalis pedis
  a. ductus thoracici
  a. glossopalatinus
  a. iliopectineus
  a. inguinalis
  a. juvenilis
  a. lipoides corneae
  a. lipoides myringis
  a. palatini
  a. palatoglossus
  a. palatopharyngeus
  a. palmaris profundus
  a. palmaris superficialis
  a. palpebrales
  a. palpebralis inferior
  a. palpebralis superior
  a. parieto-occipitalis
  a. pedis longitudinalis
  a. pedis transversalis
  a. pharyngopalatinus
  a. plantaris profundus
  a. plantaris superficialis
  a. posterior atlantis
  a. presenilis
  a. pubicus
  a. pubis
  a. senilis
  a. superciliaris
  a. tarseus inferior
  a. tarseus superior
  a. tendineus
  a. venae azygou
  a. venosus dorsalis pedis
  a. venosus jugularis
  a. venosus palmaris profundus
  a. venosus palmaris
    superficialis
  a. venosus plantaris
  a. vertebrae
  a. zygomaticus
ARD—
  acute respiratory disease
  acute respiratory distress
  anorectal dressing
  arthritis and rheumatic disease
ARDMS—American Registry of
  Diagnostic Medical Sonographers
ardor urinae

ARDS—
  acute respiratory distress
    syndrome
  adult respiratory distress
    syndrome
area (areae, areas)
  alisphenoid a.
  anterior amygdaloid a.
  aortic a.
  apical a.
  areae gastricae
  associative a.
  asthmagenic a.
  auditory cortical a.
  auditory projection a.
  auditory psychic a.
  autonomic a.
  axial a.
  Bamberger a.
  bare a. of liver
  basal seat a.
  B-dependent a.
  body surface a. (BSA)
  Broca motor speech a.
  Broca parolfactory a.
  Brodmann a.
  buccopharyngeal a.
  cardiogenic a.
  catchment a.
  a. centralis
  central speech a.
  a. choroidea
  cingulate a.
  a. cochleae
  Cohnheim a's
  contact a.
  a. contingens dentis
  cortical 4S a.
  cortical gustatory a.
  cortical oculomotor a.
  cortical speech a.
  cortical tactile a.
  cortico-oculocephalogyric a.
  cribriform a. of renal papilla
  a. cribrosa papillae renalis
  a. of critical definition
  denture-bearing a.
  denture foundation a.
  denture-supporting a.
  dermatomic a.
  donor a.
  dorsal hypothalamic a.
  embryonic a.
  entorhinal a.
  excitable a.
  excitomotor a.

area (areae, areas) *(continued)*
    extrapyramidal motor a.
    first motor speech a.
    Flechsig a.
    a. of Forel
    frontal a.
    fronto-orbital a.
    fusion a.
    gastric a's
    areae gastricae
    genital a's
    glove a.
    gustatory receiving a.
    Hines strip a.
    hypoglossal a.
    impression a.
    insular a.
    intercondylar a's of tibia
    interglobular a's
    Kiesselbach a.
    Laimer-Haeckerman a.
    language a.
    lateral hypothalamic a.
    Little a.
    a. of Martegiani
    a. medullovasculosa
    mesobranchial a.
    mirror a.
    mitral valve a.
    a. nervi facialis
    a. nuda hepatis
    Obersteiner-Redlich a.
    olfactory a.
    optic a.
    Panum a.
    parastriate a.
    a. paraterminalis
    parolfactory a. of Broca
    Patrick trigger a's
    a. pellucida
    a. perforata
    pericruciate a.
    peristriate a.
    piriform a.
    portal a.
    postcentral a.
    posterior hypothalamic a.
    posterior palatal seal a.
    a. postrema
    postrolandic a.
    prefrontal a.
    premotor a.
    preoptic a., a. preoptica
    pressure a.
    pretectal a.
    a. pretectalis

area (areae, areas) *(continued)*
    primary receptive a's
    projection a's
    psychomotor a.
    a. pterygoidea
    pulmonary valve a.
    pyriform a.
    receptive a's
    relief a.
    rest a.
    rugae a.
    saddle a.
    sensorimotor a.
    sensory a's
    septal a.
    silent a.
    somatosensory a.
    somesthetic a.
    stress-bearing a.
    striate a.
    strip a.
    a. subcallosa
    subcallosal a.
    supplementary a's
    supporting a.
    suppressor a's
    T-dependent a.
    temporal a.
    thenar a.
    thymus-dependent a.
    thymus-independent a.
    T-independent a.
    triangular a.
    tricuspid valve a.
    vagus a.
    ventral tegmental a. of Tsai
    vestibular a.
    vocal a.
    Wernicke second motor
      speech a.
areata
    alopecia a.
areflexia
aregenerative
arenaceous
arenavirus
arenoid
areola (areolae)
    a. mammae
    a. of mammary gland
    a. of nipple
    primary a.
    second a.
areolar
    a. incision
    a. pityriasis versicolor

areolate
areolitis
Arey's rule
ARF—
    acute renal failure
    acute respiratory failure
Argamaso-Lewin composite flap
argamblyopia
argema
argentaffin
argentaffinoma of bronchus
argentation
argentic
argentum
argillaceous
arginase deficiency
arginine
    a. carboxypeptidase
    suberyl a.
argininemia
argininosuccinase
argininosuccinate lyase deficiency
    (ASAL deficiency; ASL
    deficiency)
argininosuccinate synthetase
    deficiency (ASAS deficiency, ASS
    deficiency)
argininosuccinic acid (ASA)
argininosuccinicacidemia
argon (Ar)
argon laser trabeculoplasty
Argonz-del Castillo syndrome
Argyle
    catheter
    chest tube
    endotracheal tube
Argyll Robertson
    pupil
    sign
    suture
argyremia
argyria nasalis
argyric
argyrophil
Arias-Stella
    cells
    effect
    phenomenon
    reaction
ariboflavinosis
Aries-Pitanguy
    mammaplasty
    operation
    procedure
aristolochic acid
Aristotle anomaly

arithmomania
ARL—average remaining lifetime
Arloing-Courmont test
Arlt (von Arlt)
    disease
    line
    operation
    recess
    scoop
    sinus
    suture
    trachoma
Arlt-Jaesche operation
ARM—artificial rupture of
    membranes
arm
    bar clasp a.
    bird a.
    chromosome a.
    circumferential clasp a.
    glass a.
    golf a.
    Krukenberg a.
    prolapsed a.
    reciprocal a.
    retentive a.
    scanning a.
    stabilizing a.
armadillo
armamentarium
Armanni-Ebstein
    cell(s)
    change
    degeneration
    kidney
    lesion
armature
armpit
Armstrong disease
Army-Navy retractor
Arndt-Gottron
    disease
    syndrome
Arneth
    classification
    count
    formula
    index
    stages
    syndrome
arnica
Arnold
    ganglion
    bodies
    bundle
    canal

Arnold *(continued)*
  fold
  foramen
  ligament
  nerve
  nerve reflex cough syndrome
  syndrome
  tract
Arnold-Chiari
  deformity
  malformation
  syndrome
Arnold and Gunning method
AROA—autosomal recessive ocular
  albinism
aroma
aromatase inhibitors
aromatics
aromatization
arousal
ARP—at-risk period
arrangement
  anterior tooth a.
  tooth a.
array
  annular a.
  linear switched a.
  phase steered a.
  transducer a.
arrector (arrectores)
  a. pili
  arrectores pilorum
arrest
  cardiac a.
  circulatory a.
  deep transverse a.
  developmental a.
  epiphyseal a.
  heart a.
  a. of labor
  maturation a.
  metaphase a.
  pelvic a.
  sinus a.
  sudden cardiac a.
arrested
  a. descent of fetal head
  a. growth and development
  a. labor
arrestin
arrhaphia
arrhythmia
  chronic a.
  compound a.
  continuous a.
  inotropic a.

arrhythmia *(continued)*
  juvenile a.
  nodal a.
  nonphasic a.
  perpetual a.
  phasic a.
  respiratory a.
  sinus a., nonrespiratory
  sinus a., respiratory
  supraventricular a.
  vagal a.
  ventricular a.
arrhythmic
arrhythmogenic
arrhythmokinesis
arrowroot
Arroyo sign
ARRS—American Roentgen Ray
  Society
Arruga
  expressor
  forceps
  implant
  operation
  protector
  trephine
arsenic (As)
  a. acid
  a. chloride
  a. disulfide
  fuming liquid a.
  red a. sulfide
  a. trichloride
  a. trioxide
  a. trisulfide
  white a.
  a. yellow
arsenical
arsenicalism
arsenide
  hydrogen a.
arsenism
arsenite
arsenotherapy
arsenous
arsine
arsinic acid
Arslan operation
arsonic acid
arsonium
ART—automated reagin test
Artemisia absinthium
arteralgia
arteria (arteriae)
  a. anastomotica
  a. angularis

arteria (arteriae) *(continued)*
- a. appendicularis
- a. ascendens
- a. axillaris
- arteriae azygoi vaginae
- a. basilaris
- a. brachialis
- a. buccalis
- a. bulbi penis
- a. bulbi vestibuli
- a. caecalis anterior
- a. caecalis posterior
- a. callosomarginalis
- a. canalis pterygoidei
- arteriae caroticotympanicae
- a. carotis communis
- a. carotis externa
- a. carotis interna
- a. caudae pancreatis
- a. cervicalis ascendens
- a. choroidea anterior
- arteriae conjunctivales anteriores
- arteriae conjunctivales posteriores
- a. coronaria dextra
- a. coronaria sinistra
- a. cremasterica
- a. cystica
- a. ductus deferentis
- arteriae episclerales
- a. facialis
- a. femoralis
- a. fibularis
- a. frontobasalis lateralis
- a. frontobasalis medialis
- a. gyri angularis
- arteriae helicinae penis
- a. hyaloidea
- a. hypophysialis inferior
- a. hypophysialis superior
- a. ileocolica
- a. iliaca communis
- a. iliaca externa
- a. iliaca interna
- a. iliolumbalis
- a. infraorbitalis
- arteriae insulares
- arteriae intrarenales
- arteriae jejunales
- a. labyrinthi
- a. labyrinthina
- a. lacrimalis
- a. laryngea inferior
- a. laryngea superior
- a. lienalis

arteria (arteriae) *(continued)*
- a. lingualis
- a. lobi caudati
- arteriae lumbales
- a. lusoria
- a. masseterica
- a. maxillaris
- a. media genus
- a. meningea media
- a. meningea posterior
- arteriae mesencephalicae
- a. musculophrenica
- a. nasales septi
- a. nutricia
- a. obturatoria
- a. occipitalis
- a. ophthalmica
- a. ovarica
- a. paracentralis
- arteriae perforantes
- a. pericardiacophrenica
- a. perinealis
- a. peronea
- a. pharyngea ascendens
- a. plantaris lateralis
- a. plantaris medialis
- a. plantaris profunda
- arteriae pontis
- a. poplitea
- a. profunda femoris
- a. pulmonalis dextra
- a. pulmonalis sinistra
- a. radialis
- a. radicularis magna
- a. rectae spuriae
- a. rectae verae
- a. renalis
- arteriae retroduodenales
- arteriae sigmoideae
- a. sphenopalatina
- a. spinalis anterior
- a. spinalis posterior
- a. splenica
- a. stylomastoidea
- a. subclavia
- a. subcostalis
- a. sublingualis
- a. submentalis
- a. subscapularis
- a. sulci centralis
- a. sulci postcentralis
- a. sulci precentralis
- a. supraduodenalis
- a. suprascapularis
- a. supratrochlearis
- arteriae surales

arteria (arteriae) *(continued)*
  a. temporalis anterior
  a. temporalis profunda anterior
  a. temporalis profunda posterior
  a. temporalis superficialis
  a. testicularis
  a. thalamostriatae
    anteromediales arteriae
    cerebri anterioris
  a. thoracalis lateralis
  a. thoracalis suprema
  a. thoracica interna
  a. thoracica lateralis
  a. thoracica suprema
  a. thoracoacromialis
  a. thoracodorsalis
  a. thyroidea ima
  a. thyroidea inferior
  a. thyroidea superior
  a. tibialis anterior
  a. tibialis posterior
  a. transversa faciei
  a. ulnaris
  a. umbilicalis
  a. urethralis
  a. uterina
  a. vaginalis
  a. vertebralis
  a. zygomaticoorbitalis
arterial
  a. blood flow
  a. blood gases (ABGs)
  a. calcification
  a. catheter
  a. coupling
  a. line (A-line)
  a. oxygen saturation
  a. pressure
  a. pulse
  a. thrombosis
arterialization of portal vein
arteriectasis
arteriectomy
arteriectopia
arteriocapillary
arteriodilating
arteriogenesis
arteriogram
  coronary a.
  femoral a.
  pruned-tree a.
  subclavian a.
  wedge a.
arteriography
  axillary a.
  brachiocephalic a.

arteriography *(continued)*
  carotid a.
  catheter a.
  celiac a.
  cerebral a.
  cine coronary a.
  completion a.
  coronary a.
  digital subtraction a. (DSA)
  femoral a.
  mesenteric a.
  operative a.
  peripheral a.
  pulmonary a.
  renal a.
  selective a.
  spinal a.
  vertebral a.
  visceral a.
arteriola (arteriolae)
  a. ellipsoideae
  a. glomerularis afferens
  a. glomerularis efferens
  a. macularis inferior
  a. macularis superior
  a. medialis retinae
  a. nasalis retinae inferior
  a. nasalis retinae superior
  a. precapillaris
  arteriolae rectae renis
  arteriolae rectae spuriae
  arteriolae rectae verae
  a. temporalis retinae inferior
  a. temporalis retinae superior
  a. vaginatae
arteriolar
arteriole
  afferent glomerular a.
  central a.
  efferent glomerular a.
  ellipsoid a's
  glomerular a., afferent
  glomerular a., efferent
  Isaacs-Ludwig a.
  macular a., inferior
  macular a., superior
  medial a. of retina
  nasal a. of retina, inferior
  nasal a. of retina, superior
  postglomerular a.
  precapillary a.
  preglomerular a.
  renal a.
  sheathed a's
  straight a's of kidney, false
  straight a's of kidney, true

arteriole *(continued)*
  temporal a. of retina, inferior
  temporal a. of retina, superior
arteriolith
arteriolitis
arteriolonecrosis
arteriolosclerosis
arteriolosclerotic
arteriomotor
arterionecrosis
arteriopathy
  hypertensive a.
  idiopathic medial a.
  Takayasu a.
arterioplasty
arteriorenal
arteriorrhaphy
  lateral a.
arteriorrhexis
arteriosclerosis
  cerebral a.
  coronary a.
  diffuse a.
  hyaline a.
  hypertensive a.
  infantile a.
  intimal a.
  medial a.
  Mönckeberg a.
  nodose a.
  nodular a.
  a. obliterans
  peripheral a.
  presenile a.
  retinal a.
  senile a.
arteriosclerotic
arteriospasm
arteriospastic
arteriostenosis
arteriosteogenesis
arteriostosis
arteriosus
  patent ductus a.
  truncus a.
arteriotomy
arteriovenous
  a. fistula
  a. oxygen difference
  a. shunt
arteritis (arteritides)
  brachiocephalic a.
  coronary a.
  cranial a.
  a. deformans

arteritis (arteritides) *(continued)*
  giant cell a.
  granulomatous a.
  a. hyperplastica
  infantile a.
  localized visceral a.
  necrosing a.
  necrotizing a.
  a. nodosa
  a. obliterans
  rheumatic a.
  syphilitic a.
  Takayasu a.
  temporal a.
  tuberculous a.
  a. umbilicalis
  a. verrucosa
artery
  accompanying a. of median
    nerve
  accompanying a. of sciatic nerve
  accompanying a. of vein of
    Marshall
  acetabular a.
  acromial a.
  a. of Adamkiewicz
  adipose a's of kidney
  afferent a. of glomerulus
  alveolar a., inferior
  alveolar a's, superior, anterior
  alveolar a., superior, posterior
  anastomotic atrial a.
  angular a.
  a. of angular gyrus
  appendicular a.
  arch a.
  arcuate a. of foot
  arcuate a's of kidney
  ascending cervical a.
  atrial anastomotic a.
  atrioventricular nodal a.
  auditory a., internal
  auricular a., deep
  auricular a., left
  auricular a., posterior
  auricular a., right
  auricular a's, anterior
  axial a.
  axillary a.
  azygos a's of vagina
  basilar a.
  basilic a.
  brachial a., deep
  brachial a., superficial
  brachiocephalic a.

artery *(continued)*
- bronchial a's
- buccal a.
- buccinator a.
- a. of bulb of penis
- a. of bulb of vestibule
- bulbourethral a.
- calcareous a.
- calcarine a.
- callosomarginal a.
- capsular a., inferior
- capsular a., middle
- caroticotympanic a's
- carotid a., common
- carotid a., external
- carotid a., internal
- caudal a.
- caudal pancreatic a.
- a. of caudate lobe
- cecal a., anterior
- cecal a., posterior
- celiac a.
- central a's, anterolateral
- central a's, anteromedial
- central a's, posterolateral
- central a. of retina
- central a's of spleen
- a. of central sulcus
- cephalic a.
- cerebellar a., anterior inferior
- cerebellar a., posterior inferior
- cerebellar a., superior
- cerebral a., anterior
- cerebral a., middle
- cerebral a., posterior
- cervical a., ascending
- cervical a., deep
- cervical a., deep descending
- cervical a., superficial
- cervical a., transverse
- cervicovaginal a's
- a. of Charcot
- a. of Charpy
- choroid a., anterior
- choroidal a.
- ciliary a's, anterior
- ciliary a's, long
- ciliary a's, long posterior
- ciliary a's, short
- ciliary a's, short posterior
- cilioretinal a.
- circumflex a., anterior humeral
- circumflex a., deep iliac
- circumflex a. of the heart
- circumflex a., internal deep

artery *(continued)*
- circumflex a., lateral femoral
- circumflex a., medial femoral
- circumflex a., posterior humeral
- circumflex a. of scapula
- circumflex a., superficial iliac
- a. of clitoris, dorsal
- coccygeal a.
- cochlear a.
- Cohnheim a.
- coiled a's
- colic a., accessory superior
- colic a., inferior right
- colic a., left
- colic a., middle
- colic a., right
- collateral a., inferior ulnar
- collateral a., middle
- collateral a., radial
- collateral a., superior ulnar
- collateral digital a's
- a. to colliculi
- communicating a., anterior
- communicating a., posterior
- companion a. to sciatic nerve
- conal a.
- conducting a's
- conjunctival a's, anterior
- conjunctival a's, posterior
- conus a., left
- conus a., right
- conus a., third
- copper-wire a's
- corkscrew a's
- cornual a.
- coronary a., left
- coronary a., posterior descending
- coronary a., right
- coronary a., of stomach, left
- coronary a. of stomach, right
- a. to corpus cavernosum
- cortical a's
- costocervical a.
- cremasteric a.
- cricothyroid a.
- crural a.
- cystic a.
- deep a. of clitoris
- deep palmar a.
- deep a. of penis
- deferential a.
- dental a's, anterior
- dental a., inferior
- dental a., posterior

artery *(continued)*

a. of dentate nucleus
diaphragmatic a.
digital a's, collateral
digital a's, common palmar
digital a's, common plantar
digital a's, common volar
digital a's of foot, dorsal
digital a's of hand, dorsal
digital a's, proper palmar
digital a's, proper plantar
digital a's, proper volar
distributing a's
dorsal a. of clitoris
dorsal a. of foot
dorsal a. of nose
dorsal a. of penis
dorsal a. of tongue
dorsal carpal a.
dorsalis pedis a.
a. of Drummond
a. of ductus deferens
duodenal a's
efferent a. of glomerulus
elastic a's
emulgent a.
end a.
epicardial coronary a.
a. of epididymis
epigastric a., external
epigastric a., inferior
epigastric a., superficial
epigastric a., superior
episcleral a's
esophageal a.
ethmoidal a., anterior
ethmoidal a., posterior
facial a., deep
facial a., transverse
fallopian a.
femoral a., common
femoral a., deep
femoral a., superficial
fetal umbilical a's
fibular a.
fifth lumbar a.
a. of foot, dorsal
frontal a.
frontobasal a., lateral
frontobasal a., medial
funicular a.
gastric a., left
gastric a., left inferior
gastric a., posterior
gastric a., right

artery *(continued)*

gastric a., right inferior
gastric a's, short
gastroduodenal a.
gastroepiploic a., left
gastroepiploic a., right
gastro-omental a., left
gastro-omental a., right
genicular a., descending
genicular a., lateral inferior
genicular a., lateral superior
genicular a., medial inferior
genicular a., medial superior
genicular a., middle
glaserian a.
a. of glomerulus
gluteal a., inferior
gluteal a., superior
gonadal a's
helicine a.
hemorrhoidal a., inferior
hemorrhoidal a., middle
hemorrhoidal a., superior
hepatic a., common
hepatic a. proper
Heubner a.
humeral a.
hyaloid a.
a's of hybrid type
hyoid a.
hypogastric a.
hypophysial (hypophyseal) a.,
    inferior
hypophysial (hypophyseal) a.,
    superior
ileal a's
ileocolic a.
ileocolic a., ascending
iliac a., anterior
iliac a., common
iliac a., external
iliac a., internal
iliac a., small
ilioinguinal a.
iliolumbar a.
incisor a.
inferior profunda a.
infracostal a.
infraorbital a.
infrascapular a.
inguinal a's
innominate a.
insular a's
intercostal a's, anterior
intercostal a., first posterior

artery *(continued)*

- intercostal a., highest
- intercostal a's, posterior
- intercostal a., second posterior
- intercostal a., superior
- interlobar a's of kidney
- interlobular a's of kidney
- interlobular a's of liver
- intermediate atrial a., left
- intermediate atrial a., right
- intermetacarpal a's, palmar
- interosseous a., anterior
- interosseous a., common
- interosseous a., dorsal
- interosseous a., posterior
- interosseous a., recurrent
- interosseous a., volar
- intersegmental a's
- interventricular a., anterior
- interventricular septal a's, anterior
- interventricular septal a's, posterior
- intestinal a's
- intramural a.
- jejunal a's
- Kugel a.
- labial a., inferior
- labial a., superior
- labial a's of vulva, anterior
- labial a's of vulva, posterior
- a. of labyrinth
- labyrinthine a.
- lacrimal a.
- laryngeal a., inferior
- laryngeal a., superior
- left ventral paramedian a.
- lenticulostriate a.
- lingual a., deep
- long posterior ciliary a.
- lumbar a's, fifth
- lumbar a's, lowest
- malleolar a., lateral anterior
- malleolar a., lateral posterior
- malleolar a., medial anterior
- malleolar a., medial posterior
- mammary a., external
- mammary a., internal
- mandibular a.
- marginal a., left
- marginal a. of colon
- marginal a. of Drummond
- marginal a., right
- masseteric a.
- mastoid a.

artery *(continued)*

- maxillary a., external
- maxillary a., internal
- medial a. of foot, superficial
- medial calcaneal a.
- median a.
- mediastinal a's, anterior
- mediastinal a's, posterior
- medullary a.
- meningeal a., accessory
- meningeal a., anterior
- meningeal a., middle
- meningeal a., posterior
- mental a.
- mesencephalic a's
- mesenteric a., inferior
- mesenteric a., superior
- metacarpal a., deep volar
- metacarpal a's, dorsal
- metacarpal a's, palmar
- metacarpal a's, ulnar
- metatarsal a's, dorsal
- metatarsal a's, plantar
- a's of mixed type
- a's of Mueller
- muscular a's
- musculophrenic a.
- mylohyoid a.
- myomastoid a.
- nasal a., dorsal
- nasal a., external
- nasal a's, posterior lateral
- nasopalatine a.
- Neubauer a.
- nodal a.
- a. of nose, dorsal
- nutrient a's of femur
- nutrient a. of fibula
- nutrient a's of humerus
- nutrient a's of kidney
- nutrient a. of tibia
- obliterated hypogastric a.
- obturator a.
- obturator a., accessory
- obtuse marginal coronary a.
- occipital a., lateral
- occipital a., medial
- omphalomesenteric a.
- ophthalmic a.
- a. of optic chiasma
- ovarian a.
- palatine a., ascending
- palatine a., descending
- palatine a., greater
- palatine a's, lesser

artery *(continued)*
- palmar carpal a.
- palmar intermetacarpal a's
- palpebral a's, lateral
- palpebral a's, medial
- pancreatic a., dorsal
- pancreatic a., great
- pancreatic a., inferior
- pancreaticoduodenal a., anterior superior
- pancreaticoduodenal a., posterior superior
- pancreaticoduodenal a's, inferior
- paracentral a.
- paramedian a's
- parietal a., anterior
- parotid a.
- pelvic a., posterior
- a. of penis, dorsal
- perforating a's
- pericallosal a.
- pericardiac a's, posterior
- pericardiacophrenic a.
- perineal a.
- peripheral a.
- peroneal a., perforating
- pharyngeal a., ascending
- phrenic a., great
- phrenic a., inferior
- phrenic a., superior
- phrenicopericardial a.
- plantar a., deep
- plantar a., external
- plantar a., lateral
- plantar a., medial
- pontine a's
- popliteal a.
- a. of postcentral sulcus
- posterior conjunctival a.
- posterior intercostal a's
- posterior intercostal a's I-XI
- a. of precentral sulcus
- precuneal a's
- preventricular a.
- princeps pollicis a.
- principal a. of thumb
- profunda brachii a.
- profunda femoris a.
- pterygoid a's
- a. of pterygoid canal
- pubic a.
- pudendal a.
- pudendal a., deep external
- pudendal a., internal

artery *(continued)*
- pulmonary a., left
- pulmonary a., right
- a. of the pulp
- pyloric a.
- quadriceps a. of femur
- radial a., collateral
- radial a. of index finger
- radial a. of index finger, volar
- radialis indicis a.
- radiate a's of kidney
- radicular a's
- rectal a., inferior
- rectal a., middle
- rectal a., superior
- rectosigmoid a.
- recurrent a., anterior tibial
- recurrent a. of Heubner
- recurrent a., posterior tibial
- recurrent a., radial
- recurrent a., ulnar
- renal a.
- retinal a.
- retrocostal a.
- retroduodenal a's
- right dorsocaudal a.
- right ventral paramedian a.
- a. of round ligament of uterus
- sacral a's, lateral
- sacral a., median
- sacrococcygeal a.
- saphenous a.
- scapular a., descending
- scapular a., dorsal
- scapular a., transverse
- sciatic a.
- screw a's
- scrotal a's, anterior
- scrotal a's, posterior
- segmental a. of kidney, anterior inferior
- segmental a. of kidney, anterior superior
- segmental a. of kidney, inferior
- segmental a. of kidney, superior
- segmental a. of liver, anterior
- segmental a. of liver, lateral
- segmental a. of liver, medial
- segmental a. of liver, posterior
- septal a's, anterior
- sheathed a's
- short central a.
- short posterior ciliary a.
- sigmoid a's

artery *(continued)*
    silver-wire a's
    sinoatrial nodal a.
    sinuatrial nodal a.
    sinus node a.
    somatic a's
    spermatic a., external
    spermatic a., internal
    sphenopalatine a.
    spigelian a.
    spinal a., anterior
    spinal a., posterior
    spiral a's
    splenic a.
    sternal a's, posterior
    sternocleidomastoid a.
    sternocleidomastoid a., superior
    straight a's of kidney
    striate a's, lateral
    striate a's, medial
    stylomastoid a.
    subclavian a.
    subcostal a.
    sublingual a.
    submental a.
    subscapular a.
    sulcal a's
    superficial antebrachial a.
    superficial volar a.
    supraduodenal a.
    suprahyoid a.
    supraorbital a.
    suprarenal a., aortic
    suprarenal a., inferior
    suprarenal a., middle
    suprarenal a's, superior
    suprascapular a.
    supratrochlear a.
    sural a's
    sylvian a.
    tarsal a., lateral
    tarsal a's, medial
    temporal a., anterior
    temporal a., anterior deep
    temporal a's, deep
    temporal a., middle
    temporal a., posterior
    temporal a., posterior deep
    temporal a., superficial
    terminal a.
    testicular a.
    thalamogeniculate a.
    thalamoperforate a.
    thalamostriate a's, anterolateral

artery *(continued)*
    thalamostriate a's, anteromedial
    thoracic a., highest
    thoracic a., internal
    thoracic a., lateral
    thoracicoacromial a.
    thoracoacromial a.
    thoracodorsal a.
    thymic a's
    thyroid a. of Cruveilhier, inferior
    thyroid a., inferior
    thyroid a., lowest
    thyroid a., superior
    thyroidea ima a.
    tibial a., anterior
    tibial a., posterior
    tonsillar a.
    a's to orbital muscles
    transverse cervical a.
    transverse a. of face
    transverse a. of neck
    tubo-ovarian a.
    tympanic a., anterior
    tympanic a., inferior
    tympanic a., posterior
    tympanic a., superior
    ulnar a.
    ulnar collateral a., inferior
    ulnar collateral a., superior
    umbilical a.
    urethral a.
    uterine a.
    vaginal a.
    venous a's
    ventral splanchnic a's
    ventromedian a's
    vermiform a.
    vertebral a.
    vesical a., inferior
    vesical a's, superior
    vestibular a., anterior
    vidian a.
    vitelline a.
    volar a.
    volar interosseous a.
    a. of Zinn
    zygomatico-orbital a.
arthralgia
    acromegalic a.
    nonspecific a.
    periodic a.
    a. saturnina

arthralgic
arthrectomy
arthresthesia
arthritic
arthritide
arthritis (arthritides)
    acromegalic a.
    acute a.
    acute gouty a.
    acute rheumatic a.
    acute suppurative a.
    atypical mycobacterial a.
    bacterial a.
    Bekhterev (Bechterew) a.
    candidal a.
    chronic inflammatory a.
    chronic villous a.
    chylous a.
    climacteric a.
    colitic a.
    cricoarytenoid a.
    crystal-induced a.
    a. deformans
    degenerative a.
    dysenteric a.
    enteropathic reactive a.
    erosive a.
    exudative a.
    fungal a.
    a. fungosa
    gonococcal a.
    gonorrheal a.
    gouty a.
    gram-negative bacilli a.
    hemochromatotic a.
    hemophilic a.
    hemorrhagic a.
    a. hiemalis
    hypertrophic a.
    infectious a.
    inflammatory a.
    Jaccoud a.
    juvenile chronic a.
    juvenile rheumatoid a.
    Lyme a.
    Marie-Strümpell a.
    meningococcal a.
    menopausal a.
    monoarticular a.
    a. mutilans
    mycobacterial a.
    mycotic a.
    navicular a.
    neurogenic a.
    neuropathic a.

arthritis (arthritides) *(continued)*
    a. nodosa
    nonarticular a.
    nondeforming a.
    nongonococcal bacterial a.
    noninflammatory a.
    ochronotic a.
    palindromic a.
    periosteal a.
    postinfectious a.
    proliferative a.
    psoriatic a.
    purulent a.
    pyogenic a.
    reactive a.
    rheumatoid a.
    rubella a.
    sarcoid a.
    senescent a.
    septic a.
    suppurative a.
    syphilitic a.
    traumatic a.
    tuberculous a.
    urethral a.
    a. urethritica
    venereal a.
    vertebral a.
    villous a.
    viral a.
    vital a.
arthrocele
arthrocentesis
arthrochalasis multiplex
    congenita
arthrochondritis
arthroclasia
arthrodesis
    Charnley a.
    extra-articular a.
    Moberg a.
    triple a.
arthrodia
arthrodial
arthrodynia
arthrodysplasia
    hereditary a.
arthroempyesis
arthroereisis
arthrogenous
arthrogram
arthrography
    air a.
    double-contrast a.
    opaque a.

arthrogryposis
    congenital multiple a.
    a. multiplex congenita
arthrokatadysis
arthrolith
arthrolithiasis
arthrolysis
arthroncus
arthroneuralgia
arthro-onychodysplasia
arthro-ophthalmopathy
    hereditary progressive a.
arthropathia
    a. ovaripriva
    a. psoriatica
arthropathic
arthropathy
    Charcot a.
    chondrocalcific a.
    degenerative vertebral a.
    diabetic a.
    dislocating a.
    disuse a.
    gonococcal a.
    Heberden a.
    hemophilic a.
    inflammatory a.
    neurogenic a.
    neuropathic a.
    ochronotic a.
    osteopulmonary a.
    palindromic a.
    psoriatic a.
    pyrophosphate a.
    static a.
    stationary a.
    syphilitic a.
    tabetic a.
arthrophyma
arthrophyte
arthroplastic
arthroplasty
    Aufranc-Turner a.
    Austin Moore a.
    Bechtol a.
    cementless a.
    Charnley hip a.
    Charnley-Mueller a.
    Crawford-Adams cup a.
    interposition a.
    intracapsular
      temporomandibular joint a.
    Keller a.
    Lacey rotating-hinge a.
    Magnuson-Stack a.

arthroplasty *(continued)*
    McAtee-Tharias-Blazina a.
    McKee-Farrar hip a.
    New England Baptist a.
    Putti-Platt a.
    Schlein-type elbow a.
    Stanmore shoulder a.
    Thompson a.
    total hip a.
    total knee a.
arthropneumoradiography
arthropyosis
arthrosclerosis
arthroscope
arthroscopic
arthroscopy
arthrosis
    Charcot a.
    a. deformans
    temporomandibular a.
arthrostomy
arthrosynovitis
arthrotome
arthrotomy
    Magnuson-Stack shoulder a.
arthrotropic
arthroxesis
Arthus phenomenon
articular
articulare
articularis cubiti muscle
articulate
articulated
articulatio (articulationes)
    a. acromioclavicularis
    a. atlantoaxialis mediana
    a. atlantooccipitalis
    a. bicondylaris
    a. calcaneocuboidea
    a. capitis costae
    a. carpometacarpea pollicis
    articulationes costochondrales
    a. costotransversaria
    articulationes costovertebrales
    a. coxae
    a. cricoarytenoidea
    a. cricothyroidea
    a. cubiti
    a. cuneonavicularis
    a. ellipsoidea
    a. genu
    a. genus
    a. humeri
    a. humeroradialis
    a. humeroulnaris

articulatio (articulationes)
  (continued)
    a. incudomallearis
    a. incudostapedialis
    articulationes interchondrales
    a. lumbosacralis
    a. ossis pisiformis
    a. radiocarpea
    a. sacrococcygea
    a. sacroiliaca
    a. sternoclavicularis
    articulationes sternocostales
    a. subtalaris
    a. talocalcanea
    a. talocruralis
    a. tarsi transversa
    a. temporomandibularis
    a. tibiofibularis
    a. trochoidea
    articulationes vertebrales
    articulationes zygapophysiales
articulation
    acromioclavicular a.
    articulator a.
    atlantoaxial a., lateral
    atlantoaxial a., median
    atlantoepistrophic a.
    atlantooccipital a.
    atloid a.
    a. of auditory ossicles
    balanced a.
    ball-and-socket a.
    bicondylar a.
    brachiocarpal a.
    brachioradial a.
    brachioulnar a.
    calcaneoastragaloid a.
    calcaneocuboid a.
    capitular a.
    carpal a.
    carpometacarpal a., first
    carpometacarpal a. of thumb
    chondrosternal a.
    Chopart a.
    cochlear a.
    composite a.
    compound a.
    condylar a.
    confluent a.
    congruent a.
    costocentral a.
    costochondral a's
    costosternal a
    costotransverse a.
    costovertebral a.

articulation *(continued)*
    coxal a.
    coxofemoral a. of Buisson
    craniovertebral a.
    cricoarytenoid a.
    cricothyroid a.
    crurotalar a.
    cubital a.
    cubitoradial a., inferior
    cubitoradial a., superior
    cuneocuboid a.
    cuneonavicular a.
    dentoalveolar a.
    a. of elbow
    ellipsoidal a.
    false a.
    femoral a.
    fibrous a's
    a's of free inferior limb
    a's of free inferior member
    freely movable a.
    a's of girdle of inferior member
    gliding a.
    a. of head of humerus
    a. of head of rib
    hinge a.
    a. of hip
    humeroradial a.
    humeroulnar a.
    a. of humerus
    iliosacral a.
    immovable a.
    incongruent a.
    incudomalleolar a.
    incudostapedial a.
    intercarpal a's
    interchondral a's
    intercostal a's
    intercuneiform a's
    intermetacarpal a.
    intermetatarsal a.
    interphalangeal a.
    intertarsal a's
    a. of knee
    lumbosacral a.
    mandibular a.
    manubriosternal a.
    maxillary a.
    mediocarpal a.
    metacarpocarpal a's
    metacarpophalangeal a.
    metatarsophalangeal a.
    occipital a.
    occipitoatlantal a.
    ovoid a.

articulation *(continued)*
 patellofemoral a.
 petrooccipital a.
 phalangeal a.
 a. of pisiform bone
 pisocuneiform a.
 pivot a.
 plane a.
 a. of pubis
 radiocarpal a.
 radioulnar a., distal
 radioulnar a., inferior
 radioulnar a., proximal
 radioulnar a., superior
 reciprocal a.
 sacrococcygeal a.
 sacroiliac a.
 saddle a.
 scapuloclavicular a.
 sellar a.
 a. of shoulder
 simple a.
 slightly movable a.
 spheroidal a.
 sternochondral a's
 sternoclavicular a.
 sternocostal a's
 subtalar a.
 synovial a.
 synovial a's of cranium
 talocalcaneonavicular a.
 talocrural a.
 talonavicular a.
 tarsometatarsal a
 temporomandibular a.
 temporomaxillary a.
 tibiofibular a.
 a's of toes
 transverse tarsal a.
 trochoidal a.
 a. of tubercle of rib
 zygapophyseal a's
articulationes (plural of articulatio)
articulator
 adjustable a.
 anatomic a.
 dental a.
 plain-line a.
articulatory
articulo mortis
artifact
 aliasing a.
 mosaic a.
 pessary ring a.
artifactitious

artificial sweeteners
 (sugar substitutes)
  acesulfame potassium
  aspartame
  Equal
  neotame
  saccharin
  sorbitol
  Splenda
  stevia
  sucralose
  sugar alcohols
  Sweet and Low
  xylitol
Artificial Tears wetting drops
artiodactylous
arylamine
arylarsonic acid
arylesterase
arylformamidase
arylsulfatase
arylsulfatase B (ARSB) deficiency
arytenoepiglottic
arytenoid
arytenoidectomy
arytenoideus
arytenoiditis
arytenoidopexy
As.—astigmatism
AS—
  antistreptolysin
  aortic stenosis
  arteriosclerosis
A.S.—left ear (L. auris sinistra)
ASA—
  acetylsalicylic acid
  argininosuccinic acid
asacria
asafetida
ASAS—American Society of
 Abdominal Surgeons
ASAT—aspartate transaminase
asbestiform
asbestos
  amphibole a.
  blue a.
  chrysotile a.
  crocidolite a.
  white a.
asbestosis
Asboe-Hansen disease
A-scan
ascariasis
ascaricidal
ascaricide

ascarid
ascarides
Ascaris
    A. lumbricoides
    A. ovis
    A. suis
    A. suum
ascendens
ascending
    a. aorta
    a. pyelography
    a. urography
    a. venography
ascensus uteri
ascertain, ascertained
ascertainment
    complete a.
    incomplete a.
    multiple a.
    single a.
    truncate a.
Asch
    forceps
    operation
    splint
ASCH—American Society of
    Clinical Hypnosis
aschelminth
Ascher
    aqueous influx phenomenon
    blood-influx phenomenon
    negative glass rod
        phenomenon
    positive glass rod phenomenon
    syndrome
Ascherson
    membrane
    vesicles
Aschner
    phenomenon
    reflex
    sign
    test
Aschoff
    bodies
    cell
    node
    nodule
ascites
    a. adiposus
    bile a.
    bloody a.
    chyliform a.
    a. chylosus
    chylous a.

ascites *(continued)*
    dialysis a.
    exudative a.
    fatty a.
    gelatinous a.
    hemorrhagic a.
    hydremic a.
    milky a.
    nephrogenic a.
    a. praecox
    preagonal a.
    pseudochylous a.
    transudative a.
ascitic
ascitogenous
ASCLS— American Society for
    Clinical Laboratory Science
ASCO—
        American Society of Clinical
            Oncology
        American Society
            of Contemporary
            Ophthalmology
Ascoli
    reaction
    test
    treatment
ascorbate
ascorbemia
ascorbic acid
ascorburia
ascorbyl palmitate
ASCP—American Society of
    Clinical Pathologists
ASCUS—atypical squamous cells
    of uncertain significance
ASCVD—
        arteriosclerotic cardiovascular
            disease
        atherosclerotic cardiovascular
            disease
ASD—atrial septal defect
asecretory
Aselli
    glands
    pancreas
asemia
    a. graphica
    a. mimica
    a. verbalis
asepsis
aseptic-antiseptic
asepticism
asexual
asexuality

ASF—aniline, sulfur, formaldehyde
ASGE—American Society for
    Gastrointestinal Endoscopy
AsH—hyperopic astigmatism
ASH—American Society of
    Hematology
ASHA—American Speech and
    Hearing Association
Ash Split Cath
ASHD—
    arteriosclerotic heart disease
    atherosclerotic heart disease
Asherman syndrome
Asherson syndrome
Ashford
    mammaplasty
    mammilliplasty
    retracted nipple operation
Ashhurst splint
Ashley breast prosthesis
ASIA—American Spinal Injury
    Association
asialo
asiaticoside
asiderosis
as-if personality
ASIM—American Society of
    Internal Medicine
asiminine
ASIS—anterior superior iliac spine
Askanazy cell
Ask-Upmark
    kidney
    syndrome
ASL—antistreptolysin
as low as reasonably achievable
    (ALARA)
AsM—myopic astigmatism
ASO—
    antistreptolysin O (test, titer)
    arteriosclerosis obliterans
asomatognosia
aspalasoma
asparaginase
    C-a.
asparagine
asparaginyl
asparagus
aspartame
aspartate
    a. aminotransferase
    a. carbamoyl transferase
    a. kinase
    a. transaminase
    a. transcarbamylase

asparthione
aspartic acid
aspartylglycosaminidase
aspartylglycosaminuria
aspecific
aspect
    anterior a.
    dorsal a.
    facial a.
    frontal a.
    inferior a.
    lateral a.
    occipital a.
    sagittal a.
    superior a.
    temporal a.
    ventral a.
    vertical a.
aspergillar
aspergilli (plural of *Aspergillus*)
aspergillic acid
aspergillosis
    allergic bronchopulmonary a.
    aural a.
    bronchopneumonic a.
    pulmonary a.
Aspergillus
    A. amstelodami
    A. clavatus
    A. flavus
    A. fumigatus
    A. glaucus
    A. nidulans
    A. niger
    A. niveus
    A. ochraceus
    A. parasiticus
    A. repens
    A. restrictus
    A. terreus
    A. versicolor
aspermatism
aspermatogenesis
aspermia
aspheric
    a. lens
    a. lenticular spectacles
asphygmia
asphyxia
    autoerotic a.
    blue a.
    a. cyanotica
    fetal a.
    intrauterine a.
    a. livida

asphyxia *(continued)*
    local a.
    a. neonatorum
    a. pallida
    secondary a.
    sexual a.
    symmetric a.
    traumatic a.
    white a.
asphyxial
asphyxiant
asphyxiate, asphyxiated
asphyxiation
aspirate
aspirating
aspiration
    Cavitron a. unit
    endometrial a.
    meconium a.
    a. pneumonia
    vacuum a.
aspirator
    blue-tip a.
    Broyles a.
    Dieulafoy a.
    Gottschalk a.
    red-tip a.
    Thorek a.
    vacuum a.
    yellow-tip a.
aspirin
asplenia
    functional a.
asplenic
ASRT—American Society of
  Radiologic Technologists
ASS—
    anterior superior spine
    argininosuccinate synthetase
assault
    felonious a.
assaultive
assay
    biologic a., biological a.
    blastogenesis a.
    cancer antigen 125 (CA 125) a.
    CA15-3 RIA
      (radioimmunoassay)
    cell-mediated lympholysis a.
      (CML a.)
    CH50 a.
    competitive protein-binding a.
    complement a., hemolytic
    complement a., total
    complement a., whole

assay *(continued)*
    C-terminal a.
    D-dimer a.
    EAC rosette a.
    enzyme-linked immunosorbent
      a. (ELISA)
    E rosette a.
    erythropoietin a.
    estrogen receptor a. (ERA)
    factor III multimer a.
    fluorescent a.
    four-point a.
    glycosylated hemoglobin a.
    hemagglutination inhibition a.
      (HAI a.; HI a.)
    hemoglobin A_{1c} a. (A1C)
    hemolytic plaque a.
    HI a.
    immune a.
    immune adherence
      hemagglutination a. (IAHA)
    immunofluorescence a. (IFA)
    immunoradiometric a. (IRMA)
    Jerne plaque a.
    leukotactic a.
    Limulus a.
    lymphocyte proliferation a.
    microbiological a.
    microcytotoxicity a.
    microhemagglutination–
      Treponema pallidum
      (MHA-TP) a.
    mixed lymphocyte culture a.
    MLC a.
    plaque-forming cell a.
    polyethylene glycol
      precipitation a.
    radioimmunoprecipitation a.
      (RIPA)
    radioligand a.
    radiometric a.
    radioreceptor a.
    Raji cell a.
    staphylococcal protein A
      binding a.
    stem cell a.
    thyroxine radioisotope a.
    Treponema pallidum
      hemagglutination (TPHA) a.
assessment
    Ballard gestational a.
    Dubowitz Neurological A.
    psychological a.
Assézat triangle
assident

assimilable
assimilation
    genetic a.
assistant
    physician's a. (PA)
Assmann
    focus
    infiltrate
    tuberculous
      infiltrate
association
    clang a.
    controlled a. test
    dream a's
    free a.
    individual practice a.
assortment
assumption
    a. of care
    a. of risk
Ast.—astigmatism
AST—aspartate transaminase
astasia
    a.-abasia
    atonia-a.
astatic
astatine (At)
astaxanthin
asteatosis
astereognosis
asterion
asterixis
asternal
asternia
asteroid hyalosis
Asth.—asthenopia
asthenia
    muscle a.
    myalgic a.
    neurocirculatory a.
    neurotic a.
    periodic a.
    tropical
      anhidrotic a.
asthenic
asthenocoria
asthenope
asthenopia
    accommodative a.
    hysterical a.
    muscular a.
    nervous a.
    retinal a.
    tarsal a.
asthenopic

asthma
    abdominal a.
    allergic a.
    alveolar a.
    atopic a.
    bacterial a.
    bronchial a.
    bronchitic a.
    cardiac a.
    cat a.
    catarrhal a.
    Cheyne-Stokes a.
    a. convulsivum
    cotton dust a.
    cutaneous a.
    diisocyanate a.
    dust a.
    Elsner a.
    emphysematous a.
    essential a.
    extrinsic a.
    food a.
    grinders' a.
    Heberden a.
    horse a.
    humid a.
    infective a.
    intrinsic a.
    isocyanate a.
    Kopp a.
    miller's a.
    miners' a.
    nasal a.
    nervous a.
    occupational a.
    platinum a.
    pollen a.
    potters' a.
    reflex a.
    Rostan a.
    spasmodic a.
    stone a.
    strippers' a.
    symptomatic a.
    thymic a.
    true a.
    Wichmann a.
asthmatic
asthmatiform
asthmogenic
astigmagraph
astigmatic
    a. axis
    a. clock
    a. dial

astigmatism
    acquired a.
    a. against the rule
    compound a.
    congenital a.
    corneal a.
    direct a.
    hypermetropic a., compound
    hyperopic a., compound
    hyperopic a., simple
    inverse a.
    irregular a.
    lenticular a.
    mixed a.
    myopic a., compound
    myopic a., simple
    oblique a.
    physiological a.
    regular a.
    retinal a.
    a. with the rule
    simple a.
astigmatometry
astigmatoscopy
Astler-Coller
    modification of Dukes
      classification
    staging system
astomia
astomus
Aston rule
Astra-8
astragalar
astragalectomy
astragalocalcanean
astragalocrural
astragaloscaphoid
astragalotibial
astragalus
astral
astraphobia
astriction
astringent
astroblast
astroblastoma
astrocyte
    atypical a.
    fibrillary a's
    fibrous a's
    gemistocytic a.
    plasmatofibrous a's
    protoplasmic a's
astrocytoma
    anaplastic a.
    cerebellar a.

astrocytoma *(continued)*
    diffuse cerebellar a.
    a. diffusum
    a. fibrillare
    fibrillary a.
    gemistocytic a.
    grades I through IV a's
    juvenile pilocytic a.
    malignant a.
    pilocytic a.
    piloid a.
    a. protoplasmaticum
    protoplasmic a.
    subependymal giant cell a.
astrocytosis
astroglia
astrophobia
astrophorous
Astrup method
asulfurosis
asyllabia
asylum
asymbolia
    pain a.
    tactile a.
asymmetric, asymmetrical
asymmetry
    chromatic a.
    encephalic a.
asymphytous
asymptomatic
asynapsis
asynchronism
asynchronous
asynchrony
asynclitism
    anterior a.
    posterior a.
asyndesis
asynechia
asynergia
asynergia major
asynergic
asynergy
    appendicular a.
    axial a.
    axioappendicular a.
    progressive cerebellar a.
    progressive locomotor a.
    truncal a.
    verbal a.
asynovia
asyntaxia dorsalis
asystemic
asystole

asystolic
AT—atrial tachycardia
atactic
atactiform
atactilia
ataractic
ataraxia
atavism
atavistic
ataxia
  acute cerebellar a.
  acute tabetic a.
  adult onset a.
  alcoholic a.
  appendicular a.
  a.-telangiectasia
  autonomic a.
  Briquet a.
  Broca a.
  Bruns frontal a.
  bulbar a.
  central a.
  cerebellar a.
  cerebellofugal degeneration a.
  cerebral a.
  cervical a.
  dentate cerebellar a.
  diphtheric a.
  dynamic a.
  enzootic a.
  equilibratory a.
  family a.
  Fergusson and Critchley a.
  Friedreich a.
  frontal a.
  hereditary a.
  hereditary cerebellar a.
  Holmes a.
  hysterical a.
  intermittent a.
  intrapsychic a.
  kinetic a.
  labyrinthic a.
  Leyden a.
  limb kinetic a.
  locomotor a.
  Marie a.
  motor a.
  nonequilibratory a.
  nutritional spinal a.
  ocular a.
  optic a.
  periodic a.
  polyneuritic spinocerebellar a.
  postural a.

ataxia *(continued)*
  professional a.
  progressive a.
  proprioceptive a.
  pseudotabetic a.
  psychomotor a.
  Sanger Brown a.
  sensory a.
  spastic a.
  spinal a.
  spinocerebellar a.
  static a.
  a.-telangiectasia
  thermal a.
  truncal a.
  vasomotor a.
  vestibular a.
ataxiagram
ataxiaphasia
ataxia-telangiectasia syndrome
ataxophobia
ATC—addictions treatment center
ATCC—American Type Culture
  Collection
ATD—asphyxiating thoracic
  dystrophy
atelectasis
  absorption a.
  acquired a.
  compression a.
  congenital a.
  congestion a.
  discoid a.
  initial a.
  lobar a.
  lobular a.
  a. of middle ear
  obstructive a.
  patchy a.
  platelike a.
  postnatal asphyxia a.
  primary a.
  relaxation a.
  resorption a.
  rounded a.
  secondary a.
  segmental a.
atelectatic
atelencephalia
atelencephaly
atelia
ateliosis
ateliotic
atelocardia
atelocephalous

atelocephaly
atelocheilia
atelocheiria
ateloencephaly, atelencephalia
ateloglossia
atelognathia
atelomyelia
atelopodia
ateloprosopia
atelorachidia
atelostomia
ATG—antithymocyte globulin
athelia
atherectomy
athermosystaltic
atheroembolism
atheroembolus
atherogenesis
atherogenic
atheroma
    cerebral a.
    a. cutis
atheromatosis
atheromatous
atherosclerosis
    coronary a.
    a. obliterans
atherosclerotic
atherothrombosis
athetoid
athetosis
    bilateral a.
    congenital a.
    double a.
    double congenital a.
    posthemiplegic a.
    pupillary a.
    unilateral a.
athetotic
athiaminosis
athlete
athrepsia
athreptic
athymia
athymism
athyria
athyroidemia
Atkins-Cannard tracheotomy tube
Atkinson technique
Atkinson-type lid block
Atkins-Tucker laryngoscope
ATL—
    adult T-cell leukemia/lymphoma
    antitension line
atlantad

atlantal
atlantoaxial
atlantobasilaris internus
atlantoid
atlantomastoid
atlanto-occipital
atlanto-odontoid
atlas
Atlee
    clamp
    dilator
atloaxoid
atm—atmosphere(s)
atmolysis
atmospheric
ATN—
    acute tubular necrosis
    tyrosinase-negative (ty-neg)
        oculocutaneous albinism
atocia
atolide
atom
atomic
    a. number
    a. weight (at. wt.)
atomization
atomizer
    DeVilbiss a.
atonia
    a.-astasia
    choreatic a.
atonic
atonicity
atony
    chronic intestinal a.
    muscle a.
    primary ureteral a.
    uterine a.
atopen
atopic
atopognosia
atopy
atoxic
atoxigenic
ATP—adenosine triphosphate
ATPase—adenosine triphosphatase
Atraloc suture
atransferrinemia
atraumatic suture
atresia
    acquired a. of external
        auditory meatus
    anal a.
    a. ani
    aortic a.

atresia *(continued)*
    aural a.
    biliary a.
    choanal a.
    congenital a.
    duodenal a.
    esophageal a.
    a. of external auditory canal
    follicular a.
    a. folliculi
    ileal a.
    intestinal a.
    a. iridis
    meatal a.
    mitral a.
    prepyloric a.
    pulmonary a.
    pyloric a.
    tricuspid a.
    vaginal a.
atretic
atretoblepharia
atretocephalus
atretocormus
atretogastria
atretopsia
atretorrhinia
atretostomia
atria (plural of atrium)
atrial
    balloon a. septostomy
    a. contraction
    a. enlargement
    a. fibrillation
    a. flutter
    a. infarction
    a. kick
    a. myocardial cell
    a. natriuretic peptide
    a. pacing
    percutaneous transluminal a.
      valvuloplasty (PTAV)
    a. premature contraction
      (APC)
    a. rhythm
    a. septal defect (ASD)
    a. septostomy
    a. septum
    a. standstill
    a. tachycardia
atrialized
atrichia
atrichosis
atrichous
Atricor pacemaker

atriocommissuropexy
atrio-His
    pathway
    tract
atriomegaly
atriopeptin
atrioseptopexy
atrioseptoplasty
atriotomy
atrioventricular
    a. block (AVB)
    a. bundle
    a. canal defect
    a. conduction
    a. dissociation
    a. flow rambling murmurs
    a. junction
    a. junctional escape beat
    a. junctional rhythm
    a. nodal reentrant tachycardia
    a. nodal reentry
    a. node artery
    a. septal defect
    a. valve
atrioventricularis communis
atrium (atria)
    a. alveolare
    common a.
    a. cordis dextrum
    a. cordis sinistrum
    a. glottidis
    a. of glottis
    a. of heart
    a. of infection
    a. laryngis
    a. of larynx
    left a. of heart
    a. meatus medii
    a. pulmonale
    pulmonary a.
    right a. of heart
    single a.
    a. sinistrum
    a. vaginae
atrophia
    a. bulborum hereditaria
    a. cerebri senilis simplex
    a. choroideae et retinae
    a. cutis senilis
    a. dolorosa
    a. gyrata of choroid
    a. maculosa
    a. musculorum lipomatosa
    a. senilis
    a. striata et maculosa

atrophia *(continued)*
    a. testiculi
    a. unguinum
atrophic striae
atrophie
    a. blanche
    a. noire
atrophied
atrophoderma
    a. biotripticum
    follicular a.
    idiopathic a. of Pasini and
      Pierini
    macular a.
    a. maculatum
    neuritic a.
    a. neuriticum
    a. of Pasini and Pierini
    a. reticulatum symmetricum
      faciei
    senile a.
    a. striatum et maculatum
    a. vermicularis
    vermiculate a. of cheeks
atrophodermatosis
atrophodermia vermiculata
atrophy
    acute yellow a.
    alcoholic cerebral a.
    alveolar a.
    Aran-Duchenne muscular a.
    arthritic a.
    Behr a.
    black a.
    blue a.
    bone a.
    brown a.
    cardiac a.
    cerebellar a.
    Charcot-Marie a.
    Charcot-Marie-Tooth a.
    circumpapillary chorioretinal a.
    circumscribed a. of brain
    circumscribed cerebral a.
    compensatory a.
    compression a.
    concentric a.
    convolutional a.
    correlated a.
    corticostriatospinal a.
    Cruveilhier a.
    cutaneous a.
    cyanotic a.
    degenerative a.
    Dejerine-Sottas a.

atrophy *(continued)*
    Dejerine-Thomas a.
    denervated muscle a.
    a. of disuse
    Duchenne-Aran muscular a.
    eccentric a.
    Eichhorst a.
    endocrine a.
    endometrial a.
    Erb a.
    essential a. of iris
    exhaustion a.
    facial a.
    facioscapulohumeral a.
    familial spinal muscular a.
    fat replacement a.
    fatty a.
    Fazio-Londe a.
    Fuchs a.
    gastric a.
    gastric mucosal a.
    gauntlet a.
    gingival a.
    granular a. of kidney
    gray a.
    healed yellow a.
    hemifacial a.
    hemilingual a.
    Hoffmann a.
    Hunt a.
    hypoglossal a.
    idiopathic muscular a.
    inactivity a.
    infantile a.
    inflammatory a.
    interstitial a.
    ischemic muscular a.
    Jadassohn muscular a.
    lactation a.
    lamellar cerebellar a.
    Landouzy-Dejerine a.
    leaping a.
    linear a.
    lobar a.
    macular a.
    multisystem a.
    muscular a.
    myelopathic muscular a.
    myopathic a.
    myotonic a.
    neural a.
    neuritic muscular a.
    neurogenic a.
    neuropathic a.
    neurotic a.

atrophy *(continued)*
 neurotrophic a.
 numeric a.
 olivopontocerebellar a.
 optic a.
 pallidal a.
 paraneoplastic cerebellar a.
 Parrot a. of the newborn
 pathologic a.
 periodontal a.
 peroneal a.
 physiologic a.
 Pick convolutional a.
 pigmentary a.
 postmenopausal a.
 posttraumatic a. of bone
 pressure a.
 primary optic a.
 progressive choroidal a.
 progressive diffuse
  cerebrocortical a.
 progressive muscular a.
 progressive neural muscular a.
 progressive neuromuscular a.
 progressive neuropathic
  muscular a.
 progressive nuclear muscle a.
 progressive spinal muscular a.
 progressive unilateral facial a.
 pseudohypertrophic muscular a.
 pseudomyopathic spinal
  muscular a.
 pulp a.
 red a.
 renal a.
 reversionary a.
 rheumatic a.
 scapuloperoneal muscular a.
 Schnabel a.
 Schweninger-Buzzi macular a.
 secondary optic a.
 segmental sensory dissociation
  with brachial muscular a.
 senile a.
 senile a. of lung
 senile a. of skin
 serous a.
 simple a.
 spinal muscular a.
 spinoneural a.
 spinopontine a.
 striate a. of skin
 subacute a. of liver
 subchronic a. of liver
 Sudeck a.

atrophy *(continued)*
 syphilitic spinal muscular a.
 testicular a.
 Tooth a.
 toxic a.
 traction a.
 traumatic a.
 trophoneurotic a.
 tubular a.
 unilateral facial a.
 vascular a.
 von Leber a.
 Vulpian a.
 Werdnig-Hoffmann a.
 Werdnig-Hoffmann spinal
  muscular a.
 white a.
 yellow a.
 Zimmerlin a.
atropinic
atropinism
atropinization
ATS—
 antitetanic serum
 anxiety tension state
attachment
 bar a.
 edgewise a.
 extracoronal a.
 Gottlieb epithelial a.
 internal a.
 intracoronal a.
 key-and-keyway a.
 muscle-tendon a.
 orthodontic a.
 parallel a.
 precision a.
 semiprecision a.
 slotted a.
attack
 adversive a.
 anxiety a.
 apnea a.
 apoplectiform a.
 cataplectic a.
 centrencephalic a.
 cerebellar a.
 cyclical epileptic a.
 decerebrate a.
 drop a's
 epileptic a.
 epileptiform a.
 focal a.
 heart a.
 myoclonic a.

attack *(continued)*
    panic a.
    posterior a.
    Stokes-Adams a.
    tonic cerebellar a.
    transient carotid ischemic a.
    transient ischemic a. (TIA)
    uncinate a.
    vagal a.
    vasovagal a.
attar of roses
attention
    a. deficit disorder (ADD)
    a. deficit disorder with
      hyperactivity (ADDH)
    a. deficit hyperactivity
      disorder (ADHD)
attenuant
attenuate
attenuation coefficient
attenuator
attic
    a. disease
    tympanic a.
atticitis
atticoantral
atticoantrotomy
atticomastoid
atticotomy
    transmeatal a.
attitude
    abstract a.
    a. of combat
    Devergie a.
    discobolus a.
    fetal a.
    forced a.
    pugilistic a.
attractant
attraction
    a. of affinity
    capillary a.
    chemical a.
    electric a.
    magnetic a.
attribute
attrition
Atwater-Benedict
    calorimeter
    chamber
at. wt.—atomic weight
atypia
atypical
    a. monochromacy
    a. monochromat

Au—Australia antigen
AUA—American Urological
   Association
Aub-Dubois
    standards
    table
Auberger blood group
Aubert phenomenon
Auchincloss
    modified radical mastectomy
    operation
audile
audioanalgesia
audiogenic
audiogram
    cortical a.
    pure tone a.
    self-recording a.
    serial a.
    speech a.
audiologist
audiology
audiometer
    evoked potential a.
    evoked response a.
    Langenbeck (von Langenbeck)
     noise a.
    pure tone a.
    semiautomatic pure tone a.
audiometric
audiometrician
audiometry
    air-conduction a.
    Békésy a.
    bone-conduction a.
    brain stem evoked response
     (BSER) a.
    cortical a.
    electrocochleographic a.
    electrodermal a.
    impedance a.
    industrial a.
    localization a.
    psychogalvanic
     skin-response a.
    pure tone a.
    speech a.
audioscope
audiovisual
audition
    chromatic a.
    a. colorée
    gustatory a.
    thought a.
auditive

auditognosis
auditory
    a. canal
    a. hallucinations
    a. meatus
    a. nerve
    a. nuclei
    a. tube
Auenbrugger sign
Auer
    bodies
    rods
Auerbach
    ganglion (ganglia)
    node
    plexus
Aufranc-Turner
    arthroplasty
    cup
    hip prosthesis
    operation
Aufrecht
    disease
    sign
Aufricht
    elevator
    rasp
    retractor
    speculum
Aufricht-Lipsett rasp
AUG—acute ulcerative gingivitis
Auger
    effect
    electron
augmentation
    a. mammaplasty
    a. rhinoplasty
augmentor
Augustine nail
AUL—acute undifferentiated
   leukemia
aura
    a. asthmatica
    autonomic a.
    dysmnesic a.
    electric a.
    generalized somatic a.
    a. hysterica
    illusional a.
    kinesthetic a.
    myoclonic a.
    neuralgic a.
    paramnesic a.
    a. procursiva
    reminiscent a.

aura *(continued)*
    sensory a.
    somatosensory a.
    a. vertiginosa
    vertiginous a.
    visceral a.
    visual a.
aural speculum
aurantia
aureolin
aures (plural of auris)
auric
auricle
    accessory a.
    cervical a.
auricula (auriculae)
auricular
auriculare
auricularis
auriculocranial
auriculotemporal
auriculotherapy
aurid
auriform
aurin
aurinarium
aurinasal
auripigment
auris (aures)
    a. dextra (AD) (L. right ear)
    a. externa
    a. interna
    a. media
    a. sinistra (AS) (L. left ear)
    a. utraque (AU) (L. each ear)
aurochromoderma
ausc.—auscultation
auscultate
auscultation
    direct a.
    immediate a.
    Korányi a.
    mediate a.
    obstetric a.
auscultatory
auscultoplectrum
auscultoscope
Austin
    knife
    retractor
Austin Flint
    cavernous respiration
    murmur
    phenomenon
    respiration

Austin Moore
    arthroplasty
    femoral head remover
    hip prosthesis
    inside-outside calipers
    mortising chisel
    prosthesis
    rasp
    straight-stem endoprosthesis
Australia antigen (Au)
Australian X disease virus
autemesia
autism
    akinetic a.
    early infantile a.
    infantile a.
autistic
autoagglutination
autoagglutinin
autoallergic
autoamputation
autoanalysis
autoantibody
    antiplatelet a.
    Donath-Landsteiner cold a.
    incomplete a.
    warm a.
autoanticomplement
autoantigen
autoantisepsis
autoantitoxin
autobiotic
autobody
autocatalysis
autocatalyst
autocatalytic
autocatharsis
autocholecystectomy
autochthonous
autoclasis
autoclave
Autoclip
autocorrelation function
autocrine
autocytotoxin
autodermic
autodestruction
autodigestion
autodrainage
autoecholalia
autoeczematization
autoepilation
autoerotic
autoeroticism
autoerythrophagocytosis

autofundoscope
autofundoscopy
autogenous
autograft
autografting
autogram
autohemagglutination
autohemagglutinin
autohemolysin
autohemolysis
autohemolytic
autohemotherapy
autohypnosis
autohypnotic
autoimmune
autoimmune disease (AID)
autoimmunity
autoimmunization
autoinfection
autoinflation
autoinfusion
autoinoculable
autoinoculation
autoisolysin
autokeratoplasty
autokinesis
    visible light a.
autokinetic visible light
   phenomenon
autolavage
autolesion
autoleukoagglutinin
autologous
    a. clot
    a. fat graft
    a. transfusion
autolysate
autolysin
autolysis
    postmortem a.
autolysosome
autolytic
autolyze
automatic
Automatic Clinical Analyzer
automatic implantable
   cardioverter-defibrillator (AICD)
automatism
    alcohol a.
    ambulatory a.
    command a.
    epileptic a.
    postepileptic a.
    postictal a.
    vigil ambulatory a.

automatograph
automaton
Automeris io
automysophobia
autonephrectomy
autonephrotoxin
autonomic
autonomotropic
autonomous
autonomy
auto-oxidation
autopathography
autophagia
autophagy
autopharmacologic
autopharmacology
autophobia
autophonometry
autophony
autoplast
autoplastic
autoplasty
Auto-Plot
autopolymer
autopolymerization
autoprothrombin IIa
autopsy
    forensic a.
    medicolegal a.
    psychological a.
autopsychic
autoradiography
    contact a.
    dip-coating a.
    film-stripping a.
    thick-layer a.
    two-emulsion a.
autoregulation
    heterometric autoradiography
    homeometric autoradiography
autoreinfection
autoreinfusion
autosensitization
    erythrocyte a.
autosensitized
autosepticemia
autoserum
autosite
autositic
autosmia
autosomal
    a. dominant
    a. recessive
autosomatognosis
autosome

autospermotoxin
autosplenectomy
autospray
autostimulation
autosuggestibility
autosuggestion
autosynthesis
autotherapy
autothromboagglutinin
autotomography
autotopagnosia
autotransfusion
    intraoperative a.
    postoperative a.
autotransplantation
    pancreatic a.
autotrepanation
autotuberculin
autotuberculinization
autovaccination
autovaccine
autovaccinia
Auvard
    cranioclast
    weighted vaginal
    speculum
Auvard-Remine speculum
Auvray incision
auxanography
auxesis
auxetic
auxiliary
    torquing a.
auxiliomotor
auxilytic
auxocyte
auxodrome
auxogluc
auxometric
auxometry
auxotonic
auxotype
AV—aortic valve
AV, A-V (arteriovenous)
    AV anastomosis
    AV fistula
AV, A-V (atrioventricular)
    AV bundle
    AV conduction delay
    AV dissociation
    AV heart block
    AV refractory period
availability
    biologic a.
    physiologic a.

avalanche
  Townsend a.
avalvular
avascular
avascularization
Avellis
  hemiplegia
  paralysis
  syndrome
Avellis-Longhi syndrome
avenin
avenolith
average
  a. life
  moving a.
  spatial a. temporal a.
    (SATA)
  spatial peak temporal a.
    (SPTA)
  time-weighted a.
averaging
  signal a.
  spike-triggered a.
aversive
avian
avidity
Avila operation
avirulence
avirulent
avitaminosis
avitaminotic
Avitene microfibrillar collagen
  hemostat
AVM—
  Adriamycin, vincristine,
    methotrexate
  arteriovenous malformation
AVN—atrioventricular node
avoidance
  a. behavior
  phobic a.
avoidant
avoirdupois
AVP—arginine vasopressin
AVR—aortic valve
  replacement
avulsion
  nerve a.
  phrenic a.
  scalp a.
  tooth a.
A&W—alive and well
awakening
  delayed a.
AWI—anterior wall infarction

awl
  Carroll a.
  curved a.
  Rochester a.
  Wangensteen a.
  Wilson a.
awu, AWU—atomic weight unit
Axenfeld
  anomaly
  loop
  suture
  syndrome
Axenfeld-Krukenberg spindle
axenic
Axer operation
axes (plural of axis)
axial
  a. hyperopia
  a. length
  a. myopia
  a. transverse tomography
axifugal
axilla (axillae)
axillary arteriography
axillobifemoral
axillofemoral
axillopopliteal
axiobuccal
axiobuccocervical
axiobuccogingival
axiobuccolingual
axiocervical
axiodistal
axiodistocervical
axiodistogingival
axiodistoincisal
axiodisto-occlusal
axiogingival
axioincisal
axiolabial
axiolabiogingival
axiolabiolingual
axiolingual
axiolinguocervical
axiolinguogingival
axiolinguo-occlusal
axiomesial
axiomesiocervical
axiomesiodistal
axiomesiogingival
axiomesioincisal
axiomesio-occlusal
axio-occlusal
axiopulpal
axipetal

axis (axes)
    anteroposterior (AP) a.
    basibregmatic a.
    basicranial a.
    basifacial a.
    binauricular a.
    celiac a.
    cephalocaudal a.
    condylar a.
    costocervical
        arterial a.
    craniocaudal a.
    craniofacial a.
    a. cylinder
    dorsoventral a.
    Downs Y a.
    electrical a. of heart
    external a. of eye
    a. externus bulbi oculi
    facial a.
    a. of Fick
    frontal a.
    group Ia a.
    a. of heart
    hinge a.
    horizontal a.
    HPA a.
    hypothalamic-pituitary-
        adrenal a.
    internal a. of eye
    a. internus bulbi oculi
    a. of lens
    a. lentis
    long a. of body
    longitudinal a.
    mandibular a.
    normal a.
    opening a.
    optic a., optical a.
    a. opticus
    a. pelvis
    pituitary-adrenocortical a.
    pituitary-gonadal a.
    pituitary-thyroid a.
    a. of preparation
    principal a.
    pupillary a.
    renal a.
    renin-aldosterone a.
    renin-angiotensin a.
    right a.
    sagittal a. of eye
    secondary a.
    T a.
    thoracic a.

axis (axes) *(continued)*
    thyroid a.
    uterine a.
    vertical a.
    visual a.
    X a.
    Y a.
axoaxonic
axodendritic
axoid
axolemma
axolotl
axolysis
axometer
axon
    giant a.
    group Ia a.
    naked a.
    unmyelinated a.
axonal
axonopathy
axonotmesis
axophage
axosomatic
Ayala
    equation
    index
    quotient
Ayerst knife
Ayer test
Ayer-Tobey test
Ayerza
    disease
    syndrome
Ayre
    brush
    cervical spatula
    cone knife
    tube
azalide
azide
azobenzene
azobilirubin
azocarmine
azoic
azole
azolitmin
azoospermatism
azoospermia
azopigment
azoprotein
Azorean disease
azotemia
    extrarenal a.
    postrenal a.

azotemia *(continued)*
    prerenal a.
    renal a.
azotemic osteodystrophy
azotometer
azotorrhea
azoturia
azoturic
azoxybenzene
azure
    a. A
    a. B
    a. C

azure *(continued)*
    a. I
    a. II
    methylene a.
azuresin
azurin
azurophil
azurophilia
azurophilic
azygogram
azygography
azygos vein
azygous

B

β—beta (Greek letter)
b—
    base
    born
B—
    bacillus
    boron
B—magnetic flux density
Ba—barium
BA, B.A.—Bachelor of Arts
Baastrup
    disease
    syndrome
Babbitt metal
Babcock
    clamp
    forceps
    needle
    operation
    suture
Baber syndrome
Babès
    nodes
    nodules
    treatment
    tubercles
Babès-Ernst
    bodies
    corpuscles
    granules
Babesia
    B. argentina
    B. bigemina

Babesia (continued)
    B. caballi
    B. canis
    B. cati
    B. divergens
    B. equi
    B. felis
    B. gibsoni
    B. major
    B. microti
    B. motasi
    B. ovis
    B. perroncitoi
    B. trautmanni
    B. vogeli
babesiasis
babesiosis
Babinski
    law
    phenomenon
    reflex
    sign
    syndrome
Babinski-Fröhlich (Babinski-
    Froehlich) syndrome
Babinski-Nageotte syndrome
Babinski-Vaquez syndrome
baby
    blue b.
    collodion b.
    test-tube b.
BABYbird respirator
baccate

B

Baccelli
mixture
sign
bacciform
Bachmann bundle
bacillary
bacille Calmette-Guérin (BCG)
vaccine
bacillemia
bacilli
bacilliferous
bacilliform
bacillin
bacillosis
bacilluria
Bacillus
B. anthracis
B. cereus
B. megaterium
B. stearothermophilus
B. subtilis
B. tularense
bacillus (bacilli)
acid-fast b. (AFB)
Bang b.
Battey b.
Boas-Oppler b.
Bordet-Gengou b.
Calmette-Guérin
(Calmette-Guerin) b.
coliform bacilli
DF-2 b.
diphtheria b.
Döderlein (Doderlein) b.
Ducrey b.
dysentery bacilli
enteric b.
Escherich b.
Flexner b.
Friedländer b.
fusiform b.
Gartner b.
Ghon-Sachs b.
Hansen b.
Hofmann b.
influenza b.
Klebs-Löffler (Klebs-Loeffler) b.
Koch b.
Koch-Weeks b.
lepra b.
Morax-Axenfeld b.
Morgan b.
Newcastle-Manchester b.
paracolon b.
plague b.

bacillus (bacilli) *(continued)*
Preisz-Nocard b.
rhinoscleroma b.
Schmitz b.
Schmorl b.
Shiga b.
smegma b.
Sonne-Duval b.
Stanley b.
Strong b.
swine rotlauf b.
tubercle b.
typhoid b.
Vincent b.
Weeks b.
Welch b.
Whitmore b.
back
flat b.
functional b.
hollow b.
hump b.
hunch b.
old man's b.
poker b.
saddle b.
static b.
sway b.
(swayback)
backalgia
back-and-forth suture
backbleeding
backbone
back-calculation
backcross
double b.
backcut incision
backfiltration
backflow
pyelolymphatic b.
pyelorenal b.
pyelosinus b.
pyelotubular b.
pyelovenous b.
background
b. activity
b. count
b. erase
b. radiation
Backhaus
forceps
towel clamp
backing
backknee
backlighting

back-raking
backscatter
    b. factor
    b. peak
Bacon
    anoscope
    forceps
Bact.—*Bacterium*
bacterascites
    monomicrobial non-
      neutrocytic b.
    polymicrobial b.
bacteremia
    puerperal b.
bacteremic
bacteria (plural of bacterium)
bacterial
    b. endocarditis
    b. myocarditis
    b. pericarditis
bactericidal
bactericide
    specific b.
bactericidin
bacterid
    pustular b.
bacteriform
bacterin
bacterin-toxoid
bacteriochlorophyll
bacteriocin
bacteriocinogen
bacteriocinogenic
bacteriofluorescin
bacteriogenic
bacterioid
bacteriologic, bacteriological
bacteriologist
bacteriology
    clinical diagnostic b.
    medical b.
    pathological b.
    public health b.
    sanitary b.
    systematic b.
bacteriolysin
bacteriolysis
    immune b.
bacteriolytic
Bacterionema
bacterio-opsonin
bacteriophage
    lambda b.
    mature b.
    temperate b.

bacteriophage *(continued)*
    vegetative b.
    virulent b.
bacteriophagia
bacteriophagic
bacteriophagology
bacteriophytoma
bacterioplasmin
bacterioprecipitin
bacterioprotein
bacteriopsonic
bacteriopsonin
bacteriopurpurin
bacteriorhodopsin
bacteriosis
bacteriospermia
bacteriostasis
bacteriostat
bacteriostatic
bacteriotherapy
bacteriotoxemia
bacteriotoxic
bacteriotoxin
bacteriotropic
bacteriotropin
bacteritic
Bacterium
    B. aerogenes
    B. aeruginosum
    B. anitratum
    B. cholerae suis
    B. cloacae
    B. coli
    B. dysenteriae
    B. sonnei
    B. tularense
    B. typhosum
bacterium (bacteria)
    acid-fast b.
    autotrophic b.
    beaded b.
    bifid b.
    blue-green b.
    chemoautotrophic b.
    chemoheterotrophic b.
    chromogenic b.
    coliform b.
    coryneform b.
    Dar es Salaam b.
    denitrifying b.
    gram-negative b.
    gram-positive b.
    hemophilic b.
    heterotrophic b.
    higher bacteria

B

bacterium (bacteria) *(continued)*
 hydrogen b.
 lactic acid b.
 lysogenic b.
 mesophilic b.
 nonsulfur b., purple
 parasitic b.
 pathogenic b.
 photoautotrophic b.
 photoheterotrophic b.
 photosynthetic b.
 phototrophic b.
 propionic acid b.
 psychrophilic b.
 purple b.
 pyogenic acid b.
 pyrogenetic b.
 resistant b.
 rough b.
 saprophytic b.
 smooth b.
 sulfur b.
 thermophilic b.
 toxigenic b.
 toxinogenic b.
 water b.
bacteriuria
bacteriuric
bacteroid
Bacteroides
 B. asaccharolyticus
 B. bivius
 B. buccae
 B. capillosus
 B. corporis
 B. corrodens
 B. denticola
 B. disiens
 B. distasonis
 B. eggerthii
 B. endodontalis
 B. fragilis
 B. funduliformis
 B. gingivalis
 B. heparinolyticus
 B. intermedius
 B. melaninogenicus
 B. melaninogenicus subsp.
  intermedius
 B. melaninogenicus subsp.
  melaninogenicus
 B. nodosus
 B. ochraceus
 B. oralis
 B. oris

Bacteroides (continued)
 B. ovatus
 B. pneumosintes
 B. praeacutus
 B. putredinis
 B. ruminicola
 B. splanchnicus
 B. thetaiotaomicron
 B. uniformis
 B. ureolyticus
 B. vulgatus
bacteroidosis
bactroprenol
baculovirus
baculum
Badal operation
badge
 film b.
Badgley
 operation
 plate
Baelz
 disease
 syndrome
BAEP—brain stem auditory evoked
 potential
Baer (von Baer)
 cavity
 follicle
 law
 nystagmus
 vesicle
Baerensprung erythrasma
Baffe anastomosis
baffle
 intra-atrial b.
 pericardial b.
 Senning type intra-atrial b.
Bäfverstedt (Baefverstedt)
 syndrome
bag
 Ambu b.
 Barnes b.
 bolus b's
 Bunyan b.
 Champetier de Ribes b.
 colostomy b.
 Douglas b.
 Hagner b.
 ice b.
 ileostomy b.
 micturition b.
 nuclear b.
 Perry b.
 Petersen b.

bag *(continued)*
    Pilcher b.
    Pilcher hemostatic b.
    Politzer b.
    reservoir b.
    testicular b.
    Tucker dilatable b.
    Voorhees b.
    b. of waters
    Whitmore b.
bagassosis
Baggish hysteroscope
Bagolini lenses
Bahnson clamp
Bailey
    catheter
    clamp
    conductor
    leukotome
    rib contractor
Bailey-Glover-O'Neill knife
Bailey-Morse knife
Bailey-Williamson forceps
Baillarger
    bands
    lines
    sign
    striae
    stripes
    syndrome
Bainbridge
    anastomosis clamp
    hemostatic forceps
    reflex
Bair-Hugger Convective Warming
  Unit
Bakamjian flap
Baker
    Act
    cyst
    jejunostomy tube
    self-sumping tube
    velum
Bakes
    bile duct dilator
    dilator
    probe
Bakwin-Eiger syndrome
BAL—
    British antilewisite
    bronchoalveolar lavage
balance
    acid-base b.
    analytical b.
    calcium b.

balance *(continued)*
    carbon b.
    electrolyte b.
    energy b.
    fluid b.
    genic b.
    glomerulotubular b.
    heat b.
    metabolic b.
    microchemical b.
    mineral b.
    nitrogen b.
    occlusal b.
    protein b.
    semimicro b.
    thermal b.
    torsion b.
    water b.
balanced
    b. electrolyte solution
    b. salt solution
balanic
β-alaninemia
balanitis
    amebic b.
    b. circinata
    b. circumscripta
      plasmacellularis
    b. diabetica
    erosive b.
    Follmann b.
    b. gangraenosa
    gangrenous b.
    phagedenic b.
    plasma cell b.
    b. plasmacellularis
    b. xerotica obliterans
balanoblennorrhea
balanocele
balanochlamyditis
balanoplasty
balanoposthitis
    b. chronica circumscripta
      plasmocellularis
    specific gangrenous and
      ulcerative b.
balanoposthomycosis
balanopreputial
balanorrhagia
balantidial
balantidiasis
Balantidium
    B. coli
    B. suis
balanus

B

Balbiani
  body
  nucleus
  ring
bald gastric fundus
baldness
  common male b.
  male pattern b.
Baldwin operation
Baldy operation
Balfour
  bladder blade
  gastroenterostomy
  retractor
  retractor with fenestrated
    blade
  self-retaining retractor
Bálint (Balint) syndrome
Balkan
  frame
  B. nephritis
  B. nephropathy
  splint
Balke protocol
Ball [eponym]
  method
  operation
ball
  chondrin b.
  fatty b. of Bichat
  food b.
  b. of foot
  fungus b.
  hair b.
  Marchi b's
  oat hair b.
  pleural fibrin b's
  b.-valve prosthesis
  wool b.
Ballance sign
Ballantine
  clamp
  hemilaminectomy retractor
  hysterectomy forceps
  uterine curet
Ballantyne syndrome
Ballantyne-Runge syndrome
Ballard gestational assessment
Ballenger
  curet
  elevator
  forceps
  swivel knife
Ballenger-Sluder tonsillectome
Ballentine forceps

Baller-Gerold syndrome
Ballet
  disease
  sign
balling
Ballingall disease
ballism
ballismus
ballistic
ballistics
  drug b.
  forensic b.
  wound b.
ballistocardiogram
ballistocardiograph
ballistocardiography
balloon
  ACS b.
  b. angioplasty
  b. atrial septectomy
  b. atrial septostomy
  b. biliary catheter
  b. catheter
  b. catheterization
  catheter b. valvuloplasty
    (CBV)
  b. defecation
  b. dilatation, b. dilation
  Fogarty b.
  Garren b.
  Grüntzig (Gruentzig) b.
  Grüntzig-type b.
  Honan b.
  Hunter b.
  Hunter-Sessions b.
  image data intra-aortic
    counter-pulsation b.
  intranasal b.
  b. manometry
  pilot b.
  pneumatic b. dilator
  Shea-Anthony antral b.
  sinus b.
  b. tamponade
  b. tuboplasty
  b. valvuloplasty
ballooning
  b. mitral cusp
  b. mitral cusp syndrome
ballotable
ballottement
  abdominal b.
  indirect b.
  kidney b.
  renal b.

balm
        b. of Gilead
Balme cough
balneology
balneotherapeutics
balneotherapy
Baló
        concentric encephalitis
        concentric sclerosis
        concentric syndrome
        disease
        syndrome
Baloser hysteroscope
balsam
        Canada b.
        friars' b.
        b. of Gilead
        Holland b.
        Mecca b.
        b. of Peru
        St. Thomas b.
        silver b.
        tolu b.
        Turlington b.
        Wade b.
balsamic
balsamum peruvianum
balsa wood block
balteum venereum
Bamatter syndrome
Bamberger
        albuminuria
        area
        bulbar pulse
        disease
        hematogenic albuminuria
        sign
Bamberger-Marie
        disease
        syndrome
bambermycins
bamnidazole
banana
        b. bag
        b. blade
        b. sign
Bancroft filariasis
bancroftian filariasis
bancroftiasis
bancroftosis
band
        A b.
        absorption b's
        amniotic b's
        anchor b.

band *(continued)*
        angiomesenteric b.
        Angle b.
        anisotropic b.
        anogenital b.
        anterior b. of colon
        atrioventricular b.
        auriculoventricular b.
        axis b.
        b's of Baillarger
        Bekhterev (Bechterew) b.
        belly b. (bellyband)
        b. of Broca
        Broca diagonal b.
        Bungner b's
        C b.
        cholecystoduodenal b.
        chorioamniotic b's
        chromosome b.
        Clado b.
        clamp b.
        confidence b.
        contoured b.
        contraction b.
        coronary b.
        dentate b.
        diagonal b. of Broca
        elastic b.
        elastic b. fixation [of fracture]
        episternal b.
        Essick cell b.
        forbidden b.
        furrowed b.
        G b.
        genitomesenteric b.
        b. of Gennari
        Giacomini b.
        H b.
        Hall b.
        Harris b.
        Henle b.
        His b.
        Hunter-Schreger b's
        hymenal b.
        I b.
        iliotibial b.
        incisal b.
        b. keratopathy
        Ladd b.
        Lane b.
        Leonardo b.
        limbic b's
        lip furrow b.
        Maissiat b.
        Matas b.

B

band *(continued)*
- matrix b.
- MB b.
- Meckel b.
- mesocolic b.
- MM b.
- moderator b.
- molar b.
- oligoclonal b.
- omental b.
- omphalomesenteric b.
- orthodontic b.
- Parham b.
- perioplic b.
- periosteal b.
- phonatory b's
- preformed b.
- premolar b.
- Q b.
- R b.
- Reil b's
- retention b.
- Schreger b's
- Sébileau b's
- Silastic b.
- silicone b.
- Soret b.
- b. and spur retainer
- sternal b.
- Tarin b.
- valence b.
- Vicq d'Azyr b.
- Z b.
- zonular b.

bandage
- Ace b.
- adhesive b.
- barrel b.
- Barton b.
- Baynton b.
- Borsch b.
- Buller b.
- butterfly b.
- capeline b.
- Champ elastic b.
- circular b.
- compression b.
- cotton elastic b.
- cotton-wool b.
- cravat b.
- crepe b.
- crucial b.
- Curad plastic b.
- demigauntlet b.
- Desault b.

bandage *(continued)*
- E cotton b.
- elastic b.
- Elasticon b.
- Elastomull b.
- Elastoplast b.
- Esmarch b.
- figure-of-eight b.
- fixation b.
- Flexilite b.
- four-tailed b.
- Fricke b.
- gauntlet b.
- gauze b.
- Gibney b.
- hammock b.
- Hueter b.
- Hydron Burn B.
- immobilizing b.
- Kerlix b.
- Kling b.
- many-tailed b.
- Marlex b.
- Martin b.
- oblique b.
- plaster b.
- POP (plaster of Paris) b.
- pressure b.
- recurrent b.
- reversed b.
- roller b.
- Sayre b.
- Scultetus b.
- Seutin b.
- b. shears
- spica b.
- spiral b.
- spiral reverse b.
- stockinette b.
- suspensory b.
- T b.
- Theden b.
- triangular b.
- Velpeau b.
- Y b.

Band-Aid
bandaletta
- b. diagonalis
- b. diagonalis of Broca

bandeau (bandeaus)
bandelette
bandicoot
banding
- chromosome b.
- high-resolution b.

banding *(continued)*
     prophase b.
     pulmonary artery b.
     tooth b.
Bandl ring
bandwidth
Bane forceps
banewort
Bang bacillus
Bangerter
     graded occluder
     method
banian
banisterine
banjo curet
bank
Bankart
     lesion
     operation
     reconstruction
     retractor
Bannayan-Zonana syndrome
Bannister disease
Banti
     disease
     splenic anemia
     syndrome
BAO—basal acid output
Baptisia
     B. leucantha
bar
     arch b.
     b. of bladder
     chromatoid b.
     connector b.
     Dolder b.
     Erich arch b.
     fixation arch b.
     House b.
     hyoid b's
     interureteric b.
     Jelanko arch b.
     Kazanjian T b.
     Kennedy b.
     labial b.
     lingual b.
     lumbar b.
     median b.
     Mercier b.
     metatarsal b.
     occlusal rest b.
     palatal b.
     Passavant b.
     sternal b.

bar *(continued)*
     sublingual b.
     tarsal b.
     terminal b's
     thyroid b.
     Winters arch b.
Bar [eponym]
     incision
     syndrome
baragnosis
baralyme
Bárány
     drum
     noise apparatus whistle
     pointing test
     positional vertigo
     sign
     symptom
     syndrome
     test
barba (barbae)
     eczema barbae
     folliculitis barbae
     pseudofolliculitis
          barbae
     sycosis barbae
     tinea barbae
     trichophytosis barbae
barbaralalia
Barber [eponym]
     dermatosis
     psoriasis
barberry
barbital
barbiturate
barbituric acid
barbotage
barbula hirci
Barclay niche
Barcoo
     disease
     rot
Barcroft apparatus
Bard
     catheter
     sign
     syndrome
Bardelli operation
Bardenheuer
     extension
     incision
Bardet-Biedl syndrome
Bardex catheter
Bardic cannula

Bard-Parker
    blade
    dermatome
    knife
bare, bared
baresthesia
baresthesiometer
Bargen streptococcus
Barger method
bariatrics
baric
baritosis
barium (Ba)
    b. cyanoplatinate
    b. enema
    b. hydrate
    b. hydroxide
    b. meal
    b. oxide
    b. platinocyanide
    b. sulfate
    b. sulfide
    b. swallow
    b. titanate
    b. vaginography
bark
    bearberry b.
    bitter b.
    buckthorn b.
    calisaya b.
    casca b.
    chittem b.
    cinchona b.
    cramp b.
    dita b.
    dogwood b.
    eleuthera b.
    elm b.
    grape b.
    Jesuit b.
    Mancona b.
    Persian b.
    Peruvian b.
    Purshiana b.
    quillay b.
    sacred b.
    white oak b.
    wild black cherry b.
Barkan
    knife
    operation
Barker
    operation
    point

Barkman reflex
Barkow
    colliculus of B.
    ligaments
barley
Barley-Gibbon rib contractor
Barlow
    disease
    forceps
    syndrome
Barnes
    bag
    cervical dilator
    common duct dilator
    curve
    dilator
    trocar
    zone
Barnes-Crile forceps
Barnhill curet
baroagnosis
barodontalgia
baroelectroesthesiometer
barognosis
baromacrometer
baropacer
barophilic
baroreceptor
baroscope
barosensitive
barosinusitis
barospirator
barostat
barotalgia
barotaxis
barotitis media
barotrauma
    odontalgia b.
    otic b., otitic b.
    pulmonary b.
    sinus b.
barotropism
Barr
    anal speculum
    body
    bolt
    chromatin body
    crypt hook
    fistula hook
    fistula probe
    rectal hook
    rectal probe
    rectal speculum
    self-retaining rectal retractor

Barraquer
    brush
    ciliary forceps
    corneal forceps
    disease
    irrigator spatula
    keratoplasty knife
    method
    microkeratome
    needle holder
    operation
    scissors
    speculum
    suture
    trephine
Barraquer-Colibri speculum
Barraquer-DeWecker iris scissors
Barraquer-Krumeich-Swinger
    refractive set
Barraquer-Simons syndrome
Barraya forceps
Barré
    pyramidal sign
    sign
bar reader
Barré-Guillain syndrome
barrel
    b. chest
    b. distortion
    b. dressing
barrel hoop
    b.h. sign
Barré-Liéou syndrome
barreling distortion
barren
Barrett
    epithelium
    esophagus
    forceps
    syndrome
    tenaculum
    ulcer
Barrett-Adson retractor
Barrett-Allen forceps
barrier
    architectural b.
    blood-air b.
    blood-aqueous b.
    blood-brain b.
    blood–cerebrospinal fluid b.
    blood-gas b.
    blood–ocular fluid b.
    blood-testis b.
    blood-thymus b.
    energy b.

barrier *(continued)*
    filtration b.
    gastric mucosal b.
    hematoencephalic b.
    histohematic connective
        tissue b.
    Mercier b.
    placental b.
    protective b.
    radiation b.
Barrio operation
barsati
Barsky
    elevator
    operation
Bársony-Polgár syndrome
Bársony-Teschendorf syndrome
Barth hernia
Bartholin
    anus
    cyst
    duct
    duct abscess
    gland
bartholinitis
Barton
    bandage
    forceps
    fracture
    operation
    tongs
    traction handle
Barton-Cone tongs
Bartonella
    B. bacilliformis
    B. elizabethae
    B. henselae
    B. koehlerae
    B. quintana
    B. vinsonii
bartonellemia
bartonellosis
Bartonia bodies
Bärtschi-Rochaix
    (Baertschi-Rochaix) syndrome
Bart syndrome
Bartter syndrome
Bartter-Schwartz syndrome
baruria
Barwell operation
barye
barylalia
baryta
    synthetic b.
basad

basal
>   b. body temperature
>   b. iridectomy
>   b. lamina

basalis

basaloid

basaloma

base
>   acidifiable b.
>   acrylic resin b.
>   b. of bladder
>   b. of brain
>   Brønsted b.
>   buffer b.
>   cement b.
>   b. of cerebrum
>   conjugate b.
>   data b. (database)
>   denture b.
>   denture b., tinted
>   b. excess
>   extension b.
>   film b.
>   free-end b.
>   hexone b's
>   histone b's
>   b. of iris
>   Lewis b.
>   metal b.
>   b. of metatarsal
>   b. of nail
>   nitrogenous b.
>   ointment b.
>   b. pair
>   plastic b.
>   purine b's
>   pyrimidine b's
>   rare b's
>   record b.
>   b. of renal pyramid
>   b. of sacrum
>   Schiff b.
>   Schreiner b.
>   shellac b's
>   b. of skull
>   b. of stapes
>   temporary b.
>   time b.
>   tinted denture b.
>   tooth-borne b.
>   trial b.
>   whole blood buffer b.
>   whole-body buffer b.
>   wobble b.
>   xanthine b's

baseball
>   b. lens
>   b. suture

basedoid

Basedow
>   disease
>   goiter
>   pseudoparaplegia
>   syndrome
>   triad

basedowiform

baseline
>   b. film
>   Reid b.

basement membrane

baseplate
>   stabilized b.

bases (plural of basis)

bas-fond

basial

basialis

basialveolar

basiarachnitis

basiarachnoiditis

basibranchial

basic

basically

basicaryoplastin

basichromatin

basichromiole

basicity

basicranial

basicytoparaplastin

basidia

basidiobolomycosis

Basidiobolus
>   *B. haptosporus*
>   *B. meristosporus*
>   *B. ranarum*

basidiocarp

Basidiomycetes

basidiomycetous

basidiospore

basidium (basidia)

basifacial

basigenous

basihyoid

basil

basilad

basilar suture

basilaris cranii

basilateral, basolateral

Basile hip screw

basilemma

basilic

basiloma
basilomental
basilopharyngeal
basin
    kidney b.
basinasial
basioccipital
basioglossus
basion
basiotic
basiparachromatin
basiparaplastin
basipetal
basipharyngeal
basipresphenoid
basirhinal
basis
    b. cartilaginis arytenoideae
    b. cochleae
    b. cordis
    b. cranii externa
    b. cranii interna
    b. mandibulae
    b. modioli
    b. ossis sacri
    b. patellae
    b. pedunculi cerebri
    b. phalangis manus
    b. phalangis pedis
    b. prostatae
    b. pulmonis
    b. stapedis
basisphenoid
basisylvian
basitemporal
basivertebral
basket
    Browne b.
    Burhenne stone b. technique
    Councill b.
    cytopharyngeal b.
    Dormia b.
    Ferguson b.
    fiber b's
    Howard b.
    Johnson b.
    Mitchell b.
basket cells
basketing
basket procedure
basograph
basolateral, basilateral
basometachromophil
Basommatophora

basophil
    beta b.
    Crooke-Russell b's
    delta b.
basophilia
    pituitary b.
    punctate b.
basophilic
basophilism
    Cushing b.
    pituitary b.
basophobia
basophobiac
basoplasm
basosquamous
Bassen-Kornzweig
    disease
    syndrome
Basset operation
Bassini operation
bassorin
basswood
bastard suture
Basterra operation
Bastian
    law
    syndrome
Bastian-Bruns
    law
    sign
basting stitch
    Parker-Kerr b.s.
bastion
BAT—blunt abdominal trauma
Bateman
    disease
    operation
    prosthesis
    purpura
    syndrome
Bates operation
bath
    acid b.
    air b.
    alcohol b.
    alkaline b.
    alum b.
    antipyretic b.
    antiseptic b.
    aromatic b.
    astringent b.
    Aveeno b.
    borax b.
    bran b.

B

bath *(continued)*
  Brand b.
  bubble b.
  cabinet b.
  camphor b.
  carbon dioxide b.
  cold b.
  colloid b.
  continuous b.
  contrast b.
  cool b.
  creosote b.
  douche b.
  drip-sheet b.
  earth b.
  Finnish b.
  Finsen b.
  foam b.
  full b.
  gas-bubble b.
  gelatin b.
  glycerin b.
  graduated b.
  grease b.
  half b.
  herb b.
  hip b.
  hot b.
  hot-air b.
  hyperthermal b.
  immersion b.
  infrared b.
  iron b.
  kinetotherapeutic b.
  light b.
  linseed b.
  lukewarm b.
  medicated b.
  milk b.
  moor b.
  mud b.
  Nauheim b.
  needle b.
  oatmeal b.
  oil b.
  oxygen b.
  pack b.
  paraffin b.
  peat b.
  sand b.
  sauna b.
  Schott b.
  sedative b.
  sheet b.

bath *(continued)*
  sitz b.
  sponge b.
  stimulating b.
  sweat b.
  tepid b.
  transcutan b.
  vapor b.
  warm b.
  water b.
  wax b.
  whirlpool b.
bathmotropic
  negatively b.
  positively b.
bathmotropism
bathochrome
bathochromic
bathochromy
bathoflore
bathomorphic
bathorhodopsin
bathrocephaly
bathyanesthesia
bathycardia
bathyesthesia
bathyhyperesthesia
bathyhypesthesia
bathypnea
batonet
Batson
  plexus
  system
battalion
Batten disease
Batten-Mayou disease
battery of tests
Battey bacilli
Battle
  incision
  operation
  sign
Battle-Jalaguier-Kammerer incision
Baudelocque
  diameter
  line
  operation
Bauhin
  gland
  valve
Baumann angle
Baumé
  law
  scale

Baumgarten
- cirrhosis
- glands
- murmur
- syndrome

Baumrucker resectoscope

Bausch & Lomb
- cleaner
- lubricant
- solution

bauxite pneumoconiosis

bay
- lacrimal b.

Bayle
- disease
- granulations

Bayley Scales of Infant Development

Bayliss theory

Baylor
- amniotome
- splint
- sump

Baynton
- bandage
- operation

bayonet
- b. forceps
- b. incision

Bazette formula

Bazin
- disease
- ulcer

BB—
- blue bloater
- breakthrough bleeding
- breast biopsy

BBA—born before arrival [of doctor or midwife]

BBB—
- blood-brain barrier
- bundle branch block

BBBB—bilateral bundle branch block

B-B graft

BBT—basal body temperature

BC—
- bactericidal concentration
- birth control
- bone conduction
- Bowman capsule
- buccocervical

BCAF—basophil chemotaxis augmentation factor

BCDF—B cell differentiation factors

B-cell
- B-c. antibody
- B-c. antigen receptors
- B-c. lymphoma

BCG—
- bacille Calmette-Guérin (vaccine)
- ballistocardiogram
- bicolor guaiac test

BCGF—B cell growth factors

BCNU—bis-chloroethyl-nitrosourea

BCP, BCPs—birth control pills

BD—buccodistal

BDA—British Dental Association

BDE—bile duct exploration

Bdella cardinalis

bdellium

Bdellovibrio, bdellovibrio

BE—
- barium enema
- base excess

Beacham amniotome

bead
- b. chain cystography
- rachitic b's

beaded

beading of ribs

Beadle

beak of sphenoid bone

beaker

Beale ganglion cells

Beall mitral valve prosthesis

beam
- b. barrier
- broad b.
- cantilever b.
- continuous b.
- b. CT scanner
- electron b.
- b. flattening filter
- b. monitor
- narrow b.
- neutron b.
- primary b.
- b. quality comparison
- restrained b.
- simple b.
- b. splitter
- b. therapy applicator
- useful b.
- x-ray b.

bean
- broad b.
- Calabar b.

bean *(continued)*
    castor b.
    jequirity b.
    ordeal b.
    St. Ignatius b.
    soja b.
beanbag
bearberry, bear berry
Beard
    disease
    syndrome
Beard-Cutler operation
Beardsley
    aortic dilator
    cecostomy trocar
    empyema tube
    esophageal retractor
    intestinal clamp
bearing
    central b.
bearing down
Bearn-Kunkel-Slater
  syndrome
bear tracks
bearwood
beat
    apex b.
    atrial b.
    automatic b.
    capture b.
    ciliary b.
    combination b.
    coupled b's
    coupled b's
    dependent b.
    dropped b.
    echo b.
    ectopic b.
    escape b.
    escaped b.
    forced b.
    fusion b.
    idioventricular b.
    interference b.
    mixed b's
    nodal b.
    paired b's
    paired b's
    premature b.
    premature auricular b.
    reciprocal b.
    retrograde b.
    summation b.
    ventricular fusion b.
    ventricular premature b.

Beatson
    operation
    ovariotomy
Beatty-Bright friction sound
Beau
    disease
    lines
    syndrome
Beaupre forceps
Beauvais disease
Beaver
    blade
    handle
    keratome
    knife
Beaver-DeBakey blade
Beccaria sign
bechic
Bechtol
    arthroplasty
    hip prosthesis
Beck
    clamp
    disease
    gastrostomy
    gastrostomy scoop
    knife
    operation (I, II)
    rasp
    syndrome
    triad
Becker
    astigmatism test
    dystrophy
    nevus
    operation
    phenomenon
    sign
    test
Becker-type muscular dystrophy
Beck-Jianu gastrostomy
Beckman
    adenoid curet
    goiter retractor
    nasal speculum
    retractor
    self-retaining retractor
Beckman-Adson laminectomy
  retractor
Beckman-Colver nasal speculum
Beckman-Eaton laminectomy
  retractor
Beck-Mueller tonsillectome
Beck-Schenck tonsillectome
Beckwith syndrome

Beckwith-Wiedemann syndrome
Béclard
    amputation
    anastomosis
    hernia
    nucleus
    point
    sign
    suture
    triangle
becquerel (Bq)
bed
    air b.
    air-fluidized b.
    capillary b.
    circle b.
    CircOlectric b.
    Clinitron b.
    collateral vascular b.
    fracture b.
    Gatch b.
    hydrostatic b.
    Klondike b.
    metabolic b.
    mud b.
    nail b.
    placental b.
    plaster b.
    rocking b.
    Roto-Rest b.
    Sanders b.
    Sanders oscillating b.
    sawdust b.
    stomach b.
    vascular b.
    water b.
bedbug
    Mexican b.
    Oriental b.
    Texas b.
bedewing
bedlam
bedlamism
Bednar aphtha
bedpan
bedrest, bed rest
bedridden
bedsore
bedwetting
Beebe forceps
Beer
    canaliculus knife
    cataract knife
    ciliary forceps
    collyrium

Beer *(continued)*
    knife
    operation
beerwort
beeswax
    bleached b.
    unbleached b.
beetle
    blister b.
Beevor sign
Begbie disease
Begg
    appliance
    light-wire differential force
        technique
    paralleling
    straight-wire combination
        bracket
    technique
    torque
begma
Béguez César disease
behavior
    adaptive b.
    attachment b.
    automatic b.
    avoidance b.
    collective b.
    displacement b.
    impulsive b.
    instinctive b.
    invariable b.
    operant b.
    respondent b.
    species-specific b.
    variable b.
behaviorism
Behçet
    disease
    syndrome
    triple symptom complex
behenic acid
Behier-Hardy
    sign
    symptom
Behr
    atrophy
    disease
    pupil
    syndrome
Behring (von Behring)
    law
    serum
BEI—butanol-extractable iodine
Beigel disease

beikost
bejel
Békésy
    audiometry
    calibration
Bekhterev (Bechterew)
    arthritis
    band
    deep reflex
    disease
    layer
    line
    nucleus
    nystagmus
    reaction
    reflex
    rheumatoid spondylitis
    sign
    spondylitis
    test
Bekhterev-Mendel reflex
Bekhterev-Strümpell
    spondylitis
bel
belching
belemnoid
Belfield
    operation
    wire retractor
Bell
    delirium
    law
    mania
    muscle
    nerve
    operation
    palsy
    paralysis
    phenomenon
    sign
    suture
bell-crowned
belle indifférence, la belle
    indifférence
Bellini
    ducts
    ligaments
    tubules
Bell-Magendie law
Bellocq
    cannula
    sound
    tube
bellows
Bellucci scissors

belly
    anterior b. of digastric muscle
    Delhi b.
    drum b.
    frontal b. of occipitofrontal
        muscle
    inferior b. of omohyoid muscle
    muscle b.
    occipital b. of occipitofrontal
        muscle
    posterior b. of digastric muscle
    prune b.
    prune-b. syndrome
    spider b.
    swollen b.
    wooden b.
bellyache
bellyband
bellybutton
belonephobia
belonoid
belonoskiascopy
Belsey
    Mark II fundoplication
    Mark IV operation
    Mark V operation
    repair
bemegride
Benaron forceps
Bence Jones
    albumin
    albumosuria
    body
    cylinders
    globulin
    myeloma
    protein
    protein method
    protein test
    proteinuria
    reaction
    test
    urine
bench method
bend
    first order b's
    head b.
    iliac b. of ureter
    labyrinthine b's
    neck b.
    second order b's
    third order b's
    V b's
    varolian b.
bendazac

Bender
  Gestalt test
  test
  Visual-Motor Gestalt test
bendiocarb
bends
bene
beneceptor
Beneckea
Benedict
  gastroscope
  method
  retractor
  solution
  test
Benedict and Franke method
Benedict and Osterberg method
Benedict-Roth
  apparatus
  spirometer
Benedikt syndrome
beneficence
beneficial
beneficiary
benefit
  indemnity b.
  maximum hospital b.
  maximum medical b.
  service b.
benefited
Bengolea forceps
benign
benignancy
benignant
Béniqué
  catheter
  dilator
  sound
Bennett
  angle
  Differential Aptitude Test
  disease
  dislocation
  elevator
  forceps
  fracture
  leukemia
  movement
  operation
  posterior shoulder approach
  retractor
benorterone
benoxaprofen
Bensley specific granules
Benson disease

Bent operation
bentiromide
bentonite flocculation test
benzalin
benzalkonium chloride
benzamine
Benzamycin
benzanthracene
benzene
  dimethyl b.
  b. hexachloride
  methyl b.
  b. ring
benzene hexachloride
benzenoid
benzestrofol
benzethonium chloride
benzhexol hydrochloride
benzhydramine hydrochloride
benzin, benzine
benzine
  petroleum b.
benzisoxazole
benzoate
benzoated
benzoctamine
benzolism
benzopurpurine
1,2-benzopyran
benzo[*a*]pyrene
benzoquinone
benzoquinonium chloride
benzotherapy
benzothiadiazine
benzoxiquine
benzoyl
  b. ecgonine
  hydrous b. peroxide
  b. peroxide
benzoylglycine
benzoylmethylecgonine
benzoylphenylcarbinol
benzpyrinium bromide
benzpyrrole
benzurestat
benzydamine hydrochloride
benzydroflumethiazide
benzyl
  b. bromide
  b. carbinol
benzylidene
benzyloxycarbonyl
p-benzyloxyphenol [p-, para-]
benzylpenicillin
  b. potassium

benzylpenicillin *(continued)*
- b. procaine
- b. sodium

bepascum

beractant

Bérard
- aneurysm
- ligament

Berardinelli syndrome

Béraud valve

berberine bisulfate

Berberis vulgaris

bereavement

Berens
- 3-character test
- dilator
- forceps
- implant
- keratome
- lid everter
- muscle clamp
- operation
- punch
- retractor
- scissors
- scoop
- spatula
- speculum

Berens-Rosa implant

Berger
- amputation
- disease
- focal glomerulonephritis
- method
- operation
- paresthesia
- rhythm
- sign
- space
- symptom
- wave

Bergeron
- chorea
- disease

Bergey classification

Bergman sign

Bergmann
- cells
- cords
- fibers
- incision

Bergmann-Israel incision

Bergmeister papilla

Bergonié
- method

Bergonié *(continued)*
- treatment

Bergonié-Tribondeau law

beriberi
- atrophic b.
- cerebral b.
- dry b.
- infantile b.
- paralytic b.
- ship b.
- wet b.

beriberic

Berke
- double-end lid everter
- operation
- ptosis clamp
- ptosis forceps

Berkefeld filter

berkelium (Bk)

Berke-Motais operation

Berlin
- disease
- edema

Berlind-Auvard speculum

Berman locator

Berna infant abdominal retractor

Bernard
- canal
- duct
- layer
- puncture
- syndrome

Bernard-Burrows operation

Bernard-Horner syndrome

Bernard-Soulier
- disease
- syndrome

Bernay
- sponge
- tracheal retractor
- uterine gauze packer

Berne
- forceps
- rasp

Bernhardt
- disease
- paresthesia

Bernhardt-Roth
- disease
- syndrome

Bernheim
- syndrome
- therapy

Bernheimer fibers

Bernoulli
    distribution
    law
    principle
    theorem
    trial
Bernstein
    gastroscope
    test
Berotec
berry
    bear b.
    buckthorn b.
    fish b.
    horse nettle b.
    Indian b.
    ligament
    uterine-elevating forceps
Berthelot
    reaction
    reagent
Bertiella
    B. satyri
    B. studeri
bertielliasis
Bertin
    bone
    column
    ligament
    ossicles
Bertolotti syndrome
Bertrand method
berylliosis
beryllium (Be)
β-erythroidine
beseech, beseeched
besiclometer
Besnier
    prurigo
    rheumatism
Besnier-Boeck disease
Bespaloff sign
Best
    carmine stain
    clamp
    common duct stone
        forceps
    direct forward-vision
        telescope
    disease
    gallstone forceps
    intestinal forceps
    macular degeneration
    operation
bestiality

beta
    Greek letter
        (β; alphabetized as b)
    b.-*N*-acetylgalactosaminidase
    b.-*N*-acetylglucosaminyl-
        glycopeptide β-1,4-
        galactosyltransferase
    b. adrenoceptor
    b.-2 agonist
    b.-aminoisobutyricaciduria
    b.-cholestanol
    b. decay
    b. emitter
    b.-endorphin
    b.-erythroidine
    b.-estradiol
    b.-galactosidase
    b. globulin
    b. globulin, pregnancy-specific
    b.-glucuronidase
    b. hCG (human chorionic
        gonadotropin)
    11-b.-hydroxyandrostenedione
        [11-beta-]
    b.-hydroxybutyric acid
    17-b.-hydroxycorticosterone
        [17-beta-]
    3-b.-hydroxy-delta-5-steroid
        dehydrogenase
    b.-interferon
    b.-lactamase negative
    b.-lactamase positive
    b.-lactose
    b.-lipoprotein
    b.-lipotropin
    b.-methylcrotonylglycinuria
    b.-2-microglobulin
    b.-naphtholsulfonic acid
    b.-nicotyrine
    b. oxybutyric acid
    b. particle
    b.-pleated sheet
    b. quick strep test
    b. radiation
    b. ray
    b. ray microscope
    b.-sitosterolemia
    b. thromboglobulin
    b. transition
betacism
Betadine
betaine
    b. hydrochloride
beta-lysin
    b. acetate

beta-lysin *(continued)*
    b. sodium phosphate
betanaphthol
betanaphthyl
    b. benzoate
    b. salicylate
betapropiolactone
betaquinine
betatron
bete
betel nut
bethanechol
Bethea
    method
    sign
Bethune
    lung tourniquet
    periosteal elevator
    phrenic retractor
    rib cutter
    rib shears
Betula
    B. alba
    B. lenta
Betz
    cell area
    cells
Buettner method
Bevan
    gallbladder forceps
    hemostatic forceps
    incision
    Lewis cells
    operation
bevel
bex convulsiva
Beyer
    forceps
    rongeur
Beziehungswahn sensitiver
bezoar
Bezold (von Bezold)
    abscess
    ganglion
    mastoiditis
    perforation
    reflex
    sign
    symptom
    triad
BF—
    blastogenic factor
    bouillon filtrate (tuberculin)
    lymphocyte blastogenic factor
BFP—biologic false-positive

BG—
    bone graft
    Bordet-Gengou (test)
    buccogingival
B graft
BI—burn index
Bial
    reagent
    test
Bianchi
    nodule
    syndrome
    valve
biarticular
biarticulate
bias
    Berkson b.
    Neyman b.
biauricular
biaxial
biballism
bibasally
bibasic
bibasilar
    b. crackles
    b. rales
Biber-Haab-Dimmer
    degeneration
    dystrophy
bibeveled
Bibliofilm
bibliotherapy
bibulous
bicalutamide
bicameral
bicapsular
bicarbonate
    blood b.
    plasma b.
    b. of soda, sodium b.
    standard b.
bicarbonatemia
bicaudal
bicellular
bicephalus
biceps
    b. brachii
    b. femoris
Bichat
    canal
    fat pad
    fissure
    foramen
    fossa
    ligament

Bichat *(continued)*
    membrane
    protuberance
    tunic, tunica
bichromate
bicipital
bicistronic
Bickel ring
bicollis
biconcave
biconvex
bicornuate
bicorporate
bicoudate
bicristal
bicuspid
bicuspidal
bicuspidate
bicuspidization
bicuspoid
b.i.d.—twice a day (L. bis in die)
bidactyly
Bidder
    ganglia
    organ
bidental
bidentate
bidermal
bidermoma
biduotertian
biduous
Biederman sign
Biedl
    disease
    syndrome
Bielschowsky
    disease
    method
    operation
    sign
    syndrome
    test
Bielschowsky-Jansky disease
Bielschowsky-Lutz-Cogan
  syndrome
Biemond syndrome (type I, type II)
Bier
    amputation
    anesthesia
    block anesthesia
    method
    operation
    passive hyperemia
    spots
    syndrome

Biermer
    anemia
    change
    disease
    sign
Biernacki sign
Biesenberger
    mammaplasty
    operation
Biesiadecki fossa
Bietti
    dystrophy
    syndrome
bifascicular
bifid
Bifidobacterium
    B. adolescentis
    B. bifidum
    B. eriksonii
    B. infantis
bifidus
bifixate
bifixation
bifocal
bifocals
biforate
biformyl
bifoveal
bifrontal
bifurcate
bifurcatio
    b. aortae
    b. aortica
    b. carotidis
    b. tracheae
    b. trunci pulmonalis
bifurcation
    b. of aorta
    b. of bundle of His
    carotid b.
    b. of pulmonary trunk
    tracheal b.
bifurcationes
Bigelow
    ligament
    litholapaxy
    lithotrite
    operation
    septum
bigeminal
bigeminum (bigemina)
bigeminy
    atrial b.
    atrioventricular nodal b.
    escape-capture b.

B

bigeminy *(continued)*
  nodal b.
  reciprocal b.
  ventricular b.
bigerminal
bigonial
bi-ischial
bilabe
bilateral
  b. lithotomy
  b. vagotomy
bilateralism
bilayer
  lipid b.
bile
  A b.
  B b.
  C b.
  cystic b.
  gallbladder b.
  hepatic b.
  limy b.
  milk of calcium b.
  ox b.
  white b.
bilharzial
bilharziasis
bilharzioma
bilharziosis
biliary
  b. angiography
  b. atresia
  b. cirrhosis
  b. hypoplasia
  b. prosthesis
biliation
bilicyanin
bilifaction
biliflavin
bilifulvin
bilifuscin
biligenesis
biligenetic
biligenic
biligulate
bilihumin
Bili-Labstix
Bili mask
bilin
bilinoid
bilious
biliousness
biliprasin
bilipurpurin
bilirachia

bilirubin
  conjugated b.
  direct b.
  indirect b.
  unconjugated b.
bilirubinate
bilirubinemia
bilirubinic
bilirubinuria
bilis
biliuria
biliverdin
biliverdinate
bilixanthin, bilixanthine
Billeau ear wax curet
Billroth
  anastomosis (I, II)
  cord
  disease
  forceps
  gastrectomy
  gastroduodenoscopy
  gastroenterostomy (I, II, III)
  gastrojejunostomy
  hypertrophy
  operation (I, II)
  ovarian retractor
  strands
  uterine tumor forceps
  venae cavernosae
Bill traction handle
bilobate b. placenta
bilobular
bilocular
biloculation
biloma
bilophodont
bimalar
bimalleolar
bimanual
bimastoid
bimaxillary
bimodal therapy
bimolecular
binangle, binangled
binary
binasal
binaural stethoscope
binauricular
bind
  bipolar double b.
  double b.
  unipolar double b.
binder
  Velcro b.

binding
    b. constant
    b. energy
    b. protein
binegative
Binet test
Binet-Simon test
Bing
    reflex
    sign
    test
binge
bingeing and purging
Bing-Neel syndrome
Binkhorst
    implant
    lens
binocular
    b. indirect ophthalmoscopy
    b. microscope
    b. ophthalmoscope
binocularity
binomial
binophthalmoscope
binoscope
binotic
binovular
Binswanger
    dementia
    disease
    encephalitis
binuclear
binucleation
binucleolate
bioaccumulation
bioactive
bioaeration
bioallethrin
bioamine
bioaminergic
bioassay
    erythropoietin b.
bioastronautics
bioavailability
Biobrane
    adhesive
    glove
    synthetic skin
      substitute
biocatalyst
biocenosis
biocenotic
Biocept-G test
biochemistry
biochemorphic

biochemorphology
biocidal
bioclimatologist
bioclimatology
biocolloid
biocompatibility
biocompatible
biocybernetics
biocycle
biocytin
biodegradable
biodegradation
biodetritus
biodialysis
biodynamics
bioelectricity
bioelectronics
bioelement
bioenergetics
bioengineering
bioequivalence
bioequivalent
bioethics
biofeedback
    alpha b.
biofilm
bioflavonoid
biogenesis
biogenetic
biogenic
biogenous
biogeochemistry
biogeography
bioglass
Biograft
biograph
biohazard
biohydraulic
bioimplant
biokinetics
biologic, biological
biological half-life
biological
    lyophilized b's
biologist
biology
    cell b.
    descriptive b.
    mathematical b.
    molecular b.
    population b.
    radiation b.
bioluminescence
biolysis
biolytic

biomarker
biomass
biomaterial
biomathematics
    dental b.
biome
biomechanics
biomedical
    b. engineering
    b. radiography
biomedicine
biomembrane
biomembranous
biometeorologist
biometeorology
biometer
biometrician
biometry
biomicroscope
    slit-lamp b.
biomicroscopy
biomodulation
biomolecule
biomotor
bion
bionecrosis
bionics
bionomics
bionomy
bionucleonics
bio-osmotic
biophagism
biophagous
biopharmaceuticals
biophotometer
biophylaxis
biophysical
biophysics
biophysiography
biophysiology
bioplasia
bioplasm
bioplasmic
biopoiesis
biopolymer
biopotential
bioprosthesis
biopsy
    aspiration b.
    biochemical b.
    bite b.
    bone marrow b.
    brush b.
    cervical b.
    cervical punch b.

biopsy *(continued)*
    chorionic villus b.
    cold cone b.
    cold knife conization b.
    cone b.
    cytologic b.
    endometrial b.
    endoscopic b.
    excisional b.
    exploratory b.
    fine-needle b.
    fine-needle aspiration b.
    four point b.
    fractional b.
    incisional b.
    lung b.
    muscle b.
    needle b.
    b. needle
    nerve b.
    open b.
    percutaneous b.
    punch b.
    renal b.
    ring b.
    scalene lymph node b.
    shave b.
    sponge b.
    sternal b.
    surface b.
    total b.
    transbronchial lung b.
    transperineal b.
    transrectal b.
    transurethral b.
    trephine b.
    wedge b.
    wound b.
biopsychic
biopsychology
biopterin
bioptic
bioptome
    Stanford b.
biopyoculture
bioradiography
biorational
biorbital
Biörck syndrome
Biörck-Thorson syndrome
bioresmethrin
bioreversible
biorgan
biorheology
biorhythm

bios
>   b. I
>   b. II
bioscience
biosis
biosmosis
biospectrometry
biospectroscopy
biosphere
biostatics
biostatistician
biostatistics
biostereometrics
biosynthesis
biosynthetic
Biot
>   breathing
>   breathing sign
>   respiration
>   sign
biota
biotaxis
biotechnology
biotelemetry
biothesiometer
biotic
biotics
biotinyl enzyme
biotoxication
biotoxicology
biotoxin
biotransformation
biotrepy
biotype
biotypology
Biox
bipalatinoid
BiPAP—bilateral positive airway
>   pressure
biparasitic
biparasitism
biparental
biparietal
>   b. suture
>   b. diameter
biparous
bipartite
biped
bipedal
bipennate
bipenniform
biperforate
biperiden
>   b. hydrochloride
>   b. lactate

biphasic
biphenyl
>   polychlorinated b. (PCB)
biplane angiocardiography, rapid
bipolar
>   b. affective psychosis
>   augmented b. limb leads
>   b. cautery
>   b. disorder
>   b. double bind
>   b. electrocardiogram (ECG,
>   EKG)
>   b. lead
>   b. limb lead
>   b. pacemaker
>   b. psychosis
>   b. version
bipolarity
bipositive
bipotential
bipotentiality
>   b. of the gonad
bipus
biramous
Birbeck granule
Bircher operation
Birch-Hirschfeld
>   entropion operation
>   lamp
Bird
>   formula
>   respirator
>   sign
bird-arm
bird-leg
bird-lime
birdshot
>   b. chorioretinopathy
>   b. retinochoroidopathy
bird's nest filter
birefractive
birefringence
>   crystalline b.
>   flow b.
>   form b.
>   intrinsic b.
>   strain b.
>   streaming b.
birefringent
birhinia
Birkett hernia
Birnberg bow
Birtcher
>   cautery
>   Hyfrecator cautery wire

B

birth
    breech b.
    dead b.
    immature b.
    live b.
    b. membranes
    multiple b.
    b. order
    b. palsy
    b. paralysis
    partial b.
    postterm b.
    premature b.
    spontaneous breech b.
    b. trauma
    viable b.
birthing
    alternative b.
    b. center
    b. chair
    b. room
birthmark
    port wine stain b.
    strawberry b.
birthweight tannex
bisacromial
bisalbuminemia
bisaxillary
bischloromethyl ether
Bischof
    corona
    crown
    myelotomy
    operation
    test
biscuit
    hard b.
    medium b.
    soft b.
biscuiting
bisection
bisegmentectomy
biseptate
bisexual
bisexuality
bisferious
Bishop
    score
    sphygmoscope
    tendon tucker
Bishop-Black tendon tucker
Bishop-Harmon
    anterior chamber irrigating
      cannula
    bladebreaker

Bishop-Harmon *(continued)*
    forceps
    Superblade
Bishop-Peter tendon tucker
bisiliac
bismuth subnitrate
bismuthia
bismuthism
bismuthosis
bisoxatin acetate
2,3-bisphosphoglycerate
bisphosphoglycerate mutase
bisphosphoglycerate phosphatase
bisphosphoglyceromutase
bispore
bisque
    hard b.
    high b.
    low b.
    medium b.
    soft b.
bistable
bistephanic
Biston
    B. betularia
bistoury
    b. blade
    Brophy b.
    Jackson b.
bistratal
bite
    balanced b.
    check b. (checkbite, check-bite)
    close b.
    closed b.
    convenience b.
    cross b. (crossbite, cross-bite)
    deep b.
    edge-to-edge b.
    end-to-end b.
    locked b.
    open b.
    over b.
    raised b.
    rest b.
    scissors b.
    stork b.
    underhung b.
    wax b.
    X-b.
biteblock, bite-block, bite block
bite gauge, bitegage, bite-gage
bitelock, bite-lock, bite lock
bitemporal
biteplate, bite-plate, bite plate

bite-rim, bite rim
biterminal
bitewing, bite-wing, bite wing
bithinolate sodium
bithionol
    b. sulfoxide
Bithynia fuchsiana
bitolterol mesylate
bitoric contact lens
Bitot
    patches
    spots
bitrochanteric
bitropic
bitter
bitters; bitter tonics
    aromatic b.
Bittner
    milk factor
    virus
Bittorf reaction
bituberal
bitumen
bituminosis
biurate
biuret
bivalency
    monogamous b.
bivalent
bivalve, bivalved
    b. incision
    b. speculum
biventer
    b. cervicis
biventral
biventricular
bixin
bizarre behavior
bizygomatic
Bizzarri-Giuffrida laryngoscope
Bizzozero
    cells
    corpuscles
    platelets
Bjerrum
    scotoma
    scotometer
    screen
    sign
Björk-Shiley
    aortic valve prosthesis
    convexoconcave 60-degree
     valve prosthesis
    floating-disk prosthesis
    heart valve

Björnstad syndrome
B-K—below-knee
β-ketoacyl-ACP reductase [beta-]
β-ketobutyric acid
β-keto-reductase
β-ketothiolase
BL—
    baseline
    blood loss
    buccolingual
black
    fat b. HB
    indulin b.
    ivory b.
    lamp b.
    Paris b.
    solvent b. 3
    Sudan b. B
Black [eponym] classification
Blackberg and Wanger test
black braided suture
Blackett-Healy position
Blackfan-Diamond
    anemia
    syndrome
blackfly
black hairy tongue
blackhead
black lung disease
blackout
black silk suture
blacksnake
black sunburst
Black-Wylie obstetric dilator
β-lactam antibiotic [beta-]
β-lactamase [beta-]
bladder
    allantoic b.
    atonic b.
    atonic neurogenic b.
    automatic b.
    autonomic b.
    autonomous b.
    b. blade
    chyle b.
    cord b.
    denervated b.
    dome of b.
    double b.
    encysted b.
    fasciculated b.
    b. flap
    gall b.
    hypertonic b.
    hypotonic b.

B

bladder *(continued)*
    ileocecal b.
    irritable b.
    motor paralytic b.
    nervous b.
    neurogenic b.
    nonreflex b.
    paralytic b.
    reflex b.
    sacculated b.
    sensory paralytic b.
    spastic b.
    spinal shock b.
    stammering b.
    tabetic b.
    trabeculated b.
    transurethral resection of b.
      (TURB)
    uninhibited neurogenic b.
    urinary b.
BladderScan
bladderworm
blade
    banana b.
    Bard-Parker b.
    Beaver b.
    Beaver-DeBakey b.
    bistoury b.
    bladder b.
    Cooley-Pontius b.
    DeBakey b.
    Macintosh b.
    Macintosh fiberoptic
      laryngoscope b.
    McPherson-Wheeler b.
    shoulder b.
    Superblade b.
bladebreaker knife
bladevent
Blainville ears
Blair
    cleft palate knife
    modification of Gellhorn pessary
    nasal chisel
    operation
    palate hook
    serrefine
    stiletto
Blair-Brown
    graft
    knife
    operation
Blake
    disk
    ear forceps

Blake *(continued)*
    embolus forceps
    forceps
    gallstone forceps
    uterine curet
Blakemore
    esophageal tube
    nasogastric tube
Blakemore-Sengstaken tube
Blakesley forceps
Blalock operation
Blalock-Hanlon operation
Blalock-Taussig
    operation
    shunt
blanc
Blanchard
    cryptotome
    hemorrhoidal forceps
    pile clamp
Blancophor
Blandin
    ganglion
    glands
Blandin and Nuhn gland
blanket
    hypothermic b.
    b. suture
blankophore
Blasius
    duct
    operation
Blaskovics operation
blast
    bechic b.
    b. chest
    b. effect
    lung b.
    b. transformation
blastid
blastide
blastochyle
blastocoele
blastocoelic
blastocyst
Blastocystis hominis
blastocyte
blastoderm
    bilaminar b.
    embryonic b.
    extraembryonic b.
    trilaminar b.
blastodermal
blastodermic
blastodisc

blastogenesis
blastogenic
blastogeny
blastokinin
blastolysis
blastolytic
blastoma
    pluricentric b.
    pulmonary b.
    unicentric b.
blastomatoid
blastomatosis
blastomatous
blastomere
    formative b.
blastomogenic
blastomogenous
Blastomyces
    B. brasiliensis
    B. coccidioides
    B. dermatitidis
blastomycete
blastomycetes
blastomycin
blastomycosis
    Brazilian b.
    cutaneous b.
    European b.
    keloidal b.
    North American b.
    South American b.
    systemic b.
blastomycotic
blastoneuropore
blastophthoria
blastophthoric
blastophyllum
blastophyly
blastopore
blastosphere
blastospore
blastostroma
blastozooid
blastula (blastulae)
blastular
blastulation
Blasucci
    curved-tip ureteral catheter
    pigtail ureteral catheter
Blatin
    sign
    syndrome
Blattella germanica
BLB—Boothby-Lovelace-Bulbulian
  (mask)

bleaching
    coronal b.
bleb
    filtering b.
    nuclear b.
    subpleural b.
bleeder
bleeding
    dysfunctional uterine b.
    implantation b.
    midcyclical b.
    occult b.
    placentation b.
    postmenopausal b.
    punctate b.
    summer b.
bleeding time
    Duke method b.t.
    Ivy method b.t.
blennadenitis
blennemesis
blennogenic
blennogenous
blennoid
blennorrhagia
blennorrhagic
blennorrhea
    b. adultorum
    inclusion b.
    b. neonatorum
    Stoerk b.
blennorrheal
blennostasis
blennostatic
blennothorax
blennuria
bleomycin sulfate
blepharadenitis
blepharal
blepharectomy
blepharelosis
blepharism
blepharitis
    b. angularis
    b. ciliaris
    b. marginalis
    nonulcerative b.
    seborrheic b.
    b. squamosa
    squamous b.
    b. ulcerosa
blepharoadenoma
blepharoatheroma
blepharochalasis
blepharochromidrosis

blepharoclonus
blepharocoloboma
blepharoconjunctivitis
blepharodiastasis
blepharon
blepharoncus
blepharopachynsis
blepharophimosis
blepharoplast
blepharoplasty
    Ammon b.
blepharoplegia
blepharoptosis
blepharopyorrhea
blepharorrhaphy
blepharospasm
    essential b.
    symptomatic b.
blepharosphincterectomy
blepharostat
blepharostenosis
blepharosynechia
blepharotomy
Blessig
    cysts
    groove
    lacunae
    spaces
Blessig-Iwanoff cysts
blind
    color b.
blindgut
blindism
blindness
    amnesic color b.
    apperceptive b.
    blue b.
    blue-yellow b.
    Bright b.
    central b.
    color b.
    concussion b.
    cortical b.
    cortical psychic b.
    day b.
    eclipse b.
    electric light b.
    epidemic b.
    flash b.
    flight b.
    functional b.
    green b.
    hysterical b.
    legal b.
    letter b.

blindness *(continued)*
    mind b.
    moon b.
    musical b.
    night b.
    note b.
    pure word b.
    red b.
    red-green b.
    river b.
    sign b.
    snow b.
    solar b.
    soul b.
    syllabic b.
    taste b.
    text b.
    total b.
    twilight b.
    word b.
    yellow b.
blink reflex
β-lipotropin
blister
    blood b.
    burn b.
    fever b.
    Marochetti b's
    water b.
BLM—buccal-lingual-masticatory
BLN—bronchial lymph nodes
bloat
bloater
    blue b.
Bloch
    method
    reaction
    scale
Bloch-Siemens-Sulzberger
    syndrome
Bloch-Stauffer syndrome
Bloch-Sulzberger syndrome
block
    adrenergic b.
    affect b.
    air b.
    alveolar-capillary b.
    anesthetic b.
    ankle b.
    anodal b.
    antegrade b.
    anterograde b.
    arborization b.
    articular b.
    Atkinson-type lid b.

block *(continued)*
- atrioventricular b.
- balsa wood b.
- Bier b.
- bite b. (biteblock, bite-block)
- brachial b.
- brachial plexus b.
- bundle-branch b.
- caudal b.
- cerebrospinal fluid b.
- cervical plexus b.
- comparator b.
- complete heart b.
- cryogenic b.
- dynamic b.
- ear b.
- elbow b.
- entrance b.
- epidural b.
- exit b.
- fascicular b.
- femoral b.
- field b.
- first-degree atrioventricular (AV) b.
- ganglionic b.
- heart b.
- incomplete heart b.
- infraorbital b.
- intercostal nerve b.
- interventricular b.
- intra-atrial b.
- intranasal b.
- intraspinal b.
- intravenous b.
- intraventricular b.
- lumbar plexus b.
- meningeal b.
- mental b.
- metabolic b.
- methadone b.
- nerve b.
- neuromuscular b.
- O'Brien b.
- b. osteotomy
- paracervical b.
- paraneural b.
- parasacral b.
- paravertebral b.
- partial b.
- perineural b.
- portal b.
- presacral b.
- pudendal b.

block *(continued)*
- regional b.
- b. resection
- retrobulbar b.
- sacral b.
- saddle b.
- sinoatrial b.
- sinus b.
- sphenopalatine b.
- spinal b.
- spinal subarachnoid b.
- splanchnic b.
- stellate b.
- subarachnoid b.
- sympathetic b.
- transsacral b.
- tubal b.
- uterosacral b.
- vagal b.
- vagus nerve b.
- van Lint b.
- ventricular b.
- vertebral b.
- Wilson b.
- wrist b.

blockade
- adrenergic b.
- adrenergic neuron b.
- alpha-b.
- alpha-adrenergic b.
- beta-b.
- beta-adrenergic b.
- cholinergic b.
- lymphatic b.
- narcotic b.
- neuromuscular b.
- renal b.
- reticuloendothelial b.
- sympathetic b.
- virus b.

blockage

blocker
- α-b.
- alpha-adrenergic b.
- alpha-adrenoceptor b.
- β-b. [beta-]
- bronchial b.
- calcium channel b.
- neuromuscular b.
- renin-angiotensin b.
- starch b.

blocking
- adrenergic b.
- thought b.

B

blockout
Blocq disease
Blom-Singer
    puncture
    valve
    voice prosthesis
Blondlot rays
blood
    arterial b.
    b. bank
    banked b.
    cord b.
    defibrinated b.
    deoxygenated b.
    laky b.
    occult b.
    oxalated b.
    peripheral b.
    sludged b.
    splanchnic b.
    strawberry-cream b.
    venous b.
    whole b.
blood bank
blood-brain barrier
blood flow study
    cerebral b.f.s.
    pulmonary b.f.s.
Bloodgood
    disease
    operation
blood group
    ABO b.
    Auberger b.
    Bombay b.
    Cartwright b.
    CDE b.
    Diego b.
    Dombrock b.
    Duffy b.
    high frequency b.
    Ii b.
    Kell b.
    Kidd b.
    Lewis b.
    low frequency b.
    Lutheran b.
    MNSs b.
    P b.
    Rh b.
    Sutter b.
    Xg b.
bloodless operation
bloodletting

blood patch
blood plasma
blood pool
    b.p. imaging
    b.p. scan
blood pressure
bloodroot
blood serum
    glycerin b.
    Loeffler (Löffler) b.s.
    Lorrain Smith b.s.
blood stream
blood type
blood volume measurements
bloom
Blot perforator
blotch
    palpebral b.
blotchy
blotting
    Northern b.
    Southern b.
    Western b.
Blount
    brace
    disease
    operation
    osteotome
    plate
    retractor
    stapler
blow
    diastolic b.
blow-by oxygen
blowfly
blow-in fracture
blown pupil
blow-out fracture
blowpipe
BLS—basic life support
blue
    alcian b.
    alizarin b.
    alkali b.
    aniline b.
    aniline b. WS
    anthracene b.
    azidine b.
    benzamine b.
    benzo b.
    Berlin b.
    b. bloater
    Borrel b.
    brilliant b. C

blue *(continued)*
    brilliant cresyl b.
    bromchlorphenol b.
    bromphenol b.
    bromthymol b.
    china b.
    chlorazol b.
    Congo b.
    cresyl b.
    cyanol b.
    diamine b.
    dianil b., H. 3 G.
    Evans b.
    Helvetia b.
    indigo b.
    indophenol b.
    isamine b.
    isosulfan b.
    Kühne methylene b.
    Löffler (Loeffler) methylene b.
    marine b.
    methylene b. O
    naphthamine b., 3 B. X.
    new methylene b., N.
    Niagara b.
    Nile b. A
    Nile b. sulfate
    polychrome methylene b.
    Prussian b.
    pyrrole b.
    quinaldine b.
    soluble indigo b.
    spirit b.
    sulfan b.
    Swiss b.
    tetrabromophenol b.
    thymol b.
    toluidine b.
    toluidine b. O
    trypan b.
    Victoria b.
    b. vitriol
    water b.
blue diaper syndrome
blue sclera
bluestone
Blumberg sign
Blumenau
    nucleus
    test
Blumenbach
    clivus
    plane
    process
Blumenthal disease

Blumer shelf
Blundell-Jones operation
blur
    spectacle b.
blurting
blush
    angiographic b.
    tumor b.
BM—
    body mass
    bone marrow
    bowel movement
    buccomesial
BMET—basic metabolic (panel, profile)
BMG—benign monoclonal gammopathy
BMI—body mass index
BMP—basic metabolic panel (profile)
BMR—basal metabolic rate
BMT—
    behavioral marital therapy
    bone marrow transplantation
BNA—Basle Nomina Anatomica
β-nicotyrine
BO—bucco-occlusal
BOA—British Orthopaedic Association
board
    alphabet b.
    angle b.
    back b.
    bed b.
    powder exercise b.
    spine b.
    transfer b.
board certified, board-certified
board eligible, board-eligible
Boari
    button
    flap
    operation
Boas
    algesimeter
    point
    sign
    test
    test meal
Boas-Oppler
    bacillus
    lactobacillus
Bobath method
bobbing

Bochdalek
    canal
    duct
    flower basket (flower basket of
      Bochdalek)
    foramen
    foramen (of Bochdalek) hernia
    ganglion
    gap
    hernia
    muscle
    nerve
    pseudoganglion
    sinus
    valve
Bock
    ganglion
    nerve
Bockhart impetigo
Bodansky unit
Bodechtel-Guttmann disease
Bodenheimer anoscope
bodenplatte
Bodian
    copper-Protargol stain
    method
Bodian-Schwachman syndrome
Bodo
    B. caudatus
    B. saltans
    B. urinaria
    B. urinarius
body (bodies)
    acetone b's
    adipose b. of cheek
    adipose b. of ischiorectal fossa
    adipose b. of orbit
    adrenal b.
    Alder-Reilly b's
    alkapton b's
    Amato b's
    amygdaloid b.
    amylaceous b's
    amyloid b's
    anococcygeal b.
    anti-immune b.
    aortic b's
    apical b.
    apoptotic b's
    b's of Arantius
    Arnold b's
    asbestos b's
    Aschoff b.
    asteroid b.
    Auer b.

body (bodies) *(continued)*
    bacillary b.
    Balbiani b.
    bamboo b's
    Barr b.
    Bartonia b.
    basal b.
    Behla b's
    Bence Jones b's
    Bichat fatty b. of cheek
    Bollinger b's
    Borrel b's
    Bracht-Wächter b's
    brassy b.
    bull's eye b.
    Cabot ring b.
    Call-Exner b.
    cancer b's
    carotid b.
    cavernous b. of clitoris
    cavernous b. of penis
    cell b.
    central fibrous b. of heart
    chromaffin b.
    chromatin b.
    chromatinic b.
    chromatoid b.
    chromophilous b's
    ciliary b.
    Civatte b.
    coccoid x b's
    coccygeal b.
    colloid b.
    colostrum b's
    compressible cavernous b.
    Councilman b's
    Cowdry intranuclear inclusion
      b. (type A, type B)
    Cowdry type I inclusion b's
    creola b.
    crystalloid b.
    cytoid b.
    cytomegalic inclusion b.
    cytoplasmic inclusion b.
    demilune b.
    dense b's
    Döhle (Doehle) inclusion b's
    Donné b's
    Donovan b.
    Dutcher b.
    elementary b.
    Elschnig b's
    Elzholz b.
    embryoid b.
    b. of epididymis

body (bodies) *(continued)*
- epithelial b.
- falciform b.
- fat b. of ischioanal fossa
- fatty b. of acetabular fossa
- fatty b. of orbit
- ferruginous b's
- fibrin b's of pleura
- filling b's
- foreign b.
- fruiting b.
- fuchsin b.
- b. of gallbladder
- Gamna-Favre b.
- Gamna-Gandy b.
- gastric b.
- geniculate b.
- geniculate b., lateral
- Giannuzzi b's
- glass b.
- glomus b.
- Golgi b.
- Gordon elementary b.
- Guarnieri b's
- habenular b.
- Halberstaedter-Prowazek b's
- Harting b's
- Hassall b's
- Hassall-Henle b's
- Heinz b.
- Heinz-Ehrlich b.
- hematoxylin b.
- Hensen b.
- Herring b's
- b. of Highmore
- Hirano b.
- Hollenhorst b.
- Howell b.
- Howell-Jolly b.
- hyaline b's
- hyaloid b.
- b. of hyoid bone
- b. of ilium
- immune b.
- inclusion b.
- infrapatellar fatty b.
- infundibular b.
- inner b's
- interrenal b.
- intravertebral b's
- b. of ischium
- Jaworski b's
- Joest b's
- Jolly b.
- jugular b.

body (bodies) *(continued)*
- jugulotympanic b.
- juxtaglomerular b.
- juxtarestiform b.
- ketone b.
- Kurloff b's
- Kurlov b's
- Lafora b's
- Lallemand b's
- Lallemand-Trousseau b's
- Laveran b.
- LCL b's
- Leishman-Donovan b.
- Levinthal-Coles-Lillie b's
- Lewy b's
- Lieutaud b.
- Lindner initial b's
- Lipschütz (Lipschuetz) b.
- Lostorfer b's
- Luschka b.
- b. of Luys
- lyssa b's
- Mallory b.
- malpighian b.
- malpighian b's of kidney
- malpighian b's of spleen
- mamillary b.
- mammillary b.
- b. of mandible
- Marchal b's
- Masson b's
- b. of maxilla
- medullary b.
- melon seed b.
- metachromatic b's
- Michaelis-Gutmann b's
- mitochondrial b.
- Miyagawa b.
- molluscum b's
- Mooser b's
- Mott b's
- multilamellar b.
- multivesicular b.
- Negri b.
- Neill-Mooser b's
- nemaline b's
- nigroid b.
- Nissl b.
- Nothnagel b's
- no-threshold b's
- Odland b.
- Oken b.
- olivary b.
- onion b's
- orbital fat b.

body (bodies) *(continued)*
    oryzoid b's
    pacchionian b
    pampiniform b.
    b. of pancreas
    Pappenheimer b's
    para-aortic b's
    parabasal b.
    paraphysial b.
    pararenal fat b.
    paraterminal b.
    parathyroid b.
    parietal b.
    parolivary b's
    Paschen b's
    pearly b's
    penile b.
    perineal b.
    pheochrome b.
    Pick b's
    pineal b.
    pituitary b.
    platelet dense b.
    Plimmer b's
    polar b's
    postbranchial b's
    presegmenting b's
    Prowazek b's
    Prowazek-Greeff b.
    psammoma b.
    psittacosis inclusion b.
    b. of pubis
    purine b's
    pyknotic b's
    quadrigeminal b's
    b. of radius
    Reilly b's
    Renaut b's
    residual b.
    residual b. of Regaud
    restiform b.
    reticulate b.
    b. of Retzius
    b. of rib
    rice b's
    Ross b's
    Russell b.
    sand b's
    Sandström b's
    Savage perineal b.
    Schaumann b's
    Schmorl b.
    Seidelin b's
    semilunar b's
    b. of sphenoid

body (bodies) *(continued)*
    spongy b.
    b. of sternum
    Stieda b.
    b. of stomach
    striate b.
    suprarenal b.
    b. of sweat gland
    Symington b.
    b. of talus
    telobranchial b's
    threshold b's
    thyroid b.
    b. of tibia
    tigroid b's
    tingible b.
    Todd b.
    b. of tongue
    Torres-Teixeira b's
    trachoma b's
    trapezoid b.
    Trousseau-Lallemand b's
    turbinated b.
    tympanic b.
    b. of ulna
    ultimobranchial b's
    b. of uterus
    vagal b's
    vermiform b's
    Verocay b's
    vertebral b., body of vertebra
    b. of Vicq d'Azyr
    Virchow-Hassall b.
    vitelline b.
    vitreous b.
    Winkler b's
    wolffian b.
    xanthine b's
    X chromatin b.
    yellow b. of ovary
    zebra b.
    Zuckerkandl b's
body rocking
body section
    b.s. radiography
    b.s. roentgenography
Boeck
    disease
    itch
    sarcoid, sarcoidosis
    scabies
Boehm
    anoscope
    proctoscope
    sigmoidoscope

Boerhaave
  sweat glands
  syndrome
boggy
  b. mucous membranes
  b. prostate
  b. uterus
Bogros space
Bogrov fiber
Böhler
  calcaneal angle
  clamp
  splint
Böhler-Braun splint
Bohlman pin
Böhm (Boehm) operation
Bohr
  atom
  effect
  equation
  isopleth method
  magneton
  radius
  theory
Boies forceps
boil
  Aleppo b.
  Baghdad b.
  Biskra b.
  blind b.
  Delhi b.
  gum b.
  Jericho b.
  Madura b.
  Oriental b.
  salt water b.
  sea water b.
  shoe b.
boldenone undecylenate
boldine
boldo
bolenol
Boletus satanas
Bolk retardation theory
Bollinger
  bodies
  granules
bolometer
bolster suture
Bolt sign
bolt
  Webb b.
  Wilson b.
Bolton
  plane

Bolton *(continued)*
  point
  triangle
Bolton-nasion
  line
  plane
bolus
  b. alba
  alimentary b.
  b. dressing
BOM—bilateral otitis media
bomb
bombard
bombardment
bombé
bombesin
bombicesterol
bombykol
Bombyx mori
Bonaccolto
  forceps
  scleral ring
Bonaccolto-Flieringa operation
bond
  conjugated double b's
  coordinate covalent b.
  covalent b.
  disulfide b.
  energy rich b.
  glycosidic b's
  high-energy b.
  high-energy phosphate b.
  high-energy sulfur b.
  hydrogen b.
  hydrophobic b.
  ionic b.
  isopeptide b.
  pair b.
  peptide b.
  phosphodiester b.
  pi b.
  sigma b.
  van der Waals b.
Bond [eponym]
  forceps
  splint
bonding
  direct b.
  tooth b.
Bondy
  mastoidectomy
  operation
bone
  accessory b.
  acetabular b.

bone *(continued)*
- acromial b.
- b. age
- alar b.
- Albers-Schönberg (Albers-Schoenberg) b.
- Albers-Schönberg marble b's
- Albrecht b.
- alisphenoid b.
- alveolar b.
- ankle b.
- astragaloid b.
- astragaloscaphoid b.
- basal b.
- basihyal b.
- basilar b.
- basioccipital b.
- basiotic b.
- basisphenoid b.
- Bertin b.
- blade b.
- breast b.
- bregmatic b.
- Breschet b.
- brittle b.
- bundle b.
- calcaneal b.
- calf b.
- cancellated b.
- cancellous b.
- capitate b.
- carpal b.
- cartilage b.
- cavalry b.
- central b.
- b. of cerebral cranium
- chalky b.
- cheek b.
- b. clamp
- coccygeal b.
- collar b.
- compact b.
- b. conduction
- cortical b.
- costal b.
- cotyloid b.
- cranial b.
- b's of cranium
- cribriform b.
- cuboid b.
- cuckoo b.
- cuneiform b.
- b.-cutting forceps
- b. depression
- dermal b.

bone *(continued)*
- ectethmoid b.
- ectocuneiform b.
- endochondral b.
- entocuneiform b.
- epactal b.
- epactal b., proper
- epihyal b.
- epipteric b.
- episternal b.
- ethmoid b.
- exercise b.
- exoccipital b.
- exocranial wormian b.
- facial b's
- femoral b.
- fetal b.
- fibular b.
- flank b.
- flat b.
- Flower b.
- b. forceps
- frontal b.
- funny b.
- Goethe b.
- hamate b.
- haunch b.
- b. head
- heterotopic b.
- humeral b.
- hyoid b.
- iliac b.
- inca b.
- incarial b.
- incisive b.
- innominate b.
- intermaxillary b.
- intermediate b.
- interparietal b.
- intrachondrial b.
- irregular b.
- ischial b.
- ivory b.
- jaw b., lower
- jaw b., upper
- jugal b.
- Krause b.
- lacrimal b.
- lamellated b.
- lenticular b.
- lenticular b. of hand
- lentiform b.
- lingual b.
- long b.
- lunate b.

bone *(continued)*
  malar b.
  marble b's
  mastoid b.
  maxillary b.
  maxillary b., inferior
  maxillary b., superior
  maxilloturbinal b.
  membrane b.
  mesethmoid b.
  mesocuneiform b.
  metacarpal b.
  metatarsal b.
  mosaic b.
  multangular b.
  multangular b., accessory
  multangular b., larger
  multangular b., smaller
  nasal b.
  navicular b.
  navicular b. of foot
  navicular b. of hand
  b.-nibbling forceps
  nonlamellated b.
  occipital b.
  odontoid b.
  orbital b.
  orbitosphenoidal b.
  palatine b.
  parietal b.
  pelvic b.
  perichondral b.
  periosteal b.
  petrous b.
  phalangeal b.
  Pirie b.
  pisiform b.
  b. plug
  pneumatic b.
  postsphenoidal b.
  postulnar b.
  prefrontal b.
  preinterparietal b.
  premaxillary b.
  presphenoidal b.
  primary b.
  primitive b.
  b. processes
  pterygoid b.
  pubic b.
  pyramidal b.
  radial b.
  replacement b.
  resurrection b.
  reticulated b.

bone *(continued)*
  rider's b.
  Riolan b's
  rudimentary b.
  sacral b.
  b. scan
  scaphoid b.
  scapular b.
  scroll b's
  secondary b.
  secondary cuboid b.
  b. seeker
  semilunar b.
  septal b.
  sesamoid b.
  sesamoid b. of lateral head of
    gastrocnemius muscle
  shank b.
  shin b.
  short b.
  shoulder b.
  sieve b.
  solid b.
  sphenoid b.
  sphenoturbinal b.
  splint b's
  spongy b.
  squamo-occipital b.
  squamosal b.
  squamous b.
  subperiosteal b.
  substitution b.
  supernumerary b.
  suprainterparietal b.
  supraoccipital b.
  suprapharyngeal b.
  suprasternal b's
  supreme ethmoid b.
  supreme nasal b.
  sutural b.
  tabular b.
  tarsal b.
  temporal b.
  tibia b.
  tongue b.
  trabecular b.
  trapezium b.
  trapezoid b.
  trapezoid b. of Henle
  trapezoid b. of Lyser
  triangular b.
  triquetral b.
  turbinate b.
  tympanic b.
  ulna b.

bone *(continued)*
    ulnar b.
    ulnar carpal b.
    ulnar styloid b.
    unciform b.
    uncinate b.
    vesalian b.
    vomer b.
    b. wax
    whettle b.
    whirl b.
    wormian b.
    woven b.
    xiphoid b.
    zygomatic b.
bone graft
    diamond inlay b.g.
    dual inlay b.g.
    hemicylindrical b.g.
    inlay b.g.
    intramedullary b.g.
    medullary b.g.
    onlay b.g.
    osteoperiosteal b.g.
    peg b.g.
    sliding inlay b.g.
bonelet
bone marrow
    b.m. scanning
    b.m. transplant
Bonhoeffer
    sign
    symptom
Bonine bone
Bonn forceps
Bonner position
bonnet
    gluteal b.
Bonnet [eponym]
    capsule
    sign
    syndrome
Bonnet-Dechaume-Blanc
  syndrome
Bonnevie-Ullrich syndrome
Bonney
    clamp
    forceps
    hysterectomy
    test
Bonnier syndrome
Bonnot gland
Bonwill
    crown
    triangle

bony
    b. island
    b. processes
    b. prominence
    b. suture
Bonzel operation
Boo-Chai craniofacial cleft
BOOP—bronchiolitis obliterans
    organizing pneumonia
Boorman gastric cancer typing
    system (I–IV)
booster
boot
    air b.
    bunny b.
    gelatin compression b.
    Gibney b.
    Jobst b.
    moon b.
    pneumatic b.
    Unna b.
    Unna paste b.
Boothby mask
borate
borated
borax
borborygmus (borborygmi)
bordeaux B
border
    b. of acetabulum
    alveolar b. of mandible
    alveolar b. of maxilla
    anterior b.
    brush b.
    denture b.
    b. detection method
    external b. of tibia
    inferior b. of mandible
    interosseous b.
    lacrimal b.
    lambdoid b.
    lateral b.
    left b. of cardiac dullness
    medial b.
    mucocutaneous b.
    orbital b. of sphenoid bone
    b. of oval fossa
    peripheral b.
    posterointernal b. of fibula
    superior b. of patella
    vermilion b.
borderline
Bordetella
    B. bronchiseptica
    B. parapertussis

Bordetella (continued)
    B. pertussis
Bordet-Gengou
    agar
    bacillus
    culture medium
    phenomenon
    reaction
Bordier-Fränkel sign
borism
Bornholm disease
Born method
bornyl salicylate
borocain
boron (B)
    b. carbide
Borrelia
    B. afzelii
    B. anserina
    B. berbera
    B. buccalis
    B. burgdorferi
    B. carteri
    B. caucasica
    B. crocidurae
    B. duttonii
    B. garinii
    B. hermsii
    B. hispanica
    B. kochii
    B. latyschewii
    B. mazzottii
    B. neotropicalis
    B. parkeri
    B. persica
    B. recurrentis
    B. refringens
    B. theileri
    B. turicatae
    B. venezuelensis
    B. vincentii
borreliosis
Borrmann
    classification
    gastric cancer typing system
      (types I–IV)
Borsieri
    line
    sign
Borthen operation
Bose
    operation
    tracheostomy hook
Bosher knife

boss
    frontal b.
    parietal b.
    sanguineous b.
Bossalino operation
bosselated
bosselation
bossing of cranium
Bostock
    catarrh
    disease
Boston sign
Bosworth
    coracoclavicular screw
    nasal snare
    operation
    procedure
bot
Botallo
    duct
    foramen
    ligament
botanic
botany
    medical b.
botfly
bothridium
bothriocephaliasis
Bothriocephalus
    B. mansoni
    B. mansonoides
bothrium (bothria)
bothropic
Bothrops atrox
botogenin
botryoid
botryomycoma
botryomycosis
botryomycotic
botrytimycosis
Botrytis bassiana
Böttcher (Boettcher)
    canal
    cells
    crystals
    forceps
    ganglion
    hook
    scissors
    space
bottle
    Castaneda b.
    Junker b.
    spritz b.

bottle *(continued)*
    wash b.
    Woulfe b.
bottom
bottromycin
botuliform
botulin
botulinal
botulinogenic
botulism
    food-borne b.
    infant b.
    wound b.
bouba
Bouchard
    coefficient
    disease
    nodes
    nodules
    sign
Bouchardat
    test
    treatment
bouche de tapir
Boucheron speculum
Bouchut
    respiration
    laryngeal tube
    tubes
boufée délirante
bougie
    b. á boule
    acorn-tipped b.
    bulbous b.
    common duct b.
    conic b.
    coudé b.
    cylindrical b.
    dilating b.
    elastic b.
    elbowed b.
    filiform b.
    fusiform b.
    Hurst b.
    Jackson b.
    Le Fort b.
    Maloney b's
    olive-tip b., olive-tipped b.
    Otis b.
    Phillips b.
    Plummer b.
    polyvinyl b.
    Ruschelit b.
    soluble b.

bougie *(continued)*
    Trousseau b.
    tunneled b.
    wax-tipped b.
    whip b.
    whistle b.
bougienage
Bouillaud
    disease
    sign
    syndrome
    tinkle
bouillon
Bouin
    fixative
    fluid
    solution
boundary
    ego b.
bouquet of Riolan
Bourgery ligament
Bourneville
    disease
    phakomatosis
    syndrome
Bourneville-Brissaud disease
Bourneville-Pringle syndrome
bout
bouton
    b. de Baghdad
    b. de Biskra
    b. d' Orient
    b. en chemise
    b. en passage
    b. en passant
boutonneuse
boutonniére
Bouveret
    disease
    syndrome
    tachycardia
Bouveret-Duguet ulcer
bovied
Bovie unit
bovine heterograft
bow
    Birnberg b.
    Cupid's b.
    hypochordal b.
    labial b.
    Logan b.
Bowditch
    effect
    law

Bowditch *(continued)*
 phenomenon
bowel
 gangrenous b.
 greedy b.
 b. movement (BM)
 b. obstruction
 b. sounds
Bowen
 disease
 osteotome
 precancerous dermatosis
Bowen-Grover
 meniscotome
 meniscotomy
bowenoid
bowie
bowl
 mastoid b.
 mastoidectomy b.
Bowlby splint
bowleg
 nonrachitic b.
bowlegged
Bowman
 capsule
 disks
 eye knife
 glands
 iris needle
 iris scissors
 lacrimal dilator
 lacrimal probe
 lamina
 membrane
 muscle
 needle
 operation
 probe
 space
 strabismus scissors
 theory
 tubes
box
 anatomical snuff-b.
 Bárány b.
 black b.
 brain b.
 CAT b.
 glove b.
 Hogness b.
 homeo b.
 hot air b.
 obstruction b.

box *(continued)*
 Pribnow b.
 Skinner b.
 Stockholm b.
 TATA b.
 voice b.
 Yerkes discrimination b.
boxcarring
boxidine
boxing
box-note
Boyce
 position
 sign
Boyd
 implant
 operation
Boyden
 sphincter
 test
 test meal
Boyer
 bursa
 cyst
Boyes-Goodfellow hook
Boyle law
Boynton needle holder
Boys-Allis forceps
Bozeman
 catheter
 forceps
 operation
 position
 speculum
 suture
Bozeman-Fritsch catheter
Bozzolo sign
bp—base pair
BP—
 bathroom privileges
 birthplace
 blood pressure
b.p.—boiling point
BPA—British Paediatric
 Association
BPD—biparietal diameter
B Ph—British Pharmacopoeia
BPH—
 benign prostatic hyperplasia
 benign prostatic hypertrophy
BPIG—bacterial polysaccharide
 immune globulin
bpm—beats per minute
Bq—becquerel(s)

Braasch
- bulb catheter
- cystoscope
- forceps

brace
- Bledsoe b.
- Blount b.
- Boston b.
- chair-back b.
- clam-shell b.
- drop foot b.
- Fisher b.
- 49'er knee b.
- Goldthwait b.
- Hudson b.
- ischial weightbearing (weight-bearing) b.
- Jewett b.
- Jones b.
- Klenzak b.
- Knight b.
- Knight-Taylor b.
- Kydex b.
- Lenox Hill b.
- long leg b.
- LSU reciprocation–gait orthosis b.
- Lyman-Smith b.
- McKee b.
- Milwaukee b.
- Moe b.
- Roylan tibia fracture b.
- Seton hip b.
- Taylor b.
- toe drop b.
- UBC (University of British Columbia) b.
- weightbearing (weight-bearing) b.

bracelet
- Nageotte b's

Brachet mesolateral fold
brachia (plural of brachium)
brachial
brachialgia statica paresthetica
brachial plexus
brachiation
brachiform
brachiocephalic arteriography
brachiocrural
brachiocubital
brachiocyllosis
brachiocyrtosis
brachiofaciolingual

brachiogram
brachio-thoraco-omphalo-ischiopagus bipus
brachium (brachia)
- anterior conjunctival b.
- b. cerebelli
- b. cerebri
- b. colliculi inferioris
- b. colliculi superioris
- b. of colliculus
- b. conjunctivum
- b. conjunctivum cerebelli
- b. of inferior colliculus
- b. of mesencephalon
- b. opticum
- b. pontis
- b. quadrigeminum
- b. of superior colliculus

Brachmann-de Lange syndrome
Bracht maneuver
Bracht-Wachter lesion
brachybasia
brachycephalic
brachycephaly
brachycheilia
brachychronic
brachycranic
brachydactyly
brachydontia
brachyesophagus
brachyfacial
brachyglossal
brachygnathia
brachygnathous
brachykerkic
brachyknemic
brachymetacarpia
brachymetapody
brachymetatarsia
brachymetropia
brachymetropic
brachymorphic
brachyphalangia
brachypodous
brachyrhinia
brachyrhyncus
brachyskelous
brachystaphyline
brachystasis
brachytherapy
- interstitial b.
- intracavitary application b.
- remote afterloading b.

brachyuranic

bracing
Bracken forceps
bracket
Brackin
    incision
    ureterointestinal anastomosis
      technique
    technique
bract
Bradford
    forceps
    frame
Bradley disease
Bradshaw-O'Neill clamp
bradyacusia
bradyauxesis
bradycardia
    Branham b.
    cardiomuscular b.
    central b.
    clinostatic b.
    essential b.
    fetal b.
    nodal b.
    physiologic b.
    postinfective b.
    sinoatrial b.
    sinus b. (SB)
    true b.
    vagal b.
bradycardiac
bradycrotic
bradydiastole
bradyecoia
bradyesthesia
bradygenesis
bradyglossia
bradykinesia
bradykinetic
bradykinin
bradylalia
bradylexia
bradylogia
bradymenorrhea
bradyphagia
bradyphasia
bradyphrasia
bradyphrenia
bradypnea
bradypragia
bradyrhythmia
bradyspermatism
bradytachycardia
bradyteleokinesis
bradytocia

bradytrophia
bradytrophic
bradyuria
bradyzoite
Bragard sign
Bragg
    curve
    peak
Bragg-Paul pulsator
braided
    black b. suture
    b. suture
    white b. suture
Braid strabismus
Brailey operation
braille
Brain [eponym]
    airway
    quadrupedal reflex
    reflex
brain
    b. abscess
    base of b.
    b. cicatrix
    cyclopean b.
    b. death
    b. disorder
    hernia of b.
    isolated b.
    b. laceration
    organic b. syndrome
    b. pressure
    primitive b.
    b. purpura
    b. sand
    b. scan
    b. scanning
    softening of the b.
    b. stem
    b. swelling
    b. syndrome
    b. wave
brain-damaged
brain-dead
brain death protocol
    electroencephalogram (EEG)
brain stem
    b.s. auditory evoked potential
      (BAEP)
    b.s. crisis
    b.s. evoked response (BSER)
    b.s. evoked response (BSER)
      audiometry
    b.s. infarction
    b.s. ischemia

B

brainwashing
braking radiation
branch
  branches of bundle of His
  gluteal b. of MacAlister
  left bundle b.
  right bundle b.
  branches of suprascapular
    artery
  sural communicating b.
  thenar b. of median nerve
  branches of vertebral
    artery
branched-chain α-keto acid
  dehydrogenase [alpha-]
branched-chain 2-keto acid
  dehydrogenase
brancher deficiency
brancher enzyme, branching
  enzyme
branchial
  b. arch
  b. cleft
branching
  b. decay
  b. fraction
  b. ratio
branching enzyme
branchiogenic
branchiogenous
branchioma
branchiomere
branchiomeric
branchiomerism
branch vein occlusion
Brand bath
Brandt
  brassiere
  syndrome
  technique
  treatment
Brandt-Andrews maneuver
Branham
  bradycardia
  sign
Branhamella catarrhalis
Brant aluminum splint
Brantley-Turner retractor
brash
  water b.
  weaning b.
Brassica
  B. napus
  B. nigra
brassidic acid

brassiere
  Brandt b.
  b.-type dressing
BRAT—bananas, rice cereal,
  applesauce, toast (diet)
Brauer operation
Braun
  anastomosis
  canal
  cranioclast
  graft
  hook
  operation
  scissors
  tenaculum
  von Ferwald sign
Braune
  canal
  muscle
  valve
  vein
Braun-Fernwald (Braun-von
  Fernwald) sign
Braun and Jaboulay
  gastroenterostomy
Braunwald
  prosthesis
  sign
Braun-Wangensteen
  graft
  operation
Bravais-jacksonian epilepsy
Brawley retractor
brawny
  b. edema
  b. induration
Braxton-Hicks
  contraction
  sign
  version
brayera
brazilin
breach
breadth
  b. of accommodation
  bizygomatic b.
break
  chromatid b.
  isochromatid b.
  single chain b.
  single strand b.
breakage and reunion
breakdown
  nervous b.
breakoff

breast
  broken b.
  caked b.
  chicken b.
  Cooper irritable b.
  cystic b.
  funnel b.
  gathered b.
  keeled b.
  pigeon b.
  proemial b.
  shoemakers' b.
  shotty b.
  supernumerary b.
  thrush b.
breast-fed
breast-feed, breast-feeds
breast-feeding
breath
  bad b.
  lead b.
  liver b.
  saturnine b.
Breathalyzer
breath-holding
  blue b.
  white b.
breathiness
breathing
  apneustic b.
  ataxic b.
  autonomous b.
  Biot b.
  bronchial b.
  Cheyne-Stokes b.
  cogwheel b.
  continuous positive-pressure
    b. (CPPB)
  diaphragmatic b.
  frog b.
  glossopharyngeal b.
  intermittent positive-pressure
    b. (IPPB)
  Kussmaul b.
  labored b.
  mouth-to-mouth b.
  periodic b.
  shallow b.
  suppressed b.
  vesicular b.
breathless
breathlessness
breathy
Breda disease
bredouillement

breech
  complete b.
  b. delivery
  b. extraction
  frank b.
  incomplete b.
  b. presentation
  single footling b.
breeder reactor
breeding
  random b.
  selective b.
  b. true
bregma
bregmatic
bregmatodymia
bregmatomastoid suture
Brehmer
  method
  treatment
brei
Breisky
  disease
  pelvimeter
bremsstrahlung
Brennemann syndrome
Brenner
  nodules
  oophoroma folliculare
  operation
  tumor
Brent eyebrow reconstruction
brephic
brephoplastic
brephotrophic
Breschet
  bones
  canals
  hiatus
  sinus
  veins
Brescia-Cimino fistula
Breslow
  classification
  thickness
Bretonneau
  angina
  disease
Brett operation
Breus mole
Brevibacterium linens
brevicollis
breviflexor
brevilineal
breviradiate

Brewer
   infarcts
   point
   speculum
brewer's yeast
Brewster retractor
Bricker operation
bridge
   anaphase b.
   arteriolovenular b.
   Bellevue b.
   cantilever b.
   cell b's
   chromatid b.
   chromosome b.
   conjugative b.
   cytoplasmic b.
   dentin b.
   disulfide b.
   extension b.
   fixed b.
   fixed b. with rigid
      connectors
   fixed b. with rigid and
      nonrigid connectors
   fixed-fixed b.
   fixed-movable b.
   b. flap
   Gaskell b.
   intercellular b.
   malleus-footplate b.
   malleus-stapes b.
   protoplasmic b.
   removable b.
   salt b.
   stationary b.
   tarsal b.
   b. of the nose
   ureteric b.
   b. of Varolius
   Wheatstone b.
bridgework
   fixed b.
   removable b.
bridging
   myocardial b.
   b. osteophytes
bridle suture
bridou
Briggs
   law
   operation
Bright
   blindness
   disease

Bright (continued)
   eye
   murmur
brightfield
bright-field microscopy
brightic
brightism
Brill disease
Brill-Zinsser disease
brim
Brinkerhoff
   anoscope
   rectal speculum
Brinton disease
Brion-Kayser disease
Briquet
   ataxia
   syndrome
brisement forcé
Brissaud
   dwarf
   infantilism
   reflex
   scoliosis
Brissaud-Marie syndrome
Brissaud-Sicard syndrome
Bristow
   operation
   periosteal elevator
   procedure
Bristowe syndrome
Brittain operation
brittle diabetes
broach
   barbed b.
   pathfinder b.
   root-canal b.
   smooth b.
broad-beam scattering
Broadbent
   apoplexy
   inverted sign
   law
   sign
Broadbent-Bolton plane
Broca
   amnesia
   aphasia
   area
   ataxia
   band
   center
   convolution
   convolution fissure
   fissure

Broca *(continued)*
    formula
    gyrus
    motor speech area of the brain
    plane
    point
    pouch
    region
    space
Brock
    incision
    infundibulectomy
    knife
    punch
    syndrome
Brockenbrough
    catheter
    sign
Brockman operation
Brocq
    disease
    erythrose péribuccale
      pigmentaire
    lupoid sycosis
    pseudopelade
Brödel (Broedel)
    bloodless line
    white line
Broden position
Broders
    classification
    index (1–4)
Brodie
    abscess
    disease
    knee
    ligament
Brodmann areas
Brodney clamp
Broesike fossa
bromated
bromatology
bromatotherapy
bromatotoxin, bromatotoxismus
bromatoxism
bromhidrosis
bromic
bromide
    hydrogen b.
    methyl b.
bromidism
brominated
bromindione
bromine (Br)
brominized

bromism
bromisovalum
bromization
bromized
bromobenzene
bromoiodism
bromomania
bromomenorrhea
bromomethane
bromophos
bromopnea
brompheniramine maleate
bromphenol blue
Brompton
    cocktail
    mixture
    solution
bromsalans
bromsulphalein
bromthymol blue
bromurated
bromuret
bronchadenitis
bronchi (plural of bronchus)
bronchia (plural of bronchium)
bronchial
    b. adenoma
    b. brushing
    b. challenge test
    b. circulation
    b. lavage
    b. obstruction
    b. reactivity
    b. stenosis
    b. tube
bronchiarctia
bronchiectasis
    capillary b.
    chemical b.
    cylindrical b.
    cystic b.
    dry b.
    follicular b.
    pseudocylindrical b.
    saccular b.
bronchiectatic
bronchiloquy
bronchiocele
bronchiocrisis
bronchiolar
    b. lavage
    b. stenoses
bronchiole
    alveolar b.
    lobular b.

bronchiole *(continued)*
    respiratory b.
    terminal b.
bronchiolectasis
bronchioli (plural of bronchiolus)
bronchiolitis
    acute obliterating b.
    b. exudativa
    b. fibrosa obliterans
    vesicular b.
    viral b.
bronchioloalveolar
bronchiolus (bronchioli)
    acute obliterating b.
    bronchioli exudativa
    bronchioli respiratorii
    vesicular b.
bronchitic
bronchitis
    acute b.
    acute laryngotracheal b.
    acute suppurative b.
    arachidic b.
    asthmatic b.
    capillary b.
    Castellani b.
    catarrhal b.
    cheesy b.
    chronic b.
    chronic obstructive b.
    croupous b.
    dry b.
    epidemic capillary b.
    ether b.
    exudative b.
    fibrinous b.
    hemorrhagic b.
    infectious asthmatic b.
    laryngotracheal b.
    mechanic b.,
      mechanical b.
    membranous b.
    b. obliterans
    parasitic b.
    phthinoid b.
    plastic b.
    polypoid b.
    productive b.
    pseudomembranous b.
    putrid b.
    secondary b.
    staphylococcal b.
    streptococcal b.
    suffocative b.
    summer b.

bronchitis *(continued)*
    vanadium b.
    vesicular b.
bronchium (bronchia)
bronchoadenitis
bronchoalveolar lavage
bronchoalveolitis
bronchoaspergillosis
bronchobiliary
bronchoblastomycosis
bronchoblennorrhea
bronchocandidiasis
bronchocavernous
bronchocavitary
bronchocele
bronchocentric granulomatosis
bronchoconstriction
bronchoconstrictor
bronchodilatation
bronchodilation
bronchodilator
bronchoegophony
bronchoesophageal fistula
bronchoesophagology
bronchoesophagoscopy
bronchofiberscope
bronchofibroscopy
bronchogenic
bronchogram
    air b.
    tantalum b.
bronchographic
bronchography
    Cope-method b.
    percutaneous transtracheal b.
broncholith
broncholithiasis
bronchologic
bronchology
bronchomalacia
bronchomoniliasis
bronchomotor
bronchomucotropic
bronchomycosis
bronchonocardiosis
broncho-oidiosis
bronchopancreatic fistula
bronchopathy
bronchophony
    pectoriloquous b.
    sniffling b.
    whispered b.
bronchoplasty
bronchoplegia
bronchopleural

bronchopleuropneumonia
bronchopneumonia
    inhalation b.
    postoperative b.
    subacute b.
    virus b.
bronchopneumonic
bronchopneumonitis
bronchopneumopathy
bronchopulmonary
    b. aspergillosis
    b. dysplasia
    b. lavage
    b. markings
bronchoradiography
bronchorrhagia
bronchorrhaphy
bronchorrhea
bronchoscope
    ACMI b.
    Albert b.
    Broyles b.
    Bruening b.
    Chevalier Jackson b.
    coagulation b.
    costophrenic b.
    Davis b.
    double-channel irrigating b.
    Emerson b.
    fiberoptic b.
    Foregger b.
    Haslinger b.
    Holinger b.
    Holinger-Jackson b.
    hook-on b.
    Jackson b.
    Jesberg b.
    Moersch b.
    Negus b.
    Overholt-Jackson b.
    Pilling b.
    Riecker b.
    Safar b.
    Staple b.
    Storz b.
    telescope b.
    Tucker b.
    ventilation b.
    Waterman b.
    Yankauer b.
bronchoscopic
bronchoscopy
    fiberoptic b.
    nonfiberoptic b.
bronchosinusitis

bronchospasm
bronchospirochetosis
bronchospirography
bronchospirometer
bronchospirometry
    differential b.
bronchostaxis
bronchostenosis
bronchostomy
bronchotome
bronchotomy
bronchotracheal
bronchovesicular
bronchus (bronchi)
    anterior basal segmental b.
    anterior segmental b.
    anteromedial basal
      segmental b.
    apical b.
    apical segmental b.
    apicoposterior segmental b.
    cardiac b.
    bronchi cardiacus
    dorsal b.
    eparterial b.
    esophageal b.
    extrapulmonary b.
    hyparterial b.
    inferior lingular b.
    intermediate b.
    intrapulmonary b.
    intrasegmental bronchi
    bronchi intrasegmentales
    lateral basal segmental b.
    lateral segmental b.
    left inferior lobar b.
    left main b.
    left primary b.
    left superior lobar b.
    left superior ventral b.
    lingular b.
    b. lingularis
    b. lingularis inferior
    b. lingularis superior
    lobar b.
    bronchi lobares
    b. lobaris inferior dexter
    b. lobaris inferior sinister
    b. lobaris medius
    b. lobaris superior dexter
    b. lobaris superior sinister
    lower lobe b.
    main bronchi, right and left
    main stem b.
    medial basal segmental b.

B

bronchus (bronchi) *(continued)*
    medial segmental b.
    middle lobar b.
    middle lobe b.
    posterior basal segmental b.
    posterior segmental b.
    primary bronchi, right and left
    b. principalis dexter
    b. principalis sinister
    right inferior lobar b.
    right main b.
    right primary b.
    right superior lobar b.
    right ventral b.
    secondary bronchi
    segmental bronchi
    bronchi segmentales
    b. segmentalis anterior
    b. segmentalis apicalis
    b. segmentalis apicoposterior
    b. segmentalis basalis
    b. segmentalis basalis anterior
    b. segmentalis basalis lateralis
    b. segmentalis basalis medialis
    b. segmentalis basalis posterior
    b. segmentalis lateralis
    b. segmentalis medialis
    b. segmentalis posterior
    b. segmentalis superior
    stem b.
    subapical b.
    superior lingular b.
    superior segmental b.
    tracheal b.
    upper lobe b.
Brønsted
    acid
    base
brontophobia
bronzed disease
Brooke
    disease
    epithelioma
    tumor
Brooks scissors
Brophy
    bistoury
    forceps
    knife
    operation
    plate
broth
    brain-heart infusion b.
    carbohydrate b.
    dextrose b.

broth *(continued)*
    heart infusion b.
    hippurate b.
    indole-nitrate b.
    infusion b.
    laurel sulfate b.
    Middlebrook b.
    Mueller-Hinton b.
    nitrate b.
    nutrient b.
    selenite b.
    Stuart b.
    sugar b.
    thioglycolate (THIO) b.
    Todd-Hewitt b.
    Voges-Proskauer b.
Brouha test
brow
brown
    aniline b.
    Bismarck b.
    Bismarck b. R
    Bismarck b. Y
    Manchester b.
    phenylene b.
Brown [eponym]
    applicator
    dermatome
    forceps
    graft
    knife
    needle
    operation
    retractor
    snare
    splint
    tendon sheath syndrome
    tonsillectome
Brown-Adson forceps
Brown-Blair operation
Brown-Buerger cystoscope
Brown-Dohlman implant
Browne
    basket
    operation
brownian
    b. movement
    b.-Zsigmondy movement
Browning vein
Brown-Kelly sign
brown lung disease
Brown-McHardy dilator
Brown-Séquard
    lesion
    paralysis

Brown-Séquard *(continued)*
    syndrome
    treatment
Brown-Symmers disease
Brown-Vialetto-van Laere
  syndrome
Broxolin
Broyles
    aspirator
    bronchoscope
    dilator
    esophagoscope
    forceps
    laryngoscope
    nasopharyngoscope
    telescope
    tube
BRP—
    bathroom privileges
    bilirubin production
BRS—British Roentgen
  Society
Bruce
    septicemia
    stages I–VI
    tract
    treadmill protocol
Brucella
    B. abortus
    B. bronchiseptica
    B. canis
    B. melitensis
    B. ovis
    B. suis
brucellar
Brucellergen
brucellin
brucellosis
Bruch
    glands
    layer
    membrane
brucine
Bruck
    disease
    test
Brücke (Bruecke)
    fibers
    lens
    lines
    muscle
    reagent
    test
    tunic, tunica nervea
Bruckner test

Brudzinski
    reflex
    sign
Bruening
    bronchoscope
    esophagoscope
    forceps
    otoscope
    snare
Brugia
    B. malayi
    B. microfilariae
    B. pahangi
    B. timori
brugian
Bruhat maneuver
Brühl (Bruehl) disease
bruise
    stone b.
bruissement
bruit
    abdominal b.
    aneurysmal b.
    aortic b.
    carotid b.
    cranial b.
    b. d'airain
    b. de bois
    b. de canon
    b. de choc
    b. de clapotement
    b. de claquement
    b. de craquement
    b. de cuir neuf
    b. de diable
    b. de drapeau
    b. de froissement
    b. de frottement
    b. de galop
    b. de grelot
    b. de lime
    b. de moulin
    b. de parchemin
    b. de piaulement
    b. de pot fêlé
    b. de rape
    b. de rappel
    b. de Roger
    b. de scie
    b. de soufflet
    b. de tabourka
    b. de tambour
    false b.
    femoral b.
    Roger b.

bruit *(continued)*
  seagull b.
  b. skodique
  spinal b.
  systolic b.
  Verstraeten b.
Brun curet
Bruner line
brunescent
Brunn (von Brunn)
  epithelial nests
  membrane
  nests
Brunner
  dissector
  forceps
  gland hamartoma
  glands
Bruns
  ataxia
  disease
  sign
  syndrome
Brunschwig operation
Brunsting syndrome
Brunton otoscope
brush
  Ayre b.
  Barraquer b.
  b. biopsy
  electrical b.
  Haidinger b.
  b. of Ruffini
  stomach b.
Brushfield spot
Brushfield-Wyatt
  disease
  syndrome
brushing
  bronchial b.
brushite
Bruton
  agammaglobulinemia
  disease
brux
bruxism
  centric b.
bruxomania
BRW—Brown-Roberts-Wells
BRW CT stereotaxic guide
Bryant
  ampulla
  line
  operation
  sign

Bryant *(continued)*
  traction
  triangle
Bryce-Teacher ovum
Bryobia praetiosa
bryonia
BS—
  Babinski sign
  Bachelor of Surgery
  blood sugar
  bowel sounds
B/S—breath sounds
BSA—
  bismuth-sulfite agar
  body surface area
BSAER—brain stem auditory
  evoked response
BSB—body surface burned
B scan ultrasonogram
BSE—
  bilateral, symmetrical, and
    equal
  breast self-examination
BSER—brain stem evoked
  response
BSF—
  backscatter factor
  basal skull fracture
  B lymphocyte stimulatory
    factors
BSI—bound serum iron
BSN—bowel sounds normal
BSO—bilateral salpingo-
  oophorectomy
BSP—bromsulfophthalein (test)
BSS—
  balanced salt solution
  black silk suture
  buffered saline solution
BST—brief stimulus therapy
BSV—binocular single vision
BT—
  bladder tumor
  brain tumor
BTB—breakthrough bleeding
BTE—behind the ear
β-thromboglobulin
BThU, BTU—British thermal unit
BTL—bilateral tubal ligation
BTR—Bezold-type reflex
BTU—British thermal unit
BU—
  base (of prism) up
  Bodansky unit
  burn unit

B

bubble
    Garren-Edwards gastric b.
    b. ventriculography
bubble-like
bubo
    bullet b.
    chancroidal b.
    climatic b.
    Frei b.
    gonorrheal b.
    indolent b.
    malignant b.
    nonvenereal b.
    pestilential b.
    strumous b.
    syphilitic b.
    tropical b.
    venereal b.
    virulent b.
bubon d'emblée
bubonic plague
bubonocele
bubonulus
bucainide maleate
bucardia
bucca (buccae)
buccal
    b. mucosa
    b. smear
    b. tube
buccally
buccinator
buccoaxial
buccoaxiocervical
buccoaxiogingival
buccocervical
buccoclusal
buccoclusion
buccodistal
buccofacial
buccogingival
buccoglossopharyngitis sicca
buccolabial
buccolingual
buccolingually
buccomaxillary
buccomesial
bucco-occlusal
buccopharyngeal
buccoplacement
buccopulpal
buccoversion
Büchner
    extract
    tuberculin

buchu
Buck
    curet
    extension
    fascia
    hook
    knife
    operation
    splint
    traction
Buckberg
    blood-cardioplegia
    method
    solution
    cardioplegia
buckeye
buckle
    b. fracture
    scleral b.
buckling
    scleral b.
Bucky
    diaphragm
    grid
    rays
Bucky-Potter
    diaphragm
buclizine hydrochloride
bucrylate
Bucy
    knife
    retractor
Bucy-Frazier cannula
bud
    appendage b.
    appendicular b.
    bronchial b.
    end b.
    epidermal b.
    epithelial b.
    gustatory b.
    hepatic b.
    limb b.
    liver b.
    lung b.
    mammary b.
    metanephric b.
    periosteal b.
    placental syncytial b's
    skin b.
    tail b.
    tooth b.
    ureteric b.
    b. of urethra
    vascular b.

B

bud *(continued)*
 wing b.
Budd
 cirrhosis
 jaundice
Budd-Chiari
 disease
 syndrome
budding
buddy splint
Budge center
budgerigar, budgie
Budin
 joint
 obstetric joint
 pelvimeter
 rule
Budinger operation
BUE—both upper
 extremities
Buerger
 disease
 exercises
 symptom
Buerger-McCarthy forceps
bufadienolide
bufagin
bufanolide
buffalo hump
buffer
 bicarbonate b.
 cacodylate b.
 phosphate b.
 protein b.
 TRIS b.
 veronal b.
buffering
buffy coat, buffy-coated
 b.c. cells
 b.c. smear
bufilcon A
bufin
buformin
bufotalin
bufotenin
bufotherapy
bufotoxin
bufylline
bug
 assassin b.
 barley b.
 blister b.
 blue b.
 cocaine b.
 cone-nose b.

bug *(continued)*
 Croton b.
 harvest b.
 hematophagous b.
 kissing b.
 Malay b.
 miana b.
 Mianeh b.
 red b.
 wheat b.
Bugbee electrode
Buhl
 desquamative pneumonia
 disease
Buhl-Dittrich law
buiatrics
Buie
 clamp
 forceps
 irrigator
 position
 probe
 procedure
 rectal suction tube
 scissors
 sigmoidoscope
 technique
Buie-Hirschman
 anoscope
 clamp
Buie-Smith
 retractor
 speculum
bulb
 b. of aorta
 auditory b.
 b. of corpus cavernosum
 dental b.
 duodenal b.
 end b.
 end b's of Krause
 b. of eye
 gustatory b.
 b. of hair
 b. of heart
 inferior b. of
  jugular vein
 b. of Krause
 Krause end b.
 b. of occipital horn of lateral
  ventricle
 olfactory b.
 onion b.
 b. of ovary
 b. of penis

bulb *(continued)*
- b. of posterior horn of lateral ventricle
- Rouget b.
- sinovaginal b.
- spinal b.
- superior b. of jugular vein
- taste b.
- terminal b. of Krause
- vaginal b.
- b. of vestibule of vagina
- b. of vestibule of vulva
- vestibulovaginal b.

bulbar
bulbi (plural of bulbus)
bulbiform, bulboid
bulbitis
bulboatrial
bulbocapnine
bulbocavernosus
bulbogastrone
bulboid
bulbomembranous
bulbonuclear
bulbopontine
bulbospinal
bulbospinal tract
bulbospongiosus
bulbourethral
bulbous
Bulbulian mask
bulbus (gen. and pl. bulbi)
- b. aortae
- b. arteriosus
- b. caroticus
- b. cordis
- b. cornus occipitalis ventriculi lateralis
- b. cornus posterioris ventriculi lateralis
- b. duodeni
- b. inferior venae jugularis
- b. oculi
- b. olfactorius
- b. penis
- b. pili
- b. rhombencephali
- b. superior venae jugularis
- b. urethrae
- b. venae jugularis
- b. vestibuli vaginae

bulesis
bulimia nervosa
bulimic

bulimorexia
Bulimus
- *B. africanus*
- *B. fuchsianus*
- *B. leachii*
- *B. truncatus*

bulkage
bulky dressing
bulla (bullae)
- emphysematous b.
- ethmoidal b.
- b. ethmoidalis
- b. ethmoidalis cavi nasi
- b. ethmoidalis ossis ethmoidalis
- b. ossea

Bull angle
bullate
bullation
bulldog clamp
bullectomy
Buller
- bandage
- shield

bullneck
bullosis
- diabetic b.
- b. diabeticorum

bullous
- b. congenital ichthyosiform erythroderma
- b. dermatosis
- b. erythema multiforme
- b. impetigo
- b. pemphigoid

bull's eye lesion
bumblefoot
Buminate
Bumke pupil
Bumm curet
bump
- goose b.
- pump b.

Bumpus
- forceps
- resectoscope

BUN—blood urea nitrogen
bunamidine hydrochloride
bunching suture
bundle
- aberrant b's
- Arnold b.
- atrioventricular (AV) b.
- a-v. b.
- axial b. of muscle spindle
- Bachmann b.

B

bundle *(continued)*
    b. branch block
    b. branch reentry
    Bruce b.
    central tegmental b.
    circumolivary b. of pyramid
    comb b.
    common b.
    cornucommissural b.
    crossed olivocochlear b.
    b. of Flechsig
    forebrain b., medial
    hair b.
    Helweg b.
    b. of His
    Keith b.
    Kent b.
    Kent-His b.
    Killian b.
    lateral pontine b.
    longitudinal medial b.
    Mahaim b.
    mammillotegmental b.
    marginal b.
    medial forebrain b.
    Meynert b.
    Monakow b.
    muscle b.
    neurovascular b.
    olfactory b.
    olivocochlear b. of Rasmussen
    b. of Oort
    oval b.
    papillomacular b.
    posterior longitudinal b.
    precommissural b.
    proprius b's of spinal cord
    b. of Rasmussen
    Schütz b.
    sinoatrial b.
    solitary b.
    b. of Stanley-Kent
    subcallosal b.
    tendon b.
    thalamomammillary b.
    Thorel b.
    transverse b's of palmar
      aponeurosis
    Türck b.
    uncinate b.
    b. of Vicq d'Azyr
    Weissmann b.
bungarotoxin
Bunge
    amputation

Bunge *(continued)*
    sponge
    spoon
bungeye
Bungner
    bands
    cell
    cordons
Bunim forceps
buniodyl
bunion
    tailor's b.
bunionectomy
    Akin b.
    Keller b.
    Mitchell b.
    Silver b.
    Stone b.
bunionette
Bunker implant
Bunnell
    anvil
    drill
    flap
    needle
    operation
    probe
    splints
    suture
    tendon transfer
bunodont
bunolol hydrochloride
bunolophodont
bunoselenodont
Bunsen
    burner
    coefficient
Bunyaviridae
bunyavirus
BUO—bleeding of undetermined
    origin
buphthalmia
buphthalmos
buphthalmus
bupicomide
bur
    Adson b.
    Burwell b.
    D'Errico b.
    diamond b.
    Hall b.
    b.-hole incision
    Hudson b.
    Jordan-Day b.
    Lempert b.

bur *(continued)*
McKenzie b.
round b.
Wullstein b.
buramate
Burch
calipers
operation
pick
Burchard-Liebermann
reaction
test
Burch-Greenwood tendon tucker
Burdach
bundle
columns
cuneate fasciculus
fasciculus
fibers
fissure
nucleus
tract
Bureau of Radiological Health
buret, burette
Burford rib spreader
Bürger-Grütz (Buerger-Gruetz)
syndrome
Burghart
sign
symptom
Burhenne stone basket technique
buried suture
burimamide
Burkholderia
B. cepacia
B. mallei
B. pseudomallei
Burkitt
lymphoma
tumor
burn
arc b.
brush b.
chemical b.
closed space b.
coagulation b.
contact b.
corneal b.
electrical b.
first-degree b.
flash b.
fourth-degree b.
friction b.
full-thickness b.
high-tension b.

burn *(continued)*
immersion b.
partial-thickness b.
powder b.
radiation b.
respiratory b.
second-degree b.
sun b.
thermal b.
third-degree b.
x-ray b.
burner
Burnett
disinfecting fluid
solution
syndrome
Burnham scissors
burn-in
burnisher
burnishing
burn-out
Burns
amaurosis
ligament
space
Burow
operation
solution
triangle
vein
burping
bursa (bursae)
Achilles b.
b. of Achilles tendon
acromial b.
adventitious b.
anconeal b.
anconeal b. of triceps muscle
b. anserina
anserine b.
anterior genual b.
anterior thyrohyoid b.
b. of biceps brachii muscle
bicipital b.
bicipitofibular b.
bicipitoradial b.
b. bicipitoradialis
Boyer b.
Brodie b.
calcaneal b.
Calori b.
common peroneal b.
b. copulatrix
coracobrachial b.
coracoid b.

bursa (bursae) *(continued)*
    b. cubitalis interossea
    deep infrapatellar b.
    deep patellar b.
    deep postcalcaneal b.
    deltoid b.
    epiploic b.
    external inferior genual b.
    external infracondyloid b.
    external postgenual b.
    b. of Fabricius
    fibular b.
    Fleischmann b.
    gastro-
      cnemiosemimembranous b.
    genual b.
    gluteal b.
    gluteofascial bursae
    gluteofemoral bursae
    gluteotuberosal b.
    His b.
    humeral b.
    hyoid b.
    b. iliopectinea
    b. of iliopsoas muscle
    inferior subtendinous b. of
      biceps femoris muscle
    infracardiac b.
    infragenual b.
    infrahyoid b.
    b. infrahyoidea
    infrapatellar b.
    b. infrapatellaris profunda
    intermuscular gluteal bursae
    internal superior genual bursae
    internal supracondyloid b.
    interosseous cubital b.
    intertubercular b.
    b. intratendinea olecrani
    ischiadic b.
    ischiogluteal b.
    lateral subtendinous b. of
      gastrocnemius muscle
    Luschka b.
    medial subtendinous b. of
      gastrocnemius muscle
    medial supracondyloid b.
    middle patellar b.
    middle prepatellar b.
    Monro b.
    multilocular b.
    nasopharyngeal b.
    olecranon b.
    omental b.
    b. omentalis

bursa (bursae) *(continued)*
    patellar b.
    b. of pectoralis major muscle
    pharyngeal b.
    popliteal b.
    postcalcaneal b.
    posterior genual b.
    prepatellar b.
    prespinous patellar b.
    pretibial b.
    radial b.
    radiohumeral b.
    retrocalcaneal b.
    retrocondyloid b.
    retrohyoid b.
    b. retrohyoidea
    retromämmary b.
    rider's b.
    sacral b.
    scapulohumeral b.
    semimembranosus b.
    semitendinous b.
    sternohyoid b.
    subachilleal b.
    subacromial b.
    b. subacromialis
    subacromiodeltoid b.
    subcalcaneal b.
    subcoracoid b.
    subcrural b.
    b. subcutanea
    b. subcutanea acromialis
    b. subcutanea calcanea
    b. subcutanea infrapatellaris
    b. subcutanea olecrani
    b. subcutanea prepatellaris
    b. subcutanea sacralis
    b. subcutanea trochanterica
    subcutaneous acromial b.
    subcutaneous calcaneal b.
    subcutaneous infrapatellar b.
    subcutaneous patellar b.
    subcutaneous prepatellar b.
    subcutaneous synovial b.
    subcutaneous trochanteric b.
    subdeltoid b.
    b. subdeltoidea
    subfascial b.
    b. subfascialis
    b. subfascialis prepatellaris
    subfascial prepatellar b.
    subhyoid b.
    subiliac b.
    subligamentous b.
    b. sublingualis

bursa (bursae) *(continued)*
    submuscular b.
    b. submuscularis
    subpatellar b.
    b. subtendinea
    b. subtendinea iliaca
    b. subtendinea prepatellaris
    subtendinous b.
    subtendinous iliac b.
    subtendinous b. of iliacus
    subtendinous prepatellar b.
    superficial inferior
      infrapatellar b.
    supragenual b.
    suprapatellar b.
    b. suprapatellaris
    synovial b.
    b. synovialis
    b. tendinis calcanei
    Thornwaldt b.
    thyrohyoid b.
    Tornwaldt (Thornwaldt) b.
    b. of trapezius muscle
    trochlear synovial b.
    tuberoischiadic b.
    ulnar b.
    ulnoradial b.
bursal
bursectomy
bursitis
    Achilles b.
    adhesive b.
    anserine b.
    calcaneal b.
    calcific b.
    Duplay b.
    iliopectineal b.
    ischial b.
    ischiogluteal b.
    olecranon b.
    omental b.
    pharyngeal b.
    popliteal b.
    prepatellar b.
    radiohumeral b.
    retrocalcaneal b.
    scapulohumeral b.
    septic b.
    subacromial b.
    subdeltoid b.
    superficial calcaneal b.
    Tornwaldt (Thornwaldt) b.
    traumatic b.
    trochanteric b.
bursocentesis

bursolith
bursopathy
bursotomy
burst
    bilaterally synchronous b.
    metabolic b.
    respiratory b.
Burton
    line
    sign
Burwell bur
BUS—Bartholin, urethral, Skene
    (glands)
Busacca nodule
Buschke
    disease
    scleredema
Buschke-Löwenstein (Buschke-
    Lowenstein; Buschke-
    Loewenstein) tumor
Buschke-Ollendorff syndrome
bushmaster
Busquet disease
Busse-Buschke disease
busulfan
BUT—breakup time
butabarbital sodium
butacaine sulfate
butacetin
butaclamol hydrochloride
butadiazamide
butalbital
butallylonal
butamben
butamirate citrate
butamisole hydrochloride
butamoxane hydrochloride
    normal b.
butane
butanoic acid
butaperazine maleate
butethal
butethamine hydrochloride
buthiazide
Buthus
    B. occitanus
    B. quinquestriatus
butirosin sulfate
butonate
butoprozine hydrochloride
butopyronoxyl tartrate
butorphanol
butoxamine hydrochloride
butriptyline hydrochloride
Bütschli nuclear spindle

B

butt balm
butt butter
butter
Butterfield cystoscope
butterfly
    b. bandage
    b. drain
    b. dressing
    b. needle
    b. rash
buttock
button
    Aleppo b.
    belly b. (bellybutton)
    Biskra b.
    Boari b.
    bone b.
    bromide b.
    dog b.
    iodide b.
    Jaboulay b.
    mescal b's
    Moore tracheostomy b.
    Murphy b.
    Oriental b.
    Panje voice b.
    peritoneal b.
    polyethylene collar b.
    quaker b.
    b. suture
    synaptic b.
    terminal b.
buttonhole
    b. incision
    b. iridectomy
    mitral b.
    b. operation
    b. suture
butyl
    b. acetate
    b. aminobenzoate
    b. chloride
    b. formate
    b. hydride
butylene
butylparaben
butyraceous
butyrate
butyric
butyric acid
butyrin
butyrine
butyroid
butyromel
butyrometer

butyrophenone
butyroscope
butyrous
butyryl-CoA
    dehydrogenase
Buxton clamp
Buzzi operation
BV—
    biologic value
    blood vessel
    blood volume
    bronchovesicular
BVA—best corrected visual acuity
BVAD—biventricular assist device
BVH—biventricular hypertrophy
BVI—blood vessel invasion
BW—
    biological warfare
    birthweight
b-wave
B-W graft
Bx—biopsy
Byers flap
Byford retractor
Byler disease
bypass
    aortobifemoral b.
    aortocoronary b.
    aortocoronary vein b.
    aortofemoral b.
    aortoiliac b.
    aortorenal b.
    axillo-axillary b.
    axillobifemoral b.
    axillofemoral b.
    axillopopliteal b.
    cardiopulmonary b.
    carotid-subclavian b.
    coronary b.
    coronary artery b. (CAB)
    distal b.
    extra-anatomic b.
    extracranial/intracranial b.
    fem-fem b.
    femoral-femoral b.
    femoral-popliteal b.
    femorofemoral b.
    femorofemoropopliteal b.
    femoropopliteal b.
    gastric b.
    ileojejunal b.
    infrapopliteal b.
    in situ b.
    intestinal b.
    jejunal b.

bypass *(continued)*
    jejunoileal b.
    left heart b.
    obturator b.
    partial b.
    partial ileal b.
    percutaneous biliary b.
    right heart b.
    saphenous vein b.
    subclavian carotid b.
    subclavian-subclavian b.

by-product
byssaceous
byssinosis
byssinotic
byssocausis
byssoid
byssus
bystander
Bywaters syndrome

C

c—
    centi-
    homeopathic symbol for
      centesimal scale of potencies
      $(1/100^c)$
    small calorie
$\bar{c}$ —L. cum (with)
C—
    calculus
    carbohydrate
    carbon
    Caucasian
    Celsius
    centigrade
    certified
    cervical
    chest
    clearance rate
    complement
    contraction
    contracture
    correct
    cytidine
    cytosine
    hundred
C—
    capacitance
    clearance
C.—
    Clostridium
    Cryptococcus
C1–C7—cervical vertebrae 1–7
C1–C9—complement components
    1–9 (CR1, CR2, CR3, CR4, C1qR,
    C3aR, C5aR; C1q, C1r, C1s to
    C9q, C9r, C9s)

C1 INH—C1 inhibitor
C3 NeF—C3 nephritic factor
C3PA—C3 proactivator
Ca—calcium
Ca, CA—
    cancer
    carcinoma
CA—
    cardiac arrest
    cardiac arrhythmia
    carotid artery
    cervicoaxial
    chronologic(al) age
    cold agglutinin
    corneal abrasion
    coronary angiography
    coronary arrest
    coronary artery
    croup-associated
      (virus)
CA15-3 RIA—CA15-3
    radioimmunoassay
CAB—coronary artery
    bypass
CABG—coronary artery bypass
    graft
cable wire suture
Cabot
    ring bodies
    splint
cabufocon A, B
cacao
Cacchi-Ricci syndrome
CACG—cineangiocardiogram
cachectic
cachet

C

cachexia
    addisonian c.
    amyotrophic c.
    Brieger c.
    cancer c.
    cardiac c.
    c. exophthalmica
    fluoric c.
    Grawitz c.
    hypophysial (hypophyseal) c.
    c. hypophysiopriva
    hypothalamic pituitary c.
    malarial c.
    c. mercurialis
    neurogenic c.
    pituitary c.
    psychogenic c.
    saturnine c.
    c. suprarenalis
    uremic c.
    urinary c.
cachinnation
cacodemonomania
cacodyl
    c. cyanide
    c. hydride
cacodylic acid
cacogenics
cacogeusia
cacosmia
cacuminal
CAD—
    computer-assisted design
    coronary artery disease
cadaver
cadaveric
cadaverine
cadaverous
cadmiosis
cadmium (Cd)
    c. bromide
CAD prosthesis
caduceus
caecum
    cupular c. of cochlear duct
    c. cupulare ductus cochlearis
    vestibular c. of cochlear duct
    c. vestibulare ductus cochlearis
caecus minor ventriculi
caeruleus, ceruleus, coeruleus
CAF—
    continuous atrial fibrillation
    coronary arteriovenous fistula
    cyclophosphamide,
        Adriamycin, fluorouracil

café au lait spot
café coronary
caffeinated
caffeine
    c. benzoate
    c. citrate
    citrated c.
caffeinism
Caffey
    disease
    syndrome
Caffey-Kenny disease
Caffey-Silverman syndrome
CAG—chronic atrophic gastritis
cage
    Faraday c.
    thoracic c.
caged-ball valve
CAH—
    chronic active hepatitis
    congenital adrenal
        hyperplasia
CAHC—chronic active hepatitis
  with cirrhosis
CAHD—
    coronary arteriosclerotic heart
        disease
    coronary atherosclerotic heart
        disease
CAI—computer-assisted
  instruction
Cairns
    forceps
    operation
    syndrome
caisson disease
Cajal
    astrocyte
    cells
    interstitial nucleus
    stain
Cal—large calorie
Cal, Kcal—kilocalorie
CAL—computer-assisted learning
Calabar
    bean
    edema
    swellings
calamus scriptorius
Calandruccio compression apparatus
C_{alb}—albumin clearance
calcaneal
calcaneitis
calcaneoapophysitis
calcaneocavus

calcaneocuboid
calcaneodynia
calcaneofibular
calcaneonavicular
calcaneoplantar
calcaneoscaphoid
calcaneotibial
calcaneovalgocavus
calcaneus
calcar
    c. avis
    c. femorale
    c. pedis
calcareous
calcarine fissure
calcariuria
calcaroid
calcibilia
calcic
calcicosilicosis
calcicosis
calcific shadows
calcification
    aortic c.
    conjunctival metastatic c.
    coronary c.
    dystrophic c.
    eggshell c.
    habenular c.
    intracranial c.
    metastatic c.
    Mönckeberg c.
    myocardial c.
    parentheses-like c's
    periarticular c.
    pericardial c.
    pulmonary c.
    valvular c.
calcified
calcigerous
calcineurin
calcinosis
    c. circumscripta
    c. cutis
    c. interstitialis
    c. intervertebralis
    tumoral c.
    c. universalis
calciokinesis
calciokinetic
calciorrhachia
calcipectic
calcipenia
calcipenic
calcipexy

calciphilia
calciphylactic
calciphylaxis
    systemic c.
    topical c.
calciprivia
calciprivic
calcitonin
calcium (Ca)
    c. 45, c. 47 (radiocalcium)
    c. alginate dressing
      (bead system)
    c. acetate
    c. ascorbate
    c. carbimide
    c. carbonate ($CaCO_3$)
    c. caseinate
    c. chloride ($CaCl_2$)
    c. cyanamide
    cyclamate c.
    c. disodium edathamil
    c. disodium edetate
    c. disodium
      ethylenediaminetetraacetate
    edetate calcium disodium
      (c. EDTA)
    c. fluoride
    c. glubionate
    c. gluceptate
    c. gluconate
    c. glycerophosphate
    c. hydroxide
    c. ion(s)
    c. lactate
    c. levulinate
    c. oxalate
    c. oxide
    c. pantothenate
    c. paradox
    c. phosphate
    c. polycarbophil
    c. propionate
    c. pyrophosphate
    radioactive c. (radiocalcium)
    c. stearate
    c. sulfate
    c. transient
    c. trisodium pentetate
    c. undecylenate
calciuria
calcoglobulin
calcospherite
calculary
calculation
calculi (plural of calculus)

C

calculous cholecystitis
calculus (calculi)
    alternating c.
    alvine c.
    articular c.
    biliary c.
    branched c.
    bronchial c.
    calcareous renal c.
    calcium oxalate c.
    cholesterol c.
    combination c.
    coral c.
    cystic c.
    cystine c.
    decubitus c.
    dendritic c.
    dental c.
    encysted c.
    fibrin c.
    fusible c.
    gastric c.
    gonecystic c.
    hemic c.
    hemp seed c.
    hepatic c.
    indigo c.
    intestinal c.
    joint c.
    lacrimal c.
    lacteal c.
    lung c.
    mammary c.
    matrix c.
    metabolic c.
    mulberry c.
    nasal c.
    nephritic c.
    noncalcareous renal c.
    oxalate c.
    pancreatic c.
    phosphate c.
    pocketed c.
    preputial c.
    prostatic c.
    renal c.
    salivary c.
    serumal c.
    shellac c.
    spermatic c.
    staghorn c.
    stomachic c.
    struvite c.
    subgingival c.
    submorphous c.

calculus (calculi) *(continued)*
    supragingival c.
    tonsillar c.
    urate c.
    ureteral c.
    urethral c.
    uric acid c.
    urinary c.
    urostealith c.
    uterine c.
    vesical c.
    vesicoprostatic c.
    xanthic c.
Caldani ligament
Caldwell
    position
    protection
Caldwell-Luc operation
Caldwell-Moloy
    classification
    method
calefacient
calf (calves)
caliber
calibrate, calibrated
calibration
    Békésy c.
    E-dial c.
    pure tone c.
calibrator
    digital isotope c.
    dose c.
    radioisotope c.
caliceal, calyceal
calicectasis
calicectomy
calices, calyces (plural of
  calix, calyx)
calicine
calicivirus
caliculus (caliculi)
    c. gustatorius
    c. ophthalmicus
caliectasis
California encephalitis (CE)
californium (Cf)
caligo lentis
calipers
    Austin Moore inside-outside c.
    Burch c.
    Castroviejo c.
    Green c.
    Jameson c.
    Ladd c.
    Lange skinfold c.

calipers *(continued)*
    Machemer c.
    Oscher c.
    skinfold c.
    Stahl c.
    Thorpe c.
    ultrasonic c.
    Vernier c.
    walking c.
calisthenics
calix, calyx (calices, calyces)
    renal calices
    calices renales
    calices renales majores
    calices renales minores
    c. superior renis
Calkins sign
CALLA—common acute
  lymphoblastic leukemia antigen
Callahan
    method
    operation
Callander amputation
Callaway test
Calleja
    islands
    islets
Call-Exner body
Calliphora vomitoria
Callison fluid
callosal
callosity
callosomarginal
callosum
    corpus c.
callous
callus
    bony c.
    central c.
    definitive c.
    ensheathing c.
    external c.
    inner c.
    intermediate c.
    internal c.
    medullary c.
    myelogenous c.
    permanent c.
    provisional c.
    temporary c.
Calmette
    conjunctival reaction
    ophthalmic reaction
    ophthalmoreaction
    vaccine

Calmette-Guérin bacillus
calmodulin
calor
    c. febrilis
    c. fervens
    c. innatus
    c. internus
    c. mordax
    c. mordicans
Calori bursa
caloric
    c. nystagmus
    c. testing
caloricity
calorie
    gram c.
    International Table (IT) c.
    large c.
    mean c.
    small c.
    standard c.
    thermochemical c.
calorifacient
calorific
calorigenic
calorimetry
    direct c.
    indirect c.
    partitional c.
Calot
    operation
    triangle
calotte
calpain
calsequestrin
Caltagirone knife
calvaria (calvariae)
calvarial
Calvé disease
Calvé-Legg-Perthes syndrome
Calvé-Perthes disease
calvities
calx
calyceal, caliceal
Calymmatobacterium granulomatis
calyx, calix
C_{am}—amylase clearance
CAM—
    Caucasian adult male
    chorioallantoic membrane
    computer-assisted
      myelography
    contralateral axillary
      metastasis
cambium

camera (camerae) [chamber
  or cavity]
    c. anterior bulbi oculi
    camerae bulbi oculi
    c. oculi anterior
    c. oculi posterior
    c. posterior bulbi oculi
    c. pulpi
    c. vitrea bulbi
    c. vitrea bulbi oculi
camera
    Anger c.
    cine c.
    electron diffraction c.
    gamma c.
    Isocon c.
    c. lucida
    Medx c.
    multicrystal c.
    c. obscura
    Orthicon c.
    positron scintillation c.
    powder c.
    radioisotope c.
    radionuclide c.
    recording c.
    scintillation c.
    video display c.
Camerer law
Cameron-Haight elevator
Camey ileocystoplasty
Camino intracranial catheter
camisole
Cammann stethoscope
CA (cardiac-apnea) monitor
CAMP—computer-assisted menu
  planning
cAMP—cyclic adenosine
  monophosphate
Campbell
    catheter
    elevator
    forceps
    ligament
    operation
    osteotome
    procedure
    retractor
    sound
    trocar
Camp-Coventry position
Camper
    angle
    chiasm
    fascia

Camper *(continued)*
    ligament
    plane
Camp-Gianturco method
camphene
camphor
    carbolated c.
    carbolic c.
    gum c.
    mentholated c.
    phenol c.
    c. salicylate
    salol c.
camphoraceous
camphorated
camphorism
campimetry
campotomy
3′,5′-cAMP synthetase
camptocormia
camptodactyly
camptomelia
camptomelic
campus of Wernicke
Campylobacter
    C. coli
    C. fennelliae
    C. fetus enteritis
    C. fetus subsp. *fetus*
    C. fetus subsp. *intestinalis*
    C. fetus subsp. *jejuni*
    C. jejuni
    C. rectus
    C. sputorum subsp. *sputorum*
campylobacteriosis
Camurati-Engelmann diaphyseal
  dysplasia
Canada-Cronkhite syndrome
Canadian crutch
canal
    abdominal c.
    accessory palatine c's
    adductor c.
    Alcock c.
    alimentary c.
    alisphenoid c.
    alveolar c.
    alveolodental c's
    anal c.
    c. of Arantius
    Arnold c.
    arterial c.
    atrioventricular c.
    auditory c., external
    auditory c., internal

canal *(continued)*

- basipharyngeal c.
- Bichat c.
- biliary c's, interlobular
- biliary c's, intralobular
- birth c.
- c. of Bochdalek
- bony c's of ear
- Böttcher (Boettcher) c.
- branching c.
- Braun c.
- Breschet c's
- calciferous c's
- caroticotympanic c's
- carotid c.
- carpal c.
- c's of cartilage
- central c. of modiolus
- central c. of spinal cord
- central c. of Stilling
- central c. of vitreous
- cerebrospinal c.
- cervical c. of uterus
- chordal c.
- ciliary c's
- Civinini c.
- Cloquet c.
- cochlear c.
- collateral pulp c.
- condylar c.
- condyloid c.
- connecting c.
- corneal c.
- c. of Corti
- c. of Cotunnius
- craniopharyngeal c.
- craniovertebral c.
- crural c. of Henle
- c. of Cuvier
- dental c., inferior
- dental c's, posterior
- dentinal c's
- digestive c.
- diploic c's
- Dorello c.
- endocervical c.
- c. of epididymis
- ethmoidal c., anterior
- ethmoidal c., posterior
- eustachian c., osseous
- external acoustic c.
- facial c.
- fallopian c.
- femoral c.
- Ferrein c.

canal *(continued)*

- flexor c.
- c. for facial nerve
- c. for Jacobson nerve
- ganglionic c.
- Gartner c.
- gastric c.
- genital c.
- gubernacular c's
- c. of Guidi
- Guyon c.
- gynecophoral c.
- hair c.
- Hannover c.
- haversian c.
- hemal c.
- Henle c.
- Hensen c.
- c. of Hering
- hernial c.
- Hirschfeld c's
- His c.
- c. of Hovius
- Huguier c.
- Hunter c.
- Huschke c.
- hyaloid c.
- hypoglossal c.
- iliac c.
- incisive c's
- infraorbital c.
- inguinal c.
- intercellular c.
- interdental c's
- interfacial c.
- internal acoustic c.
- intersacral c's
- Jacobson c.
- Kovalevsky c.
- lacrimal c.
- Laurer c.
- Lauth c.
- Leeuwenhoek c.
- longitudinal c's of modiolus
- Löwenberg c.
- lumbrical c's of Kanavel
- mandibular c.
- maxillary c., superior
- medullary c.
- mental c.
- c. of midbrain
- Müller c.
- musculotubal c.
- nasal c.
- nasolacrimal c.

canal *(continued)*

- nasopalatine c's
- neural c.
- neurenteric c.
- notochordal c.
- c. of Nuck
- nutrient c.
- obstetric c.
- obturator c.
- c. of Oken
- olfactory c.
- omphalomesenteric c.
- optic c.
- orbital c's
- osseous cochlear c.
- osseous eustachian c.
- palatine c's, accessory
- palatine c's, anterior
- palatine c's, lesser
- palatine c's, posterior
- palatomaxillary c.
- palatovaginal c.
- parturient c.
- pelvic c.
- peritoneovaginal c.
- perivascular c.
- persistent common atrioventricular c.
- Petit c.
- pharyngeal c.
- pharyngotracheal c.
- plasmatic c.
- pleural c's
- pleuropericardial c.
- pleuroperitoneal c.
- portal c.
- pterygoid c.
- pterygopalatine c.
- pudendal c.
- pulmoaortic c.
- pulp c.
- pyloric c.
- c's of Recklinghausen
- recurrent c.
- Reichert c.
- c's of Rivinus
- root c., accessory
- sacculocochlear c.
- sacculoutricular c.
- sacral c.
- Santorini c.
- Scarpa c.
- c. of Schlemm
- scleral c.
- scleroticochoroidal c.

canal *(continued)*

- semicircular c.
- seminal c.
- serous c.
- sheathing c.
- Sondermann c
- spermatic c.
- sphenopalatine c.
- sphenopharyngeal c.
- spinal c.
- spiral c.
- spiral c. of Rosenthal
- spiroid c.
- Steno c.
- Stensen c.
- c. of Stilling
- c. of stomach
- subsartorial c.
- Sucquet-Hoyer c.
- supraciliary c.
- supraoptic c.
- supraorbital c.
- tarsal c.
- Theile c.
- thymopharyngeal c.
- tubal c.
- tubotympanic c.
- tympanic c. of cochlea
- umbilical c.
- urogenital c.
- uterine c.
- uterocervical c.
- uterovaginal c.
- utriculosaccular c.
- vaginal c.
- vaginoperitoneal c.
- van Hoorne (van Hoorn, van Horne) c.
- Velpeau c.
- ventricular c.
- Verneuil c's
- vertebral c.
- vesicourethral c.
- vestibular c.
- vidian c.
- Volkmann c's
- vomerine c.
- vomerobasilar c., lateral inferior
- vomerobasilar c., lateral superior
- vomerorostral c.
- vomerovaginal c.
- vulvar c.
- vulvouterine c.
- c's of Walther
- c's of Wearn

canal *(continued)*
    c. of Wirsung
    zygomaticofacial c.
    zygomatico-orbital c.
    zygomaticotemporal c.
canalicular scissors
canaliculi (plural of canaliculus)
canaliculitis
canaliculization
canaliculodacryocystostomy
canaliculorhinostomy
canaliculus (canaliculi)
    apical c.
    auricular c.
    bile canaliculi
    biliary canaliculi
    c. bilifer
    bone canaliculi
    caroticotympanic canaliculi
    canaliculi caroticotympanici
    c. chordae tympani
    canaliculi cochleae
    cochlear c.
    dental canaliculi
    canaliculi dentales
    haversian c.
    incisor c.
    innominate c.
    c. innominatus
    intercellular canaliculi of
      parietal cells
    c. lacrimalis
    c. laqueiformis
    mastoid c. for Arnold nerve
    c. mastoideus
    c. of osteocytes
    c. petrosus
    petrous c.
    pseudobile c.
    secretory c.
    Thiersch c.
    tympanic c. for Jacobson
      nerve
    c. tympanicus
    vestibular c.
    c. vestibuli
canalis (canales)
    c. adductorius
    c. analis
    c. caroticus
    c. carpi
    c. centralis medullae spinalis
    c. cervicis uteri
    c. condylaris
    canales diploici
    c. facialis

canalis (canales) *(continued)*
    c. femoralis
    c. gastricus
    c. hyaloideus
    c. hypoglossalis
    canales incisivi
    c. infraorbitalis
    c. inguinalis
    canales longitudinales
      modioli
    c. mandibulae
    c. musculotubarius
    c. nasolacrimalis
    c. nervi facialis
    c. nervi hypoglossi
    c. nutricius
    c. nutriens
    c. obturatorius
    c. opticus
    canales palatini minores
    c. palatinus major
    c. palatovaginalis
    c. pterygoideus
    c. pudendalis
    c. pyloricus
    c. radicis dentis
    c. reuniens
    c. spiralis cochleae
    c. spiralis modioli
    c. vertebralis
    c. vomerorostralis
    c. vomerovaginalis
canalization
canalplasty
canal wall
    intact c.w. tympanoplasty
Canavan
    disease
    sclerosis
    spongy degeneration
Canavan-van Bogaert-Bertrand
    disease
cancellated
cancellous
cancellus
cancer
    c. à deux
    aniline c.
    arsenic c.
    asbestos c.
    cerebriform c.
    chimney sweeps' c.
    colloid c.
    contact c.
    cystic c.
    dendritic c.

cancer *(continued)*
    dermoid c.
    duct c.
    dye workers' c.
    encephaloid c.
    c. en cuirasse
    endothelial c.
    epithelial c.
    glandular c.
    hereditary nonpolyposis
        colorectal c. (HNPCC)
    c. in situ
    latent c.
    medullary c.
    melanotic c.
    metastatic c.
    nonmelanoma skin c's
    non–small-cell lung c.
    occult c.
    Schneeberg c.
    scirrhous c.
    soft c.
    soot c.
    spindle cell c.
    tar c.
    testicular c.
    tubular c.
    ulcerated c.
canceremia
cancericidal
cancerous
cancerphobia
cancriform
cancroid
cancrum
    c. nasi
    c. oris
Candida
    C. albicans
    C. krusei
    C. lusitaniae
    C. parapsilosis
    C. pseudotropicalis
    C. stellatoidea
    C. stomatitis
    C. tropicalis
candidal
candidemia
candidiasis
    acute pseudomembranous c.
    atrophic c.
    bronchial c.
    chronic mucocutaneous c.
    cutaneous c.
    endocardial c.
    oral c.

candidiasis *(continued)*
    pulmonary c.
    vaginal c.
candidid
candidin skin test
    antigen
candiduria
candle
    Chamberland c.
    foot c.
    meter c.
    vaginal c.
candle-guttering
candle power
candlewax drippings
cane
    adjustable c.
    broad-based c.
    English c.
    glider c.
    quadripod c.
    tripod c.
canescent
Canfield
    knife
    operation
canine
canities
canker sore
cannabinoid
cannabis
Cannizzaro reaction
Cannon
    endarterectomy loop
    law
    point
    ring
    syndrome
    theory
Cannon-Bard theory
cannula
    Abelson c.
    Abraham c.
    Adson c.
    Bardic c.
    Bellocq c.
    Bishop-Harmon anterior
        chamber irrigating c.
    Bucy-Frazier c.
    Castroviejo c.
    Coakley c.
    Concorde suction c.
    Cone c.
    Cooper c.
    Day c.
    Flexicath c.

cannula *(continued)*
  Floyd c.
  Frazier c.
  Goldstein c.
  Goodfellow c.
  Haynes c.
  Holman-Mathieu c.
  infusion c.
  Ingals c.
  irrigation c.
  Jarcho c.
  Kahn c.
  Kanavel brain-exploring c.
  Karman c.
  Krause c.
  Lifemed c.
  Mayo c.
  Mercedes tip c.
  Moncrieff irrigating c.
  Morris c.
  nasal c.
  Neal c.
  Packo pars plana c.
  Padgett shark-mouth c.
  Paterson laryngeal c.
  perfusion c.
  Polystan c.
  Portnoy c.
  Pritchard c.
  Randolph c.
  Rockey c.
  Roper c.
  Rubin c.
  Sachs c.
  Scheie c.
  Scott c.
  Seletz c.
  Silastic coronary artery c.
  Soresi c.
  Tulevech c.
  USCI c.
  Veirs c.
  venous c.
  ventricular c.
  Veress c.
  washout c.
cannulate
cannulation
cannulization
cant of mandible
Cantelli sign
canthal
canthectomy
canthi (plural of canthus)
canthitis

cantholysis
canthoplasty
  Ammon c.
canthorrhaphy
canthotomy
canthus (canthi)
  inner c.
  c. inversus
  lateral c.
  medial c.
  nasal c.
  outer c.
  temporal c.
Cantlie cannula
Cantor tube
CAO—chronic airway obstruction
CAP—College of American
  Pathologists
cap
  bishop's c.
  chin c.
  cradle c.
  Dumas c.
  duodenal c.
  enamel c.
  fibrin c.
  fibrinoid c.
  knee c.
  phrygian c.
  pyloric c.
  skull c.
  c. of Zinn
capacious
capacitance
capacitation
capacitor
capacity
  antigen-binding c.
  carbon monoxide–diffusing c.
  cranial c.
  diffusing c.
  diffusion c.
  forced vital c. (FVC)
  functional residual c.
  inspiratory c.
  maximal breathing c.
  maximal tubular excretory c.
  maximal tubular reabsorptive c.
  maximal tubular secretory c.
  maximum lung c.
  mental c.
  oxygen c.
  oxygen-diffusing c.
  respiratory c.
  testamentary c.

capacity *(continued)*
    timed vital c.
    total iron-binding c. (TIBC)
    total lung c.
    virus neutralizing c.
    vital c. (VC)
CAPD—continuous ambulatory
  peritoneal dialysis
capeline
Capetown
    aortic prosthetic valve
    aortic valve prosthesis
Capgras
    phenomenon
    symptom
    syndrome
capillarectasia
capillariasis
    intestinal c.
capillariomotor
capillaritis
capillarity
capillaropathy
capillaroscopy
capillary (capillaries)
    arterial c.
    arteriolar c.
    bile c's
    continuous c's
    erythrocytic c's
    fenestrated c's
    glomerular c.
    c. hemangioma
    lymph c.
    lymphatic c.
    Meigs c.
    c. microscope
    peritubular c.
    secretory c.
    sheathed c's
    sinusoidal c.
    c. tube
    venous c.
capillovenous
capillus (capilli)
capita (plural of caput)
capitate
capitation
capitatum
capitellum
capitonnage suture
capitular
capitulum (capitula)
    c. humeri
    c. stapedis

Caplan
    nodules
    syndrome
Capnocytophaga canimorsus
capnography
capnometry
capotement
capping
    pulp c.
Capps
    reflex
    sign
capriloquism
caprylic acid
CAPS—
    caffeine, alcohol, pepper, spicy
      foods
    carbamoyl phosphate
      synthetase
capsaicin
CAPS-free diet
capsicum
capsitis
capsula (capsulae)
    c. adiposa renis
    c. articularis
    c. bulbi
    c. cordis
    c. externa
    c. extrema
    c. fibrosa renis
    c. ganglii
    c. glomeruli
    c. interna
    c. lentis
    c. pancreatis
    c. prostatica
    c. tonsillaris
capsular
capsulation
capsule
    acoustic c.
    adherent c.
    adipose c.
    adrenal c's, accessory
    anthrax c.
    articular c.
    auditory c.
    biopsy c.
    Bonnet c.
    Bowman c.
    cartilage c.
    cartilaginous ear c.
    cricoarytenoid
      articular c.

capsule *(continued)*
    cricothyroid articular c.
    Crosby c.
    Crosby-Kugler c.
    crystalline c.
    dental c.
    enteric c.
    external c.
    extreme c.
    fibrous c.
    fibrous articular c.
    fibrous c. of corpora cavernosa
      penis
    c. forceps
    Gerota c.
    Glisson c.
    glomerular c.
    hepatobiliary c.
    internal c.
    joint c.
    c. of labyrinth
    malpighian c.
    Müller c.
    nasal c.
    ocular c.
    olfactory c.
    otic c.
    perinephric c.
    periotic c.
    perivascular
      fibrous c.
    radiotelemetering c.
    renal c's
    serous c. of spleen
    sodium iodide ^{131}I c's
    suprarenal c.
    synovial c.
    telemetering c.
    c. of Tenon
    c. of thymus
    tonsillar c.
capsulectomy
capsulitis
    adhesive c.
    hepatic c.
capsulolenticular
capsuloplasty
capsulorrhaphy
capsulorrhexis
capsulotome
    Darling c.
capsulotomy
    renal c.
capture
    atrial c.
    ventricular c.

caput (capita)
    c. coli
    c. costae
    c. deformatum
    c. distortum
    c. epididymidis
    c. femoris
    c. fibulae
    c. humeri
    c. mallei
    c. mandibulae
    c. medusae
    c. metacarpale
    c. metatarsale
    c. musculi
    c. nuclei caudati
    c. ossis femoris
    c. pancreatis
    c. planum
    c. quadratum
    c. radii
    c. stapedis
    c. succedaneum
    c. tali
    c. ulnae
Carabelli
    aspirator
    cusp
    endobronchial tube
    lumen finder
    sign
    tubercle
caramel
carat
caraway
carbamic acid
carbaminohemoglobin
carbamoylaspartic acid
carbamoylation
carbamoyl phosphate
carbamoyl-phosphate synthase
    (ammonia)
carbamoyl phosphate synthetase
    (CPS) deficiency
carbamoyl-phosphate
    synthetase (glutamine-
    hydrolyzing)
carbinol
    acetylmethyl c.
    dimethyl c.
carbogaseous
carbogen
carbohydrate
    reserve c's
carbohydraturia
carbohydrogenic

Carbo-Jet bone-cleaning device
carbolate
carbolfuchsin
    Ziehl-Neelsen c.
carbolic acid
carbolism
carbolize
carboluria
carbolxylene
carbon (C)
    c. 12
    c. 13
    c. 14
    c. dioxide (CO_2)
    c. disulfide
    c. monoxide
    c. tetrachloride
carbonaceous
carbonate
carbonate-apatite
carbonate dehydratase
carbonic acid
carbonic anhydrase
carbonize
Carborundum grinding wheel
γ-carboxyglutamate [gamma-]
carboxyhemoglobin (HbCO)
carboxyhemoglobinemia
carboxyl (acid) proteinase
carboxylase
    amino acid c.
    multiple c. deficiency (MCD)
carboxylate
carboxylation
    reductive c.
carboxylesterase
carboxyltransferase
carboxymyoglobin
carboxypeptidase A (B, N)
carbuncle
    malignant c.
    renal c.
carbuncular
carbunculoid
Carcassonne perineal ligament
carcinoembryonic antigen (CEA)
carcinogen
    direct-reacting c.
carcinogenesis
carcinogenic
carcinogenicity
carcinoid
    bronchial c.
    c. of bronchus
    enterochromaffin c.
    G-cell c.

carcinoid *(continued)*
    c. heart disease
    c. plaque
    c. syndrome
    c. tumor
    c. valve disease
carcinolysis
carcinolytic
carcinoma (carcinomas,
    carcinomata)
    acinar c.
    acinic cell c.
    acinous c.
    adenocystic c.
    adenoid cystic c.
    c. adenomatosum
    adenosquamous c.
    adrenal c.
    adrenocortical c.
    alveolar cell c.
    ampullary c.
    anaplastic c.
    apocrine c.
    argentaffin c.
    basal cell c.
    basaloid c.
    basosquamous cell c.
    bile duct c.
    biliary c.
    bronchioalveolar c.
    bronchiolar c.
    bronchogenic c.
    cavitated c.
    cerebriform c.
    chorionic c.
    clear cell c.
    cloacogenic c.
    colloid c.
    colorectal c.
    comedo c.
    corpus c.
    cribriform c.
    c. cuniculatum
    c. cutaneum
    cylindrical cell c.
    desmoplastic c.
    ductal c.
    ductal papillary c.
    embryonal c.
    encephaloid c.
    c. en cuirasse
    endometrial c.
    endometrioid c.
    epidermoid c.
    epithelial c.
    esophageal c.

C

carcinoma (carcinomas, carcinomata)
(continued)
    fibrosing basal cell c.
    c. fibrosum
    follicular c.
    fungating c.
    gelatiniform c.,
      gelatinous c.
    giant cell c.
    glandular c.
    granular cell c.
    hepatocellular c.
    hilar c.
    Hürthle cell c.
    hyaline c.
    hypernephroid c.
    infantile embryonal c.
    infiltrating ductal cell c.
    inflammatory c.
    c. in situ
    intraductal c.
    intraepidermal c.
    intraepithelial c.
    invasive c.
    islet cell c.
    Kulchitsky cell c.
    large cell c.
    laryngeal c.
    lenticular c.
    lobular c.
    lymphoepithelial c.
    medullary c.
    melanotic c.
    Merkel cell c.
    metastatic c.
    metatypical c.
    c. molle
    mucinous c.
    c. muciparum
    c. mucocellulare
    mucoepidermoid c.
    mucoid c.
    c. mucosum
    nasopharyngeal c.
    oat cell c.
    occult c.
    c. ossificans
    osteoid c.
    pancreatic c.
    papillary serous c.
    parafollicular thyroid c.
    parenchymatous c.
    peritoneal c.
    preinvasive c.

carcinoma (carcinomas, carcinomata)
(continued)
    prickle cell c.
    pseudomucinous c.
    radiogenic c.
    renal cell c.
    schneiderian c.
    scirrhous c.
    sebaceous c.
    seminal c.
    signet-ring cell c.
    c. simplex
    small-cell c.
    spindle cell c.
    c. spongiosum
    squamous cell c.
    teratoid c.
    tonsillar c.
    trabecular c.
    transitional cell c.
    tuberous c.
    undifferentiated c.
    verrucous c.
    villous c., c. villosum
carcinomatoid
carcinomatosis
    meningeal c.
    c. peritonei
    c. pleurae
carcinomatous
carcinophobia
carcinosarcoma
    embryonal c.
    Flexner-Jobling c.
    Walker c. 256
carcinostatic
Cardarelli
    sign
    symptom
Carden amputation
cardia
    incompetent c.
    c. of stomach
cardiac
    c. catheterization
    c. output
    c. risk factors (CRFs)
    c. shunt detection
    c. tube
    c. ventriculography
cardial
cardiectasis
cardiectomized
cardiectomy

cardinal
    c. movements
    c. points
    c. sign
cardioaccelerator
cardioactive
cardioangiography
    retrograde c.
cardioangiology
Cardiobacterium hominis
cardiocele
cardiocentesis
cardiochalasia
cardiodilator
cardiodiosis
cardiodynamics
cardiodynia
cardioesophageal
cardiogenesis
cardiogenetic
cardiogenic
cardiogram
    apex c.
    esophageal c.
    negative c.
    precordial c.
    vector c.
cardiographic
cardiography
    apex c.
    M-mode c.
    radionuclide c.
    ultrasonic c.
    vector c.
cardiohepatic
cardiohepatomegaly
cardioid
cardioinhibitor
cardiokinetic
cardiokymographic
cardiolipin
cardiologist
cardiology
cardiolysis
cardiomalacia
cardiomegaly
    glycogenic c.
    idiopathic c.
cardiomelanosis
cardiometry
cardiomotility
cardiomyoliposis
    infiltrative c.
    peripartum c.

cardiomyoliposis *(continued)*
    restrictive c.
cardiomyopathy
    alcoholic c.
    Becker c.
    beer-drinkers' c.
    cobalt c.
    congestive c.
    dilated c.
    end-stage c.
    familial c.
    fatty c.
    hypertrophic c. (HCM)
    hypertrophic obstructive c.
      (HOCM)
    idiopathic dilated c.
    infectious c.
    infiltrative c.
    ischemic c.
    nephropathic c.
    nonobstructive hypertrophic c.
    obliterative c.
    obstructive hypertrophic c.
    peripartum c.
    postpartum c.
    primary c.
    restrictive c.
    right ventricular c.
    secondary c.
    thyrotoxic c.
    toxic c.
cardiomyopexy
cardiomyotomy
cardionephric
cardioneural
cardiopathic
cardiopathy
    endocrine c.
    infarctoid c.
cardiopericardiopexy
cardiopericarditis
cardiophobia
cardiophrenic
cardioplasty
cardioplegia
    antegrade blood c.
    Buckberg c.
    cold blood c.
    cold crystalloid c.
    intermittent antegrade c.
    isothermic blood c.
    leukocyte-depleted blood c.
    normothermic c.
    retrograde continuous c.

C

cardioplegia *(continued)*
    tepid blood c.
    warm blood hyperkalemic c.
cardioplegic solution
cardiopneumatic
cardiopneumograph
cardiopneumonopexy
cardioprotectant
cardioprotective
cardioptosis
cardiopulmonary
cardiopyloric
cardiorenal
cardiorespiratory arrest
cardiorrhaphy
cardiorrhexis
cardiosclerosis
cardioselective
cardiospasm
cardiotachometry
cardiotherapy
cardiothymic silhouette
cardiothyrotoxicosis
cardiotocography
cardiotomy
cardiotonic
cardiotopometry
cardiotoxic
cardiotoxicity
cardiovalvular
cardiovalvulitis
cardiovalvulotome
cardiovalvulotomy
cardiovascular
cardioversion
cardiovert
cardioverter
    automatic implantable
    c.-defibrillator (AICD)
cardiovirus
carditis
    Lyme c.
    rheumatic c.
    streptococcal c.
    verrucous c.
care
    acute c.
    ambulatory c.
    continuity of c.
    custodial c.
    extended c.
    follow-up c.
    home health c.
    primary c.
    respiratory c.

care *(continued)*
    secondary c.
    skilled nursing c.
    tertiary c.
Carey-Coombs murmur
Cargile membrane
Carhart notch
caricous
caries
    arrested c.
    backward c.
    cemental c.
    central c.
    dental c.
    dentinal c.
    dry c.
    enamel c.
    c. fungosa
    internal c.
    lateral c.
    necrotic c.
    pit c.
    rampant c.
    senile dental c.
    c. sicca
    spinal c.
carina (carinae)
    c. fornicis
    c. tracheae
    c. urethralis vaginae
carinate
cariogenic
cariogenicity
cariosity
carious
Carlens
    catheter
    mediastinoscope
    tube
Carleton spots
Carmack ear curet
Carmalt
    arterial forceps
    clamp
    hemostatic forceps
    hysterectomy forceps
    splinter forceps
    thoracic forceps
carmalum
Carman
    meniscus sign
    rectal tube
C-arm fluoroscopy
Carmichael crown
carminative

carmine
    alizarin c.
    indigo c.
    lithium c.
    Schneider c.
carminic acid
carminophil
Carmody forceps
carnal
carneous
carnification
carnitine
carnitine palmitoyl transferase
carnivorous
Carnochan operation
carnosinase deficiency
carnosine
carnosinuria
carnosity
Carnot
    function
    test
Caroli disease
carotene
    beta c.
carotenoid
caroticotympanic
carotid
    c. angiography
    c. artery
    c. cavernous fistula
    c. compression tonography
    c. endarterectomy (CEA)
    c. ischemia
    c. pulse
    c. shudder
    c. sinus
carotidynia
carpal
    c. tunnel syndrome (CTS)
carpale
    os c.
carpectomy
Carpenter
    dissector
    knife
    syndrome
Carpentier
    heart valve
    rings
    stent
Carpentier-Edwards valve
carphology
carpitis
carpocarpal

carpogonium
carpometacarpal
carpopedal
carpophalangeal
carpoptosis
Carpue
    operation
    rhinoplasty
carpus curvus
Carrel
    clamp
    method
    mosquito forceps
    operation
    patch
    suture
    treatment
    tube
Carrel-Dakin
    fluid
    treatment
Carrel-Girard screw
Carrel-Lindberg pump
carrier
    active c.
    amalgam c.
    chronic c.
    contact c.
    convalescent c.
    Deschamps c.
    enteric c.
    c.-free radioisotope
    gametocyte c.
    healthy c.
    hemophilia c.
    incubation c.
    intermittent c.
    intestinal c.
    isotopic c.
    Lahey c.
    lentulo paste c.
    ligature c.
    Mayo c.
    oxygen c.
    paste c.
    urinary c.
    Wangensteen c.
carrier-free
Carrión disease
Carroll
    awl
    bone-holding forceps
    bone hook
    finger goniometer
    forearm tendon stripper

Carroll *(continued)*
    hook curet
    osteotome
    periosteal elevator
    self-retaining spring retractor
    tendon-passing forceps
    tendon-pulling forceps
    tendon retriever
Carroll-Legg osteotome
Carroll-Smith-Petersen osteotome
Carr-Price test
Carr-Purcell-Meiboom-Gill
    sequence
Carson catheter
Carswell grapes
cart
    crash c.
    dressing c.
    resuscitation c.
Carter
    clamp
    introducer
    mycetoma
    operation
    retractor
    splint
cartilage
    alar c's
    anular c.
    aortic c.
    arthrodial c.
    articular c.
    arytenoid c.
    c. of auditory tube
    auricular c.
    basal c.
    branchial c.
    calcified c.
    cariniform c.
    cellular c.
    circumferential c.
    conchal c.
    condylar c.
    connecting c.
    corniculate c.
    costal c.
    cricoid c.
    cuneiform c.
    dentinal c.
    diarthrodial c.
    ectethmoid c.
    elastic c.
    embryonic c.
    ensiform c.
    epiglottic c.

cartilage *(continued)*
    epiphyseal c.
    episternal c.
    eustachian c.
    falciform c.
    fetal c.
    floating c.
    gingival c.
    growth c.
    guttural c.
    hyaline c.
    innominate c.
    interarticular c.
    interarytenoid c.
    intermediary c.
    interosseous c.
    intervertebral c.
    intrathyroid c.
    investing c.
    Jacobson c.
    laryngeal c's
    laryngeal c. of Luschka
    lateral c's
    mandibular c.
    meatal c.
    Meckel c.
    mesethmoid c.
    minor c's of nose
    c. of Morgagni
    nasal c's
    obducent c.
    ossifying c.
    parachordal c's
    paranasal c.
    paraseptal c.
    parenchymatous c.
    periotic c.
    permanent c.
    posterior cricoarytenoid c.
    precricoid c.
    precursory c.
    pulmonary c.
    pyramidal c.
    Reichert c.
    reticular c.
    Santorini c.
    semilunar c.
    septal c.
    sesamoid c.
    sigmoid c's
    slipping rib c.
    sphenobasilar c.
    spheno-occipital c.
    sternal c.
    stratified c.

cartilage *(continued)*
    subvomerine c.
    supra-arytenoid c.
    suprascapular c.
    synarthrodial c.
    temporary c.
    tendon c.
    thyroid c.
    tracheal c's
    triangular c. of nose
    triquetral c.
    triradiate c.
    triticeal c.
    tubal c.
    tympanomandibular c.
    uniting c.
    vomerian c. of Hirschfeld
    vomerian c. of Huschke
    vomerine c.
    vomeronasal c.
    Weitbrecht c.
    Wrisberg c.
    xiphoid c.
    Y c.
    yellow c.
cartilagin
cartilagines (plural of cartilago)
cartilaginification
cartilaginiform
cartilaginous
cartilago (cartilagines)
    cartilagines alares minores
    c. alaris major
    c. articularis
    c. arytenoidea
    c. auriculae
    c. auricularis
    c. corniculata
    c. costalis
    c. cricoidea
    c. cuneiformis
    c. ensiformis
    c. epiglottica
    c. epiphysialis
    cartilagines falcatae
    c. jacobsoni
    cartilagines laryngeales
    cartilagines laryngis
    c. meatus acustici
    cartilagines nasales accessoriae
    cartilagines nasi
    c. nasi lateralis
    c. santorini
    c. septi nasi
    cartilagines sesamoideae nasi

cartilago (cartilagines) *(continued)*
    c. sesamoidea laryngis
    c. sesamoidea ligamenti vocalis
    c. thyroidea
    cartilagines tracheales
    c. triquetra
    c. triticea
    c. tubae auditivae
    c. vomeronasalis
    c. wrisbergi
Cartwright prosthesis
caruncle
    c. epicanthus
    hymenal c.
    lacrimal c.
    major c. of Santorini
    Morgagni c.
    morgagnian c.
    myrtiform c.
    salivary c.
    sublingual c.
    urethral c.
caruncula (carunculae)
    carunculae hymenales
    c. lacrimalis
    c. salivaris
    c. sublingualis
caruncular
Carus
    circle
    curve
Carvallo sign
carver
caryophil
CAS—chronic alcohol syndrome
Casal
    collar
    necklace
cascade
    extrinsic coagulation c.
    intrinsic coagulation c.
cascara
    c. amarga
    c. sagrada
case
    borderline c.
    index c.
    primary c.
    secondary c.
    trial c.
caseation
casebook
case history
casein
caseinate

caseogenous
caseous necrosis
caseum
Casoni
    intradermal test
    reaction
Caspar ring opacity
cassava
Casselberry position
Casser (Casserio, Casserius)
    fontanelle
    ligament
    muscle
casserian
cassette
Cassidy syndrome
Cassidy-Brophy forceps
Cassidy-Scholte syndrome
CAST—
    Cardiac Arrhythmia
      Suppression Trial
    color allergy screening test
cast
    bacterial c.
    blood c.
    Cotrel c.
    decidual c.
    dental c.
    diagnostic c.
    epithelial c.
    false c.
    fatty c.
    fibrinous c.
    gnathostatic c.
    granular c.
    hair c.
    hanging c.
    hemoglobin c.
    Hexcelite c.
    hyaline c.
    investment c.
    Külz (Kuelz) c.
    leukocyte c.
    long arm c.
    long leg c.
    master c.
    mucous c.
    pigmented c's
    plaster of Paris c.
    preextraction c.
    preoperative c.
    pus c.
    quarter c.
    red cell c.
    refractory c.

cast *(continued)*
    renal c.
    Risser localizer c.
    Sarmiento c.
    short arm c.
    short leg c.
    spica c.
    spiral c.
    spurious tube c.
    study c.
    urate c.
    urinary c.
    wax c.
Castallo retractor
Castaneda
    bottle
    forceps
Castellani
    bronchitis
    disease
    paint
    test
Castellani-Low symptom
Castelli tube
casting
Castle intrinsic factor
Castleman disease
castrate
castration
    chemical c.
    female c.
    male c.
    radiologic c.
cast room
Castroviejo
    calipers
    cannula
    dilator
    forceps
    holder
    keratome
    knife
    needle holder
    operation
    punch
    retractor
    scissors
    spatula
    speculum
    trephine
Castroviejo-Arruga forceps
Castroviejo-Kalt needle
    holder
casualty
casuistics

CAT—
　　Children's Apperception Test
　　computerized axial
　　　tomography
CAT scan
catabasial
catabolism
　　antibody c.
catacrotism
catadicrotic
catagen
catalase
catalepsy
cataleptic
cataleptiform
catalysis
catalyst
catalytic
catalyze
catamenia
catamenial
catamnesis
catamnestic
catapasm
cataphoresis
cataphoretic
cataphoria
cataphylaxis
cataplasm
cataplectic
cataplexie du réveil
cataplexy
catapophysis
cataract
　　adherent c.
　　adolescent c.
　　after-c.
　　aminoaciduria c.
　　arborescent c.
　　atopic c.
　　axial fusiform c.
　　axillary c.
　　black c.
　　blue c., blue dot c.
　　brown c.
　　brunescent c.
　　calcareous c.
　　capsular c.
　　capsulolenticular c.
　　caseous c.
　　cerulean c.
　　cheesy c.
　　choroidal c.
　　complete c.
　　complicated c.

cataract *(continued)*
　　congenital c.
　　contusion c.
　　coralliform c.
　　coronary c.
　　cortical c.
　　cuneiform c.
　　cupuliform c.
　　cystic c.
　　dermatogenic c.
　　developmental c.
　　diabetic c.
　　discission c.
　　dry-shelled c.
　　duplication c.
　　electric c.
　　embryonal nuclear c.
　　embryopathic c.
　　evolutionary c.
　　extracapsular c.
　　fibroid c.
　　floriform c.
　　fluid c.
　　fusiform c.
　　galactosemic c.
　　glass blowers' c.
　　glaucomatous c.
　　gray c.
　　hard c.
　　heterochromic c.
　　hypermature c.
　　hypocalcemic c.
　　immature c.
　　incipient c.
　　infantile c.
　　intracapsular c.
　　intumescent c.
　　irradiation c.
　　juvenile c.
　　lamellar c.
　　lenticular c.
　　mature c.
　　membranous c.
　　metabolic c.
　　milky c.
　　morgagnian c.
　　c. needle
　　nuclear c.
　　nutritional deficiency c.
　　occupational c.
　　overripe c.
　　perinuclear c.
　　peripheral c.
　　polar c.
　　postinflammatory c.

cataract *(continued)*
    c's of prematurity
    presenile c.
    primary c.
    progressive c.
    punctate c.
    pyramidal c.
    radiation c.
    ringform congenital c.
    ripe c.
    rubella c.
    secondary c.
    sedimentary c.
    senile c.
    senile nuclear sclerotic c.
    snowflake c., snowstorm c.
    Soemmering ring c.
    spindle c.
    stationary c.
    stellate c.
    subcapsular c.
    subtotal c.
    sunflower c.
    supranuclear c.
    sutural c.
    syndermatotic c.
    syphilitic c.
    thermal c.
    total c.
    toxic c.
    traumatic c.
    unripe c.
    zonular c.
cataracta
    c. accreta
    c. brunescens
    c. cerulea
    c. complicata
    c. congenita membranacea
    c. coronaria
    c. electrica
    c. membranacea accreta
    c. nigra
    c. ossea
cataractogenic
cataractous
catarrh
    atrophic c.
    autumnal c.
    Bostock c.
    epidemic c.
    hypertrophic c.
    Laënnec c.
    postnasal c.
    sinus c.

catarrh *(continued)*
    spring c.
    suffocative c.
    summer c.
    vernal c.
catarrhal
catarrhine
catastaltic
catastrophe
catastrophic
catathymia
catathymic
catatonia
catatonic
catatricrotic
catecholamine
catecholaminergic
category
catelectrotonus
catenating
catenoid
cat-eye, cat's eye
    c-e. amaurosis
    c-e. pupil
    c-e. reflex
    c-e. syndrome
catgut
    carbolized c.
    chromic c. suture
    IKI c.
    iodine c.
    iodochromic c.
    silverized c.
    c. suture
catharsis
cathartic
    bulk c.
    lubricant c.
    saline c.
    stimulant c.
    c. acid
cathectic
Cathelin
    method
    segregator
cathemoglobin
cathepsin
catheresis
catheretic
catheter
    Abramson c.
    acorn-tip c., acorn-tipped c.
    Alcock c.
    Amplatz c.
    angiographic c.

catheter *(continued)*

aortic flush pigtail c.
Argyle c.
arterial c.
Ash Split Cath hemodialysis c.
atherectomy c.
Bailey c.
balloon c.
balloon-tip c.
c. balloon valvuloplasty (CBV)
Bard c.
Bardex c.
bicoudate c.
c. bicoudé
biliary c.
Blasucci curved-tip ureteral c.
Blasucci pigtail ureteral c.
Bozeman c.
Bozeman-Fritsch c.
Braasch bulb c.
Brockenbrough transseptal c.
Broviac c.
butterfly c.
Camino intracranial c.
Campbell c.
cardiac c.
Carlens c.
Carson c.
Castillo c.
central venous pressure
    (CVP) c.
c. clip
closed end-hole c.
coaxial counterflow single-
    needle blood access c.
condom c.
conical c.
Cook c.
Cope loop c.
coudé c.
Councill c.
Cournand c.
CVP (central venous
    pressure) c.
DeLee c.
de Pezzer c.
directional atherectomy c.
double-channel c.
double-current c.
double-J stent c.
double-lumen c.
Drew-Smythe c.
dual-lumen c.
Edwards c.
elbowed c.

catheter *(continued)*

electrode c.
Emmett-Foley c.
end-hole c.
eustachian c.
female c.
femoral c.
filiform c.
filiform-tipped c.
flexible c.
fluid-filled c.
Fogarty c.
Foley c.
Foley-Alcock c.
French polyethylene c.
French-Robinson c.
Fritsch c.
Furniss c.
Garceau c.
Gensini coronary c.
Goodale-Lubin c.
Gouley c.
Grollman pigtail c.
Groshong c.
Grüntzig (Gruentzig)
    balloon-tip c.
headhunter c.
hemodialysis c.
Hickman c.
c.-induced thrombosis
indwelling c.
Ingram trocar c.
internal jugular c.
intracardiac c.
Intracath c.
intraluminal c.
intraperitoneal c.
Itard c.
Jackson-Pratt c.
Judkins coronary c.
Judkins pigtail left
    ventriculography c.
Karman c.
KISS (kidney internal
    splint/stent) c.
Lane c.
latex c.
Le Fort c.
left coronary c.
Lehman c.
Lloyd c.
Malecot c.
manometer-tipped c.
Metras c.
Mixter c.

catheter *(continued)*
  multipurpose c.
  mushroom c.
  nasogastric c.
  nasotracheal c.
  needle c. jejunostomy
  Nélaton c.
  nephrostomy c.
  NIH (National Institutes of Health) c.
  Nutricath c.
  Nycore pigtail c.
  olive-tip c.
  opaque c.
  oropharyngeal c.
  Owen c.
  pacing c.
  percutaneous c.
  peripherally inserted central c. (PICC)
  Pezzer c.
  Phillips c.
  pigtail angiographic c.
  polyethylene c.
  preformed c.
  prostatic c.
  pulmonary artery c.
  radiopaque c.
  red Robinson c.
  red rubber c.
  retention c.
  retrograde c.
  return flow hemostatic c.
  right coronary c.
  Ring-McLean c.
  Robinson c.
  self-retaining c.
  sheathed c.
  sidewinder c.
  Silastic mushroom c.
  Simmons c.
  snare c.
  Sones coronary c.
  spiral-tip c.
  split-sheath c.
  subclavian c.
  Swan-Ganz c.
  swan neck c.
  Teflon c.
  Tenckhoff peritoneal c.
  Texas c.
  thermodilution c.
  Thompson c.
  Tiemann c.
  toposcopic c.

catheter *(continued)*
  tracheal c.
  transluminal endarterectomy c.
  transtracheal oxygen c.
  trocar c.
  tunneled c.
  two-way c.
  umbilical c.
  ureteral c.
  urethral c.
  venous c.
  ventricular c.
  vertebrated c.
  von Sonnenberg c.
  Weber c.
  whip c.
  whistle-tip c.
  Winer c.
  winged c.
  Yankauer c.
catheterization
  balloon c.
  cardiac c.
  eustachian c.
  hepatic vein c.
  laryngeal c.
  retrourethral c.
  Seldinger c.
  suprapubic c.
  transseptal c.
cathexis
cathode-ray tube (CRT)
cation
cationic
catlin, catling
cat-scratch disease
cat's cry syndrome
Cattani serum
Cattel Infant Intelligence Scale
Cattell
  operation
  tube
Caucasian
caucasoid
cauda (caudae)
  c. cerebelli
  c. corporis striati
  c. epididymidis
  c. equina
  c. helicis
  c. nuclei
  c. pancreatis
caudad
caudal
caudalward

caudate
caudatolenticular
caudocephalad
caul
cauliflower ear
Caulk punch
caumesthesia
causal
causalgia
causation
    legal c.
causative
cause
    constitutional c.
    contributory c. of death
    c. of death
    exciting c.
    immediate c.
    local c.
    precipitating c.
    predisposing c.
    primary c.
    proximate c.
    remote c.
    secondary c.
    specific c.
    ultimate c.
    underlying c. of death
caustic
    Churchill iodine c.
    Filhos c.
    Landolfi c.
    Lugol c.
    lunar c.
    mitigated c.
    Plunket c.
    Rousselot c.
    Vienna c.
    zinc c.
causticize
cauterant
cauterization
    cold c.
    c. by points
    punctuate c.
cauterize
cautery
    actual c.
    bicap c.
    bipolar c.
    Birtcher c.
    chemical c.
    cold c.
    Corrigan c.
    electric c.

cautery *(continued)*
    galvanic c.
    gas c.
    Graefe c. (von Graefe c.)
    Mils c.
    Mueller c.
    Percy c.
    potential c.
    Scheie c.
    virtual c.
    Wadsworth-Todd c.
    wet-field c.
    Ziegler c.
cautionary
CAV—
    congenital absence of
        vagina
    congenital adrenal virilism
    croup-associated virus
    cyclophosphamide,
        Adriamycin, vincristine
cava (plural of cavum)
caval
CAVB—complete atrioventricular
    block
Cave operation
caveola
cavern
caverna (cavernae)
    cavernae corporis spongiosi
        penis
    cavernae corporum
        cavernosorum penis
caverniloquy
cavernitis
    fibrous c.
cavernoscopy
cavernostomy
cavernous
    c. hemangioma
    c. lymphangioma
    c. sinus
    c. sinus thrombosis
Cave-Rowe operation
CAVH—continuous arteriovenous
    hemofiltration
cavitary lesion
cavitas (cavitates)
    c. abdominalis
    c. articularis
    c. conchae
    c. conchalis
    c. coronalis
    c. cranii
    c. dentis

cavitas (cavitates) *(continued)*
- c. epiduralis
- c. glenoidalis
- c. infraglottica
- c. laryngis
- c. medullaris ossium
- c. nasi ossea
- c. oris externa
- c. oris propria
- c. pelvis
- c. pericardialis
- c. peritonealis
- c. pharyngis
- c. pleuralis
- c. pulparis
- c. septi pellucidi
- c. subarachnoidea
- c. subarachnoidealis
- c. thoracis
- c. tympanica
- c. uteri

cavitation of septum pellucidum

cavitis

Cavitron
- aspiration unit
- dissector
- ultrasonic aspirator (CUSA)

cavity
- abdominal c.
- absorption c's
- allantoic c.
- alveolar c.
- amniotic c.
- articular c.
- body c.
- buccal c.
- complex c.
- compound c.
- cotyloid c.
- cranial c.
- dental c.
- distal c.
- ectoplacental c.
- endometrial c.
- epidural c.
- epiploic c.
- faucial c.
- fibrotic c's
- fissure c.
- gastrovascular c.
- gastrulation c.
- glandular c.
- glenoid c.
- incisal c.
- infraglottic c.

cavity *(continued)*
- ischioanal c.
- ischiorectal c.
- joint c.
- labial c.
- laryngeal c.
- laryngopharyngeal c.
- lingual c.
- lymph c's
- marrow c.
- mastoid c.
- Meckel c.
- mediastinal c.
- medullary c.
- mesial c.
- c. of middle ear
- nasal c.
- occlusal c.
- oral c.
- orbital c.
- pectoral c.
- pelvic c.
- pericardial c.
- pericardiopleuroperitoneal c.
- peritoneal c.
- pharyngeal c.
- pharyngolaryngeal c.
- pharyngonasal c.
- pharyngo-oral c.
- c. of pharynx
- pit c.
- pleural c.
- pleuroperitoneal c.
- popliteal c.
- prepared c.
- proximal c.
- pulp c.
- rectoischiadic c.
- Retzius c.
- Rosenmüller c.
- segmentation c.
- serous c.
- sigmoid c.
- simple c.
- smooth surface c.
- somatic c.
- splanchnic c.
- Stafne c.
- subarachnoid c.
- subdural c.
- synovial c.
- tension c's
- thoracic c.
- trigeminal c.
- tympanic c.

C

cavity *(continued)*
    uterine c.
    visceral c.
cavography
cavosurface
cavovalgus
cavum (cava)
    c. conchae
    c. dentis
    c. epidurale
    c. oris externum
    c. psalterii
    c. pulpae
    c. septi pellucidi
    c. subarachnoideum
    c. trigeminale
cavus foot
cayenne
Cazenave
    disease
    lupus
    vitiligo
CB—chronic bronchitis
C&B—crown and bridge
CBA—chronic bronchitis with
    asthma
CBBB—complete bundle branch
    block
CBC—complete blood count
CBD—common bile duct
CBF—
    cerebral blood flow
    coronary blood flow
CBG—
    corticosteroid-binding globulin
    cortisol-binding globulin
CBI—continuous bladder irrigation
CBP—complete breech
    presentation
CBS—chronic brain syndrome
CBV—
    catheter balloon valvuloplasty
    central blood volume
    circulating blood volume
    corrected blood volume
CBW—chemical and biological
    warfare
c, cc—correction with glasses
cc, cm³, cu cm—cubic centimeter(s)
CC—
    cardiac cycle
    clinical course
    closing capacity
    cord compression
    costochondral

CC— *(continued)*
    cradle cap
    current complaints
CC, C/C—chief complaint
CC, C$_{cr}$—creatinine clearance
CCA—
    circumflex coronary artery
    common carotid artery
    congenital contractural
    arachnodactyly
CCAT—conglutinating complement
    absorption test
CCC—chronic calculous
    cholecystitis
CCF—
    carotid cavernous fistula
    cephalin-cholesterol
    flocculation
    compound comminuted
    fracture
    congestive cardiac failure
    crystal-induced chemotactic
    factor
CCK—cholecystokinin
C-clamp
CCN—coronary care nursing
CCP—chronic calcifying
    pancreatitis
CCPD—continuous cycled
    peritoneal dialysis
C$_{cr}$, CC—creatinine clearance
CCS—casualty clearing station
CCT—
    composite cyclic therapy
    cranial computed tomography
CCU—
    coronary care unit
    critical care unit
CCW—counterclockwise
CD—
    cadaver donor
    cardiac disease
    cardiac dullness
    common duct
    consanguineous donor
    curative dose
    cystic duct
C/D, C/d—cigarettes per day
C&D—cystoscopy and
    dilatation
CDC—
    calculated date of confinement
    Centers for Disease Control
    and Prevention
    chenodeoxycholate

CDCA—chenodeoxycholic acid
CDD—certificate of disability for discharge
CDE—common duct exploration
CDH—
    congenital diaphragmatic hernia
    congenital dislocation of the hip
CDI—Children's Depression Inventory
CDILD—chronic diffuse interstitial lung disease
cDNA—
    complementary DNA
    copy DNA
CDP—
    comprehensive discharge planning
    cytidine diphosphate
CDR—
    clinical dementia rating
    computed digital radiography
    cup-to-disk ratio
CDSS—clinical decision support system
CDU—chemical dependency unit
CE—
    cardiac enlargement
    cerebral edema
    cholesterol esters
    contractile element
CEA—
    carcinoembryonic antigen
    carotid endarterectomy
ceasmic
cebocephalus
cebocephaly
ceca (plural of cecum)
cecal
cecectomy
Cecil
    operation
    repair
Cecil-Culp repair
cecitis
cecocele
cecocolic
cecocolon
cecocolopexy
cecocolostomy
cecocystoplasty
cecoileostomy
cecopexy
cecoplication

cecoptosis
cecorectal
cecorrhaphy
cecosigmoidostomy
cecostomy
    Beardsley c. trocar
cecotomy
CECT—contrast-enhanced computed tomography
cecum (ceca)
    cupular c. of cochlear duct
    c. cupulare ductus cochlearis
    hepatic c.
    high c.
    mobile c.
    vestibular c. of cochlear duct
    c. vestibulare ductus cochlearis
CEG—chronic erosive gastritis
Celestin tube
celiac
    c. arteriography
    c. disease
    c. sprue
celiectomy
celiocolpotomy
celioenterotomy
celiogastrotomy
celiohysterectomy
celiohysterotomy
celioma
celiomyomectomy
celiomyomotomy
celiomyositis
celioparacentesis
celiopathy
celiopyosis
celiorrhaphy
celiosalpingectomy
celiosalpingotomy
celiotomy
    c. incision
    vaginal c.
    ventral c.
celitis
cell
    A c.
    Abbe-Zeiss counting c.
    acanthoid c.
    accessory c.
    acidophilic c.
    acinar c., acinous c.
    acoustic hair c.
    activated reticular c.
    adherent c.

cell *(continued)*

adipose c.
adventitial c.
agger nasi c's
agranular c.
air c's of Mosher
albuminous c.
algoid c's
alpha c.
alveolar c's, type I and type II
Alzheimer c.
amacrine c.
ameboid c.
amine precursor uptake and
  decarboxylation c's
amphophilic c.
anaplastic c.
aneuploid c.
Anitschkow (Anichkov) c.
anterior ethmoidal air c's
anterior horn c.
antigen-presenting c.
antigen-reactive c's
antigen-sensitive c's
apocrine c's
APUD c's
argentaffin c.
argyrophilic c's
Arias-Stella c's
Armanni-Ebstein c.
Aschoff c.
Askanazy c.
atypical c.
auditory c.
autologous lymphokine
  activated killer c.
B c.
balloon c.
band c.
bank c.
basal c.
basal granular c's
basilar c.
basket c.
basophilic c.
beaker c.
Beale ganglion c's
Bergmann c's
berry c.
beta c.
Betz c's
Bevan-Lewis c.
bipolar retinal c's
Bizzozero c.
bladder c's

cell *(continued)*

blast c.
blood c.
bone marrow c.
border c's
Böttcher (Boettcher) c's
breviradiate c's
bristle c's
bronchic c.
buffy coat c., buffy-coated c.
burr c.
C c.
Cajal c.
caliciform c.
cameloid c.
capsule c's
cardiac failure c's
cartilage c.
castration c's
caudate c's
caveolated c's
CD4 c's, CD4+ c's
CD8 c's, CD8+ c's
cement c.
central c.
centroacinar c's
chalice c.
chief c's
Chinese hamster ovary
  (CHO) c's
chromaffin c.
chromophobe c's,
  chromophobic c's
ciliated c.
Clara c's
Clarke c's
Claudius c's
clear c's
clonogenic c.
clue c.
clump c's
columnar c.
commissural c's
committed c.
companion c.
cone c., cone bipolar c.
connective tissue c's
contractile fiber c's
contrasuppressor c's
corneal c.
cornified c.
c. of Corti
corticotrope c., corticotroph c.
corticotroph-lipotroph c.
counting c.

cell *(continued)*

cover c.
crenated c.
crescent c's
cribrate c.
Crooke c's
cuboid c.
Custer c's
cylindric c.
cytomegalic c.
cytotoxic c., cytotoxic T c's
D c's
daughter c.
Davidoff (Davidov) c's
decidual c.
deep c.
Deiters c's
delta c.
demilune c's
dendritic c's
dentin c.
c. differentiation
diploid c.
displaced ganglion c.
c. division
dome c's
Dorothy Reed c's
Downey c.
dust c.
effector c.
embryonic stem c.
emigrated c.
enamel c.
encasing c.
endocervical c.
endocrine c.
endometrial c.
endothelial c., endothelioid c.
enterochromaffin c.
ependymal c.
epidermic c's
epithelial c., epithelioid c.
erythroid c.
ethmoidal c's
eukaryotic c.
F c.
c. of Fañanás (Fananas)
fat c.
fat-storing c. of liver
fiber c.
fixed c.
flagellate c.
c. and flare
flat bipolar c.
foam c.

cell *(continued)*

follicle c's, follicular c's
follicular dendritic c.
follicular epithelial c's
foreign body giant c's
free c.
fuchsinophil c.
fusiform c.
G c's
gametoid c's
gamma c.
ganglion c.
Gaucher c.
Gegenbaur c.
germ c's
germinal c.
ghost c.
Giannuzzi c's
giant c.
giant pyramidal c's
Gierke c's
glandular c.
Gley c's
glia c.
glitter c.
glomerular c.
glomus c.
goblet c.
Golgi c.
gonadotroph c.
Goormaghtigh c's
granular c.
granulosa c.
granulosa-lutein c's
grape c.
ground-glass c.
gustatory c's
H c.
hair c's
hairy c.
Hammar myoid c's
haploid c.
heart disease c's
heart failure c's
heart lesion c's
hecatomeral c's
heckle c.
Heidenhain c's
HEK (human embryo kidney) c.
HEL (human embryo lung) c.
HeLa c.
helmet c.
helper c's, helper T c's
hematopoietic precursor c.
hematopoietic stem c.

cell *(continued)*

Hensen c's
hepatic c.
heteromeral c's, heteromeric c's
hilum c's
Hodgkin c's
Hofbauer c's
homozygous typing (HTC) c's
horizontal c.
horizontal c. of Cajal
horn c., horny c.
Hortega c.
human embryo kidney c. (HEK c.)
human embryo lung c. (HEL c.)
Hürthle c.
hybrid c.
hyperchromatic c.
I-c.
immunocompetent c.
immunologically competent c.
incasing c.
inclusion c.
indifferent c.
inducer c.
inflammatory c.
initial c's
integrator c.
intercalary c.
intercalated c's
intercapillary c's
interdental c's
interdigitating c's
interfollicular c's
internuncial c.
interstitial c., interstitial c's of Cajal
intestinal absorptive c.
intracytoplasmic inclusion c.
islet c.
juvenile c.
juxtaglomerular c's
K c.
keratinized c.
killer c., killer T c's
Kulchitsky c's
Kupffer c.
L c's
lacis c.
lacrimoethmoid c's
lacunar c.
Langerhans c.
Langhans giant c's
large cleaved follicular center c.
large granule c's

cell *(continued)*

large noncleaved follicular center c.
LE c.
Leishman chrome c's
lepra c.
Leydig c.
light c's
Lipschütz (Lipschuetz) c.
littoral c's
liver c.
lupus erythematosus (LE) c.
luteal c's, lutein c., luteum c.
lymph c.
lymphoid c.
lymphoreticular c.
M c.
macroglial c.
malpighian c.
Marchand c.
marginal c's
marrow c.
Martinotti c's
mast c.
mastoid c's
matrix c's
maturation B c.
Mauthner c.
c.-mediated immunity
mediator c.
medullary interstitial c.
medulloepithelial c.
melanotropic c.
memory c's
Merkel-Ranvier c's
Merkel tactile c's
mesangial c's
mesenchymal c's
mesothelial c.
metallophil c.
metaplastic c.
Mexican hat c.
Meynert c's
microglial c.
Mikulicz c's
mitral c.
mononuclear c.
Mooser c.
morular c.
mossy c.
mother c.
motor c.
Mott c.
mouth c's
mucoalbuminous c's

cell *(continued)*

    mucous c., mucous neck c's
    mulberry c.
    c's of Müller
    multipolar c.
    mural c.
    muscle c.
    myeloid c.
    myeloma c.
    myoepithelial c's
    myoepithelioid c's
    myoid c's
    myointimal c.
    Nageotte c's
    natural killer (NK) c.
    nerve c.
    neuroepithelial c.
    neuroglia c's, neuroglial c's
    neuromuscular c.
    neurosecretory c.
    neutrophilic c.
    nevus c.
    Niemann-Pick c's
    NK (natural killer) c.
    noble c.
    nonadherent c.
    noncleaved follicular
      center c.
    normal c.
    nucleated red blood c.
    null c.
    nurse c's
    oat c's
    olfactory c.
    oligodendroglial c.
    osseous c.
    osteoprogenitor c's
    oxyntic c's
    oxyphil c's, oxyphilic c's
    P c.
    packed c's
    packed human blood c's
    packed red blood c's
    Paget c., pagetoid c.
    palatine c's
    palisade c's
    Paneth c.
    parabasal c.
    parafollicular c.
    paraluteal c's, paralutein c's
    parenchymal hepatic c.,
      parenchymal liver c
    parent c.
    parietal c's
    pathologic c.

cell *(continued)*

    pavement c's
    pediculated c's
    peg c's
    Pelger-Huët c.
    peptic c's
    pericapillary c.
    peripheral blood precursor c.
    peripheral blood stem c.
    perithelial c.
    peritubular contractile c's
    perivascular c.
    pessary c.
    phagocytic c.
    phalangeal c's, phalangeal c. of
      Deiters
    phantom c.
    pheochrome c's
    photoreceptor c's
    physaliferous c's,
      physaliphorous c's
    Pick c's
    pigment c.
    pillar c's
    pineal c.
    plaque-forming c's
    plasma c.
    pluripotent c.
    pneumatic c.
    PNH c's
    polychromatic c's,
      polychromatophil c's
    polygonal c.
    PP c's
    pre-B c.
    prefollicle c's
    pregnancy c.
    pregranulosa c.
    pre-T c.
    prickle c.
    primary c.
    primordial germ c.
    principal c's
    progenitor c.
    prokaryotic c.
    prolactin c.
    pulmonary epithelial c's
    pulpar c's
    pyramidal c.
    RA c.
    radial c's of Müller
    Raji c's
    red c's, red blood c's (RBCs)
    Reed c's
    Reed-Sternberg giant c.

cell *(continued)*

- renal c., renal tubular c.
- Renshaw c's
- reserve c's
- residential c.
- resting c., resting wandering c.
- reticular c's, reticulum c.
- reticuloendothelial c.
- Rieder c.
- rod c's
- Rohon-Beard c's
- Rolando c's
- root c.
- Rouget c.
- round c.
- S c's
- Sala c's
- sarcogenic c.
- satellite c's
- scavenger c.
- Schultze c's
- Schwann c.
- segmented c.
- seminal c's
- seminoma c.
- sensitized c.
- sensory c.
- sentinel c's
- septal c's
- serous c.
- Sertoli c.
- sexual c's
- Sézary c.
- shadow c.
- sickle c.
- signet c., signet ring c.
- skeletogenous c.
- small cleaved follicular center c.
- small granule c's
- small noncleaved follicular center c.
- smooth muscle c.
- smudge c.
- somatic c.
- somatostatin c's
- somatotropic c.
- sperm c.
- spermatogonial c.
- sphenoid c.
- spider c.
- spindle c., spindle-shaped c.
- spur c.
- squamous c.
- stab c.
- staff c.

cell *(continued)*

- star c's
- stave c's
- stellate c.
- stem c.
- Sternberg giant c's
- Sternberg-Reed c's
- stippled c.
- superficial c.
- supporting c's
- suppressor c.
- sustentacular c's
- sympathicotrophic c's
- sympathochromaffin c's
- syncytial c.
- synovial c's
- T c's
- tactile c.
- tadpole c.
- tagged red c's
- target c.
- tart c.
- taste c's
- tautomeral c's
- T-cytotoxic c.
- TDTH c's
- teardrop c.
- tegmental c's
- tendon c's
- Tγ (T-gamma) c's
- theca c., theca-lutein c.
- thymus-dependent c., thymus-derived c.
- thyroidectomy c's
- Tμ [T-mu] c's
- totipotential c.
- Touton giant c.
- transducer c.
- transitional c.
- trisomic c.
- trophochrome c's
- T-suppressor c.
- tubal air c's
- tube c.
- Türk c.
- tympanic c's
- Tzanck c.
- ultimobranchial c's
- umbrella c.
- undifferentiated c.
- unipolar c.
- vacuolated c.
- c's of van Gehuchten
- van Hansemann c's
- vasofactive c.

cell *(continued)*
 veil c's, veiled c.
 ventricular c.
 Vero c's
 vestibular hair c's
 veto c's
 Vignal c's
 Virchow c.
 visual c's
 von Kupffer c's
 Walthard c.
 wandering c.
 Warthin-Finkeldey c.
 wasserhelle c's
 water-clear c.
 Wedl c's
 white c's, white blood c's
  (WBCs)
 wing c's
 xanthoma c.
 Zander c's
 zymogenic c.
cella (cellae)
 c. lateralis ventriculi lateralis
 c. media ventriculi lateralis
cell body
cell-free
cell-mediated immunity (CMI)
cellobiuronic acid
celloidin
Cellolite
cellophane
 c. dressing
 c. retinopathy
Cell Saver Haemolite
cell saver transfusion
cellula (cellulae)
 cellulae anteriores
  ethmoidales
 cellulae ethmoidales mediae
 cellulae ethmoidales osseae
 cellulae ethmoidales
  posteriores
 cellulae lentis
 cellulae mastoideae
 cellulae pneumaticae tubae
  auditivae
 cellulae pneumaticae tubariae
 c. sensoria pilosa
 cellulae tympanicae
cellular
 c. immune deficiency
 c. immunity
cellularity
cellule claire

cellulifugal
cellulipetal
cellulitis
 anaerobic c.
 cervical c.
 clostridial c.
 clostridial anaerobic c.
 dissecting c. of scalp
 eosinophilic c.
 facial c.
 finger c.
 gangrenous c.
 gaseous c.
 indurated c.
 necrotizing c.
 nonclostridial
  anaerobic c.
 orbital c.
 pelvic c.
 peritonsillar c.
 periurethral c.
 phlegmonous c.
 streptococcal c.
 ulcerative c.
celluloid suture
cellulose
 absorbable c.
 c. acetate
 c. acetate phthalate
 hydroxyethyl c.
 hydroxypropyl c.
 microcrystalline c.
 oxidized c.
 c. sodium phosphate
 starch c.
 c. tetranitrate
cellulosic acid
cellulosity
celoschisis
celosomia
celosomus
celozoic
Celsius (C)
 degrees (°C)
 thermometer
Celsus
 kerion
 operation
 papules
 vitiligo
cement
 calcium hydroxide c.
 dental c.
 c. dressing
 glass ionomer c.

cement *(continued)*
    methylmethacrylate c.
    oxyphosphate c.
    polycarboxylate c.
    polymethacrylate c.
    resin c.
    root canal c.
    silicate c.
    zinc oxide–eugenol c.
    zinc phosphate c.
cementation
cementicle
    adherent c.
    attached c.
    free c.
    interstitial c.
cementin
cementitis
cementless arthroplasty
cementoblastoma
cementoclasia
cementogenesis
cementoid
cementoma
    gigantiform c.
    true c.
cementopathia
cementosis
cementum
    acellular c.
    afibrillar c.
    cellular c.
    uncalcified c.
cenadelphus
cenesthopathy
cenopsychic
censor
    freudian c.
    psychic c.
censorship
center
    accelerating c.
    acoustic c.
    active c.
    anospinal c's
    appetite c.
    association c.
    auditory c.
    basioccipital c.
    basiotic c.
    basisphenoid c.
    Béclard ossification c.
    birthing c.
    brain c.
    Broca c.

center *(continued)*
    Budge cell
    bulbar respiratory c.
    burn c.
    cardioaccelerating c.
    cardioinhibitory c.
    cardiomotor c.
    cell c.
    chiral c.
    c's of chondrification
    ciliospinal c.
    community mental health c.
      (CMHC)
    convergence c.
    coordination c.
    correlation c.
    cortical c.
    costal c.
    coughing c.
    defecation c.
    deglutition c.
    dentary c.
    ejaculation c.
    epiotic c.
    feeding c.
    Flemming c.
    genital c., genitospinal c.
    germinal c.
    glossokinesthetic c.
    gustatory c.
    health c.
    heat-regulating c's
    hunger c.
    inactivation c.
    inhibitory c.
    interim accommodation c.
    interparietal c.
    Kerckring (Kerkring) c.
    kinesthetic c.
    kinetic c.
    Kronecker c.
    Kupressoff c.
    Lumsden c.
    medullary c. of cerebellum
    medullary respiratory c.
    micturition c's
    motor c.
    negative reward c.
    nerve c.
    olfactory c.
    optic c.
    ossification c.
    pacemaker c.
    panting c.
    parturition c.

C

center *(continued)*
    phrenic c.
    plantar reflex c.
    pneumotaxic c.
    poison control c.
    polypneic c.
    pontine c. for lateral
        gaze
    pteriotic c.
    punishment c.
    reaction c.
    rectovesical c.
    reflex c.
    respiratory c's
    reward c.
    rotation c.
    salivary c.
    satiety c.
    sex-behavior c.
    speech c.
    sphenotic c.
    splenial c.
    sudorific c's
    swallowing c.
    sweat c's
    taste c.
    thermoregulatory c's
    thirst c.
    vasoconstrictor c.
    vasodilator c.
    vesical c's
    vesicospinal c's
    vital c's
    vomiting c.
    Wernicke c.
    winking c.
    word c., auditory
    word c., visual
center of rotation
Centers for Disease Control and
    Prevention (CDC)
centesimal (c)
centesis
centigrade (C)
centigray (cGy)
centiliter (cL)
centimeter (cm)
    cubic c. (cm^3, cu cm)
    c. squared (cm^2, sq cm)
centimorgan (cM)
centipede
centipoise
centra (plural of centrum)
centrad
centrage

central
    c. fixation
    c. fusion
    c. nervous system
        (CNS)
    c. retinal artery, c. retinal
        artery occlusion
    c. retinal vein, c. retinal vein
        occlusion
    c. scotoma
    c. serous
        chorioretinopathy
    c. suppression
    c. visual acuity
centralis
central nervous system (CNS)
    disease
central venous pressure (CVP)
    catheter
centraphose
centration
centraxonial
centrencephalic
centric
    c. occlusion
    power c.
    c. relation
    true c.
centriciput
centrifugal
centrifugate
centrifugation
centrifuge microscope
centrilobular
centriole
    anterior c.
    distal c.
    posterior c.
    proximal c.
    ring c.
centripetal
centroblast
centrocecal
centrocyte
centromere
centromeric
centrophose
centrosclerosis
centrosome
centrosphere
centrum (centra)
    c. semiovale
    c. vertebrae
CEOM—chronic exudative otitis
    media

CEP—
    congenital erythropoietic
        porphyria
    cortical evoked potential
    counterelectrophoresis
cephalad
cephalalgia
    histamine c.
    pharyngotympanic c.
    quadrantal c.
cephaledema
cephalgia
cephalhematocele
    Stromeyer c.
cephalhematoma deformans
cephalhydrocele traumatica
cephalic
cephalocaudad
cephalocentesis
cephalodactyly
    Vogt c.
cephalodiprosopus
cephalodymus
cephalogram
cephalogyric
cephalomegaly
cephalomelus
cephalomenia
cephalomeningitis
cephalometric
cephalometry
    fetal c.
    radiographic c.
    ultrasonic c.
cephalomotor
cephalonia
cephalopathy
cephalopelvic disproportion
cephalopharyngeus
cephaloplegia
cephalorhachidian
cephalosporin
    first-generation c.
    fourth-generation c.
    second-generation c.
    third-generation c.
cephalostat
cephalostyle
cephalothoracoiliopagus
cephalothoracopagus
cephalothorax
cephalotomy
cephalotropic
CER—central episiotomy and
    repair

CERA—
    continuous erythropoietin
        receptor activator
    cortical evoked response
        audiometry
ceraceous
ceramic
    dental c's
    glass c.
    c. head of hip prosthesis
ceramidase glucoside deficiency
ceramide
    c. trihexoside
    c. trihexosidase deficiency
ceratocricoid
ceratocricoideus
ceratohyal
ceratopharyngeus
Ceratophyllus
    C. gallinae
cercarienhullenreaktion
cerclage
Cercospora apii
cercosporamycosis
cerea flexibilitas
cereal
cerebella (plural of cerebellum)
cerebellar
cerebellifugal
cerebellipetal
cerebellitis
cerebello-olivary
cerebellopontine angle tumor
cerebellorubral
cerebellorubrospinal
cerebellospinal
cerebellum
cerebra (plural of cerebrum)
cerebral
    c. angiography
    c. arteriography
    c. dyschromatopsia
    c. ventriculography
cerebration
    unconscious c.
cerebriform
cerebrifugal
cerebripetal
cerebritis
cerebrocardiac
cerebrocerebellar
cerebrocuprein
cerebroid
cerebromalacia
cerebromedullary tube

cerebromeningeal
cerebromeningitis
cerebronic acid
cerebro-ocular
cerebropathia psychica toxemica
cerebropathy
cerebropontile
cerebrorachidian
cerebrosclerosis
cerebroside sulfatase
cerebrosidosis
cerebrosis
cerebrospinal fluid (CSF)
cerebrostomy
cerebrotendinous
cerebrotonia
cerebrovascular accident (CVA)
cerebrum
cerecloth
Cerenkov
    counter
    radiation
cereolus (cereoli)
cerium (Ce)
ceroid lipofuscin
ceroid lipofuscinosis
    Jansky-Bielschowsky–
      type c.
    Kufs-type c.
ceroplasty
certifiable
cerulean
ceruleus
cerumen
    impacted c.
    inspissated c.
ceruminal
ceruminolysis
ceruminolytic
ceruminoma
ceruminosis
ceruminous
cervical
    anterior c. diskectomy and
      fusion (ACDF)
    c. biopsy
    c. canal
    c. caps
    c. collar
    c. conization
    c. os
    c. fascia
    c. incision
    c. laminectomy
    c. plexus

cervical *(continued)*
    c. punch biopsy clamp
    c. sympathectomy
cervicalis
cervicectomy
cervices (plural of cervix)
cervicitis
    granulomatous c.
    traumatic c.
cervicoaxillary
cervicobrachial
cervicobrachialgia
cervicobuccal
cervicocolpitis emphysematosa
cervicodorsal
cervicodynia
cervicofacial
cervico-occipital
cervicopexy
cervicoplasty
cervicoscapular
cervicothoracic
cervicotomy
cervicovaginal
cervicovaginitis
cervicovesical
cervix (cervices)
    c. of axon
    conglutination of c.
    c. dentis
    double c.
    c. glandis penis
    incompetent c.
    c. mallei
    tapiroid c.
    c. uteri
    c. vesicae urinariae
CES—clitoral engorgement
  syndrome
cesarean section
    cervical c.s.
    classic c.s.
    corporeal c.s.
    extraperitoneal c.s.
    Kerr c.s.
    Latzko c.s.
    low c.s., low-cervical c.s.
    lower segment c.s.
    Munro-Kerr c.s.
    Porro c.s.
    postmortem c.s.
    radical c.s.
    transperitoneal c.s.
    transverse c.s.
    Waters c.s.

CESD—cholesteryl ester storage
  disease
CES-D—Center for Epidemiological
  Studies of Depression
CES-D scale
cesium (Cs)
  c. with barium 137m
Cestan
  sign
  syndrome
Cestan-Chenais syndrome
Cestan-Raymond syndrome
cesticidal
cestode
cestodiasis
cestoid
CF—
  carbolfuchsin
  cardiac failure
  Caucasian female
  Christmas factor
  citrovorum factor
  complement fixation;
    complement-fixing
  contractile force
  count fingers
  cystic fibrosis
CFA—
  common femoral artery
  complement-fixation antibody
  complement-fixing antibody
  complete Freund adjuvant
  craniofacial abnormality
CF antibody titer
CFF—
  critical flicker fusion test
  critical fusion frequency
CFIDS—chronic fatigue immune
  deficiency syndrome
CFP—
  chronic false-positive
  cystic fibrosis of pancreas
CFS—chronic fatigue syndrome
CFT—
  clinical full-time
  complement fixation test
cfu—colony-forming unit(s)
CG—
  choking gas (phosgene)
  chorionic gonadotropin
  chronic glomerulonephritis
  colloidal gold
CGD—chronic granulomatous
  disease
CGI—clinical global impression

CGL—chronic granulocytic leukemia
cGMP, 3′,5′-GMP—cyclic guanosine
  monophosphate
CGN—chronic glomerulonephritis
CG/OQ—cerebral glucose oxygen
  quotient
CGP—
  choline glycerophosphatide
  chorionic growth hormone
    prolactin
  circulating granulocyte pool
CGRP—calcitonin gene-related
  peptide
CGS—catgut suture
cgs—centimeter-gram-second
CGT—chorionic gonadotropin
CGTT—cortisone glucose tolerance
  test
cGy—centigray
χ—chi (Greek letter)
CH—
  conversion hysteria
  crown-heel (length)
CH50—total serum hemolytic
  complement
CHA—
  congenital hypoplastic anemia
  cyclohexylamine
CHAD—cold hemolytic
  antibody disease
Chaddock
  reflex
  sign
Chadwick sign
chafe
Chaffin-Pratt tube
Chagas disease
Chagas-Cruz disease
chagasic
chagoma
chain
  α c. [alpha]
  A c.
  β c. [beta]
  branched c.
  closed c.
  c. cystourethrography
  δ c. [delta]
  ε c. [epsilon]
  food c.
  γ c. [gamma]
  H c.
  heavy c.
  immunoglobulin c.
  J c.

chain *(continued)*
    κ c. [kappa]
    L c.
    λ c. [lambda]
    lateral c.
    light c.
    μ c. [mu]
    nascent polypeptide c.
    nuclear c.
    open c.
    ossicular c.
    respiratory c.
    side c.
    c. suture
    sympathetic c.
chair
    birthing c.
    Gardner c.
    pendular c.
chair-back brace
chakra
chalasia
chalazion (chalazia)
chalazodermia
chalcosis
    c. corneae
    c. lentis
    c. oculi
chalicosis
chalk
    precipitated c.
    prepared c.
chalkitis
challenge
    fluid c.
    oxytocin c. test (OCT)
chamaecephalic
chamaecephaly
chamaeprosopic
chamaeprosopy
chamber
    Abbe-Zeiss counting c.
    acoustic c.
    air-equivalent ionization c.
    altitude c.
    anterior c.
    aqueous c.
    Atwater c.
    Atwater-Benedict c.
    Boyden c.
    cardiac c's
    counting c.
    decompression c.
    diffusion c.
    c's of eye

chamber *(continued)*
    free-air ionization c.
    c's of the heart
    hyperbaric c.
    ionization c.
    Petroff-Hauser counting c.
    pocket c.
    posterior c. of eye
    pulp c.
    relief c.
    Sandison-Clark c.
    Storm van Leeuwen c.
    thimble c.
    Thoma-Zeiss counting c.
    tissue-equivalent
      ionization c.
    vitreous c.
    Wilson c.
    Zappert c.
Chamberland
    candle
    filter
Chamberlen forceps
chamfer reamer
chamomile
Champetier de Ribes bag
Chance fracture
chancre
    erosive c.
    fungating c.
    hard c.
    hunterian c.
    indurated c.
    mixed c.
    monorecidive c.
    Nisbet c.
    c. redux
    Ricord c.
    Rollet c.
    soft c.
    sulcus c.
    tuberculous c.
    tularemic c.
chancriform
chancroid
    phagedenic c.
    serpiginous c.
chancroidal
chancrous
chandelier sign
Chandler
    disease
    elevator
    forceps
    retractor

Chandler *(continued)*
    splint
    syndrome
change
    Alzheimer neurofibrillary c's
    Armanni-Ebstein c.
    Biermer c.
    Crooke c's
    Crooke-Russell c's
    E to A c's
    fatty c.
    free energy c.
    Gerhardt c. of sound
    harlequin color c.
    QRS c.
    QRST c.
    ST-segment c.
    tubular hydropic c.
    T-wave c.
ch'ang shan
channel
    acetylcholine c.
    amiloride-sensitive sodium c.
    ATP-gated c's
    blood c's
    calcium c.
    calcium-sodium c.
    central c.
    chloride c.
    epithelial sodium c.
    fast c.
    gated c.
    c. of Haller
    inward rectifier potassium c's
    ion c.
    ligand-gated c.
    lymph c's
    mechanosensitive c.
    perineural c.
    perivascular c.
    potassium c.
    protein c.
    slow c.
    sodium c.
    thoroughfare c.
    voltage-gated c.
    water c.
Chantemesse reaction
Chaoul
    therapy
    tube
chapped
Chaput
    operation
    method

character
    acquired c.
    compound c.
    dominant c.
    epileptic c.
    imvic c's
    mendelian c.
    monogenic c.
    polygenic c.
    primary sex c's
    quantitative c.
    recessive c.
    secondary sex c's
    sex-influenced c.
    sex-limited c.
    sex-linked c.
    unit c.
characteristic
    demand c's
charcoal
    activated c.
    animal c.
    dextran-coated c.
    purified animal c.
Charcot
    arthropathy
    arthrosis
    bath
    cirrhosis
    disease
    fever
    foot
    gait
    joint
    syndrome
    triad
Charcot-Böttcher crystalloid
Charcot-Bouchard aneurysm
Charcot-Leyden crystals
Charcot-Marie
    atrophy
    type
Charcot-Marie-Tooth
    atrophy
    disease
    type
    syndrome
Charcot-Marie-Tooth-Hoffmann
    disease
    syndrome
Charcot-Neumann crystals
Charcot-Weiss-Baker syndrome
charlatan
Charles operation
charley horse

Charlin syndrome
Charlouis disease
Charnley
    arthrodesis
    hip arthroplasty
    total hip prosthesis
Charnley-Mueller
    arthroplasty
    hip prosthesis
Charriére bone saw
charring
chart
    alignment c.
    Amsler c's
    Donder c.
    Duane accommodative c.
    E-type c.
    exposure c.
    flow c.
    Guibor c.
    Landolt ring c.
    Liley c.
    pseudoisochromatic c.
    reading c.
    Reuss color c.
    Snellen c.
chartaceous
chartreuse
chartula
Chassaignac tubercle
Chassard-Lapiné projection
Chauffard syndrome
Chauffard-Still syndrome
Chausse III projection
    (third projection of Chausse)
CHB—complete heart block
CHD—
    childhood disease
    congenital heart disease
    congestive heart disease
    coronary heart disease
Cheadle disease
Cheatle-Henry hernia
Cheatle slit
checkbite, check-bite,
   check bite
checkerboard
Chédiak-Higashi
    disease
    syndrome
Chédiak-Steinbrinck-Higashi
   anomaly
cheek
    cleft c.
cheekbone

cheek-tooth
cheesy
cheilectomy
cheilectropion
cheilitis
    actinic c.
    c. actinica
    allergic c.
    angular c.
    apostematous c.
    commissural c.
    exfoliativa c.
    c. glandularis
    glandularis apostematosa c.
    c. granulomatosa
    impetiginous c.
    Miescher granulomatous c.
    migrating c.
    mycotic c.
    solar c.
    c. venenata
cheiloangioscopy
cheilocarcinoma
cheilognathopalatoschisis
cheilognathoprosoposchisis
cheilognathoschisis
cheilognathouranoschisis
cheilophagia
cheiloplasty
    Abbe c. (stage I, stage II)
cheilorrhaphy
cheiloschisis
cheilosis
    angular c.
cheilostomatoplasty
cheilotomy
cheiragra
cheiralgia paresthetica
cheirarthritis
cheirokinesthesia
cheirokinesthetic
cheirology
cheiromegaly
cheiroplasty
cheiropodalgia
cheiroscope
cheirospasm
chelate
chelation
Chelsea-Eaton speculum
chemabrasion
chemexfoliation
chemical
    c. castration
    c. hysterectomy

chemical *(continued)*
    radiomimetic c.
    c. sympathectomy
chemicogenesis
chemiluminescence
chemist
chemistry (chemistries)
    blood c. studies
    clinical c.
    forensic c.
    histological c.
    medical c.
    metabolic c.
    pharmaceutical c.
chemobiotic
chemocautery
chemocoagulation
chemodectoma
chemodifferentiation
chemoembolization
chemohormonal
chemokine
chemokinesis
chemokinetic
chemolysis
chemonucleolysis
chemopallidectomy
chemopallidothalamectomy
chemopharmacodynamics
chemoprophylaxis
    primary c.
    secondary c.
chemoprotectant
chemopsychiatry
chemoreception
chemoreceptor
chemoresistance
chemosensitive
chemosensory
chemosis
chemostat
chemosterilant
chemosterilization
chemosuppression
chemosurgery
    Mohs c.
chemosynthesis
chemosynthetic
chemotactic
chemotaxin
chemotaxis
chemothalamectomy
chemotherapeutic
chemotherapy
    adjuvant c.

chemotherapy *(continued)*
    combination c.
    induction c.
    neoadjuvant c.
    preoperative c.
    primary c.
    regional c.
    sequential c.
chemotic
chemotropism
chenodeoxycholate
chenodeoxycholic acid (chenodiol)
chenodeoxycholylglycine
chenodeoxycholyltaurine
Cherney incision
Chernez incision
Cherry
    osteotome
    retractor
    tongs
Cherry-Kerrison forceps
cherubism
chest
    alar c.
    AP (anteroposterior) c. x-ray
    barrel c.
    blast c.
    cobbler's c.
    emphysematous c.
    fissured c.
    flail c.
    flat c.
    foveated c.
    funnel c.
    hourglass c.
    keeled c.
    PA (posteroanterior) and
      lateral c. x-ray
    paralytic c.
    pendelluft c.
    phthinoid c.
    pigeon c.
    pterygoid c.
    rachitic c.
    stove-in c.
    tetrahedron c.
    c. tube
chestnut
Chevalier Jackson
    bronchoscope
    esophagoscope
    laryngoscope
    operation
    speculum
    tube

chevron
    c. osteotomy
    c.-shaped incision
Cheyne
    nystagmus
    operation
Cheyne-Stokes
    asthma
    breathing
    nystagmus
    psychosis
    respiration
CHF—congestive heart failure
CHH—cartilage-hair hypoplasia
chi—Greek letter (χ; alphabetized
    as ch)
CHI—closed head injury
Chiari
    disease
    network
    reticulum
    syndrome
Chiari-Arnold syndrome
Chiari-Frommel
    disease
    syndrome
Chiari-type malformation
chiasm
    campers' c.
    optic c.
    tendinous c. of fingers
chiasma (chiasmata)
    c. arachnoiditis
    c. opticum
    c. syndrome
    c. tendinum digitorum manus
chiasmal
chiasmatic
chiasmatypy
Chiba needle
chickenpox
Chiene
    incision
    operation
    test
Chievitz
    layer
    organ
chigger bite
chignon
Chilaiditi
    sign
    syndrome
chilblain
    necrotized c.

childbirth
Child hepatic risk classification
    (A–C)
childhood
Child-Phillips needle
childproof
chill
    brass c.
    brazier's c.
    creeping c.
    shaking c.
    spelter's c.
    urethral c.
    zinc c.
chilomastigiasis
Chilomastix mesnili
chimera
    heterologous c.
    homologous c.
    isologous c.
    radiation c.
    tetraparental c.
chimerism
    blood group c.
chin
    galoche c.
chincap
chinch bug
chionablepsia
chip
    bone c's
chiral
chirality
chiropractic
chiropractor
chisel
    Adson c.
    Alexander c.
    Converse c.
    Derlacki c.
    Derlacki-Shambaugh c.
    Fomon c.
    Freer c.
    guarded c.
    Hajek c.
    House c.
    Killian c.
    Moore c.
    periodontal c.
    Sewall c.
    Shambaugh-Derlacki c.
    Sheehan c.
    Troutman c.
chitin
chitinous

chitosan
CHL—crown-heel length
chlamydemia
Chlamydia
    C. trachomatis
chlamydia sepsis
Chlamydiazyme test
chloasma
chloracetic acid, chloroacetic acid
chloracne
chlorate
chlordane
chlordecone
chlorhexidine
    c. acetate
    c. gluconate
    c. hydrochloride
chloric acid
chloride
    acid c.
    ferric c.
    mercuric c.
    mercurous c.
    stannous c.
    thallous c. Tl 201
chloridimetry
chloridorrhea
    familial c.
chlorinated
chlorine (Cl)
    c. dioxide
chloriodized
chlorite
chloroacetic acid
chloroform
chloroleukemia
chloroma
p-chloromercuribenzoate [p-, para-]
chlorometry
chlorophane
chlorophyll
chlorophyllin
chloroprene
chloropsia
chlorosis
chlorostigmine
chlorosulfonic acid
chlorothen citrate
chlorothenium citrate
chlorothymol
chlorotic
chlorous
chloroxine
chloroxylenol
chloruresis, chloruria

chloruretic
choana (choanae)
    primary c.
    secondary c.
choanal atresia
chocolate
choke
    ophthalmovascular c.
    thoracic c.
    water c.
choked disk
chol.—cholesterol
cholagogic
cholagogues
cholaneresis
cholangiectasis
cholangioadenoma
cholangiocarcinoma
cholangiodrainage
    percutaneous transhepatic c.
cholangioenterostomy
cholangiogastrostomy
cholangiogram
cholangiographic
cholangiography
    cystic duct c.
    delayed operative c.
    direct percutaneous
      transhepatic c.
    endoscopic retrograde c. (ERC)
    fine-needle transhepatic c.
      (FNTC)
    intraoperative c.
    intravenous c. (IVC)
    operative c.
    percutaneous hepatobiliary c.
    percutaneous transhepatic c.
      (PTC)
    postoperative c.
    retrograde c.
    transabdominal c.
    transhepatic c. (TC)
    transjugular c.
    T-tube c.
cholangiohepatitis
cholangiohepatoma
cholangiojejunostomy
    intrahepatic c.
cholangiolar
cholangiole
cholangiolitis
cholangioma
cholangiopancreatography
    endoscopic retrograde c. (ERCP)
cholangiostomy

C

cholangiotomy
cholangitis
    chronic nonsuppurative
      destructive c.
    c. lenta
    primary sclerosing c.
    progressive nonsuppurative c.
cholanic acid
cholanopoiesis
cholanopoietic
cholanthrene
cholate
cholebilirubin
cholecalciferol
cholechromopoiesis
cholecyanin
cholecyst
cholecystalgia
cholecystatony
cholecystectasia
cholecystectomy
cholecystenteric
cholecystenteroanastomosis
cholecystenterorrhaphy
cholecystenterostomy
cholecystic
cholecystitis
    acute c.
    acute acalculous c.
    chronic c.
    c. cystica
    c. emphysematosa
    emphysematous c.
    follicular c.
    gaseous c.
    c. glandularis proliferans
cholecystnephrostomy
cholecystocholangiogram
cholecystocolonic
cholecystocolostomy
cholecystocolotomy
cholecystoduodenostomy
cholecystoenterostomy
cholecystogastric
cholecystogastrostomy
cholecystogram
cholecystography
    intravenous c.
    oral c.
    post–fatty meal c.
cholecystoileostomy
cholecystointestinal
cholecystojejunostomy
cholecystokinetic

cholecystokinin (CCK)
cholecystolithiasis
cholecystolithotomy
cholecystolithotripsy
cholecystopathy
cholecystopexy
cholecystoptosis
cholecystopyelostomy
cholecystorrhaphy
cholecystosis
    hyperplastic c.
cholecystotomy
choledochal sphincterotomy
choledochectomy
choledochitis
choledochocele
choledochocholedochostomy
choledochoduodenostomy
choledochoenterostomy
choledochogastrostomy
choledochogram
choledochography
choledochohepatostomy
choledochoileostomy
choledochojejunostomy
choledocholith
choledocholithiasis
choledocholithotomy
choledocholithotripsy
choledochoplasty
choledochorrhaphy
choledochoscope
choledochostomy
choledochotomy
choledochus
choleglobin
cholehematin
choleic
cholelith
cholelithiasis
cholelithic
cholelithotomy
cholelithotripsy
cholelithotrity
cholemesis
cholemia
    familial c.
    Gilbert c.
cholemic
cholemimetry
choleperitoneum
cholepoiesis
cholepoietic
choleprasin

cholera
 Asiatic c.
 dry c.
 pancreatic c.
 c. sicca
choleragen
choleraic
choleresis
choleretic
choleria
choleric
cholerigenic
cholescintigram
cholescintigraphy
 radionuclide c.
cholestane
cholestanol
 beta-c.
cholestasia, cholestasis
 familial intrahepatic c.
cholesteatoma
 congenital c.
 intracranial c.
 paranasal sinus c.
 primary acquired c.
 secondary acquired c.
 c. tympani
cholesteatomatous
cholesteatosis
cholesterogenesis
cholesterol
 c. acyltransferase
 c. desmolase
 c. emboli syndrome
 c. esterase
 high-density–lipoprotein
   (HDL) c.
 low-density–lipoprotein (LDL) c.
 c. monooxygenase (side-chain
   cleaving)
 c. sulfatase
cholesteroleresis
cholesterolopoiesis
cholesterolosis
cholesteroluria
cholesterosis
 c. cutis
 extracellular c.
cholesteryl ester storage disease
cholestyramine resin
cholic acid
choline
 acetyl glyceryl ether
   phosphoryl c.

choline *(continued)*
 c. magnesium trisalicylate
 c.-*O*-acetyltransferase
 phosphatidyl c.
 c. salicylate
cholinergic
cholinesterase
cholinolytic
chologenetic
cholohemothorax
cholothorax
cholylglycine
cholyltaurine
chondral
chondralgia
chondrectomy
chondric
chondrification
chondritis
 auricular c.
 costal c.
 c. intervertebralis calcanea
chondroangioma
chondroblast
chondroblastoma
chondrocalcinosis
chondroclast
chondrocostal
chondrocranium
chondrocyte
 isogenous c's
chondrodermatitis nodularis
  chronica helicis
chondrodynia
chondrodysplasia
 genotypic c.
 hereditary deforming c.
 hyperplastic c.
 McKusick-type metaphyseal c.
 metaphyseal c.
 c. punctata
 rhizomelic-type c.
chondrodystrophia
 c. calcificans congenita
 c. congenita punctata
 c. fetalis calcificans
chondrodystrophy
 familial c.
 hereditary deforming c.
 hyperplastic c.
 hypoplastic c.
 hypoplastic fetal c.
 c. malacia
chondroendothelioma

chondroepiphyseal
chondroepiphysitis
chondrofibroma
chondrogenesis
chondrogenic
chondroglossus
chondroid syringoma
chondroitic
chondroitinuria
chondrolipoma
chondrolysis
chondroma (chondromas,
  chondromata)
    joint c.
    juxtacortical c.
    periosteal c.
    synovial c.
    true c.
chondromalacia
    c. fetalis
    c. patellae
chondromatosis
    Reichel c.
    synovial c.
chondromatous
chondrometaplasia
    synovial c.
    tenosynovial c.
chondromucoprotein
chondromyoma
chondromyxoma
chondromyxosarcoma
chondronecrosis
chondro-osseous
chondro-osteodystrophy
chondropathia tuberosa
chondropathy
chondrophyte
chondroplasia punctata
chondroplast, chondroblast
chondroplastic
chondroplasty
chondroporosis
chondrosamine
chondrosarcoma
    central c.
    clear cell c.
    dedifferentiated c.
    juxtacortical c.
    mesenchymal c.
    myxoid c.
    periosteal c.
    peripheral c.
    spindle cell c.
chondrosarcomatosis

chondrosarcomatous
chondroseptum
chondrosin
chondrosternal
chondrosternoplasty
chondrotome
chondrotomy
chondrotrophic
CHOP—cyclophosphamide,
  hydroxydaunomycin, Oncovin,
  prednisone
Chopart
    amputation
    articulation
    joint
    operation
chord
chorda (chordae)
    c. dorsalis
    c. gubernaculum
    c. magna
    c. spermatica
    c. spinalis
    c. tendineae cordis
    c. tympani
    c. umbilicalis
    c. vertebralis
    c. vocalis
    chordae Willisii
chordal
chordee
chorditis
    c. fibrinosa
    c. nodosa
    c. tuberosa
    c. vocalis
    c. vocalis inferior
chordoblastoma
chordocarcinoma
chordoepithelioma
chordoid
chordoma
chorea
    acute c.
    atonic c.
    automatic c.
    Bergeron c.
    button-maker's c.
    chronic c.
    chronic progressive
      nonhereditary c.
    c. cordis
    c. cruciata
    dancing c.
    degenerative c.

C

chorea *(continued)*
    diaphragmatic c.
    c. dimidiata
    Dubini c.
    electric c.
    epidemic c.
    c. festinans
    fibrillary c.
    c. gravidarum
    c. gravis
    habit c.
    hemilateral c.
    hemiplegic c.
    Henoch c.
    hereditary c.
    Huntington c.
    hyoscine c.
    hysterical c.
    imitative c.
    infective c.
    jumping c.
    juvenile c.
    laryngeal c.
    limp c.
    local c.
    c. major
    malleatory c.
    maniacal c.
    methodic c.
    mimetic c.
    c. minor
    c. mollis
    Morvan c.
    c. nocturna
    c. nutans
    one-sided c.
    paralytic c.
    polymorphous c.
    posthemiplegic c.
    prehemiplegic c.
    procursive c.
    rheumatic c.
    rhythmic c.
    rotary c.
    saltatory c.
    school-made c.
    Schrötter (Schroetter) c.
    c. scriptorium
    senile c.
    simple c.
    Sydenham c.
    tetanoid c.
    tic c.
choreal, choreic
choreiform

choreoathetoid
choreoathetosis
    familial paroxysmal c.
    paroxysmal kinesigenic c.
choreoid
choreomania
chorial
chorioadenoma destruens
chorioallantoic
chorioallantois
chorioamnionic
chorioamnionitis
chorioangiofibroma
chorioangioma
chorioangiopagus
    parasiticus
chorioblastosis
choriocapillaris
choriocarcinoma
choriocele
chorioepithelioma malignum
choriogenesis
chorioma
choriomammotropin
choriomeningitis
    lymphocytic c.
chorion
    c. frondosum
    c. laeve
    primitive c.
    shaggy c.
chorionic
    c. villi
    c. villus biopsy (CVB)
chorionic gonadotropin
  (CG)
    human c.g. (hCG)
chorioplacental
chorioretinal
chorioretinitis
    c. sclopetaria
    toxoplasmic c.
chorioretinopathy
    birdshot c.
chorista
choristoblastoma
choristoma
choroid, choroidea
choroidal
    c. detachment
    c. flush
    c. hemorrhage
    c. nevus
choroidectomy
choroideremia

choroiditis
    anterior c.
    areolar c.
    central c.
    diffuse c.
    disseminated c.
    Doyne familial honeycombed c.
    exudative c.
    focal c.
    Förster c.
    c. guttata senilis
    Jensen c.
    juxtapapillary c.
    macular c.
    metastatic c.
    senile macular exudative c.
    c. serosa
    suppurative c.
    syphilitic c.
    Tay c.
    toxoplasmic c.
choroidocyclitis
choroidoiritis
choroidopathy
    areolar c.
    guttate c.
choroidoretinitis
Chotzen syndrome
Choyce
    implant
    Mark VIII lens
CHP—
    child psychiatry
    comprehensive health
      planning
Christensen-Krabbe
    disease
    poliodystrophy
Christian
    disease
    syndrome
Christian-Weber
    disease
Christmas
    disease
    factor
    C.-tree pattern
Christ-Siemens-Touraine
    syndrome
chromaffin, chromaffinity
chromaffinoma
    medullary c.
chromaffinopathy
chromargentaffin
chromate

chromatic
    c. aberration
    c. dispersion
    c. perimetry
chromatid-type aberration
chromatin
    nucleolar-associated c.
    nucleolus-associated c.
    sex c.
chromatinic
chromatin-negative
chromatin-positive
chromatism
chromatize
chromatoblast
chromatogenous
chromatography
    adsorption c.
    affinity c.
    antibody affinity c.
    column c.
    electric c.
    filter paper c.
    gas c. (GC)
    gas-liquid c. (GLC)
    gas-solid c. (GSC)
    gel filtration c.
    gel permeation c.
    high-performance liquid c.
      (HPLC)
    high-pressure liquid c. (HPLC)
    instant thin-layer c. (ITLC)
    ion exchange c.
    liquid-liquid c.
    molecular sieve c.
    paper c.
    partition c.
    thin-layer c. (TLC)
    two-dimensional c.
chromatoid
chromatokinesis
chromatolysis
chromatophagus
chromatophil
chromatophilia, chromatophilic
chromatophore
chromatophorotropic
chromatoplasm
chromatoptometry
chromatoscopy
    gastric c.
chromatosis
chromatotaxis
chromatotropism
chromaturia

C

chromesthesia
chromhidrosis
chromic catgut suture
chromic acid
chromium (Cr)
    c. Cr 51 serum albumin
    c. trioxide
Chromobacterium violaceum
chromoblastomycosis
chromocholoscopy
chromoclastogenic
chromocystoscopy
chromocyte
chromodacryorrhea
chromodiagnosis
chromogen
    Porter-Silber c's
chromogenesis
chromogenic
chromogranin
chromohydrotubation
chromoisomerism
chromolipoid
chromomere
chromometer
chromomycosis
chromoparic
chromopectic
chromopertubation
chromopexy
chromophil
chromophilic
chromophobe
chromophobia
chromophose
chromoprotein
chromoretinography
chromorhinorrhea
chromosomal markers
chromosome
    accessory c's
    acentric c.
    acrocentric c.
    B c.
    bivalent c.
    daughter c's
    dicentric c.
    fragile X c.
    gametic c.
    giant c.
    heteromorphic c.
    heterotypical c's
    homologous c's
    late replicating X c.
    metacentric c.

chromosome *(continued)*
    mitochondrial c. (m-c.)
    mitotic c.
    monocentric c.
    nonhomologous c's
    nucleolar c's
    odd c's
    Philadelphia c. (Ph1 c.)
    polytene c.
    ring c.
    sex c's
    small c.
    somatic c.
    submetacentric c.
    subtelocentric c.
    supernumerary c.
    telocentric c.
    c.-type aberration
    W c's
    c. walking
    X c.
    Y c.
    Z c's
chromospermism
chromotherapy
chromotoxic
chromotrichia
chromotrichial
chromotropic
chronic
chronicity
chronobiologic, chronobiological
chronognosis
chronometry
    mental c.
chronophobia
chronotaraxis
chronotropic
chronotropism
chrysiasis
chrysoderma
Chrysops
    C. cecutiens
    C. discalis
chrysotherapy
chrysotile
CHS—compression hip screw
chthonophagia, chthonophagy
Churg-Strauss
    syndrome
    vasculitis
Chvostek
    anemia
    sign
    symptom

Chvostek *(continued)*
    test
Chvostek-Weiss sign
chylangioma
chylaqueous
chyle
chylectasia
chylemia
chylifacient
chylifaction
chyliferous
chylification
chyliform
chylocele
    parasitic c.
chylocyst
chyloderma
chyloid
chylomediastinum
chylomicron
chylomicronemia
chylopericarditis
chylopericardium
chyloperitoneum
chylopneumothorax
chylopoiesis
chylopoietic
chylorrhea
chylosis
chylothorax
chylous
chyluria
chymase
chyme
chymification
chymorrhea
chymosin
chymotrypsin
chymotrypsinogen
chymous
Ci—curie(s)
CI—
    cardiac index
    cardiac insufficiency
    cerebral infarction
    colloidal iron
    complete iridectomy
    coronary
      insufficiency
    crystalline insulin
Ciaccio
    glands
    method
    stain
Ciarrocchi disease

CIBD—chronic inflammatory
    bowel disease
cicatrectomy
cicatrices (plural of cicatrix)
cicatricial alopecia
cicatricotomy
cicatrix (cicatrices)
    filtering c.
    hypertrophic c.
    vicious c.
cicatrizant
cicatrization
cicatrize
CICE—combined intracapsular
    cataract extraction
Cicherelli forceps
CICU—
    cardiac intensive care unit
    coronary intensive care unit
cicutoxin
CID—
    combined immunodeficiency
      disease
    cytomegalic inclusion disease
CIDP—chronic inflammatory
    demyelinating polyneuropathy
CIDS—
    cellular immune deficiency
      syndrome
    continuous insulin delivery
      system
CIE, CIEP—
    counterimmunoelectrophoresis
cig.—cigarettes
cigarette drain
CIHD—chronic ischemic heart
    disease
Ci-hr—curie-hour
CIL—center for independent living
cilia (plural of cilium)
ciliaris
ciliarotomy
ciliary
    c. arteries
    c. body
    c. flush
    c. ganglion
    c. hyperemia
    c. muscle
    c. nerve
    c. process
    c. spasm
    c. vein
    c. zonule
ciliate, ciliated

ciliation
ciliectomy
ciliogenesis
cilioretinal
    c. artery
    c. vein
cilioscleral
ciliospinal
ciliotomy
cilium (cilia)
cillosis
cimbia
Cimex
    C. lectularius
    C. rotundatus
cimicosis
C_{in}—insulin clearance
CIN—cervical intraepithelial
  neoplasia (I–III)
cinching
cinchona bark
cinchonic
cinchonism
cinclisis
cinctured
cine
    c. camera
    c. coronary arteriography
    c. CT scan
    c. study
cineangiocardiography
cineangiogram
cineangiography
    radionuclide c.
cinedensigraphy
cinefluorography
cinefluoroscopy
cinemicrography
    time-lapse c.
cineol, cineole
cinephlebography
cineradiography
cinerea
cinereal
cineritious
cinesalgia
cineurography
cingulate
cingulectomy
cingulotomy
cingulum (cingula)
    c. membri inferioris
    c. membri superioris
    c. pectorale
    c. pelvicum

cinnabar
cinnamon
CIOH—chronic idiopathic
  orthostatic hypotension
CIPN—chronic idiopathic
  peripheral neuropathy
circ.—circulation
circadian
    c. heterotropia
    c. rhythm
circellus
circinate
    c. exudate
    c. retinopathy
circle
    arterial c.
    Berry c's
    c. of confusion
    defensive c.
    c. of dispersion
    c. of dissipation
    c. of Haller
    Huguier c.
    Latham c.
    Minsky c's
    Robinson c.
    sensory c.
    vascular c.
    venous c. of mammary gland
    Vieth-Müller c.
    c's of Weber
    c. of Willis
    c. of Zinn
circlet
CircOlectric bed
circuit
    Bain c.
    breathing c.
    closed c. anesthesia
    constant potential c.
    gate c.
    Papez c.
    reentrant c., reentry c.
    reflex c.
    reverberating c.
circuitous
circuitry
circular
    c. incision
    Livaditis c. myotomy
    c. suture
    c. tomography
circulation
    allantoic c.
    assisted c.

C

circulation *(continued)*
    chorionic c.
    collateral c.
    compensatory c.
    coronary c.
    cross c.
    derivative c.
    embryonic c.
    enterohepatic c.
    extracorporeal c.
    fetal c.
    first c.
    fourth c.
    greater c.
    hypophysioportal c.
    intervillous c.
    lesser c.
    lymph c.
    omphalomesenteric c.
    persistent fetal c.
    placental c.
    plasmatic c.
    portal c.
    portoumbilical c.
    primitive c.
    pulmonary c.
    sinusoidal c.
    systemic c.
    thebesian c.
    umbilical c.
    vertebral-basilar c.
    vitelline c.
circulatory
    c. arrest
    c. failure
circulus (circuli)
    c. arteriosus
    c. arteriosus cerebri
    c. arteriosus halleri
    c. articuli vasculosus
    c. umbilicalis
    c. vasculosus
    c. venosus halleri
    c. willisii
    c. zinnii
circumanal
circumareolar incision
circumarticular
circumaxillary
circumbuccal
circumbulbar
circumcallosal
circumcise
circumcision
    female c.

circumcision *(continued)*
    c. incision
    pharaonic c.
    Sunna c.
    c. suture
circumcorneal
circumcrescent
circumduction
circumference
    articular c.
    occipitofrontal c. (OFC)
circumferentia
    c. articularis
    c. articularis capitis radii
    c. articularis capitis ulnae
    c. articularis capituli ulnae
circumferential incision
circumflex artery
circumflexus
circuminsular
circumintestinal
circumlental
circumlimbal incision
circumnuclear
circumocular
circumolivary
circumoral
circumorbital
circumrenal
circumscribed
circumscribing incision
circumscriptus
circumstantiality
circumvallate
circumvascular
circumvolute
circus senilis
cirrhogenous
cirrhonosus
cirrhosis
    acholangic biliary c.
    acute juvenile c.
    alcoholic c.
    atrophic c.
    bacterial c.
    biliary c.
    Budd c.
    calculus c.
    cardiac c.
    Charcot c.
    congenital hepatic c.
    congestive c.
    Cruveilhier-Baumgarten c.
    cryptogenic c.
    decompensated c.

cirrhosis *(continued)*
    fatty c.
    Laënnec c.
    macronodular c.
    malarial c.
    metabolic c.
    micronodular c.
    multilobular c.
    obstructive c.
    periportal c.
    pigment c.
    pigmentary c.
    pipestem c.
    portal c.
    posthepatitic c.
    postnecrotic c.
    primary biliary c.
    secondary biliary c.
    stasis c.
    syphilitic c.
    Todd c.
    toxic c.
    unilobular c.
    vascular c.
cirrhotic
cirsomphalos
cirsophthalmia
CIS—
    carcinoma in situ
    central inhibitory state
cistern
    anterolateral cerebellar c.
    basal c.
    cerebellomedullary c.
    chiasmatic c.
    chyle c.
    c. of corpus callosum
    c. of fossa of Sylvius
    Golgi c's
    great c.
    c. of great cerebral vein
    interpeduncular c.
    c. of lateral fossa of cerebrum
    lumbar c.
    c. of Pecquet
    pontine c.
    posterior cerebellomedullary c.
    subarachnoid c's
    supracallosal c.
    c. of Sylvius
    terminal c.
cisterna (cisternae)
    c. ambiens
    c. basalis
    c. caryothecae

cisterna (cisternae) *(continued)*
    c. chiasmatica
    c. chiasmatis
    c. corporis callosi
    c. fossae lateralis cerebri
    c. fossae Sylvii
    c. intercruralis profunda
    c. interpeduncularis
    c. laminae terminalis
    c. lateralis pontis
    c. lumbalis
    c. magna
    perinuclear c.
    c. subarachnoidales
    c. sulci lateralis
    c. Sylvii
    c. valleculae lateralis cerebri
    c. venae magnae cerebri
cisternal
    c. arachnoiditis
    c. puncture
cisternogram
cisternography
    metrizamide c.
    oxygen c.
    radionuclide c.
CIT—crisis intervention therapy
Citelli
    rongeur
    syndrome
Citelli-Meltzer atticus punch
citrate
    ferric c.
    c. lyase
    synthase
citreoviridin
citric acid
Citrobacter
    C. amalonaticus
    C. diversus
    C. freundii
citronella
citrophosphate
citrovorum rescue
citrulline
citrullinemia
citrullinuria
citta
cittosis
Civatte
    bodies
    poikiloderma
Civiale operation
Civinini
    canal

Civinini *(continued)*
    ligament
    process
    spine
CIXU—constant infusion excretory
    urogram
CJD—Creutzfeldt-Jakob disease
CK—creatine kinase
Cl—
    chloride
    chlorine
CL—chest and left arm (ECG lead)
Clado
    anastomosis
    band
cladosporiosis
Cladosporium
    C. bantianum
    C. carrionii
    C. trichoides
Clagett operation
clairvoyance
clamp
    Allen c.
    Allis c.
    Alyea c.
    anastomosis c.
    aortic cross-c.
    Atlee c.
    Babcock c.
    Backhaus towel c.
    Bahnson c.
    Bailey c.
    Bainbridge anastomosis c.
    Ballantine c.
    Beardsley intestinal c.
    Beck c.
    Berens muscle c.
    Berke ptosis c.
    Best c.
    Blanchard pile c.
    Böhler c.
    bone c.
    Bonney c.
    Bradshaw-O'Neill c.
    Brodney c.
    Buie c.
    Buie-Hirschman c.
    bulldog c.
    Buxton c.
    C c.
    Carmalt c.
    Carrel c.
    Carter c.
    cervical punch biopsy c.

clamp *(continued)*
    circumscribed c.
    Cooley c.
    Cope c.
    cord c.
    Cottle c.
    cotton roll rubber dam c.
    Craafoord c.
    Crile c.
    crushing c.
    Crutchfield c.
    Cunningham c.
    Daniel c.
    Davidson c.
    Davis c.
    DeBakey c.
    DeMartel-Wolfson c.
    Dennis c.
    Derra c.
    Diethrich shunt c.
    Dixon-Thomas-Smith c.
    Doyen c.
    Eastman c.
    Edwards c.
    Fehland c.
    fenestrated c.
    Forrester c.
    Foss c.
    Friedrich-Petz c.
    Furniss c.
    Furniss-Clute c.
    Furniss-McClure-Hinton c.
    Gandy c.
    Gant c.
    gingival c.
    Glassman c.
    Glover c.
    Goldblatt c.
    Gomco c.
    Gross c.
    Guyon c.
    Guyon-Péan c.
    Halsted c.
    Hayes c.
    Heaney c.
    hemostatic c.
    Herbert-Adams c.
    Herff c.
    Herrick c.
    Hey Groves c.
    Hopkins c.
    Hudson c.
    Hufnagel c.
    Hume c.
    Humphries c.

clamp *(continued)*
    Hunt c.
    Hurwitz c.
    Hyams c.
    Jackson c.
    Jacobson c.
    Jarvis c.
    Javid bypass c.
    Jesberg c.
    Johns Hopkins c.
    Joseph c.
    Juevenelle c.
    Kane c.
    Kantor c.
    Kantrowitz c.
    Kapp-Beck c.
    Kelly c.
    Kinsella-Buie c.
    Kocher c.
    Lahey c.
    Lambotte c.
    Lane c.
    Lee c.
    lever-compression c.
    Liddle aorta c.
    Linton c.
    Lockwood c.
    Lowman c.
    MacDonald c.
    Martel c.
    Mastin c.
    Mattox c.
    Mayo c.
    microvascular c.
    Mikulicz c.
    Moreno c.
    mosquito c.
    Moynihan c.
    Mueller c.
    Nichols c.
    Noon AV fistula c.
    Nussbaum c.
    occlusion c.
    Ochsner c.
    Ockerblad c.
    Parker c.
    Payr c.
    Péan c.
    pedicle c.
    Pemberton c.
    penile c.
    Pennington c.
    Phillips c.
    Poppen c.
    Poppen-Blalock c.

clamp *(continued)*
    Potts c.
    Potts-Niedner c.
    Potts-Smith c.
    Price-Thomas c.
    Ralks c.
    Rankin c.
    Ranzewski c.
    Reich c.
    Reich-Nechtow c.
    Rienhoff c.
    Rockey c.
    Roosevelt c.
    rubber dam c.
    rubber-shod c.
    Rubin c.
    Rumel c.
    Salibi c.
    Sarot c.
    Satinsky c.
    Schoemaker c.
    Scudder c.
    Sehrt c.
    Selverstone c.
    serrefine c.
    Shoemaker c.
    splenectomy c.
    Stevenson c.
    Stille c.
    Stockman c.
    Stone c.
    Stone-Holcombe c.
    Tatum c.
    Thomson c.
    towel c.
    Trendelenburg-Crafoord c.
    vascular c.
    Verbrugge c.
    von Petz c.
    Walther c.
    Walther-Crenshaw c.
    Wangensteen c.
    Watts c.
    Wertheim c.
    Wertheim-Cullen c.
    Wertheim-Reverdin c.
    Wester c.
    Willett c.
    Williams c.
    Wilman c.
    Wilson c.
    Wolfson c.
    Yellen c.
    Young c.
    Zipser c.

C

clamping
clanging
clap
clapotement
claquement
Clara cells
clarificant
clarification
clarify
Clark classification of malignant
   melanoma (levels I–V)
Clark-Collip method
Clarke
      cells
      collateral bundle
      column
      dorsal nucleus
      nucleus
Clarke-Hadfield syndrome
Clarke-Monakow nucleus
CLAS—congenital localized
   absence of skin
clasmatosis
clasp
      Adams c.
      arrow c.
      arrowhead c.
      ball c.
      bar c.
      circumferential c.
      continuous lingual c.
      Crozat c.
      wrought c.
classification
      Angle c. of malocclusion
      Astler-Coller modification of
         Dukes c.
      Bergey c. of bacteria
      Berman c. of pelves
      Black c. of dental caries
      Borrmann c. of gastric
         carcinoma
      Breslow c.
      Caldwell-Moloy c. of female
         pelves
      Chicago c. of human
         chromosomes
      Child c. of hepatic risk
      Clark c. of malignant
         melanoma (levels I–V)
      DeBakey c. of aortic dissection
         (types I–III, IIIA, IIIB)
      Duane c. of strabismus
      Dukes c. of colorectal
         carcinoma (A, B, B_2, C_1, C_2)
         [B2, C1, C2]

classification *(continued)*
      FAB (French-American-
         British) c. of acute leukemia
      FIGO c. of endometrial
         carcinoma (stages 0–IV)
      Frankel c. of spinal cord
         injuries (groups A–E)
      Gell and Coombs c. of allergic
         reactions (types I–IV)
      International C. of Diseases
         (ICD)
      Jewett c. of bladder carcinoma
         (stages 0, A–D)
      Jewett and Strong c. of
         bladder carcinoma (stages
         0, A–D)
      Karnofsky performance status
         c. (score 0–100)
      Keith-Wagener-Barker
         c. of hypertension and
         arteriosclerosis (groups 1–4)
      Keith-Wagener (K-W) c.
      Kennedy c. of partially
         edentulous conditions
      Kiel c. of non-Hodgkin
         lymphoma
      Killip c. of cardiac function
         (I–IV)
      Lancefield serologic c. of
         hemolytic streptococci
         (groups A–O)
      Lennert c. of non-Hodgkin
         lymphoma
      Lukes-Collins c. of non-
         Hodgkin lymphoma
      Lund-Browder c. of burn
         severity in children
      McNeer c. of gastric carcinoma
      multiaxial c. (axes I–V)
      Neer c. of shoulder fracture
         (I–III)
      New York Heart Association
         (NYHA) c. (classes I–IV,
         A–D)
      Paris modification of the
         Chicago c. of human
         chromosomes
      REAL (Revised European
         American Lymphoma) c.
      Reese-Ellsworth c. of
         retinoblastoma
      Runyon c. of mycobacteria
      Rye histopathologic c. of
         Hodgkin disease
      Salter-Harris c. of epiphyseal
         plate injuries

classification *(continued)*
    Skinner c. of partially
      edentulous conditions
    Tessier c. for clefts
    TNM (tumor, node,
      metastasis) c.
    van Heuven anatomical c. of
      diabetic retinopathy
    White c. of maternal diabetes
      mellitus (classes A–H, R, T)
    Wiberg c. of patellar types
class-interval
clastic
clastothrix
clathrate
Claude
    hyperkinesis sign
    syndrome
Claude-Lhermitte syndrome
claudicant
claudication
    intermittent c.
    jaw c.
    venous c.
Claudius
    cells
    fossa
claustral
claustrophobia
claustrum (claustra)
clava
claval
clavate
clavicle
clavicotomy
clavicula
clavicular
claviculectomy
claviculus
clavipectoral
clavus (clavi)
    c. durus
    c. hystericus
    c. mollis
    c. syphiliticus
clawfoot
clawhand
clay shoveler's fracture
Clayton osteotome
CLD—chronic lung disease
clean-catch urine specimen
clearance
    aerosol c.
    blood urea c.
    creatinine c.
    fractional c. of dextran

clearance *(continued)*
    free water c.
    hepatic c.
    immune c.
    indocyanine green c.
    interocclusal c.
    inulin c.
    mucociliary c.
    occlusal c.
    osmolal c.
    p-aminohippurate c. (PAH c.)
    plasma iron c.
    renal c.
    sodium p-aminohippuric
      (PAH) acid c. [p-, para-]
    total c., total body c.
    urea c.
    whole-body c.
cleavage
    accessory c.
    adequal c.
    complete c.
    determinate c.
    discoidal c.
    equal c.
    equatorial c.
    holoblastic c.
    incomplete c.
    indeterminate c.
    latitudinal c.
    meridional c.
    meroblastic c.
    partial c.
    radial c.
    spiral c.
    superficial c.
    total c.
    unequal c.
Cleaves position
Cleeman sign
cleft
    anal c.
    branchial c.
    cervical c's
    cholesterol c.
    clunial c.
    corneal c.
    facial c.
    fetal c.
    genital c.
    gingival c.
    gluteal c.
    hyoid c.
    interdental c.
    intergluteal c.
    Lanterman c's

C

cleft *(continued)*
    Larrey c.
    laryngotracheoesophageal c.
    c. lip
    c. of mandible
    Maurer c's
    middle ear c.
    natal c.
    oblique facial c.
    orbitonasal c.
    c. palate
    pharyngeal c.
    posthyoidean c.
    pudendal c.
    Santorini c.
    Schmidt-Lanterman c's
    Sondergaard c.
    Stillman c.
    submucous c.
    synaptic c.
    tubotympanic c.
    visceral c.
    vulval c.
cleft palate prosthesis
cleidagra
cleidal
cleidarthritis
cleidocostal
cleidocranial
cleidomastoid
cleidotomy
clenching
cleoid
Clérambault-Kandinsky
    complex
    syndrome
Clerf
    laryngoscope
    saw
Cleveland procedure
click
    ejection c's
    midsystolic c.
    mitral c.
    Ortolani c.
    systolic c.
clicking
climacteric
climacterium praecox
climactic
climax
clinarthrosis
clinic
    ambulatory care c.
    free medical c.

clinic *(continued)*
    mental health c.
    pain c.
    urgent care c.
    walk-in c.
clinical microscopy
clinical pathology
clinician
clinicogenetic
clinicopathologic
Clinistix
Clinitest
Clinitron bed
clinocephaly
clinodactyly
    factitious c.
    traumatic c.
clinoid process
clinostatic
clinotherapy
CLIP—corticotropin-like
    intermediate lobe peptide
clip
    Acland c.
    Adson c.
    catheter c.
    Cushing c.
    dura c.
    Halberg c.
    Heifitz c.
    Hulka c.
    Mayfield c.
    McKenzie c.
    Michel c.
    Olivecrona c.
    Paterson long-shank brain c.
    Raney c.
    Schütz c.
    Schwartz c.
    Scoville c.
    Scoville-Lewis c.
    skin c.
    Smith c.
    Sugar c.
    tantalum c.
    towel c.
    Weck c.
    Yasargil c.
clition
clitoral
clitoralgia
clitoridauxe
clitoridectomy
clitoriditis
clitoridotomy

clitorimegaly
clitoris
  bifid c.
  crura of c.
  prepuce of c.
clitorism
clitoritis
clitoroplasty
clitorotomy
clival
clivus
  basilar c.
  c. basilaris
  Blumenbach c.
  c. monticuli
  c. ossis occipitalis
  c. ossis sphenoidalis
CLL—chronic lymphocytic
  leukemia
CLO—cod liver oil
cloaca (cloacae)
  congenital c.
  persistent c.
cloacal
clock
  aging c.
  biological c.
  c. dial
clonal
clonality
clone
clonic
clonicity
clonicotonic
cloning
  DNA c.
clonism
clonorchiasis
clonospasm
clonotype
clonus
  ankle c.
  drawn ankle c.
  foot c.
  patellar c.
  toe c.
  wrist c.
C-loop of duodenum
Cloquet
  canal
  fascia
  ganglion
  hernia
  ligament
  node

Cloquet *(continued)*
  pseudoganglion
  septum
clostridia
clostridial myonecrosis
Clostridium
  C. bifermentans
  C. botulinum
  C. butyricum
  C. cadaveris
  C. clostridioforme
  C. difficile
  C. histolyticum
  C. innocuum
  C. novyi
  C. perfringens
  C. piliforme
  C. ramosum
  C. septicum
  C. sordellii
  C. sphenoides
  C. sporogenes
  C. subterminale
  C. tertium
  C. tetani
closure
  delayed primary c.
  flask c.
  Latzko c.
  Smead-Jones c.
  Tom Jones c.
  velopharyngeal c.
clot
  agonal c.
  antemortem c.
  autologous c.
  blood c.
  chicken fat c.
  currant jelly c.
  distal c.
  external c.
  heart c.
  internal c.
  laminated c.
  marantic c.
  muscle c.
  passive c.
  plasma c.
  plastic c.
  postmortem c.
  proximal c.
  Schede c.
  spider-web c.
  stratified c.
  washed c.

clot *(continued)*
    white c.
CLOtest
clouding of consciousness
Cloudman melanoma S91
Clouston syndrome
clove-hitch knot
cloverleaf skull
Cloward
    back fusion
    drill
    operation
    osteotome
    retractor
    rongeur
Cloward-Hoen retractor
clubbing of digits
clubfoot
clubhand
    radial c.
    ulnar c.
clump, clumping
cluneal
clunis (clunes)
Clute incision
cluttering
Clutton joint
clysis
cm—centimeter
cm^2 [sq cm]—square centimeter
cm^3 [cu cm, cc]—cubic centimeter
CM—
    cochlear microphonic
        (potential)
    costal margin
CMA—
    Certified Medical Assistant
    chronic metabolic acidosis
CMAP—compound muscle action
    potential
CMB—carbolic methylene blue
CMC—
    carpometacarpal (joint)
    critical micellar concentration
CMD—cerebromacular
    degeneration
CME—cystoid macular edema
CMET—comprehensive metabolic
    panel (profile)
CMF—
    chondromyxoid fibroma
    cyclophosphamide,
        methotrexate, 5-fluorouracil
CMGN—chronic membranous
    glomerulonephritis

CMHC—community mental health
    center
cm H_2O [cm H2O]—centimeter(s)
    of water
CMI—
    cell-mediated immunity
    cellular-mediated immune
        (response)
    cytomegalic inclusion
c/min—cycle(s) per minute
CML—
    cell-mediated lympholysis
    chronic myelocytic leukemia
    chronic myelogenous leukemia
    chronic myeloid leukemia
CMM—cutaneous malignant
    melanoma
CMN—cystic medial necrosis
CMN-AA—cystic medial necrosis of
    the ascending aorta
CMO—
    cardiac minute output
    comfort measures only
C-MOPP—cyclophosphamide,
    mechlorethamine, Oncovin,
    procarbazine, prednisone
CMP—
    complete metabolic panel
        (profile)
    comprehensive metabolic
        panel (profile)
CMR—
    carpometacarpal ratio
    cerebral metabolic rate
    crude mortality ratio
CMRG—cerebral metabolic rate of
    glucose
CMRO—cerebral metabolic rate of
    oxygen
CMS—Clyde Mood Scale
CMT—
    California mastitis test
    Certified Medical
        Transcriptionist
    Charcot-Marie-Tooth (atrophy,
        disease, syndrome)
CMV—
    continuous mechanical
        ventilation
    cytomegalovirus
CN—
    clinical nursing
    cranial nerve
    cyanogen
CNA—Certified Nurse Anesthetist

CND—congenital neuromuscular disorder
CNE—chronic nervous exhaustion
cnemial
cnemis
cnemitis
cnemoscoliosis
CNH—community nursing home
CNM—Certified Nurse-Midwife
CNPAP—continuous nasal positive airway pressure
CNS—central nervous system
CNSD—chronic nonspecific diarrhea
CNV—conduction nerve velocity
c/o—complains of
Co—cobalt
CO—
    carbon monoxide
    cardiac outpouching
    cardiac output
    castor oil
    cervicoaxial
    coenzyme
    corneal opacity
    coronary occlusion
    court order
CO_2 [CO2]—carbon dioxide
^{60}Co—radioactive cobalt [cobalt Co 60]
CoA—coenzyme A
COAD—chronic obstructive airway disease
coadaptation
coag.—coagulation
COAG—chronic open-angle glaucoma
coagglutination
coagulability
coagulable
coagulant effect
coagulase
coagulate
coagulation
    blood c.
    diffuse intravascular c. (DIC)
    disseminated intravascular c. (DIC)
    electric c.
    infrared c.
    massive c.
coagulative
coagulator
    Malis c.
coagulogram

coagulopathy
    consumption c.
    disseminated intravascular c. (DIC)
coagulum
    closing c.
Coakley
    cannula
    curet
    forceps
    operation
    speculum
    suture
    trocar
coalesce
coalescence
coapt
coaptation suture
coarctate
coarctation
    c. of aorta, adult type
    c. of aorta, infantile type
    reversed c.
coarctectomy
coarse
    c. gravel
    c. markings
    c. material
    c. texture
coarsening
coarticulation
CoA-SH—coenzyme A
coat
    adventitial c., adventitious c.
    adventitious c. of uterine tube
    albugineous c.
    buffy c.
    cremasteric c. of testis
    dartos c.
    dry c.
    external c. of capsule of graafian follicle
    external c. of ureter
    external c. of vessels
    external c. of viscera
    fibrous c.
    fibrous c. of corpus cavernosum of penis
    fibrous c. of eye
    fibrous c. of ovary
    fibrous c. of pharynx
    fibrous c. of testis
    fuzzy c.
    inner c. of vessels

C

coat *(continued)*
    internal c. of capsule of
      graafian follicle
    internal elastic c. of artery
    middle c. of vessels
    mucous c.
    mucous c. of tympanic cavity
    mucous c. of urinary bladder
    muscular c. of colon
    muscular c. of gallbladder
    muscular c. of large intestine
    muscular c. of rectum
    muscular c. of renal pelvis
    muscular c. of small intestine
    muscular c. of stomach
    muscular c. of urinary
      bladder
    outer c. of vessels
    pharyngobasilar c.
    proper c.
    sclerotic c.
    serous c. of esophagus
    serous c. of gallbladder
    serous c. of large intestine
    serous c. of liver
    serous c. of small intestine
    serous c. of stomach
    serous c. of urinary bladder
    spore c.
    subendothelial c.
    submucous c.
    subserous c.
    uveal c.
    vaginal c. of testis
    vascular c. of eyeball
    vascular c. of viscera
    white c. syndrome
coating
    enteric c.
CoA-transferase
Coats
    disease
    retinitis
    ring
coaxial counterflow single-needle
  blood access catheter
cobalamin concentrate
cobalt (Co)
    c. 57, c. 58, c. 60
    radioactive c.
cobaltosis
Coban wrap
Cobb
    elevator
    gouge

Cobb *(continued)*
    method
    osteotome
cobbler's suture
cobblestones, cobblestoning
cobralysin
cobra retractor
COC—
    calcifying odontogenic cyst
    combination-type oral
      contraceptive
cocaine
    crack c.
    c. hydrochloride (HCl)
cocarcinogen
cocarcinogenesis
coccal
coccerin
cocci (plural of coccus)
coccidia
coccidial
coccidian
coccidioidal
Coccidioides immitis
coccidioidin
coccidioidoma
coccidioidomycosis
    disseminated c.
    latent c.
    primary extrapulmonary c.
coccidiosis
coccigenic
coccobacteria
coccode
coccoid
coccus (cocci)
    gram-negative cocci
    gram-positive cocci
    pyogenic cocci
coccycephalus
coccygeal
coccygectomy
coccygerector
coccygodynia
coccygotomy
coccyx
cochlea (cochleae)
    membranous c.
    Mondini c.
cochlear
    c. duct
    c. implant
    c. nerve
cochleariform
cochleitis

cochleography
   acoustic c.
cochleostomy
cochleotopic
cochleovestibular
Cochliomyia hominivorax
Cock operation
Cockayne
   disease
   syndrome
cockroach
cocktail
   cytokine c.
   drug c.
   GI c.
   lytic c.
cocoa
coconsciousness
coconut
cocoon dressing
coction
coctoantigen
coctolabile
coctoprecipitin
coctoprotein
coctostabile
cocultivation
COD—
   cause of death
   condition on discharge
code
   genetic c.
   molecular c.
coded-aperture imaging
Codivilla
   extension
   operation
Codman
   exercise
   incision
   sign
   triangle
codominance
codominant
codon
COE—court-ordered examination
coefficient
   absorption c.
   activity c.
   c. of consanguinity
   creatinine c.
   dilution c.
   extinction c.
   homogeneity c.
   isometric c. of lactic acid

coefficient *(continued)*
   linear absorption c.
   linear attenuation c.
   mass absorption c.
   mass attenuation c.
   c. of relationship
   urohemolytic c.
   urotoxic c.
   c. of utilization of oxygen
coenurosis
Coenurus cerebralis
coenzyme
   c. A (CoA)
   c. Q 10 (CoQ 10)
Coe-Pak dressing
coeur en sabot
coexcitation
cofactor
   platelet c. I and II
coffee enema
coffee-grounds
   c.-g. vomit
   c.-g. vomitus
Coffey
   incision
   operation
   suspension
   technique
Coffey-Humber treatment
coffin
COG—closed angle glaucoma
Cogan
   disease
   dystrophy
   syndrome
cognate
   c. interaction
   c. recognition
cognition
cognitive
cognizant
cog tooth of malleus
COGTT—cortisone-primed oral
  glucose tolerance test
cogwheel
   c. breathing
   c. gait
   c. phenomenon
   c. rigidity
   c. sign
cogwheeling
COHb—carboxyhemoglobin
Cohen forceps
coherent
cohesion

cohesive
Cohnheim theory
Cohn solution
cohoba
cohobation
cohort
cohosh
coil
    c. array
    birdcage c.
    breast c.
    butterfly c.
    choke c.
    chromosome c.
    crossed c.
    Gianturco wool-tufted wire c.
    Golay c.
    helical c.
    Helmholtz c.
    induction c.
    Margulies c.
    paranemic c.
    plectonemic c.
    random c.
    relational c.
    resistance c.
    spark c.
coincidence
    c. circuit
    c. counting
    c. detection
    c. loss
    c. sum peak
coin-counting tremor
coindication
coinfection
coin lesion
coinlike
coital
coitophobia
coitus
    c. incompletus
    c. interruptus
    c. reservatus
Coker technique
COLD—chronic obstructive lung
   disease
cold
    allergic c.
    common c.
    June c.
    c. lesion
    rose c.
    c. spot
cold-blooded

cold punch resectoscope
coldsore
cold water calories test
Cole
    operation
    retractor
colectomy
Coleman-Shaffer diet
Cole sign
colibacillemia
colibacillosis
    enteric c., enterotoxigenic c.
    c. gravidarum
colibacilluria
colibacillus
Colibri forceps
colic
    appendicular c.
    biliary c.
    bilious c.
    copper c.
    crapulent c.
    cystic c.
    Devonshire c.
    endemic c.
    flatulent c.
    gallstone c.
    gastric c.
    hepatic c.
    infantile c.
    intestinal c.
    kidney c.
    lead c.
    milk c.
    mucous c.
    nephric c.
    ovarian c.
    painters' c.
    pancreatic c.
    Poitou c.
    pseudomembranous c.
    renal c.
    salivary c.
    saturnine c.
    stercoral c.
    tubal c.
    ureteral c.
    uterine c.
    vermicular c.
    verminous c.
    wind c.
    worm c.
    zinc c.
colicky pain
colicoplegia

coliform
colitis (colitides)
    adaptive c.
    amebic c.
    antibiotic-associated c.
    balantidial c.
    cathartic c.
    collagenous c.
    Crohn c.
    c. cystica profunda
    c. cystica superficialis
    diversion c.
    fulminating c.
    granulomatous c.
    c. gravis
    infectious c.
    irradiation c.
    ischemic c.
    mucous c.
    c. polyposa
    pseudomembranous c.
    radiation c.
    regional c.
    segmental c.
    transmural c.
    tuberculous c.
    c. ulcerativa
    ulcerative c.
    uremic c.
colitoxemia
colitoxicosis
colitoxin
colla (plural of collum)
collacin
collagen
    c. disease
    fibrous long-spacing c.
    FLS c.
    intimal c.
    segment long-spacing c.
    SLS c.
    c. suture
    c. vascular disease
collagenase
    Clostridium histolyticum c.
    vertebrate c.
collagenation
collagenoblast
collagenocyte
collagenolysis
collagenolytic
collagenoma
    familial cutaneous c.
collagenosis
    reactive perforating c.

collagenous plaques
collapse
    alveolar c.
    circulatory c.
    heat c.
    hemodynamic c.
    c. of lung
    massive c.
collapsed lung
collar
    abrasion c.
    Biett c.
    Casal c.
    c. dressing
    four-poster c.
    c. incision
    c. of pearls
    perichondral bony c.
    periosteal bone c.
    renal c.
    Spanish c.
    c. of Stokes
    Thomas c.
    venereal c.
    c. of Venus
collarbone, collar bone
collarette
    iris c.
collastin
collateral
    Schaffer c's
collecting
    c. system
    c. tubes
Colles
    fascia
    fracture
    ligament
    space
    splint
Collet syndrome
Collet-Sicard syndrome
colliculectomy
colliculitis
colliculus (colliculi)
    c. abducentis
    c. of arytenoid cartilage
    c. of Barkow
    bulbar c.
    c. cartilaginis arytenoideae
    caudal c.
    c. caudalis
    c. caudatus
    cervical c. of female urethra
    facial c.

C

colliculus (colliculi) *(continued)*
- c. facialis
- inferior c.
- rostral c.
- c. rostralis
- seminal c.
- c. seminalis
- c. superior laminae
  quadrigeminate

Collier sign
collimation
collimator
- automatic c.
- converging c.
- diverging c.
- focusing c.
- multihole c.
- parallel-hole c.
- pin-hole c.
- single-hole c.
- thick-septa c.
- thin-septa c.

Collin
- forceps
- osteoclast
- pelvimeter
- speculum
- test

Collin-Beard operation
collinear
Collins respirometer-spirometer
Collip unit
colliquation
- ballooning c.
- reticulating c.

colliquative
collision
- elastic c.
- scattering c.

Collison screw
collodiaphyseal
collodion
- c. baby
- c. dressing
- c. elastique
- flexible c.
- hemostatic c.
- salicylic acid c.
- simple c.
- styptic c.

colloid
- antimony trisulfide c.
- association c.
- bovine c.
- dispersion c.

colloid *(continued)*
- emulsion c.
- hydrophilic c.
- hydrophobic c.
- irreversible c.
- lyophilic c.
- lyophobic c.
- lyotropic c.
- protective c.
- reversible c.
- stable c.
- stannous sulfur c.
- suspension c.
- technetium-sulfur c.
- thyroid c.

colloidal
colloidin
colloidophagy
collum (colla)
- c. anatomicum humeri
- c. chirurgicum humeri
- c. cosine
- c. costae
- c. dentis
- c. distortum
- c. femoris
- c. fibulae
- c. folliculi pili
- c. glandis penis
- c. mallei
- c. mandibulae
- c. processus condyloidei
  mandibulae
- c. radii
- c. scapulae
- c. tali
- c. valgum
- c. vesicae biliaris
- c. vesicae felleae

collyrium
coloboma
- atypical c's
- c. auriculae
- bridge c.
- c. of choroid
- c. of ciliary body
- complete c.
- facial c.
- Fuchs c.
- c. of fundus
- c. iridis
- c. of iris
- c. of lens
- c. lentis
- c. lobuli

coloboma *(continued)*
    c. of optic disk
    c. of optic nerve
    c. at optic nerve entrance
    c. palpebrale
    peripapillary c.
    c. of retina
    c. retinae
    retinochoroidal c.
    typical c.
    c. of vitreous
colocecostomy
colocentesis
colocholecystostomy
coloclysis
coloclyster
colocolic
colocolostomy
colocutaneous
colodyspepsia
coloenteritis
colofixation
colohepatopexy
coloileal
cololysis
colon
    c. ascendens
    ascending c.
    c. descendens
    descending c.
    distal c.
    giant c.
    iliac c.
    irritable c.
    lead-pipe c.
    left c.
    pelvic c. of Waldeyer
    proximal c.
    redundant c.
    c. resection (CR)
    right c.
    sigmoid c.
    c. sigmoideum
    spastic c.
    thrifty c.
    transverse c.
    c. transversum
    unstable c.
colonalgia
colonic
colonization
Colonna operation
colonopathy
colonorrhagia
colonoscope

colonoscope *(continued)*
    adult c.
    fiberoptic c.
    forward-viewing c.
    high-resolution c.
    pediatric c.
colonoscopy
    fiberoptic c.
    virtual c.
colony count
colopexostomy
colopexotomy
colopexy
coloplication
coloptosis
color
    complementary c's
    confusion c's
    contrast c.
    incidental c.
    metameric c's
    Munsell c's
    primary c's
    pseudoisochromatic c's
    pure c.
    saturation c.
Colorado tick fever
coloration
colorblind, color-blind
color-contrast microscope
colorectal
colorectitis
colorectostomy
colorectum
colorimetrically
colorimetry
colorrhaphy
colorrhea
colosigmoidostomy
colostomy
    dry c.
    end c.
    end-to-side ileotransverse
      c.
    Hartmann c.
    ileotransverse c.
    Mikulicz c.
    Wangensteen c.
    wet c.
colostric
colostrorrhea
colostrous
colostrum
    c. gravidarum
    c. puerperarum

C

colotomy
    Allingham c.
colovaginal
colovesical fistula
colpalgia
colpatresia
colpectasia
colpectomy
colpedema
colpeurysis
colpismus
colpitis
    c. emphysematosa
    emphysematous c.
    c. granulosa
    c. mycotica
colpocele
colpoceliocentesis
colpoceliotomy
colpocleisis
colpocystitis
colpocystocele
colpocystoplasty
colpocystotomy
colpocystourethropexy
colpocytogram
colpocytology
colpodynia
colpohyperplasia
    cystica
colpohysterectomy
colpohysteropexy
colpohysterotomy
colpomicroscope
colpomicroscopy
colpomyomectomy
colpomyomotomy
colpoperineoplasty
colpoperineorrhaphy
colpopexy
colpoplasty
colpopoiesis
colpoptosis
colporectopexy
colporrhagia
colporrhaphy
colporrhexis
colposcope
colposcopy
colpospasm
colpostat
colpostenosis
colpostenotomy
colposuspension
    Pereyra c.

colpotomy
    posterior c.
colpoureterocystotomy
colpoureterotomy
colpoxerosis
columella (columellae)
    c. cochleae
    c. nasi
column
    c's of abdominal ring
    anal c's
    anterolateral c.
    Bertin c.
    Burdach c.
    Clarke c.
    dorsal c.
    enamel c's
    fat c's
    fleshy c's of heart
    c. of fornix
    fractionating c.
    fundamental c.
    Goll c.
    Gowers c.
    gray c's of spinal cord
    Kölliker (Koelliker) c.
    Lissauer c.
    Morgagni c.
    muscle c.
    c. of nose
    positive c.
    posteroexternal c.
    posterovesicular c. of Clarke
    Prosorba c.
    Rathke c's
    rectal c's
    renal c's of Bertin
    c. of Rolando
    c. of Sertoli
    somatic motor c.
    somatic sensory c.
    spinal c.
    Spitzka-Lissauer c.
    Stilling c.
    striomotor c.
    thoracic c.
    Türck c.
    ventral c. of spinal cord
    vertebral c.
    visceral motor c.
    visceral sensory c.
columna (columnae)
    c. adiposae
    columnae anales
    columnae ani

columna (columnae) *(continued)*
    columnae bertini
    columnae carneae cordis
    c. fornicis
    columnae griseae medullae
        spinalis
    c. nasi
    c. posterolateralis
        posteromediana
    columnae rectales
    columnae renales
    c. thoracica
    c. vertebralis
columnar
columnization
Colver
    forceps
    knife
coma
    alcoholic c.
    alpha c.
    deanimate c.
    diabetic c.
    epileptic c.
    hepatic c.
    c. hepaticum
    hyperosmolar nonketotic c.
    hypoglycemic c.
    hypopituitary c.
    hypothermic c.
    irreversible c.
    Kussmaul c.
    metabolic c.
    myxedema c.
    thyrotoxic c.
    uremic c.
    c. vigil
comatose
Comberg lens
combined approach
    c.a. mastoidectomy
    c.a. tympanoplasty
combined immunodeficiency
    disease
Combitube
combustion
Comby sign
comedo (comedones)
    closed c.
    open c.
    solar c.
comedocarcinoma
comedogenic
comedomastitis
comes (comites)

comfortization
comitance
comitant
Commando operation
commensurate
comminuted
comminution
commissura (commissurae)
    c. alba medullae spinalis
    c. anterior
    c. anterior cerebri
    c. bulborum vestibuli
    c. of bulbs of vestibule of vagina
    c. cerebelli
    c. colliculi caudalis
    c. colliculi rostralis
    c. colliculi superioris
    c. colliculorum cranialium
    c. colliculorum inferiorum
    c. epithalamica
    c. fornicis
    c. grisea medullae spinalis
    c. habenularis
    c. habenularum
    c. hippocampi
    c. inferior guddeni
    c. labiorum anterior
    c. labiorum oris
    c. labiorum posterior
    c. labiorum pudendi
    c. magna cerebri
    c. media cerebri
    c. mollis
    c. olivarum
    c. optica
    c. palpebrarum lateralis
    c. palpebrarum medialis
    c. palpebrarum nasalis
    c. palpebrarum temporalis
    c. posterior
    c. rostralis
    c. superior Meynerti
    c. supraoptica dorsalis
    c. supraopticae
    c. supraoptica ventralis
commissural myelotomy
commissure
    anterior c.
    anterior hypothalamic c.
    arcuate c.
    c. of bulb
    c. of caudal colliculus
    chiasmatic posterior c.
    c. of cranial colliculi
    dorsal supraoptic c.

commissure *(continued)*
    c. of epithalamus
    Forel c.
    c. of fornix
    Ganser c.
    gray c.
    great c.
    Gudden c.
    c. of habenulae
    habenular c.
    hippocampal c.
    c. of inferior colliculus
    interthalamic c.
    intrachiasmatic c.
    laryngeal c.
    c. laryngoscope
    lateral c. of eyelids
    lateral palpebral c.
    c. of lips of mouth
    medial c. of eyelids
    medial palpebral c.
    Meynert c.
    middle c. of cerebrum
    optic c.
    palpebral c.
    posterior c.
    rostral c.
    c. of rostral colliculus
    c. of superior colliculus
    supraoptic c., dorsal
    ventral supraoptic c.
    c. of vestibule
commissurorrhaphy
commissurotomy
    mitral c.
    percutaneous mitral c. (PMC)
commitment
common duct bougie
commotio
    c. cerebri
    c. retinae
    c. spinalis
communicable disease
communicans
communis
    atrioventricularis c.
community
    therapeutic c.
Comolli sign
comorbid
comorbidity
compact
compaction
compages
comparison microscope

comparison view
compartimentum superficiale
    perinei
compartment
    extracellular c.
    intracellular c.
    muscular c.
    vascular c.
compartmental analysis
compartmentalization
compatibility
    ABO c.
compatible
compendium (compendia)
    drug c.
compensated
compensation
    attenuation c.
    Bekhterev (Bechterew) c.
    broken c.
    dosage c.
    electronic distance c.
    time gain c.
    Worker's Compensation
compensatory
Compere
    operation
    pin
competence
    embryonic c.
    immunologic c.
competency
competent
    c. bladder
    c. bowel
    mentally c.
    c. vessel
competition
    antigenic c.
competitive
    c. behavior
    c. blood flow
complaint
    chief c.
complement
    c. activation
    chromosome c.
    component of c.
    c. deficiency
    c. deviation
    c. fixation
    c. level
    c.-mediated anaphylaxis
    normal c. of cells
    c. receptors

complement *(continued)*
   c. sequence
   c. test
complementarity
complementary
   c. afterimage
   c. chromaticities
   c. colors
complementation
   interallelic c.
   intercistronic c.
   intergenic c.
   intracistronic c.
   intragenic c.
   in vitro c.
complete
   c. colectomy
   c. hysterectomy
   c. iridectomy (CI)
   c. laryngotomy
completion arteriography
complex
   abortive c.
   adrenochrome
      monosemicarbazone sodium
      salicylate c.
   AIDS-related c. (ARC)
   amniotic band disruption c.
   amygdaloid c.
   amyotrophic lateral sclerosis–
      parkinsonism–dementia c.
   antigen-antibody c.
   apical c.
   atrial c.
   basal c. of choroid
   Behçet triple symptom c.
   calcarine c.
   castration c.
   chlormerodrin-cysteine c.
   Clérambault-Kandinsky c.
   diphasic c.
   EAHF (eczema, asthma, hay
      fever) c.
   Eisenmenger c.
   Electra c.
   equiphasic c.
   factor IX c.
   father c.
   flocculonodular c.
   Friedmann c.
   gene c.
   Ghon c.
   Golgi c.
   H-2 c.
   hapten-carrier c.

complex *(continued)*
   hemoglobin-haptoglobin c.
   HLA c.
   hydrocodone resin c.
   immune c.
   inclusion c.
   inferiority c.
   inferior olivary c.
   iron-dextran c.
   jumped process c.
   junctional c.
   K c.
   α-ketoglutarate
      dehydrogenase c. [alpha-]
   α-ketoisovalerate
      dehydrogenase c. [alpha-]
   Lutembacher c.
   major histocompatibility c.
      (MHC)
   membrane attack c. (MAC)
   Meyenburg c's
   oculomotor nuclear c.
   Oedipus c.
   Parkinson dementia c.
   perihypoglossal c.
   primary inoculation c.
   primary tuberculous c.
   QRS c.
   QRST c.
   QS c.
   Ranke c.
   ribosome-lamella c.
   rSr c.
   Schilder-Addison c.
   sicca c.
   soluble c.
   spike-wave c.
   Steidele c.
   symptom c.
   synaptonemal c.
   ternary c.
   ureterotrigonal c.
   urobilin c.
   ventricular c. (Q, R, S, T waves)
   ventricular depolarization c.
   Wilks symptom c.
complexion
complexus basalis choroideae
compliance
   motor c.
   patient c.
   pulmonary c.
   somatic c.
complicated
complication

C

component
    anterior c.
    complement c's
    G c.
    group-specific c.
    M c.
    plasma thromboplastin c. (PTC)
    secretory c. (SC)
    somatic motor c.
    somatic sensory c.
    splanchnic motor c.
    splanchnic sensory c.
    Woodbridge c's of anesthesia
composite
    resin matrix c.
composition
compos mentis
compound
    acyclic c.
    addition c.
    aliphatic c.
    APC c.
    aromatic c.
    benzene c's
    binary c.
    clathrate c.
    closed-chain c.
    coal-tar c.
    condensation c.
    cyclic c.
    diazo c.
    c. dressing
    endothermic c.
    energy-rich c's
    exothermic c.
    fatty c.
    c. G-11
    genetic c.
    Grignard c.
    heterocyclic c.
    Hurler-Scheie c.
    impression c.
    inorganic c.
    isocyclic c.
    isopropyl alcohol rubbing c.
    low-energy c's
    methonium c's
    c. microscope
    nonpolar c's
    occlusion c's
    open-chain c.
    organic c.
    organometallic c.
    polar c's
    quaternary c., quaternary
        ammonium c.

compound *(continued)*
    ring c.
    saturated c.
    substitution c.
    sulfonylurea c's
    c. suture
    tertiary c.
    unsaturated c.
compress
    cribriform c.
    fenestrated c.
compressibility
compression
    cardiac c.
    c. of cauda equina
    cerebral c.
    digital c.
    c. dressing
    fluffy c. dressing
    instrumental c.
    jugular c.
    c. of nerve roots
    renal artery c.
    spinal c.
    spinal cord c.
    sponge stick c.
    c. stockings
compressor
    Anthony c.
    aortic c.
    Deschamps c.
    c. naris
    Sehrt c.
    shot c.
    c. urethrae
    c. vaginae
    c. venae dorsalis
compressorium
compromise
Compton
    edge
    effect
    electron
    photon
    scatter
    scattering
    wavelength
compulsion
    repetition c.
compulsive
computed
    cranial c. tomography (CCT)
    emission c. tomography (ECT)
    c. myelography
    quantitative c. tomography
    c. tomography (CT)

computer
    c.-assisted design (CAD)
computerized
    c. axial tomography (CAT)
    dynamic c. tomography
    c. fluoroscopy
    c. radiography
    c. tomography (CT)
COMS—chronic organic mental
  syndrome
COMT—catechol-*O*-methyl
  transferase
conalbumin
conation
conative
conavanine
concatenate
concatenation
Concato disease
concave
concavity
concavoconcave
concavoconvex
concede
conceive
concentrate
    liver c.
    lyophilized c.
    plant protease c.
    vitamin c.
concentration
    bicarbonate ion c.
    hydrogen ion c.
    ionic c.
    limiting isorrheic c. (LIC)
    mass c.
    maximum allowable c. (MAC)
    maximum cell c. (MC c.)
    maximum urinary c.
      (MUC)
    mean corpuscular
      hemoglobin c.
    minimal alveolar c. (MAC)
    minimal bactericidal c.
      (MBC)
    minimal inhibitory c. (MIC)
    minimal isorrheic c. (MIC)
    minimal lethal c. (MLC)
    minimum alveolar c. (MAC)
    molar c.
    selective c.
    substance c.
concentric pantomography
concept
    no-threshold c.
    ring of bone c.

conception
conceptive
conceptus
concerted
concha (conchae)
    c. of auricle
    c. auriculae
    c. bullosa
    c. of cranium
    ethmoidal c.
    nasal c.
    c. nasalis inferior ossea
    c. nasalis media ossea
    c. nasalis superior ossea
    c. nasalis suprema ossea
    nasoturbinal c.
    Santorini c.
    sphenoidal c.
    c. sphenoidalis
    superior nasal c.
conchiform
conchiolin
conchiolinosteomyelitis
conchitis
conchoidal
conchoscope
conchotome
conchotomy
conclination
concoction
concomitant
    c. chemotherapy
    c. condition
    c. disease
    c. medical problem
    c. metabolic acidosis
    c. procedure
    c. radiation
      therapy
concomitantly
concordance
concordant
concrement
concrescence
concretio
    c. cordis
    c. pericardii
concretion
    alvine c.
    calculous c.
    preputial c.
    prostatic c's
    tophic c.
concretism
concretization
concurrent

concussion
　　acceleration c.
　　c. of the brain
　　compression c.
　　hydraulic abdominal c.
　　c. of the labyrinth
　　pulmonary c.
　　c. of the retina
　　c. of the spinal cord
condensation
　　aldol c.
condenser
　　Abbe c.
　　amalgam c.
　　automatic c.
　　back-action c.
　　cardioid c.
　　darkfield c.
　　foil c.
　　foot c.
　　gold c.
　　mechanical c.
　　paraboloid c.
　　reverse c.
condition
　　preexisting c.
conditioner
　　tissue c.
conditioning
　　aversive c.
　　avoidance c.
　　classical c.
　　higher-order c.
　　instrumental c.
　　operant c.
　　pavlovian c.
　　physical c.
　　reinforcement c.
　　respondent c.
condom
conduct
conductance
　　airway c.
conduction
　　aberrant c.
　　accelerated c.
　　aerial c.
　　aerotympanal c.
　　air c.
　　anomalous c.
　　anterograde c.
　　atrial c.
　　atrioventricular c.
　　avalanche c.
　　bone c.

conduction *(continued)*
　　cardiac c.
　　concealed c.
　　cranial c.
　　c. velocity
　　decremental c.
　　ephaptic c.
　　forward c.
　　His-Purkinje c.
　　intra-atrial c.
　　intraventricular c.
　　nerve c.
　　osteotympanic c.
　　retrograde c.
　　saltatory c.
　　synaptic c.
　　tissue c.
　　ventricular c.
　　ventriculoatrial c.
conductivity
　　thermal c.
conductor
　　Adson c.
　　Bailey c.
　　Davis c.
　　Kanavel c.
conduit
　　ileal c.
conduplicate
conduplicato corpore
condurangin
condurango
condylar
condylarthrosis
condyle
　　extensor c. of humerus
　　external c. of femur
　　external c. of humerus
　　external c. of tibia
　　fibular c. of femur
　　flexor c. of humerus
　　internal c. of femur
　　internal c. of humerus
　　internal c. of tibia
　　lateral c. of femur
　　lateral c. of humerus
　　lateral c. of tibia
　　c. of mandible
　　medial c. of femur
　　medial c. of humerus
　　medial c. of tibia
　　occipital c.
　　radial c. of humerus
　　c. of scapula
　　tibial c. of femur

condyle *(continued)*
  ulnar c. of humerus
condylectomy
condyli (plural of condylus)
condylicus
condylion
condyloid
condyloma (condylomata)
  c. acuminatum (condylomata
    acuminata)
  flat c.
  giant c.
  c. latum (condylomata
    lata)
  pointed c.
  c. subcutaneum
condylomatoid
condylomatosis
condylomatous
condylotomy
condylus (condyli)
Cone cannula
  needle
  retractor
cone
  acrosomal c.
  adjusting c's
  arterial c.
  attraction c.
  bifurcation c.
  cerebellar pressure c.
  Dunham c's
  c. dystrophy
  ectoplacental c.
  elastic c.
  fertilization c.
  graduated c.
  growth c.
  gutta-percha c.
  Haller c's
  c. of light
  long c.
  medullary c.
  c. monochromacy
  c. monochromat
  ocular c.
  pilar c.
  Politzer c.
  pressure c.
  primitive c.
  pulmonary c.
  retinal c.
  sarcoplasmic c.
  short c.
  silver c.

cone *(continued)*
  tentorial pressure c.
  terminal c. of spinal cord
  treatment c.
  twin c.
  Tyndall c.
  ureteral c.
  vascular c's
  visual c.
cone biopsy
coned-down view
cone-monochromat
cone-nose
confabulation
confection
conference
confertus
confidentiality
configuration
  arcuate c.
  cis c.
  trans c.
confinement
confirmatory incision
conflict
  approach-approach c.
  approach-avoidance c.
  avoidance-avoidance c.
  extrapsychic c.
  intrapersonal c.
  intrapsychic c.
confluence of sinuses
confluens sinuum
confluent
confocal
conformation
conformational determinant
Conform dressing
conformer
  Fox c.
  neck c.
confrication
confrontation
confrontation fields
confusion
confusional
congelation
congener
congeneric
congenerous
congenital
congested
congestin
congestion
  active c.

congestion *(continued)*
    cerebral c.
    circulatory c.
    functional c.
    hypostatic c.
    neuroparalytic c.
    neurotonic c.
    passive c.
    physiologic c.
    pleuropulmonary c.
    pulmonary c.
    rebound c.
    renal c.
    venous c.
congestive heart failure (CHF)
conglobate
conglobation
conglomerate
conglutin
conglutinant
conglutination of cervix
conglutinatio orificii externi
conglutinin
    immune c.
conglutinogen
congophilic
Congo red
    stain
    test
congruence
congruent
    affect was c. with mood
    c. articular surface
    mood c. psychosis
congruous
coni (plural of conus)
conical
coniine
coniism
coniofibrosis
coniolymphstasis
coniophage
coniosis
coniotoxicosis
conization
    cold c.
    cold knife c.
conjoined
conjoining
conjugal
conjugant
conjugata
    anatomic c.
    c. anatomica pelvis
    diagonal c.

conjugata *(continued)*
    c. diagonalis pelvis
    c. externa pelvis
    c. interna pelvis
    obstetric c.
    c. obstetrica
    true c.
    c. vera obstetrica
    c. vera pelvis
conjugate
    anatomical c. of pelvis
    available c.
    diagonal c.
    effective c.
    external c. of pelvis
    false c.
    c. of inlet
    internal c.
    median c. of pelvis
    obstetric c.
    c. of outlet
    pelvic c.
    straight c. of pelvis
    true c.
conjugation
conjunctiva (conjunctivae)
    bulbar c.
    injected conjunctivae
    irritation of conjunctivae
    pale conjunctivae
    pallor of conjunctivae
    palpebral c.
    pink conjunctivae
conjunctival incision
conjunctivitis
    acne rosacea c.
    actinic c.
    allergic c.
    anaphylactic c.
    angular c.
    arc-flash c.
    atopic c.
    atropine c.
    bacterial c.
    blennorrheal c.
    calcareous c.
    catarrhal c.
    chemical c.
    chronic c.
    contact c.
    croupous c.
    diphtheritic c.
    diplobacillary c.
    eczematous c.
    Elschnig c.

C

conjunctivitis *(continued)*
  epidemic c.
  follicular c.
  glare c.
  gonococcal c.
  gonorrheal c.
  granular c.
  hypertrophic c.
  inclusion c.
  infantile purulent c.
  infectious c.
  Koch-Weeks c.
  larval c.
  lithiasis c.
  c. medicamentosa
  membranous c.
  meningococcus c.
  molluscum c.
  Morax-Axenfeld c.
  mucopurulent c.
  c. necroticans infectiosus
  necrotic infectious c.
  neonatal c.
  c. nodosa
  nodular c.
  parasitic c.
  Parinaud c.
  Pascheff c.
  c. petrificans
  phlyctenular c.
  prairie c.
  pseudomembranous c.
  purulent c.
  scrofular c.
  shipyard c.
  simple c.
  spring c.
  swimming pool c.
  trachomatous c.
  tularemic c.
  c. tularensis
  uratic c.
  vaccinial c.
  vernal c.
  viral c.
  welder's c.
  Widmark c.
conjunctivodacryocystostomy
conjunctivoma
conjunctivoplasty
conjunctivorhinostomy
Conn operation
connection
  clamp c.
  intertendinous c's

connection *(continued)*
  major c.
  minor c.
  saddle c.
  thalamostriate c.
connective tissue disease
connector
  major c.
  minor c.
  Rochester c.
  saddle c.
Connell suture
connexus
  c. intertendinei
  c. intertendineus
Conn syndrome
conoid
  Sturm c.
conomyoidin
conophthalmus
Conradi
  disease
  line
  syndrome
consanguineous
consanguinity
conscience
conscious
consciousness
conscious sedation
consensual
consensus
consent
  informed c.
conservation
conservative mastoidectomy
conserve
consistency
consolidation
consolidative
conspecific
constancy
  cell c.
  object c.
constant
  absorption c.
  affinity c.
  association c.
  Avogadro c.
  binding c.
  Boltzmann c.
  catalytic c.
  decay c.
  dielectric c.
  diffusion c.

constant *(continued)*
    disintegration c.
    flotation c.
    gas c.
    gravitational c.
    growth rate c.
    Lapicque c.
    Michaelis c.
    newtonian c. of gravitation
    permeability c.
    Planck c.
    quantum c.
    radioactive c.
    sedimentation c.
    specific gamma-ray c.
    specificity c.
    velocity c.
constellation of symptoms
constipated
constipation
    atonic c.
    gastrojejunal c.
    proctogenous c.
    spastic c.
constituent
constitution
    ideo-obsessional c.
    lymphatic c.
    psychopathic c.
    vasoneurotic c.
    XXX sex chromosome c.
    XYY chromosome c.
constitutional
constrict
constricted
constriction
    congenital ring c's
    duodenopyloric c.
    primary c.
    pyloric c.
    Ranvier c's
    secondary c.
constrictive
constrictor
    c. isthmi faucium
    c. naris
    c. urethrae
    c. vaginae
constringent
constructive
consult
consultant
consultation
consumption
consumptive

contact
    c. autoradiography
    balancing c.
    centric c.
    complete c.
    deflective c.
    direct c.
    immediate c.
    indirect c.
    initial c.
    mediate c.
    occlusal c.
    premature c.
    proximal c.
    proximate c.
    weak c.
    working c.
contactant
contagion
    psychic c.
contagiosity
contagious
contaminant
contamination
content
    carbon dioxide c.
    effective radium c.
    equivalent
        radium c.
    latent c.
    manifest c.
    polymorphism information c.
        (PIC)
contiguity
contiguous
continence
    fecal c.
    urinary c.
continent
continuity
continuous
    c. passive motion (CPM)
    c. positive airway pressure
        (CPAP)
    c. suture
contortion
contour
    equal loudness c.
    height of c.
    c. retractor
contoured
contouring
    occlusal c.
contra-angle
contra-aperture

contraception
    intrauterine c.
    rhythm method of c.
contraceptive
    barrier c.
    chemical c.
    emergency c.
    intrauterine c.
    oral c.
    postcoital c.
contract
contractile
contractility
    cardiac c.
    galvanic c.
    idiomuscular c.
    neuromuscular c.
contraction
    aerobic c.
    anaerobic c.
    anisometric c.
    atrial c.
    atrial premature c. (APC)
    automatic ventricular c.
    bladder neck c.
    blocked arterial c.
    Braxton-Hicks c.
    cardiac c.
    carpopedal c.
    cathodal closure c.
    cathodal opening c.
    cicatricial c.
    clonic c.
    concentric c.
    Dupuytren c.
    escaped ventricular c.
    false uterine c.
    fibrillary c's
    Gowers c.
    Hicks c's
    hunger c.
    idiomuscular c.
    isokinetic c.
    isometric c.
    isotonic c.
    lengthening c.
    myoclonic c.
    myotatic c.
    nodal premature c.
    palmar c.
    paradoxical c.
    postural c.
    premature c.
    premature ventricular c. (PVC)
    premonitory c.

contraction *(continued)*
    R-on-T premature ventricular c.
    segmentation c.
    shortening c.
    supraventricular premature c.
    tetanic c.
    tone c.
    tonic c.
    tumultuous c's
    twitch c.
    uterine c.
    wound c.
contracture
    burn scar c.
    Dupuytren c.
    extrapyramidal c.
    flexion c.
    functional c.
    hypertonic c.
    hysterical c.
    ischemic c.
    muscle c.
    organic c.
    postpoliomyelitic c.
    Volkmann c.
contraincision
contraindicant
contraindicate
contraindication
contrainsular
contralateral
    c. antagonist
    c. synergist
contrasexual
contrast
    film c.
    high c.
    c. laryngography
    long-scale c.
    low c.
    object c.
    positive c. encephalography
    radiographic c.
    c. radiography
    short-scale c.
    c. studies
    subject c.
    c. ventriculography
contrastimulant
contrastimulus
contrecoup
contrectation
control
    associative automatic c.
    astigmatism c.

control *(continued)*
    automatic gain c.
    aversive c.
    biologic c.
    birth c.
    chin c.
    Diack c.
    feedback c.
    fine c.
    idiodynamic c.
    multivalent c.
    reflex c.
    relaxed c.
    Schick test c.
    sex c.
    stimulus c.
    stringent c.
    synergic c.
    tonic c.
    vestibuloequilibratory c.
    volitional c.
    voluntary c.
Controlled Substances Act
contuse
contusion
    brain c.
    cerebral c.
    contrecoup c.
contusive
conular
conus (coni)
    c. arteriosus
    coni epididymidis
    coni vasculosi
    distraction c.
    c. elasticus
    c. elasticus laryngis
    c. medullaris
    myopic c.
    supertraction c.
    c. terminalis
convalesce
convalescence
convalescent
convection
convergence
    accommodative c.
    amplitude of c.
    c. amplitudes
    conjugate c.
    far point of c.
    fusional c.
    c. insufficiency
    near point of c.
    negative c.

convergence *(continued)*
    positive c.
    proximal c.
    relative c.
    c. spasm
    tonic c.
    voluntary c.
convergent
Converse
    chisel
    line
    operation
    osteotome
    rongeur
    speculum
conversion
    c. coefficient
    c. disorder
    gene c.
    hysterical c.
    internal c.
    lysogenic c.
    Mantoux c.
    phage c.
    c. reaction
    somatic c.
    wound c.
convertase
convertin
convex
convexity
convex lens
convexobasia
convexoconcave lens
convexoconvex
convoluted
convolution
    Broca c.
    callosal c.
    c. of cerebrum
    c's of Gratiolet
    Heschl c.
    occipitotemporal c.
    transitional c.
    Zuckerkandl c.
convolutional
convulsant
convulsibility
convulsion
    audiogenic c.
    central c.
    choreic c.
    clonic c.
    coordinate c.
    crowing c.

convulsion *(continued)*
    epileptiform c.
    essential c.
    febrile c.
    hypoglycemic c.
    hysterical c.
    hysteroid c.
    infantile c.
    jackknife c.
    lightning major c.
    local c.
    mimetic c.
    mimic c.
    myoclonic c.
    puerperal c.
    salaam c.
    spontaneous c.
    static c.
    tetanic c.
    tonic c.
    tonic-clonic c.
    toxic c.
    traumatic c.
    uremic c.
convulsive
Conway
    mammaplasty
    operation
Cook speculum
coolant
Cooley
    anemia
    clamp
    dilator
    disease
    forceps
    prosthesis
    retractor
    scissors
Cooley-Pontius blade
Cooley-Tukey algorithm
Coolidge x-ray tube
Coombs test
    direct
    indirect
Coons method
Cooper
    cannula
    disease
    fascia
    hernia
    irritable breast
    irritable testis
    ligament
    neuralgia

Cooper *(continued)*
    operation
cooperation
    T lymphocyte–B lymphocyte c.
    T lymphocyte–T lymphocyte c.
cooperative
cooperativity
Coopernail sign
coordinate
coordination
coossification
coossify
COP—cyclophosphamide, Oncovin,
  prednisone
copal
COPD—chronic obstructive
  pulmonary disease
Cope
    clamp
    needle
Copeland
    implant
    retinoscope
Cope-method bronchography
coping
    transfer c.
copiopia
copious
copolymer
copper
    c. sulfate
    c. wire effect
    c. wiring
copperas
copperhead
copper storage disease
Coppridge forceps
copracrasia
coprecipitation
coprecipitin
copremesis
coproantibody
coprolagnia
coprolalia
coprolith
coprophagous
coprophagy
coprophilia
coprophilic, coprophiliac
coprophilous
coprophobia
coproporphyria
    erythropoietic c.
    hereditary c.
coproporphyrin

C

coproporphyrinogen oxidase
coproporphyrinuria
copropraxia
coprostanol
coprostasis
copula linguae
copulation
copulatory
CoQ 10 (coenzyme Q 10)
coquille plano lens
COR—conditioned orientation
   response
cor
     c. adiposum
     c. arteriosum
     c. biloculare
     c. bovinum
     c. pulmonale
     c. dextrum
     c. juvenum
     c. mobile
     c. pendulum
     c. pseudotriloculare biatriatum
     c. pulmonale
     c. sinistrum
     c. taurinum
     c. tomentosum
     c. triatriatum
     c. triloculare biatriatum
     c. triloculare biventriculare
     c. venosum
     c. villosum
CORA—conditioned orientation
   reflex audiometry
coracidium (coracidia)
coracoacromial
coracobrachialis
coracoclavicular
coracohumeral
coracoid
coracoiditis
coracoradialis
coracoulnaris
coralliform
corallin
     yellow c.
Corbett
     forceps
     spud
Corbin technique
Corbus disease
cord
     Bergmann c's
     Billroth c's
     c. blood

cord *(continued)*
   c. clamp
   clamping c.
   c. compression
   condyle c.
   dental c.
   enamel c.
   Ferrein c's
   ganglionated c.
   genital c.
   germinal c.
   gubernacular c.
   hepatic c's
   c. of Hippocrates
   lateral c. of brachial plexus
   lumbosacral c.
   lymph c's
   medullary c.
   mesonephrogenic c.
   metanephrogenic c.
   nasolacrimal c.
   nephrogenic c.
   nerve c.
   oblique c. of elbow joint
   ovigerous c.
   Pflüger c's
   posterior c.
   primary sex c.
   pronephrogenic c.
   psalterial c.
   red pulp c's
   rete c's
   scirrhous c.
   sex c's
   sexual c's
   spermatic c.
   spinal c.
   splenic c's
   tendinous c.
   testis c's
   umbilical c.
   urogenital c.
   vocal c., false
   vocal c., true
   Weitbrecht c.
   Willis c's
cordal
cordate
cordectomy
Cordes forceps
Cordes-New forceps
cordial
cordiform
corditis
cordopexy

cordotomy
core
    cast c.
    c. vesicles
coreclisis
corectasis
corectome
corectomedialysis
corectomy
corectopia
coredialysis
corediastasis
coregonin
corelysis
coremorphosis
corenclisis
coreometer
coreometry
coreoplasty
corepexy
corepressor
corestenoma congenitum
coretomedialysis
coretomy
Corey forceps
Cori
    cycle
    disease
    ester
coriaceous
coriamyrtin
coriander
coriin
corium
    lingual c.
CORLA—clusters of radiolucent
  areas
corn
    hard c.
    seed c.
    soft c.
cornea
    conical c.
    c. farinata
    flat c.
    c. globata
    c. globosa
    c. guttata
    c. opaca
    c. plana
    sugar-loaf c.
    c. verticillata
    Vogt c.
corneal
    c. abrasion

corneal *(continued)*
    c. apex
    c. astigmatism
    c. bedewing
    c. button
    c. cap
    c. dellen
    c. dystrophy
    c. erosion
    c. lens
    c. microscope
    c. reflex
    c. scraping
    c. transplant
    c. tubes
    c. ulcer
corneal graft
    lamellar c.g.
    mushroom c.g.
    penetrating c.g.
corneitis
Cornelia de Lange syndrome
corneoblepharon
corneoiritis
corneosclera
corneoscleral
    c. incision
    c. scissors
corneous
Corner tampon
Corner-Allen
    test
    unit
Cornet forceps
corneum
corniculate
corniculum
cornification
cornified
Corning
    anesthesia
    method
    puncture
Cornish wool dressing
cornoid
cornu (cornua)
    c. ammonis
    c. anterius ventriculi lateralis
    c. coccygeale
    c. coccygeum
    c. cutaneum
    c. descendens
    ethmoid c.
    c. inferius ventriculi lateralis
    c. majus ossis hyoidei

C

cornu (cornua) *(continued)*
    c. medullae spinalis
    c. minus ossis hyoidei
    sacral c.
    c. sacrale
    cornua of spinal cord
    cornua of the uterus
cornual
cornuate
cornucommissural
cornucopia
corona (coronae)
    c. capitis
    c. ciliaris
    c. clinica
    dental c.
    c. dentis
    c. glandis penis
    c. of glans penis
    c. radiata
    c. seborrheica
    c. veneris
    Zinn c.
coronad
coronal suture
coronale
coronalis
coronary
    c. angiography (CA)
    c. angioplasty
    c. arterial reserve
    c. arteriography
    c. artery bypass graft (CABG)
    c. artery disease (CAD)
    c. artery ectasia
    c. artery occlusion
    c. atherosclerosis
    c. bifurcation
    c. bypass surgery
    café c.
    cine c. arteriography
    c. heart disease (CHD)
    c. insufficiency
    c. ostial stenosis
    percutaneous transluminal c.
      angioplasty (PTCA)
    c. sinus
    c. steal
    c. stenosis
    c. thrombolysis
    c. thrombosis
    c. vascular resistance
coronavirus
corone
coroner

coronet
coronion
coronitis
coronoid
coronoidectomy
coroparelcysis
coroplasty
coroscopy
corotomy
corpora (plural of corpus)
corporeal
corporic
corporis (genitive of corpus)
corps
    medical c.
    c. ronds
corpse
corpulency
corpus (corpora)
    c. adiposum
    c. adiposum fossae ischioanalis
    c. adiposum orbitae
    c. albicans
    corpora allata
    c. amygdaloideum
    corpora amylacea
    corpora arantii
    c. atretica
    corpora bigemina
    c. calcanei
    c. callosum
    corpora cavernosa
    c. cavernosum clitoridis
    c. cavernosum penis
    c. cavernosum urethrae virilis
    c. cerebelli
    c. ciliare
    c. ciliaris
    c. claviculae
    c. clitoridis
    c. coccygeum
    c. costae
    c. delicti
    c. dentatum
    c. epididymidis
    c. femoris
    c. fibrosum
    c. fibulae
    c. fimbriatum
    corpora flava
    c. fornicis
    c. gastricum
    c. geniculatum
    c. glandulae bulbourethralis
    c. glandulae sudoriferae

corpus (corpora) *(continued)*
    c. glandulare prostatae
    c. granulosum
    c. hemorrhagicum
    c. Highmori
    c. highmorianum
    c. humeri
    c. hypothalamicum
    c. incudis
    c. interpedunculare
    c. linguae
    corpora lutea atretica
    c. luteum
    c. Luysii
    c. mammae
    c. mammillare
    c. mandibulae
    c. maxillae
    c. medullare cerebelli
    c. medullare vermis
    c. metacarpale
    c. metatarsalis
    c. nuclei caudati
    c. of Oken
    corpora oryzoidea
    c. ossis femoris
    c. ossis hyoidei
    c. ossis ilii
    c. ossis ischii
    c. ossis metacarpalis
    c. ossis metatarsalis
    c. ossis pubis
    c. ossis sphenoidalis
    c. pampiniforme
    c. pancreatis
    corpora para-aortica
    c. paraterminalis
    c. penis
    c. pineale
    c. pontobulbare
    c. pyramidale medullae
    corpora quadrigemina
    c. radii
    c. restiforme
    corpora restiformis
    c. rhomboidale
    c. santorianum
    c. sphenoidale
    c. spongiosum penis
    c. spongiosum urethrae
      muliebris
    c. sterni
    c. striatum
    c. subthalamicum
    c. tali

corpus (corpora) *(continued)*
    c. tibiae
    c. trapezoideum
    c. triticeum
    c. ulnae
    c. unguis
    corpora uteri
    uterine c.
    c. ventriculare
    c. ventriculi
    c. vertebrale
    c. vesicae biliaris
    c. vesicae felleae
    c. vesicae urinariae
    c. vesiculae seminalis
    c. vitreum
    c. Wolffi
corpuscallostomy
corpuscle
    amylaceous c's
    amyloid c's
    articular c.
    Babès-Ernst c.
    basal c.
    Bennet large c's
    Bennet small c's
    Bizzozero c.
    blood c.
    bridge c.
    bulboid c.
    cartilage c.
    cement c.
    chorea c's
    chromophil c's
    chyle c.
    colloid c's
    colostrum c's
    concentrated human red
      blood c.
    concentric c's
    corneal c's
    Dogiel c.
    Donné c's
    Drysdale c's
    dust c's
    genital c's
    Gierke c's
    Gluge c's
    Golgi-Mazzoni c's
    Grandry c's
    Grandry-Merkel c's
    Guarnieri c's
    Hassall c.
    Hayem elementary c.
    Herbst c's

C

corpuscle *(continued)*
  Jaworski c's
  Krause c.
  lamellar c's
  lamellated c's
  Laveran c's
  Leber c's
  lingual c.
  Lostorfer c's
  lymph c's
  lymphoid c's
  malpighian c.
  Mazzoni c's
  meconium c's
  Meissner c.
  Merkel c.
  milk c's
  mucous c's
  Norris c's
  Nunn gorged c's
  oval c.
  Pacini c.
  pacinian c's
  Paschen c's
  pessary c.
  phantom c.
  Purkinje c's
  pus c's
  Rainey c.
  red c.
  renal c.
  reticulated c.
  Röhl (Roehl) marginal c's
  Ruffini c's
  Russell c's
  salivary c.
  Schwalbe c.
  splenic c's
  tactile c.
  taste c's
  tendon c's
  terminal nerve c.
  thymus c's
  Timofeew c.
  touch c.
  Toynbee c's
  Tröltsch (Troeltsch) c's
  typhic c's
  Valentin c's
  Vater c's
  Vater-Pacini c.
  Virchow c's
  Wagner c's
  Weber c.
  white c.

corpuscular
corpusculum (corpuscula)
  corpuscula articularia
  c. bulboideum
  c. genitale
  c. lamellosum
  c. nervosum acapsulatum
  c. nervosum terminale
  c. renale
  corpuscula renis
  c. tactus
correction
  Yates c.
corrective
corrector
  function c.
correlation
  zero c.
correspondence
  anomalous retinal c.
  harmonious retinal c.
  normal retinal c.
  retinal c.
corresponding ray
Corrigan
  cautery
  disease
  line
  pneumonia
  pulse
  respiration
  sign
corrigent
corrin
corrinoid
corrosion
corrosive
corrugation
corrugator
corset
  Milwaukee c.
cortex (cortices)
  aberrant suprarenal c.
  adrenal c.
  agranular c.
  auditory c.
  cerebellar c.
  c. cerebelli
  c. of cerebellum
  cerebral c.
  c. cerebri
  c. of cerebrum
  cingulate c.
  driftwood c.
  entorhinal c.

cortex (cortices) *(continued)*
    fetal adrenal c.
    frontal premotor c.
    c. glandulae suprarenalis
    c. of hair shaft
    heterotypical c.
    homotypical c.
    interpyramidal c.
    c. lentis
    limbic c.
    motor c.
    c. nodi lymphatici
    nonolfactory c.
    occipital c.
    olfactory c.
    c. ovarii
    periamygdaloid c.
    piriform c.
    precentral motor c.
    premotor c.
    provisional c.
    renal c.
    c. renis
    sensorimotor c.
    somatosensory c.
    somesthetic c.
    striate c.
    supplementary motor c.
    tertiary c.
    c. thymi
    visual c.
Corti
    arches
    canal
    cell
    fiber
    ganglion
    organ
    rod
    tunnel
cortiadrenal
cortical
    c. hyperostosis
    c. incision
    c. mastoidectomy
    c. nephron
    c. spoking
    c. thumb
corticalization
corticalosteotomy
corticate
corticectomy
cortices (plural of cortex)
corticifugal
corticipetal

corticis (genitive of cortex)
corticoadrenal
corticoafferent
corticoautonomic
corticobulbar
corticocancellous
corticocerebral
corticodiencephalic
corticoefferent
corticoid
corticomedullary
corticomesencephalic
corticopeduncular
corticopleuritis
corticopontine
corticopontocerebellar
corticoreticular
corticorubral
corticospinal
corticosteroid
corticosterone
corticostriate
corticotensin
corticothalamic
corticotroph
corticotropic
corticotropinoma
cortilymph
cortisol
cortisone acetate
Cortrosyn stimulation test
corundum
coruscation
Corvisart
    disease
    facies
Corwin hemostat
corydaline
Coryllos
    raspatory
    retractor
corymbiform
corynebacteria
Corynebacterium
    C. diphtheriae
    C. minutissimum
    C. parvum
    C. pseudodiphtheriticum
    C. pyogenes
    C. tenuis
    C. ulcerans
    C. xerosis
corynebacterium
    group JK c.
coryneform

corytuberine
coryza
    allergic c.
    c. foetida
cosensitize
cosmesis
cosmetic operation
cosmid
cosmopolitan
costa (costae)
    c. cervicalis
    c. fluctuans decima
    costae fluctuantes
    costae fluitantes
    c. prima
    costae spuriae
    costae verae
costal margin
costalgia
costalis
costectomy
Costen syndrome
costicartilage
costicervical
costiferous
costiform
costispinal
costive
costiveness
costoabdominal
costocentral
costocervical
costocervicalis
costochondral
costochondritis
costoclavicular
costocoracoid
costogenic
costoinferior
costolumbar
costophrenic
costoplasty
costopleural
costopneumopexy
costoscapular
costoscapularis
costosternal
costosternoplasty
costosuperior
costotome
    Tudor-Edwards c.
costotomy
costotransverse
costotransversectomy
costoversion thoracoplasty

costovertebral
    c. angle (CVA)
    c. angle tenderness
      (CVAT)
costoxiphoid
cosyntropin stimulation test
COT—critical off-time
Cotard syndrome
cothromboplastin
cotinine
Cotrel cast
Cotrel-Dubousset spinal
    instrumentation
Cotte operation
Cotting operation
Cottle
    clamp
    elevator
    forceps
    knife
    osteotome
    rasp
    retractor
    saw
    scissors
    speculum
    tenaculum
Cottle-Arruga forceps
Cottle-Jansen forceps
Cottle-Kazanjian forceps
Cottle-Neivert retractor
cotton
    absorbent c.
    capsicum c.
    collodion c.
    gun c., soluble
    purified c.
    salicylated c.
    styptic c.
Cotton fracture
cottonmouth
cottonoid patty
cottonpox
cotton-wool
    c.-w. appearance
    c.-w. bandage
    c.-w. exudates
    c.-w. patches
    c.-w. spots
Cotugno disease
Cotunnius
    aqueduct (aqueduct of
      Cotunnius)
    canal
    nerve

Cotunnius *(continued)*
    space
coturnism
co-twin
cotyledontoxin
cotyloid
cotylosacral
cotype
couching
coudé
    c. bougie
    c. catheter
cough
    aneurysmal c.
    Balme c.
    barking c.
    brassy c.
    compression c.
    dog c.
    dry c.
    ear c.
    extrapulmonary c.
    habit c.
    hacking c.
    mechanical c.
    minute gun c.
    Morton c.
    nonproductive c.
    paroxysmal c.
    privet c.
    productive c.
    psychogenic c.
    reflex c.
    c. response
    smoker's c.
    stomach c.
    Sydenham c.
    tea taster's c.
    c. threshold
    trigeminal c.
    weavers' c.
    wet c.
    whooping c.
    winter c.
coumaric acid
Councill
    basket
    catheter
    stone dislodger
counseling
    genetic c.
    nondirective c.
count
    Addis c.
    Arneth c.

count *(continued)*
    bleeding point c.
    blood c.
    complete blood c.
    c. density
    differential leukocyte c.
    dust c.
    filament-nonfilament c.
    kick c's
    leukocyte c.
    neutrophil lobe c.
    platelet c., direct
    platelet c., indirect
    pollen c.
    red cell c.
    reticulocyte c.
    ridge c.
    Schilling blood c.
    total white c.
counter
    automated differential
      leukocyte c.
    boron c.
    Cerenkov c.
    colony c.
    Coulter c.
    crystal c.
    electronic cell c.
    end-window c.
    gamma scintillation c.
    gamma well c.
    gas-flow c.
    Geiger c.
    Geiger-Müller c.
    immersion c.
    liquid-flow c.
    proportional c.
    radiation c.
    scintillation c.
    whole-body c.
counteraction
counterbalance
    renal c.
countercurrent
   immunoelectrophoresis
counterdepressant
counterextension
counterfissure
counterimmunoelectrophoresis (CIE)
counterincision
counterinvestment
counterirritant
counterirritation
counteropening
counterphobia

counterphobic
counterpoison
counterpulsation
    intra-aortic balloon c.
counterpuncture
counter-rolling
counterstain
counterstroke
countertraction
countertransference
counting rate meter
count rate
coup
    c. de fouet
    c. de sabre
    c. de sang
    c. de soleil
    en c. de sabre
    c. Highmori
    c. sur c.
coupler
    acoustic c.
coupling
    contact c.
    electrochemical c.
    excitation-contraction c.
    fixed c.
    immersion c.
    liquid c.
Cournand
    catheter
    needle
course
    arterial c.
    c. of artery
    c. of convalescence
    convalescent c.
    downhill c.
    treatment c.
    c. of vein
    venous c.
coursing
Courtois sign
Courvoisier
    gallbladder
    gastroenterostomy
    incision
    law
    sign
Courvoisier-Terrier syndrome
couvade
Couvelaire uterus
couvercle
covalence
covalent

covariance
covariate
Coventry
    osteotomy
    screw
coverglass
coverslip
cover-uncover test
cowage
Cowden
    disease
    syndrome
Cowdry inclusion bodies (type A,
    type B)
Cowper gland
cowperian
cowperitis
cowpox
Cox
    line
    vaccine
coxa
    c. adducta
    c. flexa
    c. magna
    c. plana
    c. valga
    c. vara
    c. vara luxans
coxalgia
    Mediterranean c.
coxarthria
coxarthritis
coxarthrocace
coxarthropathy
coxarthroplasty
coxarthrosis
Coxiella burnetii
coxitis
    c. fugax
    senile c.
    transient c.
coxodynia
coxofemoral
coxotomy
coxotuberculosis
coxsackieviral
coxsackievirus (group A, group B)
CP—
    cerebral palsy
    chest pain
    chloroquine and primaquine
    chronic pyelonephritis
    cochlear potential
    combination product

C

CP— *(continued)*
  combining power
  coproporphyrin
  cor pulmonale
C/P—cholesterol-phospholipid ratio
C&P—compensation and pension
C~pah~—para-aminohippurate
  clearance
CPAP—continuous positive airway
  pressure
CPB—cardiopulmonary bypass
CPBS—cardiopulmonary bypass
  surgery
CPC—
  cetylpyridinium chloride
  chronic passive congestion
  clinicopathological conference
  clinicopathologic conference
CP&C—cast post and core
CPD—
  calcium pyrophosphate
    dihydrate (crystals)
  cephalopelvic disproportion
  citrate-phosphate-dextrose
  congenital polycystic disease
CPDA-1—citrate phosphate
  dextrose adenine
CPDD—calcium pyrophosphate
  deposition disease
CPE—
  cardiogenic pulmonary edema
  chronic pulmonary emphysema
CPEO—chronic progressive
  external ophthalmoplegia
CPH—Certificate in Public Health
CPI—
  congenital pain indifference
  constitutional psychopathic
    inferiority
  coronary prognostic index
CPID—chronic pelvic inflammatory
  disease
cpm, c.p.m.—counts per minute
CPM—
  central pontine myelinolysis
  continuous passive motion
CPN—chronic pyelonephritis
CPPB—continuous positive-
  pressure breathing
CPPD—calcium pyrophosphate
  dihydrate (crystals)
CPR—
  cardiopulmonary resuscitation
  cerebral-cortex perfusion rate
  cortisol production rate

CPS—
  carbamoyl phosphate
    synthetase
  carbamoyl phosphate
    synthetase II
  clinical performance score
  cumulative probability of
    success
CPT—chest physiotherapy
CQ—
  chloroquine-quinine
  circadian quotient
C1q (to C9q) assay
CR—
  calculus removed
  chest and right arm (ECG
    lead)
  colon resection
  complete remission
  conditioned reflex
  conversion reaction
  corneal reflex
  crown-rump (length)
^{51}Cr—radioactive chromium
  (chromium Cr 51)
^{51}Cr-heated RBC
crab louse
Crabtree effect
crack cocaine
cracked heels
cracked pot note
crackle
  pleural c's
cradle
  electric c.
  heat c.
  ice c.
Crafoord
  clamp
  forceps
  scissors
Crafts test
Craig
  forceps
  needle
  scissors
  test
Craigies tube
Cramer splint
cramp
  accessory c.
  heat c.
  menstrual c's
  muscle c.
  nocturnal c's

cramp *(continued)*
    occupational c.
    professional c.
    recumbency c's
    seamstresses' c.
    stoker's c.
    tailors' c.
    writers' c.
Crampton
    muscle
    test
Crane
    flap
    mallet
    osteotome
craniad
cranial
    c. computed tomography (CCT)
    c. sutures
cranialis
craniamphitomy
craniectomy
cranioacromial
cranioaural
craniobuccal
craniocaudal
craniocele
craniocerebral
craniocervical
cranioclasis
cranioclast
    Auvard c.
    Braun c.
    Zweifel-DeLee c.
cranioclasty
craniodidymus
craniofacial
craniofacial cleft
    Boo-Chai c.c.
    Tessier c.c.
craniofenestria
craniognomy
craniography
craniolacunia
craniology
craniomalacia
craniomandibular
craniomeningocele
craniometer
craniometric
craniometry
craniopagus
    c. frontalis
    c. occipitalis
    c. parasiticus
    c. parietalis

craniopathy
    metabolic c.
craniopharyngeal
craniopharyngioma
craniophore
cranioplasty
craniopuncture
craniorachischisis totalis
craniosacral
cranioschisis
craniosclerosis
cranioscopy
craniospinal
craniostenosis
craniostosis
craniosynostosis
craniotabes
craniotome
craniotomy scissors
craniotonoscopy
craniotopography
craniotrypesis
craniotympanic
craniovertebral
cranium
    c. bifidum
    c. bifidum occultum
    cerebral c.
    c. cerebrale
    visceral c.
    c. viscerale
crank amphetamine
CRAO—central retinal artery
  occlusion
crapulent, crapulous
crater
    ulcer c.
crateriform
craterization
cravat
Crawford
    operation
    retractor
Crawford-Adams
    acetabular cup
    arthroplasty
    cup arthroplasty
Crawford-Cooley tunneler
crazing
CRBBB—complete right bundle
  branch block
CRC—crisis resolution center
CRD—
    chronic renal disease
    chronic respiratory disease
    crown-rump distance

C

cream
    aluminum hydroxide c.
    antibiotic c.
    barrier c.
    cold c.
    c. of magnesia
    c. of tartar
crease
    ear lobe c.
    flexion c.
    gluteofemoral c.
    palmar c.
    Sidney c.
    simian c.
    sole c.
creatine
    c. kinase (CK)
    c. phosphate
    c. phosphotransferase
creatinemia
creatinuria
creatorrhea
creatotoxism
crèche
Credé prophylaxis
Credo operation
Creech technique
Creevy evacuator
CREG—cross-reactive group
cremaster
    internal c. of Henle
cremasteric
cremation
crematorium
cremor
crena (crenae)
    c. ani
    c. clunium
    c. cordis
crenate, crenated
crenation
crenilabrin
crenocyte
crenocytosis
Crenshaw forceps
creophagism
creosol
creosote carbonate
crepitant
crepitation
crepitus
    articular c.
    bony c.
    false c.
    c. indux
    joint c.

crepitus (continued)
    c. redux
    silken c.
    c. uteri
crepuscular
crescendo
crescendo-decrescendo murmur
crescent
    articular c.
    blastoporal c.
    cellular c.
    congenital c. of choroid
    epithelial c.
    fibrous c.
    Giannuzzi c's
    gray c.
    c. incision
    malarial c's
    myopic c.
    sublingual c.
crescentic
cresol
cresolphthalein
cresorcin
crest
    acoustic c.
    acusticofacial c.
    alveolar c.
    anterior c. of fibula
    anterior c. of tibia
    arcuate c. of arytenoid cartilage
    basilar c. of cochlear duct
    buccinator c.
    cerebral c's of cranial bone
    c. of cochlear window
    conchal c. of body of maxilla
    conchal c. of palatine bone
    deltoid c.
    dental c.
    dermal c's
    ethmoid c. of maxilla
    ethmoid c. of palatine bone
    falciform c.
    femoral c.
    fimbriated c.
    frontal c.
    ganglionic c.
    gingival c.
    glandular c. of larynx
    gluteal c.
    iliac c.
    iliopectineal c. of iliac bone
    iliopectineal c. of pelvis
    iliopectineal c. of pubis
    infratemporal c.
    infundibuloventricular c.

crest *(continued)*
- inguinal c.
- c. of insertion
- interosseous c.
- intertrochanteric c.
- interureteric c.
- jugular c. of greater wing of sphenoid bone
- lacrimal c., anterior
- lacrimal c., posterior
- lateral c. of fibula
- marginal c.
- c. of matrix of nail
- medial c. of fibula
- mental c., external
- mitochondrial c's
- nasal c. of maxilla
- nasal c. of palatine bone
- nasopalatine c.
- neural c.
- oblique c. of thyroid cartilage
- obturator c.
- occipital c., external
- occipital c., internal
- orbital c.
- papillary c.
- pectineal c. of femur
- pharyngeal c. of occipital bone
- radial c.
- c. of ridge
- rough c. of femur
- sacral c.
- c. of scapular spine
- seminal c.
- sphenoidal c.
- spinal c. of Rauber
- spiral c.
- supracondylar c.
- supramastoid c.
- supraventricular c.
- temporal c. of frontal bone
- terminal c. of right atrium
- tibial c.
- triangular c.
- trigeminal c.
- turbinal c.
- ulnar c.
- urethral c.
- zygomatic c. of greater wing of sphenoid bone

CREST—calcinosis cutis, Raynaud phenomenon, esophageal dysfunction/hypermotility, sclerodactyly, telangiectasia (syndrome)

cresyl blue
cresylic acid
cresyl violet
Creutzfeldt-Jakob
- disease
- syndrome

crevice
- gingival c.

crevicular

CRF—
- cardiac risk factor(s)
- chronic renal failure
- corticotropin-releasing factor

CRH—corticotropin-releasing hormone

CRI—
- cardiac risk index
- chronic renal insufficiency

crib
- clinical c.
- c. death
- Jackson c.

cribra (plural of cribrum)
cribral
cribrate
cribriform
- c. ligament
- c. plate
- c. spot

cribrum (cribra)
- cribra orbitalia of Welcker

Crichton-Browne sign
cricoarytenoid
cricoid
cricoidectomy
cricoidynia
cricopharyngeal myotomy
cricopharyngeus
cricothyreotomy
cricothyroid
cricothyroidotomy
cricothyrotomy
cricotomy
cricotracheotomy
cri-du-chat syndrome
Crigler-Najjar
- disease
- syndrome

Crikelair otoplasty
Crile
- clamp
- forceps
- knife

Crile *(continued)*
    retractor
criminalistics
criminology
crinin
crinis (crines)
Cripps
    obturator
    operation
crisis (crises)
    abdominal c.
    adolescent c.
    adrenal c.
    adrenocortical c.
    anaphylactoid c.
    aplastic c.
    blast c.
    brain stem c.
    bronchial c.
    cardiac c.
    cataleptic c.
    catathymic c.
    celiac c.
    cholinergic c.
    clitoris c.
    decerebrate c.
    deglobulinization c.
    developmental c.
    Dietl c.
    false c.
    febrile c.
    gastric c.
    genital c. of newborn
    glaucomatocyclitic c.
    hemolytic c.
    hepatic c.
    hypertensive c.
    identity c.
    intestinal c.
    laryngeal c.
    myasthenic c.
    nefast c.
    nephralgic c.
    ocular c.
    oculogyric c.
    parkinsonian c.
    Pel crises
    pharyngeal c.
    physiologic c.
    posterior c.
    rectal c.
    reflex anoxic c.
    reflex hypoxic c.
    renal c.
    salt depletion c.

crisis (crises) *(continued)*
    salt-losing c.
    sickle cell c.
    situational c.
    tabetic c.
    thoracic c.
    utricular c.
    vesical c.
    visceral c.
crispation
crisscross heart
crista (cristae)
    c. acustica
    c. ampullaris
    c. anterior fibulae
    c. anterior tibiae
    c. arcuata
    c. arcuata cartilaginis
        arytenoideae
    c. basilaris ductus cochlearis
    c. buccinatoria
    c. capitis costae
    c. colli costae
    c. conchalis corporis maxillae
    c. conchalis maxillae
    c. conchalis ossis palatini
    cristae cutis
    c. dividens
    c. ethmoidalis maxillae
    c. ethmoidalis ossis palatini
    c. falciformis
    c. femoris
    c. fenestrae cochleae
    c. frontalis
    c. galli
    c. helicis
    c. iliaca
    c. infratemporalis
    c. interossea fibulae
    c. interossea radii
    c. interossea tibiae
    c. interossea ulnae
    c. intertrochanterica
    c. lacrimalis anterior
    c. lacrimalis posterior
    c. lateralis fibulae
    c. marginalis
    c. matricis unguis
    c. medialis fibulae
    c. musculi supinatoris
    c. nasalis maxillae
    c. nasalis ossis palatini
    c. obturatoria
    c. occipitalis externa
    c. occipitalis interna

crista (cristae) *(continued)*
    c. palatina ossis palatini
    c. pubica
    c. sacralis intermedia
    c. sacralis lateralis
    c. sphenoidalis
    c. spiralis
    c. spiralis cochleae
    c. supramastoidea
    c. supraventricularis
    c. temporalis
    c. terminalis atrii dextri
    c. transversalis
    c. transversa meati acustici
      interni
    c. triangularis
    c. tuberculi majoris
    c. tuberculi minoris
    c. tympanica
    c. ulnae
    c. urethralis
    c. urethralis femininae
    c. urethralis masculinae
    c. urethralis muliebris
    c. urethralis virilis
    c. vestibuli
cristal
cristobalite
Critchett operation
criterion (criteria)
    Cooke criteria
    Hyams criteria
    Jones criteria
    Ranson criteria for severity of
      acute pancreatitis
    Spiegelberg criteria for
      ovarian pregnancy
critical
criticality
critical mass
CRL—crown-rump length
CRM—cross-reacting material
CRNA—Certified Registered Nurse
  Anesthetist
crocein
crocidolite
crocodile tears
Crocq disease
Crohn disease
cromoglycate
cromoglycic acid
Cronin
    method
    operation
    prosthesis

Cronkhite-Canada syndrome
Crookes
    lens
    space
    tube
CROS—contralateral routing of
  signals
cross
    occipital c.
    phage c.
    Ranvier c's
    silver c.
    two-factor c.
    yellow c.
cross-absorption
crossbite, cross-bite, cross bite
    anterior c.
    buccal c.
    lingual c.
    posterior c.
cross-bridges
cross-clamp
cross-dressing
crossed coil
crossed reflex
cross-eyed
cross-fire
    c-f. radiation therapy
    c-f. treatment
crossfoot
crosshatch incision
cross hearing
crossing over
    unequal c.o.
cross-leg Patrick maneuver
cross-linking
crossmatching
crossover
cross-over vasectomy
cross-reaction
cross-reactivation
cross-reactivity
cross-section
    capture c.
    nuclear c.
    total atomic attenuation c.
cross-sectional echocardiography
cross-sensitivity
cross-sensitization
cross-striations
crosstalk
cross-tolerance
crossway
crotalin
crotalism

crotalotoxin
crotamine
crotamiton
crotaphion
crotch
crotin
crotonic acid
crotonism
croton oil
crotoxin
croup
    bacterial c.
    catarrhal c.
    diphtheritic c.
    false c.
    membranous c.
    pseudomembranous c.
    spasmodic c.
croupette
croupous
croupy
Crouzon
    disease
    syndrome
crowding
Crowe-Davis mouth gag
crown
    anatomical c.
    artificial c.
    basket c.
    bell c.
    Bischoff c.
    Bonwill c.
    cap c.
    Carmichael c.
    celluloid c.
    ciliary c.
    clinical c.
    collar c.
    complete c.
    Davis c.
    dental c.
    dowel c.
    extra-alveolar c.
    faced c.
    half-cap c.
    c. of head
    jacket c.
    open-face c.
    overlay c.
    physiological c.
    pinledge c.
    post c.
    radiating c.
    Richmond c.

crown *(continued)*
    c. saw
    shell c.
    steel c.
    tapered c.
    three-quarter c.
    c. of tooth
    veneered c.
    window c.
crown-heel (length of fetus)
crowning
Crozat appliance
CRP—C-reactive protein
CRS—
    Chinese restaurant syndrome
    colorectal surgery
CRT—cathode ray tube
CRU—clinical research unit
cruces (plural of crux)
crucial
cruciate incision
crucible
cruciform suture
crude
crunch
    mediastinal c.
    xiphisternal c.
cruor
crura (plural of crus)
crural
crureus
cruris (genitive of crus)
cruritis
crurogenital
cruroscrotal
crurotomy
crus (crura)
    c. I, c. II
    ampullary osseous
        crura
    anterior c. of stapes
    c. anterius stapedis
    c. anthelicis
    c. of anthelix
    c. breve incudis
    c. cerebelli ad pontem
    c. cerebri
    c. clitoridis
    c. of clitoris
    common osseous c.
    c. commune
    c. dextrum diaphragmatis
    diaphragmatic crura
    c. fasciculi atrioventricularis
        dextrum

crus (crura) *(continued)*
    c. fasciculi atrioventricularis
      sinistrum
    c. fornicis
    c. glandis clitoridis
    c. helicis
    c. of helix
    c. laterale
    left c. of diaphragm
    long c. of incus
    c. longum incudis
    c. mediale
    crura membranacea
    membranous crura
    crura ossea
    crura ossea ampullaria
    osseous crura
    c. osseum commune
    c. osseum simplex
    c. penis
    posterior c. of stapes
    c. posterius stapedis
    right c. of diaphragm
    short c. of incus
    simple osseous c.
    c. sinistrum diaphragmatis
crust
    buffy c.
    milk c.
crusta (crustae)
    c. inflammatoria
    c. lactea
    c. petrosa dentis
    c. phlogistica
    c. radicis
crustacean
crustal
crustosus
crutch
    Canadian c.
    jocked stand c.
    perineal c.
Crutchfield
    clamp
    drill
    operation
    tongs
Crutchfield-Raney tongs
Cruveilhier
    atrophy
    disease
    fascia
    fossa
    joint
    ligaments

Cruveilhier *(continued)*
    paralysis
    sign
    ulcer
Cruveilhier-Baumgarten
    cirrhosis
    syndrome
crux (cruces)
    c. of heart
    cruces pilorum
Cruz trypanosomiasis
Cruz-Chagas disease
CRV—central retinal vein
CRVO—central retinal vein
    occlusion
cry
    cat's c. syndrome
    cephalic c.
    epileptic c.
    hydrocephalic c.
    joint c.
    night c.
cryalgesia
cryanesthesia
Cryer elevator
cryesthesia
crymodynia
crymophilic
crymophylactic
cryoablation
cryoanalgesia
cryoanesthesia
cryobank
cryobiology
cryocardioplegia
cryocautery
cryocrit
cryodestruction
cryoextraction
cryoextractor
    Amoils c.
    Bellows c.
cryofibrinogen
cryofibrinogenemia
cryogammaglobulin
cryogelification
cryogen, cryogenic
cryoglobulin
cryoglobulinemia
cryohydrate
cryohypophysectomy
cryomagnet
cryometer
cryopallidectomy
cryopathy

cryopexy
cryophile
cryophilic
cryophylactic
cryoprecipitability
cryoprecipitate
cryoprecipitation
cryopreservation
cryoprobe
 Amoils c.
cryoprotective
cryoprotein
cryoscope
cryoscopical
cryoscopy
cryospasm
cryostat
 Ames Lab-Tek c.
cryosurgery
cryothalamectomy
cryothalamotomy
cryotherapy
cryothermia
cryotolerant
cryotome
cryoultramicrotomy
crypt
 anal c.
 bony c.
 dental c.
 enamel c.
 c's of Fuchs
 c's of Haller
 c's of iris
 c's of Lieberkühn
 lingual c's
 c's of Littre
 Luschka c's
 c. of Morgagni
 mucous c's of duodenum
 multilocular c.
 odoriferous c's of prepuce
 synovial c.
 c's of tongue
 tonsillar c's of palatine tonsil
 tonsillar c's of pharyngeal tonsil
 tonsillar c's of tubal tonsil
 tooth c.
 Tyson c's
crypta (cryptae)
 cryptae mucosae
 cryptae tonsillares tonsillae
  lingualis
 cryptae tonsillares tonsillae
  palatinae

crypta (cryptae) *(continued)*
 cryptae tonsillares tonsillae
  pharyngealis
 cryptae tonsillares tonsillae
  tubariae
cryptectomy
cryptic
crypticity
cryptitis
 anal c.
cryptocephalus
cryptococcal
 c. meningitis
 c. meningoencephalitis
cryptococcoma
cryptococcosis
 cutaneous c.
 pulmonary c.
Cryptococcus
 C. albidus
 C. neoformans
 C. terreus
cryptodeterminant
cryptodidymus
cryptoempyema
cryptogenetic
cryptogenic drop
 attacks
cryptoglandular
cryptoglioma
cryptolith
cryptomenorrhea
cryptomere
cryptomerorachischisis
cryptomnesia
cryptomnesic
cryptomonad
cryptophthalmos
cryptoplasmic
cryptopodia
cryptoporous
cryptopyic
cryptorchid
cryptorchidectomy
cryptorchidism
cryptorchidopexy
cryptoscope
 Satvioni c.
cryptoscopy
cryptosporidiosis
 biliary c.
Cryptosporidium listeria
Cryptostroma corticale
cryptostromosis
cryptotia

cryptotome
   Blanchard c.
cryptotoxic
cryptozoite
cryptozygous
crypt
crystal
   asthma c's
   blood c's
   Böttcher (Boettcher) c's
   calcium pyrophosphate
      dihydrate c's (CPPD c's)
   Charcot-Leyden c.
   Charcot-Neumann c's
   coffin lid c's
   CPPD c's
   dumbbell c's
   ear c.
   hedgehog c's
   hydroxyapatite c.
   knife rest c's
   Leyden c's
   liquid c's
   Lubarsch c's
   Platner c's
   c's of Reinke
   scintillation c.
   Teichmann c's
   thorn-apple c's
   c. violet
   Virchow c's
   whetstone c's
crystalbumin
crystallin
crystalline
crystallitis
crystallization
   fern-leaf c.
crystallography
   x-ray c.
crystalloid
   c. cardioplegia
   Charcot-Böttcher (Charcot-
      Boettcher) c.
   c's of Reinke
crystalluria
CS—
   Central Service
   Central Supply
   cesarean section
   chondroitin sulfate
   conditioned stimulus
   coronary sinus
   corticosteroid
   current strength

C&S—
   conjunctiva and sclera
   culture and sensitivity
CSA— criminal sexual assault
CSC—blow-on-blow (Fr. coup sur
   coup)
C-section—cesarean section
CSF—
   cerebrospinal fluid
   colony-stimulating factor
CSF rhinorrhea
CSH—
   chronic subdural hematoma
   cortical stromal hyperplasia
CSIU—cardiac surgery
   intermediate unit
CSL—cardiolipin synthetic lecithin
CSLR—crossed straight leg raising
   (test)
CSM—
   cerebrospinal meningitis
   corn-soy milk
CSMT—capillary refill, sensation,
   motor function, temperature
CSN—carotid sinus nerve
CSR—
   Cheyne-Stokes respiration
   corrected sedimentation rate
   cortisol secretion rate
CSS—carotid sinus stimulation
CST—contraction stress test
CT—
   cardiothoracic
   carotid tracing
   carpal tunnel
   cerebral thrombosis
   circulation time
   clotting time
   coagulation time
   collecting tubule
   computed tomography
   computerized tomography
   connective tissue
   contraction time
   coronary thrombosis
   corrected transposition
   corrective therapy
   cover test
   crest time
   cytotechnologist
CTAP—clear to auscultation and
   percussion
CT body scanner
CTD—
   carpal tunnel decompression

CTD— *(continued)*
    congenital thymic dysplasia
Ctenocephalides
    C. canis
    C. felis
ctenoids
ctenophore
C-terminal
CTF—Colorado tick fever
CTL—cytotoxic T lymphocyte(s)
CTR—cardiothoracic ratio
CT scan
CTS—carpal tunnel syndrome
CTx—chemotherapy
CTZ—
    chemoreceptor trigger zone
    chlorothiazide
cu—cubic
C_u—urea clearance
CU—convalescent unit
Cubbins operation
cubic centimeters (cu cm, cm^3, cc)
cubicle
cubic millimeter(s) (cu mm, mm^3)
cubital tunnel syndrome
cubitocarpal
cubitoradial
cubitus
    c. valgus
    c. varus
cuboid, cuboidal
cuboideonavicular
cuboides
cu cm, cm^3, cc—cubic centimeter(s)
cucoline
cucullaris
cucurbitol
cue
    distance c's
    verbal c's
cuff
    epithelial c.
    Honan c.
    musculotendinous c.
    rotator c.
cuffed tube
cuffing
    peribronchial c.
CUG—cystourethrogram
cuirass
    tabetic c.
cul-de-sac
    conjunctival c.d.s..
    Douglas c.d.s.
    dural c.

cul-de-sac *(continued)*
    Gruber c.
    inferior c.
    lesser c.
culdocentesis
culdolaparoscopy
culdoplasty
culdoscope
    Decker c.
culdoscopy
culdotomy
culicide
culicifuge
Cullen sign
culling
culmen (culmina)
    c. cerebelli
    c. of cerebellum
    c. of left lung
    c. monticuli
Culp ureteropelvioplasty
Culp-DeWeerd
    pyeloplasty
    ureteropelvioplasty
culprit
    c. lesion
    c. organism
    c. vessel
cultivation
culturable
cultural
culture
    asynchronous c.
    attenuated c.
    blood c.
    cell c.
    chorioallantoic c.
    continuous flow c.
    direct c.
    embryo c.
    enrichment c.
    flask c.
    hanging-block c.
    hanging-drop c.
    histologic c. of wound sections
    mixed c.
    mixed lymphocyte c. (MLC)
    needle c.
    organ c.
    plate c.
    primary c.
    pure c.
    quantitative c.
    radioisotopic c.
    roll-tube c.

culture *(continued)*
    secondary c.
    selective c.
    sensitized c.
    shake c.
    slant c.
    slope c.
    smear c.
    sputum c.
    stab c.
    stock c.
    streak c.
    stroke c.
    surface c.
    suspension c.
    synchronized c.
    thrust c.
    tissue c.
    tracheal aspirate c.
    tube c.
    type c.
culture medium
    Bordet-Gengou c.m.
    defined c.m.
    indicator c.m.
    N.N.N. (Novoy, McNeal,
      Nicolle) c.m.
    Thayer-Martin c.m.
cu mm, mm^3—cubic millimeter(s)
cumulative
cumulus (cumuli)
    c. oophorus
    ovarian c.
    c. ovaricus
cuneate
cunei
cuneiform
    c. osteotomy
cuneocuboid
cuneonavicular
cuneoscaphoid
cuneus
cunicular
cuniculus (cuniculi)
    c. externus
    c. internus
    c. medius
cunnilingus
Cunningham clamp
cunnus
cup
    acetabular
    Aufranc-Turner c.
    chin c.
    Crawford-Adams acetabular c.
    Diogenes c.

cup *(continued)*
    dry c.
    eye c.
    favus c.
    glaucomatous c.
    McKee-Farrar acetabular c.
    optic c.
    perilimbal suction c.
    physiologic c.
    Silastic c.
    wet c.
cup-and-ball osteotomy
cupped disk
cupping
    c. of calix
    pathologic c.
cupremia
cupric
cupriuria
cuprophane
cuprous
cupruresis
cupruretic
cup-to-disk ratio
cupula (cupulae)
    c. ampullaris
    c. of ampullary crest
    c. of cochlea
    c. cochleae
    c. cristae ampullaris
    c. of pleura
    c. pleurae
    c. pleuralis
cupular
cupuliform
cupulogram
cupulolithiasis
cupulometry
curare
curaremimetic
curariform
curarization
curative
curb tenotomy
curcumin
    alum c. of Riverius
curd
Curdy sclerotome
cure
curet, curette
    adenoid c.
    Ballenger c.
    banjo c.
    Barnhill c.
    Beckmann c.
    Billeau ear wax c.

curet, curette *(continued)*
    Brun c.
    Buck c.
    Bumm c.
    Carmack ear c.
    Coakley c.
    Delstanche c.
    Derlacki c.
    Faulkner c.
    Fox c.
    Freimuth c.
    Gifford c.
    Goldman c.
    Gottstein c.
    Govons c.
    Gracey c.
    Gross c.
    Gusberg c.
    Halle c.
    Hannon c.
    Hartmann c.
    Hayden c.
    Heaney c.
    Heath c.
    Hibbs c.
    Holden c.
    Holtz c.
    House c.
    Hunter c.
    Ingersoll c.
    Jones c.
    Kelly c.
    Kelly-Gray c.
    Kevorkian c.
    Kushner-Tandatnick c.
    Lempert c.
    Lounsbury c.
    McCaskey c.
    Meyerding c.
    Meyhoeffer c.
    Middleton c.
    Mosher c.
    Moult c.
    Myles c.
    Novak c.
    Piffard c.
    Pratt c.
    Randall c.
    Raney c.
    Récamier c.
    Reich-Nechtow c.
    Richards c.
    Ridpath c.
    Rosenmüller c.
    St. Clair-Thompson c.
    Schaeffer c.

curet, curette *(continued)*
    serrated c.
    Shapleigh c.
    Shea c.
    Sims c.
    Skeele c.
    Skene c.
    Spratt c.
    Stubbs c.
    Tabb c.
    Thomas c.
    Vogel c.
    Volkmann c.
    Walsh c.
    Weisman c.
    Whiting c.
    Yankauer c.
curettage
    apical c.
    fractional c.
    gentle c.
    gingival c.
    medical c.
    periapical c.
    root c.
    sharp c.
    subgingival c.
    suction c.
    surgical c.
    ultrasonic c.
    vacuum c.
curetted
curettement
    physiologic c.
    root c.
curie(s) (Ci)
curie-hour (Ci-hr)
curing
    denture c.
curiosity
curious
curium (Cm)
curling
Curling ulcer
current
    abnerval c.
    action c.
    alternating c.
    anelectrotonic c.
    anionic c.
    anodal c.
    ascending c.
    axial c.
    blaze c.
    catelectrotonic c.
    centrifugal c.

C

current *(continued)*
- centripetal c.
- coagulating c.
- combined c.
- compensating c.
- damped c.
- d'Arsonval c.
- demarcation c.
- depolarization c.
- descending c.
- direct c.
- eddy c.
- electric c.
- electrotonic c.
- ephaptic c.
- fault c.
- fulguration c.
- galvanic c.
- high-frequency c.
- induced c.
- interaxonal c.
- inverse c.
- ionization c.
- K c.
- monophasic action c.
- nerve-action c.
- oscillating c.
- Oudin c.
- pulsating c.
- resting c.
- rising c.
- saturation c.
- sine-wave c.
- single-phase c.
- sinusoidal c.
- static-wave c.
- surgical c.
- three-phase c.
- undamped c.
- unidirectional c.

curriculum (curricula)

Curry
- needle
- splint

Curschmann
- disease
- spirals

curse
- Ondine's c.

Curtis forceps

Curtis and Fitz-Hugh syndrome

Curtius syndrome

curvatura

curvature
- anterior c.

curvature *(continued)*
- backward c.
- compensating c.
- c. of field
- gastric c., greater
- gastric c., lesser
- greater c. of stomach
- hyperopia of c.
- lateral c.
- lesser c. of stomach
- occlusal c.
- Petzval c.
- Pott c.
- spinal c.

curve
- alignment c.
- anti-Monson c.
- audibility c.
- auditory c.
- Barnes c.
- bell-shaped c.
- biphasic c.
- Bragg c.
- buccal c.
- camel c.
- c. of Carus
- compensating c.
- cystometric c.
- Damoiseau c.
- decay c.
- dental c.
- diabetic glucose tolerance c.
- diphasic c.
- dromedary c.
- c. of Ellis and Garland
- Frank-Starling c.
- Friedman c.
- Garland c.
- gaussian c.
- Gompertz c.
- growth c.
- Harrison c.
- indicator-dilution c.
- intracardiac pressure c.
- inverted-U c. of arousal
- isodose c's
- isoresponse c.
- isovolume pressure-flow c.
- Kaplan-Meier survival c.
- labial c.
- learning c.
- logistic c.
- luetic c.
- modified exponential c.
- Monson c.

curve *(continued)*
    muscle c.
    c. of occlusion
    oxygen dissociation c.
    paretic c.
    photopic sensitivity c.
    Price-Jones c.
    pulse c.
    regression c.
    reverse c.
    ROC (receiver operating
      characteristics) c.
    saddleback temperature c.
    Starling c.
    stress-strain c.
    survival c.
    temperature c.
    tension c's
    titration c.
    Traube c's
    visibility c.
    Wunderlich c.
curved incision
curvilinear incision
CUSA—Cavitron ultrasonic
  aspirator
cuscamidine
cuscamine
Cusco speculum
Cushing
    basophilism
    clip
    depressor
    disease
    drill
    effect
    forceps
    medulloblastoma
    needle
    operation
    phenomenon
    pituitary basophilism
    reaction
    response
    retractor
    spatula
    spoon
    suture
    syndrome
    syndrome medicamentosus
    tumor
    ulcer
cushingoid
Cushing-Rokitansky
  ulcer

cushion
    air c.
    atrioventricular canal c.
    coronary c.
    digital c.
    endocardial c's
    c. of epiglottis
    intimal c's
    levator c.
    Passavant c.
    plantar c.
    polar c. of glomerulus
    sucking c.
cushioning suture
cusp
    aortic c.
    Carabelli c.
    dental c.
    c. of mitral valve
    plunger c.
    semilunar c.
    shearing c.
    stamp c.
    c. of tricuspid valve
cuspid
cuspidate
cuspis (cuspides)
    c. anterior valvae
      atrioventricularis dextrae
    c. anterior valvae
      atrioventricularis sinistrae
    c. anterior valvulae
      bicuspidalis
    c. anterior valvulae
      tricuspidalis
    c. coronae
    c. dentales
    c. dentalis
    c. dentis
    c. medialis valvulae
      tricuspidalis
    c. posterior valvae
      atrioventricularis sinistrae
    c. posterior valvulae
      bicuspidalis
    c. posterior valvulae
      tricuspidalis
    c. septalis valvae
      atrioventricularis dextrae
Custodis operation
cut
    tomographic c.
cutaneous
    c. anthrax
    c. larva migrans

cutaneous *(continued)*
  c. leishmaniasis
  c. mucormycosis
  c. nevi
  c. suture
  c. suture of palate
  c. ureterostomy
  c. vasculitis
  c. vesicostomy
cutdown
cuticle
  dental c.
  enamel c.
  Gottlieb c.
  keratose c.
  primary c.
  prism c.
  c. of root sheath
  secondary c.
cuticula (cuticulae)
  c. dentis
cuticular suture
cuticulum
  Flechsig c.
Cutie Pie ion chamber
cutin
cutireaction
  von Pirquet c.
cutis
  c. anserina
  c. elastica
  c. hyperelastica
  c. laxa
  c. marmorata
  c. marmorata telangiectatica
    congenita
  c. pendula
  c. pensilis
  c. rhomboidalis nuchae
  c. testacea
  c. unctuosa
  c. vera
  c. verticis gyrata
Cutler operation
Cutler-Beard operation
Cutlet implant
Cutter-SCDK prosthesis
Cutter-Smeloff cardiac valve
  prosthesis
cutting loops
cuvette
CV—
  cardiovascular
  central venous
  cerebrovascular

CV— *(continued)*
  color vision
  conjugata vera
  conversational voice
  corpuscular volume
  cresyl violet
CVA—
  cardiovascular accident
  cerebrovascular accident
  costovertebral angle
CVAT—costovertebral angle
  tenderness
CVB—chorionic villus biopsy
CVC—central venous catheter
CVD—
  cardiovascular disease
  cerebrovascular disease
  collagen vascular disease
CVF—
  central visual field
  cobra venom factor
CVH—
  combined ventricular
    hypertrophy
  common variable
    hypogammaglobulinemia
CVI—
  cerebrovascular insufficiency
  common variable
    immunodeficiency
CVIU—cardiovascular
  intermediate unit
CVOD—cerebrovascular occlusive
  disease
CVP—
  central venous pressure
  cyclophosphamide, vincristine,
    prednisone
CVP catheter
CVR—
  cardiovascular-respiratory
  cerebrovascular resistance
CVRD—cardiovascular renal disease
CVS—
  cardiovascular surgery
  cardiovascular system
  chorionic villus sampling
  clean-voided specimen
CW—
  cardiac work
  case work
  chemical warfare
  chest wall
  continuous wave
CWP—childbirth without pain

CWS—cotton-wool spot
cx—
    cervix
    convex
CX, CXr—chest x-ray
CxMT—cervical motion tenderness
Cy—cyanogen
cyanalcohol
cyanamide
cyanate
cyanhematin
cyanhemoglobin
cyanide
cyanmethemoglobin
cyanmetmyoglobin
cyanoacrylate
cyanoalcohol
cyanocobalamin
    c. Co 57
    c. Co 58
    c. Co 60
    radioactive c.
cyanocrystallin
cyanoform
cyanogen
    c. bromide
    c. chloride
cyanogenesis
cyanogenetic
cyanohydrin
cyanolabe
cyanophil
cyanophilous
cyanophoric
cyanophose
cyanophytes
cyanopsia
cyanopsin
cyanose
cyanosis
    autotoxic c.
    c. bulbi
    central c.
    compression c.
    enterogenous c.
    false c.
    hereditary
      methemoglobinemic c.
    c. lienis
    peripheral c.
    pulmonary c.
    c. retinae
    shunt c.
    tardive c.
    toxic c.

cyanotic
cyanuria
cyanuric acid
cyanurin
cybernetics
Cybex ergometer
Cybex test
cycasin
cyclamate
cyclamate calcium
cyclamic acid
cyclamin
cyclandelate
cyclarthrodial
cyclarthrosis
cyclase
    adenyl c.
    adenylate c.
cycle
    aberrant c.
    anovulatory c.
    asexual c.
    biliary c.
    breakage-fusion-bridge c.
    Calvin c.
    carbon c.
    cardiac c.
    cell c.
    chewing c.
    citrate-pyruvate c.
    citric acid c.
    Cori c.
    cytoplasmic c.
    Embden-Meyerhof c.
    endogenous c.
    endometrial c.
    estrous c.
    exogenous c.
    fatty acid oxidation c.
    forced c.
    futile c.
    gastric c.
    genesial c.
    glucose-lactate c.
    glycine succinate c.
    glyoxylate c.
    gonadotropic c.
    gonotrophic c.
    growth c.
    hair c.
    Hodgkin c.
    isohydric c.
    Krebs c.
    Krebs-Henseleit urea c.
    lactation c.

C

cycle *(continued)*
    life c.
    mammary c.
    menstrual c.
    mitotic c.
    mosquito c.
    myometrial c.
    nasal c.
    nitrogen c.
    oogenetic c.
    ornithine c.
    ovarian c.
    pentose c.
    pentose phosphate c.
    pregnancy c.
    reproductive c.
    restored c.
    returning c.
    Ross c.
    Schiff biliary c.
    sexual c.
    tricarboxylic c.
    urea c.
    uterine c.
    vaginal c.
    visual c.
cyclectomy
cycle-length window
cyclencephalus
cyclencephaly
cyclic
    c. adenosine monophosphate (cAMP; $3',5'$-AMP)
    c. guanosine monophosphate (cGMP, $3',5'$-GMP)
    c. nucleotides
    c. phosphate
$3',5'$-cyclic AMP synthetase
cyclicotomy
cyclin
cyclindole
cyclitic
cyclitis
    heterochromic c.
    plastic c.
    pure c.
    purulent c.
    serous c.
cyclization
cyclo—
    cyclophosphamide
    cyclopropane
cycloartenol
cyclobutanol
cyclocephalus

cycloceratitis
cyclochoroiditis
cyclocryotherapy
cyclocytidine
cyclodamia
cyclodeviation
cyclodextrin
    beta c.
cyclodialysis
cyclodiathermy
cycloduction
cycloelectrolysis
cycloergometer
cyclogeny
cyclogram
cycloguanide embonate
cycloguanil pamoate
cyclohexanehexol
cyclohexanesulfamic acid
cyclohexanol
cycloheximide
cycloid
cycloisomerase
cyclokeratitis
cyclo-ligase
cyclomastopathy
cyclooxygenase, cyclo-oxygenase
cyclopean
cyclopentane
cyclopentanophenanthrene
cyclophoria
    accommodative c.
    minus c.
    plus c.
cyclophorometer
cyclophosphamide
cyclopia
cyclopin
cycloplegia
cycloplegic
cyclopropane
cyclops hypognathus
cyclose
cycloserine
cyclosis
cyclospasm
cyclostat
cyclotate
cyclotherapy
cyclothyme
cyclothymia
cyclothymiac
cyclothymic
cyclothymosis
cyclotia

C

cyclotol
cyclotome
cyclotomy
cyclotorsion
cyclotron
cyclotropia
cyclozoonosis
cyesis
cyestein
cyesthein
cyl.—cylindrical lens
cylinder
    axis c.
    Bence Jones c's
    crossed c's
    Külz c.
    Leydig c's
    Ruffini c.
    terminal c.
    urinary c.
cylindrarthrosis
cylindraxile
cylindrical
cylindrocellular
cylindrodendrite
cylindroid
cylindroma
    eccrine dermal c.
cylindromatous
cylindruria
cylite
cyllosis
cyllosoma
cymarose
cymba (cymbae)
    c. conchae auriculae
    c. conchalis auriculae
cymbiform
cymbocephalic
cymbocephalous
cymbocephaly
cyme
cymograph
cynanche
    c. maligna
    c. tonsillaris
cynanthropy
cynic
cynocephalic
cynocephaly
cynodont
cynodontism
cynomolgus
cynophobia
cyogenic

cyophoria
cyophoric
cyopin
cyotrophy
cypermethrin
cypothrin
cyprinin
cyproterone acetate
cyrtograph
cyrtoid
cyrtometer
cyrtos
cyrtosis
cyst
    adnexal c.
    adrenal c.
    adventitious c.
    allantoic c.
    alveolar c.
    alveolar hydatid c.
    amnionic c.
    aneurysmal bone c.
    angioblastic c.
    antral c.
    apical c.
    apoplectic c.
    arachnoid c.
    atheromatous c.
    Baker c.
    Bartholin c.
    Blessig c.
    Blessig-Iwanoff c.
    blue dome c.
    bone c.
    Boyer c.
    branchial c.
    bronchial c.
    bronchogenic c.
    bronchopulmonary c.
    bursal c.
    cervical c.
    cervical
      lymphoepithelial c.
    chocolate c.
    choledochal c.
    choledochus c.
    chorionic c.
    chyle c.
    colloid c.
    compound c.
    congenital preauricular c.
    congenital c. of prostate
    congenital c. of urethra
    corpus luteum c.
    Cowper c.

cyst *(continued)*

   craniobuccal c.
   craniopharyngeal
     duct c.
   cutaneous c.
   cuticular c.
   daughter c.
   dental c.
   dentigerous c.
   dermoid c.
   dermoid c. with malignant
     transformation
   dilatation c.
   distention c.
   duplication c.
   echinococcus c.
   embryonal c.
   endometrial c.
   endothelial c.
   enteric c.
   ependymal c.
   epidermal c.
   epidermal inclusion c.
   epidermoid c.
   c. of epididymis
   epithelial c.
   eruption c.
   extra-axial
     leptomeningeal c.
   extravasation c.
   exudation c.
   false c.
   fissural c.
   follicular c.
   ganglionic c.
   gartnerian c.
   gas c.
   germinal inclusion c.
   gingival c.
   globulomaxillary c.
   glomerular c.
   granddaughter c.
   granulosa lutein c.
   hemorrhagic c.
   heterotopic oral
     gastrointestinal c.
   hydatid c.
   hymenal c.
   implantation c.
   incisive canal c.
   inclusion c.
   inflammatory c.
   intracranial parasitic c.
   intraepithelial c's

cyst *(continued)*

   intraluminal c's
   intrapituitary c's
   involution c.
   Iwanoff c's
   Klestadt c.
   lacteal c.
   laryngeal c.
   lateral periodontal c.
   leptomeningeal c.
   lutein c.
   lymphoepithelial c.
   median anterior
     maxillary c.
   median mandibular c.
   median palatal c.
   medullary c.
   meibomian c.
   mesenteric c.
   milk c.
   c. of Morgagni
   morgagnian c.
   mother c.
   mucous c.
   multilocular c.
   myxoid c.
   Naboth c.
   nabothian c.
   nasoalveolar c.
   nasopalatine c.
   nasopalatine duct c.
   necrotic c.
   neural c.
   neurenteric c.
   nevoid c.
   odontogenic c.
   oil c.
   omental c.
   oophoritic c.
   osseous hydatid c.
   ovarian c.
   pancreatic c.
   c. of paramesonephric
     duct
   parapyelitic c's
   parasitic c.
   paratracheal c.
   paratubal c.
   parovarian c.
   pearl c.
   pedicled c.
   periapical c.
   pericardial c.
   perinephric c.

C

cyst *(continued)*
  perineurial c.
  periodontal c.
  perirenal c.
  perisalpingian c.
  phaeomycotic c.
  pheomycotic c.
  pilar c.
  pilonidal c.
  placental c.
  polycystic c.
  popliteal c.
  porencephalic c.
  post-traumatic
    leptomeningeal c.
  primordial c.
  proligerous c.
  pyelogenic c.
  pyelogenic renal c.
  radicular c.
  radiculodental c.
  Rathke c's
  renal c.
  residual c.
  retention c.
  retroperitoneal c.
  root c.
  root-end c.
  sacral c.
  sacrococcygeal c.
  Sampson c.
  sanguineous c.
  sarcosporidian c.
  sebaceous c.
  secretory c.
  seminal vesicle c.
  septal c.
  sequestration c.
  serous c.
  simple bone c.
  soapsuds c.
  solitary bone c.
  c. of spermatic cord
  springwater c.
  steatoid c.
  sterile c.
  subchondral c.
  sublingual c.
  subsynovial c.
  suprasellar c.
  synovial c.
  Tarlov c.
  tarry c.
  tarsal c.

cyst *(continued)*
  testicular c.
  thecal c.
  theca-lutein c.
  thymic c.
  thyroglossal c.
  tissue c.
  Tornwaldt
    (Thornwaldt) c.
  traumatic bone c.
  trichilemmal c.
  true c.
  tubo-ovarian c.
  tubular c.
  umbilical c.
  unicameral c.
  unilocular c.
  urachal c.
  urinary c.
  vaginal c.
  vaginal inclusion c.
  vitelline duct c.
  vitellointestinal c.
  wolffian c.
cystadenofibroma
  c. adamantinum
  mucinous c.
  pseudomucinous c.
  serous c.
cystadenolymphoma
cystadenoma
  c. adamantinum
  apocrine c.
  bile duct c.
  eccrine c.
  mucinous c.
  papillary c.
  c. phyllodes
  c. phylloides
  pseudomucinous c.
  serous c.
cystadenosarcoma
cystalgia
cystathionase
cystathionine
  c. β-synthase [beta-]
  c. γ-lyase [gamma-]
cystatrophia
cystauchenitis
cystauchenotomy
cysteamine
cystectasia
cystectasy
cystectomy

cysteic acid
cysteinyl
cystelcosis
cystencephalus
cysterethism
cysthypersarcosis
cystic
    c. fibrosis
    c. duct
      cholangiography
    c. fibrosis
    c. hygroma
    c. mastitis
cysticerci
cysticercoid
cysticercosis
    racemose
      form c.
    spinal c.
cystic
    microphthalmia
cysticolithectomy
cysticolithotripsy
cysticorrhaphy
cysticotomy
cystides
cystidoceliotomy
cystidolaparotomy
cystidotrachelotomy
cystifellotomy
cystiferous
cystiform
cystigerous
cystine
cystinemia
cystinosis
    benign c.
    intermediate c.
    nephrogenic c.
cystinuria
    familial c.
cystinuric
cystirrhea
cystis fellea
cystistaxis
cystitis
    acute catarrhal c.
    allergic c.
    bacterial c.
    catarrhal c.
    chemical c.
    c. colli
    croupous c.
    cystic c.

cystitis (continued)
    c. cystica
    diphtheritic c.
    c. emphysematosa
    eosinophilic c.
    exfoliative c.
    c. follicularis
    gangrenous c.
    glandular c.
    c. glandularis
    hemorrhagic c.
    incrusted c.
    interstitial c.
    mechanical c.
    panmural c.
    papillary c.
    c. papillomatosa
    postpartum c.
    c. senilis feminarum
    subacute c.
    submucous c.
    ulcerative c.
cystitome
cystitomy
cysto—cystoscopy
cystoblast
cystoblastema
cystocarcinoma
    pseudomucinous c.
cystocele
cystochrome
cystochromoscopy
cystocolostomy
cystodiaphanoscopy
cystoduodenostomy
cystodynia
cystoelytroplasty
cystoenterocele
cystoepiplocele
cystoepithelioma
cystofibroma
    papillare
cystogastrostomy
cystogenesis
cystogram
    air c.
    excretory c.
    gravity c.
    postvoiding c.
    triple-voiding c.
    voiding c.
cystography
    bead chain c.
    delayed c.

cystography *(continued)*
    radionuclide c.
    retrograde c.
    triple-voiding c.
    voiding c.
cystoid
cystoid macular edema
cystojejunostomy
    Roux-en-Y c.
cystolith
cystolithectomy
cystolithiasis
cystolithic
cystolithotomy
cystolutein
cystoma
    colloid ovarian c.
    myxoid c.
    c. serosum simplex
cystomatitis
cystomatous
cystometer
    Lewis c.
cystometric
cystometrogram
cystometrography
cystometry
    flow c.
cystomorphous
cystonephrosis
cystoneuralgia
cystoparalysis
cystoparesis
cystopexy
cystophorous
cystophotography
cystophthisis
cystoplasty
    augmentation c.
    cecal c.
cystoplegia
cystoproctostomy
cystoprostatectomy
cystoptosis
cystopyelitis
cystopyelogram
cystopyelography
cystopyelonephritis
cystoradiography
cystorectocele
cystorectostomy
cystorrhagia
cystorrhaphy
cystorrhea

cystosarcoma
    c. phyllodes
    c. phylloides
cystoschisis
cystosclerosis
cystoscope
    Braasch c.
    Brown-Buerger c.
    Butterfield c.
    fiberoptic c.
    Kelly c.
    Lowsley-Peterson c.
    McCarthy c.
    McCarthy-Campbell c.
    McCarthy-Peterson c.
    National c.
    Ravich c.
    Storz c.
    Wappler c.
cystoscopic urography
cystoscopy and
   dilatation (C&D)
cystose
cystospasm
cystospermitis
cystosphincterometry
cystostaxis
cystostomy
    tubeless c.
cystotome
    Graefe (von Graefe) c.
    Wheeler c.
cystotomy
    suprapubic c.
cystotrachelotomy
cystoureteritis
cystoureterocele
cystoureterogram
cystoureterography
cystoureteropyelitis
cystoureteropyelonephritis
cystourethritis
cystourethrocele
cystourethrogram
    bead-chain c.
    micturition c.
    retrograde c.
    voiding c.
cystourethrography
    chain c.
    expression c.
    isotope voiding c.
     (IVCU)
    micturating c.

cystourethrography *(continued)*
    micturition c.
    radionuclide voiding c.
    retrograde c.
    voiding c. (VCUG)
cystourethropexy
cystourethroscope
cystourethroscopy
cystous
cystyl
cytapheresis
cytarme
cytaster
cythemolysis
cytheromania
cytidine
    c. deaminase
    c. diphosphate (CDP)
    c. diphosphate
      choline
    c. diphosphate
      ethanolamine
    c. monophosphate
      (CMP)
    c. triphosphate
      (CTP)
cytidylate
cytidylic acid
cytidylyl
cytisine
cytisism
cytoanalyzer
cytoarchitectonic
cytoarchitectural
cytoarchitecture
cytobiology
cytobiotaxis
cytoblast
cytocentrum
cytochalasin B
cytochemism
cytochemistry
cytochrome
    c. b
    c. b_5 reductase
    c. c oxidase
    c. c_1
    c. oxidase
    c. P-450 reductase
cytochylema
cytocidal
cytocide
cytoclasis
cytoclastic
cytoclesis

cytocletic
cytocrit
cytoctony
cytocuprein
cytode
cytodendrite
cytodesma
cytodiagnosis
    exfoliative c.
cytodiagnostic
cytodieresis
cytodifferentiation
cytodistal
cytoflav
cytoflavin
cytofluorimeter
cytogene
cytogenesis
cytogenetic,
    cytogenetical
cytogeneticist
cytogenetics
    clinical c.
cytogenic,
    cytogenous
cytogeny
cytoglomerator
cytoglycopenia
cytogony
cytohistogenesis
cytohistologic
cytohistology
cytohormone
cytohyaloplasm
cytoid
cyto-inhibition
cytokalipenia
cytokerastic
cytokine
cytokinesis
cytokinin
cytolemma
cytolipin H
cytologic,
    cytological
cytologist
cytology
    aspiration biopsy c.
      (ABC)
    exfoliative c.
    nuclear c.
cytolymph
cytolysate
    blood c.
cytolysin

cytolysis
    immune c.
cytolysosome
cytolytic
cytoma
cytomegalic
cytomegalic inclusion disease
  (CID, CMID)
cytomegaloviruria
cytomegalovirus
  (CMV)
cytomegaly
cytomembrane
cytomere
cytometaplasia
cytometer
    eyepiece c.
    flow c.
    stage c.
cytometry
    flow c.
    image c.
cytomicrosome
cytomitome
cytomorphology
cytomorphosis
cyton
cytonecrosis
cytopathic
cytopathogenesis
cytopathogenetic
cytopathogenic
cytopathogenicity
cytopathologic,
  cytopathological
cytopathologist
cytopathology
cytopenia
cytophagocytosis
cytophagous
cytophagy
cytopharynx
cytophil
cytophilic
cytophotometric
cytophotometry
cytophylactic
cytophylaxis
cytophyletic
cytophysics
cytophysiology
cytopigment
cytopipette
cytoplasm
cytoplasmic

cytoplast
cytopreparation
cytoproct
cytoprotectant
cytoprotective
cytoproximal
cytoreduction
cytoreticulum
cytorrhyctes
cytoscopy
cytosiderin
cytosine
    c. arabinoside
    5-hydroxymethyl c.
    c. deaminase
cytoskeletal
cytoskeleton
cytosmear
cytosol
  aminopeptidase
cytosolic
cytosome
cytost
cytostasis
cytostatic
cytosteatonecrosis
cytostome
cytostromatic
cytotactic
cytotaxigen
cytotaxin
cytotaxis
cytotechnologist
cytotherapy
cytothesis
cytotoxic
    c. T lymphocyte
    c. T lymphocyte
      precursor
cytotoxicity
cytotoxin
cytotrophoblast
cytotropic
cytotropism
cyturia
Czapek-Dox solution
Czermak operation
Czerny
    anemia
    disease
    operation
    suture
Czerny-Lembert suture
CZI—crystalline
  zinc insulin

D

δ—
    delta (Greek letter)
    the heavy chain of IgD

d—
    day
    deci-
    deoxyribose
    diameter

d—dextro- [prefix]

D—
    daughter
    dead
    deciduous
    density
    died
    diffusing capacity
    diopter
    distal
    divorced
    dorsal
    duration
    dwarf
    mean dose
    vitamin D unit

2,4-D—dichlorophenoxyacetic
  acid

dA—deoxyadenosine

DA—
    degenerative arthritis
    dental assistant
    developmental age
    direct agglutination
    disaggregated
    dopamine
    ductus arteriosus

DAAO—D-amino acid oxidase

DAB—dimethylaminoazobenzene

d'Acosta (Acosta) disease

DaCosta syndrome

dacryoadenitis

Dacron
    D. graft
    D. prosthesis
    D. suture

dacryoadenalgia
dacryoadenectomy
dacryoadenitis
dacryoblennorrhea
dacryocanaliculitis
dacryocele
dacryocyst
dacryocystalgia
dacryocystectasia
dacryocystectomy

dacryocystis
    phlegmonous d.
    syphilitic d.
    trachomatous d.
    tuberculous d.

dacryocystitis
dacryocystitome, dacryocystotome
dacryocystoblennorrhea
dacryocystocele
dacryocystography
dacryocystoptosis
dacryocystorhinostenosis
dacryocystorhinostomy
dacryocystorhinotomy
dacryocystostenosis
dacryocystostomy
dacryocystotome
dacryocystotomy
dacryocyte
dacryogenic
dacryohelcosis
dacryohemorrhea
dacryoid
dacryolith
dacryolithiasis
dacryoma
dacryon
dacryops
dacryopyorrhea
dacryopyosis
dacryorhinocystotomy
dacryorrhea
dacryoscintigraphy
dacryosinusitis
dacryosolenitis
dacryostenosis
dacryosyrinx
dactylate
dactyledema

dactylitis
    d. strumosa
    d. syphilitica
    d. tuberculosa

dactylocampsodynia
dactylogram
dactylography
dactylogryposis
dactyloid
dactylology
dactylolysis spontanea
dactyloscopy
dactylospasm
dactylus

DAD—delayed after-depolarization

DADDS—diacetyl
  diaminodiphenylsulfone
D/A (digital-to-analog)
  converter
dADP—deoxyadenosine
  diphosphate
DAF—
    decay accelerating factor
    delayed auditory feedback
DAG—diacylglycerol
DAH—disordered action of the
  heart
Dakin
    antiseptic solution
    fluid
Dakin-Carrel method
Dale
    phenomenon
    reaction
Dalén-Fuchs nodule
Dalkon shield IUD
Dallas operation
D'Allesandro serial suture-holding
  forceps
Dalrymple
    disease
    sign
daltonism
DAM—degraded amyloid
dam
    rubber d.
D'Amato sign
damiana
dammar
damp
    after-d.
    black d.
    choke d.
    cold d.
    fire d.
    white d.
dAMP—deoxyadenosine
  monophosphate
damping
DAN—diabetic autonomic
  neuropathy
Dana operation
Danbolt-Closs syndrome
dance
    brachial d.
    hilar d.
    hilus d.
    St. Vitus d.
Dance sign
D&C—dilatation and curettage

dander
dandruff
Dandy
    hemostat
    hook
    scissors
Dandy-Walker
    deformity
    syndrome
Dane particle
Danforth
    method
    sign
Daniel
    clamp
    operation
Daniels tonsillectome
Danielssen disease
Danielssen-Boeck
    disease
    sarcoidosis
Danlos
    disease
    syndrome
Danubian endemic familial
  nephropathy
Danysz
    effect
    phenomenon
DAO—diamine oxidase
DAP—
    dihydroxyacetone phosphate
    direct agglutination pregnancy
      (test)
daphnetin
daphnin
daphnism
DAPT—direct agglutination
  pregnancy test
Dardik Biograft
Darier
    disease
    sign
Darier-Roussy sarcoid
Darier-White disease
darkfield
    d. examination
    d. microscopy
Darkschewitsch (Darkshevich)
    fibers
    nucleus
Darling
    capsulotome
    disease
Darrach operation

Darrow-Gamble syndrome
Darrow solution
d'Arsonval current
dartoic, dartoid
dartos
Darwin
 ear
 tubercle
Daseler zone
D'Assumpção (D'Assumpcao)
 rhytidoplasty marker
DAT—
 differential agglutination titer
 diphtheria antitoxin
 direct antiglobulin test
data (plural of datum)
 censored d.
 ferrokinetic d.
database
dATP—deoxyadenosine
 triphosphate
datum (data)
daturine
daturism
Daubenton
 angle
 line
 plane
daughter
 d. cell
 DES d.
 d. nuclide
Davenport stain
David
 disease
 speculum
Davidoff (Davidov)
 retractor
 cells
Davidson
 clamp
 retractor
Daviel
 operation
 scoop
 spoon
Davies-Colley operation
Davis
 bronchoscope
 clamp
 conductor
 crown
 forceps
 gag
 graft
 knife needle

Davis *(continued)*
 line
 needle
 operation
 retractor
 sound
 spatula
 splint
 spud
 stone dislodger
Davis-Crowe mouth gag
Davis-Kitlowski operation
Dawbarn sign
dawn
 d. effect
 d. phenomenon
Dawson
 encephalitis
 inclusion
Day
 cannula
 operation
dB, db—decibel
DB—
 date of birth
 dextran blue
 distobuccal
DBA—dibenzanthracene
DBC—dye-binding capacity
DBCL—dilute blood clot lysis
 (method)
DBM—
 demineralized bone matrix
 dibromomannitol
DBO—distobucco-occlusal
DBP—
 diastolic blood pressure
 distobuccopulpal
DC—
 daily census
 deoxycholate
 diagnostic code
 diphenylarsine cyanide
 direct current
 discharge
 discontinue
 distocervical
DC, D.C.—Doctor of Chiropractic
D&C, D and C—
 dilatation and curettage
 dilation and curettage
dC—deoxycytidine
DCA—
 deoxycholate-citrate agar
 deoxycholic acid
DCC; DCc—double concave

D

dCDP—deoxycytidine diphosphate
DCF—direct centrifugal flotation
DCG—disodium cromoglycate
DCHFB—diclorohexafluorobutane
dCMP—deoxycytidine
monophosphate
DCNB—dichloronitrobenzene
D_{co}, DCO—diffusing capacity for
carbon monoxide
DCOG—Diploma of the College of
Obstetricians and Gynaecologists
DCTMA—desoxycorticosterone
trimethylacetate
dCTP—deoxycytidine triphosphate
DCx—double convex
DD—
    died of the disease
    differential diagnosis
    disk diameter
D&D—Drake and Drake [medical
reference products]
DDC—direct display console
DDD—
    degenerative disk disease
    dichlorodiphenyl-
        dichloroethane
DDH—dissociated double
hypertropia
D-dimer
DDS, D.D.S.—Doctor of Dental
Surgery
DDSc—Doctor of Dental Science
DDT—dichlorodiphenyl-
trichloroethane
DE—
    dream elements
    duration of ejection
D&E—
    dilatation and evacuation
    dilation and evacuation
deacidification
deactivation
deacylase
DEAE—diethylaminoethyl
DEAE-D—diethylaminoethyl
dextran
deaf
deafferentated
deafferentation
deaf-mute
deaf-mutism
    endemic d.
deafness
    acoustic trauma d.
    Alexander d.
    apoplectiform d.

deafness *(continued)*
    bass d.
    Bing-Stibenmann–type
        genetic d.
    boilermakers' d.
    central d.
    cerebral d.
    ceruminous d.
    cochlear d.
    conduction d.
    congenital d.
    cortical d.
    familial perceptive d.
    functional d.
    genetic d.
    heredodegenerative d.
    high-frequency d.
    hysterical d.
    immune complex associated d.
    labyrinthine d.
    malarial d.
    Michel d.
    midbrain d.
    Mondini d.
    music d.
    nerve d.
    neural d.
    noise-induced d.
    organic d.
    ototoxic d.
    pagetoid d.
    paradoxic d., paradoxical d.
    perceptive d.
    postlingual d.
    prelingual d.
    retrocochlear d.
    Scheibe d.
    sensorineural d.
    syphilitic d.
    tone d.
    toxic d.
    transmission d.
    traumatic d.
    vascular d.
    word d.
dealbation
dealcoholization
deallergization
dealt
De Alvarez forceps
deamidase
deamidization
deaminase
deamination
Dean
    applicator

Dean *(continued)*
    forceps
    knife
    periosteotome
    scissors
Dean Ornish reversal diet
dearterialization
dearth
    d. of evidence
    d. of findings
    d. of symptoms
dearticulation
death
    apparent d.
    associated d.
    brain d.
    cell d.
    cot d.
    crib d.
    fetal d.
    functional d.
    genetic d.
    infant d.
    instantaneous d.
    intrauterine d.
    liver d.
    local d.
    molecular d.
    neonatal d.
    nonmaternal d.
    perinatal d.
    somatic d.
    sudden d.
    sudden infant d. (SID)
    voodoo d.
death-cap
Deaver
    incision
    retractor
    scissors
DEBA—diethylbarbituric acid
DeBakey
    blade
    clamp
    forceps
    graft
    prosthesis
    scissors
    tunneler
DeBakey-Bahnson forceps
DeBakey-Bainbridge forceps
DeBakey-Balfour retractor
DeBakey-Cooley
    dilator
    forceps

DeBakey-Cooley *(continued)*
    retractor
DeBakey-Metzenbaum scissors
debanding
Debaryomyces hansenii
debilitate
debilitated
    d. patient
    d. state
debilitating illness
debilitation
debilitative disease
debility
débouchement
Débove
    disease
    membrane
    treatment
    tube
debranching enzyme
Debré-de Toni-Fanconi syndrome
Debré-Sémélaigne syndrome
débride
débridement
    enzymatic d.
    surgical d.
    tangential d.
debrider
    Sauer d.
debris
    clots and d.
    dermal d.
    inflammatory cell d.
    loose d.
    d. of Malassez
    purulent d.
    stonelike d.
    tissue d.
    word d.
debt
    oxygen d.
debulking
decade scaler
decalcification
decalcify
decane
decannulation
decantation
decapeptide
decapitate
decapitation
decapitator
decapsulation
decarbonization
decarboxylase

decarboxylation
    oxidative d.
decay
    alpha d.
    beta d.
    branching d.
    d. constant
    dental d.
    exponential d.
    free induction d.
    isomeric level d.
    isometric d.
    d. mode
    nuclear d.
    positron d.
    d. product
    radioactive d.
    d. scheme
    tone d.
    tooth d.
decedent
deceleration
    early d.
    late d.
    variable d's
decenter
decentration
deceration
decerebellation
decerebrate rigidity
decerebration
dechloridation
decholesterolization
decibel (dB)
    A-weighted d. (dBA)
decidua
    basal d.
    d. basalis
    capsular d.
    d. capsularis
    d. compacta
    ectopic d.
    d. marginalis
    menstrual d.
    d. menstrualis
    parietal d.
    d. parietalis
    d. polyposa
    reflex d.
    d. reflexa
    d. serotina
    d. spongiosa
    d. subchorialis
    true d.
    d. tuberosa papulosa

decidua *(continued)*
    d. vera
decidual
deciduate
deciduation
deciduitis
deciduoma
    Loeb d.
    d. malignum
deciduomatosis
deciduosis
deciduous
deciliter (dL)
decipara
decision
    Brawner d.
    Durham d.
Decker
    culdoscope
    operation
declination
declinator
decline
declive monticuli cerebelli
decoagulant
decoction
decollation
décollement
decoloration
decolorize
decompensated
decompensation
    Bekhterev (Bechterew) d.
    corneal d.
decomplementize
decomposition
    anaerobic d.
    d. of movement
decompression
    abdominal d.
    cardiac d.
    cerebral d.
    explosive d.
    d. of heart
    Heyns d.
    intestinal d.
    microvascular d.
    Naffziger orbital d.
    nerve d.
    d. operation
    d. of pericardium
    d. of rectum
    d. of spinal cord
    suboccipital d.
    subtemporal d.

D

decompression *(continued)*
  trigeminal d.
decompressive laminectomy
deconditioning
decongestant
decongestive
decontamination
decorticate
decortication
  arterial d.
  chemical d.
  enzymatic d.
  d. of lung
  renal d.
decrement
decrepitate
decrepitation
decrudescence
decrustation
decubital
decubitus
  d. acutus
  Andral d.
  d. chronicus
  dorsal d.
  lateral d.
  sacral d.
  ventral d.
decurrent
decussate
decussatio (decussationes)
  d. brachii conjunctivi
  d. lemniscorum medialium
  d. motoria
  d. nervorum trochlearium
  d. pedunculorum
    cerebellarium cranialium
  d. pedunculorum
    cerebellarium superiorum
  d. pyramidum
  d. sensoria
  decussationes tegmenti
  d. trochlearis
decussation
  anterior hypothalamic d.
  d. of the brachia conjunctiva
  d. of cranial cerebellar
    peduncles
  d. of fillet
  Forel d.
  fountain d. of Meynert
  Held d.
  inferior hypothalamic d.
  d. of medial lemnisci
  motor d.

decussation *(continued)*
  optic d.
  posterior hypothalamic d.
  pyramidal d.
  d. of pyramids
  rubrospinal d.
  d. of rubrospinal tracts
  sensory d.
  d. of superior cerebellar
    peduncles
  superior hypothalamic d.
  superior supraoptic d.
  suprachiasmatic d.
  supramammillary d.
  tectospinal d.
  d. of tectospinal tracts
  tegmental d's
  trochlear d.
  d. of trochlear nerves
decussationes (plural of
  decussatio)
dedentition
dedifferentiation
Dedo laryngoscope
dedolation
Dedo-Pilling laryngoscope
deem, deemed
deep
de-epicardialization
Dees needle
deet, DEET—diethyltoluamide
de-excitation
def.—deficiency
DEF, def—decayed, extracted,
  filled
DEF, def
  D. index
  D. rate
defatigation
defatted
defecation
  fragmentary d.
defect
  acquired d.
  aorticopulmonary septal d.
  aortic septal d.
  aortopulmonary d.
  atrial septal d., atrioseptal d.
  atrioventricular septal d.
  birth d.
  congenital d.
  congenital pericardial d.
  congenital reading d.
  cortical d.
  dehalogenase d.

D

defect *(continued)*
  developmental d.
  ectodermal d., congenital
  endocardial cushion d.
  fibrous cortical d.
  filling d.
  galactokinase d.
  genetic d.
  genetic d. of folate
    metabolism
  3β-hydroxysteroid
    dehydrogenase d. [3-beta-]
  interatrial septal d.
  iodine transport d.
  iodotyrosine coupling d.
  iodotyrosine deiodinase d.
  limb reduction d.
  lucent d.
  luteal phase d.
  metaphyseal fibrous d.
  napkin-ring d.
  obstructive
    ventilatory d.
  organification d.
  ostium primum d.
  ostium secundum d.
  polytopic field d.
  restrictive ventilatory d.
  retention d.
  salt-losing d.
  septal d.
  serum iodoprotein d.
  subcortical d.
  subperiosteal cortical d.
  ventricular septal d.
defective
defeminization
defense
  character d.
  d. mechanism
  insanity d.
  muscular d.
deferens
deferent
deferentectomy
deferential
deferentitis
Defer method
defervesce, defervesced
defervescence
defervescent
defiance
defiant
defibrillated
defibrillation

defibrillator
  automatic external d.
    (AED)
  automatic implantable
    cardioverter-d. (AICD)
defibrinated
defibrination
defibrinogenation
deficiency
  acid-maltase d.
  acquired C1 inhibitor d.
  adenosine deaminase d.
  α₁-antitrypsin d. [alpha-1-]
  apolipoprotein C-II d.
  argininosuccinic acid
    synthetase d.
  C7 d.
  carnitine d.
  carnitine palmityl
    transferase d.
  cerebroside sulfatase d.
  complement d.
  congenital intrinsic factor d.
  congenital myeloperoxidase d.
  congenital
    transcobalamin II d.
  cystathionine β-synthase d.
    [beta-]
  cytochrome b d.
  debrancher d.
  disaccharidase d.
  erythrocyte glutathione
    peroxidase d.
  factor VIII d.
  factor D (H, I) d.
  familial aldosterone d.
  familial high-density
    lipoprotein (HDL) d.
  fibrinogen d.
  folic acid d.
  fructokinase d.
  fructose d.
  galactokinase d.
  α-galactosidase d. [alpha-]
  glucocerebrosidase d.
  glucose-6-phosphate
    dehydrogenase d.
  α-1,4-glucosidase d. [alpha-]
  glutathione synthetase d.
  heme synthetase d.
  hepatic phosphorylase
    kinase d.
  HGPRTase d.
  high-density lipoprotein
    (HDL) d.

deficiency *(continued)*
    21-hydroxylase enzyme d.
    3β-hydroxysteroid
      dehydrogenase d. [3-beta-]
    hypoxanthine-guanine
      phosphoribosyltransferase d.
    IgA d.
    IgM d.
    immune d.
    immunoglobulin (Ig) d.
    immunologic d.
    iron d.
    isolated IgA d.
    kappa chain d.
    lactase d.
    lecithin-cholesterol acyl
      transferase d.
    leukocyte adhesion d.
    leukocyte G6PD d.
    luteal phase d.
    mental d.
    muscle phosphofructokinase d.
    muscle phosphorylase d.
    oxygen d.
    phosphoglucomutase d.
    phytanic acid oxidase d.
    plasma thromboplastin
      antecedent d.
    pseudocholinesterase d.
    pyridoxine d.
    pyruvate-kinase d.
    riboflavin d.
    selective IgA d.
    sphingomyelinase d.
    Stuart-Prower factor d.
    thymus-dependent d.
    thymus-independent d.
    transferrin d.
    tryptophan d.
    tyrosine aminotransferase d.
    vitamin d.
    xanthine oxidase d.
    X-linked
      hypogammaglobulinemia
      with growth hormone d.
    X-linked mental d.
    xylitol dehydrogenase d.
deficit
    base d.
    oxygen d.
    pulse d.
    reversible ischemic
      neurologic d.
    saturation d.
definitely

definition
definitive
definitively
deflation
deflection
    atrial d.
    His bundle d.
    intrinsic d.
    QRS d.
    QS d.
    vesicouterine d.
defloration
deflorescence
defluvium
    postpartum d.
    d. unguium
defluxio
    d. capillorum
    d. ciliorum
defluxion
deformability
deformation
deforming
deformity
    Åkerlund (Akerlund) d.
    Arnold-Chiari d.
    boutonniére d.
    buttonhole d.
    Chiari d.
    cloverleaf d.
    cloverleaf skull d.
    coup de sabre b.
    crossbar d.
    Dandy-Walker d.
    dish-face d.
    equinus d.
    Erlenmeyer flask d.
    funnel d.
    gun stock d.
    Haglund d.
    Ilfeld-Holder d.
    intrinsic minus (or plus) d.
    J-sella d.
    lobster-claw d.
    Madelung d.
    mermaid d.
    Michel
    Mondini d.
    parachute d.
    pinched-tip d.
    pollybeak d.
    recurvatum d.
    reduction d.
    riding breeches d.
    rocker bottom d.

deformity *(continued)*
    rolled edge d.
    round back d.
    saddle d. of nose
    seal-fin d.
    silver fork d.
    simian d.
    split foot d.
    split hand d.
    Sprengel d.
    swan neck d.
    thumb-in-palm d.
    torsional d.
    trap door d.
    ulnar drift d.
    uni-tip d.
    valgus d.
    varus d.
    Velpeau d.
    Volkmann d.
    whistling d.
Dega pelvic osteotomy
deganglionate
degassing
degeneracy of code
degenerate
degeneratio micans
degeneration
    Abercrombie d.
    adipose d.
    adiposogenital d.
    albuminoid d.
    albuminous d.
    alcoholic cerebellar d.
    Alzheimer neurofibrillary d.
    amyloid d.
    angiolithic d.
    Armanni-Ebstein d.
    Armanni-Ehrlich d.
    ascending d.
    atheromatous d.
    atrophic pulp d.
    axonal d.
    ballooning d.
    basic d.
    basophilic d.
    Best macular d.
    Biber-Haab-Dimmer d.
    black d. of brain
    blastophthoric d.
    calcareous d.
    Canavan spongy d.
    carneous d.
    caseous d.
    cellulose d.

degeneration *(continued)*
    central d. of the corpus
      callosum
    cerebellar d.
    cerebellofugal d.
    cerebromacular d.
    cerebroretinal d.
    cheesy d.
    chitinous d.
    cloudy-swelling d.
    cobblestone d.
    colloid d. of choroid
    comma d.
    congenital macular d.
    corticostriatal-spinal d.
    corticostriatonigral d.
    Crooke hyaline d.
    cystic d. of adventitia
    cystoid d.
    descending d.
    disciform macular d.
    Doyne familial colloid d.
    Doyne honeycomb d.
    dystrophic d.
    earthy d.
    elastoid d.
    familial colloid d.
    fascicular d.
    fatty d.
    fibrinous d.
    fibroid d.
    fibrous d.
    floccular d.
    gelatiniform d.
    glassy d.
    glistening d.
    glycogenic d.
    Gombault d.
    granular d.
    granulovacuolar d.
    gray d.
    hematohyaloid d.
    hepatolenticular d.
    heredomacular d.
    Holmes d.
    Horn d.
    hyaline d.
    hyaloid d.
    hydropic d.
    Kozlowski d.
    Kuhnt-Junius d.
    lardaceous d.
    lattice d. of retina
    lenticular d.
    lipoidal d.

D

degeneration *(continued)*
 liquefaction d.
 macular disciform d.
 Mönckeberg d.
 mucinoid d., mucinous d.
 mucoid d., mucous d.
 multisystem d.
 myelinic d.
 myxomatous d.
 neurosomatic d.
 Nissl d.
 olivopontocerebellar d.
 pallidal d.
 paraneoplastic subacute
  cerebellar d.
 parenchymatous d.
 paving stone d.
 pigmental d.
 pigmentary d. of globus pallidus
 polychromatophilic d.
 polypoid d.
 primary progressive
  cerebellar d.
 progressive
  pyramidopallidal d.
 Quain d.
 red d.
 retinal lattice d.
 retrograde d.
 rim d.
 Rosenthal d.
 sclerotic d.
 secondary d.
 senile d.
 senile disciform macular d.
 senile exudative macular d.
 spinocerebellar d.
 spongiform d.
 spongy d. of central nervous
  system
 spongy d. of white matter
 Stock pigmentary d.
 striatonigral d.
 subacute combined d. of spinal
  cord
 system d.
 tapetoretinal d.
 Terrien d.
 trabecular d.
 transneuronal d.
 traumatic d.
 turbid-swelling d.
 Türck d.
 uratic d.
 vacuolar d.

degeneration *(continued)*
 van Bog familial axonal
  spongy d.
 Virchow d.
 vitelliform d. of Best
 vitelliform macular d.
 vitelline macular d.
 vitreous d.
 Vogt d.
 wallerian d.
 waxy d.
 Wilson d.
 Zenker d.
degenerative
degenerative joint disease
degenitalize
degerm
degloving
deglutible
deglutition
deglutitory
Degos
 disease
 syndrome
degradable
degradation
degranulation
degree
 d. absolute
 d's Celsius
 d's Fahrenheit
 d's of freedom
 prism d.
degrowth
degustation
dehematized
dehemoglobinized
dehepatized
Dehio test
dehiscence
 d. of alveolar process
 iris d.
 root d.
 d. of uterus
 wound d.
 Zuckerkandl d.
dehumanization
dehumidifier
dehydrant
dehydratase
dehydrate
dehydration
 absolute d.
 hypernatremic d.
 relative d.

dehydration *(continued)*
 voluntary d.
dehydroascorbic acid
dehydrocholaneresis
dehydrocholate
dehydrocholesterol
 7-d., activated
dehydrocholic acid
11-dehydrocorticosterone
dehydroepiandrosterone sulfate
 (DHEA sulfate)
dehydrogenase
 isocitric d.
 lactate d. (LDH)
 lactic d.
dehydrogenate
dehydrogenation
dehypnotize
deiodination
deionization
deiteral
Deiters
 cells
 frame
 nucleus
 phalanges
 phalanx
 process
 tract
déjà entendu
déjà éprouvé
déjà fait
déjà pensé
déjà raconté
déjà vécu
déjà voulu
déjà vu
Dejean syndrome
dejection
Dejerine
 disease
 sign
 syndrome
 type
Dejerine-Klumpke
 palsy
 paralysis
 syndrome
Dejerine-Landouzy
 dystrophy
 type
Dejerine-Lichtheim phenomenon
Dejerine-Roussy syndrome
Dejerine-Sottas
 atrophy

Dejerine-Sottas *(continued)*
 disease
 syndrome
Dejerine-Thomas atrophy
de Kleijn neck reflex
Deknatel suture
delacrimation
delactation
Delafield
 fluid
 hematoxylin
delamination
de Lange syndrome
delay
 interventricular conduction d.
 pulse d.
 synaptic d.
delayed
 d. operative cholangiography
 d. primary suture
Delbet sign
del Castillo syndrome
DeLee
 catheter
 forceps
 maneuver
 pelvimeter
 retractor
 suction
 tenaculum
DeLee-Hillis obstetric stethoscope
deleterious effects
deletion
 antigenic d.
 intercalary d.
 terminal d.
delimitation
delimiting keratotomy
delineate
delineation
delinquency
delinquent
 juvenile d.
deliquescence
deliquescent
délire
 d. ambitieux
 d. á quatre
 d. chronique
 d. de toucher
 d. ecmnesique
 d. en partie double
 d. de négation
 d. onirique
 d. terminal

délire *(continued)*
 d. tremblant
deliria (plural of delirium)
deliriant
delirifacient
delirious
delirium (deliria)
 acute d.
 alcohol withdrawal d.
 Bell d.
 collapse d.
 d. cordis
 febrile d.
 d. grandiosum
 d. grave
 low d.
 d. mussitans
 oneiric d.
 organic d.
 postcardiotomy d.
 senile d.
 substance-induced d.
 substance
  intoxication d.
 substance withdrawal d.
 toxic d.
 traumatic d.
 d. tremens (DTs)
delitescence
deliver
delivery
 abdominal d.
 breech d.
 forceps d.
 forceps d., high
 forceps d., outlet
 low-forceps d.
 midforceps d.
 normal spontaneous vaginal d.
  (NSVD)
 postmature d.
 postmortem d.
 premature d.
 spontaneous d.
 vaginal d.
delle
dellen
delling
Delmege sign
delomorphous
Delorme operation
De Lorme boot
delousing
Delphian node
Delstanche curet

delta
 Greek letter
  (δ; alphabetized as d)
 d.-aminolevulinic acid (ALA)
 d. antigen
 Galton d.
 d. hepatitis
 d. mesoscapulae
 d. ray
 d. wave
deltoid
deltopectoral incision
Del Toro operation
delusion
 autochthonous d.
 d. of being controlled
 bizarre d.
 d. of control
 depressive d.
 encapsulated d.
 erotomaniacal d.
 expansive d.
 fragmentary d's
 d. of grandeur
 grandiose d.
 d. of influence
 messianic d.
 d. of misidentification
 mood-congruent d.
 mood-incongruent d.
 d. of negation
 nihilistic d.
 paranoid d's
 d. of persecution
 persecutory d.
 d. of poverty
 primary d.
 d. of reference
 secondary d.
 self-referential d.
 shared d.
 somatic d.
 systematized d's
delusional
demarcation
 no line of d.
 shell-like d.
 surface d.
Demarquay sign
DeMartel-Wolfson clamp
demasculinization
dement
demented
dementia
 alcoholic d.

dementia *(continued)*
    Alzheimer d.
    arteriosclerotic d.
    Binswanger d.
    boxer's d.
    catatonic d.
    chronic d.
    dialysis d.
    epileptic d.
    hebephrenic d.
    hydrocephalic d.
    d. infantilis
    multi-infarct d.
    d. myoclonica
    myxedematous d.
    paralytic d.
    d. paralytica
    d. paranoides
    paretic d.
    post-traumatic d.
    d. praecocissima
    d. praecox
    d. praesenilis
    presenile d.
    primary degenerative d.
      of the Alzheimer type
    progressive d.
    d. pugilistica
    semantic d.
    senile d.
    static d.
    subcortical d.
    terminal d.
    toxic d.
    vascular d.
    Wernicke d.
demethylation
Demianoff sign
demifacet
    inferior d. for head of rib
    superior d. for head of rib
demigauntlet
demilune
    d's of Adamkiewicz
    Giannuzzi d's
    Heidenhain d's
demimonstrosity
demineralization
demipenniform
demise
demodectic
Demodex folliculorum
demodulation
demography
    dynamic d.

demography *(continued)*
    static d.
demoniac
demonomania
demonophobia
demonstrator
De Morgan spots
demorphinization
de Morsier syndrome
de Morsier-Gauthier syndrome
Demours membrane
demucosation
demulcent
de Musset sign
de Mussy
    point
    sign
demustardization
demutization
demyelinate
demyelinating disease
demyelination
demyelinization
denarcotize
denasality
denaturant
denaturation
    protein d.
denatured
dendriform
dendrite
    apical d.
    basal d.
dendritic
dendritum
    d. apicale
    d. basale
dendrodendritic
dendroid
dendrophagocytosis
denervate
denervation
dengue
    hemorrhagic d.
Denhardt mouth gag
Denhardt-Dingman mouth gag
denial
denidation
Denis Browne
    clubfoot splint
    needle
    operation
    pouch
    technique
Denis method

D

denitrification
denitrifier
denitrify
denitrogenation
Denker operation
Denman
    method
    spontaneous evolution
    version
Dennie-Marfan syndrome
Dennie sign
Dennis
    clamp
    forceps
Denny-Brown
    sensory radicular neuropathy
    syndrome
Denonvilliers
    aponeurosis
    fascia
    operation
dens (dentes)
    dentes acustici
    d. acutus
    dentes angulares
    d. axis
    dentes canini
    d. caninus
    dentes de Chiaie
    dentes decidui
    d. epistrophei
    dentes incisivi
    d. incisivus
    d. in dente
    d. invaginatus
    dentes molares
    d. molaris
    dentes permanentes
    dentes premolares
    d. premolaris
    d. sapientiae
    d. serotinus
dense-deposit disease
densitometry
    dual-photon d.
    Norland-Cameron photon d.
    photon d.
    quantitative CT d.
density
    absolute d.
    arciform d.
    background d.
    buoyant d.
    calcific d.
    conglomerate d.

density *(continued)*
    count information d.
    flux d.
    inherent d.
    ionization d.
    ocular d.
    optical d. (OD)
    relative d.
    scan information d.
    superhelix d.
dentagra
dental prosthesis
dentalgia
dentata
dentate suture
dentatothalamic
dentatum
dentes (plural of dens)
dentia
    d. praecox
    d. tarda
dentibuccal
denticle
    adherent d.
    attached d.
    embedded d.
    false d.
    free d.
    interstitial d.
    true d.
denticulate suture
denticulated
dentification
dentiform
dentifrice
dentigerous
dentilabial
dentilingual
dentin
    adventitious d.
    calcified d.
    circumpulpal d.,
      circumpulpar d.
    cover d.
    functional d.
    hereditary opalescent d.
    hypoplastic d.
    interglobular d.
    intermediate d.
    irregular d.
    mantle d.
    opalescent d.
    peritubular d.
    primary d.
    reparative d.

dentin *(continued)*
    sclerotic d.
    secondary irregular d.
    secondary regular d.
    sensitive d.
    tertiary d.
    transparent d.
dentinal
dentinalgia
dentinoblast
dentinogenesis imperfecta
dentinogenic
dentinoid
dentinoma
dentinosteoid
dentinum
dentiparous
dentist
dentistry
    cosmetic d.
    esthetic d.
    forensic d.
    four-handed d.
    geriatric d.
    legal d.
    operative d.
    pediatric d.
    preventive d.
    prosthetic d.
    psychosomatic d.
    restorative d.
dentition
    artificial d.
    deciduous d.
    delayed d.
    first d.
    mixed d.
    natural d.
    permanent d.
    precocious d.
    predeciduous d.
    premature d.
    primary d.
    retarded d.
    secondary d.
    temporary d.
    transitional d.
dentoalveolar
dentoalveolitis
dentofacial
dentography
dentomechanical
dentosurgical
dentotropic
dentulous

denture
    clasp d.
    complete d.
    conditioning d.
    distal extension partial d.
    Every d.
    fixed partial d.
    full d.
    immediate d.
    immediate-insertion d.
    implant d.
    interim d.
    overlay d.
    partial d.
    provisional d.
    removable partial d.
    skeleton d.
    spoon d.
    telescopic d.
    temporary d.
    tooth-borne partial d.
    transitional d.
    trial d.
    unilateral partial d.
denturism
denturist
Denucé quadrate ligament
denucleated
denudation
denutrition
Denver Developmental Screening Test
Denver shunt
deodorant
deodorize
deodorizer
deoppilant
deoppilation
deorsumduction
deorsumvergence
deorsumversion
deossification
deoxidation
deoxyadenosine
    d. diphosphate (dADP)
    d. monophosphate (dAMP)
    d. triphosphate (dATP)
5′-deoxyadenosyl transferase
deoxyadenylate
deoxyadenylic acid
deoxyadenylyl
deoxycholaneresis
deoxycholate
deoxycholic acid
deoxycholylglycine

deoxycholyltaurine
11-deoxycorticosterone (DOC)
    d. acetate
    d. pivalate
deoxycortone
deoxycytidine
    d. diphosphate (dCDP)
    d. monophosphate (dCMP)
    d. triphosphate (dCTP)
deoxycytidylate
deoxycytidylic acid
deoxycytidylyl
6-deoxy-1-galactose
deoxygenate
deoxygenation
2-deoxy-D-glucose
deoxyguanosine
    d. diphosphate (dGDP)
    d. monophosphate (dGMP)
    d. triphosphate (dGTP)
deoxyguanylate
deoxyguanylic acid
deoxyguanylyl
deoxyhemoglobin
deoxynucleoside
deoxyribonucleic acid (DNA)
deoxyribonucleoprotein
deoxyribonucleoside
deoxyribonucleotide
deoxyribose
deoxythymidine
    d. diphosphate (dTDP)
    d. monophosphate (dTMP)
    d. triphosphate (dTTP)
deoxythymidylate
deoxythymidylic acid
deoxythymidylyl
deoxyuridine (dU)
    d. monophosphate
      (dUMP)
    d. triphosphate (dUTP)
Depage position
DePalma
    prosthesis
    staple procedure
depatterning
dependence
    drug d.
    emotional d.
    physical d.
    physiologic d., physiological d.
    polysubstance d.
    psychoactive substance d.
    pyridoxine d.
    substance d.

dependency
    drug d.
    psychological d.
    pyridoxine d.
dependent
    d. drainage
    d. edema
depepsinized
depersonalization
de Pezzer catheter
dephosphorylation
depigmentation
depilate
depilation
depilatory
deplasmolysis
deplasmolyze
deplete
depletion
    plasma d.
depolarization
    atrial premature d. (APD)
    ventricular premature d.
      (VPD)
depolarize
depolarizer
depolymerization
depolymerize
deposit
    active d.
    bismuth d.
    dense d's
    glomerular d's
    hyaline d.
    mesangial d.
    para-amyloid d.
    renal amyloid d.
    subendothelial d.
    subepithelial d.
    tooth d.
depot
    fat d.
depravation
depraved
depressant
    cardiac d.
depressed
depression
    agitated d.
    anaclitic d.
    congenital chondrosternal d.
    endogenous d.
    freezing point d.
    involutional d.
    Leão spreading d.

depression *(continued)*
    major d.
    neurotic d.
    otic d.
    pacchionian d.
    postdormital d.
    postpartum d.
    precordial d.
    psychotic d.
    pterygoid d.
    radial d.
    reactive d.
    retarded d.
    situational d.
    ST d.
    ST-segment d.
    supratrochlear d.
    systolic d.
    tooth d.
    unipolar d.
    ventricular d.
depressive
depressomotor
depressor
    d. anguli oris
    Cushing d.
    d. epiglottidis
    d. labii inferioris
    tongue d.
deprimens oculi
deprivation
    emotional d.
    maternal d.
    psychosocial d.
    sensory d.
    thought d.
deproteinization
depside
depsipeptide
depth
    focal d.
    d. of focus
    d. of perception
depurant
depurate
depuration
depurative
depurator
DePuy
    orthopedic implant
    prosthesis
    splint
de Quervain
    disease
    fracture

de Quervain *(continued)*
    syndrome
    tenosynovitis
    thyroiditis
deradelphus
derailment
deranencephalia
derangement
    Hey internal d.
Derby operation
Dercum disease
derealization
dereism
dereistic
derencephalocele
derencephalus
derepression
    gene d.
Derf needle holder
derivant
derivation
derivative
    benzisoxazole d.
    hematoporphyrin d.
    purified protein d. .
    tricyclic d.
Derlacki
    chisel
    curet
    gouge
    knife
    mobilizer
    operation
Derlacki-Shambaugh chisel
DermaBond topical adhesive
dermabraded
dermabrader
    Iverson d.
    sandpaper d.
dermabrasion
dermacarrier
Dermacentor andersoni
dermad
dermal suture
Dermalene suture
Dermalon suture
dermatitis (dermatitides)
    actinic d.
    d. aestivalis
    allergic contact d.
    d. ambustionis
    ammonia d.
    ancylostome d.
    arsphenamine d.
    d. artefacta

D

dermatitis (dermatitides) *(continued)*
 ashy d.
 atopic d.
 d. atrophicans
 autosensitization d.
 bathers' d.
 berlock d., berloque d.
 brown-tail moth d.
 d. bullosa striata pratensis
 d. calorica
 carcinomatous d.
 caterpillar d.
 cement d.
 cercarial d.
 chemical d.
 chigger d.
 chromate d.
 chronic bullous d.
 d. combustionis
 d. congelationis
 contact d.
 contagious pustular d.
 d. contusiformis
 cosmetic d.
 cumulative insult d.
 diaper d.
 eczematous d.
 d. epidemica
 d. erythematosa
 d. escharotica
 d. excoriativa infantum
 d. exfoliativa epidemica
 d. exfoliativa neonatorum
 exudative discoid and
  lichenoid d.
 factitial d.
 d. gangrenosa infantum
 grass d.
 d. herpetiformis
 d. hiemalis
 industrial d.
 infectious eczematous d.
 insect d.
 interdigital d.
 io-moth d.
 irritant d.
 Jacquet d.
 Leiner d.
 livedoid d.
 marine d.
 meadow d., meadow-grass d.
 d. medicamentosa
 moth d.
 d. multiformis
 mycotic d.

dermatitis (dermatitides) *(continued)*
 napkin d.
 nasal solar d.
 nickel d.
 d. nodosa
 d. nodularis necrotica
 nummular eczematous d.
 occupational d.
 onion mite d.
 d. papillaris capillitii
 papular d.
 d. pediculoides ventricosus
 Pelodera d.
 perfume d.
 periocular d.
 perioral d.
 photoallergic contact d.
 photocontact d.
 phototoxic d.
 phytophototoxic d.
 pigmented purpuric lichenoid d.
 poison ivy d.
 poison oak d.
 poison sumac d.
 precancerous d.
 primary irritant d.
 d. psoriasiformis nodularis
 purpuric pigmented lichenoid d.
 radiation d.
 rat mite d.
 d. repens
 rhabditic d.
 rhus d.
 roentgen-ray d.
 schistosome d.
 seborrheic d., d. seborrheica
 d. simplex
 d. solaris
 stasis d.
 d. striata pratensis bullosa
 swimmer's d.
 d. traumatica
 trefoil d.
 uncinarial d.
 d. vegetans
 d. venenata
 verminous d.
 d. verrucosa
 verrucose d., verrucous d.
 vesicular d.
 weeping d.
 x-ray d.
dermatoarthritis
 lipid d., lipoid d.
dermatoautoplasty

Dermatobia hominis
dermatobiasis
dermatochalasis
dermatoconjunctivitis
dermatodysplasia verruciformis
dermatofibroma
    d. protuberans
dermatofibrosarcoma
    progressive recurrent d.
    d. protuberans
dermatofibrosis lenticularis
  disseminata
dermatoglyphics
dermatographic
dermatographism
    black d.
    white d.
dermatoheteroplasty
dermatologic, dermatological
dermatologist
dermatology
dermatolysis palpebrarum
dermatome
    Bard-Parker d.
    Brown d.
    Castroviejo d.
    drum d.
    Hall d.
    Hood d.
    Meek-Wall d.
    Padgett d.
    Reese d.
    Stryker d.
dermatomegaly
dermatomere
dermatomic
dermatomycosis
    blastomycetic d.
    d. furfuracea
    d. microsporina
    d. trichophytina
dermatomyiasis
dermatomyoma
dermatomyositis
dermatoneurology
dermato-ophthalmitis
dermatopathic
dermatopathology
dermatopathy
dermatopharmacology
dermatophiliasis
dermatophilosis
dermatophyte
dermatophytid
dermatophytosis

dermatoplastic
dermatoplasty
    Thompson d.
dermatopolyneuritis
dermatorrhagia parasitica
dermatorrhexis
dermatosclerosis
dermatosis (dermatoses)
    acarine d.
    acute febrile neutrophilic d.
    angioneurotic d.
    ashy d. of Ramirez
    Auspitz d.
    Bowen precancerous d.
    d. cenicienta
    cholinogenic d.
    chronic bullous d. of childhood
    chronic hemosideric d.
    contact d.
    dermatolytic bullous d.
    industrial d.
    juvenile plantar d.
    lichenoid d.
    meadow grass d.
    menstrual d.
    neutrophilic d.
    occupational d.
    palmoplantar d.
    d. papulosa nigra
    precancerous d.
    progressive pigmentary d.
    purpuric d.
    radiation d.
    rhythmical d.
    Schamberg d.
    seborrheic d.
    stasis d.
    subcorneal pustular d.
    transient acantholytic d.
    Unna d.
    d. vegetans
    vulvar d.
dermatosparaxis
dermatotherapy
dermatotropic
dermatozoon (dermatozoa)
dermic
dermis
    reticular d.
dermohygrometer
dermoid
    corneal d.
    d. cyst
    implantation d.
    inclusion d.

D

dermoid *(continued)*
    intracranial d.
    intramedullary d.
    thyroid d.
    tubal d.
dermoidectomy
dermolipectomy
dermolipoma
dermolysin
dermometry
dermomyotome
dermoneurotropic
dermopathic
dermopathy
    diabetic d.
    infiltrative d.
dermoreaction
dermosynovitis
dermotoxin
dermovascular
Derra
    clamp
    dilator
    knife
D'Errico
    bur
    drill
    forceps
    retractor
D'Errico-Adson retractor
derriengue
DES—
    diethylstilbestrol
    diffuse esophageal spasm
DES daughter
desalination
desalivation
De Sanctis-Cacchione syndrome
desaturation
Desault
    apparatus
    bandage
    ligation
    sign
Descemet membrane
descemetitis
descemetocele
descendens
    d. cervicalis
    d. cervicis
descending
    d. colon
    d. root tractotomy
    d. urography
    d. venography

descensus
    d. testis
    d. uteri
    uterine d.
    d. ventriculi
descent
    d. of testis
    x d.
    y d.
Deschamps
    carrier
    compressor
    needle
desensitization
    anaphylactic d.
    systematic d.
desensitize
desexualize
deshydremia
desiccant
desiccate
desiccation
    electric d.
desiccative
Desjardins
    forceps
    point
    probe
    scoop
desmalgia
Desmarres
    clamp
    forceps
    knife
    lid elevator
    retractor
    scarifier
desmectasis
desmepithelium
desmin
desmiognathus
desmitis
desmocranium
desmocyte
desmocytoma
desmodontium
desmodynia
desmogenous
desmography
desmohemoblast
17,20-desmolase
desmoma
desmopathy
desmoplasia
desmoplastic trichoepithelioma

desmorrhexis
desmose
desmosine
desmosis
    half d.
desmosterol
desmotomy
Desnos
    disease
    pneumonia
desoleolecithin
desorb
desorption
DeSouza exercises
despair
despairing
despeciate
despeciation
despecification
desperate
desperation
d'Espine sign
desquamate
desquamation
    furfuraceous d.
    lamellar d. of the newborn
    membranous d.
    siliquose d.
desquamative
desthiobiotin
desulfhydrase
desultory labor
desynapsis
desynchronization
desynchrony
detachment
    annular d.
    epiphyseal d.
    exudative retinal d.
    retinal d.
    rhegmatogenous retinal d.
    vitreous d.
detection
detector
    collimation scintillation d.
    crystalline phosphor d.
    Doppler fetal heart d.
    flame ionization d.
    flame photometric d.
    flame thermoionic d.
    radiation d.
    scintillation d.
    semiconductor d.
    thermoluminescent d.
    threshold d.

detector *(continued)*
    x-ray d.
deter
detergent
    anionic d.
    cationic d.
deterioration
    d. of affect
    emotional d.
    schizophrenic d.
    simple senile d.
determinant
    allotypic d.
    antigenic d.
    hidden d.
    immunogenic d.
    sequential d.
determination
    embryonic d.
    sex d.
    sweat chloride d.
determinism
    psychic d.
deterrent
detonation
de Toni-Debré-Fanconi syndrome
de Toni-Fanconi syndrome
de Toni-Fanconi-Debré syndrome
detorsion
detoxification
    metabolic d.
detoxify
detrition
detritus
detruncation
detrusor
    d. urinae
    d. vesicae
detrusorrhaphy
detubation
detumescence
deutan
deuteranomal
deuteranomalous
deuteranomaly
deuteranope
deuteranopia
deuteranopic
deuteropathic
deuteropathy
deuteropine
deutonephron
Deutschländer disease
DEV—duck embryo vaccine
devascularization

devastation
  senile cortical d.
DeVega annuloplasty
development
  arrested d.
  cognitive d.
  mosaic d.
  postnatal d.
  prenatal d.
  psychomotor d.
  psychosexual d.
  psychosocial d.
  regulative d.
developmental milestones
Deventer
  diameter
  pelvis
Devergie disease
deviance
deviant
  sexual d.
deviation
  axis d.
  complement d.
  conjugate d.
  Hering-Hellebrand d.
  immune d.
  latent d.
  manifest d.
  minimum d.
  ocular conjugate d.
  primary d.
  right axis d.
  sample standard d.
  secondary d.
  sexual d.
  skew d.
  squint d.
  standard d.
  strabismic d.
  ST-T d.
  d. to the left
  d. to the right
  ulnar d.
Devic
  disease
  syndrome
device
  Adams-DeWeese d.
  arachnophlebectomy surgical d.
  central-bearing tracing d.
  contraceptive d.
  emergency infusion d. (EID)
  Fletcher-Suit afterloading d.
  intrauterine d. (IUD)

device *(continued)*
  left ventricular assist d.
  MediPort vascular access d.
  static imaging d.
DeVilbiss
  atomizer
  forceps
  irrigator
  nebulizer
  rongeur
  speculum
  trephine
devisceration
devitalization
  pulp d.
devitalize
devolution
De Vries theory
Dewar flask
DeWecker
  iris scissors
  operation
Dewey forceps
Dew sign
DEXA—dual energy x-ray
  absorptiometry (scan)
dexiotropic
Dexon
  mesh
  suture
dexter
dextrad
dextral
dextrality
dextranomer
dextrates
dextraural
dextriferron
dextrin
  limit d.
dextrinase
dextrinize
dextrinosis
dextrinuria
dextrocardia
  isolated d.
  mirror-image d.
  secondary d.
dextrocerebral
dextroclination
dextrocompound
dextrocular
dextrocularity
dextrocycloduction
dextroduction

dextrogastria
dextrogyration
dextromanual
dextropedal
dextroposition
dextrorotation
dextrorotatory
dextrose
dextrosinistral
Dextrostix
dextrosuria
dextrotorsion
dextrotropic
dextroversion
dextroverted
Deyerle
    drill
    plate
    punch
DF—
    decapacitation factor
    deficiency factor
    degree of freedom
    diabetic father
    discriminant function
    disseminated foci
DFA—direct fluorescent antibody
    (test)
DFDT—difluoro-diphenyl-
    trichloroethane
D-film
dg—decigram
DG—
    deoxyglucose
    diastolic gallop
    distogingival
DG, Dx—diagnosis
dG—deoxyguanosine
dGDP—deoxyguanosine
    diphosphate
dGMP—deoxyguanosine
    monophosphate
dGTP—deoxyguanosine
    triphosphate
DH—delayed hypersensitivity
DHA—docosahexaenoic acid
DHE—dihydroergotamine
DHEA—dehydroepiandrosterone
DHEAS—dehydroepiandrosterone
    sulfate
DHE 45 protocol
d'Herelle phenomenon
DHFR—dihydrofolate reductase
DHIA—dehydroisoandrosterone
DHL—diffuse histiocytic lymphoma

DHPG—
    3,4-dihydroxyphenylglycol
    dihydroxy-
      propoxymethylguanine
DHT—dihydrotestosterone
DI—
    diabetes insipidus
    diagnostic imaging
diabetes
    adult-onset d. mellitus
    d. alternans
    brittle d.
    bronze d.
    central d. insipidus
    chemical d.
    class A d.
    gestational d.
    growth-onset d.
    d. insipidus
    insulin-dependent d. mellitus
      (IDDM)
    juvenile-onset d.
    ketosis-prone d. mellitus
    ketosis-resistant d.
    latent d.
    lipoatrophic d.
    maturity-onset d. mellitus
    maturity-onset d. of youth
      (MODY)
    d. mellitus (DM)
    nephrogenic d. insipidus
    new-onset d. mellitus
    non–insulin-dependent d.
      mellitus (NIDDM)
    obesity-associated d.
    overt d.
    pancreatic d.
    piqûre d.
    preclinical d.
    pregnancy d., d. of pregnancy
    renal d.
    secondary d.
    starvation d.
    steroid d., steroidogenic d.
    subclinical d.
    thiazide d.
    type 1 d.
    type 2 d.
    vasopressin-resistant d.
      insipidus
    Young d.
diabetic
    d. autonomic neuropathy
    d. gastroparesis
    d. ketoacidosis

D

diabetic *(continued)*
    d. retinopathy
diabetogenic
diabetogenous
diabrosis
diabrotic
diacetemia
diacetic acid
diaceturia
diacetyl peroxide
diaclasis
diacrinous
diacrisis
diacritic
diactinic
diactinism
diacylglycerol
diadochokinesia
diadochokinetic
diagnose
diagnosis
    biological d.
    clinical d.
    cytohistologic d.
    cytologic d.
    differential d.
    direct d.
    d. by exclusion
    d. ex juvantibus
    laboratory d.
    niveau d.
    pathologic d.
    physical d.
    provocative d.
    quick-section d.
    roentgen d.
    serum d.
diagnostic dilatation and curettage
   (D&C)
diagnostician
diagnostics
diagram
    burn d.
diagrammatic radiography
diagraph
Diakiogiannis sign
dial
    astigmatic d.
    clock d.
    fan d.
    Lancaster Regan d.
    sunburst d.
dial-a-flow IV line
diallyl
dialysance

dialysate
dialysis
    chronic d.
    continuous ambulatory
      peritoneal d. (CAPD)
    continuous cycling
      peritoneal d.
    cross d.
    Drake-Willock d.
    equilibrium d.
    intermittent peritoneal d.
     (IPD)
    kidney d.
    lymph d.
    maintenance d.
    periodic d.
    peritoneal d.
    renal d.
    single-needle d.
dialyzable
dialyze, dialyzed
dialyzer
    coil d.
    Terumo d.
diameter
    anatomical conjugate d.
    anterior sagittal d.
    anteroposterior d.
    anterotransverse d.
    Baudelocque d.
    biischial d.
    biparietal d.
    bisacromial d.
    bisiliac d.
    bispinous d.
    bitemporal d.
    buccolingual d.
    cervicobregmatic d.
    coccygeopubic d.
    d. conjugata pelvis
    conjugate d. of pelvis
    cranial d.
    craniometric d.
    Deventer d.
    diagonal conjugate d.
    external conjugate d.
    extracanthic d.
    frontomental d.
    fronto-occipital d.
    intercanthic d.
    intercristal d.
    internal conjugate d.
    interspinous d.
    intertrochanteric d.
    intertuberal d.

D

diameter *(continued)*
    Löhlein d.
    longitudinal d., inferior
    mean corpuscular d.
    mento-occipital d.
    mentoparietal d.
    d. obliqua pelvis
    oblique d. of pelvis
    obstetric conjugate d.
    occipitofrontal d.
    occipitomental d.
    parietal d.
    pelvic d.
    posterior sagittal d.
    posterotransverse d.
    pubosacral d.
    pubotuberous d.
    sacropubic d.
    sagittal d.
    suboccipitobregmatic d.
    suboccipitofrontal d.
    suprasubparietal d.
    temporal d.
    d. transversa pelvis
    transverse d. of pelvic outlet
    transverse d. of pelvis
    true conjugate d.
    vertebromammary d.
    vertical d.
diamide
diamidine
diamine
diamine oxidase
diaminoacridine
diaminodiphenylsulfone
diaminuria
diamnionic
Diamond-Blackfan
    anemia
    syndrome
diamond bur
diamond-shaped
diamylene
dianhydroantiarigenin
dianoetic
diantebrachia
diapedesis
diapedetic
diaphane
diaphaneity
diaphanography
diaphanometry
diaphanoscope
diaphanoscopy
diaphanous

diaphemetric
diaphorase
diaphoresis
diaphoretic
diaphragm
    accessory d.
    Akerlund d.
    All-Flex d.
    Bucky d.
    Bucky-Potter d.
    compression d.
    condensing d.
    contraceptive d.
    epithelial d.
    filtration slit d. of glomerulus
    graduating d.
    iris d.
    d. of mouth
    oral d.
    pelvic d.
    polyarcuate d.
    Potter-Bucky d.
    respiratory d.
    secondary d.
    d. of sella turcica
    thoracoabdominal d.
    urogenital d.
    vaginal d.
diaphragma (diaphragmata)
    d. oris
    d. pelvis
    d. sellae
    d. urogenitale
diaphragmalgia
diaphragmatic
    d. excursion
    d. pacing
    d. paralysis
diaphragmatocele
diaphragmitis
diaphyseal
diaphysectomy
diaphysis (diaphyses)
    distal d.
    epiphysis-d. angle
    femoral d.
    humeral d.
    proximal d.
    radial d.
    tibial d.
    true anatomic d.
diaphysitis
    tuberculous d.
diaplacental
diapnoic

diapophysis
diapyesis
diapyetic
diarrhea
    cachectic d.
    congenital chloride d.
    dysenteric d.
    epidemic d.
    familial chloride d.
    infantile d.
    inflammatory d.
    mechanical d.
    mucous d.
    neonatal d.
    osmotic d.
    secretory d.
    stercoral d.
    summer d.
    toxigenic d.
    travelers' d.
    viral d., virus d.
    watery d.
diarrheal
diarrheogenic
diarthric
diarthrodial
diarthrosis (diarthroses)
    planiform d.
    d. rotatoria
diaschisis
diascope
diaspironecrobiosis
diaspironecrosis
diastalsis
diastase
    pancreatic d.
diastasis
    d. cordis
    iris d.
    d. recti
    d. recti abdominis
diastasuria
diastatic
diastema (diastemata)
    anterior d.
diastematocrania
diastematomyelia
diastematopyelia
diastereoisomeric
diastereoisomerism
Diastix
diastole
    atrial d.
    end d.
    ventricular d.

diastolic
    d. filling
    d. function
    d. motion
    d. overload
    d. pressure-time index
    d. pressure-volume relation
    d. reserve
    d. stiffness
diastrophic
diataxia
    cerebral d.
    d. cerebralis infantilis
diathermal
diathermic
diathermocoagulation
diathermy
    conventional d.
    long wave d.
    microwave d.
    pulsed d.
    short wave d.
    surgical d.
    ultrashort wave d.
diathesis
    allergic d.
    atopic d.
    autoimmune d.
    bleeding d.
    explosive d.
    exudative d.
    fibroplastic d.
    genetic d.
    gouty d.
    hemorrhagic d.
    lipogenic d.
    ossifying d.
    spasmodic d.
    thrombogenic d.
diathetic
diatomaceous earth
diatomite fibrosis
diauchenos
diauxic
diauxie
diaxon
diazine
diazobenzenesulfonic acid
diazoma
diazomethane
diazonal
diazone
diazosulfobenzol
diazotization
dibasic

dibenzanthracene
dibrachia
dibrachius
dibutyl
DIC—
    diffuse intravascular
      coagulation
    disseminated intravascular
      coagulation
dicalcic
dicentric
dicephalous
dicephalus
    d. dipus dibrachius
    d. dipus tetrabrachius
    d. dipus tribrachius
    d. tripus tribrachius
dicephaly
dicheilia
dicheiria
dicheirus
dichloride
    carbonic d.
dichlorodiethyl sulfide
dichlorodifluoromethane
1,1-dichloroethane
2,4-dichlorophenoxyacetic acid
    (2,4,-D)
dichlorotetrafluoroethane
dichorionic
dichotomy
dichroic
dichroism
dichromacy
dichromat
dichromate
dichromatic
dichromatism
dichromatopsia
dichromic
dichromophil
dichromophilism
Dick
    dilator
    reaction
    test
    toxin
Dickson operation
Dickson-Diveley operation
dicroceliasis
Dicrocoelium dendriticum
dicrotic
dicrotism
dicyclic
didactic

didactylism
didactylous
didelphia
didelphic
didermoma
Didiée projection
didymitis
didymous
didymus
die
    amalgam d.
    electroformed d.
    electroplated d.
    plated d.
    stone d.
    waxing d.
Dieffenbach operation
Dieffenbach-Warren
  operation
Diego blood group
dieldrin
dielectric
dielectrolysis
diembryony
diencephalic syndrome
diencephalohypophysial,
    diencephalohypophyseal
diencephalon
diener
Dienst test
Dientamoeba fragilis
dieresis
diesophagus
diesterase
diet
    absolute d.
    acid-ash d.
    adequate d.
    alkali-ash d.
    antiketogenic d.
    Atkins d.
    balanced d.
    basal d.
    basic d.
    Beverly Hills d.
    bland d.
    BRAT (bananas, rice cereal,
      applesauce, toast) d.
    CAPS-free d.
    convalescent d.
    crash d.
    DASH (Dietary Approach to
      Stop Hypertension) d.
    Dean Ornish reversal d.
    diabetic d.

D

diet *(continued)*
  Dr. Phil's Ultimate Weight Loss Solution d.
  Eat Right for Your Type d.
  elemental d.
  elimination d.
  Feingold d.
  Gerson d.
  gluten-free d.
  glycemic d.
  gouty d.
  high-calorie d.
  high-fat d.
  high-fiber d.
  high-protein d.
  high-sodium d.
  Jenny Craig d.
  ketogenic d.
  light d.
  low-calorie d.
  low-carbohydrate d.
  low-fat d.
  low-oxalate d.
  low-purine d.
  low-residue d.
  low-salt d., low-sodium diet
  macrobiotic d.
  Mediterranean d.
  Meulengracht d.
  optimal d.
  paleolithic d.
  Perricone d.
  Pritikin d.
  protein-sparing d.
  provocative d.
  purine-free d.
  reducing d.
  rice d.
  salt-free d.
  smooth d.
  Sonoma d.
  South Beach d.
  subsistence d.
  Sugar Busters! d.
  Weight Watchers d.
  Zone d.
dietary
dietetic
dietetics
Diethrich shunt clamp
diethylstilbestrol (DES)
diethyltoluamide
diethyltryptamine
dieting
  yo-yo d.

dietitian
Dietl crisis
Dieulafoy
  aspirator
  disease
  erosion
  triad
  ulcer
difference
  alveolar-arterial oxygen d.
  arteriovenous oxygen d.
  cation-anion d.
  interaural intensity d.
  interaural time d.
  just-noticeable d.
  linking d.
  d. threshold
differential
  d. contractility
  d. diagnoses
  d. effects
  d. response
  d. stethoscope
differentiate
differentiation
  cellular d.
  correlative d.
  dependent d.
  functional d.
  invisible d.
  regional d.
  response d.
  self d.
  sexual d.
  thymus cell d.
diffluence
diffluent
Diff-Quik
diffraction
  d. grating
  x-ray d.
diffusate
diffuse
diffusible
diffusion
  alveolar capillary d.
  d. components
  d. limitation
  double d. in one dimension
  double d. in two dimensions
  exchange d.
  facilitated d.
  free d.
  gel d.
  impeded d.

diffusion *(continued)*
    single d.
    single radial d.
    thermal d.
DiGeorge syndrome
digest
digestant
digestives
digestion
    artificial d.
    biliary d.
    gastric d.
    gastrointestinal d.
    intercellular d.
    intestinal d.
    intracellular d.
    lipolytic d.
    pancreatic d.
    parenteral d.
    peptic d.
    primary d.
    salivary d.
    secondary d.
digestive tract
digit
    sausage d.
    d. span task
digital
    d. autofluoroscope
    d. fibromatosis
    d. fluoroscopy
    d. radiography
    d. subtraction angiography
      (DSA)
    d. subtraction arteriography
      (DSA)
digital-to-analog (D/A) converter
digitalgia paresthetica
digitalis
    d. effect
digitalization
digitaloid
digitate warts
digitatio (digitationes)
    digitationes hippocampi
digitation
digitiform
digitigrade
digitize
digitonin
digitoplantar
digitoxigenin
digitoxose
digitus (digiti)
    d. anularis

digitus (digiti) *(continued)*
    d. demonstrativus
    d. extensus
    d. hippocraticus
    d. malleus
    digiti manus
    d. medius
    d. minimus manus
    d. minimus pedis
    d. mortuus
    digiti pedis
    d. postminimus
    d. primus manus
    d. primus pedis
    d. quartus manus
    d. quartus pedis
    d. quintus manus
    d. quintus pedis
    d. secundus manus
    d. secundus pedis
    d. tertius manus
    d. tertius pedis
    d. valgus
    d. varus
diglossia
diglyceride
dignathus
Di Guglielmo
    disease
    syndrome
diheterozygote
dihybrid
dihydrate
dihydrated
dihydric
dihydrobiopterin synthetase
  deficiency
dihydrocholesterol
dihydrofolate reductase (DHFR)
  deficiency
dihydrofolic acid
dihydroindolone
dihydrol
dihydrolipoamide acyltransferase
dihydrolipoamide dehydrogenase
dihydrolipoamide
    S-succinyltransferase
dihydrolutidine
dihydroorotase
dihydropteridine reductase (DHPR)
  deficiency
dihydrotestosterone
dihydrouridine
dihydroxyacetone phosphate
dihydroxycholecalciferol

3,4-dihydroxyphenylalanine
3,4-dihydroxyphenylglycol (DHPG)
dihysteria
diiodide
3,5-diiodosalicylic acid
3,5-diiodothyronine
diiodotyrosine
diisocyanate
diisopropyliminodiacetic acid
  (DISIDA)
dikaryote
dikaryotic
diketone
diketopiperazine
diktyoma
dikwakwadi
dilaceration
dilatation
    balloon d.
    d. of cervix
    d. and curettage (D&C)
    digital d.
    esophageal d.
    d. and evacuation (D&E)
    gastric d.
    d. of the heart
    idiopathic d.
    intraluminal d.
    poststenotic d.
    prognathic d.
    prognathion d.
    sinusoidal d.
    d. of the stomach
    supradiaphragmatic
      esophageal d.
dilatation and curettage (D&C)
    diagnostic D&C
    fractional D&C
    suction D&C
dilatator
dilate, dilated
dilating urethrotome
dilation
    digital d.
dilator
    anal d.
    Atlee d.
    Bakes d.
    Barnes d.
    Beardsley aortic d.
    Berens d.
    Black-Wylie obstetric d.
    Brown-McHardy d.
    Broyles d.
    Castroviejo d.

dilator *(continued)*
    Cooley d.
    DeBakey-Cooley d.
    Derra d.
    Dick d.
    Einhorn d.
    esophageal d.
    Ferris d.
    French d. Nos. 8 to 36
    Gohrbrand d.
    Goodell d.
    Guyon d.
    Hank d.
    Hank-Bradley d.
    Heath d.
    Hegar d.
    Jackson d.
    Jackson-Mosher d.
    Jackson-Trousseau d.
    Jolly d.
    Jones d.
    Kelly d.
    Kollmann d.
    Kron d.
    Laborde d.
    laryngeal d.
    Leader-Kollmann d.
    Maloney d.
    Mixter d.
    Mosher d.
    Muldoon d.
    Murphy d.
    d. muscle
    d. naris
    Negus hydrostatic d.
    Nettleship-Wilder d.
    Ottenheimer d.
    Palmer d.
    Patton d.
    Plummer d.
    Plummer-Vinson d.
    pneumatic balloon d.
    Pratt d.
    d. pupillae
    Ramstedt d.
    Reich-Nechtow d.
    Savary-Gilliard d.
    Starck d.
    Steele d.
    tracheal d.
    Trousseau d.
    Trousseau-Jackson d.
    Tubbs d.
    Tucker d.
    Van Buren d.

dilator *(continued)*
    Wales d.
    Walther d.
    Wylie d.
    Young d.
dilecanus
dilemma
diluent
dilute
dilution
    doubling d.
    nitrogen d.
    serial d.
    triple isotope d.
DIM—divalent ion metabolism
dimelia
dimelus
dimension
    contact vertical d.
    occlusal vertical d.
    postural vertical d.
    rest vertical d.
    vertical d.
dimensionless
dimer
    D-d.
    ionic d.
    nonionic d.
    thymine d.
    UV-induced d.
dimeric
dimerization
dimerous
Dimer X
dimetallic
dimethicone
    d. 350
    activated d.
2,5-dimethoxy-4-
    methylamphetamine (DOM)
3,4-dimethoxyphenylethylamine
dimethylamine
p-dimethylaminoazobenzene
    [p-, para-]
7,12-dimethylbenz[*a*]anthracene
    (DMBA)
dimethylbenzene
5,6-dimethylbenzimidazole
dimethyl carbate
dimethylethylpyrrole
dimethylformamide (DMF)
dimethylketone
dimethylnitrosamine
dimethylphenanthrene
dimethyl phthalate

dimethyl sulfate
dimethyl sulfoxide
dimethyltryptamine
diminution
Dimitri
    disease
    syndrome
Dimmer keratitis
DIMOAD—diabetes insipidus,
    diabetes mellitus, optic atrophy,
    deafness (syndrome)
dimorphism
    physical d.
    sexual d.
dimorphobiotic
dimorphous
dimple
    anal d.
    Fuchs d.
    postanal d.
    sacrococcygeal d.
dimpling
Dinamap
dineric
Dingman
    elevator
    forceps
    osteotome
    retractor
dinitrate
dinitrated
dinitroaminophenol
dinitrobenzene
dinitrochlorobenzene
dinitrofluorobenzene
dinitrogen monoxide
dinitro-*o*-cresol
dinitrophenol
dinitroresorcinol
dinitrotoluene
dinoflagellate
dinogunellin
diode
    light-emitting d.
Diogenes syndrome
diopter
    prism d.
dioptometry
dioptoscopy
dioptric
diovulatory
dioxane
dioxide
dioxin
dioxybenzone

dioxygen
dioxygenase
DIP—
     desquamative interstitial
          pneumonia
     desquamative interstitial
          pneumonitis
     distal interphalangeal
dipentene
dipeptidase
dipeptide
dipeptidyl I carboxypeptidase
dipeptidyl peptidase I
diperodon
diphallia
diphallus
diphasic
diphenadione
diphenyl
diphenylamino-azo-benzene
diphenylchlorarsine
diphonia
diphosgene
diphosphonate
diphosphotransferase
diphtheria
     Bretonneau d.
     cutaneous d.
     faucial d.
     d. gravis
     laryngeal d.
     laryngeotracheal d.
     malignant d.
     nasal d.
     nasopharyngeal d.
     pharyngeal d.
     scarlatinal d.
     septic d.
     surgical d.
     umbilical d.
     wound d.
diphtherin
diphtheritic
diphtheroid
diphthong
diphthongia
diphyllobothriasis
Diphyllobothrium
     D. cordatum
     D. latum
     D. parvum
diphyodont
DIPJ—distal interphalangeal joint
diplacusis
     binaural d.

diplacusis *(continued)*
     d. binauralis dysharmonica
     d. binauralis echoica
     disharmonic d.
     echo d.
     monaural d.
     d. monauralis
diplasmatic
diplegia
     atonic-astatic d.
     facial d.
     facial d., congenital
     flaccid d.
     Förster d.
     hypotonic d.
     infantile d.
     infantile cerebrocerebellar d.
     masticatory d.
     spastic d.
     tonic d.
diplegic
diploalbuminuria
diplobacillus (diplobacilli)
     Morax-Axenfeld d.
diplobacterium (diplobacteria)
diplococcal
diplococcemia
diplococcoid
diplococcus (diplococci)
     d. of Morax-Axenfeld
     d. of Neisser
     Weichselbaum d.
diploë
diploetic
diplogenesis
Diplogonoporus grandis
diploic
diploid
     Sappinia d.
diploidy
diplomate
diplomyelia
diplopagus
diplopia
     binocular d.
     crossed d.
     direct d.
     facial fracture d.
     heteronymous d.
     homonymous d.
     horizontal d.
     incongruous d.
     intranasal tumor d.
     monocular d.
     paradoxical d.

diplopia *(continued)*
    pathologic d.
    physiologic d.,
      physiological d.
    stereoscopic d.
    torsional d.
    uncrossed d.
    vertical d.
diplosomatia
diplosome
dipodia
dipole
    magnetic d.
dipotassium phosphate
dipping
diprosopus tetrophthalmus
diprotrizoate
dipsesis
dipsetic
dipsia
dipsogen
dipsogenic
dipsomania
dipsosis
dipsotherapy
dipstick
dipus
dipygus parasiticus
dipylidiasis
dire
    d. consequences
    d. straits
direct
    d. laryngoscopy
    d. ophthalmoscopy
    d. percutaneous transhepatic
      cholangiography
    d. vision spectroscope
directive
    advance d.
director
    grooved d.
    Larry d.
    Pratt d.
dirhinic
dirigomotor
Dirofilaria repens
dirofilariasis
disability
    developmental d.
    learning d.
    major d.
    partial d.
    permanent d.
disable

disaccharidase
    intestinal d. deficiency
disaccharide
    reducing d's
disacchariduria
disacidify
disarticulation
disc
discharge
    brush d.
    conductive d.
    convective d.
    delta d.
    diencephalic autonomic d.
    disruptive d.
    electroencephalographic d.
    epileptic d.
    hypersynchronous neuronal d.
    myotonic d.
    nervous d.
    neural d.
    periodic lateralized
      epileptiform d's (PLEDs)
    polysynaptic reflex d.
    pseudomyotonic d.
    systolic d.
    d. tube
disci (genitive and plural of discus)
disciform
disciplinary
discission
    d. of cataract
    d. of pleura
    d. of lens
    posterior d.
disclination
disclosing
disclusion
discoblastic
discogenic
discoid
    d. aortic prosthesis
    d. lupus erythematosus
discoloration
disconjugate gaze
disconnection
discontinuity
    ossicular d.
discopathy
    traumatic d.
discophorous
discoplacenta
discord
discordance
    atrioventricular d.

D

discordance *(continued)*
    ventriculoarterial d.
discordant
discrepancy
    tooth size d.
discrete
    d. area of consolidation
    d. area of effusion
    d. disease
    d. downward drifting
    d. focal stenosis
    d. lesion
    d. masses
    d. narrowing
    d. nodule
    d. organ enlargement
    d. plaque
    d. slowing
    d. thyromegaly
    d. weakness
discrimination
    pitch d.
    speech d.
    tactile d.
    tonal d.
    two-point d.
discriminator
    pulse-height d.
discus (disci)
    d. articularis
    d. interpubicus
    d. intervertebralis
    d. nervi optici
    d. oophorus
    d. opticus
    d. ovigerus
discutient
disdiaclast
disease
    Abrami d.
    Acosta d.
    acute demyelinating d.
    Adams d.
    Adams-Stokes d.
    d's of adaptation
    Addison d.
    Addison-Gull d.
    adenocystic d.
    adult celiac d.
    airflow obstruction d.
      (AOD)
    air space d.
    akamushi d.
    Akureyri d.
    Åland eye d.

disease *(continued)*
    Albers-Schönberg
      (Albers-Schoenberg) d.
    Albert d.
    Albright d.
    Alexander d.
    Alibert d.
    alkali d.
    allogeneic d.
    Almeida d.
    Alpers d.
    alpha chain d.
    Alport d.
    Alström (Alstrom) d.
    altitude d.
    alveolar hydatid d.
    Alzheimer d.
    amyloid d.
    Anders d.
    Andersen d.
    Anderson-Fabry d.
    Andes d.
    Andrews d.
    angiospasmodic d.
    anti–glomerular basement
      membrane (anti-GBM)
      antibody d.
    aortoiliac occlusive d.
    apatite deposition d.
    Apert d.
    Apert-Crouzon d.
    Aran-Duchenne d.
    arc welders' d.
    Arlt d.
    Armenian d.
    Armstrong d.
    Arndt-Gottron d.
    Asboe-Hansen d.
    atheroembolic renal d.
    atopic d.
    attic d.
    Aufrecht d.
    Australian X d.
    autoimmune d. (AID)
    autologous immune complex d.
    aviators' d.
    Ayerza d.
    Azorean d.
    Baastrup d.
    Baelz d.
    Ballet d.
    Ballingall d.
    Baló d.
    Bamberger d.
    Bamberger-Marie d.

disease *(continued)*
  Bannister d.
  Banti d.
  Barclay-Baron d.
  Barcoo d.
  Barlow d.
  barometer-makers' d.
  Barraquer d.
  Basedow d.
  Bassen-Kornzweig d.
  Bateman d.
  Batten d.
  Batten-Mayou d.
  bauxite workers' d.
  Bayle d.
  Bazin d.
  Beck d.
  Béguez César d.
  Behçet d.
  Behr d.
  Bekhterev (Bechterew) d.
  Bennett d.
  Benson d.
  Berger d.
  Berlin d.
  Bernard-Soulier d.
  Bernhardt d.
  Bernhardt-Roth d.
  Besnier-Boeck d.
  Besnier-Boeck-Schaumann d.
  Best d.
  Bettlach May d.
  Biedl d.
  Bielschowsky d.
  Bielschowsky-Jansky d.
  Bilderbeck d.
  Binswanger d.
  bird-breeders' d.
  black d.
  black lung d.
  bleeders' d.
  Blocq d.
  Bloodgood d.
  Blount d.
  Blumenthal d.
  Bodechtel-Guttmann d.
  Boeck d.
  Bornholm d.
  Bostock d.
  Boston exanthem d.
  Bouchard d.
  Bouchet-Gsell d.
  Bouillaud d.
  Bourneville d.
  Bourneville-Brissaud d.

disease *(continued)*
  Bourneville-Crouzon d.
  Bouveret d.
  Bowen d.
  Bradley d.
  brass-founders' d.
  Breda d.
  Breisky d.
  Bretonneau d.
  Breutsch d.
  bridegrooms' d.
  Bright d.
  Brill d.
  Brill-Symmers d.
  Brill-Zinsser d.
  Brinton d.
  Brion-Kayser d.
  broad-beta d.
  Brodie d.
  Brooke d.
  Brown-Séquard d.
  Brown-Symmers d.
  Bruck d.
  Brühl (Bruehl) d.
  Brushfield-Wyatt d.
  Bruton d.
  Budd-Chiari d.
  Buerger d.
  Buhl d.
  Buschke d.
  Busquet d.
  Buss d.
  Busse-Buschke d.
  Byler d.
  Cacchi-Ricci d.
  Caffey d.
  Caffey-Kenny d.
  caisson d.
  calcium hydroxyapatite
    deposition d.
  calcium pyrophosphate
    deposition d. (CPDD)
  California d.
  Calvé d.
  Calvé-Perthes d.
  Camurati-Engelmann d.
  Canavan d.
  Canavan-van Bogaert-
    Bertrand d.
  candle wax d.
  Cannon d.
  carcinoid heart d.
  Caroli d.
  Carrión d.
  Castellani d.

D

disease *(continued)*

cat-bite d.
cat-scratch d.
Cavare d.
Cazenave d.
celiac d.
central core d. of muscle
central nervous system d.
Chagas d.
Chagas-Cruz d.
Chandler d.
Charcot d.
Charcot-Marie-Tooth d.
Charcot-Marie-Tooth-Hoffman d.
Charlouis d.
Cheadle d.
Chédiak-Higashi d.
Cherchewski d.
Chester d.
Chiari d.
Chiari-Frommel d.
Chicago d.
cholesteryl ester storage d. (CESD)
Christensen-Krabbe d.
Christian-Weber d.
Christmas d.
chronic granulomatous d. (CGD)
Ciarrocchi d.
coast d.
Coats d.
Cogan d.
cold agglutinin d.
cold hemolytic antibody d.
collagen d.
collagen vascular d.
combined immunodeficiency d.
combined system d.
communicable d.
complicating d.
compressed-air d.
Concato d.
congenital d.
congenital cystic d. of liver
congenital heart d. (CHD)
congestive heart d. (CHD)
connective tissue d.
Conor d.
Conradi d.
constitutional d.
contagious d.
Cooley d.
Cooper d.

disease *(continued)*

copper storage d.
Corbus d.
Cori d.
coronary artery d. (CAD)
coronary heart d. (CHD)
Corridor d.
Corrigan d.
Corvisart d.
Cotugno d.
Cowden d.
CPPD (calcium pyrophosphate deposition) d.
creeping d.
Creutzfeldt-Jakob d.
Crigler-Najjar d.
Crocq d.
Crohn d.
Crouzon d.
Cruveilhier d.
Cruz-Chagas d.
Curschmann d.
Cushing d.
cyanotic heart d.
cystic d. of breast
cystic d. of kidney, acquired
cystic d. of lung
cysticercus d.
cystine d.
cystine storage d.
cytomegalic inclusion d. (CID, CMID)
cytomegalovirus d.
Czerny d.
Daae d.
Daae-Finsen d.
Dalrymple d.
Danielssen d.
Danielssen-Boeck d.
Danlos d.
Darier d.
Darier-White d.
Darling d.
David d.
Debove d.
debrancher glycogen storage d.
decompression d.
deficiency d.
degenerative joint d.
Degos d.
Dejerine d.
Dejerine-Sottas d.
demyelinating d.
dense-deposit d.
deprivation d.

disease *(continued)*
    de Quervain d.
    Dercum d.
    Desnos d.
    Deutschländer d.
    Devergie d.
    Devic d.
    Dieulafoy d.
    Dimitri d.
    disappearing bone d.
    diverticular d.
    Döhle d.
    Down d.
    Dressler d.
    drug d.
    Dubini d.
    Dubois d.
    Duchenne d.
    Duchenne-Aran d.
    Duchenne-Griesinger d.
    Ducrey d.
    Duhring d.
    Dukes d.
    Duncan d.
    Duplay d.
    Dupré d.
    Dupuytren d. of foot
    Durand d.
    Durand-Nicolas-Favre d.
    Durante d.
    Duroziez d.
    Dutton d.
    Eales d.
    Ebola virus d.
    Ebstein d.
    echinococcus d.
    Economo (von Economo) d.
    Edsall d.
    Ehlers-Danlos d.
    Eisenmenger d.
    elevator d.
    endemic d.
    endocrine d.
    end-stage renal d. (ESRD)
    Engelmann d.
    Engel-Recklinghausen d.
    Engman d.
    eosinophilic endomyocardial d.
    epidemic d.
    Epstein d.
    Erb d.
    Erb-Charcot d.
    Erb-Goldflam d.
    Erb-Landouzy d.
    Erichsen d.

disease *(continued)*
    Eulenburg d.
    euthyroid Graves d.
    extramammary Paget d.
    extrapyramidal d.
    Fabry d.
    factor X deficiency d.
    Fahr d.
    Fahr-Volhard d.
    Fallot d.
    familial hypophosphatemic
      bone d.
    Fanconi d.
    Farber d.
    fat-deficiency d.
    Fauchard d.
    Favre d.
    Favre-Durand-Nicolas d.
    Fazio-Londe d.
    Feer d.
    Fenwick d.
    fibrocystic d.
    fibrocystic d. of breast
    fibrocystic d. of the pancreas
    fibromuscular d.
    Fiedler d.
    fifth d.
    Filatov (Filatow) d.
    Filatov-Dukes d.
    file-cutters' d.
    Flajani d.
    Flatau-Schilder d.
    flax-dressers' d.
    flecked retina d.
    Flegel d.
    Fleischner d.
    flint d.
    fluke d.
    focal d.
    Foix-Alajouanine d.
    Fölling d.
    foot process d.
    Forbes d.
    Fordyce d.
    Forestier d.
    Förster d.
    Fothergill d.
    Fournier d.
    fourth d.
    Fox d.
    Fox-Fordyce d.
    Franceschetti d.
    Francis d.
    Frankl-Hochwart d.
    Franklin d.

D

disease *(continued)*
  Frei d.
  Freiberg d.
  Friedländer d.
  Friedmann d.
  Friedreich d.
  Frommel d.
  functional d.
  functional cardiovascular d.
  Fürstner (Fuerstner) d.
  Gaisböck d.
  gamma chain d.
  gamma heavy chain d.
  Gamna d.
  Gamstorp d.
  Gandy-Gamna d.
  Gandy-Nanta d.
  ganglioside storage d.
  Garré d.
  Gastaut d.
  gastroesophageal reflux d.
    (GERD)
  Gaucher d.
  Gayet d.
  Gee d.
  Gee-Herter d.
  Gee-Herter-Heubner d.
  Gee-Thaysen d.
  genetic d.
  genetotrophic d.
  Gerhardt d.
  Gerlier d.
  giant platelet d.
  Gibert d.
  Gibney d.
  Gierke d.
  Gilbert d.
  Gilchrist d.
  Gilles d.
  Gilles de la Tourette d.
  Glanzmann d.
  Glasser d.
  Glénard d.
  Glisson d.
  glomerular epithelial cell d.
  glycogen storage d.
  Goldflam d.
  Goldflam-Erb d.
  Goldstein d.
  Gowers d.
  Graefe d.
  graft-versus-host d. (GVHD;
    GVH d.)
  Graves d.
  Greenfield d.

disease *(continued)*
  grinders' d.
  Grisel d.
  Gross d.
  Guinon d.
  Gull d.
  Gumboro d.
  Günther d.
  GVH (graft-versus-host) d.
  Habermann d.
  Haff d.
  Hageman d.
  Haglund d.
  Hailey-Hailey d.
  Halban d.
  Hallervorden-Spatz d.
  Hallopeau d.
  Hamman d.
  Hamman-Rich d.
  Hammond d.
  Hand d.
  Hand-Schüller-Christian d.
  Hanot d.
  Hansen d.
  Harada d.
  hard metal d.
  Harley d.
  Hartnup d.
  Hashimoto d.
  heart d.
  heavy chain d.
  Heberden d.
  Hebra d.
  Heerfordt d.
  Heine-Medin d.
  Heller d.
  Heller-Döhle d.
  helminthic d.
  hemoglobin d.
  hemoglobin C–thalassemia d.
  hemoglobin E–thalassemia d.
  hemolytic d. of the newborn
  hemorrhagic d. of the newborn
  Henderson-Jones d.
  Henneberg d.
  Henoch d.
  hepatic venous web d.
  hepatobiliary tract d.
  hepatolenticular d.
  hepatorenal glycogen storage d.
  hereditary d.
  heredoconstitutional d.
  heredodegenerative d.
  Herlitz d.
  Hers d.

disease *(continued)*

    Herter d.
    Herter-Heubner d.
    Heubner d.
    Heubner-Herter d.
    HIB (*Haemophilus influenzae* type b) d.
    Hildenbrand d.
    hip-joint d.
    Hippel d.
    Hippel-Lindau d.
    Hirschsprung d.
    His d.
    His-Werner d.
    Hodgkin d.
    Hodgson d.
    Hoffa d.
    Hoffa-Kastert d.
    holoendemic d.
    homozygous hemoglobin S d.
    hookworm d.
    Horton d.
    Huchard d.
    Hünermann d.
    hungry d.
    Hunt d.
    Huntington d.
    Hurler d.
    Hurst d.
    Hutchinson d.
    Hutchinson-Boeck d.
    Hutchinson-Gilford d.
    Hutinel d.
    hyaline membrane d.
    hydatid d.
    hydatid d., alveolar
    hydatid d., unilocular
    Hyde d.
    hyperendemic d.
    hypertensive heart d.
    hypertensive renal d.
    hypertensive vascular d.
    hypopigmentation-immunodeficiency d.
    Iceland d.
    I-cell d.
    idiopathic d.
    immune-complex d's
    immunodeficiency d.
    immunoproliferative small intestine d.
    inborn lysosomal d's
    inclusion d.
    infantile celiac d.
    infectious d.

disease *(continued)*

    inflammatory bowel d. (IBD)
    inherited d.
    intercurrent d.
    interstitial d. (ID)
    interstitial lung d.
    iron storage d.
    irritable bowel d. (IBD)
    ischemic bowel d.
    ischemic heart d. (IHD)
    itai-itai d.
    Itsenko d.
    Jadassohn d.
    Jaffe d.
    Jaffe-Lichtenstein d.
    Jakob d.
    Jakob-Creutzfeldt d.
    Janet d.
    Jansen d.
    Jansky-Bielschowsky d.
    Jensen d.
    Jessner-Kanof d.
    Johne d.
    Johnson-Stevens d.
    Joseph d.
    jumper d. of Maine
    juvenile Paget d.
    Kahlbaum d.
    Kahler d.
    Kaiserstuhl d.
    Kalischer d.
    Kaposi d.
    Kartagener d.
    Kashin-Bek (Kaschin-Beck) d.
    Kawasaki d.
    Kienböck d.
    Kimmelstiel-Wilson d. (K-W d.)
    Kimura d.
    Kinnier Wilson d.
    Kirkland d.
    kissing d.
    Klebs d.
    Klemperer d.
    Klippel d.
    Köbner (Koebner) d.
    Koeppe d.
    Köhler bone d.
    Köhler-Pellegrini-Stieda d.
    Köhler second d.
    Kohlmeier-Degos d.
    König (Koenig) d.
    Korsakoff d.
    Kostmann d.
    Kozhevnikov (Koshevnikoff, Koschewnikow) d.

D

disease *(continued)*
    Krabbe d.
    Krishaber d.
    Kufs d.
    Kugelberg-Welander d.
    Kuhnt-Junius d.
    Kümmell d.
    Kümmell-Verneuil d.
    Kussmaul d.
    Kussmaul-Maier d.
    Kyasanur Forest d.
    Kyrle d.
    laboratory d.
    Laënnec d.
    Lancereaux-Mathieu d.
    Landouzy d.
    Landry d.
    Lane d.
    Langdon Down d.
    Larrey-Weil d.
    Larsen d.
    Larsen-Johansson d.
    Lauber d.
    laughing d.
    Leber d.
    Lederer d.
    Legal d.
    Legg d.
    Legg-Calvé d.
    Legg-Calvé-Perthes d.
    Legg-Calvé-Waldenström d.
    legionnaires' d.
    Leigh d.
    Leiner d.
    Leloir d.
    Lemierre d.
    Lenègre d.
    Leriche d.
    Letterer-Siwe d.
    Lev d.
    Lewandowsky-Lutz d.
    Leyden d.
    Libman-Sacks d.
    Lichtheim d.
    Lignac d.
    Lignac-Fanconi d.
    Lindau d.
    Lindau-von Hippel d.
    lipid storage d.
    Lipschütz (Lipschuetz) d.
    Little d.
    Lobo d.
    Lobstein d.
    local d.
    Löffler d.

disease *(continued)*
    Lorain d.
    Lortat-Jacobs d.
    Louis-Bar d.
    Lowe d.
    L-S (Letterer-Siwe) d.
    Lucas-Championnière d.
    Luft d.
    lunger d.
    lung fluke d.
    Lutembacher d.
    Lutz-Miescher d.
    Lutz-Splendore-Almeida d.
    Lyell d.
    Lyme d.
    lysosomal storage d.
    MAC (*Mycobacterium avium* complex) d.
    Machado-Joseph d.
    Mackenzie d.
    MacLean-Maxwell d.
    Madelung d.
    Majocchi d.
    malabsorption d.
    Malassez d.
    Malibu d.
    mammary Paget d.
    Manson d.
    maple bark d.
    maple syrup urine d. (MSUD)
    marble bone d.
    Marburg d.
    March d.
    Marchiafava-Bignami d.
    Marchiafava-Micheli d.
    Marek d.
    Marie-Bamberger d.
    Marie-Strümpell d.
    Marie-Tooth d.
    Marion d.
    Maroteaux-Lamy d.
    Marsh d.
    Martin d.
    mast cell d.
    Mathieu d.
    McArdle d.
    medullary cystic d.
    Meige d.
    Meleda d.
    Melnick-Needles d.
    Ménétrier d.
    Ménière d.
    Menkes d.
    mental d.
    Merzbacher-Pelizaeus d.

disease *(continued)*
    metabolic d.
    metazoan d.
    Meyenburg d.
    Meyer d.
    Meyer-Betz d.
    Miana d.
    Mianeh d.
    Mibelli d.
    microcystic d.
    microdrepanocytic d.
    Mikulicz d.
    Miller d.
    Mills d.
    Milroy d.
    Milton d.
    Minamata d.
    minimal change d.
    Minor d.
    Mitchell d.
    mixed connective tissue d.
    mixed cryoglobulin d.
    Möbius d.
    Moeller-Barlow d.
    molecular d.
    Molten d.
    Mondor d.
    Monge d.
    Morel-Kraepelin d.
    Morquio d.
    Morquio-Ullrich d.
    Mortimer d.
    Morton d.
    Morvan d.
    Moschcowitz d.
    motor neuron d.
    Mouchet d.
    moyamoya d.
    Mozer d.
    Mucha d.
    Mucha-Habermann d.
    mu chain d.
    mu heavy chain d.
    multisystem d.
    Münchmeyer d.
    Murray Valley d.
    mushroom pickers' d.
    mushroom workers' d.
    Mycobacterium avium
        complex d.
    Neumann d.
    Newcastle d.
    Nicolas-Favre d.
    Niemann d.
    Niemann-Pick d.

disease *(continued)*
    nil d.
    Nonne-Milroy d.
    Norrie d.
    Norum-Gjone d.
    nosocomial d.
    notifiable d.
    obstructive small airways d.
    occupational d.
    Oguchi d.
    Ohara d.
    oid-oid d.
    Ollier d.
    Ondiri d.
    ophthalmic Graves d.
    Opitz d.
    Oppenheim d.
    organic d.
    Oriental lung fluke d.
    Ormond d.
    Osgood-Schlatter d.
    Osler d.
    Osler-Vaquez d.
    Osler-Weber-Rendu d.
    Otto d.
    Owren d.
    Paas d.
    Paget d.
    Paget d. of bone
    Paget d., extramammary
    Paget d. of the nipple
    Paget d. of penis
    Panner d.
    parenchymatous d.
    Parkinson d.
    Parry d.
    Parsons d.
    Pavy d.
    Payr d.
    pearl-workers' d.
    Pel-Ebstein d.
    Pelizaeus-Merzbacher d.
    Pellegrini d.
    Pellegrini-Stieda d.
    pelvic inflammatory d.
    Pendred d.
    peptic ulcer d. (PUD)
    periodic d.
    periodontal d.
    Perrin-Ferraton d.
    Perthes d.
    Peyronie d.
    Pfeiffer d.
    Phocas d.
    phytanic acid storage d.

disease *(continued)*

Pick d.
Pictou d.
pigeon breeders' d.
pink d.
plaster-of-Paris d.
Plummer d.
pneumatic hammer d.
policeman's d.
polycystic hydatid d.
polycystic d. of kidneys
polycystic ovary d.
polycystic renal d.
polyendocrine autoimmune d.
Pompe d.
Poncet d.
Portuguese-Azorean d.
Posadas-Wernicke d.
Pott d.
Potter d.
Preiser d.
Profichet d.
pseudo-Hurler d.
pseudo-Pott d.
psychosomatic d.
pulmonary embolic d.
pulmonary heart d.
pulseless d.
Purtscher d.
Pyle d.
pyramidal d.
Quervain (de Quervain) d.
Quincke d.
ragpickers' d.
ragsorters' d.
Ramsay Hunt d.
Rayer d.
Raynaud d.
Recklinghausen d.
Recklinghausen-Applebaum d.
Recklinghausen d. of bone
Reclus d.
Reed-Hodgkin d.
Refsum d.
Reichmann d.
Reis-Bücklers d.
Reiter d.
renal artery d.
renal cystic d.
Rendu-Osler-Weber d.
reportable d.
rheumatic heart d.
rheumatoid d.
Ribas-Torres d.
rice d.

disease *(continued)*

Riedel d.
Riga-Fede d.
Riggs d.
Ritter d.
Robinson d.
Robles d.
Roger d.
Rokitansky d.
Romberg d.
Rossbach d.
Roth (Rot) d.
Roth-Bernhardt d.
Rougnon-Heberden d.
Roussy-Lévy d.
Royal Free d.
Rubarth d.
Rummo d.
Runeberg d.
Rust d.
Ruysch d.
Sachs d.
sacroiliac d.
salivary gland d.
Sanders d.
Sandhoff d.
sandworm d.
Sanfilippo d.
San Joaquin Valley d.
Saunders d.
Schamberg d.
Schanz d.
Schaumann d.
Scheuermann d.
Schilder d.
Schimmelbusch d.
Schlatter d.
Schlatter-Osgood d.
Schmorl d.
Scholz d.
Scholz-Greenfield d.
Schönlein d.
Schönlein-Henoch d.
Schottmüller (Schottmueller) d.
Schroeder d.
Schüller d.
Schüller-Christian d.
Schultz d.
Schwediauer d.
sclerocystic d.
secondary d.
Seitelberger d.
self-limited d.
Selter d.
Senear-Usher d.

disease *(continued)*
   senecio d.
   septic d.
   Sever d.
   severe combined
     immunodeficiency d. (SCID)
   sexually transmitted d. (STD)
   Shaver d.
   Sheehan d.
   sickle cell d.
   sickle cell–hemoglobin C d.
   sickle cell–hemoglobin D d.
   sickle cell–thalassemia d.
   silo fillers' d.
   Simmonds d.
   Simons d.
   Sinding-Larsen-Johansson d.
   sixth d.
   Sjögren d.
   Skevas-Zerfus d.
   sleeping d.
   small airways d.
   small-vessel d.
   Smith-Strang d.
   Sneddon-Wilkinson d.
   Sottas d.
   specific d.
   Spencer d.
   Spielmeyer-Vogt d.
   spinocerebellar degenerative d.
   sponge-divers' d.
   Stanton d.
   Stargardt d.
   Steinert d.
   Sternberg d.
   Stevens-Johnson d.
   Sticker d.
   Stieda d.
   Still d.
   Stokes-Adams d.
   storage d.
   storage pool d.
   Strachan d.
   structural d.
   Strümpell d.
   Strümpell-Leichtenstern d.
   Strümpell-Marie d.
   Stuart-Bras d.
   Stuart-Prower factor
     deficiency d.
   Stühmer (Stuehmer) d.
   Sturge d.
   Sturge-Weber d.
   Sturge-Weber-Dimitri d.
   Stuttgart d.

disease *(continued)*
   Sudeck d.
   Sutton d.
   Swediaur d.
   Swift d.
   Swift-Feer d.
   swineherders' d.
   Sylvest d.
   Symmers d.
   systemic d.
   Taenzer d.
   Takahara d.
   Takayasu d.
   Talfan d.
   Talma d.
   Tangier d.
   Tarui d.
   Taussig-Bing d.
   Tay d.
   Tay-Sachs d. (TSD)
   Teschen d.
   thalassemia–sickle cell d.
   Thaysen d.
   Theiler d.
   Thiemann d.
   Thomsen d.
   Thomson d.
   thyrocardiac d.
   thyrotoxic heart d.
   Tietze d.
   Tillaux d.
   Tommaselli d.
   Tornwaldt (Thornwaldt) d.
   Tourette d.
   transplantation d.
   Traum d.
   Trevor d.
   Trinidad d.
   tubotympanic d.
   tunnel d.
   Underwood d.
   unilocular hydatid d.
   Unna-Thost d.
   Unverricht d.
   Urbach-Oppenheim d.
   Urbach-Wiethe d.
   uremic bone d.
   uremic medullary cystic d.
   Usher d.
   vagabonds' d.
   vagrants' d.
   valvular d.
   valvular heart d.
   van Bogaert-Bertrand d.
   van Bogaert-Nyssen-Peiffer d.

D

disease *(continued)*
- van Buchem d.
- Vaquez d.
- Vaquez-Osler d.
- venereal d.
- veno-occlusive d. of the liver
- Verneuil d.
- Verse d.
- vibration d.
- Vincent d.
- vinyl chloride d.
- Virchow d.
- Vogt d.
- Vogt-Spielmeyer d.
- Volkmann d.
- Voltolini d.
- von Economo d.
- von Gierke d.
- von Hippel-Lindau d.
- von Recklinghausen d.
- von Willebrand d.
- Voorhoeve d.
- Vrolik d.
- Waardenburg d.
- Wagner d.
- Waldenström d.
- Wartenberg d.
- Wassilieff d.
- wasting d.
- Weber d.
- Weber-Christian d.
- Weber-Dimitri d.
- Wegner d.
- Weil d.
- Weir Mitchell
- Wenckebach d.
- Werdnig-Hoffmann d.
- Werlhof d.
- Werner d.
- Werner-His d.
- Werner Schultz d.
- Wernicke d.
- Wesselsbron d.
- Westphal-Strümpell d.
- Wetherbee d.
- Whipple d.
- White d.
- Whitmore d.
- Whytt d.
- Widal-Abrami d.
- Wilkins d.
- Willis d.
- Wilson d.
- Winiwarter-Buerger d.
- Winkelman d.

disease *(continued)*
- Winkler d.
- Winton d.
- Witkop d.
- Witkop-Von Sallmann d.
- Wolman d.
- woolsorters' d.
- Woringer-Kolopp d.
- x d.
- X-linked lymphoproliferative d.
- Zahorsky d.
- Ziehen-Oppenheim d.

disengagement

disequilibration

disequilibrium
- linkage d.

disesthesia

dish
- culture d.
- dappen d.
- evaporating d.
- Petri d.
- Stender d's

disharmony
- maxillomandibular d.
- occlusal d.

DISI—dorsiflexion intercalated segment instability

DISIDA—diisopropyliminodiacetic acid

disinfect

disinfectant
- coal tar d.

disinfection
- concomitant d.
- concurrent d.
- terminal d.

disinfestation

disinhibition

disinsertion of the retina

disintegration
- radioactive d.
- spontaneous d.
- d. rate

disintegrator

disjoint

disjunction
- craniofacial d.

disjunctive

disk
- A d.
- abrasive d.
- acromioclavicular d.
- Amici d.
- anangioid d.

disk *(continued)*
    anisotropic d.
    anisotropous d.
    articular d.
    Bardeen primitive d.
    bilaminar embryonic d.
    Blake d.
    blastodermic d.
    blood d.
    Bowman d's
    Carborundum d.
    cartilaginous d.
    choked d.
    ciliary d.
    cloth d.
    contained d.
    cupped d.
    cutting d.
    cuttlefish d.
    dental d.
    d. diameter
    diamond d.
    d. drusen
    ectodermal d.
    embryonic d.
    emery d.
    Engelmann d.
    epiphyseal d.
    equatorial d.
    extruded d.
    floppy d.
    gelatin d.
    germinal d.
    growth d.
    hair d.
    Hensen d.
    herniated d.
    I d.
    interarticular d.
    intercalated d's
    intermediate d.
    interpubic d.
    intervertebral d.
    intra-articular d.
    isotropic d.
    J d.
    M d.
    mandibular d.
    Merkel d's
    micrometer d.
    Miller d.
    Newton d.
    noncontained d.
    nuclear d.
    optic d.

disk *(continued)*
    pinhole d.
    Placido d.
    polishing d.
    proligerous d.
    protruded d.
    Q d.
    Ranvier tactile d's
    Rekoss d.
    ruptured d.
    sandpaper d.
    sarcous d.
    Schiefferdecker d.
    sequestered d.
    slipped d.
    stenopeic d.
    sternoclavicular d.
    d. of striated muscle fibers
    stroboscopic d.
    tactile d.
    thin d.
    transverse d.
    triangular d. of wrist
    Z d.
diskectomy
    anterior cervical d. and fusion
      (ACDF)
    automatized percutaneous d.
    cervical d.
    lumbar d.
    microscopic d.
    percutaneous transforaminal
      endoscopic d. (PTED)
    spinal d.
diskiform
diskitis
diskography
diskopathy, discopathy
disk valve prosthesis
dislocate, dislocated
dislocatio erecta
dislocation
    anterior d.
    anterior shoulder d.
    d. of articular processes
    Bell-Dally d.
    Bennett d.
    central d.
    Chopart d.
    closed d.
    complete d.
    complicated d.
    compound d.
    congenital d.
    consecutive d.

dislocation *(continued)*
  divergent d.
  fracture-d.
  frank d.
  habitual d.
  incomplete d.
  incudomallear d.
  incudostapedial d.
  intrauterine d.
  Kienböck d.
  Lisfranc d.
  Monteggia d.
  Nélaton d.
  obturator d.
  old d.
  open d.
  paralytic d.
  partial d.
  pathologic d.
  perilunate d.
  posterior d.
  posterior shoulder d.
  primitive d.
  recent d.
  recurrent d.
  sciatic d.
  simple d.
  Smith d.
  subastragalar d.
  subclavicular d.
  subcoracoid d.
  subglenoid d.
  subspinous d.
  d. of the lens
  traumatic d.
  unifacet d.
  unreduced d.
  vertebral d.
  voluntary d.
dislodger
  stone d.
dismemberment
dismutation
disocclude
disorder
  adjustment d.
  affective d.
  aggressive behavior d.
  alcoholic brain d's
  amnestic d's
  antisocial personality d.
  anxiety d.
  appetite d.
  arteriosclerotic brain d.
  attention deficit d. (ADD)

disorder *(continued)*
  attention deficit hyperactivity
    d. (ADHD)
  attention deficit d. with
    hyperactivity (ADDH)
  autistic d.
  autonomic d.
  avoidant d. of childhood or
    adolescence
  avoidant personality d.
  behavior d.
  bipolar d.
  body dysmorphic d.
  borderline personality d.
  brain d.
  cerebelloparenchymal d.
  character d's
  character impulse d.
  collagen d.
  conduct d.
  consumptive
    thrombohemorrhagic d.
  conversion d.
  cycloid personality d.
  cyclothymic d.
  delusional d.
  delusional paranoid d.
  dependent personality d.
  depersonalization d.
  dissociative d.
  dysthymic d.
  eating d.
  emotional d.
  epileptoid personality d.
  equilibratory d.
  extrapyramidal d.
  factitious d.
  functional d.
  generalized anxiety d.
  genetic d.
  gnostic d's
  habit d.
  hereditary d.
  histrionic personality d.
  hyperkinetic impulse d.
  identity d.
  immunodeficiency d.
  immunoproliferative d.
  impulse d.
  induced psychotic d.
  intermittent explosive d.
  isolated explosive d.
  late luteal phase dysphoric d.
  LDL-receptor d.
  major mood d's

disorder *(continued)*
   manic-depressive d.
   mendelian d.
   mental d.
   monogenic d.
   mood d's
   motility d.
   multifactorial d.
   multiple personality d.
   narcissistic personality d.
   neurotic depressive d.
   obsessive-compulsive d. (OCD)
   obsessive-compulsive
     personality d.
   organic mental d.
   overanxious d.
   panic d.
   panic d. without agoraphobia
   paranoid d.
   paranoid personality d.
   passive-aggressive
     personality d.
   personality d.
   pervasive developmental d's
   post-traumatic personality d.
   post-traumatic stress d. (PTSD)
   psychoactive substance use d's
   psychogenic pain d.
   psychophysiologic d.
   psychosexual d.
   psychosomatic d.
   sadistic personality d.
   schizoaffective d.
   schizoid personality d.
   schizophrenic d.
   schizophreniform d.
   schizothymic personality
   schizotypal personality d.
   seasonal mood d.
   self-defeating personality d.
   separation anxiety d.
   shared paranoid d.
   single-gene d.
   sleep terror d.
   sleepwalking d.
   somatization d.
   somatoform d.
   somatoform pain d.
   stress d.
   substance use d's
   thought d.
   Tourette d.
   transient situational
     personality d.
   unipolar d's

disorder *(continued)*
   vibration d.
disorganization
disorientation
   right-left d.
   spatial d.
disoxidation
dispar
disparate
disparity
dispensary
dispense
dispermy
dispersal
   flash d.
dispersate
disperse
dispersible
dispersion
   chromatic d.
   colloid d.
   d. of light
   molecular d.
   optical rotatory d.
displaceability
displacement
   condylar d.
   fetal d.
   fish-hook d.
   gallbladder d.
   mesial d.
   d. osteotomy
   Proetz d.
   tissue d.
display
   real-time d.
disposable sigmoidoscope
disposition
disproportion
   borderline pelvic d.
   cephalopelvic d.
   fiber-type d.
disruption
disruptive
dissecans
   Cahill type 2-C
     osteochondritis d.
   esophagitis d.
   osteochondritis d.
dissect
dissecting
   d. aortic aneurysm
   d. cellulitis
   d. hematoma
   d. microscope

D

dissection
    aortic d.
    arterial d.
    axillary lymph node d.
    block d.
    blunt d.
    lymph node d.
    radical neck d.
    sharp d.
    suprahyoid neck d.
    supraomohyoid neck d.
dissector
    Brunner d.
    Cavitron d.
    Fisher d.
    Green d.
    Holinger d.
    Hurd d.
    Kocher d.
    Lewin d.
    Lynch d.
    Oldberg d.
    Pierce d.
    Roger d.
    Sheldon-Pudenz d.
    ultrasonic d.
    Walker d.
    Wangensteen d.
    water-jet d.
Dissectron
disseminated lupus erythematosus
    (DLE)
Disse spaces
dissimilate
dissimilation
dissipate
dissociable
dissociated
    d. nystagmus
    d. position
    d. vertical deviation
    d. vertical divergence (DVD)
dissociation
    albuminocytologic d.
    atrial d.
    atrioventricular (AV) d.
    electromechanical d.
    interference d.
    longitudinal d.
    Mobitz-type atrioventricular d.
    peripheral d.
    syringomyelic d.
    tabetic d.
dissociative
    d. disorder

dissociative *(continued)*
    d. identity disorder
    d. trance disorder
dissolution
dissolve
dissolvent
dissonance
    cognitive d.
distad
distal
distalis
distally
distance
    angular d.
    cone-surface d.
    focal d.
    focal skin d.
    infinite d.
    interarch d.
    interocclusal d.
    interocular d.
    interorbital d.
    interpediculate d.
    interpupillary d.
    interridge d.
    map d.
    object-film d.
    source-skin d.
    target-skin d.
    vertex d.
    working d.
distend, distended
distensibility
distention
distichiasis
distichous
distill
distillate
distillation
    cold d.
    destructive d.
    dry d.
    fractional d.
    molecular d.
    vacuum d.
distoaxiogingival
distoaxioincisal
distoaxio-occlusal
distobuccal
distobucco-occlusal
distobuccopulpal
distocervical
distoclination
distoclusion
distogingival

distolabial
distolabioincisal
distolingual
distolinguoincisal
distolinguo-occlusal
distolinguopulpal
distomia
distomiasis
    hepatic d.
    intestinal d.
    pulmonary d.
distomolar
distomus
disto-occlusal
distoplacement
distopulpal
distopulpolabial
distopulpolingual
distortion
    apperceptive d.
    parataxic d.
    pin-cushion d.
distortor
    d. oris
distoversion
distractibility
distraction
distraught
distress
    acute respiratory d.
    fetal d.
    idiopathic respiratory d. of
      newborn
distribution
    age d.
    continuous d.
    depth dose d.
    discontinuous d.
    discrete d.
    dose d.
    isodose d.
    saddle d.
    spatial dose d.
    stocking-glove d.
districhiasis
distrix
disturbance
    emotional d.
    personality pattern d.
    personality trait d.
    sexual orientation d.
    transient situational d.
disulfate
disulfide
dithiol

Dittel
    operation
    sound
diurese
diuresis (diureses)
    alcohol d.
    osmotic d.
    tubular d.
    water d.
diuretic
    cardiac d.
    d. effect
    high-ceiling d's
    loop d.
    mercurial d's
    osmotic d's
    potassium-sparing d.
    thiazide d's
diuria
diurnal
divagation
divarication
divergence
    d. amplitudes
    beam d.
    dissociated vertical d. (DVD)
    d. excess
    d. insufficiency
    negative vertical d. (−V.D.)
    positive vertical d. (+V.D.)
divergent
diversion
    antigenic d.
    ileal conduit d.
    ileocecal cutaneous d.
    jejunal cutaneous urinary d.
    Leadbetter ileal loop d.
    urinary d.
diversity
diverticula (plural of diverticulum)
diverticular
diverticularization
diverticulectomy
diverticulitis
diverticulogram
diverticuloma
diverticulopexy
diverticulosis
    jejunal d.
diverticulum (diverticula)
    acquired d.
    d. ampullae ductus deferentis
    bladder d.
    caliceal d., calyceal d.
    cervical d.

diverticulum (diverticula)
   (continued)
      colonic diverticula
      congenital d.
      false d.
      functional d.
      ganglion d.
      Ganser d.
      Graser d.
      Heister d.
      hepatic d.
      intestinal d.
      jejunal d.
      Kirchner d.
      laryngeal d.
      Meckel d.
      midesophageal d.
      Nuck d.
      pancreatic diverticula
      Pertik d.
      pharyngeal d.
      pharyngoesophageal d.
      pituitary d.
      pressure d.
      pulsion d.
      Rokitansky d.
      supradiaphragmatic d.
      synovial d.
      thyroid d.
      tracheal d.
      traction d.
      ureteric d.
      urethral d.
      d. of utricle
      vesical d.
      Zenker d.
divisio (divisiones)
division
      anterior d's of brachial plexus
      autonomic d. of peripheral
         nervous system
      cell d.
      craniosacral d.
      dorsal d's of trunks of brachial
         plexus
      equational d.
      indirect nuclear d.
      mandibular d.
      maturation d.
      maxillary d.
      multiplicative d.
      posterior d's of brachial plexus
      reduction d.
      Remak d.
      thoracolumbar d.

division (continued)
      ventral d's of trunks of
         brachial plexus
divulse
divulsion
divulsor
Dix-Hallpike test
Dixon-Thomas-Smith clamp
Dix spud
dizygotic
dizziness
DJD—degenerative joint disease
djenkolic acid
djenkolism
DKA—diabetic ketoacidosis
dL, dl—deciliter
DL—
      danger list
      distolingual
      Donath-Landsteiner (test)
D_L, DL—diffusing capacity of lung
DLA—distolabial
DLAI—distolabioincisal
D_LCO, DLCO—diffusing capacity of
   lung for carbon monoxide
DLE—
      discoid lupus erythematosus
      disseminated lupus
         erythematosus
DLI—distolinguoincisal
DLO—distolinguo-occlusal
DLP—distolinguopulpal
DM—
      diabetes mellitus
      diabetic mother
      diastolic murmur
DMA—dimethyladenosine
DMARD—disease-modifying
   antirheumatic drug
DMBA—
   7,12-dimethylbenz[a]anthracene
DMD, D.M.D.—Doctor of Dental
   Medicine
DMF—
      decayed, missing, or filled
         (teeth)
      dimethylformamide
DMF index
DMN—dimethylnitrosamine
DMPE—3,4-
   dimethoxyphenylethylamine
DMS, DMSO—dimethyl sulfoxide
DN—dicrotic notch
D/N—dextrose-nitrogen ratio
   (quotient)

D&N—distance and near (vision)
DNA—deoxyribonucleic acid
DNA
  complementary DNA
  double-stranded DNA
  DNA library
  DNA ligase
  linker DNA
  native DNA
  DNA nucleotidyltransferase
  DNA polymerase
  recombinant DNA
  repetitive DNA
  satellite DNA
  single-copy DNA
  single-stranded DNA
  DNA topoisomerase
  transferred DNA
  unique DNA
  Z DNA
DNAase—deoxyribonuclease
DNA-directed DNA polymerase
DNA-directed RNA
  polymerase
DNB—dinitrobenzene
DNCB—dinitrochlorobenzene
DND—died a natural death
DNFB—dinitrofluorobenzene
DNP—deoxyribonucleoprotein
DNPH—dinitrophenylhydrazine
DNR—do not resuscitate
DNT—did not test
DO—
  diamine oxidase
  disto-occlusal
DO, D.O.—Doctor of
  Osteopathy
DOA—dead on arrival
DOB—date of birth
Dobbhoff feeding tube
Dobie
  globule
  layer
  line
DOC—
  deoxycholate
  died of other causes
Docke murmur
docking needle
DOCs—deoxycorticoids
DOD—
  date of death
  dead of disease
Döderlein (Doderlein)
  bacillus

Döderlein (Doderlein) *(continued)*
  laparoscopic-assisted
    hysterectomy
    operation
DOE—dyspnea on exertion
Doerfler-Stewart test
doffing
  donning and d.
Dogiel corpuscles
dogma
  central d.
Doherty implant
Döhle
  disease
  inclusion bodies
Döhle-Heller aortitis
Dohlman operation
dolabrate
Doléris operation
dolichocephalic
dolichocephaly
dolichocolon
dolichocranial
dolichoderus
dolichofacial
dolichohieric
dolichokerkic
dolichoknemic
dolichomorphic
dolichopellic
dolichopelvic
dolichoprosopic
dolichostenomelia
doll's eye
  reflex
  sign
  test
doll's head
  maneuver
  phenomenon
dolor (dolores)
  d. capitis
  d. coxae
  d's praesagientes
  d. vagus
dolorific
dolorimetry
DOM—
  deaminated-*o*-methyl
    metabolite
  2,5-dimethoxy-4-
    methylamphetamine
DOMA—dihydroxymandelic acid
domain
Dombrock blood group

dome
    d. osteotomy
    pleural d.
Domeboro
domiciliary
dominance
    cerebral d.
    conditioned d.
    incomplete d.
    lateral d.
    ocular d.
    one-sided d.
    partial d.
    reversed d. of eyes
dominance-submission
dominant
Donald operation
Donald-Fothergill operation
Donaldson tube
Donath test
Donath-Landsteiner
    antibody
    phenomenon
    syndrome
    test
Donders
    chart
    glaucoma
    law
    line
donee
Donné
    bodies
    corpuscles
donning
    d. and doffing
Donohue syndrome
donor
    d.-specific
    general d.
    universal d.
Donovan body
dopamine β-hydroxylase [beta-]
dopamine β-monooxygenase [beta-]
dopaminergic
Doppler
    directional Doppler
    echocardiography
    effect
    interrogation
    operation
    phenomenon
    principle
    pulse Doppler
    study

Doppler *(continued)*
    ultrasonography
    ultrasound
Dorello canal
Dorendorf sign
Dorian rib stripper
dormancy
dormant
Dormia
    basket
    stone dislodger
dormifacient
Dornavac
Dorn-Sugarman test
Dorothy Reed cells
Dorrance operation
dorsa (plural of dorsum)
dorsad
dorsal
    d. lithotomy position
    d. rhizotomy
dorsalgia
dorsalis pedis
dorsi (genitive of dorsum)
dorsiduct
dorsiflex
dorsiflexion
dorsiflexor
dorsispinal
dorsoanterior
dorsocephalad
dorsointercostal
dorsolateral incision
dorsolumbar
dorsomedial thalamotomy
dorsomedian
dorsomesial
dorsonasal
dorsonuchal
dorsoposterior
dorsoradial
dorsosacral
dorsoscapular
dorsoventrad
dorsoventral
dorsum (dorsa)
    d. of foot
    d. of hand
    d. ilii
    d. linguae
    d. manus
    d. nasi
    d. pedis
    d. penis, d. of penis
    d. of scapula, d. scapulae

dorsum (dorsa) *(continued)*
  d. sellae
  d. of testis
  d. of tongue
dosage
dose
  absorbed d.
  air d.
  average d.
  booster d.
  broken d.
  central axis depth d.
  cumulative d.
  curative d.
  daily d.
  depth d.
  divided d.
  doubling d.
  effective d.
  entrance d.
  epilating d.
  erythema d.
  d. estimate
  exit d.
  exposure d.
  fatal d.
  fractional d., fractionated d.
  fractionation d.
  immunizing d.
  infective d.
  integral absorbed d.
  invariably lethal d.
  lethal d.
  loading d.
  maintenance d.
  maximum d.
  maximum permissible d.
  mean effective d.
  mean lethal d.
  median curative d.
  median effective d.
  median infective d.
  median lethal d.
  median tissue culture
    infective d.
  minimal hemagglutinating d.
  minimal hemolytic d.
  minimal reacting d.
  minimum lethal d.
  nominal single d.
  organ tolerance d.
  permissible d.
  preventative d.
  preventive d.
  priming d.

dose *(continued)*
  radiation absorbed d.
  reacting d.
  refractive d.
  sensitizing d.
  skin d. (SD)
  therapeutic d.
  threshold d.
  threshold erythema d.
  tissue d.
  tissue tolerance d.
  tolerance d.
  toxic d.
  unit d.
  volume d.
dosimeter
dosimetric
dosimetry
dosis
  d. curativa
  d. efficax
  d. refracta
  d. tolerata
dossier
dot
  Gunn d's, Marcus Gunn d's
  Maurer d's
  Mittendorf d.
  d. scan
  Schüffner d.
  Trantas d.
dotage
Dott
  mouth gag
  operation
Dotter tube
double-armed suture, doubly armed
  suture
double-blind
  d.-b. clinical trial
  d.-b. experiment
  d.-b. study
  d.-b. test
double-bubble appearance
double-button suture
double-channel irrigating
  bronchoscope
double-contrast
  d.-c. arthrography
  d.-c. barium enema
  d.-c. radiography
  d.-c. roentgenography
double-J stent catheter
double lip
double-lumen catheter

double pyloroplasty
double-stranded
doublet
douche
    air d.
    alternating d.
    Betadine d.
    fan d.
    jet d.
    nasal d.
    Scotch d.
    Tivoli d.
    transition d.
    vinegar d.
doughnut sign
doughy
    d. abdomen
    d. consistency
Douglas
    bag
    bag spirometer
    cul-de-sac
    fold
    graft
    knife
    ligament
    line
    mechanism
    method
    operation
    pouch
    septum
    space
douglascele
douglasitis
dowager's hump
Dow-Corning implant
dowel
down
downbeat nystagmus
Downey cell
down-gaze
downgoing
Downing knife
downstream
Down syndrome
Doyen
    clamp
    elevator
    forceps
    gag
    operation
    retractor
    scissors
    vaginal hysterectomy

Doyère
    eminence
    hillock
Doyne
    colloid degeneration
    familial honeycombed
      choroiditis
    iritis
DP—
    dementia praecox
    diastolic pressure
    distopulpal
    Doctor of Podiatry
DPA—dipropylacetate
DPC—delayed primary closure
DPDL—diffuse poorly
  differentiated lymphoma
DPG—
    diphosphoglycerate
    displacement placentogram
DPGM—diphosphoglyceromutase
DPGP—diphosphoglycerate
  phosphatase
DPH—Diploma in Public Health
DPI—disposable personal
  income
DPL—distopulpolingual
dpm—disintegrations per
  minute
DPM—Diploma in Psychological
  Medicine
DPM, D.P.M.—Doctor of Podiatric
  Medicine
DPN—diphosphopyridine
  nucleotide
DPS—dimethylpolysiloxane
DPT—
    diphtheria, pertussis, and
      tetanus (vaccine)
    dipropyltryptamine
DPVNS—diffuse pigmented
  villonodular synovitis
DQ—developmental quotient
Dr.—doctor
DR—diabetic retinopathy
dracuncular
dracunculiasis
Dracunculus medinensis
Draeger tonometer
draft
drag
    solvent d.
dragée
Dragstedt
    graft

Dragstedt *(continued)*
    operation
drain
    accordion d.
    butterfly d.
    cigarette d.
    controlled d.
    Hemovac d.
    latex d.
    Malecot d.
    Mikulicz d.
    Penrose d.
    Pezzer d.
    polyethylene d.
    polyvinyl d.
    quarantine d.
    Redivac d.
    rubber dam d.
    stab wound d.
    suction d.
    sump d.
    sump-Penrose d.
    whistle-tip d.
drainage
    anomalous pulmonary
      venous d.
    basal d.
    button d.
    capillary d.
    closed d.
    continuous suction d.
    dependent d.
    duodenal d.
    d. headache
    open d.
    percutaneous d.
    percutaneous transhepatic
      biliary d. (PTBD)
    postural d.
    Roux-Y d.
    suction d.
    through d.
    tidal d.
    d. tube
    ventriculoatrial d.
    Wangensteen d.
    water-seal d.
drainage system
    closed water-seal d.s.
    continuous suction d.s.
    Glover d.s.
    Monaldi d.s.
    postural d.s.
    Redivac d.s.
    Snyder Surgivac d.s.

drainage system *(continued)*
    sump d.s.
    Surgivac suction d.s.
    three-bottle d.s.
    tidal d.s.
    two-bottle d.s.
    vacuum d.s.
    waterseal d.s.
Drake-Willock dialysis
dramatic
dramatization
drape
drapetomania
drastic
draught
drawer sign
drawn ankle clonus
dream
    clairvoyant d.
    day d.
    d. interpretation
    wet d.
drench
Dresbach
    anemia
    syndrome
dresser
dressing
    absorbable d.
    Adaptic gauze d.
    adhesive d.
    adhesive absorbent d.
    Aeroplast d.
    antiseptic d.
    Band-Aid d.
    barrel d.
    biologic d., biological d.
    bolus d.
    brassiere-type d.
    bulky d.
    butterfly d.
    cellophane d.
    cement d.
    cocoon d.
    Coe-Pak d.
    collar d.
    collodion d.
    compound d.
    compression d.
    Conform d.
    Cornish wool d.
    cross d.
    dry d.
    dry pressure d.
    felt d.

dressing *(continued)*
    fine mesh d.
    fixed d.
    fluff d.
    fluffy compression d.
    foam rubber d.
    four-tailed d.
    Fricke scrotal d.
    Gelfilm d.
    Gelfoam d.
    Gelocast d.
    impregnated d.
    iodoform d.
    Lister d.
    many-tailed d.
    Mersilene gauze d.
    mustache d.
    Nu Gauze d.
    occlusive d.
    paraffin d.
    patch d.
    petrolatum gauze d.
    plastic d.
    pressure d.
    propylene d.
    protective d.
    Ray-Tec d.
    sheepskin d.
    stent d.
    stockinette d.
    Styrofoam d.
    surgical gauze d.
    Surgicel gauze d.
    Telfa d.
    tie-over d.
    tulle gras d.
    Vaseline gauze d.
    Velcro d.
    Vioform d.
    Wangensteen d.
    wet-to-dry d.
    Xeroform gauze d.
Dressler
    beat
    syndrome
DREZ (dorsal root entry zone) lesion
DRG—diagnosis-related group
DRI—Discharge Readiness
    Inventory
dribbling
drift
    mesial d.
    physiologic d.
    radial d.
    ulnar d.

drill
    Adson d.
    Amico d.
    Bunnell d.
    cannulated d.
    Cloward d.
    Crutchfield d.
    Cushing d.
    D'Errico d.
    Deyerle d.
    Hall air d.
    Hall surgical d.
    Hudson d.
    intramedullary d.
    Jordan-Day d.
    Lentulo spiral d.
    McKenzie d.
    mirror d.
    Ralks d.
    Raney d.
    Shea d.
    Smedberg d.
    Stille d.
    Stryker d.
    Vitallium d.
drilling
drink
drinker
    problem d.
    social d.
drinking
    binge d.
    episodic excessive d.
    habitual excessive d.
    periodic d.
    social d.
drip
    heparin d.
    d. infusion pyelography
    d. infusion urography
    intravenous d.
    Murphy d.
    nasal d.
    pitocin d.
    postnasal d.
    d. pyelography
    succinylcholine d.
drive
    aggressive d.
    exploratory d.
    learned d.
    secondary d.
    sexual d.
driver
    Küntscher d.

dromotropic
dromotropism
    negative d.
    positive d.
drooling
drop
    ankle d.
    d. attacks
    capsular d.
    ear d's
    enamel d.
    eye d's
    d. foot [also: footdrop]
    d. foot brace
    hanging d.
    Hoffmann d's
    lid d.
    nose d's
    d. phalangette
    d. spells
    steel d's
    wrist d.
dropacism
droplet
    Flügge (Fluegge) d.
    hyaline d.
    lipid d.
    protein d.
dropper
dropping
dropsy
    abdominal d.
    articular d.
    d. of belly
    d. of chest
    cutaneous d.
    epidemic d.
    peritoneal d.
    salpingian d.
    wet d.
drowning
    near d.
    secondary d.
drug
    antagonistic d.
    controlled d.
    crude d.
    designer d.
    generic d.
    illicit d.
    investigational d.
    licit d.
    over-the-counter d.
    prescription d.
    proprietary d.

druggist
drug-resistant
drum
    Bárány d.
    blue d.
drumhead
Drummond
    marginal artery
    sign
Drummond-Morison operation
drumstick
drunkenness
drusen
    giant d. of macula
dry eye syndrome
dry pressure dressing
Drysdale corpuscles
DS—
    dead space
    dextrose-saline
    dry swallow
DSA—
    digital subtraction
      angiography
    digital subtraction
      arteriography
DSAP—disseminated superficial
    actinic porokeratosis
dT—diphtheria (booster) and
    tetanus toxoids (vaccine)
DT—
    deoxythymidine
    diphtheria (vaccine) and
      tetanus toxoids (vaccine)
    distance test
    duration tetany
    dye test
DT, DTs—delirium tremens
dTDP—
    deoxyribose diphosphate
    deoxythymidine diphosphate
DTH—delayed-type
    hypersensitivity
D time—dream time
DTM—dermatophyte test medium
dTMP—deoxyribose
    monophosphate
DTMP—deoxythymidine
    monophosphate
DTN—diphtheria toxin normal
DTNB—dithiobisnitrobenzoic acid
DTP—
    diphtheria and tetanus
    (toxoids) and pertussis
    (vaccine)

DTP— *(continued)*
 distal tingling on pressure
DTR—deep tendon reflex
dTTP—
 deoxyribose triphosphate
 deoxythymidine triphosphate
DU—
 deoxyuridine
 diagnosis undetermined
Dua antireflux valve
dualism
dual-photon
 d. absorptiometry
 d. densitometry
Duane
 accommodative chart
 syndrome
 test
DUB—dysfunctional uterine
 bleeding
Dubini
 chorea
 disease
Dubin-Johnson syndrome
Dubois
 abscess
 disease
 method
 sign
DuBois-Reymond law
Dubos
 crude crystals
 enzyme
 lysin
Duboscq colorimeter
Dubowitz
 evaluation
 examination
 infant maturity scale
 Neurological Assessment
 score
 syndrome
Dubreuilh precancerous
 melanosis
Duchenne
 muscular dystrophy
 paralysis
 sign
 type
Duchenne-Aran
 muscular atrophy
 sign
 type
Duchenne-Erb paralysis
Duchenne-Landouzy dystrophy

Duchenne-Landouzy–type
 dystrophy
Duchenne-type muscular dystrophy
duckbill, duck-billed
 d. speculum
duck waddle test
Ducrey
 bacillus
 disease
 test
duct
 aberrant d.
 accessory bile d's
 acoustic d.
 adipose d.
 alimentary d.
 alveolar d.
 arterial d.
 Bartholin d.
 Bellini d.
 Bernard d.
 bile d.
 bile d's, interlobular
 biliary d.
 Blasius d.
 Bochdalek d.
 d. of Botallo
 canalicular d's
 cervical d.
 choledochal d.
 chyliferous d.
 cochlear d.
 collecting d.
 common bile d.
 common hepatic d.
 common pharyngobranchial d.
 cowperian d.
 craniopharyngeal d.
 d's of Cuvier
 cystic d.
 deferent d.
 d. of Rivinus
 dorsal pancreatic d.
 efferent d.
 efferent d's of testis
 ejaculatory d.
 endolymphatic d.
 d. of epididymis
 epigenital d.
 d. of epoöphoron
 excretory d. of bulbourethral
  gland
 excretory d. of lacrimal gland
 extrahepatic bile d.
 frontonasal d.

duct *(continued)*

- galactophorous d's
- Gartner d.
- gasserian d.
- genital d.
- Guérin d.
- guttural d.
- Haller aberrant d.
- Hensen d.
- hepaticopancreatic d.
- hepatocystic d.
- d. of His
- hypophyseal d.
- incisive d.
- incisor d.
- intercalated d.
- interlobular d's
- lacrimal d.
- lacrimonasal d.
- lactiferous d.
- left d. of caudate lobe
- Leydig d.
- lingual d.
- longitudinal d. of epoöphoron
- Luschka d's
- lymphatic d's
- mammary d.
- mammillary d's
- milk d's
- d. of Müller
- müllerian d.
- nasal d.
- nasofrontal d.
- nasolacrimal d.
- nasopharyngeal d.
- nephric d.
- omphalomesenteric d.
- ovarian d.
- pancreatic d., accessory
- pancreatic d., minor
- papillary d.
- paragenital d's
- paramesonephric d's of female urethra
- paraurethral d's of female urethra
- paraurethral d's of male urethra
- parotid d.
- d. of Pecquet
- perilymphatic d.
- persistent craniopharyngeal d.
- persistent mesonephric d.
- persistent omphalomesenteric d.

duct *(continued)*

- persistent thyroglossal d.
- prostatic d.
- Rathke d.
- Reichel cloacal d.
- renal d.
- right d. of caudate lobe
- d's of Rivinus
- Rokitansky-Aschoff d's
- sacculoutricular d.
- salivary d.
- d. of Santorini
- Schüller d's
- sebaceous d.
- secretory d.
- segmental d.
- semicircular d.
- seminal d's
- d. of seminal gland
- Skene d.
- spermatic d.
- d. of Steno
- Stensen d.
- striated d's
- sublingual d's, major
- sublingual d's, minor
- submandibular d.
- submaxillary d. of Wharton
- sudoriferous d.
- sweat d.
- tear d.
- testicular d.
- thoracic d.
- thyrocervical d.
- thyroglossal d.
- thyrolingual d.
- thyropharyngeal d.
- umbilical d.
- urogenital d's
- utriculosaccular d.
- d. of Vater
- ventral pancreatic d.
- vitelline d.
- vitellointestinal d.
- Walther d.
- Wharton d.
- d. of Wirsung
- d. of Wolff
- wolffian d.

ductal

ductile

ductility

duction

- d's and versions
- forced d's

ductless
ductography
   peroral retrograde
     pancreaticobiliary d.
ductular
ductule
   aberrant d's
   alveolar d's
   bile d's
   biliary d's
   cranial aberrant d.
   efferent d's of testis
   excretory d's of lacrimal gland
   Haller aberrant d.
   inferior aberrant d.
   interlobular d's
   d's of prostate
   superior aberrant d.
   transverse d's of epoöphoron
ductulus (ductuli [genitive and
  plural])
    d. aberrans inferior
    d. aberrans superior
    ductuli aberrantes
    ductuli alveolares
    ductuli biliferi
    ductuli efferentes testis
    ductuli excretorii glandulae
     lacrimalis
    ductuli interlobulares
    ductuli prostatici
    ductuli transversi epoöphori
    ductuli transversi
     epoöphorontis
ductus (ductus)
    d. aberrans halleri
    d. aberrantes
    d. Arantii
    d. arteriosus bilateralis
    d. arteriosus, patent
    d. arteriosus, reversed
    d. biliaris
    d. biliferi
    d. choledochus
    d. cochlearis
    d. cuvieri
    d. cysticus
    d. deferens vestigialis
    d. ejaculatorius
    d. endolymphaticus
    d. epididymidis
    d. epoöphori longitudinalis
    d. epoöphorontis longitudinalis
    d. excretorius glandulae
     bulbourethrales

ductus (ductus) *(continued)*
    d. excretorius vesiculae
     seminalis
    d. glandulae bulbourethralis
    d. hepaticus communis
    d. hepaticus dexter
    d. hepaticus sinister
    d. incisivus
    d. interlobulares bilifer
    d. lacrimalis
    d. lactiferi
    d. lingualis
    d. lobi caudati dexter
    d. lobi caudati sinister
    d. longitudinalis
    d. lymphatici
    d. lymphaticus dexter
    d. mesonephricus
    d. Muelleri
    d. nasolacrimalis
    d. pancreaticus accessorius
    d. papillaris
    d. paramesonephricus
    d. paraurethrales urethrae
     femininae
    d. paraurethrales urethrae
     masculinae
    d. parotideus
    d. perilymphatici
    d. perilymphaticus
    d. prostatici
    d. reuniens
    d. semicirculares
    d. spermaticus
    d. sublinguales minores
    d. sublingualis major
    d. submandibularis
    d. sudoriferus
    d. thoracicus dexter
    d. thyroglossalis
    d. utriculosaccularis
    d. venosus
    d. wolffi
Duddell membrane
Dudley
   hook
   operation
Dudley-Smith speculum
Duffy
   antigen
   blood antibody type
   blood group
Dufourmental
   forceps
   rongeur

D

Dugas
    sign
    test
Duguet siphon
Duhamel operation
Duhring
    disease
    pruritus
Dührssen (Duehrssen)
    incision
    operation
    tampon
Duke
    method
    test
    trocar
Duke-Elder
    lamp
    operation
Dukes classification (A, B, B$_2$, C$_1$, C$_2$ [B2, C1, C2])
dulcitol
dull
dullness
    Gerhardt d.
    Grocco triangular d.
    shifting d.
    tympanitic d.
Dulox suture
dumbbell of Schäfer
dummy
DUMP—deoxyuridine monophosphate
dumping syndrome
Duncan
    disease
    syndrome
    ventricle
Dunfermline scale
Dunham
    cones
    fans
    triangles
Dunhill hemostat
Dunn-Brittain operation
duodenal
    d. atresia
    d. bulb
    d. diverticula
    d. drainage
    d. ileus
    d. loop
    d. obstruction
    d. papilla
    d. tube

duodenal (continued)
    d. ulcer
duodenectomy
duodenitis
duodenocholangeitis
duodenocholecystostomy
duodenocholedochotomy
duodenocolic
duodenocystostomy
duodenoduodenostomy
duodenoenterostomy
duodenogram
duodenography
    hypotonic d.
duodenohepatic
duodenoileostomy
duodenojejunostomy
duodenolysis
duodenopancreatectomy
duodenoplasty
duodenorrhaphy
duodenoscope
duodenoscopy
duodenostomy
duodenotomy
duodenum
duoparental
Duplay
    bursitis
    disease
    hook
    operation
    speculum
    syndrome
    tenaculum
Duplay-Lynch speculum
duplication
    d. of colon
    d. of duodenum
    d. of esophagus
    d. of ileum
    incomplete d. of spinal cord
    d. of rectum
    d. of stomach
    tandem d.
duplicitas
    d. anterior
    d. asymmetros
    d. completa
    d. cruciata
    d. incompleta
    d. inferior
    d. media
    d. parallela
    d. posterior

duplicitas *(continued)*
    d. superior
    d. symmetros
Dupuy-Dutemps operation
Dupuytren
    amputation
    contracture
    enterotome
    fascia
    fracture
    hydrocele
    operation
    sign
    splint
    suture
dura clip
dural
    d. forceps
    d. hook
    d. incision
dura mater
    d.m. of brain
    d.m. encephali
    d.m. of spinal cord
    d.m. spinalis
Durand disease
Durand and Giroud vaccine
Durand-Nicolas-Favre disease
durapatite
duraplasty
duration
    pulse d.
Dürck (Duerck)
    granuloma
    nodes
Duret
    hemorrhages
    lesion
Durham
    trocar
    tube
duroarachnitis
Duromedics
    prosthesis
    valve
Duroziez
    disease
    murmur
    sign
duskiness
dusky
DUSN—diffuse unilateral subacute
  neuroretinitis
dust
    blood d.

dust *(continued)*
    chromatin d.
    ear d.
dust-borne
Dutcher body
dUTP—deoxyuridine triphosphate
Dutton
    disease
    relapsing fever
    spirochete
Duval
    intestinal forceps
    lung-grasping forceps
Duval-Crile forceps
DuVal procedure
Duverney fracture
DuVries hammer toe repair
DV—double vision
D&V—diarrhea and vomiting
DVA—distance visual acuity
DVD—
    dissociated vertical deviation
    dissociated vertical divergence
DVI—digital vascular imaging
DVT—
    deep vein thrombosis
    deep venous thrombosis
DW—
    distilled water
    dry weight
D/W—dextrose in water
D5W, D_5W, D5/W—5% dextrose in
  water
dwarf
    achondroplastic d.
    acromelic d.
    adrenal d.
    Amsterdam d.
    asexual d.
    ateliotic d.
    Brissaud d.
    camptomelic d.
    chondrodystrophic d.
    deformed d.
    diastrophic d.
    geleophysic d.
    hypophysial (hypophyseal) d.
    hypopituitary d.
    hypoplastic d.
    hypothyroid d.
    idiopathic d.
    infantile d.
    Laron d.
    Lévi-Lorain d.
    Lorain-Lévi d.

dwarf *(continued)*
    mesomelic d.
    micromelic d.
    nanocephalic d.
    normal d.
    Paltauf d.
    panhypopituitary d.
    phocomelic d.
    physiologic d.
    pituitary d.
    Pott d.
    prepubertal d.
    primordial d.
    pure d.
    rachitic d.
    renal d.
    rhizomelic d.
    Russell d.
    Seckel d.
    senile d.
    sexual d.
    thanatophoric d.
    thyroid d.
    true d.
dwarfism
    acromelic d.
    camptomelic d.
    cardiac d.
    chondrodystrophic d.
    deprivation d.
    diabetic d.
    exostotic d.
    hypophysial
      (hypophyseal) d.
    hypopituitary d.
    mesomelic d.
    micromelic d.
    myxedematous d.
    pituitary d. I,
      pituitary d. III
    polydystrophic d.
    pseudometatropic d.
    psychosocial d.
    renal d.
    rhizomelic d.
    Robinow d.
    thanatophoric d.
    thyroid d.
Dx, Dg—diagnosis
DX—dextran
DXA—dual x-ray absorptiometry
DXM—dexamethasone
DXT—deep x-ray therapy
Dy—dysprosium
dyad

dye
    acid d., acidic d.
    amphoteric d.
    aniline d.
    anionic d.
    azo d.
    basic d.
    cationic d.
    fluorescein d.
    halogenated phenolphthalein d.
    indigo carmine d.
    d. laser
    metachromatic d.
    orthochromatic d.
    rose bengal d.
    vital d.
Dyggve-Melchior-Clausen
   syndrome
Dyke-Young syndrome
dynamic
    d. computed tomography
    d. venous plethysmography
dynamics
    group d.
    topological d.
dynamogenic
dynamometer
    Collins d.
    squeeze d.
dynamopathic
dynamophore
dynamoscopy
dyne
dynein
dysacusis
dysadaptation
dysadrenalism
dysallilognathia
dysanagnosia
dysantigraphia
dysaphia
dysarteriotony
dysarthria
    ataxic d.
    cerebellar d.
    developmental d.
    d. literalis
    spastic d.
    d. syllabaris spasmodica
dysarthric
dysarthrosis
    craniofacial d.
dysautonomia
    familial d.
    Riley-Day d.

D

dysbarism
    altitude d.
dysbasia lordotica progressiva
dysbetalipoproteinemia
dysbolism
dysbulia
dysbulic
dyscalculia
dyscephaly
    mandibulo-oculofacial d.
dyschezia
dyschiasia
dyschiria
dyscholia
dyschondroplasia
    Ollier d.
dyschondrosteosis
dyschromatopsia
dyschromia
dyschronism
dyschylia
dyscontrol
    episodic d.
dyscoria
dyscorticism
dyscrasia
    blood d.
    lymphatic d.
    plasma cell d's
dyscratic
dysdiadochokinesia
dysdiadochokinetic
dysdipsia
dysecoia
dysencephalia splanchnocystica
dysenteric
dysenteriform
dysentery
    amebic d.
    asylum d.
    bacillary d.
    balantidial d.
    bilharzial d.
    catarrhal d.
    ciliary d.
    ciliate d.
    epidemic d.
    flagellate d.
    Flexner d.
    fulminant d.
    giardiasis d.
    helminthic d.
    institutional d.
    Japanese d.
    malarial d.

dysentery *(continued)*
    malignant d.
    protozoal d.
    schistosomal d.
    scorbutic d.
    Shiga d.
    Sonne d.
    spirillar d.
    sporadic d.
    viral d.
dysequilibrium
dysergia
dyserythropoiesis
dyserythropoietic
dysesthesia
    auditory d.
dysesthetic
dysfibrinogenemia
dysfluency
dysfunction
    central auditory d.
    constitutional hepatic d.
    hypertonic uterine d.
    hypotonic uterine d.
    minimal brain d.
    myocardial d.
    myofascial pain d.
    orgasmic d.
    papillary muscle d.
    placental d.
    sensorineural d.
    temporomandibular joint d.
    d. of uterus
dysfunctional uterine bleeding (DUB)
dysgalactia
dysgammaglobulinemia
dysgenesis
    disseminated nodular d.
    epiphyseal d.
    gonadal d.
    iridocorneal mesodermal d.
    mixed gonadal d.
    mosaic gonadal d.
    pure gonadal d.
    reticular d.
    Rieger d.
    seminiferous tubule d.
dysgenic
dysgenitalism
dysgerminoma
dysgeusia
dysglobulinemia
dysglycemia
dysgnathia

dysgnathic
dysgnosia
dysgonesis
dysgonic
dysgrammatism
dysgraphia
dyshematopoiesis
dyshematopoietic
dyshepatia
   lipogenic d.
dyshesion
dyshidrosis
   trichophytic d.
dysimmunoglobulinemia
dyskaryosis
dyskaryotic
dyskeratoma
   warty d.
dyskeratosis
   d. congenita
   congenital d.
   d. follicularis
   hereditary benign
     intraepithelial d.
   isolated d. follicularis
dyskeratotic
dyskinesia
   biliary d.
   buccal-lingual-masticatory
     (BLM) d.
   facial d.
   d. intermittens
   occupational d.
   orofacial d.
   phenothiazine-induced d.
   tardive d.
   tracheobronchial d.
   uterine d.
dyskinetic
dyslalia
dyslexia
   congenital d.
   developmental d.
dyslipidemia
dyslipidosis
dyslipoproteinemia
dyslochia
dyslogia
dysmature
dysmaturity
   pulmonary d.
dysmegalopsia
dysmelia
dysmenorrhea
   acquired d.

dysmenorrhea *(continued)*
   congestive d.
   essential d.
   inflammatory d.
   d. intermenstrualis
   mechanical d.
   membranous d.
   obstructive d.
   ovarian d.
   plethoric d.
   psychogenic d.
   spasmodic d.
   tubal d.
   uterine d.
   vaginal d.
dysmentia
   tardive d.
dysmetabolism
dysmetria
   ocular motor d.
dysmetropsia
dysmnesia
dysmnesic
dysmorphic
dysmorphism
dysmorphophobia
dysmorphopsia
dysmorphosis
dysmyelination
dysmyelopoietic
dysmyotonia
dysnomia
dysodontiasis
dysodynia
dysopia algera
dysopsia
dysorexia
dysorganoplasia
dysoria
dysoric
dysosmia
dysosteogenesis
dysostosis
   acrofacial d.
   cleidocranial d.
   craniofacial d.
   d. enchondralis epiphysaria
   mandibulofacial d.
   maxillonasal d.
   metaphyseal d.
   d. multiplex
   Nager acrofacial d.
   nasomaxillary d.
   orodigitofacial d.
   otomandibular d.

D

dyspareunia
dyspepsia
    acid d.
    appendicular d.
    catarrhal d.
    chichiko d.
    cholelithic d.
    colon d.
    fermentative d.
    flatulent d.
    gastric d.
    intestinal d.
    nonulcer d.
dyspeptic
dysperistalsis
dysphagia
    contractile ring d.
    d. globosa
    d. inflammatoria
    d. lusoria
    d. nervosa
    oropharyngeal d.
    d. paralytica
    sideropenic d.
    d. spastica
    tropical d.
    vallecular d.
    d. valsalviana
dysphagic
dysphasia
    dyslexia, d., and dysgraphia
    expressive d.
    high-grade d.
    overt d.
    residual d.
    transient d.
    Wernicke d.
dysphemia
dysphonia
    d. clericorum
    dysplastic d.
    d. plicae ventricularis
    d. puberum
    spasmodic d.
    spastic d.
    d. spastica
dysphonic
dysphoretic
dysphoria
    gender d.
dysphoriant
dysphoric
dysphrasia
dysphrenia
dysphylaxia

dyspigmentation
dysplasia
    anhidrotic ectodermal d.
    anteroposterior facial d.
    arteriohepatic d.
    asphyxiating thoracic d.
    atriodigital d.
    bronchopulmonary d.
    camptomelic d.
    caudal d.
    cervical d.
    d. of cervix
    chondroectodermal d.
    cleidocranial d.
    congenital alveolar d.
    congenital d. of hip
    craniocarpotarsal d.
    craniodiaphyseal d.
    craniometaphyseal d. of Pyle
    craniotelencephalic d.
    cretinoid d.
    dental d.
    dentinal d.
    dentoalveolar d.
    diaphyseal d.
    diastrophic d.
    ectodermal d.
    enamel d.
    encephalo-ophthalmic d.
    epiphyseal d.
    d. epiphysealis hemimelica
    d. epiphysealis multiplex
    d. epiphysealis punctata
    extracranial fibromuscular d.
    faciogenital d.
    familial white folded mucosal d.
    fibromuscular d.
    fibrous d. of bone
    fibrous d. of jaw
    florid osseous d.
    frontometaphyseal d.
    hereditary bone d.
    hereditary renal-retinal d.
    hidrotic ectodermal d.
    hypohidrotic ectodermal d.
    Kniest d.
    d. linguofacialis
    mammary d.
    metaphyseal d.
    metatropic d.
    Mondini d.
    monostotic fibrous d.
    multiple epiphyseal d.
    nuclear d.
    OAV d.

D

dysplasia *(continued)*
    oculoauricular d.
    oculoauriculovertebral
      (OAV) d.
    oculodentodigital
      (ODD) d.
    oculodentoosseous d.
    olfactory genital d.
    ophthalmomandibulomelic d.
    oral familial white
      folded d.
    osseous d.
    osteodental d.
    periapical cemental d.
    polyostotic fibrous d.
    progressive diaphyseal d.
    pseudoachrondroplastic d.
    punctate epiphyseal d.
    renal d.
    retinal d.
    Robinow mesomelic d.
    skeletal d.
    skeletodental d.
    spondyloepiphyseal d.
    spondylometaepiphyseal d.
    spondylometaphyseal d.
    Streeter d.
    thanatophoric d.
    thymic d.
    trichorhinophalangeal d.
    ureteral neuromuscular d.
    ventriculoradial d.
dysplastic
dysplastic coloboma
dyspnea
    cardiac d.
    exertional d.
    expiratory d.
    functional d.
    inspiratory d.
    nocturnal d.
    nonexpansional d.
    orthostatic d.
    paroxysmal d.
    paroxysmal nocturnal d.
      (PND)
    renal d.
    sighing d.
    Traube d.
    two-flight d.
dyspneic
dyspoiesis
dyspoietic
dysponderal
dysponesis

dyspragia
    d. angiosclerotica
    d. intermittens
    d. intestinalis
dyspraxia
dysprosium (Dy)
dysprosody
dysproteinemia
dysprothrombinemia
dysraphia
dysraphism
dysreflexia
    autonomic d.
    cerebral d.
    electroencephalographic d.
    esophageal d.
dysrhythmia
    cerebral d.
    cortical d.
    electroencephalographic d.
    esophageal d.
    paroxysmal cerebral d.
    d. pneumophrasia
    d. prosodia
    sinus d.
    d. tonia
dyssebacia
dyssocial
dyssomatognosia
dyssomnia
dysspermia
dysstasia
    hereditary areflexic d.
dysstatic
dyssymbolia
dyssymmetry
dyssynergia
    biliary d.
    d. cerebellaris myoclonica
    d. cerebellaris progressiva
dyssynergy
dystasia
    hereditary ataxic d.
    Roussy-Lévy hereditary
      ataxic d.
dystaxia
    d. agitans
    cerebral d.
    d. cerebralis infantilis
dystectia
dysthymia
dysthymic
dysthyroid
dysthyroidal
dysthyroidism

dystithia
dystocia
    cervical d.
    constriction ring d.
    contraction ring d.
    fetal d.
    maternal d.
    placental d.
dystonia
    attitudinal d.
    autonomic d.
    cranial d.
    d. deformans progressiva
    hypersympatheticotonic d.
    kinetic d.
    d. lenticularis
    d. musculorum
      deformans
    periodic d.
    segmental d.
    tardive d.
    torsion d.
dystonic
dystopia
    crossed d. of kidney
    simple renal d.
dystopic
dystrophia
    d. adiposa corneae
    d. adiposogenitalis
    d. brevicollis
    d. endothelialis corneae
    d. epithelialis corneae
    d. mediana canaliformis
    d. mesodermalis congenita
      hyperplastica
    d. myotonica
    d. unguium
dystrophic
    d. epidermolysis bullosa
    d. palmoplantar
      hyperkeratosis
dystrophoneurosis
dystrophy
    adiposogenital d.
    Albright d.
    arthritic d.
    asphyxiating
      thoracic d. (ATD)
    autosomal-dominant
      distal d.
    Becker-type muscular d.
    Best macular d.
    Biber-Haab-Dimmer d.
    Bietti d.

dystrophy *(continued)*
    Cogan d.
    corneal d.
    craniocarpotarsal d.
    crystalline d. of cornea
    Dejerine-Landouzy d.
    distal muscular d.
    Duchenne-Landouzy d.
    Duchenne muscular d.
    Duchenne-type
      muscular d.
    Emery-Dreifuss d.
    endothelial corneal d.
    Erb d.
    facioscapulohumeral
      muscular d.
    familial osseous d.
    Fleischer d.
    Franceschetti d.
    Francois d.
    Fröhlich
      adiposogenital d.
    Fuchs d.
    Gowers muscular d.
    Groenouw corneal d.
    gutter d. of cornea
    hereditary vitelliform d.
    hyperplastic d.
    hypophysial
      (hypophyseal) d.
    infantile neuroaxonal d.
    juvenile progressive
      muscular d.
    Landouzy d.
    Landouzy-Dejerine d.
    lattice corneal d.
    Leyden-Möbius muscular d.
    limb-girdle muscular d.
    macular corneal d.
    median canaliform d. of the nail
    Meesmann d.
    muscular d.
    myotonic d.
    neuroaxonal proteid d.
    ocular muscular d.
    oculocerebrorenal d.
    oculopharyngeal muscular d.
    progressive muscular d.
    progressive
      tapetochoroidal d.
    pseudohypertrophic
      muscular d.
    reflex sympathetic d.
    Salzmann nodular corneal d.
    scapulohumeral d.

dystrophy *(continued)*
 scapuloperoneal d.
 Schlichting d.
 Seitelberger d.
 sex-linked muscular d.
 Simmerlin d.
 speckled d. of cornea
 tapetochoroidal d.
 thoracic-pelvic-phalangeal d.
 thyroneural d.
 twenty-nail d.
 vitelliform macular d.

dystrophy *(continued)*
 wound d.
 X-linked muscular d.
dystrypsia
dysuresia
dysuria
 psychic d.
 spastic d.
dysuric
dysvitaminosis
dyszoospermia
DZ—dizygous (twins)

E

ε—
 epsilon (Greek letter)
 molar absorptivity
e⁻—electron

e^-—electron
e^+—positron
e—elementary unit of electric charge
E—
 emmetropia
 energy
 erythrocyte
 esophoria
 esotropia
 eye
E—
 elastance
 expectancy
E.—
 Entamoeba
 Escherichia
E_1—estrone
E_2—estradiol
E_3—estriol
E_4—estetrol
ea.—each
EA—
 educational age
 erythrocyte antibody
 ethacrynic acid
EAA—extrinsic allergic alveolitis
EAb, EAB—elective abortion
EAC—
 Ehrlich ascites carcinoma

EAC— *(continued)*
 erythrocyte antibody complement
 external auditory canal
EACA—epsilon-aminocaproic acid
EACD—extrinsic allergic contact dermatitis
EAD—early afterdepolarization
EAE—experimental allergic encephalomyelitis
Eagle-Barrett syndrome
EAHF—eczema, asthma, hay fever
EAHLG—equine antihuman lymphoblast globulin
EAHLS—equine antihuman lymphoblast serum
Eales disease
EAM—external auditory meatus
ear
 artificial e.
 aviator's e.
 bat e.
 beach e.
 Blainville e's
 boxer's e.
 cat's e.
 cauliflower e.
 cup e.
 Darwin e.
 dead e.
 diabetic e.
 external e.
 glue e.
 hairy e's

ear *(continued)*
    hot weather e.
    internal e.
    lop e.
    middle e.
    Morel e.
    Mozart e.
    prizefighter's e.
    satyr e.
    scroll e.
    shell e.
    swimmer's e.
    tropical e.
    Wildermuth e.
    wrestler's e.
earache
eardrum
Earle probe
earlobe
earphone
earwax
earwig
EAST—external rotation and abduction stress test
Eastman
    clamp
    retractor
easy-pulls
eating cell
Eaton
    agent
    agent pneumonia
    speculum
Eaton-Lambert syndrome
EB—
    elementary body
    epidermolysis bullosa
    Epstein-Barr (virus)
    escape beat
    estradiol benzoate
Ebbinghaus test
EBBS—equal bilateral breath sounds
Eber forceps
EBF—
    elastic band fixation
    erythroblastosis fetalis
EBF of fracture
EBI—emetine bismuth iodide
EBL—estimated blood loss
EBNA—Epstein-Barr nuclear antigen
Ebner
    gland
    line

Ebola
    E. hemorrhagic fever
    E. virus
ebonation
ébranlement
ebriety
Ebstein
    angle
    anomaly
    diet
    disease
    malformation
ebullition
ebur dentis
eburnated
eburnation of dentin
eburneous
eburnitis
EBV—Epstein-Barr virus
EC—
    ejection click
    electron capture
    entrance complaint
    Escherichia coli
    exaltation-contraction
    extracellular
    eyes closed
écarteur
ECAT—emission computerized axial tomography
ecaudate
ecbolic
ecbolium
ecbovirus
ECBV—effective circulating blood volume
ECC—
    edema, clubbing, cyanosis
    endocervical curettage
    extracapsular cataract
    extracorporeal circulation
ECCE—extracapsular cataract extraction
eccentric
    e. fixation
    e. pantomography
eccentrochondroplasia
eccentro-osteochondrodysplasia
ecchondroma (ecchondromas, ecchondromata)
ecchondrotome
ecchordosis physaliphora
ecchymoma
ecchymosed

ecchymosis (ecchymoses)
 cadaveric e.
 diffuse e's
 disseminated e's
 foot e. sign
 multiple e's
 old e.
 periorbital e.
 postoperative e.
 postrhinoplasty e's
 prominent e's
 Roederer e.
 scattered e's
 scrotal e.
 soft tissue e.
 spontaneous e's
 subcutaneous e.
 transient e's
ecchymotic
eccrine
eccrisis
eccritic
eccyesis
 uterine e.
 ipsilateral e.
ECD—endothelial corneal
 dystrophy
ecdemic
ecdemomania
ecdovirus
ecdysiasm
ECE—endocervical ecchymosis
ECF—
 eosinophil chemotactic factor
 epicanthic fold
 extended care facility
 extracellular fluid
ECFA, ECF-A—eosinophil
 chemotactic factor of
 anaphylaxis
ECG—
 electrocardiogram
 electrocardiography
ecgonine
echidnase
echidnin
Echidnophaga gallinacea
echidnotoxin
echidnovaccine
echinenone
Echinochasmus perfoliatus
echinochrome
echinococciasis
echinococcosis
echinococcotomy

Echinococcus
 E. alveolaris
 E. granulosus
 E. multilocularis
 E. vogeli
echinocyte
echinoderm
Echinolaelaps echidninus
echinophthalmia
Echinorhynchus
 E. gigas
 E. hominis
 E. moniliformis
echinosis
echinostomiasis
echinulate
echo
 amphoric e.
 cochlear e.
 e. delay time
 metallic e.
 midline e.
 e. planar imaging
 e. ranging
 e. texture
 e. time (TE)
 ventricular e.
echoacousia
echocardiogram
echocardiography
 cross-sectional e.
 Doppler e.
 M-mode e.
 real-time e.
 two-dimensional e.
 (TDE, 2-D e.)
echoencephalogram
echoencephalograph
 midline e.
echoencephalography
echogenic
echogenicity
echogram
echographia
echography
echoic
echoing
 thought e.
echokinesis
echolalia
echolaminography
echolucent
echomimia
echomotism
echo-ophthalmography

echopathy
echophonocardiography
echophony
echophotony
echophrasia
echo-planar imaging
echopraxia
echopraxis
echo-ranging
echoscope
echo time (TE)
echovirus
    e. 28
    e. serotypes 1–7, 9, 11–18,
      20–27, 29–34
ECIL—extracorporeal irradiation
  of lymph
Ecker
    fissure
    fluid
Eckhout vertical gastroplasty
eclabium
eclampsia
    cerebral e.
    puerperal e.
    superimposed e.
    uremic e.
eclampsism
eclamptic
eclamptogenic
eclectic
eclecticism
eclipse
eclysis
ECM—
    erythema chronicum migrans
    extracellular material
ecmnesia
ECMO—extracorporeal membrane
  oxygenation
ecmovirus
ecogenetics
E. coli—Escherichia coli
ecologist
ecology
ecomania
Economo (von Economo)
    disease
    encephalitis
economy
    e. of motion
    token e.
ecophobia
écorché
ecosite

ecostate
ecosystem
ecotaxis
ecotone
ecotropic
écouvillon
écouvillonage
ecphoria
ecphorize
ecphyaditis
écrasement
écraseur
ECS—electroconvulsive shock
ecsomatics
ecsovirus
ecstasy
ecstatic
ECT—
    electroconvulsive therapy
    emission computed
      tomography
ectacolia
ectad
ectal
ectasia
    alveolar e.
    annuloaortic e.
    corneal e.
    diffuse arterial e.
    hypostatic e.
    e. iridis
    mammary duct e.
    papillary e.
    scleral e.
    senile e.
    tubular e.
ectatic
ectental
ectethmoid
ecthyma
    e. contagiosum
    contagious e.
    e. gangrenosum
    e. syphiliticum
ecthymiform
ectoantigen
ectobiology
ectoblast
    primary e.
ectocardia
ectocervical
ectocervix
ectocolon
ectocommensal
ectocondyle

ectocornea
ectocranial
ectocuneiform
ectocyst
ectocytic
ectoderm
    amniotic e.
    basal e.
    blastodermic e.
    chorionic e.
    dorsal e.
    epithelial e.
    extraembryonic e.
    neural e.
    primitive e.
    superficial e.
ectodermal dysplasia
ectodermoidal
ectodermosis erosiva pluriorificialis
ectoentad
ectoenzyme
ectogenous
ectoglia
ectogony
ectohormone
ectolecithal
ectolysis
ectomeninx
ectomere
ectomesenchyme
ectomesoblast
ectomorph
ectomorphic
ectomorphy
ectomy
ectonuclear
ectopagia
ectopagus
ectoparasite
ectoparasiticide
ectoparasitism
ectopectoralis
ectoperitoneal
ectoperitonitis
ectophyte
ectopia
    e. cloacae
    e. cordis
    e. cordis abdominalis
    crossed renal e.
    e. lentis
    pectoral e. cordis
    e. pupillae congenita
    renal e.
    e. renis

ectopia (continued)
    e. testis
    e. vesicae
    visceral e.
ectopic
ectoplacenta
ectoplasm
ectoplasmatic
ectoplasmic
ectoplast
ectoplastic
ectopterygoid
ectopy
ectoretina
ectosarc
ectoscopy
ectosphere
ectosteal
ectostosis
ectosymbiont
ectotherm
ectothermic
ectothermy
ectothrix
ectotoxemia
ectozoal
ectozoon (ectozoa)
ectrocheiry
ectrochiry
ectrodactyly
ectrogenic
ectrogeny
ectromelia
    infectious e.
ectromelic
ectromelus
ectrometacarpia
ectrometatarsia
ectrophalangia
ectropion
    atonic e.
    cervical e.
    e. cicatriceum
    cicatricial e.
    flaccid e.
    e. luxurians
    mechanical e.
    paralytic e.
    e. paralyticum
    e. of pigment layer
    e. sarcomatosum
    senile e.
    e. senilis
    spastic e.
    e. spasticum

E

ectropion *(continued)*
    e. uveae
ectropionize
ectropium
ectropody
ectrosis
ectrosyndactyly
ectrotic
ectylurea
ectyonin
ectypia
ECV—extracellular volume
ECW—extracellular water
eczema
    allergic e.
    e. articulorum
    asteatotic e.
    atopic e.
    autoallergic e.
    bakers' e.
    e. barbae
    bullous e. of legs
    e. capitis
    e. craquelé
    e. crustosum
    e. diabeticorum
    dry e.
    dyshidrotic e.
    dyskeratotic e. of hand
    e. epilans
    e. epizootica
    e. erythematosum
    facial e. of ruminants
    fissured e.
    flexural e.
    follicular e.
    e. herpeticum
    e. hypertrophicum
    infantile e.
    infective e.
    intertriginous e.
    e. intertrigo
    lichenoid e.
    linear e.
    e. madidans
    e. marginatum
    e. medicamentosa
    e. neonatorum
    e. neuriticum
    nipple e.
    e. nummulare
    occupational e.
    e. papulosum
    e. parasiticum
    phlyctenular e.

eczema *(continued)*
    pustular e.
    e. pustulosum
    e. rhagadiforme
    e. rubrum
    e. scrofuloderma
    seborrheic e.
    e. seborrheicum
    e. siccum
    e. solare
    e. squamosum
    stasis e.
    e. tyloticum
    e. vaccinatum
    varicose e.
    e. verrucosum
    e. vesiculosum
    weeping e.
    xerotic e.
eczematization
eczematogenic
eczematoid
eczematous
ED—
    effective dose
    epileptiform discharge
    erythema dose
EDB—ethylene dibromide
EDC—
    estimated date of confinement
    expected date of confinement
EDD—expected date of delivery
eddies
Eddowes
    disease
    syndrome
eddy currents
Edebohls
    incision
    operation
    position
edeitis
Edelmann
    anemia
    cell
edema
    alimentary e.
    alveolar e.
    angioneurotic e.
    angioneurotic e., hereditary
    Berlin e.
    brain e.
    brawny e.
    brown e.
    e. bullosum vesicae

edema *(continued)*
  Calabar e.
  e. calidum
  cardiac e.
  cerebral e.
  circumscribed e.
  cyclic e.
  dependent e.
  epidermal e.
  famine e.
  e. frigidum
  e. fugax
  gaseous e.
  gestational e.
  giant e.
  e. glottidis
  hepatic e.
  hereditary angioneurotic e.
    (HANE)
  high-altitude pulmonary e.
  Huguenin e.
  hunger e.
  hydremic e.
  idiopathic e.
  inflammatory e.
  insulin e.
  interstitial e.
  invisible e.
  Iwanoff retinal e.
  lymphatic e.
  macular e.
  malignant e.
  menstrual e.
  Milroy e.
  Milton e.
  mucous e.
  e. neonatorum
  nephritic e.
  nephrotic e.
  noninflammatory e.
  nonpitting e.
  nutritional e.
  paroxysmal pulmonary e.
  passive e.
  pedal e.
  periodic e.
  periorbital e.
  periretinal e.
  Pirogoff e.
  pitting e.
  placental e.
  prehepatic e.
  pulmonary e.
  purulent e.
  Quincke e.

edema *(continued)*
  Reinke e.
  renal e.
  rheumatismal e.
  salt e.
  solid e.
  solid pulmonary e.
  Stellwag brawny e.
  subglottic e.
  subpleural e.
  terminal e.
  toxic e.
  tubular e.
  turban e.
  venous e.
  vernal e.
  vernal e. of lung
  war e.
  wound e.
edemagen
edematization
edematogenic
edematous
Eden-Hybbinette operation
edentia
edentulism
edentulous
Eder
    forceps
    gastroscope
    laparoscope
Eder-Chamberlin gastroscope
Eder-Hufford
    esophagoscope
    gastroscope
Eder-Palmer gastroscope
edetic acid disodium salt
edge
    Compton e.
    cutting e.
    denture e.
    incisal e.
    e. packing
edge-strength
edge-to-edge suture
EdGr—Edmondson Grading
E-dial calibration
edible
Edinger
    law
    nucleus
Edinger-Westphal nucleus
Edison effect
Edmondson Grading (EdGr)
    System

EDP—
    electronic data processing
    end-diastolic pressure
EDR—
    effective direct radiation
    electrodermal response
EDRF—endothelium-derived
  relaxing factor
Edsall disease
EDTA—
    edetic acid
    ethylenediaminetetra-acetic
     acid
educable
education
    compensatory e.
    health e.
eduction
edulcorant
edulcorate
EDV—end-diastolic volume
Edwards
    catheter
    clamp
    hook
    patch
    prosthesis
    syndrome
Edwardsiella
    E. hoshinae
    E. ictaluri
    E. tarda
EE—
    end-to-end
    eye and ear
EEA—electroencephalic audiometry
EEC—enteropathogenic
  Escherichia coli
EEE—eastern equine
  encephalomyelitis
EEG—
    electroencephalogram
    electroencephalography
EEME—ethinylestradiol methyl
  ether
EENT—eyes, ears, nose, and throat
EERP—extended endocardial
  resection procedure
EF—
    ectopic focus
    ejection fraction
    encephalitogenic factor
EFA, EFAs
    essential fatty acid(s)
    extrafamily adoptee(s)

EFC—endogenous fecal calcium
EFE—endocardial fibroelastosis
effaced
effacement
effect [verb: to produce, to bring
  about]
    to e. closure of an incision
    to e. a cure
effect [noun: result, outcome]
    accumulative e.
    additive e.
    adverse e.
    anachoretic e.
    Anrep e.
    Arias-Stella e.
    Auger e.
    Bainbridge e.
    Bezold-Jarisch e.
    blast e.
    Blinks e's
    Bohr e.
    Bowditch e.
    Bruce e.
    cis-trans position e.
    clasp-knife e.
    cohort e.
    columella e.
    Compton e.
    contrary e.
    contrast e.
    copper wire e.
    Cotton e.
    Crabtree e.
    crowding e.
    cumulative e.
    Cushing e.
    cyclosporine e.
    cytopathic e.
    cytoprotective e.
    Danysz e.
    Deelman e.
    deleterious e's
    digitalis e.
    diuretic e.
    Donnan e.
    Doppler e.
    Edison e.
    electrophonic e.
    electrotonic e.
    Emerson e.
    estrogen e., estrogenic e.
    experimenter e's
    Fahraeus-Lindqvist e.
    field e.
    founder e.

effect *(continued)*
- gene dose e.
- generation e.
- glucose e.
- graded e.
- Haldane e.
- Hallberg e.
- Hallwachs e.
- heel e.
- Hering e.
- horse-race e.
- hybrid e.
- hyperchromic e.
- hypochromic e.
- inductive e.
- interpolar e.
- isomorphic e.
- isotope e.
- jet e.
- Köbner (Koebner) e.
- Lyon e.
- mass e.
- McCollough e.
- Mierzejewski e.
- muscarinic e.
- Nagler e.
- nicotine e.
- Orbeli e.
- Pasteur e.
- photechic e.
- photoelectric e.
- piezoelectric e.
- placebo e.
- polar e.
- position e.
- pressure e.
- Purkinje e.
- quantal e.
- radiographic e.
- Raman e.
- relative biologic e., relative biological e.
- Russell e.
- scalar e.
- second gas e.
- side e's
- silver wire e.
- Somogyi e.
- Soret e.
- specific dynamic e.
- Staub-Traugott e.
- Stiles-Crawford e.
- treppe e.
- untoward e's
- variegated position e.

effect *(continued)*
- Venturi e.
- Wever-Bray e.
- Whitten e.
- Wolff-Chaikoff e.
- Zeeman e.

effective
- e. half-life
- e. renal plasma flow

effectiveness
- relative biological e.

effector
- allosteric e.

effemination

efferent
- α-e. [alpha-]
- β-e. [beta-]
- dynamic γ-e. [gamma-]
- general visceral e.
- somatic e.
- special visceral e.
- static γ-e. [gamma-]

effervescent

efficacious

efficacy

efficiency
- counting e.
- detection e.
- intrinsic counter e.
- photopeak e.
- production e.
- window e.

effleurage

effloresce

efflorescence

efflorescent

effluve

effluvium
- anagen e.
- telluric e.
- telogen e.

efflux of clear urine

effraction

effumability

effuse

effusion
- chylous e.
- hemorrhagic e.
- middle ear e.
- pericardial e.
- pleural e.
- subdural e.

EG—esophagogastrectomy

EGA—estimated gestational age

egagropilus

E

EGD—
   esophagogastroduodenoscopy
egersimeter
egest
egesta
egestion
EGF—epidermal growth factor
EGG—electrogastrogram
Eggers
   operation
   plate
   screw
   splint
egilops
eglandulous
EGM—electrogram
ego
   body e.
egocentric
ego-ideal
egoism
egomania
egophony
ego-strength
EGOT—erythrocyte glutamic-
   oxaloacetic transaminase
egotism
egotistic, egotistical
egotropic
egress
Egyptian
   conjunctivitis
   ophthalmia
EH—essential hypertension
EHBF—
   estimated hepatic blood flow
   extrahepatic blood flow
EHC—
   enterohepatic circulation
   essential hypercholesterolemia
EHF—exophthalmos-hyperthyroid
   factor
EHL—endogenous hyperlipidemia
Ehlers-Danlos
   disease
   syndrome
EHO—extrahepatic obstruction
EHP—excessive heat production
Ehrlich
   body
   granule
   reaction
   reagent
   stain
   test

Ehrlich *(continued)*
   theory
   tumor
Ehrlich-Hata
   preparation
   treatment
Ehrlich-Heinz granules
Ehrlichia
   E. canis
   E. chaffeensis
   E. ewingii
ehrlichial
ehrlichiosis
   human granulocytic e.
   human monocytic e.
E/I—expiration-inspiration ratio
EIA—enzyme immunoassay
Eicher prosthesis
Eichhorst
   atrophy
   corpuscles
   type
eicosanoate
eicosanoic acid
eicosanoid
eicosapentaenoic acid (EPA)
EID—
   egg-infective dose
   electroimmunodiffusion
   emergency infusion device
eidetic
   e. image
   e. imagery
eidogen
eidoptometry
EIEC—enteroinvasive *Escherichia
coli*
eight-ball hyphema
Eikenella corrodens
eikonometer
eiloid
Einhorn
   dilator
   saccharimeter
   string test
einsteinium (Es)
Einthoven
   formula
   galvanometer
   law
   triangle
EIP—extensor indicis proprius
eisanthema
Eisenmenger
   complex

Eisenmenger *(continued)*
    disease
    syndrome
    tetralogy
eisodic
EIT—erythrocyte iron
  turnover
ejaculate
ejaculatio
    e. deficiens
    e. praecox
    e. retardata
ejaculation
    premature e.
ejaculator seminis
ejaculatory
ejaculum
ejecta
ejection
    e. fraction (EF)
    milk e.
    e. phase indices
    e. shell image
    e. sound
ejector
    saliva e.
Ekbom syndrome
EKC—epidemic
  keratoconjunctivitis
Ekehorn operation
EKG, ECG—
    electrocardiogram
    electrocardiography
ekiri
elaborate
elaboration
elacin
elaidic acid
elaioplast
ELAM—endothelial leukocyte
  adhesion molecule
elantrine
elapid
elasmobranch
elassosis
elastance
elastase
elastic
    e. collision
    intermaxillary e.
    intramaxillary e.
    e. suture
    vertical e.
elastica
elasticity

elastin
elastoblast dorsi
elastofibroma
    e. dorsi
    perforating e.
elastogel
elastoid
elastoidosis
    nodular e.
elastolysis
    generalized e.
    perifollicular e.
    postinflammatory e.
elastolytic
elastoma
    juvenile e.
    Miescher e.
elastomer
elastometer
elastometry
elastomucin
elastopathy
Elastoplast
elastorrhexis
elastose
elastosis
    actinic e.
    e. dystrophica
    nodular e.
    nodular e. of Favre-Racouchot
    nodular e. of skin
    e. perforans serpiginosa
    perforating e.
    senile e.
    e. senilis
    solar e.
elastotic
elater
elation
elbow
    baseball pitchers' e.
    beat e.
    capped e.
    dropped e.
    golfer's e.
    little leaguers' e.
    miners' e.
    nursemaids' e.
    pulled e.
    tennis e.
elcosis
elder
Eldridge-Green lamp
elective
Electra complex

E

electrical impedance
  plethysmography
electric chromatography
electroacupuncture
electroanalgesia
electroanalysis
electroanesthesia
electroaugmentation
electrobasograph
electrobiology
electrobioscopy
electrocapillarity
electrocardiogram (ECG, EKG)
    bipolar e.
    esophageal e.
    intracardiac e.
    scalar e.
    twelve-lead e., 12-lead e.
    unipolar e.
electrocardiography (ECG, EKG)
    fetal e.
    intrabronchial e.
    intracardiac e.
    intracavitary e.
    precordial e.
    twelve-lead e., 12-lead e.
electrocatalysis
electrocauterization
electrocautery
electrocerebellogram
electrocerebral inactivity
electrochemistry
electrochromatography
electrocoagulation
electrocochleogram
electrocochleograph
electrocochleographic
electrocochleography
electrocoma
electrocontractility
electroconvulsive
electrocorticogram
electrocorticography
electrocution
electrocystography
electrode
    active e.
    ball-tip e.
    bayonet-tip e.
    Bugbee e.
    calomel e.
    carbon dioxide e.
    central terminal e.
    Clark e.
    conical-tip e.

electrode *(continued)*
    depolarizing e.
    dispersing e.
    dual e. lead
    esophageal e.
    esophageal pill e.
    exciting e.
    fixed e.
    glass e.
    Gradle e.
    Hamm e.
    impregnated e.
    indifferent e.
    ion-selective e.
    Kronfeld e.
    localizing e.
    McCarthy e.
    multi-e. lead
    multiple point e.
    Neil-Moore e.
    periaqueductal gray e.
    Pischel e.
    point e.
    return e.
    reversible e.
    scalp e.
    silent e.
    therapeutic e.
    transcutaneous oxygen e.
    ureteral meatotomy e.
    Weve e.
electrodermal
electrodermatome
electrodesiccation
electrodiagnosis
electrodiagnostic
electrodiagnostics
electrodialysis
electrodialyzer
electroencephalogram (EEG)
    brain death protocol e.
    flat e.
    isoelectric e.
electroencephalography
  (EEG)
electroencephaloscope
electroendosmosis
electroexcision
electrofocusing
electrogalvanic
electrogastrogram
electrogastrograph
electrogastrography
electrogenic
electrogoniometer

electrogram
    atrial e.
    coronary sinus (CS) e.
    esophageal e.
    high right atrial (HRA) e.
    His bundle e. (HBE)
    intra-atrial e.
    intracardiac e.
    right ventricular e.
    right ventricular apical e.
    sinus node e.
electrography
electrogustometer
electrogustometry
electrohemostasis
electrohysterogram
electrohysterography
electroimmunoassay
electroimmunodiffusion
electrokinetic
electrolaryngogram
electrolaryngograph
electrolaryngography
electrolepsy
electrolithotrity
electrolysis
electrolyte
    amphoteric e.
    colloidal e.
    e. imbalance
    protein e.
    serum e's
electrolytic
electrolyzable
electrolyzer
electromagnet
electromagnetic
    e. induction
    e. radiation
    e. spectrum
electromagnetism
electromanometer
electromanometry
electromechanical
    e. coupling
    e. dissociation
    e. interval
electrometer
    dynamic-condenser e.
    vibrating-reed e.
electrometrogram
electromigratory
electromotive
electromyogram (EMG)
    integrated e. (IEMG)

electromyogram (EMG) *(continued)*
    single-fiber e. (SFEMG)
    ureteral e.
electromyograph
    free e.
    ureteral e.
    valence e.
electromyography (EMG)
    needle e.
    single fiber e. (SFEMG)
    ureteral e.
electron
    Auger e.
    e. beam therapy
    bound e.
    e. capture
    Compton e.
    emission e.
    free e.
    e. microscope
    e. microscopy
    e. multiplier tube
    e. radiography
    scanning transmission e.
      microscopy
    secondary e.
    thermionic e.
    valence e.
    e. volt(s)
electronarcosis
electron-dense
electronegative
electronegativity
electroneurography
electroneurolysis
electroneuromyography
electronic stethoscope
electronics
electron microscope
    scanning e.m.
electron-microscopic
electron-microscopical
electron neutrino
electronograph
electron volt (eV)
electronystagmogram (ENG)
electronystagmograph
electronystagmography
electro-oculogram (EOG)
electro-oculography
electro-olfactogram (EOG)
electro-osmosis
electroparacentesis
electropathology
electropherogram

E

electrophile
electrophilic
electrophoregram
    counter e.
    lipoprotein e.
    protein e.
electrophoresis
    agarose gel e.
    cellulose acetate e.
    counter e.
    countercurrent e.
    disc e.
    gel e.
    lipoprotein e.
    moving boundary e.
    paper e.
    polyacrylamide gel e. (PAGE)
    protein e.
    pulsed-field e.
    rocket e.
    SDS–polyacrylamide gel e.
      (SDS-PAGE)
    serum protein e.
    single-cell gel e.
    starch gel e.
    two-dimensional gel e.
    zone e.
electrophoretic
electrophoretically
electrophoretogram
electrophorus
electrophotometer
electrophrenic
electrophysiologic
electrophysiology
    cardiac e.
electroplating
electroplexy
electropneumograph
electropositive
electroprosthesis
electroradiometer
electroresection
electroretinogram (ERG)
    E e.
    I e.
electroretinograph
electroretinography
electrosalivogram
electroscission
electroscope
electrosection
electroshock
electrosleep
electrosol

electrospectrogram
electrospectrography
electrospinogram
electrospinography
electrostatic
electrostenolysis
electrostimulation
electrostriatogram
electrosurgery
electrosyneresis
electrosynthesis
electrotaxis
electrothanasia
electrotherapeutics
electrotherapeutist
electrotherapist
electrotherapy
    cerebral e.
electrotherm
electrothrombosis
electrotome
    laparoscopic e.
    Stern-McCarthy e.
electrotomy
electrotonic
electrotonus
electrotransfer
electrotrephine
electrotropism
    negative e.
    positive e.
electroultrafiltration
electroureterogram
electroureterography
electrovagogram
electrovalence
electrovalent
electroversion
electrovert
electuary of senna
eledoisin
eleidin
element
    anatomic e.
    appendicular e's
    daughter e.
    electronegative e.
    electropositive e.
    formed e's of the blood
    labile e.
    morphologic e.
    parent e.
    radioactive e.
    rare earth e's
    sarcous e.

E

element *(continued)*
    stable e.
    tissue e.
    trace e's
    tracer e's
    transcalifornium e's
    transduced e.
    transition e.
    transposable e.
    transuranic e's
    transuranium e's
elementary
elemicin
eleoma
eleometer
eleoplast
eleoptene
eleosaccharum
eleotherapy
elephantiasic
elephantiasis
    e. asturiensis
    e. chirurgica
    e. congenita angiomatosa
    congenital e.
    filarial e.
    e. filariensis
    e. gingivae
    e. graecorum
    e. italica
    e. leishmaniana
    lymphangiectatic e.
    e. neuromatosa
    nevoid e.
    e. nostras
    e. oculi
    e. scroti
    e. telangiectodes
    e. of vulva
elephantoid
Elettaria cardamomum
elevation
    e. of head of bed
    serum troponin I e.
    ST e., ST-segment e.
    tactile e's
    threshold e.
    tubal e.
elevator
    Adson e.
    angular e.
    apical e.
    Aufricht e.
    Ballenger e.
    Barsky e.

elevator *(continued)*
    Bennett e.
    Cameron-Haight e.
    Campbell e.
    Chandler e.
    Cobb e.
    Cottle e.
    cross bar e.
    Cryer e.
    Cushing periosteal e.
    dental e.
    Desmarres lid e.
    Dingman e.
    e. disease
    Doyen e.
    Farabeuf e.
    Frazier e.
    Freer e.
    Hajek-Ballenger e.
    Hedblom e.
    Hibbs e.
    House e.
    Hurd e.
    Jackson e.
    joker e.
    Killian e.
    Lamont e.
    Lane e.
    Langenbeck
      (von Langenbeck) e.
    Lempert e.
    Love-Adson e.
    MacKenty e.
    malar e.
    Matson e.
    McIndoe e.
    Overholt e.
    palatal e.
    Pennington e.
    periosteal e.
    periosteum e.
    Phemister e.
    Pierce e.
    Proctor e.
    e. of prostate
    Ralks e.
    Ray-Parsons-Sunday e.
    Rochester e.
    root e.
    screw e.
    Sédillot e.
    Shambaugh e.
    Shambaugh-Derlacki e.
    Soonawalla uterine e.
    straight e.

elevator *(continued)*
    Sunday e.
    T-bar e.
    Veau e.
    wedge e.
    Woodson e.
elicit, elicited
eliminant
elimination
    immune e.
    pyelography by e.
elinin
ELISA—enzyme-linked
immunosorbent assay
ELITT—endometrial laser
intrauterine thermotherapy
elixir
    adjuvant e.
    aromatic e.
    cascara e.
    e. of diamorphine
      and terpin
    glycyrrhiza e.
    high-alcoholic e.
    iso-alcoholic e.
    lactated pepsin e.
    low-alcoholic e.
    e. of nux vomica
elkosis
Ellik evacuator
Elliot
    corneal trephination
    operation
    position
    sign
    trephine
Elliott
    forceps
    plate
    treatment
ellipse
ellipsin
ellipsis
ellipsoid of spleen
elliptic, elliptical
    e. incision
elliptocytary
elliptocyte
elliptocytosis
    hereditary e.
elliptocytotic
Ellis
    curve
    line
    needle holder

Ellis-Garland
    curve
    line
Ellis-Jones operation
Ellis-van Creveld syndrome
Ellsner gastroscope
Ellsworth-Howard test
Elmslie-Cholmeley operation
Eloesser
    flap
    operation
elongation
eloped
elopement
Elsberg incision
Elschnig
    bodies
    conjunctivitis
    forceps
    knife
    operation
    pearls
    retractor
    spatula
    spoon
    spots
    syndrome
Elschnig-O'Brien forceps
Elsner asthma
ELT—euglobulin lysis time
eluate
elucaine
elucidate
elude, eluded
eluent
elute
elution
    affinity e.
    gradient e.
    membrane e.
elutriation
Ely
    operation
    sign
    test
elytroceliotomy
elytroplasty
elytropolypus
Elzholtz bodies
Em.—
    emanation
    emmetropia
EM—
    ejection murmur
    erythrocyte mass

EM, EMC—electron microscopy
emaciated
emaciation
emailloblast
eman
emanate
emanating
emanation (Em.)
    e. 219, e. 220, etc.
emancipation
emasculate
emasculation
EMB—
    embryology
    eosin-methylene blue
embalm
embalming
embarrass
embarrassment
    e. of choices
    respiratory e.
    e. of riches
Embden ester
Embden-Meyerhof glycolytic
    pathway
Embden-Meyerhof-Parnas pathway
embed, embedded
embedding
EMB (eosin-methylene blue) agar
embole
embolectomy
emboli (plural of embolus)
embolic
emboliform
embolism
    air e.
    amniotic fluid e.
    bacillary e.
    bacterial e.
    bland e.
    bone marrow e.
    capillary e.
    cerebral e.
    coronary e.
    crossed e.
    direct e.
    fat e.
    hematogenous e.
    infective e.
    lymph e.
    lymphogenous e.
    miliary e.
    multiple e.
    oil e.
    pantaloon e.

embolism *(continued)*
    paradoxical e.
    plasmodium e.
    pulmonary e.
    retinal e.
    saddle e.
    spinal e.
    trichinous e.
    tumor e.
    venous e.
embolization
    partial vein e. (PVE)
    poppet e.
embolalia
embolomycotic
embolophrasia
embolotherapy
embolus (emboli)
    air e.
    cancer e.
    cellular e.
    cholesterol e.
    fat e.
    foam e.
    obturating e.
    pantaloon e.
    platelet e.
    pulmonary e.
    renal cholesterol e.
    riding e.
    saddle e.
    shower of emboli
    straddling e.
emboly
embouchement
embrasure
    buccal e.
    incisal e.
    interdental e.
    labial e.
    lingual e.
    occlusal e.
embrocation
embryatrics
embryectomy
embryo
    hexacanth e.
    Janošík e.
    presomite e.
    previllous e.
    somite e.
    Spee e.
embryoblast
embryocardia
embryocidal

E

embryoctony
embryogenesis
　　accelerated e.
embryogenetic
embryogenic
embryogeny
embryograph
embryography
embryoid
embryoism
embryologic
embryologist
embryology
　　causal e.
　　chemical e.
　　comparative e.
　　descriptive e.
　　experimental e.
embryoma
embryomorphous
embryonal
embryonate
embryonic fallopian tube
embryoniferous
embryoniform
embryonism
embryonization
embryonoid
embryony
embryopathia rubeolaris
embryopathology
embryopathy
　　rubella e.
embryophore
embryoplastic
embryoscope
embryotome
embryotomy
embryotoxic
embryotoxicity
embryotoxon
　　anterior e.
　　posterior e.
embryotroph
embryotrophic
embryotrophy
EMC—encephalomyocarditis
EMD—electromechanical
　dissociation
emedullate
emerge, emerged
emergency
emergent
Emerson
　　bronchoscope

Emerson (continued)
　　pump
　　stripper
emery
Emery-Dreifuss dystrophy
emesis
　　fecal e.
　　e. gravidarum
emetatrophia
emetic
　　central e.
　　direct e.
　　indirect e.
　　mechanical e.
　　systemic e.
　　tartar e.
emeticology
emetine and bismuth iodide
emetocathartic
EMF—
　　electromagnetic flowmeter
　　electromotive force
　　endomyocardial fibrosis
　　erythrocyte maturation factor
EMG—
　　electromyogram
　　electromyography
　　exophthalmos, macroglossia,
　　　gigantism (syndrome)
EMI—
　　Electric and Musical
　　　Industries (brain scanner)
　　electromagnetic interference
emigration
eminence
　　alveolar e's
　　antithenar e.
　　arcuate e.
　　articular e. of temporal bone
　　arytenoid e.
　　bicipital e.
　　capitate e.
　　caudate e. of liver
　　coccygeal e.
　　cochlear e. of sacral bone
　　collateral e. of lateral ventricle
　　collateral e. of Meckel
　　e. of concha
　　cruciate e.
　　cruciform e. of occipital bone
　　cuneiform e. of head of rib
　　deltoid e.
　　Doyère e.
　　facial e. of eminentia teres
　　frontal e.

eminence *(continued)*
 genital e.
 gluteal e. of femur
 e. of humerus
 hypobranchial e.
 hypoglossal e.
 hypothenar e.
 iliopectineal e.
 iliopubic e.
 intercondylar e.
 intercondyloid e.
 intermediate e.
 jugular e.
 lateral e's of tuber cinereum
 malar e.
 mammillary e.
 e. of maxilla
 maxillary e.
 medial e. of fourth ventricle
 medial e. of rhomboid fossa
 median e. of hypothalamus
 median e. of neurohypophysis
 median e's of tuber cinereum
 nasal e.
 oblique e. of cuboid bone
 occipital e.
 olivary e. of sphenoid bone
 orbital e. of zygomatic bone
 parietal e.
 postchiasmatic e.
 postfundibular e.
 postinfundibular e.
 pyramidal e.
 radial e. of wrist
 e. of scapha
 e. of superior semicircular
  canal
 supracondylar e.
 terete e.
 thenar e.
 thyroid e.
 triangular e.
 e. of triangular fossa of auricle
 trigeminal e.
 e. of triquetral fossa
 trochlear e.
 ulnar e. of wrist
 vagal e.
eminent
eminentia
 e. arcuata
 e. articularis ossis temporalis
 e. capitata
 e. carpi radialis
 e. carpi ulnaris

eminentia *(continued)*
 e. cinerea cuneiformis
 e. conchae
 e. cruciata
 e. cruciformis
 e. facialis
 e. fallopii
 e. fossae triangularis auriculae
 e. frontalis
 e. gracilis
 e. hypoglossi
 e. hypothenaris
 e. iliopectinea
 e. iliopubica
 e. intercondylaris
 e. jugularis
 e. maxillare
 e. medialis fossae rhomboideae
 e. orbitalis ossis zygomatici
 e. papillaris
 e. pyramidalis
 e. restiformis
 e. scaphae
 e. styloidea
 e. symphysis
 e. teres
 e. thenaris
 e. triangularis
 e. trigemina
 e. vagi
emiocytosis
EMI scan
emissarium
 e. condyloideum
 e. mastoideum
 e. occipitale
 e. parietale
emissary
emission
 e. angiography
 beta e.
 cold e.
 e. computed tomography
  (ECT)
 filament e.
 nasal e.
 nocturnal e.
 photoelectric e.
 positron e. tomography (PET)
 positron e. transverse
  tomography
 radionuclide e. tomography
 e. renography
 single photon e. computed
  tomography (SPECT)

E

emission *(continued)*
    thermionic e.
    e. tomography
emissivity
EMIT—enzyme-multiplied
    immunoassay technique
emittance
emitter
emmenagogic
emmenagogue
    direct e.
    indirect e.
emmenia
emmenic
emmeniopathy
emmenology
Emmet
    hook
    operation
    retractor
    scissors
    suture
Emmet-Gellhorn pessary
emmetrope
emmetropia (Em.)
emmetropic
Emmet-Studdiford
    method
    perineorrhaphy
emodin
emollient
emotiomotor
emotion
emotional
emotiovascular
empacho
empasma
empathic
empathize
empathy
emperipolesis
emphraxis
emphysema
    aging-lung e.
    alveolar e.
    alveolar duct e.
    atrophic e.
    bullous e.
    centriacinar e.
    centrilobular e.
    chronic hypertrophic e.
    compensating e.
    compensatory e.
    congenital lobar e.
    cutaneous e.

emphysema *(continued)*
    cystic e.
    diffuse e.
    ectatic e.
    false e.
    familial e.
    focal-dust e.
    gangrenous e.
    generalized e.
    glass blower's e.
    hypertrophic e.
    hypoplastic e.
    idiopathic unilobar e.
    infantile lobar e.
    interlobular e.
    interstitial e.
    intestinal e.
    Jenner e.
    lobar e.
    loculated e.
    mediastinal e.
    obstructive e.
    panacinar e.
    panlobular e.
    paracicatricial e.
    paraseptal e.
    pulmonary e.
    senile e.
    skeletal e.
    small-lunged e.
    subcutaneous e.
    subfascial e.
    subgaleal e.
    surgical e.
    traumatic e.
    unilateral e.
    vesicular e.
emphysematous
empiric, empirical
empiricism
emplastic
emplastration
emplastrum
emporiatrics
emprosthotonos
emptysis
empyema
    e. articuli
    e. benignum
    extradural e.
    e. of gallbladder
    interlobar e.
    latent e.
    loculated e.
    mastoid e.

empyema *(continued)*
    metapneumonic e.
    e. necessitatis
    e. of pericardium
    pneumococcal e.
    pulsating e.
    putrid e.
    sacculated e.
    streptococcal e.
    subdural e.
    synpneumonic e.
    thoracic e.
    e. tube
    tuberculous e.
empyemic
empyesis
empyocele
empyreuma
empyreumatic
EMS—emergency medical service
EMT—emergency medical
    technician
emulgent
emulsification
emulsifier
emulsify
emulsion
    bacillary e.
    benzyl benzoate e.
    e. of cod liver oil
    hexachlorophene cleansing e.
    kerosene e.
    e. of liquid paraffin with cascara
    e. of liquid paraffin with
      phenolphthalein
    liquid petrolatum e.
    mineral oil e.
    nuclear e.
    e. of peppermint
    perlsucht bacillen e. (PBE)
    photographic e.
    Pusey e.
    water-in-oil e.
emulsive
emulsoid
emulsum
emunctory
EN— erythema nodosum
ENA—extractable nuclear antigen(s)
ENaC—epithelial sodium channel
enamel
    curled e.
    dental e.
    dwarfed e.
    gnarled e.

enamel *(continued)*
    hereditary brown e.
    hypoplastic e.
    mottled e.
    nanoid e.
    straight e.
enameloblast
enameloblastoma
enamelogenesis
enameloma
enamelum
enanthema
enanthematous
enanthic acid
enantiobiosis
enantiomer
enantiomerism
enantiomorphic
enantiopathia
enarkyochrome
enarthritis
enarthrodial
enarthrosis
en bloc
encainide
encanthis
encapsidate
encapsulate
encapsulated
encapsulation
encased
encatarrhaphy
enceinte
encelialgia
enceliitis
encephalalgia
encephalatrophy
encephalauxe
encéphale isolé
encephalemia
encephalic
encephalitic
encephalitis (encephalitides)
    acute demyelinating e.
    acute disseminated e.
    acute necrotizing e.
    American e.
    arbovirus e.
    Baló concentric e.
    benign myalgic e.
    Binswanger e.
    boutonneuse e.
    bulbar e.
    Calabrian e.
    California e.

E

encephalitis (encephalitides)
(continued)

Central European e.
cerebellar e.
chronic subcortical e.
Condorelli e.
cortical e.
e. corticalis
Coxsackie e.
Dawson e.
demyelinating e.
diffuse sclerosing e.
eastern e.
eastern equine e.
eastern North American e.
Economo (von Economo) e.
epidemic e.
e. epidemica
equine e.
forest-spring e.
Hayem e.
hemorrhagic e.
hemorrhagic arsphenamine e.
e. hemorrhagica superior
herpes e.
herpes simplex e.
herpetic e.
e. hyperplastica
Ilheus e.
inclusion body e.
infantile e.
influenzal e.
Japanese B e.
Leichtenstern e.
lethargic e.
e. lethargica
limbic e.
Mengo e.
mumps e.
Murray Valley e.
e. neonatorum
otic e.
e. periaxialis concentrica
e. periaxialis diffusa
perivenous e.
postexanthematous e.
postinfectious e.
postvaccinal e.
Powassan e.
purulent e.
pyogenic e.
Russian autumnal e.
Russian endemic e.
Russian forest-spring e.
Russian spring-summer e.

encephalitis (encephalitides)
(continued)

Russian tick-borne e.
Russian vernal e.
St. Louis e.
Schilder e.
Semliki Forest e.
Sicilian e.
e. siderans
Strümpell-Leichtenstern e.
subacute inclusion body e.
e. subcorticalis chronica
summer e.
suppurative e.
tick-borne e.
torula e.
typhoid e.
van Bogaert e.
varicella e.
Venezuelan equine e.
vernal e.
vernoestival e.
Vienna e.
viral e.
von Economo e.
western e.
western equine e.
West Nile e.
woodcutter e.
encephalitogen
encephalitogenic
Encephalitozoon
E. cuniculi
E. hellem
E. intestinalis
encephalitozoonosis
encephalization
encephalocele
orbital e.
encephaloclastic
encephalocystocele
encephalocystomeningocele
encephalodialysis
encephalodysplasia
encephaloedema
encephalogram
encephalography
air e.
fractional e.
gamma e.
positive contrast e.
encephaloid
encephalolith
encephalology
encephaloma

encephalomalacia
    avian e.
    periventricular e.
encephalomeningitis
encephalomeningocele
encephalomeningopathy
encephalomere
encephalometer
encephalometry
encephalomyelitis
    acute disseminated e.
    benign myalgic e.
    disseminated e.
    eastern equine e. (EEE)
    equine e.
    experimental allergic e. (EAE)
    granulomatous e.
    Kelly e.
    Mengo e.
    parainfectious e.
    postexanthematous e.
    postimmunization e.
    postinfectious e.
    postvaccinal e.
    Venezuelan equine e. (VEE)
    viral e.
    western equine e. (WEE)
    zoster e.
encephalomyelocele
encephalomyeloneuropathy
encephalomyelopathy
    epidemic myalgic e.
    Leigh necrotizing e.
    postinfection e.
    postvaccinal e.
    subacute necrotizing e.
encephalomyeloradiculitis
encephalomyeloradiculoneuritis
encephalomyeloradiculopathy
encephalomyopathy
encephalon
encephalonarcosis
encephalopathic
encephalopathy
    acute infantile e.
    alcoholic e.
    anoxic e.
    arsenical e.
    atonic-astasic e.
    biliary e.
    bilirubin e.
    callosal demyelinating e.
    Creutzfeldt-Jakob presenile e.
    cystic multilocular e.
    demyelinating e.

encephalopathy *(continued)*
    dialysis e.
    e. and fatty degeneration of
      viscera
    hepatic e.
    hypercalcemic e.
    hypernatremic e.
    hypertensive e.
    hypoglycemic e.
    hypoxic e.
    Leigh e.
    metabolic e.
    myoclonic e. of childhood
    necrotizing e.
    palindromic e.
    para-Wernicke e.
    pertussis e.
    portal-systemic e.
    portasystemic e.
    portocaval e.
    postanoxic e.
    progressive dialysis e.
    progressive multifocal e.
    progressive subcortical e.
    punch-drunk e.
    rheumatic e.
    saturnine e.
    spongiform e.
    subacute necrotizing e.
    subacute spongiform e.
    subcortical arteriosclerotic e.
    toxic e.
    traumatic e.
    uremic e.
    Wernicke e.
    e. with forminiminotransferase
      deficiency
    e. with prolinemia
    e. with tyrosinuria
encephalopsychosis
encephalopuncture
encephalopyosis
encephalorachidian
encephaloradiculitis
encephalorrhagia
encephaloschisis
encephalosclerosis
encephaloscope
encephaloscopy
encephalosepsis
encephalosis
    azotemic e.
encephalospinal
encephalothlipsis
encephalotome

E

encephalotomy
encephalotrigeminal angiomatosis
enchondroma (enchondromas, enchondromata)
 e. petrificum
 multiple congenital enchondromas
enchondromatous
enchondrosarcoma
enchondrosis
enchylema
enchyma
enclave
enclitic
enclomiphene
enclosure
 Charnley e.
encolpism
encolpismus
encompass, encompassed
encompassing
encopresis
encounter
encranius
encyesis
encyopyelitis
encysted
encystment
end
 e. colostomy
 C-terminal e.
 distal e.
 end-terminal e.
 e. ileostomy
 reducing e.
 e.-to-side ileotransverse colostomy
 sticky e.
 taste e.
 e. tracheostome
 e. tube
endadelphos
Endamoeba blattae
endangiitis
endangium
endaortic
endaortitis
 bacterial e.
endarterectomize
endarterectomy
 Cannon e. loop
 carotid e. (CEA)
 eversion e.
 gas e.
 transaortic e.

endarterial
endarteritis
 e. deformans
 Heubner specific e.
 e. obliterans
 e. proliferans
 spinal e.
 syphilitic cerebral e.
endarterium
endarteropathy
 digital e.
endartery
endaural incision
endbrain
end-brush
end-bud
end-bulb
 cylindrical e.
 e. of Held
 e's of Krause
endchondral
end-diastolic
end-to-end anastomosis
endeictic
endemia
endemic
endemicity
endemoepidemic
endepidermis
endergic
endergonic
enderon
enderonic
end-feet of Held
end-flake
ending
 annulospiral e's
 ball-of-thread e's
 basket e's
 calyciform e.
 club e. of Bartelmez
 Dogiel e.
 encapsulated nerve e.
 en plaque e.
 epilemmal e's
 free nerve e.
 Golgi-Mazzoni e's
 grape e's
 nerve e's
 nonencapsulated e.
 pain e.
 palisade e.
 primary e.
 Ruffini e's
 secondary e.

E

ending *(continued)*
    spiral e.
    spray e's
    synaptic e.
    taste e.
    trail e.
    ultraterminal e.
    unencapsulated e.
end-nucleus, end-nuclei
endoabdominal
Endo agar
endoamylase
endoaneurysmoplasty
endoaneurysmorrhaphy
endoappendicitis
endoauscultation
endobacillary
endobiotic
endoblast
endoblastic
endobronchial tube
endobronchitis
endocardial
    e. cushion defect
    e. fibroelastosis
    e. fibrosis
    e. resection
    e. sclerosis
    e. tube
endocardiography
endocardiopathy
endocarditic
endocarditis
    abacterial thrombotic e.
    acute bacterial e.
    atypical verrucous e.
    bacterial e.
    e. benigna
    e. chordalis
    chronic e.
    constrictive e.
    Coxsackie e.
    fungal e.
    gonococcal e.
    infectious e.
    infective e.
    e. lenta
    Libman-Sacks e.
    Löffler e.
    malignant e.
    marantic e.
    mural e.
    mycotic e.
    nonbacterial thrombotic e.
    nonbacterial verrucous e.

endocarditis *(continued)*
    noninfective e.
    parietal e.
    e. parietalis fibroplastica
    plastic e.
    polypous e.
    prosthetic valve e.
    pulmonic e.
    pustulous e.
    rheumatic e.
    rickettsial e.
    right-side e.
    septic e.
    subacute bacterial e.
    syphilitic e.
    tuberculous e.
    ulcerative e.
    valvular e.
    vegetative e.
    verrucous e.
    viridans e.
endocardium
endoceliac
endocellular
endocervical
    e. canal
    e. mucosa
    e. polyp
endocervicitis
endocervix
endochondral
endochorion
endochrome
endochylema
endocolitis
endocolpitis
endocommensal
endoconidiotoxicosis
endocorpuscular
endocranial
endocraniosis
endocranitis
endocranium
endocrine
endocrinium
endocrinologist
endocrinology
endocrinopathic
endocrinopathy
endocrinosis
endocrinotherapy
endocrinotropic
endocuticle
endocyclic
endocyst

endocystitis
endocyte
endocytize
endocytosis
endodeoxyribonuclease
endoderm
    primitive e.
    primordial e.
    ventral e.
    yolk sac e.
endodermal
endodermoreaction
endodiascope
endodiascopy
endodontics
endodontist
endodontium
endodontology
endodural
endodyogeny
endoectothrix
endoelectrontherapy
endoenteritis
endoenzyme
endoepidermal
endoepithelial
endoergic
endoergic reaction
endoesophagitis
endoexoteric
endofaradism
endogalvanism
endogamous
endogamy
endogastric
endogastritis
endogenote
endogenous
endogeny
endoglobular
endognathic suture
endognathion
endogonidium
endoherniorrhaphy
endointoxication
endolabyrinthitis
endolaryngeal
endolarynx
Endolimax nana
endolymph
endolympha
endolymphangial
endolymphangitis
    proliferans
endolymphatic hydrops

endolysin
    leukocytic e.
endolysis
endomastoiditis
endomeninges
endomesoderm
endomesognathic suture
endometrectomy
endometria (plural of
    endometrium)
endometrial laser intrauterine
    thermotherapy (ELITT)
endometrioid
endometrioma
endometriosis
    e. of colon
    colonic e.
    cutaneous e.
    cystic e.
    e. externa
    e. interna
    interstitial e.
    ovarian e.
    e. ovarii
    stromal e.
    tubal e.
    e. uterina
    e. vesicae
endometriotic
endometritis
    bacteriotoxic e.
    decidual e.
    e. dissecans
    exfoliative e.
    glandular e.
    membranous e.
    postpartum e.
    puerperal e.
    syncytial e.
    tuberculous e.
    e. tuberosa
        papulosa
endometrium
    (endometria)
    hyperplastic e.
    secretory e.
    Swiss-cheese e.
endometrorrhagia
endometry
endomitosis
endomitotic
endomixis
endomorph
endomorphic
endomorphy

Endomyces
    E. albicans
    E. epidermidis
endomyelography
endomyocardial
    e. biopsy
    e. fibrosis
endomyocarditis
endomyometritis
endomysium
endonasal
endoneural
endoneurial
endoneuritis
endoneurium
endoneurolysis
end-on mattress suture
endonuclear
endonuclease
    restriction e.
endonucleolus
endoparasite
endoparasitic
endoparasitism
endopelvic
endopeptidase
endopericardial
endopericarditis
endoperimyocarditis
endoperineuritis
endoperitoneal
endoperitonitis
endoperoxide isomerase
endophasia
endophlebitis
    e. hepatica obliterans
    proliferative e.
endophthalmitis
    phacoanaphylactic e.
endophylaxination
endophyte
endophytic
endoplasm
endoplasmic
endopolygeny
endopolyploid
endopolyploidy
endopredator
endoradiography
endoradiosonde
endoradiotherapy
endoreduplication
end-organ
endorhinitis
endoribonuclease

endorphin
    α-e. [alpha-]
    β-e. [beta-]
    γ-e. [gamma-]
endorrhachis
endosalpingiosis
endosalpingitis
endosalpingoma
endosalpinx
endoscope
    Kelly e.
    Rockey e.
endoscopic
    e. cholangiography
    percutaneous e. gastrostomy
    (PEG)
    e. retrograde cholangiography
    (ERC)
    e. retrograde
    cholangiopancreatography
    (ERCP)
    e. ultrasonography
endoscopy
    fiberoptic e.
    flexible e.
    lower gastrointestinal (LGI) e.
    peroral e.
    e. suite
    transcolonic e.
    upper gastrointestinal (UGI) e.
endosecretory
endosepsis
endoskeletal prosthesis
endoskeleton
endosmometer
endosmosis
endosmotic
endosperm
endospore
endosporium
endosteal
endosteitis
endosteohyperostosis
endosteoma
endostethoscope
endosteum
endosymbiont
endosymbiosis
endotendineum
endothelia (plural of endothelium)
endothelial
endothelialization
endotheliitis
endothelin-1 receptor antagonists
endothelioblastoma

endotheliochorial
endotheliocyte
endothelioid
endotheliolysin
endotheliolytic
endothelioma
    e. angiomatosum
    e. capitis
    e. cutis
    diffuse e.
    dural e.
    perithelial e.
endotheliomatosis
endotheliosarcoma
endotheliosis
    glomerular capillary e.
endotheliotoxin
endothelium (endothelia)
    anterior e. of cornea
    e. anterius corneae
    e. camerae anterioris bulbi
    e. camerae anterioris oculi
    corneal e.
    extraembryonic e.
    vascular e.
endotherm
endothermic
endothermy
endothoracic
endothrix
endothyroidopexy
endotoxemia
endotoxic
endotoxin
endotoxoid
endotracheal (ET)
    e. intubation
    e. tube
endotracheitis
endotrachelitis
endourethral
endouterine
endovaccination
endovasculitis
endovenitis
endovenous
endozoite
endplate, end-plate, end plate
    motor e.
end-pleasure
end point
endpoint nystagmus
end product
endrin
endrysone

end-to-side anastomosis
end-stage
end-stage renal disease (ESRD)
end-systolic
    e.-s. counts
    e.-s. pressure-volume relation
    e.-s. stress-dimension relation
    e.-s. volume
end-tidal
enema (enemas, enemata)
    air contrast e.
    air contrast barium e.
    barium e.
    blind e.
    cleansing e.
    coffee e.
    contrast e.
    double-contrast e.
    Fleet e.
    high e.
    hydrocortisone e.
    Hypaque e.
    nutrient e.
    nutritive e.
    opaque e.
    pancreatic e.
    sedative e.
    small bowel e.
    soapsuds e.
    starch e.
    starch and opium e.
    theophylline olamine e.
enemator
energetics
energid
energizer
    psychic e.
energometer
energy
    activation e.
    atomic e.
    binding e.
    chemical e.
    chemical potential e.
    disintegration e.
    electrical potential e.
    electromagnetic e.
    excitation e.
    free e.
    e. frequency
    Gibbs free e. (*G*)
    kinetic e.
    latent e.
    mechanical potential e.
    nuclear e.

energy *(continued)*
    phosphate bond e.
    photon e.
    e. of position
    potential e.
    quadrant e.
    radiant e.
    recoil e.
    e. resolution
    specific nerve e.
    e. spectrum
    thermal e.
    e. wavelength
    x-ray e.
energy-rich
enervation
en face
enflagellation
enflurane
ENG—
    electronystagmogram
    electronystagmography
engagement
engastrius
Engel alkalimetry
Engelmann
    disease
    disk
    splint
Engel-Recklinghausen disease
engender, engendered
Engen extension orthosis
engine
    dental e.
engineering
    biomedical e.
    genetic e.
    human e.
English
    cane enostosis
    rhinoplasty
englobe
englobement
Engman
    dermatitis
    disease
engorge
engorged
engorgement
    breast e.
engram
engraphia
en grappe
enhancement
    acoustic e.

enhancement *(continued)*
    contrast e.
    edge e.
    immunologic e.
enhancer
enhexymal
Enhydrina schistosa
enigmatic, enigmatical
enkephalin
enkephalinergic
ENL—erythema nodosum
    leprosum
enlargement
    cardiac e.
    cervical e.
    gingival e.
    e. of heart
    tympanic e.
en masse
enniatin
enol
enolase
    neuron-specific e.
enolization
enology
enomania
enophthalmos
enophthalmus
enorganic
enostosis
enoyl-ACP reductase
enoyl-CoA hydratase
en plaque
enpromate
enrichment
Enroth sign
ensiform
ensisternum
ensomphalus
enstrophe
ENT—ear, nose, and throat
entad
ental
entamebiasis
Entamoeba
    E. buccalis
    E. dispar
    E. dysenteriae
    E. gingivalis
    E. hartmanni
    E. histolytica
    E. invadens
    E. moshkowskii
    E. nana
    E. nipponica

E

Entamoeba (continued)
    E. polecki
    E. tropicalis
    E. undulans
entasia
entelechy
entepicondyle
enteque
enteraden
enteradenitis
enteral
enteralgia
enteramine
enterectasis
enterectomy
enterepiplocele
enteric
enterically
enteric-coated
entericoid
enterics
enteritis
    bacterial e.
    choleriform e.
    chronic cicatrizing e.
    cicatrizing e.
    e. cystica chronica
    diphtheritic e.
    duck virus e.
    Escherichia coli e.
    feline e.
    granulomatous e.
    e. gravis
    infectious feline e.
    leishmanial e.
    mink viral e.
    mucous e.
    myxomembranous e.
    e. necroticans
    necrotizing e.
    e. nodularis
    pellicular e.
    phlegmonous e.
    e. polyposa
    protozoan e.
    pseudomembranous e.
    radiation e.
    regional e.
    segmental e.
    specific feline e.
    streptococcus e.
    terminal e.
    tuberculous e.
    ulcerative e.
enteroanastomosis

enteroanthelone
enteroapokleisis
Enterobacter
    E. aerogenes
    E. agglomerans
    E. alvei
    E. amnigenus
    E. cloacae
    E. gergoviae
    E. intermedium
    E. liquefaciens
    E. sakazakii
enterobacterium
    (enterobacteria)
enterobiasis
enterobiliary
Enterobius vermicularis
enterocele
enterocentesis
enteroceptor
enterochelin
enterochirurgia
enterocholecystostomy
enterocholecystotomy
enterocinesia
enterocinetic
enterocleisis
    omental e.
enteroclysis
    barium e.
    CT (computed tomographic)
      e. (CTE)
    double contrast e.
    magnetic resonance
      (MR) e.
    multidetector computed
      tomography (MDCT) e.
    small-bowel e.
enterococcemia
enterococcus
enterocoele
enterocoelic
enterocoelomate
enterocolectomy
enterocolic
enterocolitis
    antibiotic-associated e.
    hemorrhagic e.
    necrotizing e.
    pseudomembranous e.
    regional e.
enterocolostomy
enterocrinin
enterocutaneous
enterocyst

enterocystocele
enterocystoma
enterocyte
enterodynia
enteroenteric
enteroenterostomy
    Parker-Kerr e.
enteroepiplocele
enterogastric
enterogastritis
enterogastrone
enterogenous
enteroglucagon
enterogram
enterograph
enterography
enterohepatitis
enterohepatocele
enterohepatopexy
enterohydrocele
enteroidea
enterointestinal
enteroinvasive
enterokinase
enterokinesia
enterokinetic
enterokinin
enterolith
enterolithiasis
enterology
enterolysis
    excitation e.
enteromegaly
enteromenia
enteromere
enteromerocele
Enteromonas hominis
enteromycodermitis
enteromyiasis
enteromyxorrhea
enteroneuritis
enteronitis
entero-oxyntin
enteroparesis
enteropathogen
enteropathogenesis
enteropathogenic
enteropathy
    exudative e.
    gluten e.
    gluten-sensitive e.
    protein-losing e.
enteropexy
enteroplasty
enteroplex

enteroplexy
enteroptosis
enteroptotic
enteroptychia
enteroptychy
enterorenal
enterorrhagia
enterorrhaphy
    circular e.
enterorrhea
enterorrhexis
enteroscope
enterosepsis
enterospasm
enterostasis
enterostaxis
enterostenosis
enterostomal
enterostomy
    gun-barrel e.
    Witzel e.
enterotome
    Dupuytren e.
enterotomy incision
enterotoxemia
    hemorrhagic e.
    infectious e. of
      sheep
enterotoxigenic
enterotoxin
    cholera e.
    perfringens e.
enterotoxism
enterotropic
enterotyphus
enterovaginal
enterovenous
enterovesical fistula
enteroviral
enterovirus
enterozoic
enterozoon (enterozoa)
enteruria
enthalpy
enthesis
enthesitis
enthesopathy
enthetic
enthetobiosis
enthlasis
en thyrse
entire
entirety
entiris
entity

entoblast
entocele
entochondrostosis
entochoroidea
entocnemial
entocondyle
entocornea
entocuneiform
entocyte
entoderm
    primitive e.
    yolk-sac e.
entodermal
entoectad
entomere
entomion
entomogenous
entomologist
entomology
    medical e.
entomophagous
Entomophthora
    E. coronata
    E. muscae
entomophthoromycosis
ento-occipital
entophthalmia
entophyte
entopic
entoptic
entoptoscope
entoptoscopy
entoretina
entorganism
entorhinal
entotic
entotympanic
entozoa
entozoal
entozoon (entozoa)
entrapment
entripsis
entropion
    e. cicatriceum
    cicatricial e.
    spastic e.
    e. spasticum
    e. uveae
entropionize
entropium
entropy
entwicklungsmechanik
entypy
enucleate
enucleated

enucleation
enucleator
    Young e.
enuresis
    diurnal e.
    epileptic e.
    nocturnal e.
enuretic
envelope
    basilar membrane e.
    cell e.
    egg e.
    nuclear e.
envenom
envenomation
environment
    controlled e.
    external e.
    internal e.
environmental allergies
envy
    penis e.
enzootic
enzygotic
enzymatic
enzyme
    adaptive e.
    allosteric e.
    angiotensin converting e.
    biotinyl e.
    brancher e.
    branching e.
    catheptic e.
    collagenolytic e.
    constitutive e.
    cryptic e.
    debrancher e.
    debranching e.
    débridement e's
    degradative e.
    digestant e's
    early e.
    extracellular e.
    fat-splitting e.
    fibrinolytic e's
    glycolytic e.
    hydrolytic e.
    induced e.
    inducible e.
    intracellular e.
    late e.
    Lohmann e.
    malic e.
    proteolytic e.
    Q e.

enzyme *(continued)*
    receptor-destroying e. (RDE)
    redox e.
    regulatory e.
    repair e.
    repressible e.
    respiratory e.
    restriction e.
    serum e.
    terminal addition e.
    transferring e.
enzyme-linked
enzymology
enzymolysis
enzymopathy
    lysosomal e.
EO—
    eosinophil
    ethylene oxide
    eyes open
EOD—entry on duty
EOG—
    electro-oculogram
    electro-olfactogram
EOM—
    extraocular movement(s)
    extraocular muscle(s)
EOMI—extraocular muscles intact
eos—eosinophils
eosin
    e. B
    ethyl e.
    e. I bluish
    e. W
    water-soluble e.
    e. W S
    e. Y
    e. yellowish
eosinoblast
eosinopenia
    hormonal e.
eosinophil
    polymorphonuclear e.
eosinophile
eosinophilia
    hereditary e.
    Löffler e.
    pulmonary infiltration e.
    tropical e.
    tropical pulmonary e.
eosinophilic
    e. cellulitis
    e. endomyocardial disease
    e. exudates
    e. fasciitis

eosinophilic *(continued)*
    e. gastroenteropathy
    e. granuloma
    e. spongiosis
eosinophilopoietin
eosinophilotactic
eosinophiluria
eosinotactic
eosolate
EP—
    ectopic pregnancy
    erythrocyte protoporphyrin
      (test)
    evoked potential
EPA—eicosapentaenoic acid
epacmastic
epacme
epactal
epallobiosis
eparsalgia
eparterial
epaxial
EPC—epilepsia partialis continua
EPEC—enteropathogenic
    Escherichia coli
epencephalic
epencephalon
ependyma
ependymal
ependymitis
ependymoblast
ependymoblastoma
ependymocyte
ependymocytoma
ependymoma
    anaplastic e.
    myxopapillary e.
    papillary e.
    water-in-oil e.
ependymopathy
eperythrozoonosis
EPF—exophthalmos-producing
  factor
ephapse
ephaptic
epharmony
ephebiatrics
ephebic
ephebogenesis
ephebogenic
ephebology
ephelides
ephelis
ephemera
ephemeral

ephidrosis cruenta
epiallopregnanolone (EAP)
epiandrosterone
epiblast
epiblastic
epiblepharon
epiboly
epibranchial
epibulbar
epicanthal
epicanthic
epicanthus inversus
epicarcinogen
epicardia
epicardial
epicardiectomy
epicauma
epicentral
epichitosamine
epichordal
epichorion
epicillin
epicene
epicoeloma
epicomus
epicondylalgia
epicondyle
    external e. of femur
    external e. of humerus
    internal e. of femur
    internal e. of humerus
    lateral e. of femur
    lateral e. of humerus
    medial e. of femur
    medial e. of humerus
epicondyli (plural of epicondylus)
epicondylian
epicondylic
epicondylitis
    external humeral e.
    lateral e.
    radiohumeral e.
epicondylus (epicondyli)
    e. lateralis femoris
    e. lateralis humeri
    e. medialis femoris
    e. medialis humeri
epicoracoid
epicorneascleritis
epicostal
epicotyl
epicranium
epicrisis
epicritic
epicuticle

epicystitis
epicystotomy
epicyte
epidemic
epidemicity
epidemiography
epidemiologic, epidemiological
epidemiologist
epidemiology
epidermal
epidermatitis
epidermatoplasty
epidermic
epidermicula
epidermidalization
epidermides
epidermis
epidermitis
epidermization
epidermodysplasia
    verruciformis
epidermoid
    cerebrospinal e.
epidermoidoma
epidermolysin
epidermolysis
    acquired e. bullosa
    e. acquisita
    e. bullosa acquisita
    e. bullosa dystrophica,
      albopapuloid
    e. bullosa dystrophica,
      dysplastic
    e. bullosa dystrophica,
      hyperplastic
    e. bullosa dystrophica,
      polydysplastic
    e. bullosa hereditaria
    e. bullosa, junctional
    e. bullosa letalis
    e. bullosa simplex, generalized
    e. bullosa simplex, localized
    dominant e. bullosa
      dystrophica
    junctional e. bullosa
    polydysplastic e. bullosa
      dystrophica
    recessive e. bullosa
      dystrophica
    toxic bullous e.
    Weber-Cockayne e. bullosa
epidermolytic hyperkeratosis
epidermoma
epidermomycosis
epidermophytid

Epidermophyton
    E. floccosum
    E. inguinale
    E. purpureum
    E. rubrum
epidermophytosis
    e. axillaris
    e. cruris
    e. interdigitale
epidermopoiesis
epidermosis
    aural e.
epidermotropic reticulosis
epididymal
epididymectomy
epididymis
epididymitis
    spermatogenic e.
epididymodeferentectomy
epididymodeferential
epididymography
epididymo-orchitis
epididymotomy
epididymovasectomy
epididymovasostomy
epidural
    e. abscess
    e. empyema
    e. hemorrhage
epiduritis
epidurography
epiestriol
epifascial
epigamous
epigaster
epigastralgia
epigastric
epigastrium
epigastrius parasiticus
epigastrocele
epigenesis
epigenetic
epigenetics
epiglottic
epiglottidean
epiglottidectomy
epiglottiditis
epiglottis
epiglottitis
epignathous
epignathus parasiticus
epigonal
epiguanine
epihidrosis
epihyal

epihydrinaldehyde
epihyoid
epikeratomileusis
epilamellar
epilate
epilation
epilatory
epilemma
epilemmal
epilepsia
    e. arithmetica
    e. cursiva
    e. gravior
    e. major
    e. minor
    e. mitior
    e. mitis
    e. nutans
    e. partialis continua
    e. procursiva
    e. rotatoria
    e. tarda
epilepsy
    abdominal e.
    abortive e.
    absence e.
    accelerative e.
    acousticomotor e.
    acquired e.
    activated e.
    adult e.
    adversive e.
    affective e.
    akinetic e.
    alcoholic e.
    alternating e.
    ambulatory e.
    amygdaloid e.
    aphasic e.
    atonic e.
    audiogenic e.
    auditosensory e.
    auditory hallucinatory e.
    auditory illusional e.
    automatic e.
    autonomic e.
    Baltic myoclonic e.
    benign e. with centrotemporal
        spikes
    benign e. with rolandic spikes
    benign rolandic e.
    Bravais-jacksonian e.
    catamenial e.
    centrencephalic e.
    chronic focal e.

E

epilepsy *(continued)*
   cingulate e.
   conditioned e.
   contact e.
   continuous e.
   continuous partial e.
   cortical e.
   corticoreticular e.
   cryptogenic e.
   cyclical e.
   diencephalic e.
   diurnal e.
   dysmnesic e.
   enuretic e.
   essential e.
   familial e.
   febrile e.
   focal e., chronic
   focal e., minor
   fortuitous e.
   gaze e.
   gelastic e.
   generalized e.
   generalized flexion e.
   grand mal e.
   e. gravidarum
   gustatory e.
   haut mal e.
   hereditary e.
   hysterical e.
   hysteriform e.
   ideational e.
   idiopathic e.
   illusional e.
   induced e.
   insular e.
   jacksonian e.
   juvenile myoclonic e.
   kinetogenic e.
   Koshevnikoff e.
   Lafora myoclonic e.
   Lafora-type of e.
   larval e.
   laryngeal e.
   late e.
   latent e.
   limbic e.
   localized e.
   major e.
   masticatory e.
   matutinal e.
   menstrual e.
   mental e.
   metabolic e.
   midbrain e.

epilepsy *(continued)*
   minor e.
   minor focal e.
   morning e.
   morpheic e.
   movement-induced e.
   musicogenic e.
   myoclonic e.
   myoclonic e. with Lafora bodies
   myoclonus e.
   nocturnal e.
   occipital e.
   olfactory e.
   opercular e.
   opisthotonic e.
   oral e.
   organic e.
   oropharyngeal e.
   paramnesic e.
   partial e.
   Penfield e.
   petit mal e.
   pharyngeal e.
   photic e.
   photosensitive e.
   physiologic e.
   postcentral e.
   posthemiplegic e.
   postrolandic e.
   posttraumatic e.
   pregnancy e.
   primary e.
   procursive e.
   progressive myoclonic e.
   psychic e.
   psychomotor e.
   pubertal e.
   reading e.
   reflex e.
   rolandic e.
   rotatory e.
   secondary e.
   secondary generalized e.
   seesaw e.
   self-induced e.
   senile e.
   sensory e.
   serial e.
   somatomotor e.
   somatosensory e.
   somatosensory reflex e.
   somesthetic e.
   somnambulistic e.
   spinal e.
   spontaneous e.

epilepsy *(continued)*
    startle e.
    subclinical e.
    sylvian e.
    symptomatic e.
    tardy e.
    television e.
    temporal lobe e.
    tonic e.
    tornado e.
    traumatic e.
    uncinate e.
    unilateral e.
    Unverricht-Lundborg type of e.
    vertiginous e.
    visceral e.
    visual e.
    visual hallucinatory e.
    visuosensory e.
    vocal e.
    waking e.
epileptic
    e. equivalent
    e. seizure
epileptiform
epileptogenic
epileptogenous
epileptoid
epileptologist
epileptology
epileptosis
epiloia
epimandibular
epimastigote
epimenorrhagia
epimenorrhea
epimer
epimerase
epimere
epimerization
epimestrol
epimorphic
epimorphosis
epimyocardium
epimysiotomy
epimysium
epinephrinemia
epinephros
epineural suture
epineurial
epineurium
epinosic
epiorchium
epiotic
epipastic

epipericardial
epipharyngeal
epipharyngitis
epipharynx
epiphenomenon
epiphora
epiphyseal
epiphysectomy
epiphyses (plural of epiphysis)
epiphysiodesis
epiphysioid
epiphysiolisthesis
epiphysiolysis
    distraction e.
epiphysiometer
epiphysiopathy
epiphysis (epiphyses)
    capital e.
    e. cerebri
    slipped e.
    slipped capital femoral e.
    stippled e.
epiphysitis
    e. juvenilis
    vertebral e.
epiphyte
epiphytic
epipial
epipleural
epiplocele
epiploectomy
epiploenterocele
epiploic
epiploitis
    Sherlock e.
epiplomerocele
epiplomphalocele
epiploon
    greater e.
    lesser e.
epiplopexy
epiploplasty
epiplorrhaphy
epiploscheocele
epipygus parasiticus
epipyramis
epiretinal
epirizole
epirotulian
episclera
episcleral
episcleritis
    gouty e.
    e. partialis fugax
episclerotitis

E

episioperineoplasty
episioperineorrhaphy
episioplasty
episiorrhaphy
episiostenosis
episiotomy
    central e. and repair (CER)
    Matsner e.
    Matsner median e. and repair
    median e.
    mediolateral e.
episode
    acute schizophrenic e.
    hypomanic e.
    major depressive e.
    manic e.
    psycholeptic e.
    psychomotor e.
    syncopal e.
episome
epispadiac
epispadial
epispadias
    balanic e.
    balanitic e.
    clitoral e.
    complete e.
    female e.
    glandular e.
    incomplete e.
    penile e.
    penopubic e.
    subsymphyseal e.
epispastic
epispinal
episplenitis
epistasis
epistatic
epistaxis
    Gull renal e.
epistemology
episternal
episternum
episthotonos
epistropheus
episylvian
epitarsus
epitela
epitendineum
epitenon
epith—epithelium
epithalamic
epithalamus
epithalaxia
epithelia (plural of epithelium)

epithelial downgrowth
epithelialization
epithelialize, epithelialized
epitheliitis
epithelioceptor
epitheliochorial
epitheliocytus
    e. basalis gustatorius
    e. phalangeus externus
    e. phalangeus internus
    e. pilosus columnaris
    e. sensorius gustatorius
    e. sensorius pilosus externus
    e. sensorius pilosus internus
    e. sensorius pilosus piriformis
    e. sustentans gustatorius
epitheliofibril
epitheliogenetic
epitheliogenic
epithelioglandular
epithelioid
epitheliolysin
epitheliolysis
epitheliolytic
epithelioma
    e. adamantinum
    e. adenoides cysticum
    basal cell e.
    basisquamous e.
    benign calcifying e.
    calcified e.
    calcifying e.
    calcifying e. of Malherbe
    e. capitis
    chorionic e.
    columnar e.
    e. contagiosum
    e. cuniculatum
    cylindrical e.
    diffuse e.
    glandular e.
    intraepidermal e.
    e. of Malherbe
    Malherbe calcifying e.
    malignant e.
    e. molluscum
    morpheic e.
    multiple self-healing
      squamous e.
    pigmented basal cell e.
    pseudocystic e.
    self-healing squamous e.
    squamous cell e.
epitheliomatosis
epitheliomatous

epitheliomuscular
epitheliopathy
   acute multifocal placoid
      pigment e.
epitheliosis desquamativa
   conjunctivae
epitheliotoxin
epitheliotropic
epithelite
epithelium (epithelia)
   e. anterius corneae
   Barrett e.
   capsular e.
   ciliated e.
   coelomic e.
   columnar e.
   e. corneae
   corneal e.
   crevicular e.
   cubical e.
   cuboidal e.
   dental e.
   e. ductus semicircularis
   dysplastic e.
   enamel e.
   false e.
   follicular e.
   germinal e.
   gingival e.
   glandular e.
   glomerular e.
   junctional e.
   laminated e.
   e. of lens
   e. lentis
   mesenchymal e.
   e. mucosae
   muscle e.
   myxopleomorphic e.
   nerve e.
   olfactory e.
   oral e.
   pavement e.
   pigmentary e.
   pigmented e.
   pigmented e. of iris
   e. pigmentosum iridis
   e. pigmentosum partis ciliaris
      retinae
   posterior e. of cornea
   e. posterius corneae
   e. posterius pigmentosum
      partis iridicae retinae
   protective e.
   pseudostratified e.

epithelium (epithelia) *(continued)*
   pyramidal e.
   respiratory e.
   retinal pigment e.
   rod e.
   seminiferous e.
   sense e.
   sensory e.
   simple e.
   squamous e.
   stratified e.
   subcapsular e.
   sulcal e.
   sulcular e.
   e. superficiale ovarii
   surface e.
   tabular e.
   tegumentary e.
   tessellated e.
   transitional e.
   visceral e.
epithesis
epithet
epitonic
epitope
epitrichium
epitriquetrum
epitrochlea
epitrochlear
epitrochleitis
epituberculosis
epiturbinate
epitympanic
epitympanum
epitype
epityphlitis
epityphlon
epivaginitis
epizoa
epizoic
epizoicide
epizoon (epizoa)
epizoonosis
epizootic
epizootiology
EPL—extracorporeal piezoelectric
   lithotriptor
épluchage
EPM—progressive myoclonic
   epilepsy
epontic
eponychium
eponym
eponymic
eponymous

epoophorectomy
epoöphoron
epoprostenol
epornithology
epornitic
epoxide
epoxy
epoxymethamine bromide
epoxytropine tropate
EPP—
    end-plate potential
    erythropoietic protoporphyria
EPR—
    electron paramagnetic
      resonance
    electrophrenic respiration
    estradiol production rate
EPS—
    electrophysiology study
    exophthalmos-producing
      substance
    expressed prostatic secretions
    extrapyramidal signs
    extrapyramidal symptoms
epsilon
    Greek letter (ε; alphabetized
      as e)
    e.-aminocaproic acid
EPSP—excitatory postsynaptic
  potential
Epstein
    disease
    nephrosis
    osteotome
    pearls
    symptom
    syndrome
Epstein-Barr virus (EBV)
EPTE—existed prior to enlistment
EPTS—existed prior to service
epulis (epulides)
    congenital e.
    e. fibromatosa
    fibromatous e.
    e. fissurata
    giant cell e.
    e. gigantocellularis
    e. granulomatosa
    e. of newborn
    pigmented e.
    e. of pregnancy
epulofibroma
epuloid
epulosis
epulotic

eq—equivalent
equalization
    pressure e.
equate
equation
    alveolar gas e.
    Arrhenius e.
    Ayala e.
    Bloch e.
    Bohr e.
    chemical e.
    Gompertz e.
    Harden and Young e.
    Henderson-Hasselbalch e.
    Hill e.
    Larmor e.
    Lineweaver-Burk e.
    Michaelis-Menten e.
    Nernst e.
    Poiseuille e.
    Starling e.
    Ussing e.
    van't Hoff e.
equator
    e. bulbi oculi
    e. of cell
    e. of crystalline lens
    e. of eyeball
    e. of lens
    e. lentis
equatorial
    e. degeneration
    e. meridian
Equen magnet
equiaxial
equicaloric
equilateral
equilibrating operation
equilibration
    mandibular e.
    occlusal e.
equilibrator
equilibratory
equilibrium
    acid-base e.
    body e.
    calorie e.
    carbon e.
    e. constant
    e. dialysis
    Donnan e.
    dynamic e.
    fluid e.
    genetic e.
    Gibbs-Donnan e.

equilibrium *(continued)*
 Hardy-Weinberg e.
 homeostatic e.
 linkage e.
 metabolic e.
 mutational e.
 nitrogen e.
 nitrogenous e.
 nutritive e.
 physiologic e.
 protein e.
 radioactive e.
 secular e.
 transient e.
 water e.
equilin
equimolar
equimolecular
equine
equinophobia
equinovalgus
equinovarus
equinus
 talipes e.
equipotential
equipotentiality
Equisetene suture
equisetosis
equisetum
equitoxic
equivalence
 mass energy e.
equivalent
 aluminum e.
 caloric e. of oxygen
 calorie e.
 combustion e.
 concrete e.
 dose e.
 endosmotic e.
 epileptic e.
 genetic lethal e.
 gold e.
 gram e.
 isodynamic e.
 lead e.
 lethal e.
 maximum permissible
  dose e.
 neutralization e.
 nitrogen e.
 protein e.
 psychic e.
 starch e.
 toxic e.

equivalent *(continued)*
 ventilation e.
 water e.
equivocal
Er—erbium
ER—
 ejection rate
 emergency room
 endoplasmic reticulum
 estrogen receptor
 evoked response
 external resistance
ERA—
 estrogen receptor assay
 evoked response audiometry
erabutoxin
eradication
erasion of joint
Erb
 atrophy
 disease
 dystrophy
 palsy
 point
 progressive muscular
  dystrophy
 pseudohypertrophic muscular
  dystrophy
 sclerosis
 sign
 spastic paraplegia
 syndrome
Erb-Charcot disease
Erb-Duchenne paralysis
Erben
 phenomenon
 reflex
 sign
ERBF—effective renal blood flow
Erb-Goldflam disease
erbium (Er)
Erb-Landouzy disease
Erb-Oppenheim-Goldflam
 syndrome
ERC—endoscopic retrograde
 cholangiography
ERCP—endoscopic retrograde
 cholangiopancreatography
Erdheim
 cystic medial necrosis
 cystic syndrome
 disease
 syndrome
 tumor
erectile

erection
erector
eremophobia
erethism
erethistic
erethizophrenia
ERG—electroretinogram
ergasia
ergasiatry
ergasiology
ergasiophobia
ergastic
ergastoplasm
ergobasine
ergocardiogram
ergocardiography
ergodynamograph
ergoesthesiograph
ergogenesis
ergogenic
ergogram
ergograph
    Mosso e.
ergographic
ergomania
ergometer
    bicycle e.
    Cybex e.
ergometry
ergon
ergonomics
ergonovine
ergoplasm
ergosome
ergosterol
    activated e.
    irradiated e.
ergot
    hydrogenated e. alkaloids
ergotherapy
ergothioneine
ergotinin
ergotism
ergotized
ergotoxicosis
ergotoxine
ergusia
Erhard test
Erich
    arch bar
    forceps
    operation
    splint
Erichsen
    disease

Erichsen *(continued)*
    ligature
    sign
    test
Eriodictyon californicum
Eristalis tenax
Erlacher-Blount syndrome
Erlenmeyer
    flask
    flasklike deformity
Erni sign
Ernst applicator
erode
eroded
erogenous
erose
erosio interdigitalis blastomycetica
erosion
    cervical e.
    dental e.
    Dieulafoy e.
erosive
erotic
eroticomania
erotism
    anal e.
    genital e.
    muscle e.
    oral e.
erotize
erotogenesis
erotogenic
erotographomania
erotomania
erotopath
erotopathy
erotophobia
ERP—
    effective refractory period
    endocardial resection
      procedure
    equine rhinopneumonitis
    estrogen receptor protein
ERPF—effective renal plasma flow
erratic
errhine
error
    absolute e.
    biased e.
    copy e.
    experimental e.
    inborn e. of metabolism
    random e.
    sampling e.
    standard e. of the mean

error *(continued)*
    standard e. (SE)
    systematic e.
    type I e.
    type II e.
erucic acid
eructation
    nervous e.
erudite
erugation
eruption
    active e.
    bullous e.
    butterfly e.
    clinical e.
    continuous e.
    creeping e.
    crustaceous e.
    delayed e.
    demodetic e.
    drug e.
    erythematous e.
    fixed e.
    fixed drug e.
    Kaposi varicelliform e.
    maculopapular e.
    morbilliform e.
    papulosquamous e.
    partial e.
    passive e.
    petechial e.
    polymorphic light e.
    pustular e.
    sandworm e.
    seabathers' e.
    serum e.
    squamous e.
    summer e.
    surgical e.
    tooth e.
    total e.
    tubercular e.
    vaccinal e.
    vesicular e.
    vesiculopustular e.
eruptive
ERV—expiratory reserve volume
Erwinia
    E. amylovora
    E. carotovora
    E. herbicola
erysipelas
    ambulant e.
    e. bullosum
    coast e.

erysipelas *(continued)*
    gangrenous e.
    e. grave internum
    hemorrhagic e.
    idiopathic e.
    malignant e.
    e. migrans
    migrant e.
    necrotizing e.
    e. perstans
    phlegmonous e.
    e. pustulosum
    swine e.
    e. verrucosum
    e. vesiculosum
    wandering e.
    zoonotic e.
erysipelatous
erysipeloid
    Rosenbach e.
Erysipelothrix
    E. insidiosa
    E. rhusiopathiae
erysipelotoxin
erythema
    e. ab igne
    acrodynic e.
    acute infectious e.
    e. annulare
    e. annulare centrifugum
    e. annulare rheumaticum
    e. a pudore
    e. arthriticum
    e. arthriticum epidemicum
    e. bullosum
    e. caloricum
    e. chromicum figuratum
        melanodermicum
    e. chronicum migrans
    circinate syphilitic e.
    e. circinatum
    e. circinatum rheumaticum
    cold e.
    e. contusiformis
    diaper e.
    e. dyschromicum perstans
    e. elevatum diutinum
    e. endemicum
    epidemic e.
    epidemic arthritic e.
    e. exudativum
    figurate e.
    e. figuratum
    e. figuratum perstans
    e. fugax

E

erythema *(continued)*
    gyrate e.
    e. gyratum
    e. gyratum perstans
    e. gyratum repens
    e. induratum
    e. infectiosum
    e. intertrigo
    e. iris
    Jacquet e.
    e. marginatum
    e. marginatum rheumaticum
    e. migrans
    migratory e.
    Milian e.
    e. multiforme bullosum
    e. multiforme exudativum
    e. multiforme majus
    e. multiforme minus
    necrolytic migratory e.
    e. necroticans
    e. neonatorum
    e. neonatorum toxicum
    e. nodosum leprosum
    e. nodosum migrans
    e. nodosum syphiliticum
    e. nuchae
    nummular e.
    palmar e.
    e. palmare
    e. palmare hereditarium
    papuloerosive e.
    e. papulosum
    e. paratrimma
    pellagroid e.
    e. pernio
    e. perstans
    e. pudicitiae
    e. punctatum
    rheumatic e.
    e. simplex
    e. solare
    e. streptogenes
    e. subitum
    toxic e.
    e. toxicum
    e. toxicum neonatorum
    e. traumaticum
    e. urticans
    e. venenatum
erythematosus
    discoid lupus e.
    disseminated lupus e. (DLE)
    systemic lupus e. (SLE)

erythematous
erythemogenic
erythralgia
erythrasma
    Baerensprung e.
erythredema polyneuropathy
erythremia
    high-altitude e.
erythrism
erythristic
erythritol
erythrityl tetranitrate
erythroblast
    acidophilic e.
    basophilic e.
    definitive e's
    early e.
    eosinophilic e.
    intermediate e.
    late e.
    orthochromatic e.
    oxyphilic e.
    polychromatic e.
    polychromatophilic e.
    primitive e's
erythroblastemia
erythroblastic
erythroblastoma
erythroblastomatosis
erythroblastopenia
    idiopathic transitory e.
erythroblastosis
    e. fetalis
    e. neonatorum
erythroblastotic
erythrochromia
erythroclasis
erythroclast
erythroclastic
erythrocuprein
erythrocyanosis
    e. crurum puellaris
    e. frigida
    e. frigida crurum puellarum
    e. supramalleolaris
erythrocytapheresis
erythrocyte
    achromic e.
    basophilic e.
    burr e.
    crenated e.
    dichromatic e.
    hypochromic e.
    immature e.

erythrocyte *(continued)*
    Mexican hat e.
    normochromic e.
    nucleated e.
    orthochromatic e.
    polychromatic e.
    reticulated e.
    target e.
    e. transketolase
erythrocythemia
erythrocytic
erythrocytolysin
erythrocytolysis
erythrocytometer
erythrocytometry
erythrocyto-opsonin
erythrocytophagous
erythrocytophagy
erythrocytorrhexis
erythrocytoschisis
erythrocytosis
    anoxemic e.
    leukemic e.
    e. megalosplenica
    renal e.
    stress e.
erythrocyturia
erythrodegenerative
erythroderma
    atopic e.
    congenital ichthyosiform e.,
      bullous
    congenital ichthyosiform e.,
      nonbullous
    desquamative e.
    e. desquamativum
    exfoliative e.
    e. ichthyosiforme congenitum
    leukemic e.
    lymphomatous e.
    e. psoriaticum
    resistant maculopapular
      scaly e.
    Sézary e.
    e. squamosum
erythrodextrin
erythrodontia
erythrogen
erythrogenesis imperfecta
erythrogenic
erythrogone
erythrogonium
erythrogranulose
erythroid

β-erythroidine [beta-]
erythrokatalysis
erythrokeratodermia
    progressive symmetrical
      verrucous e.
    e. variabilis
erythrokinetics
erythro tetranitrate
erythrolabe
erythrolein
erythroleukoblastosis
erythroleukosis
erythroleukothrombocythemia
erythrolitmin
erythromelalgia of the head
erythrometer
erythrometry
erythromyeloblastosis
erythron
erythroneocytosis
erythronoclastic
erythroparasite
erythropenia
erythrophage
erythrophagocytosis
erythrophil
erythrophilous
erythrophobia
erythrophobic
erythrophore
erythrophose
erythrophyll
erythropia
erythroplakia
    speckled e.
erythroplasia
    e. of Queyrat
    Zoon e.
erythroplastid
erythropoiesis
erythropoietic
erythropoietin
erythroprosopalgia
erythropsia
erythropsin
erythropyknosis
erythrosarcoma
erythrose péribuccale pigmentaire
    of Brocq
erythrosedimentation
erythrosis of Bekhterev
    (Bechterew)
erythrostasis
erythrothioneine

E

erythrulose
erythruria
Es—einsteinium
ES—
    end-to-side
    Expectation Score
ESB—electrical stimulation to
    brain
Esbach method
ESC—electromechanical slope
    computer
escape
    aldosterone e.
    atrioventricular junctional e.
    nasal e.
    nodal e.
    vagal e.
    ventricular e.
Esch.—*Escherichia*
eschar
    burn e.
    neuropathic e.
escharotic
escharotomy
Escherich
    bacillus
    reflex
    sign
Escherichia
    E. aerogenes
    E. alkalescens
    E. aurescens
    E. blattae
    E. coli virulent strain O157:h7
    E. dispar
    E. dispar var. *ceylonensis*
    E. fergusonii
    E. freundii
    E. hermanii
    E. intermedia
    E. vulneris
eschew
escin
escorcin
esculapian
esculent
esculin
escutcheon
ESD—electronic summation device
eseptate
eserine
ESF—erythropoietic-stimulating
    factor
ESL—end-systolic length
ESM—ejection-systolic murmur

Esmarch
    bandage
    operation
    scissors
    tourniquet
    tube
esocataphoria
esocine
esodeviation
esoethmoiditis
esogastritis
esophagalgia
esophageal
    e. atresia
    e. dilator
    e. speculum
    e. sphincter
    e. stethoscope
    e. tube
    e. varices
esophagectasia
esophagectomy
esophagism
    hiatal e.
esophagitis
    acute corrosive e.
    Candida e.
    chronic hyperkeratotic e.
    chronic peptic e.
    e. dissecans superficialis
    herpetic e.
    infectious e.
    monilia e.
    peptic e.
    reflux e.
    thrush e.
esophagobronchial
esophagocardiomyotomy
esophagocele
esophagocologastrostomy
esophagocoloplasty
esophagoduodenostomy
esophagodynia
esophagoenterostomy
esophagoesophagostomy
esophagofundopexy
esophagogastrectomy (EG)
esophagogastric
esophagogastroanastomosis
esophagogastroduodenal
esophagogastroduodenoscopy
esophagogastromyotomy
esophagogastroplasty
esophagogastroscopy
esophagogastrostomy

esophagogram
esophagography
esophagohiatal
esophagojejunogastrostomosis
esophagojejunogastrostomy
esophagojejunoplasty
esophagojejunostomy
esophagolaryngectomy
esophagology
esophagomalacia
esophagomycosis
esophagomyotomy
    Heller e.
esophagopharyngolaryngectomy
esophagopharynx
esophagoplasty
esophagoplication
esophagoptosis
esophagorespiratory
esophagoscope
    Broyles e.
    Bruening e.
    Chevalier Jackson e.
    Eder-Hufford e.
    fiberoptic e.
    full-lumen e.
    Haslinger e.
    Holinger e.
    Jackson e.
    Jesberg e.
    Lell e.
    Moersch e.
    Mosher e.
    Moure e.
    Negus e.
    optical e.
    oval e.
    Roberts e.
    Schindler e.
    Tucker e.
    Yankauer e.
esophagoscopy
esophagospasm
esophagostenosis
esophagostoma
esophagostomiasis
esophagostomy
esophagotome
esophagotomy
esophagotracheal
esophagram
esophagus
    Barrett e.
    nutcracker e.
esophoria

esophoric
esosphenoiditis
esoteric
esotropia
esotropic
ESP—
    end-systolic pressure
    eosinophil stimulation
     promoter
    extrasensory perception
espnoic
esponja
espundia
esquillectomy
ESR—
    electron spin resonance
    erythrocyte sedimentation rate
ESS—erythrocyte-sensitizing
  substance
essence of peppermint
essential
Esser
  graft
  operation
Essex-Lopresti method
Essic cell band
EST—
    electric shock therapy
    electroshock therapy
est.—estimated
ester
    Cori e.
    Embden e.
    Harden-Young e.
    Neuberg e.
    Robison e.
esterapenia
esterification
esterify
esterize
Esterman visual function score
esterolysis
esterolytic
Estes operation
estetrol
esthematology
esthesia
esthesic
esthesioblast
esthesiogen
esthesiogenic
esthesiology
esthesiometer
esthesiometry
esthesioneure

esthesioneuroblastoma
esthesioneurocytoma
esthesioneuroepithelioma
esthesiophysiology
esthesodic
esthetic
esthetics
estimate
    biased e.
    consistent e.
    interval e.
    point e.
    product-limit e.
    unbiased e.
estimation
    magnitude e.
    numerical e.
estimator
estival
estivation
estivoautumnal
Estlander operation
    flap
eston
estradiol
    e. 6β-hydroxylase [6-beta-]
    e. 6β-monooxygenase [6-beta-]
    e.-17α [e.-17-alpha]
    e.-17β [e.-17-beta]
    e. benzoate
    e. cypionate
    e. dipropionate
    e. enanthate
    ethinyl e.
    e. undecylate
    e. valerate
estrane
estratriene
Estren-Dameshek syndrome
estrenol
estrin
estrinization
estriol
estrofurate
estrogen
    conjugated e's
    e. effect
    esterified e's
    e. glucuronides
estrogenic
estrogenicity
estrogenlike
estrogenous
estrone sulfate
estrophilin

estropipate
estrostilben
ESU—electrostatic unit
ESV—end-systolic volume
ESWL—extracorporeal shock wave
    lithotripsy
Et—ethyl
ET—
    ejection time
    endotracheal
    esotropia
    etiology
eta
    Greek letter (η; alphabetized
      as h)
ETA—ethionamide
et al.—and others (L. et alii)
état
    é. criblé
    é. dysmelinique
    é. lacunaire
    é. mammelonné
    é. marbré
    é. vermoulu
etch
    acid e.
ETEC—enterotoxic *Escherichia*
    coli
Eternod sinus
ETF—electron transfer
    flavoprotein
ethal
ethanal
ethane
ethanedial
ethanoic acid
ethanol
ethanolamine
ethanolism
ethanoyl
ethchlorvynol
ethenoid
ethenyl
ether
    anesthetic e.
    methyl tert-butyl e.
    petroleum e.
    thio e.
ethereal
etherification
etherization
etherize
etherometer
Ethibond suture
ethical

Ethicon suture
ethics
   clinical e.
   medical e.
ethidene
   e. chloride
   e. diamine
ethidium
Ethiflex suture
Ethilon suture
ethinamate
ethinyl estradiol
ethiodized oil
ethionamide
ethionine
ethisterone
ethmocarditis
ethmocephalus
ethmofrontal
ethmoid
ethmoidal
ethmoid bone
ethmoidectomy
   transantral e.
ethmoiditis
ethmoidolacrimal suture
ethmoidomaxillary suture
ethmoidopalatine
ethmoidotomy
ethmolacrimal
ethmomaxillary
ethmonasal
ethmopalatal
ethmosphenoid
ethmoturbinal
ethmovomerine
ethnic
ethnics
ethnobiology
ethnography
ethnologic
ethnology
ethnopsychiatry
ethobrom
ethocaine
ethoglucid
ethohexadiol
ethological
ethologist
ethology
ethotoin
ethyl
   e. acetate
   e. aminobenzoate
   e. biscoumacetate

ethyl *(continued)*
   e. butyrate
   e. chloride
   e. cyanide
   e. dibunate
   e. eosin
   e. ether
   e. green
   e. hydrocupreine
   e. iodophenylundecylate
   e. linoleate
   e. mercaptan
   e. oleate
   e. orange
ethylaldehyde
ethylamine
ethylate
ethylation
ethylcellulose
ethylene
   e. dibromide (EDB)
   e. dichloride
   e. glycol
   e. oxide
ethylenediamine
ethylenediaminetetraacetate
ethylenediaminetetraacetic acid
ethylenedinitrilotetraacetic acid
ethylene glycol
ethylenimine
ethylestrenol
ethylic
ethylidene chloride
ethylism
ethylmalonyl-adipicaciduria
ethylnoradrenaline
ethylnorsuprarenin
ethylparaben
ethylphenylhydantoin
ethylstibamine
ethynodiol diacetate
ethynyl
   e. estradiol
   e. testosterone
etidronic acid
etiocholanolone
etiogenic
etiol.—etiology
etiolation
etiologic, etiological
etiology
etiopathic
etiopathology
etioporphyrin
etiotropic

ETKM—every test known
to man
ETM—erythromycin
ET-NANB—enterically transmitted
non-A, non-B (hepatitis)
ETOH, EtOH—ethyl alcohol
etoprine
ETOX—ethylene oxide
ETP—entire treatment period
E trisomy
etrotomy
ETT—extrathyroidal thyroxine
ETV—educational television
Eu—europium
EU—
    Ehrlich unit(s)
    enzyme unit(s)
    excretory urogram
EUA—examination under
anesthesia
euadrenocorticism
euangiotic
eubacteria
Eubacterium
    E. alactolyticum
    E. lentum
    E. limosum
eubiotics
eubolism
eucalyptol
Eucalyptus
eucapnia
euchlorhydria
eucholia
euchromatic
euchromatin
euchromatopsy
euchylia
eucodeine
eucoelom
eucolloid
eucrasia
eudiemorrhysis
eudiometer
eudipsia
euergasia
euesthesia
euflavine
eugamy
eugenic acid
eugenicist
eugenics
    negative e.
    positive e.
eugenism

eugenol
Euglena gracilis
euglenid
euglenoid
euglobulin
euglycemia
euglycemic
eugnathia
eugnathic
eugnosia
eugnostic
eugonic
euhydration
eukaryon
eukaryosis
eukaryote
eukaryotic
eukeratin
eukinesia
eukinetic
eulaminate
Eulenburg disease
Euler number
eumenorrhea
eumetria
eumorphics
eumorphism
eumycetoma
eunuch
    fertile e.
eunuchism
    pituitary e.
eunuchoid
eunuchoidism
    female e.
    hypergonadotropic e.
    hypogonadotropic e.
euonymin
euosmia
eupancreatism
euparal
eupatheoscope
eupatorin
eupepsia
eupeptic
euperistalsis
euphenics
euphoretic
euphoria
euphoric
euphorigenic
euphoristic
euplasia
euplastic
euploid

euploidy
eupnea
eupneic
eupractic
eupraxia
eupraxic
Euproctis
    E. chrysorrhoea
    E. phaeorrhoea
eupyrene
eupyrexia
eurhythmia
europium (Eu)
Eurotium
    E. malignum
    E. repens
eurycephalic
eurycranial
eurygnathic
eurygnathism
eurymeric
euryon
euryopia
Eurypelma hentzii
eurythermal
Euscorpius italicus
eusitia
eusplanchnia
eusplenia
eustachian
    e. catheterization
    e. tube
    e. tuboplasty
eustachitis
eustachium
eusthenia
eusthenuria
eusystole
eusystolic
eutectic
eutelolecithal
euthanasia
    passive e.
euthenic
euthenics
eutherapeutic
eutherian
euthermic
euthymic
euthymism
euthyroid
euthyroidism
euthyscope
eutocia
eutopic

Eutrombicula
    E. alfreddugesi
    E. splendens
eutrophia
eutrophic
eutrophication
euvolia
eV; ev—electron-volt
EV—extravascular
evacuant
evacuate
evacuation
evacuator
    Creevy e.
    Ellik e.
    McCarthy e.
    Toomey e.
evagination
    optic e.
eval.—evaluation
evaluation
    Dubowitz e.
evanescent
Evans
    blue
    forceps
    operation
    syndrome
evaporation
evasion
evenomation
event
    ionizing e.
    positron annihilation e.
    scattering e.
eventration
    diaphragmatic e.
    umbilical e.
Everett-TeLinde operation
Eversbusch operation
eversion endarterectomy
eversion examination
    double-contrast e.e.
evert, everted
everter
    Berens lid e.
everting
    e. interrupted suture
    e. suture
evertor
Eves tonsillar snare
EVG—endovascular graft
évidement
évideur
evil

eviration
eviscerate
evisceration
evisceroneurotomy
EVLW—extravascular lung water
evocation
evocator
evoked
evolution
    bathmic e.
    convergent e.
    Denman spontaneous e.
    determinate e.
    Douglas spontaneous e.
    emergent e.
    organic e.
    orthogenic e.
    parallel e.
    saltatory e.
    spontaneous e.
evulsed
evulsio nervi optici
evulsion
EW—Emergency Ward
Ewald
    law
    tube
Ewart sign
EWB—estrogen withdrawal
  bleeding
Ewing
    sarcoma
    sign
    tumor
EWL—egg-white lysozyme
ex—
    excision
    exophthalmos
exacerbate
exacerbation
    abrupt e.
    sudden e.
    unexplained e.
exaltation
exam—examination
examination
    air-contrast e.
    bimanual e.
    darkfield e.
    double-contrast e.
    Dubowitz e.
    gastrointestinal e.
    gynecologic e.
    hanging-drop e.
    mental status e.

examination *(continued)*
    needle electromyographic e.
    physical e.
    postpartal e.
    rectovaginal e.
    slit-lamp e.
    speculum e.
examinee
examiner
exanthem
    Boston e.
    e. subitum
    vesicular e.
exanthema (exanthemata)
    Boston e.
    e. subitum
exanthematous
exanthrope
exanthropic
exarticulation
exc.—excision
excalation
excarnation
excavatio (excavationes)
    e. disci
    e. papillae nervi optici
    e. rectouterina
    e. rectovesicalis
    e. vesicouterina
excavation
    atrophic e.
    dental e.
    glaucomatous e.
    ischiorectal e.
    e. of optic disk
    physiologic e.
    rectoischiadic e.
    rectouterine e.
    rectovesical e.
    vesicouterine e.
excavationes (plural of excavatio)
excavator
    dental e.
    hatchet e.
    Schuknecht whirlybird e.
    spoon e.
excavatum
    pectus e.
exceed
excementosis
excerebration
excernent
excess
    antibody e.
    antigen e.

excess *(continued)*
    base e.
exchange
    ion e.
    plasma e.
    sister chromatid e.
exchangeable
exchanger
    anion e.
    cation e.
    heat e.
    ion e.
excipient
excise
excision
    fascial e.
    Ferris Smith e.
    narrow e.
    primary e.
    sequential e.
    tangential e.
    wide e.
    wound e.
excitability
    exteroceptive e.
    proprioceptive e.
    rhythmic e.
    seismogenic e.
    subliminal e.
excitable
excitant
excitation
    anomalous e.
    anomalous atrioventricular e.
    atrioventricular e.
    catatonic e.
    direct e.
    ephaptic e.
    indirect e.
excitatory
excitement
    anniversary e.
    catatonic e.
    psychomotor e.
excitoanabolic
excitocatabolic
excitoglandular
excitometabolic
excitomotor
excitomuscular
excitonutrient
excitor
excitosecretory
excitovascular
exclave

exclusion
    allelic e.
    competitive e.
excochleation
exconjugant
excoriation
    necrotic e.
    neurotic e.
excortication
excrement
excrementitious
excrescence
    fungating e.
    fungous e.
    Lambl e's
excrescent
excreta
excrete
excreter
excretin
excretion
    fractional e.
    pseudouridine e.
    e. pyelography
    renal tubular
      hydrogen e.
    e. urography
excretory
    e. cystogram
    e. urogram
    e. urography
excurrent
excursion
    lateral e.
    protrusive e.
    respiratory e.
    retrusive e.
excursive
excyclodeviation
excycloduction
excyclophoria
excyclotropia
excyclovergence
excyst
excystation
exelcymosis
exemia
exencephalocele
exencephalous
exencephalus
exencephaly
exenteration
    pelvic e.
exenterative
exenteritis

E

exercise
    active e.
    active assisted e.
    active resistive e.
    Codman e.
    corrective e.
    DeSouza e's
    Fournier e.
    free e.
    Frenkel e's
    graduated
      resistance e.
    isokinetic e.
    isometric e.
    isotonic e.
    Kegel e's
    muscle-setting e.
    neuromuscular
      facilitation e.
    passive e.
    Pilates e's
    static e.
    therapeutic e.
    underwater e.
    Williams e.
exeresis
exergic
exergonic
exesion
exfetation
exflagellation
exfoliate
exfoliatin
exfoliatio areata
  linguae
exfoliation
    lamellar e. of
     the newborn
exfoliative
exhalant
exhalation
exhale
exhaustion
    anhidrotic heat e.
    cold e.
    combat e.
    heat e.
    postactivation e.
    posttetanic e.
exhibition
exhibitionism
exhibitionist
exhilarant
exhilarated
exhumation

existence
existential
existentialism
exitus
exo-amylase
exobiology
exocardial
exocarp
exocataphoria
exoccipital
exocele
exocellular
exochorion
exocoelom
exocoeloma
exocolitis
exocrine
exocrinology
exocrinosity
exocuticle
exocyclic
exocytosis
exodeoxyribonuclease
exodeviation
exodontics
exodontist
exodontology
exoenzyme
exoergic
exoerythrocyte
exoerythrocytic
exogamy
exogastric
exogastritis
exogastrula
exogastrulation
exogenote
exogenous obesity
exognathia
exognathion
exognosis
exohormone
exolever
exometer
exomphalos
exomysium
exon
exonuclease
exopathic
exopathy
exopeptidase
Exophiala
    E. jeanselmei
    E. mycetoma
    E. werneckii

exophoria
exophoric
exophthalmic
exophthalmogenic
exophthalmometer
    Hertel e.
exophthalmometric
exophthalmometry
exophthalmos
    endocrine e.
    malignant e.
    pulsating e.
    thyrotoxic e.
    thyrotropic e.
exophthalmus
exophyte
exophytic
exoplasm
exorbitism
exoresis
exoribonuclease
exosepsis
exoserosis
exoskeletal
  prosthesis
exoskeleton
exosmose
exosmosis
exosomesthesia
exosplenopexy
exospore
exosporium
exostosectomy
exostosis (exostoses)
    e. bursata
    e. cartilaginea
    dental e.
    hereditary multiple
      exostoses
    ivory e.
    multiple exostoses
    multiple osteocartilaginous
      exostoses
    osteocartilaginous e.
    subungual e.
exostotic
exoteric
exothelioma
exothermic
exothymopexy
exothyropexy
exotic
exotoxic
exotoxin
exotropia

exotropic
expander
    plasma volume e.
    subperiosteal tissue e.
      (STE)
    tissue e.
expansion
    aliform e.
    e. of the arch
    clonal e.
    cubical e.
    dorsal digital e.
    extensor e.
    fibrous e's of
      eye muscles
    hygroscopic e.
    maxillary e.
    setting e.
    thermal e.
    wax e.
expansiveness
expectancy
    life e.
expectant
expectation of
  life at birth
expectorant
    liquefying e.
    stimulant e.
expectorate
expectoration
    rusty e.
expediency
expedient
expedite
expeditious
expeditiously
expel
expellant
experiment
    bulbocapnine e.
    check e.
    control e.
    cross-over e.
    crucial e.
    Cyon e.
    defect e.
    double-blind e.
    Goltz e.
    Mariotte e.
    Müller e.
    Nussbaum e.
    O'Beirne e.
    Scheiner e.
    Stensen e.

E

experiment *(continued)*
    Toynbee e.
    Valsalva e.
expirate
expiration
expiratory
expire
explant
    cellular e.
explode
exploration
exploratory
    e. incision
    e. laparotomy
    e. operation
explorer
    Rosen e.
explosion
explosive
exponent
exponential
exposure
    acute e.
    air e.
    chronic e.
    double e.
    pulp e.
express
expressate
expression
    e. cystourethrography
    Kristeller e.
    manual e. of
      placenta
expressive aphasia
expressivity
expressor
    Arruga e.
    Heath e.
    Smith e.
expulsion
    spontaneous e. of
      placenta
expulsive
exquisite
exsanguinate
exsanguination
exsanguine
exsanguinotransfusion
exsector
exsiccant
exsiccate
exsiccation
exsiccosis
exsorption

exstrophy
    e. of bladder
    e. of cloaca
    cloacal e.
exsufflation
exsufflator
ext.—
    exterior
    external
    extract
extend
extended radical
    mastectomy
extender
    artificial plasma e.
extension
    Bardenheuer e.
    Buck e.
    Codivilla e.
    nail e.
    e. per contiguitatem
    e. per continuitatem
    e. per saltam
    e. for prevention
    ridge e.
    skeletal e.
    Steinmann e.
    tectoseptal e.
extensor
    e. carpi radialis
      accessorius
    e. carpi radialis
      intermedius
    e. carpi ulnaris
    long radial e. of
      wrist
    ulnar e. of wrist
exterior
exteriorize
extern
external
    e. frontoethmoidectomy
    e. pharyngotomy
    e. proctotomy
    e. urethrotomy
externalia
externalization
externalize
external os
externus
exteroceptive
exteroceptor
exterofection
exterofective
exterogestate

extima
extinction
extinguish
extirpate
extirpation
    dental pulp e.
extorsion
extortor
extra-adrenal
extra-amnionic
extra-anatomic
extra-articular
extrabronchial
extrabuccal
extrabulbar
extracapsular
extracardial
extracarpal
extracartilaginous
extracellular
extracerebral
extrachromosomal
extracorporeal
extracorporeal shock wave
    lithotripsy (ESWL)
extracorpuscular
extracorticospinal
extracranial
extract
    alcoholic e.
    allergenic e.
    belladonna e.
    Buchner e.
    cascara sagrada e.
    cell-free e.
    Chondodendron
        tomentosum e.
    chondrus e.
    compound e.
    dry e.
    equivalent e.
    euphorbia liquid e.
    fluid e.
    glycyrrhiza e.
    henbane e.
    hydroalcoholic e.
    hyoscyamus e.
    Irish moss e.
    licorice root e.
    liver e.
    liver e., liquid
    e. of male fern
    malt e.
    meat e.
    ox bile e.

extract *(continued)*
    oxgall e., powdered
    parathyroid e.
    pilular e.
    placental e.
    poison ivy e.
    poison oak e.
    pollen e.
    powdered e.
    protein e.
    rice polishings e.
    semiliquid e.
    soft e.
    solid e.
    tikitiki e.
    trichinella e.
    yeast e.
extractant
extraction
    breech e., partial
    breech e., total
    cataract e., extracapsular
    cataract e.,
        intracapsular
    flap e.
    menstrual e.
    phenol water e.
    progressive e.
    selected e.
    serial e.
    tooth e.
    vacuum e.
extractive
extractor
    Amico e.
    basket e.
    comedo e.
    Jewett e.
    Moore e.
    Schamberg e.
    Unna e.
    vacuum e.
    Walton e.
extractum
extracystic
extradural
    venography
extraembryonic celom
extraepiphyseal
extrafascial
    hysterectomy
extrafusal
extragenital
extraglomerular
extragonadal

extrahepatic
extraligamentous
extramalleolus
extramammary
    Paget disease
extramastoiditis
extramedullary
extrameningeal
extramural
extraneous
extraneural
extranuclear
extraocular
extraosseous
extrapancreatic
extraparenchymal
extrapelvic
extrapericardial
extraperineal
extraperiosteal
extraperitoneal
extraphysiologic
extraplacental
extraplantar
extrapleural
extrapolate
extrapolation
extraprostatic
extraprostatitis
extrapsychic
extrapulmonary
    tuberculosis
extrapyramidal
extrarectus
extrarenal
extrasensory
extraserous
extrasomatic
extraspinal
extrastriate
extrasuprarenal
    infranodal e.
    nodal e.
    retrograde e.
extrasystole
    atrial e.
    atrioventricular e.
      (AV e.)
    auricular e.
    auriculoventricular e.
    AV nodal e.
    infranodal e.
    interpolated e.
    junctional e.

extrasystole *(continued)*
    nodal e.
    retrograde e.
    return e.
    supraventricular e.
    ventricular e.
extratendinous
extrathoracic
extratracheal
extratubal
extratympanic
extrauterine
extravaginal
extravasate
extravasation
    e. of contrast
    e. of dye
    punctiform e.
    pyelosinus e.
extravascular
extraventricular
extremis
extremital
extremitas (extremitates)
    e. acromialis
      claviculae
    e. anterior lienis
    e. anterior splenis
    e. inferior
    e. inferior renis
    e. inferior testis
    e. posterior lienis
    e. posterior splenis
    e. sternalis
      claviculae
    e. superior
    e. superior renis
    e. superior testis
    e. tubalis ovarii
    e. tubaria ovarii
    e. uterina ovarii
extremity (extremities)
    anterior e. of spleen
    cartilaginous e. of rib
    external e. of
      clavicle
    fimbriated e. of
      fallopian tube
    inferior e. of kidney
    inferior e. of testis
    internal e. of clavicle
    lower e.
    pelvic e. of ovary
    posterior e. of spleen

extremity (extremities) *(continued)*
    scapular e. of clavicle
    superior e. of kidney
    superior e. of testis
    tubal e. of ovary
    upper e.
    uterine e. of ovary
extrinsic
extrogastrulation
extroversion of bladder
extrovert
extrude
extrudoclusion
extrusion of tooth
extubate
extubation
exuberance
exuberant
    e. infection
    e. tumor
exudate
    catarrhal e.
    cotton-wool e's
    fibrinous e.
    gingival e.
    hemorrhagic e.
    inflammatory e.
    purulent e.
    sanguineous e.
    serofibrinous e.
    serous e.
exudation
exudative retinitis
exude
exulcerans
exulceratio simplex
exumbilication
exutory
exuviation
ex vivo
eye
    aphakic e.
    artificial e.
    black e.
    blear e.
    Bright e.
    cinema e.
    compound e.
    crab's e.
    crossed e's
    cyclopean e.
    cystic e.
    dark-adapted e.
    deviating e.

eye *(continued)*
    doll's e's
    epiphyseal e.
    exciting e.
    fixating e.
    following e.
    hare e.
    hop e.
    Klieg e.
    lazy e.
    light-adapted e.
    median e.
    monochromatic e.
    Nairobi e.
    parietal e.
    pineal e.
    pink e. (pinkeye, pink-eye)
    primary e.
    pseudophakic e.
    raccoon e's
    reduced e.
    schematic e.
    secondary e.
    shipyard e.
    Snellen reform e.
    e. speculum
    squinting e.
    sunset e.
    sympathizing e.
    wall e.
eyeball
eyebrow
eyecup
eyeglass
eyeglasses
eyeground
eyelash
eyelet
eyelid
eyepiece
    comparison e.
    compensating e.
    demonstration e.
    high-eyepoint e.
    huygenian e.
    Huygens e.
    negative e.
    positive e.
    Ramsden e.
    widefield e.
eyepoint
eyespot, eye spot
eyestrain
Eyler operation

E

F

f—
  femto-
  focal length
f—frequency
F—
  Fahrenheit
  farad
  fat
  father
  fellow
  female
  fertility
  field of vision
  filaria
  fluorine
  formula
  visual field
F—
  faraday
  force
F, Fr—French (catheter gauge)
F_1—first filial generation
F_2—second filial generation
FA—
  far advanced
  femoral artery
  field ambulance
  first aid
  fluorescence assay
  fluorescent antibody
  forearm
  free acid
Fab—fragment, antigen-binding
FAB—French-American-British
  (classification)
fabella (fabellae)
Faber
  anemia
  syndrome
fabere
  f. sign
  f. test (flexion, abduction,
    external rotation, extension)
fabrication
Fabricius bursa
Fabry
  disease
  syndrome
Facb—fragment, antigen-and-
  complement-binding
FACD—Fellow of the American
  College of Dentists
face
  adenoid f.

face *(continued)*
  bony f.
  bovine f.
  cleft f.
  cow f.
  cushingoid f.
  dish f.
  dished f.
  frog f.
  hatchet f.
  hippocratic f.
  mask-like f.
  moon f.
face-bow
  adjustable axis f.
  kinematic f.
face-lift, face lift, facelift
  f.-l. operation
faceometer
facet
  acromial f.
  anterior articular f. of talus
  articular f.
  auricular f. of sacrum
  clavicular f.
  costal f.
  costal f. of transverse process
  fibular articular f. of tibia
  lateral f's of sternum
  lateral malleolar f. of talus
  Lenoir f.
  locked f's of spine
  malleolar f. of tibia, internal
  medial malleolar f. of talus
  middle articular f. of talus
  posterior articular f. of talus
  squatting f.
  sternal articular f. of clavicle
  f. for tubercle of rib
  wear f.
facetectomy
faceted
faceting
facial
facies (facies)
  f. abdominalis
  acromegalic f.
  adenoid f.
  f. anterior antebrachii
  f. anterior brachii
  f. anterior cruris
  f. anterior femoris
  f. anterolateralis
  f. anteromedialis

facies (facies) *(continued)*
 f. articulares inferior atlantis
 f. articulares malleoli tibiae
 f. articulares superiores
  vertebrarum
 f. articularis
 f. bovina
 bovine f.
 f. buccalis
 f. cerebralis
 f. colica
 f. contactus dentis
 f. convexa cerebri
 Corvisart f.
 f. costalis
 cow f.
 cushingoid f.
 f. diaphragmatica
 f. digitales
 f. digitales dorsales
 f. digitales fibulares pedis
 f. digitales laterales
 f. digitales mediales
 f. digitales palmares
 f. digitales plantares
 f. digitales radiales
 f. digitales tibiales
 f. digitales ulnares
 f. distalis
 f. dolorosa
 f. dorsalis
 f. dorsalis digitorum pedis
 f. externa
 f. facialis
 f. frontalis
 f. gastrica
 f. glutealis ossis ilii
 f. glutea ossis ilii
 f. hepatica
 f. hippocratica
 Hutchinson f.
 f. inferior
 f. inferolateralis
 f. interlobares pulmonis
 f. interna
 f. intestinalis uteri
 f. labialis dentis
 f. lateralis
 f. lateralis brachii
 f. lateralis cruris
 f. lateralis femoris
 leonine f.
 f. leontina
 f. lingualis
 f. lunata

facies (facies) *(continued)*
 f. malaris
 f. malleolaris
 Marshall Hall f.
 f. masticatoria
 f. maxillaris
 f. medialis
 f. medialis brachii
 f. medialis cruris
 f. medialis digitorum manus
 f. medialis digitorum pedis
 f. medialis femoris
 f. mediastinalis pulmonis
 f. mesialis
 mitral f.
 mitrotricuspid f.
 moon f.
 myasthenic f.
 myopathic f.
 myxedematous f.
 f. nasalis
 f. palatina
 paralytic f.
 f. parietalis ossis parietalis
 Parkinson f.
 parkinsonian f.
 f. patellaris femoris
 f. pelvina
 f. plantares digitorum pedis
 f. poplitea femoris
 f. posterior
 f. posterior antebrachii
 f. posterior brachii
 f. posterior cruris
 f. posterior femoris
 Potter f.
 f. pulmonalis cordis
 f. renalis
 f. sacropelvina
 f. scaphoidea
 f. sphenomaxillaris alae
  magnae
 f. sternocostalis cordis
 f. superior
 f. superolateralis
 f. symphyseos
 f. symphysialis
 tabetic f.
 f. temporalis
 tortua f.
 typhoid f.
 f. urethralis penis
 f. ventralis
 f. vesicalis uteri
 f. vestibularis

F

facies (facies) *(continued)*
    f. visceralis
    f. volaris
facile
facilitation
    associative f.
    proprioceptive
      neuromuscular f.
    f. of reflexes
    Wedensky f.
facilitative
facilitatory
facilitory
facility
    acute care f. (ACF)
    adult congregate living f.
      (ACLF)
    extended care f. (ECF)
    intermediate care f. (ICF)
    skilled nursing f. (SNF)
facing
faciobrachial
faciocephalalgia
faciocervical
faciolingual
facioplasty
facioplegia
facioscapulohumeral
  dystrophy
faciostenosis
FACOG—Fellow of the American
  College of Obstetricians and
  Gynecologists
FACP—Fellow of the American
  College of Physicians
FACS—
    Fellow of the American
      College of Surgeons
    fluorescence-activated cell
      sorter
FACSM—Fellow of the American
  College of Sports Medicine
F-actin
factitial
factitious
factor
    f. VIII:c
    f. VIII:CAg
    f. VIIIR:Ag
    f. VIII T
    f. X deficiency disease
    f. A
    accelerator f.
    activated clotting f's
    activation f.

factor *(continued)*
    adrenocorticotropic releasing f.
      (ACTH-RF)
    allogeneic effect f.
    amplification f.
    angiogenesis f.
    anti–pernicious anemia f.
    antiberiberi f.
    antigen-specific T-cell
      helper f.
    antigen-specific T-cell
      suppressor f.
    antihemophilic f.,
      cryoprecipitated
    antihemophilic f., human
    antinuclear f. (ANF)
    f. B
    backscatter f.
    basophil chemotactic f.
      (BCF)
    B cell differentiation f's
      (BCDF)
    B cell growth f's (BCGF)
    Bittner milk f.
    blastogenic f. (BF)
    B lymphocyte stimulatory f's
      (BSF)
    bone f.
    buildup f.
    C f.
    C3 nephritic f. (C3 NeF)
    calibration f.
    CAMP f.
    cardiac risk f's (CRFs)
    Castle intrinsic f.
    chemotactic f.
    Christmas f.
    citrovorum f.
    clearing f.
    clonal inhibitory f.
    clumping f.
    coagulation f's I–V,
      VII–XIII
    colony-stimulating f. (CSF)
    conglutinogen activating f.
    contact f.
    contact activation f.
    cord f.
    corticotropin releasing f.
      (CRF)
    coupling f's
    crystal-induced chemotactic f.
      (CCF)
    Curling f.
    f. D

factor *(continued)*
    Day f.
    decapacitation f.
    decay-accelerating f. (DAF)
    depolarization f.
    diabetogenic f.
    diffusion f.
    Duran-Reynals
        permeability f.
    duty f.
    elongation f.
    eluate f.
    endothelium-derived
        relaxing f.
    eosinophil chemotactic f.
        (ECF)
    eosinophil chemotactic f. of
        anaphylaxis (ECF-A)
    epidermal growth f.
    epithelial thymic-activating f.
    erythropoietic stimulating f.
        (ESF)
    extrinsic f.
    F f.
    fertility f.
    fibrin stabilizing f.
    Fletcher f.
    follicle stimulating hormone–
        releasing f. (FRF; FSH-RF)
    F-prime f.
    Fy f.
    galactopoietic f.
    general f.
    geometry f.
    glass f.
    glucose tolerance f.
    gonadotropin-releasing f.
        (GnRF)
    growth f.
    growth hormone–releasing f.
        (GRF; GH-RF)
    growth inhibitory f's
    G f. of Spearman
    f. H
    Hageman f. (HF)
    Hageman f. inhibitor
    hematopoietic growth f's
    hemophilic f. A (B, C)
    hepatocyte-stimulating f.
    H f. of Lewis
    high-molecular-weight
        neutrophil chemotactic f.
        (HMW-NCF)
    histamine releasing f.
    human f. IX complex

factor *(continued)*
    hydrazine-sensitive f. (HSF)
    hyperglycemic-
        glycogenolytic f.
    f. I
    IgG rheumatoid f.
    IgM rheumatoid f.
    immunoglobulin-binding f.
        (IBF)
    inhibiting f's
    initiation f.
    insulin-antagonizing f.
    intrinsic f.
    kappa f.
    labile f.
    lactogenic f.
    Laki-Lorand f.
    LE f.
    lethal f.
    leukocyte inhibitory f. (LIF)
    leukocyte migration
        inhibition f.
    leukopenic f.
    liver filtrate f.
    LLD f.
    lupus erythematosus f.
    luteinizing
        hormone–releasing f. (LRF;
        LH-RF)
    lymph node permeability f.
        (LNPF)
    lymphocyte-activating f.
    lymphocyte blastogenic f. (BF)
    lymphocyte mitogenic f. (LMF)
    lymphocyte transforming f.
        (LTF)
    lymphocytosis-promoting f.
    lysogenic f.
    macrophage-activating f.
    macrophage chemotactic f.
        (MCF)
    macrophage-derived
        growth f.
    macrophage growth f.
        (MGF)
    macrophage inhibitory f. (MIF)
    maturation f.
    melanocyte-inhibiting f.
    migration inhibiting f.
        (MIF)
    migration inhibition f.
    migration inhibitory f.
    milk f.
    mitogenic f.
    modifying f.

F

factor *(continued)*

 mouse mammary tumor f.
 müllerian duct inhibitory f.
 müllerian regression f.
 multiple f's
 myocardial depressant f. (MDF)
 N f.
 necrotizing f.
 nephritic f.
 nerve growth f.
 neutrophil chemotactic f. (NCF)
 osteoclast-activating f. (OAF)
 f. P
 Passovoy f.
 pellagra-preventive f.
 plasma thromboplastin f.
 platelet f's (1–4)
 platelet-activating f. (PAF)
 platelet-derived growth f.
 P-P f.
 prolactin-inhibiting f. (PIF)
 prolactin-releasing f's (PRF)
 proliferation inhibitory f. (PIF)
 prothrombokinase f.
 Prower f.
 quality f.
 R f.
 recruitment f.
 reducing f.
 releasing f.
 resistance-inducing f.
 resistance transfer f.
 Reynals f.
 rhesus (Rh) f.
 rheumatoid f. (RF)
 f. rho
 risk f.
 ristocetin f.
 f. S
 secretor f.
 sex f.
 sigma f.
 Simon septic f.
 skin reactive f. (SRF)
 somatotropin-releasing f. (SRF)
 specific macrophage arming f. (SMAF)
 spreading f.
 stable f.
 Stuart f.
 Stuart-Prower f.
 T-cell growth f.
 termination f.
 thymus-replacing f.

factor *(continued)*

 thyroid-stimulating hormone–releasing f. (TSH-RF)
 thyrotoxic complement fixation f.
 thyrotropin-releasing f. (TRF)
 tissue f.
 tissue plasminogen f.
 transfer f. (TF)
 transforming f.
 transmethylation f.
 transmission f.
 Trapp f.
 tumor-angiogenesis f.
 tumor cell migration inhibitory f.
 tumor necrosis f. (TNF)
 V f.
 vascular permeability f.
 vascular tissue f.
 virulence f.
 von Willebrand f.
 f. W
 Willis f.
 X f.
 Y f.
 yeast eluate f.
 yeast filtrate f.

factorial

facultative
 f. hyperopia
 f. suppression

faculty
 fusion f.

FAD—flavin adenine dinucleotide

FADF—fluorescent antibody dark-field (examination)

fagopyrism

Fahey operation

Fahr disease

Fahraeus-Lindqvist effect

Fahrenheit (F)

failed forceps delivery

fail-safe

failure
 acute anuric renal f.
 acute oliguric renal f.
 acute polyuric renal f.
 backward heart f.
 biventricular f.
 congestive heart f. (CHF)
 forward heart f.
 heart f.
 hepatic f.
 high-output heart f.

failure *(continued)*
    high-output renal f.
    kidney f.
    left-sided heart f.
    left ventricular f.
    liver f.
    low-output heart f.
    peripheral circulatory f.
    prerenal f.
    primary (or secondary)
      adrenocortical f.
    pump f.
    renal f.
    respiratory f.
    right-sided heart f.
    right ventricular f.
    secondary glandular f.
    template f.
faint
fainting
Fajersztajn
    sign
    test
falcadina
falcate
falces
falcial
falciform
falciform fold
falcular
Falk operation
Falk-Shukuris operation
fallopian
    f. aqueduct
    f. arch
    f. artery
    embryonic f. tube
    f. hiatus
    f. ligament
    f. neuritis
    f. pregnancy
    f. tube
Fallopius
    aqueduct of F.
Fallot
    disease
    pentalogy of F.
    syndrome
    tetrad
    tetralogy of F.
    triad
    trilogy of F.
fallout
Falope ring
false-negative

false-positive
    biologic f. (BFP)
false suture
falsification
    retrospective f.
Falta
    coefficient
    triad
falx
    aponeurotic f.
    f. aponeurotica
    f. cerebelli
    f. cerebri
    inguinal f.
    f. inguinalis
    f. ligamentosa
    ligamentous f.
    f. septi
fames
familial osteochondrodystrophy
family
    extended f.
    form-f.
    Jukes f.
    Kallikak f.
    nuclear f.
    systematic f.
Family APGAR
  Questionnaire
fan
    Dunham f.
    macular f.
    sea f.
FANA—fluorescent antinuclear
  antibody
Fanconi
    anemia
    disease
    pancytopenia
    syndrome
Fanconi-Albertini-Zellweger
  syndrome
Fanconi-Petrassi
  syndrome
fango
    paraffin f.
    f. therapy
Fannia
    F. canicularis
    F. scalaris
fanning
Fansler
    anoscope
    proctoscope
    speculum

F

fantascope
fantasy
FAP—familial adenomatous polyposis
Farabeuf
 amputation
 elevator
 forceps
 triangle
Farabeuf-Lambotte forceps
farad
faraday
 constant
 dark space
 law
faradic
faradimeter
faradism
 surging f.
faradization
 galvanic f.
faradize
faradocontractility
faradomuscular
faradopalpation
far-and-near suture
Farber
 disease
 syndrome
 test
farina
farinaceous
farinometer
farmer's lung
farnesol
farnesyl pyrophosphate
farnoquinone
Farr retractor
Farre
 line
 tubercles
 white line
Farrington forceps
Farrior speculum
Farris forceps
farsighted
farsightedness
Fasanella-Servat operation
fascia (fasciae)
 abdominal f., internal
 Abernethy f.
 f. adherens
 alar f. of pharynx
 anal f.
 anoscrotal f.

fascia (fašciae) *(continued)*
 antebrachial f.
 f. antebrachii
 aponeurotic f.
 f. axillaris
 bicipital f.
 brachial f.
 f. brachialis
 f. brachii
 buccinator f.
 f. buccopharyngea
 buccopharyngeal f.
 f. buccopharyngealis
 Buck f.
 bulbar f.
 f. bulbi
 Camper f.
 cervical f.
 f. cervicalis
 cervical visceral f.
 clavipectoral f.
 f. clavipectoralis
 f. clitoridis
 Cloquet f.
 Colles f.
 f. colli
 Cooper f.
 coracoclavicular f.
 f. coracoclavicularis
 coracocostal f.
 cremasteric f.
 f. cremasterica
 cribriform f.
 f. cribrosa
 crural f.
 f. cruris
 Cruveilhier f.
 dartos f. of scrotum
 deep f.
 deep cervical f.
 deep dorsal f.
 deep f. of penis
 deltoid f.
 f. deltoidea
 Denonvilliers f.
 f. dentata hippocampi
 dentate f.
 dorsal f. of foot
 dorsal f. of hand
 f. dorsalis manus
 f. dorsalis pedis
 Dupuytren f.
 endoabdominal f.
 endopelvic f.
 f. endopelvina

fascia (fasciae) *(continued)*
  endothoracic f.
  f. endothoracica
  external intercostal f.
  external oblique f.
  extraperitoneal f.
  f. extraperitonealis
  extrapleural f.
  f. deltoidea
  f. dentata hippocampi
  femoral f.
  fibroareolar f.
  f. of forearm
  fusion f.
  Gerota f.
  gluteal f.
  f. of Godman
  hypogastric f.
  hypothenar f.
  iliac f.
  f. iliaca
  f. iliopectinea
  iliopectineal f.
  inferior f.
  infundibuliform f.
  f. of insertion
  intercolumnar f.
  investing f.
  ischiorectal f.
  lacrimal f.
  f. lata
  fasciae latae
  f. lata femoris
  f. of leg
  longitudinal f., anterior
  longitudinal f., posterior
  lumbar f.
  lumbodorsal f.
  f. lunata
  masseteric f.
  f. masseterica
  muscular f. of eye
  fasciae musculares bulbi
  f. nuchae
  nuchal f.
  f. nuchalis
  obturator f.
  f. obturatoria
  orbital fasciae
  fasciae orbitales
  palmar f.
  palpebral f.
  f. palpebralis
  parietal f. of pelvis
  parotid f.

fascia (fasciae) *(continued)*
  f. parotidea
  f. pectinea
  pectineal f.
  pectoral f.
  f. pectoralis
  pelvic f.
  pelviprostatic f.
  f. pelvis parietalis
  f. pelvis visceralis
  f. penis profunda
  f. penis superficialis
  f. perinei superficialis
  perirenal f.
  peritoneoperineal f.
  f. peritoneoperinealis
  pharyngobasilar f.
  f. pharyngobasilaris
  phrenicopleural f.
  f. phrenicopleuralis
  plantar f.
  popliteal f.
  prepubic f.
  pretracheal f.
  prevertebral f.
  f. prevertebralis
  f. profunda
  f. propria colli
  f. propria cooperi
  f. prostatae
  f. of prostate
  psoas f.
  pubic f.
  f. of quadratus lumborum
    muscle
  rectal f.
  rectoabdominal f.
  rectovaginal f.
  rectovesical f.
  renal f.
  f. renalis
  Richet f.
  scalene f.
  Scarpa f.
  semilunar f.
  Sibson f.
  f. spermatica externa
  f. spermatica interna
  spermatic f., external
  spermatic f., internal
  subcutaneous f.
  subperitoneal f.
  f. subperitonealis
  f. subscapularis
  subserous f.

F

fascia (fasciae) *(continued)*
    subvesical f.
    superficial f.
    f. superficialis
    f. superficialis perinei
    superficial f. of urogenital
      trigone
    f. of Tarin
    f. tarini
    temporal f.
    f. temporalis
    Tenon f.
    thenar f.
    thoracic f.
    f. thoracica
    f. thoracolumbalis
    thyrolaryngeal f.
    f. of Toldt
    f. transversalis
    transverse f.
    f. of Treitz
    triangular f. of Macalister
    triangular f. of Quain
    Tyrrell f.
    f. of urogenital trigone
    volar f.
fasciagram
fasciagraphy
fascial
fasciaplasty
fasciatome
    Luck f.
fascicle
    gracile f.
    longitudinal f's of cruciform
      ligament
fascicular
fasciculated
fasciculation
fasciculi
fasciculitis
fasciculus (fasciculi)
    f. aberrans of Monakow
    f. anterior proprius
    f. anterolateralis superficialis
      gowersi
    f. arcuatus
    f. atrioventricularis
    calcarine f.
    central tegmental f.
    cerebellospinal f.
    f. cerebellospinalis anterior
    f. cerebellospinalis lateralis
    f. circumolivaris pyramidalis
    crossed pyramidal f.

fasciculus (fasciculi) *(continued)*
    cuneate f. of Burdach
    cuneate f. of medulla oblongata
    cuneate f. of spinal cord
    f. cuneatus
    f. cuneatus burdachi
    direct pyramidal f.
    dorsal longitudinal f.
    dorsolateral f.
    f. dorsolateralis
    f. exilis
    extrapyramidal motor f.
    fasciculi proprii
    fastigiobulbar f.
    f. of Foville
    Goll f.
    f. of Gowers
    f. gracilis
    gyral f.
    inferior longitudinal f. of
      cerebrum
    interfascicular f.
    f. interfascicularis
    intersegmental fasciculi
    lateral cerebrospinal f.
    lenticular f.
    f. lenticularis
    longitudinal f.
    f. longitudinalis
    maculary f.
    mammillotegmental f.
    f. mammillotegmentalis
    mammillothalamic f.
    f. mammillothalamicus
    medial longitudinal f.
    medial prosencephalic f.
    medial telencephalic f.
    median triangular f.
    Meynert f.
    Monakow f.
    f. obliquus crucis cerebri
    f. obliquus pontis
    f. occipitofrontalis
    occipitothalamic f.
    olivocochlear f.
    oval f.
    f. parieto-occipitopontinus
    f. pedunculomammillaris
    perpendicular f.
    f. pontis longitudinales
    f. precommissuralis
    prerubral f.
    f. prosencephalicus medialis
    pyramidal f. of medulla
      oblongata

fasciculus (fasciculi) *(continued)*
f. pyramidalis medullae
oblongatae
f. retroflexus
f. of Rolando
semilunar f.
f. semilunaris
septomarginal f.
f. septomarginalis
solitary f.
subcallosal f.
f. subcallosus
subthalamic f.
f. subthalamicus
sulcomarginal f.
f. sulcomarginalis
superior longitudinal f. of
cerebrum
f. telencephalicus
medialis
thalamic f.
f. thalamicus
f. thalamomammillaris
thalamomammillary f.
f. triangularis
Türck f.
unciform f.
uncinate f.
f. uncinatus
Vicq d'Azyr f.
fasciectomy
fasciitis
diffuse f.
eosinophilic f.
exudative f.
exudative
calcifying f.
necrotizing f.
nodular f.
perirenal f.
proliferative f.
pseudosarcomatous f.
fasciodesis
fasciola cinerea
Fasciola
F. cervi
F. gigantica
F. hepatica
F. heterophyes
F. magna
fasciolar
fascioliasis
Fascioloides magna
fasciolopsiasis
Fasciolopsis buski

fascioplasty
fasciorrhaphy
fascioscapulohumeral
fasciotomy
fast
fast Fourier transformation
fast-glycolytic
fastidious
fastidium
fastigatum
fastigial
fastigiobulbar
fastigium
fastness
fast-oxidative glycolytic
FAT—fluorescent antibody
test
fat
bound f.
brown f.
chyle f.
corpse f.
depot f.
fetal f.
grave f.
hydrous wool f.
masked f.
milk f.
molecular f.
moruloid f.
mulberry f.
neutral f.
paranephric f.
pararenal f.
perinephric f.
perirenal f.
polyunsaturated f.
refined wool f.
saturated f.
unsaturated f.
wool f., hydrous
wool f., refined
yellow f.
fatal
fatality
fate
potential f.
prospective f.
fatigability
fatigue
auditory f.
battle f.
combat f.
flying f.
industrial f.

fatigue *(continued)*
>   pseudocombat f.
>   stance f.
>   stimulation f.

fatty acid
>   essential f.a. (EFA)
>   free f.a. (FFA)
>   medium-chain f.a. (MCFA)
>   monounsaturated f.a.
>   n-3 f.a.
>   nonesterified f.a. (NEFA)
>   ω-3 f.a. [omega-3]
>   ω-6 f.a. [omega-6]
>   ω-9 f.a. [omega-9]
>   polyunsaturated f.a. (PUFA)
>   saturated f.a.
>   short-chain f.a. (SCFA)
>   f.a. synthase
>   *trans*-f.a.
>   unsaturated f.a.

fatty meal
fauces
Fauchard disease
faucial
faucitis
Faught sphygmomanometer
Faulkner curet
fauna
fauntail
faute de mieux
Fauvel forceps
fava bean
faveolate
favic
favid
favism
Favre disease
Favre-Racouchot syndrome
favus
>   f. circinatus
>   f. herpeticus
>   f. herpetiformis
>   f. pilaris

faxen-psychosis
Fazio-Londe
>   atrophy
>   disease
>   syndrome

FB—
>   fingerbreadth
>   foreign body

FBP—
>   femoral blood pressure
>   fibrinogen breakdown product

FBS—
>   fasting blood sugar
>   fetal bovine serum

FC—
>   finger clubbing
>   finger counting

5-FC—flucytosine
FCA—
>   ferritin-conjugated antibodies
>   Freund complete adjuvant

fCi—femtocurie(s)
FD—
>   fatal dose
>   focal distance
>   foot drape
>   freeze-dried

F&D—fixed and dilated
FDA—Food and Drug
>   Administration

FDE—final drug evaluation
FDG—2-fluoro-2-deoxyglucose
FDP—
>   fibrin degradation product(s)
>   flexor digitorum profundus
>   right frontoposterior
>   (L. fronto-dextra posterior)

FDS—flexor digitorum
>   superficialis

F-duction
F-dUMP—5-fluorodeoxyuridine
>   monophosphate

Fe—iron
fear
feather analysis
feature
febantel
febricant
febricide
febricity
febricula
febrifacient
febrific
febrifugal
febrifuge
febrifugine
febrile
febris
>   f. melitensis

FEC—free erythrocyte
>   coproporphyrin

fecal
>   f. continence
>   f. fluid
>   f. impaction

fecal *(continued)*
    f. incontinence
    f. leukocytes
fecalith
    appendiceal f.
fecaloid
fecaloma
fecaluria
feces
FECG—fetal electrocardiogram
FECP—free erythrocyte
  coproporphyria
fecula
feculent
fecundate
fecundatio ab extra
fecundation
    artificial f.
fecundity
Fede disease
Federici sign
feeblemindedness
feedback
    alpha f.
    delayed auditory f. (DAF)
    negative f.
    positive f.
feed-forward
feeding
    artificial f.
    breast f.
    demand f.
    drip f.
    extrabuccal f.
    Finkelstein f.
    forced f.
    intravenous f.
    nasal f.
    f. prosthesis
    sham f.
    tube f.
feeling
Feer disease
fee-splitting
FEF—forced expiratory flow
Fegeler syndrome
Fehland clamp
Fehleisen streptococcus
Fehling
    solution
    test
Feilchenfeld forceps
Feiss line
Feist-Mankin position

FEKG—fetal electrocardiogram
feline
Felix Vi serum
Felix-Weil reaction
  (FWR)
fellatio
Fell-O'Dwyer apparatus
felo-de-se
felon
    bone f.
    deep f.
    subcutaneous f.
    subcuticular f.
    subperiosteal f.
    thecal f.
felony
felt dressing
feltwork
    Kaes f.
Felty syndrome
fem.—female
female circumcision
feminine
femininity
feminism
feminization
    testicular f.
feminize
feminizing
femme
femora (plural of femur)
femoral
    f. arteriography
    f. artery
    f. head
    f. neck
    f. shaft
    f. triangle
femorocele
femorofemoral
femorofemoropopliteal
femoroiliac
femoropopliteal
femorotibial
femtocurie(s) (fCi)
femur (femora, femurs)
    f. length
FE_{Na}—excreted fraction of filtered
  sodium
fenamate
fenchlorphos
fenclonine
fenclorac
fendosal

fenestra (fenestrae)
  f. choledocha
  f. of cochlea
  f. cochleae
  f. ovalis
  f. rotunda
  f. vestibuli
fenestrate
fenestrated tenotomy
fenestration
  alveolar plate f.
  aorticopulmonary f.
  aortopulmonary f.
  apical f.
  f. operation
fenestrel
Fenger probe
fenitrothion
fenthion
fenticlor
fenugreek
Fenwick disease
Fenwick-Hunner ulcer
FER—familial exudative
  retinopathy
feral
fer-de-lance
Fergus operation
Ferguson
  basket
  forceps
  method
  reflex
  scissors
  scoop
Ferguson-Moon retractor
Ferguson-Smith
  epithelioma
Ferguson-Smith–type
  epithelioma
Fergusson
  incision
  operation
  speculum
Fergusson and Critchley ataxia
ferment
  glycolytic f.
fermentation
  acetone-butanol f.
  alcoholic f.
  amino acid f.
  butanediol f.
  n-butanol f.
  butylene glycol f.
  butyric f.

fermentation *(continued)*
  formic f.
  heterolactic f.
  homolactic f.
  mannitol f.
  mixed acid f.
  propionic f.
  stormy f.
  f. tube
fermentum
Fermi-Dirac statistics
fermium (Fm)
Fermi vaccine
Fernandez operation
ferning
ferrate
ferrated
ferredoxin
Ferrein
  canal
  foramen
  pyramid
  tubes
  tubules
ferri-albuminic
ferric
  f. ammonium citrate
  f. ammonium sulfate
  f. citrate
  f. fructose
  f. glycerophosphate
  f. hydroxide with magnesium
    oxide
  f. hypophosphite
  f. oxide, red
  f. oxide, yellow
  f. pyrophosphate
  f. sodium edetate
ferricyanide
ferriheme
ferrihemochrome
ferrihemoglobin
ferriporphyrin
ferriprotoporphyrin
Ferris
  dilator
  forceps
  scoop
Ferris-Robb knife
Ferris-Smith
  forceps
  operation
  retractor
Ferris-Smith-Kerrison forceps
Ferris-Smith-Sewall retractor

ferritin
ferrochelatase
ferrocholinate
ferrocyanide
ferroelectric
ferroflocculation
ferrography
ferrokinetic
ferrokinetics
ferromagnetic relaxation
ferroprotein
ferrosoferric
ferrotherapy
ferroxidase
ferruginous
ferrum
Ferry-Porter law
fertile
fertility
fertilization
    cross f.
    external f.
    internal f.
    in vitro f. (IVF)
fertilizing
fervescence
FES—
    forced expiratory spirogram
    functional electrical
      stimulation
fescue
fester
festinant
festination
festoon
    gingival f.
    McCall f.
FET—forced expiratory time
fetal
    f. alcohol syndrome
    f. allograft
    f. asphyxia
    f. breathing
    f. circulation
    f. crowding
    f. distress
    f. electrocardiography
    f. head
    f. heart sound
    f. heart tone
    f. hemolysis
    f. hydantoin syndrome
    f. hydrops
    f. monitor
    f. oophoritis

fetal *(continued)*
    f. oxygenation
    f. postmaturity syndrome
    f. scalp blood sampling
    f. skull
    f. structure
    f. tachycardia
    f.-to-maternal ratio
    f. warfarin syndrome
    f. weight
    f. well-being
fetalization
fetal position
    LFA—left frontoanterior
    LFP—left frontoposterior
    LFT—left frontotransverse
    LMA—left mentoanterior
    LMP—left mentoposterior
    LMT—left mentotransverse
    LOA—left occipitoanterior
    LOP—left occipitoposterior
    LOT—left occipitotransverse
    LSA—left sacroanterior
    LScA.—left scapuloanterior
    LScP.—left scapuloposterior
    LSP—left sacroposterior
    LST—left sacrotransverse
    RFA—right frontoanterior
    RFP— right frontoposterior
    RFT— right frontotransverse
    RMA— right mentoanterior
    RMP— right mentoposterior
    RMT— right mentotransverse
    ROA— right occipitoanterior
    ROP— right occipitoposterior
    ROT— right
      occipitotransverse
    RSA— right sacroanterior
    RScA— right scapuloanterior
    RScP— right scapuloposterior
    RSP— right sacroposterior
    RST— right sacrotransverse
fetation
feticide
fetid
fetish
fetishism
    transvestic f.
fetishist
fetoamniotic
fetogram
fetography
fetologist
fetology
fetomaternal

F

fetometry
fetopathy
fetoplacental
fetoprotein
    α-f. [alpha-]
    β-f. [beta-]
    γ-f. [gamma-]
fetor
    f. hepaticus
    f. oris
fetoscope
fetoscopic
fetoscopy
fetotoxic
FETS—forced expiratory time in
  seconds
fetus
    acardiac f.
    f. acardiacus
    f. acardius
    f. amorphus
    calcified f.
    f. compressus
    harlequin f.
    f. in fetu
    macerated f.
    mummified f.
    paper-doll f.
    papyraceous f.
    f. papyraceus
    parasitic f.
    retroperitoneal f. in fetu
    f. sanguinolentis
    sireniform f.
    viable f.
Feulgen
    reaction
    stain
    test
Feulgen-positive
FEV—
    familial exudative
      vitreoretinopathy
    forced expiratory volume
FEV_1 [FEV1]—forced expiratory
  volume in one second
fever
    abortus f.
    Aden f.
    adynamic f.
    African coast f.
    African tick f.
    Andaman A f.
    aphthous f.
    apyretic typhoid f.

fever *(continued)*
    Argentine hemorrhagic f.
    artificial f.
    aseptic f.
    Assam f.
    asthenic f.
    auric f.
    Australian Q f.
    Australian tick f.
    autumn f.
    Bangkok hemorrhagic f.
    barbeiro f.
    biduotertian f.
    black f.
    blackwater f.
    blue f.
    Bolivian hemorrhagic f.
    bouquet f.
    boutonneuse f.
    brain f.
    brassfounder's f.
    Brazilian purpuric f.
    Brazilian spotted f.
    breakbone f.
    Brisbane f.
    Bullis f.
    burdwan f.
    Bushy Creek f.
    Bwamba f.
    cachectic f.
    camp f.
    cane field f.
    canicola f.
    carbuncular f.
    cat-scratch f.
    central f.
    Central Asian hemorrhagic f.
    cerebrospinal f.
    Charcot f.
    chikungunya f.
    childbed f.
    Choix f.
    Colombian tick f.
    Colorado tick f.
    Congo red f.
    continued f.
    continuous f.
    cotton-mill f.
    Crimean-Congo hemorrhagic f.
    cyclic f.
    Cyprus f.
    dandy f.
    deer fly f.
    dehydration f.
    dengue hemorrhagic f.

fever *(continued)*

- desert f.
- digestive f.
- diphasic milk f.
- drug f.
- Dutton relapsing f.
- East Coast f.
- Ebola hemorrhagic f.
- elephantoid f.
- endemic relapsing f.
- enteric f.
- entericoid f.
- ephemeral f.
- epidemic hemorrhagic f.
- eruptive f.
- essential f.
- estivoautumnal f.
- etiocholanolone f.
- exanthematous f.
- exsiccation f.
- familial Mediterranean f.
- famine f.
- Far Eastern hemorrhagic f.
- fatigue f.
- field f.
- five-day f.
- Fort Bragg f.
- foundryman's f.
- Gambian f.
- glandular f.
- Guáitara f.
- Hankow f.
- harvest f.
- Hasami f.
- Haverhill f.
- hay f., nonseasonal
- hay f., perennial
- hectic f.
- hematuric bilious f.
- hemoglobinuric f.
- hemorrhagic f.
- hemorrhagic f. with renal syndrome
- herpetic f.
- Herxheimer f.
- hospital f.
- icterohemorrhagic f.
- Ilheus f.
- inanition f.
- induced f.
- intermittent f.
- intermittent hepatic f.
- inundation f.
- island f.
- Jaccoud dissociated f.

fever *(continued)*

- jail f.
- Japanese flood f.
- Japanese river f.
- jungle f.
- jungle yellow f.
- Junin f.
- Katayama f.
- Kedani f.
- Kenya f.
- Kew Gardens spotted f.
- Kinkiang f.
- Korean hemorrhagic f.
- Korin f.
- Kyoto f.
- land f.
- leprotic f.
- Lone Star f.
- louse-borne relapsing f.
- lung f.
- macular f.
- malarial f.
- malignant tertian f.
- Malta f.
- Marburg hemorrhagic f.
- Marseilles f.
- marsh f.
- Mediterranean f.
- Mediterranean coast f.
- Mediterranean tick f.
- melanuric f.
- metabolic f.
- metal fume f.
- Meuse f.
- Mexican spotted f.
- Mianeh f.
- milk f.
- miniature scarlet f.
- mite f.
- monoleptic f.
- mosquito-borne f.
- Mossman f.
- mountain tick f.
- mud f.
- Murchison-Pel-Ebstein f.
- nanukayami f.
- neurogenic f.
- nine-mile f.
- North Queensland tick f.
- Omsk hemorrhagic f.
- o'nyong-nyong f.
- Oroya f.
- Pahvant Valley f.
- paludal f.
- pappataci f.

F

fever *(continued)*
    paramalta f.
    paratyphoid f.
    paraundulant f.
    parenteric f.
    parrot f.
    parturient f.
    Pel-Ebstein f.
    periodic f.
    Persian relapsing f.
    petechial f.
    Pfeiffer glandular f.
    pharyngoconjunctival f.
    Philippine hemorrhagic f.
    phlebotomus f.
    pinta f.
    pneumonic f.
    polyleptic f.
    polymer fume f.
    Pomona f.
    Pontiac f.
    pretibial f.
    prison f.
    protein f.
    puerperal f.
    pulmonary f.
    pythogenic f.
    Q f.
    quartan f.
    Queensland coastal f.
    Queensland tick f.
    quinine f.
    quotidian f.
    rabbit f.
    rat-bite f.
    recurrent f.
    redwater f.
    relapsing f.
    remittent f.
    rheumatic f.
    rice field f.
    Rift Valley f.
    river f. of Japan
    Rocky Mountain spotted f.
    Russian headache f.
    saddleback f.
    Sakushu f.
    salt f.
    sandfly f.
    San Joaquin f.
    São Paulo f.
    scarlet f.
    Schottmüller (Schottmueller) f.
    septic f.
    seven-day f.

fever *(continued)*
    shin bone f.
    ship f.
    shoddy f.
    Sindbis f.
    slime f.
    snail f.
    solar f.
    Songo f.
    South African tick-bite f.
    South American
        hemorrhagic f.
    Southeast Asian f.
    spelters' f.
    spiking f.
    spirillar f.
    spirillum f.
    splenic f.
    spotted f.
    sthenic f.
    stiff-neck f.
    streptobacillary f.
    sulfonamide f.
    sweat f.
    sylvan yellow f.
    tertian f.
    tetanoid f.
    Texas tick f.
    Thai hemorrhagic f.
    therapeutic f.
    thermic f.
    thirst f.
    three-day f.
    threshing f.
    tick f.
    tick-borne relapsing f.
    Tobia f.
    trench f.
    trypanosome f.
    tsutsugamushi f.
    typhoid f.
    typhomalarial f.
    typhus f.
    undulant f.
    urban yellow f.
    urethral f.
    urinary f.
    urticarial f.
    uveoparotid f.
    vaccinal f.
    valley f.
    viral hemorrhagic f's
    Volhynia f.
    war f.
    West African f.

fever *(continued)*
    West Nile f.
    Whitmore f.
    Wolhynia f.
    Yangtze Valley f.
    yellow f.
    Zika f.
    zinc fume f.
Fèvre-Languepin syndrome
FF—
    fat-free
    father factor
    fecal frequency
    filtration fraction
    finger-to-finger
    flat feet
    force fluids
    forearm flow
    foster father
FFA—free fatty acid(s)
FFDW—fat-free dry weight
FFF—flicker, fusion, frequency
FFM—fat-free mass
FFP—fresh frozen plasma
FFT—flicker fusion threshold
FFWW—fat-free wet weight
FG—fibrinogen
FGF—fresh gas flow
FH—
    family history
    fetal head
    fetal heart
FHR—fetal heart rate
FHS—fetal heart sound(s)
FHT—fetal heart tone(s)
FI—fibrinogen forced inspiration
FIA—
    fluoroimmunoassay
    Freund incomplete adjuvant
fiat
fib.—fibrinogen
fiber
    A f's
    A-alpha nerve f.
    accelerating f's
    accelerator f.
    accessory f's
    adrenergic f.
    afferent nerve f.
    alpha f's
    alveolar f's
    alveolar crest f's
    anastomosing f.
    anastomotic f.
    apical f's

fiber *(continued)*
    archiform f's
    arcuate f.
    argentaffin f's
    argentophil f's
    argyrophilic f.
    asbestos f's
    astral f.
    augmentor f's
    auxiliary f's
    axial f.
    B f's
    basilar f's
    Bergmann f's
    Bernheimer f's
    beta f's
    f's of Bogrov
    bone f's
    Brücke f.
    bulbospiral f's
    Burdach f's
    C f's
    capsular f's
    cardiac accelerator f's
    cardiac depressor f's
    cardiac pressor f's
    cemental f's
    cementoalveolar f's
    centripetal f.
    cerebrospinal f's
    chief f's
    cholinergic f's
    chromatic f.
    chromosomal f.
    cilioequatorial f's
    cilioposterocapsular f's
    circular f's
    climbing f's
    clinging f's
    collagen f's
    collateral f's of Winslow
    commissural nerve f's
    cone f.
    conjunctival f's
    continuous f's
    Corti f's
    corticobulbar f's
    corticofugal f.
    corticonuclear f's
    corticopetal f.
    corticopontine f's
    corticoreticular f's
    corticorubral f's
    corticospinal f's
    corticostriate f's

F

fiber *(continued)*

 corticothalamic f's
 dark f's
 Darkschewitsch
  (Darkshevich) f.
 daughter f.
 decussating f's
 dendritic f's
 dentatorubral f's
 dentatothalamic f's
 dentinal f's
 dentinogenic f's
 depressor f's
 dietary f.
 Dieters f's
 Edinger f's
 efferent nerve f's
 elastic f's
 endogenous f's
 exogenous f's
 extraciliary f's
 extrafusal f's
 forklike f's
 frontopontine f's
 fusimotor f.
 gamma f's
 Gerdy f's
 giant f.
 gingival f's
 gingivodental f's
 Goll f's
 Gottstein f's
 Gratiolet radiating f's
 gray f's
 hair f.
 half-spindle f's
 Henle f's
 Herxheimer f's
 heterodesmotic f's
 homodesmotic f's
 horizontal f's
 Ia f.
 Ib f.
 IF f.
 impulse-conducting f's
 inhibitory f's
 interciliary f's
 intercolumnar f's
 intercrural f's
 internuncial f's
 interzonal f's
 intrafusal f's
 isotropic f.
 James f's
 Korff f's

fiber *(continued)*

 Kühne f.
 lattice f's
 Lenhossek f's
 f's of lens
 light f's
 longitudinal f's
 Luschka f's
 Mahaim f's
 main f's
 mantle f.
 Mauthner f.
 medullated f's
 medullated nerve f's
 meridional f's of ciliary muscle
 f's of Meynert
 Monakow f's
 moss f's
 mossy f's
 motor f.
 Muller f.
 muscle f.
 myelinated nerve f's
 naked f.
 nerve f.
 neuroglial f.
 nonmedullated nerve f's
 nuclear bag f.
 nuclear chain muscle f.
 oblique f's
 odontogenic f's
 olfactory f's
 olivocerebellar f's
 optic nerve f.
 orbiculoanterocapsular f's
 orbiculociliary f's
 orbiculoposterocapsular f's
 osteocollagenous f's
 osteogenetic f's
 osteogenic f's
 oxytalan f.
 pale muscle f.
 pallidohypothalamic f's
 paraventricular f's
 parent f.
 parietotemporopontine f's
 perforating f's
 periventricular f's
 pilomotor f's
 pontocerebellar f's
 postcommissural f's
 precollagenous f's
 precommissural f's
 preganglionic nerve f's
 pressor f's

fiber *(continued)*

> principal f's
> projection nerve f's
> Prussak f's
> Purkinje f.
> pyramidal f's of medulla
>   oblongata
> radial f's of ciliary muscle
> radiating f's
> radicular f's
> ragged red f's
> ragged-red muscle f's
> Rasmussen nerve f's
> Reissner f's
> f's of Remak
> Retzius f's
> ring f's
> Ritter f.
> rod f.
> Rolando f.
> Rosenthal f's
> Sappey f.
> Schroeder f's
> sensory f.
> Sharpey f.
> short association f's
> sinospiral f's
> skeletofusimotor f.
> somatic nerve f's
> sphincter f's of ciliary muscle
> spinal parasympathetic f's
> spindle f's
> Stilling f's
> striated muscle f.
> f's of stria terminalis
> sudomotor f's
> supraoptic f's
> sustentacular f's
> T f.
> tangential nerve f's
> temporopontine f's
> tendril f's
> thalamocortical f's
> thalamoparietal f's
> thalamostriate f's
> Tomes f.
> traction f's
> transilient f's
> transseptal f's
> transverse f's of pons
> ultraterminal f.
> unmyelinated nerve f's
> varicose f's
> vasoconstrictor f's
> vasodilatory f's

fiber *(continued)*

> vasomotor f's
> visceral nerve f's
> von Monakow f.
> Weissmann f's
> white f's
> yellow f's
> zonular f's

fibercolonoscope
fibergastroscope
fiberglass
fiber-illuminated
fiberoptic

> f. angioscopy
> f. bronchoscope
> f. bronchoscopy
> f. colonoscope
> f. colonoscopy
> f. cystoscope
> f. esophagoscope
> f. gastroscope
> f. laryngoscope
> f. laryngoscopy
> f. probe
> f. sigmoidoscope
> f. tube

fiberoptics
fiberscope

> gastric f.
> Hirschowitz gastroduodenal f.
> Olympus f.

fiberscopic
fibra (fibrae)

> fibrae annulares
> fibrae arcuatae
> fibrae arcuatae cerebri
> fibrae arcuatae externae
> fibrae arcuatae internae
> fibrae cerebello-olivares
> fibrae circulares musculi
>   ciliaris
> fibrae corticonucleares
> fibrae corticopontinae
> fibrae corticoreticulares
> fibrae corticorubrales
> fibrae corticospinales
> fibrae corticothalamicae
> fibrae dentatorubrales
> fibrae frontopontinae
> fibrae intercrurales
> fibrae lentis
> fibrae longitudinales
> fibrae meridionales
> fibrae obliquae
> fibrae paraventriculares

fibra (fibrae) *(continued)*
    fibrae parietotemporopontinae
    fibrae periventriculares
    fibrae pontis longitudinales
    fibrae pontis profundae
    fibrae pontis superficiales
    fibrae pontis transversae
    fibrae pontocerebellares
    fibrae propriae
    fibrae pyramidales
    fibrae pyramidales medullae
    fibrae radiales
    fibrae striae terminalis
    fibrae supraopticae
    fibrae temporopontinae
    fibrae thalamoparietales
    fibrae zonulares
fibration
fibril
    Alzheimer f.
    anchoring f.
    axial f's
    border f's
    collagen f's
    cytoplasmic f's
    dentinal f's
    Dirck f's
    fibroglia f's
    muscle f.
    nerve f.
    side f. of Golgi
    Tomes f.
    young collagen f's
fibrilla (fibrillae)
fibrillar
fibrillary
fibrillate
fibrillated
fibrillation
    atrial f.
    auricular f.
    ventricular f.
fibrin
    stroma f.
fibrinase
fibrinemia
fibrinocellular
fibrinogen
    human f.
fibrinogenase
fibrinogenemia
fibrinogenesis
fibrinogenic
fibrinogenolysis
fibrinogenolytic

fibrinogenopenia
fibrinogenopenic
fibrinogenous
fibrinoid
    canalized f.
    f. necrosis
    placental f.
fibrinokinase
fibrinoligase
fibrinolysin
    seminal f.
fibrinolysis
fibrinolytic
fibrinopenia
fibrinopeptide
fibrinoplatelet
fibrinopurulent
fibrinorrhea
fibrinoscopy
fibrinous
fibrinuria
fibroadenoma
    giant f. of the breast
    intracanalicular f.
    pericanalicular f.
fibroadenosis
fibroadipose
fibroangioma
    nasopharyngeal f.
fibroareolar
fibroatrophy
fibroblast
    contractile f.
    pericryptal f's
fibroblastic
fibroblastoma
    meningeal f.
    perineural f.
fibrobronchitis
fibrocalcific
fibrocarcinoma
fibrocartilage
    f. of the auricle
    basal f.
    circumferential f.
    connecting f.
    cotyloid f.
    elastic f.
    glenoid f.
    interarticular f.
    intra-articular f.
    semilunar f's
    spongy f.
    sternoclavicular f.
    stratiform f.

fibrocartilage *(continued)*
    white f.
    yellow f.
fibrocartilaginous
fibrocartilago
  (fibrocartilagines)
    f. basalis
    fibrocartilagines
      intervertebrales
    f. navicularis
fibrocaseous
fibrocavitary
fibrocellular
fibrocementoma
fibrochondritis
fibrochondroma
fibrocollagenous
fibrocongestive
fibrocyst
fibrocystadenoma
fibrocystic
fibrocystic disease
fibrocystoma
fibrocyte
fibrocytogenesis
fibrodysplasia
    f. ossificans progressiva
    renal artery f.
fibroelastic
fibroelastosis
    f. cordis
    endocardial f.
    endomyocardial f.
fibroenchondroma
fibroendothelioma
fibroepithelioma
    premalignant f.
fibrofatty
fibrofibrous
fibrogenesis imperfecta
  ossium
fibrogenic
fibroglia
fibroglioma
fibrohemorrhagic
fibrohistiocytic
fibroid
fibroidectomy
fibroin
fibrokeratoma
fibrolamellar
fibrolaminar
fibroleiomyoma
fibrolipoma
fibrolipomatous

fibroma (fibromas, fibromata)
    ameloblastic f.
    calcified f.
    f. cavernosum
    cementifying f.
    cemento-ossifying f.
    chondromyxoid f.
    concentric f.
    cutaneous f.
    f. cutis
    cystic f.
    desmoplastic f.
    f. durum
    endoneural f.
    hard f.
    histiocytic f.
    intracanalicular f.
    irritation f.
    juvenile nasopharyngeal f.
    f. lipomatodes
    f. of lung
    f. molle
    f. mucinosum
    myxoid f.
    f. myxomatodes
    nonossifying f.
    nonosteogenic f.
    odontogenic f.
    ossifying f.
    osteogenic f.
    parasitic f.
    f. pendulum
    periapical f.
    perifollicular f.
    periungual f.
    recurrent digital f.
    f. sarcomatosum
    senile f.
    soft f.
    submucous f.
    telangiectatic f.
    f. of testis
    f. thecocellulare
      xanthomatodes
    f. xanthoma
fibromatogenic
fibromatoid
fibromatosis
    aggressive f.
    f. colli
    congenital generalized f.
    f. gingivae
    gingival f.
    infantile digital f.
    palmar f.

F

fibromatosis *(continued)*
  plantar f.
  subcutaneous
    pseudosarcomatous f.
  f. ventriculi
fibromatous
fibromectomy
fibromembranous adhesions
fibromuscular disease
fibromyalgia
fibromyitis
fibromyoma uteri
fibromyomectomy
fibromyositis
  nodular f.
fibromyotomy
fibromyxolipoma
fibromyxoma
fibromyxosarcoma
fibronectin
fibroneuroma
fibroneurosarcoma
fibronuclear
fibro-odontoma
  ameloblastic f.
fibro-osteoma
fibropapilloma
fibropituicyte
fibroplasia
  intimal f.
  medial f.
  myointimal f.
  retrolental f.
  subadventitial f.
fibroplastic
fibroplate
fibropolypus
fibropurulent
fibroreticulate
  odontogenic f.
fibrosarcoma
  ameloblastic f.
  f. of the nerve sheath
  odontogenic f.
  f. phyllodes
  renal f.
fibrosclerosis
  multifocal f.
fibrose
fibroserous
fibrosing
fibrosis
  African endomyocardial f.
  arteriocapillary f.
  bauxite pulmonary f.

fibrosis *(continued)*
  condensation f.
  congenital hepatic f.
  cystic f. (CF)
  diatomite f.
  diffuse interstitial pulmonary f.
  endomyocardial f.
  glomerular f.
  graphite f.
  hepatic f.
  idiopathic f.
  interstitial f.
  mediastinal f.
  neoplastic f.
  nodular subepidermal f.
  panmural f. of the bladder
  periureteral f.
  pipestem f.
  pleural f.
  postfibrinous f.
  progressive massive f.
  proliferative f.
  pulmonary f.
  renal f.
  replacement f.
  retroperitoneal f.
  root sleeve f.
  Symmers f.
  Symmers pipestem f.
  f. uteri
fibrositis
  traumatic f.
fibrosplenomegaly
  congestive f.
fibrothorax
fibrotic
fibrous
  f. dysplasia
  f. histiocytoma
  f. papule fibroxanthoma
  f. plaque
fibrovascular
fibroxanthoma
fibula
fibular
fibularis
fibulation
fibulocalcaneal
ficin
Fick
  axis
  formula
  halo
  law
  method

Fick *(continued)*
>   operation
>   position
>   principle
Ficoll-Hypaque technique
ficosis
FID—
>   flame ionization detector
>   free induction decay
fidicinales
Fiedler
>   disease
>   myocarditis
field
>   absolute f.
>   adversive f.
>   auditory f.
>   binocular f.
>   centrocecal area of f.
>   clear lung f's
>   Cohnheim f's
>   cribriform f. of vision
>   dark-f.
>   f.-dependent
>   developmental f.
>   electromagnetic f.
>   electrostatic f.
>   far f.
>   f. of fixation
>   Flechsig f.
>   f's of Forel
>   frontal eye f.
>   gamma f.
>   f. H of Forel
>   f. H$_1$of Forel
>   f. H$_2$of Forel
>   high-power f.
>   individuation f.
>   low-power f.
>   lung f's
>   magnetic f.
>   morphogenetic f.
>   myelinogenetic f.
>   near f.
>   occipital eye f.
>   penumbra f.
>   perceptual f.
>   prefrontal eye f.
>   prerubral f.
>   primary nail f.
>   receptive f.
>   relative f.
>   subicular f's
>   surplus f.
>   tactile f.

field *(continued)*
>   tegmental f.
>   f. of vision
>   visual f.
>   Wernicke f.
Fiessinger-Leroy syndrome
Fiessinger-Leroy-Reiter syndrome
Fiessinger-Rendu syndrome
FIF—forced inspiratory flow
fifth disease
5150 hold
FIGE—field inversion gel
>   electrophoresis
FIGLU—formiminoglutamic
>   acid
FIGO—Federation of International
>   Gynecology and Obstetrics
FIGO
>   classification of endometrial
>   carcinoma
>   nomenclature
>   staging
figuratum
figure
>   achromatic f.
>   chromatic f.
>   flame f.
>   fortification f.
>   Minkowski f.
>   mitotic f's
>   myelin f.
>   nuclear f.
>   Purkinje f.
>   star f.
>   Stifel f.
>   Zollner f.
figure-of-eight suture
fila (plural of filum)
filaceous
filament
>   acrosomal f.
>   actin f.
>   axial f.
>   desmin f's
>   intermediate f.
>   keratin f's
>   linin f.
>   lymphatic anchoring f's
>   meningeal f.
>   polar injecting f.
>   root f's of spinal nerve
>   spermatic f.
>   spinal f.
>   terminal f.
>   vimentin f's

F

filamentary
filamentation
filamentous adhesions
filamentum (filamenta)
filar
filaria (filariae)
    Bancroft f.
    Brug f.
Filaria
    F. bancrofti
    F. conjunctivae
    F. diurna
    F. hominis oris
    F. juncea
    F. labialis
    F. lentis
    F. lymphatica
    F. palpebralis
    F. philippinensis
    F. streptocerca
filariae (plural of filaria)
filarial
filariasis
    Bancroft f.
    f. bancrofti
    bancroftian f.
    Brug f.
    brugian f.
    lymphatic f.
    Malayan f.
    occult f.
    Ozzard f.
    periodic f.
    timorian f.
filaricidal
filaricide
filariform
filariform larvae
filarious
Filatov
    disease
    flap
    operation
Filatov-Dukes disease
Filatov-Gilles tubed pedicle
file
    endodontic f.
    root canal f.
filgrastim
filial
filicic acid
filicin
filiform
    f. catheter
    f. and follower

filiform *(continued)*
    f. tumor
    f. wart
filigree
filioparental
filipin
Filipovitch (Filipowicz) sign
fillet, filleted, filleting
filling
    complex f.
    composite f.
    compound f.
    f. defect
    direct f.
    direct resin f.
    ditched f.
    indirect f.
    permanent f.
    postresection f.
    retrograde f.
    reverse f.
    root canal f.
    root-end f.
    temporary f.
    treatment f.
film
    absorbable gelatin f.
    f. badge
    baseline f.
    bite-wing f.
    comparison f.
    f. density calibration
    fibrin f.
    fixed blood f.
    lateral decubitus f.
    lateral jaw f.
    nonscreen f.
    occlusal f.
    panoramic x-ray f.
    periapical f.
    plain f.
    port f.
    precorneal f.
    preliminary f.
    prone f.
    rapid processing f.
    scout f.
    sequential f.
    serial f.
    spot f.
    stripping f.
    sulfa f.
    x-ray f.
film-stripping autoradiography
filopodium (filopodia)

filopressure
filovaricosis
filter
 bandpass f.
 band-stop f.
 barrier f.
 Berkefeld f.
 bird's nest f.
 Chamberland f.
 collodion f.
 excitation f.
 Greenfield f.
 high-pass f.
 inferior vena cava f.
 inherent f.
 intermittent sand f.
 Kimray-Greenfield f.
 low-pass f.
 mechanical f.
 membrane f.
 Millipore f.
 Mobin-Uddin umbrella f.
 notch f.
 f. paper chromatography
 percolating f.
 roughing f.
 scrubbing f.
 sintered glass f.
 slow sand f.
 sprinkling f.
 Thoraeus f.
 trickling f.
 ultraviolet f.
 umbrella f.
 vena cava f.
 vena caval f.
 wedge f.
 Wood f.
filterable
filtrate
 bacterial f.
 Folin protein-free f.
 glomerular f.
filtration
 gel f.
 glomerular f.
filtrum
 Merkel f. ventriculi
 f. ventriculi
filum (fila)
 fila anastomotica nervi acustici
 f. durae matris spinale
 f. durae matris spinalis
 f. meningeale
 f. meningeum

filum (fila) *(continued)*
 fila olfactoria
 fila radicularia nervi spinalis
 fila radicularia nervorum
  spinalium
 f. of spinal dura mater
 f. spinale
 f. terminale
fimbria (fimbriae)
 fimbriae of fallopian tube
 f. hippocampi
 ovarian f.
 f. ovarica
 fimbriae of tongue
 fimbriae tubae uterinae
fimbrial
fimbriated
fimbriation
fimbriatum
fimbriectomy
fimbriocele
fimbriodentate
fimbrioplasty
finder
finding
fine mesh dressing
fine-needle
 f-n. aspiration biopsy
 f-n. biopsy
 f-n. transhepatic
  cholangiography
finger
 baseball f.
 blubber f.
 bolster f's
 clubbed f.
 dead f.
 drop f.
 drumstick f.
 first f.
 giant f.
 hammer f.
 hippocratic f.
 index f.
 lock f.
 Madonna f's
 mallet f.
 middle f.
 ring f.
 snapping f.
 spade f's
 spider f.
 spring f.
 stuck f.
 trigger f.

F

finger *(continued)*
    tulip f's
    vibration-induced white f's
    washerwoman's f's
    waxy f.
    webbed f.
    white f.
fingeragnosia
fingerbreadth
  (fingerbreadths)
fingerdrop
fingernail
fingerprint
Fink
    laryngoscope
    retractor
    tendon tucker
Finkelstein
    albumin milk
    feeding
    test
Finney
    operation
    pyloroplasty
Finochietto
    forceps
    rib spreader
Finsen
    apparatus
    bath
    lamp
    light
    rays
Finzi-Harmer operation
FiO$_2$ [FiO2]—fractional
  concentration of inspired
  oxygen
fire
    St. Anthony's f.
firedamp
firing
first aid
Fischer
    needle
    sign
Fish forceps
Fishberg
    concentration test
    method
Fisher
    dissector
    exact test
    knife
    spud
    syndrome

fishing
fishmouth
    f. incision
    f. laceration
    f. mitral stenosis
    f. tear
fishpox
Fiske and Subbarow method
fissile
fission
    binary f.
    bud f.
    cellular f.
    multiple f.
    nuclear f.
    simple f.
fissionable
fissiparous
fissula ante fenestram
fissura (fissurae)
    f. antitragohelicina
    f. auris congenita
    f. calcarina
    fissurae cerebelli
    f. cerebri lateralis sylvii
    f. choroidea ventriculi
      lateralis
    f. dentata
    f. dorsolateralis cerebelli
    f. hippocampi
    f. horizontalis
    f. longitudinalis
    f. obliqua
    f. orbitalis inferior
    f. orbitalis superior
    f. parietooccipitalis
    f. petro-occipitalis
    f. petrosquamosa
    f. petrotympanica
    f. pterygoidea
    f. pterygomaxillaris
    f. spheno-occipitalis
    f. sphenopetrosa
    f. transversa cerebelli
    f. transversa cerebralis
    f. tympanomastoidea
    f. tympanosquamosa
fissural
fissuration
fissure
    abdominal f.
    adoccipital f.
    Allingham f.
    Ammon f.
    amygdaline f.

fissure *(continued)*
- anal f.
- angular f.
- antitragohelicine f.
- f. of aqueduct of vestibule
- arciform f.
- f. of auricle, posterior
- auricular f. of temporal bone
- basal f.
- basilar f.
- basisylvian f.
- f. of Bichat
- branchial f.
- Broca f.
- Burdach f.
- calcarine f.
- callosal f.
- callosomarginal f.
- central f.
- cerebral f's
- cerebral f., lateral
- cervical f.
- choroid f.
- choroidal f. of eye
- Clevenger f.
- collateral f.
- corneal f.
- craniofacial f.
- decidual f.
- dentate f.
- dorsolateral cerebellar f.
- Duverney f's
- Ecker f.
- enamel f.
- entorbital f.
- ethmoid f.
- fetal f. of optic cup
- floccular f.
- f. of lung
- genitovesical f.
- glaserian f.
- great cerebral f.
- great f. of cerebrum
- great horizontal f.
- Henle f.
- hippocampal f.
- f. in ano
- inferofrontal f.
- intercerebral f.
- intercotyledonary f.
- interparietal f.
- intratonsillar f.
- lacrimal f.
- lateral f. of cerebrum

fissure *(continued)*
- linguogingival f.
- longitudinal f.
- mandibular f's
- maxillary f.
- median f.
- Monro f.
- oblique f. of lung
- occipital f.
- occipitosphenoidal f.
- optic f.
- oral f.
- orbital f., inferior
- orbital f., superior
- palpebral f.
- Pansch f.
- parafloccular f.
- parietooccular f.
- parietosphenoid f.
- petrobasilar f.
- petromastoid f.
- petrooccipital f.
- petrosal f., superficial
- petrosphenoidal f.
- petrosquamosal f.
- petrosquamous f.
- petrotympanic f.
- portal f.
- posterior f. of auricle
- posterior median f. of spinal cord
- posterolateral cerebellar f.
- postlingual f.
- postlingual cerebellar f.
- postlunate f.
- postpyramidal f.
- precentral cerebral f.
- precuneal f.
- prepyramidal f.
- presylvian f.
- primary f. of cerebellum
- pterygoid f.
- pterygomaxillary f.
- pterygopalatine f.
- pterygotympanic f.
- pudendal f.
- retrocuticular f.
- retrotonsillar f.
- rhinal f.
- Rolando f.
- f. for round ligament
- sagittal f. of liver
- Santorini f's
- Schwalbe f.
- sclerotomic f.

F

fissure *(continued)*
    secondary f. of cerebellum
    sphenoidal f.
    sphenomaxillary f.
    spheno-occipital f.
    sphenopetrosal f.
    squamotympanic f.
    subfrontal f.
    subtemporal f.
    superfrontal f.
    superior anterior f.
    supertemporal f.
    sylvian f.
    f. of Sylvius
    transtemporal f.
    transverse f.
    tympanic f.
    tympanomastoid f.
    tympanosquamous f.
    umbilical f.
    urogenital f.
    f. of venous ligament
    vestibular f. of cochlea
    f. of the vestibule
    zygal f.
    zygomaticosphenoid f.
fistula (fistulas, fistulae)
    abdominal f.
    alveolar f.
    amphibolic f.
    anal f.
    aortocaval f.
    aortoduodenal f.
    aortoenteric f.
    arteriovenous (AV) f.
    f. auris congenita
    biliary f.
    f. bimucosa
    blind f.
    branchial f.
    Brescia-Cimino f.
    bronchobiliary f.
    bronchocutaneous f.
    bronchoesophageal f.
    bronchopleural f.
    caroticocavernous f.
    cerebrospinal fluid f.
    cervical f.
    cervicoaural f.
    f. cervicovaginalis
      laqueatica
    cholecystoduodenal f.
    chylous f.
    f. cibalis
    f. colli congenita

fistula (fistulas, fistulae) *(continued)*
    colonic f.
    complete f.
    congenital coronary f.
    congenital preauricular f.
    congenital urethrorectal f.
    f. corneae
    coronary arteriovenous f.
    coronary artery f.
    craniosinus f.
    dental f.
    Eck f. in reverse
    enterocolic f.
    enterocutaneous f.
    enteroenteric f.
    enterovaginal f.
    enterovesical f.
    esophagobronchial f.
    esophagotracheal f.
    external f.
    fecal f.
    frontal sinus f.
    gastric f.
    gastrocolic f.
    gastrojejunal f.
    gastrojejunocolic f.
    gingival f.
    hepatic f.
    horseshoe f.
    f. in ano
    incomplete f.
    internal f.
    intestinal f.
    jejunocolic f.
    lacrimal f.
    f. of lip
    lymphatic f.
    f. lymphatica
    Mann-Bollman f.
    mediastinobronchial f.
    mucus f.
    oroantral f.
    oronasal f.
    parietal f.
    perilymph f.
    perirectal f.
    pharyngeal f.
    pilonidal f.
    pleurobronchial f.
    pleurocutaneous f.
    pulmonary f.
    pulmonary arteriovenous f.
    radiocephalic f.
    rectolabial f.
    rectovaginal f.

fistula (fistulas, fistulae) *(continued)*
  rectovesical f.
  salivary f.
  spermatic f.
  stercoral f.
  submental f.
  Thiry f.
  Thiry-Vella f.
  thoracic f.
  tracheal f.
  tracheoesophageal f.
  umbilical f.
  urachal f.
  ureterocervical f.
  ureterovaginal f.
  urinary f.
  uterovesical f.
  vaginoperineal f.
  Vella f.
  vesical f.
  vesicoabdominal f.
  vesicocervical f.
  vesicocolonic f.
  vesicointestinal f.
  vesicorectal f.
  vesicoumbilical f.
  vesicovaginal f.
  vulvorectal f.
fistulatome
fistulectomy
fistulization
fistulize
fistuloenterostomy
fistulogram
fistulography
fistulotomy
fistulous
fit
  running f.
FITC—fluorescein isothiocyanate
fitness
  darwinian f.
  genetic f.
  reproductive f.
Fitz
  law
  syndrome
Fitzgerald forceps
Fitz Gerald
  method
  treatment
Fitz-Hugh syndrome
Fitz-Hugh–Curtis syndrome
fixation
  arch bar f.

fixation *(continued)*
  autotrophic f.
  f. axis
  bifoveal f.
  binocular f.
  Bovin f.
  carbon dioxide f.
  complement f.
  elastic band f. (EBF) of fracture
  external pin f.
  f. forceps
  fracture f.
  freudian f.
  f. hook
  intermaxillary f.
  internal f.
  intramedullary f.
  intraosseous f.
  Luque rod f.
  maxillomandibular f.
  nasomandibular f.
  nitrogen f.
  open reduction and internal f.
    (ORIF)
  ossicular f.
  postural f.
  f. reflex
  reflex ocular f.
  skeletal f.
  f. suture
  Zickel nail f.
fixative
  Bouin f.
  denture f.
  glutaraldehyde f.
  Heidenhain Susa f.
  Helly f.
  Kaiserling f.
  lanthanum permanganate f.
  Maximow f.
  Palade f.
  paraformaldehyde f.
  potassium permanganate f.
  Rhodin f.
  Schaudinn f.
  Zenker f.
  Zenker-formol f.
fixator
  Ace-Fischer f.
fixer
fixing time
FJN—familial juvenile
  nephrophthisis
fl.—fluid
flaccid

F

flaccidity
flacherie
Flack
    node
    test
flagella (plural of flagellum)
flagellantism
flagellar
flagellate
    animal-like f.
    plantlike f.
flagellated
flagellation
flagelliform
flagellin
flagellosis
flagellospore
flagellula
flagellum (flagella)
flail
    f. chest
    f. joint
    f. mitral valve
Flajani
    disease
    operation
flame
    capillary f.
    f. figure
flammeus nevus
flange
    buccal f.
    denture f.
    labial f.
    lingual f.
flank
    f. incision
    lateral f. incision
    f. stripe
Flannery speculum
flap
    Abbe f.
    advancement f.
    Argamaso-Lewin f.
    artery island f.
    axial f.
    axilloabdominal f.
    Bakamjian f.
    bilobed f.
    bipedicle f.
    Björk f.
    bone f.
    bridge f.
    buccal f.
    Bunnell f.

flap *(continued)*
    Byers f.
    cellulocutaneous f.
    cervical f.
    cheek f.
    composite f.
    compound f.
    coronal f.
    Crane f.
    cross-arm f.
    cross-finger f.
    cross-leg f.
    cross-lip f.
    delayed f.
    delayed transfer f.
    deltopectoral f.
    direct transfer f.
    distant f.
    dorsalis pedis f.
    double-pedicle f.
    eave f.
    Eloesser f.
    envelope f.
    Estlander f.
    fan f.
    Filatov f.
    forehead f.
    free f.
    free bone f.
    French f.
    French sliding f.
    Fricke f.
    gauntlet f.
    Gillies up-and-down f.
    groin f.
    hinge f.
    Hueston spiral f.
    immediate transfer f.
    Indian rotation f.
    intercalated f.
    interpolated f.
    island leg f.
    Italian distant f.
    jump abdominal f.
    Langenbeck pedicle
        mucoperiosteal f.
    latissimus dorsi muscle f.
    Limberg f.
    lingual tongue f.
    liver f.
    local f.
    MacFee neck f.
    marsupial f.
    McGregor forehead f.
    Millard island f.

flap *(continued)*
  modified Widman f.
  Monks-Esser island f.
  mucomuscular f.
  mucoperiosteal f.
  muscle f.
  musculocutaneous f.
  myocutaneous f.
  nasolabial f.
  neurovascular f.
  New sickle f.
  f. operation
  osteoplastic f.
  over-and-out cheek f.
  pectoral muscle f.
  pedicle f.
  pericoronal f.
  pharyngeal f.
  random f.
  rope f.
  rotation f.
  sandwich f.
  scalping f.
  skin f.
  sliding f.
  split-thickness f.
  Stein-Abbe lip f.
  Stein-Kazanjian lower lip f.
  Stenstrom foot f.
  subcutaneous pedicle f.
  surgical f.
  Tagliacozzi f.
  temporal f.
  tensor fasciae latae
    muscle f.
  thoracoabdominal f.
  thoracoepigastric f.
  tongue f.
  transposition f.
  trapdoor f.
  tube f.
  tubed pedicle f.
  tumbler f.
  tunnel f.
  turnover f.
  tympanomeatal f.
  von Langenbeck bipedicle
    mucoperiosteal f.
  V-Y f.
  Widman f., modified
  Wookey neck f.
  Z-f.
  Zimany f.
  Zimany bilobed f.
  Zovickian f.

flare
  aqueous f.
  nasal f.
flaring
  alar f.
  nasal f.
flareup, flare-up, flare up
flash
FLASH—fast low-angle shot
flashblindedness
flask
  Carrel f.
  casting f.
  crown f.
  denture f.
  Dewar f.
  Erlenmeyer f.
  Erlenmeyer f.–like
    deformity
  refractory f.
  vacuum f.
  volumetric f.
flasking
flat
  optical f.
  f. suture
Flatau
  disease
  law
  syndrome
Flatau-Schilder disease
flatfoot
  rocker-bottom f.
  spastic f.
  static f.
flatness
flat plate of abdomen
flattening of diaphragm
flatulence
flatulent
flatus vaginalis
flatworm
flaunt
flavacidin
flavanone
flavanonol
flavectomy
flavescent
flavianic acid
flavicin
flavin
  f. adenine dinucleotide (FAD)
  f. mononucleotide (FMN)
  f. monooxygenase
flavivirus

F

Flavobacterium
    F. meningosepticum
    F. odoratum
flavoenzyme
flavone
flavonoid
flavonol
flavoprotein
flavor
flavoxanthin
Flaxedil suture
flaxseed
flay
flazalone
fld.—fluid
fl. dr.—fluid dram(s)
flea
    Asiatic rat f.
    burrowing f.
    cat f.
    cavy f.
    chigger f.
    chigoe f.
    common human f.
    common rat f.
    dog f.
    European mouse f.
    European rat f.
    human f.
    Indian rat f.
    jigger f.
    mouse f.
    oriental rat f.
    sand f.
    squirrel f.
    sticktight f.
    suslik f.
    tropical rat f.
    water f.
Flechsig
    area
    bundle
    cuticulum
    fasciculi
    fasciculus
    field
    law
    tract
fleck
    tobacco f's
fleckfieber
fleckmilz
fleece of Stilling
Fleischer
    dystrophy

Fleischer *(continued)*
    ring
Fleischer-Strümpell ring
Fleischman
    bursa
    follicle
Fleischner
    disease
    line
    position
Fleming
    knife
    operation
Flemming
    center
    fixing fluid
    solution
flesh
    goose f., gooseflesh
    live f.
    proud f.
Fletcher knife
fletcherism
Fletcher-Suit afterloading
    device
Fletcher-Van Doren forceps
flex
flexed incision
flexibilitas
    cerea f.
flexibility
    waxy f.
flexible
    f. catheter
    f. gastroscope
    f. shaft retractor
fleximeter
flexion
    lateral f.
    mass f.
    plantar f.
    universal f.
Flexitone suture
Flexner
    bacillus
    dysentery
    serum
Flexner-Jobling
    carcinosarcoma
Flexon suture
flexor retinaculum
flexorplasty
flexuose
flexura (flexurae)
    f. coli dextra

flexura (flexurae) *(continued)*
    f. coli sinistra
    f. duodeni inferior
    f. duodeni superior
    f. duodenojejunalis
    f. hepatica coli
    f. lienalis coli
    f. perinealis
    f. sacralis recti
flexural
flexure
    basicranial f.
    caudal f.
    cephalic f.
    cerebral f.
    cervical f.
    cranial f.
    dorsal f.
    duodenojejunal f.
    encephalic f.
    fluctuant f.
    hepatic f.
    hepatic f. of colon
    iliac f.
    inferior f. of duodenum
    left f. of colon
    lumbar f.
    mesencephalic f.
    nuchal f.
    perineal f.
    pontine f.
    right f. of colon
    sacral f.
    sacral f. of rectum
    sigmoid f.
    splenic f.
    splenic f. of colon
    superior f. of duodenum
flicker
Flieringa ring
Fliess
    therapy
    treatment
flight
    f. into disease
    f. of ideas
    topical f.
Flint
    arcade
    law
    murmur
floater
floating
floating-disk prosthesis
floccillation

floccose
floccular
flocculation
    cephalin f.
    Ramon f.
floccule
    toxoid-antitoxin f.
flocculent
flocculus (flocculi)
    accessory f.
flock of floaters
floctafenine
Flood
    ligament
    ligament of orbit
flooding
flood source
floor
    cavity f.
    f. of fourth ventricle
    inguinal f.
    f. of inguinal canal
    jugular f. of tympanic cavity
    f. of lateral ventricle
    f. of nasal cavity
    f. of orbit
    f. of pelvis
    f. of prepared cavity
    f. of third ventricle
    f. of tympanic cavity
floppy disk
flora
    intestinal f.
florantyrone
Florence reaction
Florentine iris
flores
Florey unit
florid infection
Florschütz (Florschuetz) formula
flout
flow
    axoplasmic f.
    cerebral blood f.
    effective pulmonary blood f.
    effective renal blood f.
    effective renal plasma f. (ERPF)
    gene f.
    laminar air f.
    maximal midexpiratory f.
    maximum midexpiratory f.
    peak expiratory f.
    renal blood f. (RBF)
    renal plasma f. (RPF)
    f. tract

F

Flower
  bone
  index
flower basket of Bochdalek
flowers
  f. of arsenic
  f. of benzoin
  f. of camphor
  pyrethrum f.
  f. of sulfur
flowmeter
  blood f.
  Doppler f.
  dry f.
  electromagnetic f.
  pulsed Doppler f.
flow tract
Floyd
  cannula
  needle
fl. oz.—fluid ounce(s)
FLSA—follicular lymphosarcoma
flu
  intestinal f.
flucrylate
fluctuancy
fluctuant
fluctuation
flucytosine
fludalanine
fluence
  energy f.
fluffs
fluffy compression dressing
fluid
  allantoic f.
  Altmann f.
  amniotic f.
  ascitic f.
  bleaching f.
  Bouin f.
  Callison f.
  Carrel-Dakin f.
  cerebrospinal f. (CSF)
  chlorpalladium f.
  crevicular f.
  crystalline f.
  Dakin f.
  decalcifying f.
  Delafield f.
  Ecker f.
  extracellular f.
  extravascular f.
  Flemming fixing f.
  follicular f.

fluid (continued)
  formol-Müller f.
  Gendre f.
  gingival f.
  Helly f.
  interstitial f.
  intracellular f.
  intraocular f.
  Kaiserling f.
  labyrinthine f.
  Lang f.
  Locke f.
  Müller f.
  non-newtonian f.
  Parker f.
  pericardial f.
  peritoneal f.
  Piazza f.
  Rees and Ecker diluting f.
  saline f.
  Scarpa f.
  Schaudinn f.
  seminal f.
  serous f.
  straw-colored f.
  synovial f.
  Tellyesniczky f.
  Thoma f.
  tissue f.
  Toison f.
  transcellular f.
  ventricular f.
  Waldeyer f.
  Wickersheimer f.
  xanthochromic f.
  Zenker f.
fluid dram (fl. dr.)
fluidextract
fluidglycerates
fluid ounce (fl. oz.)
fluke
  blood f.
  bronchial f.
  cat liver f.
  Chinese liver f.
  digenetic f.
  intestinal f.
  liver f.
  lung f.
  oriental f.
  sheep liver f.
flukicide
flulike
flumen (flumina)
  flumina pilorum

fluocortin butyl
fluor
    f. albus
    plastic f.
fluorane
fluorapatite
fluorescein
    f. angiography
    f. dye disappearance test
    f. fundus photography
    f. isothiocyanate (FITC)
    f. sodium
fluoresceinuria
fluorescence
    f.-activated cell sorter
    f. enhancement
    f. microscope
    f. microscopy
    natural f.
    nonspecific f.
    f. quenching
    f. retinal photography
    secondary f.
    x-ray f.
fluorescent
    f. antibody (FA)
    direct f. antibody (DFA) test
    indirect f. antibody (IFA)
    f. phosphor
    f. ray
    f. scan
    f. screen
    f. treponemal antibody (FTA)
fluorescin
fluoridation
fluoride
    stannous f.
    topical f.
fluoridization
fluorine F 18
fluoroacetate
fluoroacetic acid
fluorocarbon
fluorochrome
fluorochroming
fluorocitric acid
9α-fluorocortisol [9-alpha-]
fluorocyte
2-fluoro-2-deoxyglucose (FDG, fluorodeoxyglucose)
fluorography
    digital f.
fluoroimmunoassay (FIA)
fluorometer
fluorometry

fluoronephelometer
p-fluorophenylalanine [p-, para-]
fluorophosphate
    diisopropyl f.
fluorophotometry
    vitreous f.
fluororadiography
fluororoentgenography
fluoroscope
    biplane f.
fluoroscopic
fluoroscopical
fluoroscopy
    computerized f.
    digital f.
    image-amplified f.
fluorosilicate
fluorosis
    chronic endemic f.
    dental f.
fluoxetine
fluoxymesterone
flurothyl
flush
    atropine f.
    breast f.
    carcinoid f.
    flamingo f.
    harlequin f.
    hectic f.
    histamine f.
    limbal f.
    mahogany f.
    malar f.
    menopausal f.
    niacin f.
fluspiperone
fluspirilene
flutamide
flutiazin
flutter
    atrial f.
    auricular f.
    diaphragmatic f.
    impure f.
    mediastinal f.
    pure f.
    ventricular f.
flutter-fibrillation
fluvoxamine
flux
    bilious f.
    celiac f.
    integral neutron f.
    ionic f.

F

flux *(continued)*
    luminous f.
    menstrual f.
    neutral f.
    neutron f.
    oxidizing f.
    reducing f.
fluxion
fly
    black f.
    blackbottle f.
    bloodsucking f's
    blow f.
    bluebottle f.
    bot f.
    caddis f.
    cheese f.
    deer f.
    drone f.
    dung f.
    eye f.
    face f.
    filth f.
    flesh f.
    fruit f.
    gad f.
    greenbottle f.
    heel f.
    horn f.
    horse f.
    house f.
    hover f's
    lake f.
    latrine f.
    louse f.
    mango f.
    mangrove f.
    moth f.
    nose f.
    nostril f.
    owl f.
    ox-warble f.
    phlebotomus f.
    pomace f.
    Russian f.
    sand f.
    screw-worm f.
    Seroot f.
    snipe f.
    soldier f.
    Spanish f.
    stable f.
    tick f.
    tsetse f.
    tumbu f.
    warble f.

flying spot microscope
Flynt needle
FM—flowmeter
FME—full-mouth extraction
FMG—foreign medical graduate
FMN—flavin mononucleotide
FMR—fetal-to-maternal ratio
FMS—
    fat-mobilizing substance
    full-mouth series
FN—
    false-negative
    finger-to-nose
FNH—focal nodular
    hyperplasia
FNTC—fine-needle transhepatic
    cholangiography
FO—fronto-occipital
foam rubber dressing
FOAVF—failure of all vital forces
focal
    f. plane tomography
    f. spot
    f. zone
foci (plural of focus)
focimeter
focus (foci)
    aplanatic f.
    Assmann f.
    conjugate f.
    dysplastic f.
    epileptogenic f.
    Ghon f.
    mirror f.
    negative f.
    principal foci
    real f.
    secondary epileptogenic f.
    Simon foci
    spike f.
    virtual f.
focusing
    dynamic f.
    electronic f.
    isoelectric f.
FOD—free of disease
fog
Fogarty catheter
fogging
fogo selvagem
foil
    activation f.
    gold f.
    mat f.
    platinum f.
    tin f.

Foix
  paramedian syndrome
  syndrome
Foix-Alajouanine
  disease
  syndrome
folacin
fold
  alar f's
  amniotic f.
  aryepiglottic f.
  aryepiglottic f. of Collier
  arytenoepiglottidean f.
  axillary f.
  Brachet mesolateral f.
  bulboventricular f.
  caudal genital f.
  caval f.
  cecal f's
  cholecystoduodenocolic f.
  ciliary f's
  circular f's of Kerckring
  conjunctival f.
  costocolic f.
  cranial genital f.
  cutaneous f's of anus
  Douglas f.
  Duncan f's
  duodenojejunal f.
  duodenomesocolic f.
  epicanthal f.
  epigastric f.
  falciform f.
  falciform f. of fascia lata
  fimbriated f.
  gastric f's
  gastropancreatic f.
  gastropancreatic f's of
    Huschke
  genital f.
  glossoepiglottic f's
  gluteal f.
  Guérin f.
  Hasner f.
  head f.
  Heister f.
  Hensing f.
  hepatopancreatic f.
  horizontal f's of rectum
  ileocecal f.
  ileocolic f.
  iliopubic f. of Thompson
  incudal f.
  inferior duodenal f.
  interarticular f. of hip
  interarytenoid f.

fold *(continued)*
  interdigital f.
  interureteric f.
  iridial f's
  Jonnesco f.
  junctional f.
  Juvara f.
  Kerckring f's
  Kohlrausch f's
  lacrimal f.
  f. of laryngeal nerve
  lateral f.
  lateral nasal f.
  f. of the left vena cava
  longitudinal f. of duodenum
  mallear f.
  mammary f.
  Marshall f.
  medial nasal f.
  medullary f.
  mesolateral f.
  mesonephric f.
  mesouterine f.
  mucobuccal f.
  mucolabial f.
  mucosal f.
  mucosobuccal f.
  mucous f.
  nail f.
  nasolabial f.
  nasopharyngeal f.
  Nélaton f.
  neural f.
  opercular f.
  palantine f's
  palantine f's, transverse
  palmate f's
  palpebral f.
  palpebronasal f.
  pancreaticogastric f., left
  paraduodenal f.
  parietocolic f.
  parietoperitoneal f.
  Pawlik f's
  pharyngoepiglottic f.
  pleuroperitoneal f.
  primitive f.
  Rathke f's
  rectal f's
  rectouterine f.
  rectovaginal f.
  rectovesical f.
  retrotarsal f.
  Rindfleisch f's
  sacrogenital f.
  salpingopalatine f.

F

fold *(continued)*
    salpingopharyngeal f.
    Schultze f.
    semilunar f.
    semilunar f. of conjunctiva
    semilunar f. of fauces
    serosal f.
    serous f.
    sigmoid f's of colon
    spiral f.
    spiral f. of cystic duct
    stapedial f.
    sublingual f.
    superior duodenal f.
    synovial f.
    tail f.
    transverse f's of rectum
    Treves f.
    triangular f.
    triangular f. of His
    tubal f's of uterine tube
    umbilical f.
    f. of urachus
    urethral f.
    urogenital f's
    uterosacral f.
    vaginal f's
    vascular cecal f.
    Vater f.
    ventricular f.
    Veraguth f.
    vesical f., transverse
    vesicouterine f.
    vestibular f.
    vestigial f. of Marshall
    villous f's of stomach
    vocal f.
    vocal f., false
Foley
    catheter
    forceps
    ureteropelvioplasty
    Y-plasty
    Y-type ureteropelvioplasty
    Y-V ureteropelvioplasty
Foley-Alcock catheter
folia (plural of folium)
foliaceous
folian
folic acid
folie
    f. á deux
    f. circulaire
    f. communiquée
    f. des grandeurs

folie *(continued)*
    f. du doute
    f. du pourquoi
    f. gémellaire
    f. imitative
    f. imposée
    f. induite
    f. raisonnante
Folin
    filtrate
    gravimetric method
    method
Folin and Bell method
Folin, Benedict, and Myers method
Folin and Denis method
Folin and Farmer method
Folin and Hart method
folinic acid
Folin and Svedberg method
Folin and Wu test
Folin and Wright method
folium (folia)
    folia cerebelli
    folia of cerebellum
    lingual folia
    f. vermis
Folius
    muscle
    process
follicle
    aggregated f's
    agminated f's
    anovulvar ovarian f.
    antral f's
    atretic ovarian f.
    closed f.
    dental f.
    Fleischmann f.
    gastric f's
    germinal f.
    graafian f.
    hair f.
    intestinal f's
    laryngeal lymphatic f's
    lenticular f's
    Lieberkühn f.
    lingual f's
    lymph f.
    Montgomery f's
    mucous f's, nasal
    Naboth f.
    nabothian f.
    ovarian f.
    pilosebaceous f.
    polyovular ovarian f.

follicle *(continued)*
 primordial f.
 primordial ovarian f.
 sebaceous f.
 secondary f.
 secondary ovarian f's
 solitary f's
 splenic lymph f's
 f. of Stannius
 tertiary f.
 thyroid f's
 f's of tongue
 tooth f.
 unilaminar ovarian f.
folliclis
follicular
 f. eczema
 f. lichen planus
 f. mucinosis
 f. psoriasis
folliculi (genitive and plural of
 folliculus)
folliculitis
 f. abscedens et suffodiens
 agminate f.
 f. barbae
 f. cheloidalis
 f. cruris atrophicans
 f. decalvans
 f. decalvans cryptococcia
 f. decalvans et lichen
  spinulosus
 eosinophilic pustular f.
 f. gonorrhoeica
 gram-negative f.
 industrial f.
 keloidal f.
 f. keloidalis
 f. nares perforans
 oil f.
 f. ulerythematosa reticulata
 f. varioliformis
folliculoma lipidique
folliculosis
folliculostatin
folliculus (folliculi)
 folliculi glandulae
  thyroideae
 folliculi linguales
 folliculi lymphatici aggregati
 folliculi lymphatici aggregati
  appendicis vermiformis
 folliculi lymphatici gastrici
 folliculi lymphatici lienales
 folliculi lymphatici recti

folliculus (folliculi) *(continued)*
 folliculi lymphatici solitarii
  intestini crassi
 folliculi lymphatici solitarii
  intestini tenuis
 f. lymphaticus
 f. ovaricus primarius
 f. ovaricus vesiculosus
 f. pili
Fölling
 disease
 phenylketonuria
Follmann balanitis
follower
 filiform and f.
following
followup
follow-up care
Foltz valve
fomentation
fomes (fomites)
fomite
Fomon
 chisel
 knife
 operation
 periosteotome
 rasp
 scissors
FONAR—focused nuclear magnetic
 resonance
Fonsecaea
 F. compactum
 F. pedrosoi
fons pulsatilis
fontactoscope
Fontan operation
Fontana
 markings
 spaces
 stain
fontanel, fontanelle
 anterior f.
 anterolateral f.
 bregmatic f.
 Casser f.
 casserian f.
 Casserio f.
 cranial f's
 Gerdy f.
 lateral f's
 mastoid f.
 occipital f.
 posterior f.
 posterolateral f.

fontanel, fontanelle *(continued)*
    posterotemporal f.
    quadrangular f.
    sagittal f.
    sphenoidal f.
    triangular f.
fonticulus (fonticuli)
    f. anterior
    f. anterolateralis
    fonticuli cranii
    f. frontalis
    f. frontalis major
    f. gutturis
    f. major
    f. mastoideus
    f. minor
    f. occipitalis
    f. posterior
    f. posterolateralis
    f. quadrangularis
    f. sphenoidalis
    f. triangularis
food poisoning
    Bacillus cereus f.p.
    enterococcal f.p.
foot (feet)
    athlete's f.
    broad f.
    burning feet
    buttress f.
    Charcot f.
    cleft f.
    club f. (clubfoot, clubfeet)
    congenital convex club f.
    contracted f.
    crooked f.
    crow's feet
    dancer's f.
    dangle f.
    drop f. (footdrop)
    energy-storing f.
    flat f. (flatfoot)
    Flex-Foot
    forced f.
    Friedreich f.
    fungus f.
    Greissinger f.
    Hong Kong f.
    hot f.
    immersion f.
    f. lambert (ft. L)
    Madura f.
    march f.
    Morand f.
    Morton f.

foot (feet) *(continued)*
    mossy f.
    multiaxial f.
    multiaxis f.
    paralytic club f.
    pericapillary end f.
    perivascular f.
    pricked f.
    reel f.
    rocker-bottom f.
    SACH (solid-ankle, cushioned-heel) f.
    SAFE f.
    sag f.
    Seattle f.
    septic f.
    spatula f.
    spread f.
    sucker f.
    tabetic f.
    taut f.
    trench f.
    tropical immersion f.
    valgus club f.
    varus club f.
    warm water immersion f.
    weak f.
foot-candle
footdrop
foot-engine
foot lambert (ft. L)
footplate
    floating f.
    stapedial f.
    vascular f.
foot-pound
footprint
foramen (foramina)
    accessory f.
    alveolar foramina of maxilla
    foramina alveolaria maxillae
    aortic f.
    apical f. of root of tooth
    f. apicis dentis
    arachnoid f.
    auditory f., external
    auditory f., internal
    Bichat f.
    f. of Bochdalek
    f. of Bochdalek hernia
    Botallo f.
    f. bursae omentalis majoris
    f. caecum
    f. caecum medullae oblongatae
    caroticoclinoid f.

foramen (foramina) *(continued)*

    caroticotympanic foramina
    carotid f.
    cecal f.
    f. cecum ossis frontalis
    condyloid f., anterior
    conjugate f.
    f. costotransversarium
    costotransverse f.
    cotyloid f.
    cribroethmoid f.
    foramina cribrosa ossis
      ethmoidalis
    dental foramina
    f. diaphragmatis sellae
    Duverney f.
    emissary f.
    epiploic f.
    f. epiploicum
    esophageal f.
    ethmoidal f.
    f. ethmoidale anterius
    f. ethmoidale posterius
    foramina ethmoidalia
    f. of Fallopio
    Ferrein f.
    frontal f.
    f. frontale
    frontoethmoidal f.
    Galen f.
    glandular foramina of
      Littre
    glandular f. of Morgagni
    great f.
    greater palatine f.
    Hartigan f.
    hemal f.
    Huschke f.
    Hyrtl f.
    incisive f.
    f. incisivum
    incisor f., median
    infraorbital f.
    f. infraorbitale
    infrapiriform f.
    innominate f.
    interatrial f. secundum
    intersacral foramina
    interventricular f.
    f. interventriculare
    intervertebral f.
    f. intervertebrale
    intervertebral foramina of
      sacrum
    ischiadic f., greater

foramen (foramina) *(continued)*

    ischiadic f., lesser
    f. ischiadicum majus
    f. ischiadicum minus
    ischiopubic f.
    jugular f.
    f. of Key and Retzius
    lacerate f.
    f. lacerum anterius
    f. lacerum medium
    f. lacerum posterius
    f. of Lannelongue
    lateral f.
    lesser palatine foramina
    Luschka f.
    Magendie f.
    f. magnum
    malar f.
    f. mandibulae
    mandibular f.
    mastoid f.
    f. mastoideum
    maxillary f.
    medullary f.
    meibomian f.
    mental f.
    f. mentale
    f. of Monro
    Morand f.
    Morgagni f.
    morgagnian f.
    f. of Morgagni hernia
    nasal f.
    f. nasalia
    neural f.
    f. nutricium
    nutrient f.
    obturator f.
    f. obturatorium
    f. obturatum
    f. occipitale magnum
    occipital f., great
    occipital f., inferior
    olfactory foramina
    omental f.
    f. omentale
    optic f.
    optic f. of sclera
    f. opticum ossis sphenoidalis
    orbitomalar f.
    oval f.
    f. ovale
    f. ovale alae majoris
    f. ovale basis cranii
    f. ovale cordis

F

foramen (foramina) *(continued)*
  f. ovale ossis sphenoidalis
  oval f. of fetus
  oval f. of sphenoid bone
  f. of Pacchioni
  pacchionian f.
  foramina palatina minora
  palatine f., anterior
  palatine f., greater
  palatine foramina, accessory
  palatine foramina, lesser
  palatine f., posterior
  f. of palatine tonsil
  f. palatinum majus
  foramina papillaria renis
  parietal f.
  f. parietale
  patent f. ovale
  f. petrosum
  pleuroperitoneal f.
  f. primum
  f. processus transversi
  pterygoalar f.
  pterygopalatine f.
  pulpal f.
  quadrate f.
  f. radicis dentis
  Retzius f.
  right f.
  rivinian f.
  Rivinus f.
  root f.
  f. rotundum ossis sphenoidalis
  sacral foramina, anterior
  f. of sacral canal
  foramina sacralia anteriora
  foramina sacralia dorsalia
  foramina sacralia pelvina
  foramina sacralia posteriora
  foramina sacralia ventralia
  sacrosciatic f., great
  sacrosciatic f., small
  f. of saphenous vein
  Scarpa foramina
  Schwalbe f.
  sciatic f., greater
  sciatic f., lesser
  f. sciaticum majus
  f. sciaticum minus
  f. secundum
  f. singulare
  foramina of smallest veins of heart
  sphenopalatine f.
  f. sphenopalatinum

foramen (foramina) *(continued)*
  sphenotic f.
  spinal f.
  f. spinosum
  Spöndel (Spoendel) f.
  Stensen f.
  stylomastoid f.
  f. stylomastoideum
  suborbital f.
  supraorbital f.
  suprapiriform f.
  Tarin f.
  temporomalar f.
  thebesian foramina
  foramina thebesii
  thyroid f.
  f. thyroideum
  f. transversarium
  transverse accessory f.
  vena caval f.
  f. venae cavae
  f. venosum
  venous f.
  vertebral f.
  f. vertebrale
  vertebroarterial f.
  f. vertebroarteriale
  f. Vesalii
  f. of Vesalius
  f. of Vicq d'Azyr
  Vieussens f.
  visceral f.
  Weitbrecht f.
  f. of Winslow
  zygomatic f.
  zygomaticofacial f.
  f. zygomaticofaciale
  zygomaticoorbital f.
  f. zygomaticoorbitale
  zygomaticotemporal f.
  f. zygomaticotemporale
foraminal
foraminiferan
foraminiferous
foraminotomy
foraminulate
foraminulum
foration
Forbes
  amputation
  disease
Forbes-Albright syndrome
force
  bite f.
  catabiotic f.

force *(continued)*
    catabolic f.
    chewing f.
    electromotive f.
    extraoral f.
    field f's
    f.-frequency relation
    f.-length relation
    masticatory f.
    occlusal f.
    radiation f.
    reciprocal f.
    f. of recoil of lung
    reserve f.
    rest f.
    shearing f.
    Starling f.
    van der Waals f's
    f.-velocity relation
    vital f.
forceps
    ACMI f.
    ACMI Martin endoscopy f.
    Acufex f.
    Adair f.
    Adams f.
    adenoid f.
    Adson f.
    alligator f.
    Allis f.
    Allis-Ochsner f.
    Andrews-Hartmann f.
    f. anterior
    Arruga f.
    artery f.
    Asch f.
    axis-traction f.
    Babcock f.
    Backhaus f.
    Bacon f.
    Bailey-Williamson f.
    Bainbridge hemostatic f.
    Ballantine f.
    Ballantine hysterectomy f.
    Ballenger f.
    Bane f.
    Barlow f.
    Barnes-Crile f.
    Barraquer ciliary f.
    Barraquer corneal f.
    Barraya f.
    Barrett f.
    Barrett-Allen f.
    Barton f.
    bayonet f.

forceps *(continued)*
    Beaupre f.
    Beebe f.
    Beer ciliary f.
    Benaron f.
    Bengolea f.
    Bennett f.
    Berens f.
    Berke ptosis f.
    Berne f.
    Berry uterine-elevating f.
    Best common duct stone f.
    Best gallstone f.
    Best intestinal f.
    Bevan gallbladder f.
    Bevan hemostatic f.
    Beyer f.
    Billroth f.
    Billroth uterine tumor f.
    Bishop-Harmon f.
    Blake ear f.
    Blake embolus f.
    Blake gallstone f.
    Blakesley f.
    Blanchard hemorrhoidal f.
    Boies f.
    Bonaccolto f.
    Bond f.
    bone f.
    bone-cutting f.
    bone-nibbling f.
    Bonn f.
    Bonney f.
    Böttcher (Boettcher) f.
    Boys-Allis f.
    Bozeman f.
    Braasch f.
    Bracken f.
    Bradford f.
    Brenner f.
    Brophy f.
    Brown f.
    Brown-Adson f.
    Broyles f.
    Bruening f.
    Brunner f.
    Buerger-McCarthy f.
    Buie f.
    bulldog f.
    bullet f.
    Bumpus f.
    Bunim f.
    Cairns f.
    Campbell f.
    capsule f.

F

forceps *(continued)*

Carmalt arterial f.
Carmalt hemostatic f.
Carmalt hysterectomy f.
Carmalt splinter f.
Carmalt thoracic f.
Carmody f.
Carrel mosquito f.
Carroll bone-holding f.
Carroll tendon-passing f.
Carroll tendon-pulling f.
cartilage f.
Cassidy-Brophy f.
Castaneda f.
Castroviejo f.
Castroviejo-Arruga f.
chalazion f.
Chamberlen f.
Chandler f.
Cherry-Kerrison f.
Cicherelli f.
clamp f.
clip f.
Coakley f.
Cohen f.
Colibri f.
Collin f.
Colver f.
Cooley f.
Coppridge f.
Corbett f.
Cordes f.
Cordes-New f.
Corey f.
Cornet f.
f. of corpus callosum
Cottle f.
Cottle-Arruga f.
Cottle-Jansen f.
Cottle-Kazanjian f.
Crafoord f.
Craig f.
Crenshaw f.
Crile f.
crocodile f.
Curtis f.
Cushing f.
D'Allesandro serial suture-
    holding f.
Davis f.
De Alvarez f.
Dean f.
DeBakey f.
DeBakey-Bahnson f.
DeBakey-Bainbridge f.

forceps *(continued)*

DeBakey-Cooley f.
DeLee f.
Dennis f.
dental f.
depilatory f.
D'Errico f.
Desjardins f.
Desmarres f.
DeVilbiss f.
Dewey f.
Dingman f.
disk f.
dissecting f.
double-action f.
Doyen f.
dressing f.
Dufourmental f.
dural f.
Duval-Crile f.
ear f.
Eber f.
Eder f.
Elliot f.
Elschnig f.
Elschnig-O'Brien f.
epilating f.
Erich f.
Evans f.
extracting f.
failed f.
failed f. delivery
Farabeuf f.
Farabeuf-Lambotte f.
Farrington f.
Farris f.
Fauvel f.
Feilchenfeld f.
Ferguson f.
Ferris f.
Ferris-Smith f.
Ferris-Smith-Kerrison f.
Finochietto f.
Fish f.
Fitzgerald f.
fixation f.
Fletcher-Van Doren f.
Foerster f.
Foley f.
Förster iris f.
Foss f.
Foster-Ballenger f.
Fränkel f.
Frankfeldt f.
Fricke arterial f.

forceps *(continued)*
    f. frontalis
    Fuchs f.
    Fulpit f.
    galea f.
    Garrigue f.
    Garrison f.
    Gaylor f.
    Gellhorn f.
    Gelpi-Lowrie f.
    Gerald f.
    Gifford f.
    Glassman f.
    Glassman-Allis f.
    Glenner f.
    Glover f.
    Goldman-Kazanjian f.
    Good f.
    Goodhill f.
    Gordon f.
    gouge f.
    Graefe (von Graefe) f.
    Gray f.
    Green f.
    Gruenwald f.
    Gruenwald-Bryant f.
    Guggenheim f.
    Gutglass f.
    Haig Ferguson f.
    Hajek-Koffler f.
    Hale f.
    Halsted f.
    Harken f.
    Harrington f.
    Harrington-Mayo f.
    Harris f.
    Hartmann f.
    Hartmann-Citelli f.
    Hartmann-Gruenwald f.
    Hawkins cervical biopsy f.
    Hawks-Dennen f.
    Healy f.
    Heaney f.
    Heaney-Ballantine f.
    Heaney-Kanter f.
    Heaney-Rezek f.
    Heath f.
    hemostatic f.
    Hendren f.
    Henrotin f.
    Hess f.
    Hess-Barraquer f.
    Hess-Horwitz f.
    Hibbs f.
    high f.

forceps *(continued)*
    Hirschman f.
    Hirst-Emmett f.
    Hodge f.
    Hoffmann f.
    Holinger f.
    Holth f.
    Horsley bone-cutting f.
    House f.
    Howard f.
    Hoxworth f.
    Hudson f.
    Hunt f.
    Hurd f.
    Imperatori f.
    inlet f.
    insertion f.
    Iowa f.
    Jackson f.
    Jacobs f.
    Jacobson f.
    Jameson f.
    Jansen f.
    Jansen-Middleton f.
    Jarcho f.
    Johns Hopkins f.
    Johnson f.
    Jones f.
    Judd f.
    Judd-Allis f.
    Judd-DeMartel f.
    Juers-Lempert f.
    Julian f.
    Jurasz f.
    Kahler f.
    Kalt f.
    Katzin-Barraquer f.
    Kazanjian f.
    Kelly f.
    Kelman f.
    Kennedy f.
    Kern f.
    Kerrison f.
    Kielland (Kjelland) f.
    Kielland-Luikart f.
    Killian f.
    Kirby f.
    Kittner f.
    Knapp f.
    Knight f.
    Knight-Sluder f.
    Kocher f.
    Koeberlé f.
    Koffler f.
    Koffler-Lillie f.

F

forceps *(continued)*
    Kolb f.
    Krause f.
    Kronfeld f.
    Kuhnt f.
    Kulvin-Kalt f.
    Laborde f.
    Lahey f.
    Lahey-Péan f.
    Lambert f.
    Lambotte f.
    Lane f.
    Laufe f.
    Laufe-Barton-Kielland f.
    Laufe-Piper f.
    Lebsche f.
    Leksell f.
    Leland-Jones f.
    Lempert f.
    Leriche f.
    Levret f.
    Lewin f.
    Lewis f.
    Lewkowitz f.
    Leyro-Diaz f.
    Lillie f.
    lion-jawed f.
    Lister f.
    Liston-Stille f.
    lithotomy f.
    Littauer f.
    Littauer-Liston f.
    lock f.
    Lockwood f.
    Long f.
    Long Island f.
    Love-Gruenwald f.
    Love-Kerrison f.
    Lovelace f.
    low f.
    Löwenberg f.
    Lower f.
    Lowsley f.
    Luc f.
    Lucae f.
    Luer f.
    Luikart f.
    Luikart-Simpson f.
    Lutz f.
    Lynch f.
    Maier f.
    f. major
    Mann f.
    Marshik f.
    Martin f.

forceps *(continued)*
    Maryan f.
    Mathieu f.
    Mayo f.
    Mayo-Blake f.
    Mayo-Ochsner f.
    Mayo-Robson f.
    Mayo-Russian f.
    McCarthy f.
    McCarthy-Alcock f.
    McCullough f.
    McHenry f.
    McKay f.
    McKenzie f.
    McLane f.
    McLane-Tucker f.
    McLane-Tucker-Luikart f.
    McNealy-Glassman-Babcock f.
    McNealy-Glassman-Mixter f.
    McPherson f.
    Metzenbaum f.
    mid f.
    Millin f.
    f. minor
    Mitchell-Diamond f.
    Mixter f.
    Moersch f.
    Moritz-Schmidt f.
    mosquito f.
    Mount-Mayfield f.
    mouse-tooth f.
    Moynihan f.
    Mundie f.
    Museholdt f.
    Myerson f.
    Myles f.
    Negus ligature f.
    Nelson f.
    New f.
    Newman f.
    Noble f.
    nonfenestrated f.
    Noyes f.
    Nugent f.
    O'Brien f.
    obstetric f.
    obstetrical f.
    f. occipitalis
    Ochsner f.
    Ochsner-Dixon f.
    O'Hanlon f.
    Oldberg f.
    O'Shaughnessy f.
    Ostrom f.
    outlet f.

forceps *(continued)*

- Overstreet f.
- ovum f.
- Palmer f.
- Pang f.
- Parker-Kerr f.
- Paterson brain clip f.
- Paterson laryngeal f.
- Patterson bronchoscopic f.
- Péan f.
- Pennington f.
- Percy f.
- Perritt f.
- Phaneuf f.
- Piper f.
- Pitha f.
- placenta f.
- placental f.
- Pley f.
- point f.
- polyp f.
- Porter f.
- f. posterior
- Potts-Smith f.
- Poutasse f.
- Pratt-Smith f.
- Price-Thomas f.
- Prince f.
- Providence f.
- punch f.
- Quevedo f.
- Randall stone f.
- Raney f.
- Rankin f.
- Ratliff-Blake f.
- rat-tooth f.
- Ray f.
- Reese f.
- Reiner-Knight f.
- rib-cutting f.
- Rienhoff f.
- ring f.
- Robb f.
- Roberts f.
- Robertson f.
- Rochester f.
- Rochester-Carmalt f.
- Rochester-Ewald f.
- Rochester-Mixter f.
- Rochester-Ochsner f.
- Rochester-Péan f.
- Rochester-Rankin f.
- Rockey f.
- Roeder f.
- Rolf f.

forceps *(continued)*

- rongeur f.
- root-splitting f.
- Rowland f.
- rubber dam f.
- Rumel f.
- Ruskin f.
- Russell f.
- Russian f.
- Sam Roberts f.
- Sanders f.
- Sarot f.
- Satinsky f.
- Sauer f.
- Sauerbruch f.
- Sawtell f.
- Scheinmann f.
- Schlesinger f.
- Schoenberg f.
- Schroeder f.
- Schubert f.
- Schutz f.
- Schwartz f.
- Schweigger f.
- Schweizer f.
- Scoville f.
- Scudder f.
- Segond f.
- Seiffert f.
- Selman f.
- Semb f.
- Semken f.
- Senn f.
- sequestrum f.
- Sewall f.
- Shaaf f.
- Shallcross f.
- Shearer f.
- Simpson f.
- Simpson-Luikart f.
- Singley f.
- sinus f.
- Skene f.
- Skillern f.
- Smart f.
- Smith f.
- Smithwick f.
- Somers f.
- speculum f.
- Spence f.
- Spence-Adson f.
- Spencer Wells f.
- Spero f.
- sponge f.
- sponge-holding f.

F

forceps *(continued)*
- spring f.
- Spurling f.
- Staude f.
- Staude-Moore f.
- Steinmann f.
- Stevens f.
- Stevenson f.
- Stille f.
- Stille-Liston f.
- Stille-Luer f.
- stone f.
- Strassmann f.
- Struempel f.
- Struempel ear alligator f.
- Struempel ear punch f.
- Struyken f.
- Suker iris f.
- suture f.
- suture-holding f.
- Sweet f.
- Takahashi f.
- Tarnier f.
- Teale f.
- tenaculum f.
- Thoms f.
- Thoms-Allis f.
- Thoms-Gaylor f.
- Thorek-Mixter f.
- Thorpe f.
- thumb f.
- Tischler f.
- tissue f.
- Tivnen f.
- Tobold f.
- Tobold-Fauvel f.
- torsion f.
- towel f.
- tubular f.
- Tucker-McLane f.
- Tuttle f.
- Tydings f.
- Tydings-Lakeside f.
- uterine f.
- Van Buren f.
- Vanderbilt f.
- Van Doren f.
- Van Struyken f.
- Verhoeff f.
- Virtus f.
- volsella f.
- vulsellum f.
- Waldeau f.
- Walsham f.
- Walter f.

forceps *(continued)*
- Walther f.
- Walton f.
- Walton-Schubert f.
- Wangensteen f.
- Washam f.
- Watson-Williams f.
- Weil f.
- Weingaertner f.
- Weisman f.
- Welch-Allyn f.
- Wertheim f.
- Wertheim-Cullen f.
- White f.
- White-Lillie f.
- White-Oslay f.
- Wilde f.
- Willett f.
- Williams f.
- Wittner f.
- Wullstein f.
- Wullstein-House f.
- Yankauer f.
- Yankauer-Little f.
- Yeoman f.
- Young f.
- Zenker f.
- Ziegler f.
- Zollinger f.

Forchheimer spots
forcipate
forcipressure
Fordyce
- disease
- granule
- spot
- spots

fore-and-aft suture
forearm
foreconscious
forefinger
Foregger
- bronchoscope
- laryngoscope

forego
forehead
foreign
foreign body (FB)
- retained f.b. (RFB)

Forel
- areas
- commissure
- decussation
- fields

forensic

foreplay
fore-pleasure
foreseeability of harm
foreskin
    hooded f.
    redundant f.
Forestier disease
forewaters
fork
    replication f.
    tuning f.
Forlanini treatment
form
    accolé f.
    appliqué f.
    arch f.
    band f.
    involution f.
    juvenile f.
    L-f.
    racemic f.
    replicative f.
    resistance f.
    retention f.
    ring f.
    spherical f. of occlusion
    tooth f.
    wax f.
    young f.
    Z f.
Formad kidney
formaldehyde
formaldehyde dehydrogenase
formalin
formalinize
formant
formatio (formationes)
    f. alba
    f. grisea
    f. hippocampalis
    f. reticularis
    f. reticularis pontis
    f. vermicularis
formation
    Ammon f.
    chiasma f.
    coffin f.
    compromise f.
    endochondral bone f.
    Gothic arch f.
    hippocampal f.
    intracartilaginous bone f.
    intramembranous bone f.
    medullary reticular f.
    palisade f.

formation *(continued)*
    reaction f.
    reticular f.
    rouleau f.
    f. of rouleaux
formative
formatter
formboard
forme (formes)
    f. fruste
    formes frustes
    f. tardive
former and latter
formic acid
formicant
formication
formiciasis
formiminoglutamic acid (FIGLU)
formiminoglutamicaciduria
formiminoglycine
formocortal
formol
    f. saline
    f. sublimate
formula (formulas, formulae)
    Arneth f.
    Arrhenius f.
    autotransformer f.
    Bazette f.
    Beckmann f.
    Berkow f.
    Bernhardt f.
    Bird f.
    Black f.
    Brenner f.
    Broca f.
    Casper f.
    chemical f.
    Christison f.
    configurational f.
    constitutional f.
    Demoivre f.
    dental f.
    digital f.
    Dreser f.
    Du Bois f.
    Einthoven f.
    empirical f.
    extemporaneous f.
    Fick f.
    Florschütz (Florschuetz) f.
    Gale f.
    Gompertz f.
    Gorlin f.
    graphic f.

F

formula (formulas, formulae)
(continued)
    Guthrie f.
    Haines f.
    Hamilton-Stewart f.
    Hardy-Weinberg f.
    Häser f.
    Loebisch f.
    Long f.
    Mall f.
    molecular f.
    official f.
    paretic f.
    Pignet f.
    Poisson-Pearson f.
    projection f.
    Ranke f.
    rational f.
    Reuss f.
    Rollier f.
    Runeberg f.
    Seiler f.
    spatial f.
    stereochemical f.
    structural f.
    Trapp f.
    Van Slyke f.
    vertebral f.
    Vierdordt-Meeh f.
formulary
    National F.
formulate
formulation
    American Law Institute F.
fornical
fornicate
fornix (fornices)
    anterior f.
    f. approach
    f.-based flap
    f. cerebri
    f. conjunctivae
    f. conjunctivae inferior
    f. conjunctivae superior
    gastric f.
    f. gastricus
    inferior f.
    f. of lacrimal sac
    lateral f.
    f. longus
    f. pharyngis
    posterior f.
    f. sacci lacrimalis
    f. of stomach

fornix (fornices) *(continued)*
    superior f.
    f. vaginae
    f. ventricularis
    f. ventriculi
Foroblique panendoscope
    McCarthy F.
Forrester clamp
Forssell sinus
Forssman
    antibody
    antigen
    lipoid
    shock
Förster (Foerster)
    choroiditis
    disease
    forceps
    iris forceps
    operation
    photometer
    sign
    uveitis
Förster-Fuchs black spot
Förster-Penfield operation
fortification spectrum
fortuitous
Foss
    clamp
    forceps
    retractor
fossa (fossae)
    acetabular f.
    f. acetabuli
    adipose f.
    anconeal f.
    antecubital f.
    f. anthelicis
    articular f.
    f. axillaris
    axillary f.
    Biesiadecki f.
    Broesike f.
    f. caecalis
    f. canina
    f. capitelli
    f. capitis femoris
    cerebellar f.
    cerebral f.
    f. cerebri lateralis
    f. chordae ductus venosi
    Claudius f.
    cochleariform f.
    conchal f.

fossa (fossae) *(continued)*
    condylar f.
    f. condylaris
    condyloid f.
    f. coronoidea humeri
    coronoid f. of humerus
    f. of coronoid process
    costal f., inferior
    costal f., superior
    costal f. of transverse process
    cranial f., anterior
    cranial f., middle
    cranial f., posterior
    f. cranii anterior
    f. cranii media
    f. cranii posterior
    crural f.
    Cruveilhier f.
    cubital f.
    f. cubitalis
    f. cystidis felleae
    digastric f.
    f. digastrica
    digital f.
    f. ductus venosi
    duodenal f.
    duodenal f., inferior
    duodenal f., superior
    duodenojejunal f.
    epigastric f.
    f. epigastrica
    ethmoid f.
    f. of eustachian tube
    femoral f.
    floccular f.
    frontal f.
    f. of gallbladder
    f. of gasserian ganglion
    Gerdy hyoid f.
    f. glandulae lacrimalis
    glandular f. of frontal bone
    glenoid f.
    glenoid f. of scapula
    glossoepiglottic f.
    greater f. of Scarpa
    Gruber f.
    Gruber-Landzert f.
    harderian f.
    Hartmann f.
    f. of head of femur
    f. helicis
    f. hemielliptica
    f. hemispherica
    hyaloid f.

fossa (fossae) *(continued)*
    f. hyaloidea
    hypogastric f.
    hypophyseal f.
    f. hypophyseos
    f. hypophysialis
    ileocecal f., inferior
    ileocecal f., superior
    ileocolic f.
    iliac f.
    f. iliaca
    iliacosubfascial f.
    f. iliacosubfascialis
    f. iliopectinea
    iliopectineal f.
    implantation f.
    incisive f. of maxilla
    incudal f.
    f. incudis
    infraclavicular f.
    f. infraclavicularis
    infraduodenal f.
    f. infraspinata
    infratemporal f.
    f. infratemporalis
    inguinal f.
    f. inguinalis lateralis
    f. inguinalis medialis
    innominate f. of auricle
    intercondylar f.
    f. intercondylaris femoris
    f. intercondylica
    intercondyloid f.
    f. intercondyloidea anterior
      tibiae
    f. intercondyloidea femoris
    f. intercondyloidea posterior
      tibiae
    f. intercruralis
    interpeduncular f.
    f. interpeduncularis
    intersigmoid f.
    intrabulbar f.
    f. ischioanalis
    ischiorectal f.
    f. ischiorectalis
    Jobert f.
    f. of Jonnesco
    jugular f.
    f. jugularis
    lacrimal f.
    Landzert f.
    lateral f. of brain
    lateral f. of cerebrum

F

fossa (fossae) *(continued)*

  f. lateralis cerebri
  f. of lateral malleolus
  lateral pharyngeal f.
  lateral f. of preputial space
  lenticular f.
  lesser f. of Scarpa
  f. for ligamentum teres
  f. of little head of radius
  f. longitudinalis hepatis
  longitudinal f. of liver, right
  Luschka f.
  f. of male urethra
  Malgaigne f.
  f. malleoli lateralis
  mandibular f.
  f. mandibularis
  mastoid f.
  maxillary f.
  Merkel f.
  mesentericoparietal f.
  mesogastric f.
  middle cranial f.
  Mohrenheim f.
  f. of Morgagni
  f. of Morgagni navicular
  f. musculi biventeris
  mylohyoid f. of mandible
  myrtiform f.
  nasal f.
  navicular f.
  navicular f. of Cruveilhier
  f. navicularis
  f. navicularis urethrae
  obturator f.
  occlusal f.
  f. olecrani
  olfactory f.
  oral f.
  orbital f.
  f. ovalis cordis
  f. ovalis femoris
  ovarian f.
  f. ovarica
  f. of Pacchioni
  paraduodenal f.
  parajejunal f.
  pararectal f.
  paravesical f.
  f. paravesicalis
  parietal f.
  patellar f.
  perineal f.
  petrosal f.
  pharyngomaxillary f.

fossa (fossae) *(continued)*

  piriform f.
  pituitary f.
  f. poplitea
  popliteal f.
  postauditory f.
  postcondyloid f.
  posterior f.
  posterior f. of humerus
  f. praenasalis
  prenasal f.
  prescapular f.
  prespinous f.
  pterygoid f.
  f. pterygoidea
  pterygomaxillary f.
  f. pterygopalatina
  radial f. of humerus
  f. radialis humeri
  retrocecal f.
  retrocolic f.
  retroduodenal f.
  retromandibular f.
  f. retromandibularis
  rhomboid f.
  f. rhomboidea
  Rosenmüller f.
  f. sacci lacrimalis
  f. sagittales dextrae
    hepatis
  f. sagittales hepatis
  f. sagittalis sinistra hepatis
  scaphoid f.
  f. scaphoidea
  f. scarpae major
  sellar f.
  semilunar f. of ulna
  sigmoid f.
  sphenomaxillary f.
  splenic f. of omental sac
  subcecal f.
  f. subinguinalis
  sublingual f.
  submandibular f.
  submaxillary f.
  suborbital f.
  subpyramidal f.
  subscapular f.
  f. subscapularis
  subsigmoid f.
  supinator f.
  supraclavicular f.
  supraclavicular f., greater
  supraclavicular f., lesser
  f. supraclavicularis major

fossa (fossae) *(continued)*
    f. supraclavicularis minor
    supracondyloid f.
    supramastoid f.
    suprasphenoidal f.
    f. supraspinata
    supraspinous f.
    suprasternal f.
    supratonsillar f.
    f. supratonsillaris
    supratrochlear f., posterior
    supravesical f.
    f. supravesicalis
    sylvian f.
    f. of Sylvius
    Tarin f.
    temporal f.
    f. temporalis
    terminal f.
    tibiofemoral f.
    tonsillar f.
    f. tonsillaris
    f. transversalis hepatis
    transverse intermesocolic f.
    Treitz f.
    triangular f.
    triangular f. of auricle
    f. triangularis auriculae
    trochanteric f.
    f. trochanterica
    trochlear f.
    f. trochlearis
    ulnar f.
    umbilical f. of liver
    umbilical f., medial
    f. umbilicalis hepatis
    urachal f.
    f. venae cavae
    f. venae umbilicalis
    f. vesicae biliaris
    f. vesicae felleae
    vestibular f.
    f. of vestibule of vagina
    f. vestibuli vaginae
    f. of Waldeyer
    zygomatic f.
fossette
fossula (fossulae)
    f. of cochlear window
    f. fenestrae cochleae
    f. fenestrae vestibuli
    f. of oval window
    f. petrosa
    f. post fenestram
    f. of round window

fossula (fossulae) *(continued)*
    fossulae tonsillares
    f. of vestibular window
fossulate
Foster frame
Foster-Kennedy syndrome
Fothergill
    disease
    neuralgia
    operation
    sign
    suture
Fothergill-Donald operation
foudroyant
foundation
    denture f.
    medical f.
fourchette
four diopter base-out prism test
Fourier
    direct transformation imaging
    discrete transformation
    transformation reconstruction
    transformation
        zeugmatography
    two-dimensional imaging
    two-dimensional projection
        reconstruction
Fournier
    disease
    gangrene
    sign
    syphiloma
    teeth
    test
four-prism-diopter test
four-tailed dressing
four-valve-tube rectification
four-vessel angiography
fovea (foveae)
    articular f.
    articular f. for rib cartilages
    f. articularis
    calcaneal f.
    f. capitis femoris
    f. capitis ossis femoris
    f. capituli radii
    f. cardiaca
    caudal f.
    f. caudalis
    central f. of retina
    f. centralis
    f. centralis retinae
    f. of condyloid process
    f. of coronoid process

fovea (foveae) *(continued)*
    costal f., inferior
    f. costalis inferior
    f. costalis processus
      transversus
    f. costalis superior
    costal foveae of sternum
    costal f., superior
    costal f., transverse
    cranial f.
    f. cranialis
    crural f.
    dental f. of atlas
    f. dentis atlantis
    digastric f.
    femoral f.
    f. of fourth ventricle
    glandular foveae of Luschka
    greater anterior f. of humerus
    f. hemielliptica
    f. hemispherica
    f. inferior
    inguinal f.
    lesser anterior f. of humerus
    f. limbica
    f. of Morgagni
    f. nuchae
    f. oblonga cartilaginis
      arytenoideae
    oblong f. of arytenoid cartilage
    pterygoid f.
    f. pterygoidea mandibulae
    sublingual f.
    f. sublingualis
    submandibular f.
    f. submandibularis
    f. superior
    superior f. of sulcus limitans
    f. supravesicalis peritonaei
    f. trigemini
    trochlear f.
    f. trochlearis
foveal
foveate
foveation
foveola (foveolae)
    f. coccygea
    coccygeal f.
    f. gastricae
    granular foveolae
    foveolae granulares
    foveolae papillae
    f. retinae
    f. suprameatalis
    f. suprameatica
    triangular f.

foveolar
foveolate
Foville
    fasciculus
    syndrome
    tract
Foville-Wilson syndrome
Fowler
    incision
    operation
    position
    solution
    sound
Fowler-Murphy treatment
Fowler-Weir incision
Fox
    conformer
    curet
    disease
    impetigo
    implant
    irrigator
    operation
    shield
    splint
Fox-Fordyce disease
foxglove
    Austrian f.
    purple f.
    woolly f.
f.p.—foot-pound
FP—
    false-positive
    family practice
    freezing point
    frontoparietal
    frozen plasma
fpa—far point of accommodation
FPA—fluorophenylalanine
FPC—
    familial polyposis coli
    fish protein concentrate
FPG—fasting plasma glucose
FPM—filter paper microscopic (test)
FPP—familial paroxysmal
    polyserositis
fps—frames per second
Fr—francium
Fr, F—French (catheter gauge)
FR—
    Fisher-Race (notation)
    flocculation reaction
    flow rate
F&R—force and rhythm (of pulse)
fraction
    absorbed f.

fraction *(continued)*
    blood plasma f.
    dried human plasma
      protein f.
    ejection f.
    Fechner f.
    filtration f.
    human plasma
      protein f.
    microsome f.
    mol f.
    mole f.
    penetration f.
    plasma f's
    plasma protein f.
    recombination f.
    sampling f.
    scatter f.
    soluble f.
    substance f.
    Teicholz ejection f.
    volume f.
fractional
    f. curettage
    f. dilatation and curettage
      (D&C)
    f. encephalography
fractionate
fractionation
    cell f.
    Cohn f.
    dose f.
fractography
fracture
    abduction f.
    acute on chronic f.
    adduction f.
    agenetic f.
    apophyseal f.
    articular f.
    atrophic f.
    avulsion f.
    Barton f.
    basal neck f.
    basal skull f.
    basocervical f.
    bending f.
    Bennett f.
    bimalleolar f.
    birth f.
    blow-out f.
    boxer's f.
    bucket-handle f.
    bumper f.
    bursting f.
    butterfly f.

fracture *(continued)*
    buttonhole f.
    f. by contrecoup
    capillary f.
    cemental f.
    cementum f.
    chance f.
    chip f.
    chisel f.
    clay shoveler's f.
    cleavage f.
    closed f.
    Colles f.
    comminuted f.
    complete f.
    complex simple f.
    complicated f.
    compound f.
    compound skull f.
    compression f.
    condylar f.
    congenital f.
    cortical f.
    Cotton f.
    cough f.
    craniofacial dysjunction f.
    crush f.
    deferred f.
    dentate f.
    depressed f.
    depressed skull f.
    de Quervain f.
    diacondylar f.
    diastatic skull f.
    direct f.
    dislocation f.
    displaced f.
    double f.
    Dupuytren f.
    Duverney f.
    dyscrasic f.
    f. en coin
    endocrine f.
    f. en rave
    epiphyseal f.
    extracapsular f.
    fatigue f.
    fender f.
    fissure f.
    fissured f.
    freeze f.
    Galeazzi f.
    Gosselin f.
    greenstick f.
    grenade-thrower's f.
    Guérin f.

F

fracture *(continued)*
    gutter f.
    hairline f.
    hangman's f.
    heat f's
    hickory-stick f.
    horizontal maxillary f.
    idiopathic f.
    impacted f.
    incomplete f.
    indirect f.
    inflammatory f.
    intercondylar f.
    interperiosteal f.
    intertrochanteric f.
    intra-articular f.
    intracapsular f.
    intraperiosteal f.
    intrauterine f.
    Jefferson f.
    joint f.
    Jones f.
    lead pipe f.
    Le Fort f. (I–III)
    linear f.
    Lisfranc f.
    longitudinal f.
    loose f.
    malar f.
    mallet f.
    march f.
    midfacial f.
    Monteggia f.
    Moore f.
    multiple f.
    nasal f.
    nasomaxillary f.
    neoplastic f.
    neurogenic f.
    oblique f.
    occult f.
    open f.
    panfacial f.
    paratrooper f.
    parry f.
    pathologic f.
    perforating f.
    periarticular f.
    pertrochanteric f.
    pillion f.
    ping-pong f.
    pond f.
    posterior element f.
    Pott f.
    pressure f.

fracture *(continued)*
    puncture f.
    pyramidal f.
    Quervain (de Quervain) f.
    resecting f.
    reverse f.
    reverse Colles f.
    ring f.
    Salter f. (I–VI)
    secondary f.
    segmental f.
    shaft f.
    Shepherd f.
    silver fork f.
    simple f.
    Skillern f.
    Smith f.
    spiral f.
    splintered f.
    spontaneous f.
    sprain f.
    sprinter's f.
    stellate f.
    Stieda f.
    strain f.
    stress f.
    subcapital f.
    subcutaneous f.
    subperiosteal f.
    subtrochanteric f.
    supracondylar f.
    surgical neck f.
    temporal bone f.
    tibial plateau f.
    toms f.
    torsion f.
    torus f.
    transcervical f.
    transcondylar f.
    transverse f.
    transverse facial f.
    transverse maxillary f.
    trimalleolar f.
    trophic f.
    tuft f.
    ununited f.
    vertebra plana f.
    Wagstaffe f.
    willow f.
    zygomaticomaxillary f.
fracture-dislocation
    Monteggia f-d.
    posterior f-d.
fradicin
fragiform

fragilitas
    f. crinium
    f. ossium
    f. sanguinis
    f. unguium
fragility
    f. of blood
    capillary f.
    erythrocyte f.
    hereditary f. of bone
    mechanical f.
    osmotic f.
    red cell f.
    f. test
fragilocyte
fragilocytosis
fragment
    f. A
    f. B
    Fab f.
    Fabc f.
    Facb f.
    Fb f.
    Fc f.
    Fd f.
    fission f.
    Fv f.
    Klenow f.
    one-carbon f.
    papain f.
    restriction f.
    Spengler f.
fragmentation of
  myocardium
fragmentography
    mass f.
fraise
    diamond f.
frambesia tropica
frambesioma
framboesia, frambesia
framboesioma, frambesioma
frame
    Balkan f.
    Bradford f.
    Deiters terminal f.
    Foster f.
    freeze f.
    Hibbs f.
    occluding f.
    quadriplegic standing f.
    reading f.
    rotating f. of reference
    rubber dam f.
    Stryker f.

frame *(continued)*
    suture f.
    trial f.
    unidentified reading f. (URF)
    Whitman f.
frame shift
framework
    implant f.
    scleral f.
    uveal f.
framing
Franceschetti
    disease
    dystrophy
    operation
    syndrome
Franceschetti-Jadassohn
  syndrome
Francis
    disease
    spud
Francisella tularensis
francium (Fr)
Franco operation
François dystrophy
frange
frangulic acid
Frank
    lead system
    operation
Franke
    syndrome
    tabes operation
    triad
Frankel classification (groups A–E)
Fränkel (Fraenkel)
    forceps
    sign
    speculum
    test
    treatment
Frankfeldt
    forceps
    needle
    sigmoidoscope
    snare
Franklin disease
Franklin-Silverman needle
Frank-Starling mechanism
Franz retractor
Fraser syndrome
fraternal
fratricide
fraught
Fraunhofer zone

F

Frazier
    cannula
    elevator
    hook retractor
    osteotome
    retractor
    suction tube
    tube
Frazier-Spiller operation
FRC—
    functional reserve capacity
    functional residual capacity
freckle
    melanotic f. of Hutchinson
Frederick needle
Fredet-Ramstedt
    operation
    pyloromyotomy
free association
free ligature suture
free-living
Freeman-Sheldon syndrome
freemartin
free peritoneal air
Freer
    chisel
    elevator
    knife
freeze-cleaving
freeze-drying
freeze-etching
freeze-fracturing
freeze frame
freeze-substitution
freezing microtome
Frei
    antigen
    bubo
    disease
    test
Freiberg
    disease
    knife
Freimuth curet
Frejka pillow splint
fremitus
    bronchial f.
    friction f.
    hydatid f.
    pectoral f.
    pericardial f.
    pleural f.
    rhonchal f.
    subjective f.
    tactile f.

fremitus *(continued)*
    tussive f.
    vocal f. (VF)
frena (plural of frenum)
frenal
French-McCarthy panendoscope
French-Robinson catheter
frenectomy
frenetic, frenetical
Frenkel
    exercises
    movements
    symptoms
    tracks
    treatment
frenoplasty
frenotomy
    lingual f.
frenulum (frenula)
    f. of anterior medullary velum
    f. cerebelli
    f. clitoridis
    f. of clitoris
    f. of duodenal papilla
    f. of Giacomini
    f. of ileocecal valve
    f. of ileocolic valve
    f. of inferior lip
    f. labii inferioris
    f. labii superioris
    f. labiorum pudendi
    f. linguae
    f. linguae cerebelli
    f. of Morgagni
    f. of prepuce of penis
    f. preputii penis
    f. of pudendal labia
    f. pudendi
    f. of rostral medullary velum
    f. of superior lip
    f. of superior medullary velum
    f. synoviale
    f. of tongue
    f. valvae ilealis
    f. valvae ileocaecalis
    f. veli medullaris cranialis
    f. veli medullaris rostralis
    f. veli medullaris superioris
frenum (frena)
    buccal f.
    f. of labia
    labial f.
    f. labiorum
    lingual f.
    Macdowel (M'Dowel) f.

frenum (frena) *(continued)*
  f. of Morgagni
  synovial frena
  f. of tongue
  f. of valve of colon
frenzy, frenzied
frequency
  audio f.
  audio Doppler f.
  center f.
  class f.
  critical flicker fusion f.
  cutoff f.
  dominant f.
  gene f.
  high f.
  infrasonic f.
  Larmor f.
  low f.
  mutant f.
  nearest neighbor f.
  projection f.
  recombination f.
  relative f.
  respiratory f.
  subsonic f.
  supersonic f.
  ultrasonic f.
  urinary f.
  ventilatory f.
Frerichs theory
freshen
freshened
Fresnel
  lens
  zone
  zone plate
fressreflex
fretum (freta)
  f. halleri
Freud
  cathartic method
  theory
freudian
Freund
  adjuvant
  anomaly
  law
  operation
Frey
  gastric pits
  hairs
  implant
  syndrome
Frey-Baillarger syndrome

Freyer operation
FRF; FSH-RF—follicle-stimulating
  hormone–releasing factor
friable
fricative
Fricke
  arterial forceps
  bandage
  flap
  operation
  scrotal dressing
friction
Friderichsen-Waterhouse syndrome
Friedenwald
  operation
  ophthalmoscope
  syndrome
Friedenwald-Guyton operation
Friedländer
  bacillus
  bacillus pneumonia
  disease
  pneumobacillus
  pneumonia
Friedman
  curve
  position
  retractor
  test
Friedman-Lapham test
Friedmann
  complex
  disease
  vasomotor syndrome
Friedreich
  ataxia
  disease
  foot
  sign
  tabes
Friedrich operation
Friedrich-Petz clamp
frigid
frigidity
frigolabile
frigorific
frigostable
frigotherapy
frill
  iris f.
fringe
  subliminal f.
Fritsch
  catheter
  operation

F

Fritsch-Asherman syndrome
Fritz-Lange operation
frogleg, froglegged
    f. position
    f. projection
    f. splint
    f. view
Fröhlich (Froehlich)
    dwarfism
    dystrophy
    syndrome
Frohn
    reagent
    test
Froin syndrome
FROM—full range of motion
Froment sign
Frommel
    disease
    operation
Frommel-Chiari syndrome
frond
frondose
frons
    f. cranii
    wave f.
front
    wave f.
frontad
frontal
    f. bone
    f. lobe
    f. lobotomy
    f. suture
frontalis
frontipetal
frontocerebellar
frontoethmoidal
    f. sphenoidectomy
    f. suture
frontoethmoidectomy
    external f.
frontolacrimal suture
frontolateral partial laryngectomy
frontomalar suture
frontomaxillary suture
frontomental
frontonasal suture
fronto-occipital tract
fronto-orbital
frontoparietal suture
frontopontine
frontopontocerebellar
frontosphenoid suture
frontotemporal

frontozygomatic suture
Froriep
    ganglion
    induration
frost
    synovial f.
    urea f.
    uremic f.
Frost suture
frostbite
    deep f.
    superficial f.
    third-degree f.
Frost-Lang operation
froth of drowning
frothing
frottage
frotteur
frozen pelvis
FRP—functional refractory period
fructification
fructivorous
fructofuranose
fructopyranose
fructosamine
fructosan
fructosazone
fructose
    f. 1,6-bisphosphatase
    f. 1,6-bisphosphate
    f. 2,6-bisphosphate
    f. bisphosphate aldolase
    f. 1,6-diphosphatase
    f. 1,6-diphosphate
    f. 1-phosphate aldolase
    f. 6-phosphate
fructosidase
fructoside
fructosuria
    benign f.
    essential f.
fructosyl
fructosyltransferase
fructovegetative
frugivorous
fruit
fruitarian
fruitarianism
frustration
FS—
    full scale (IQ)
    function study
FSD—focal skin distance
FSF—fibrin-stabilizing factor
FSH—follicle-stimulating hormone

FSH/LH-RH—follicle-stimulating hormone and luteinizing hormone–releasing hormone
FSH-RF—follicle-stimulating hormone–releasing factor
FSH-RH—follicle-stimulating hormone–releasing hormone
FSPs—fibrin split products
FSR—fusiform skin revision
FSW—field service worker
ft.—foot
FT—
    false transmitter
    family therapy
    fibrous tissue
    free thyroxine
    full term
FTA—fluorescent treponemal antibody (test)
FTA-AB, FTA-ABS—fluorescent treponemal antibody absorption
FTLB—full-term live birth
FTND—full-term normal delivery
FTT—failure to thrive
FU—
    fecal urobilinogen
    fluorouracil
    follow-up
Fuchs
    atrophy
    coloboma
    crypts
    dimples
    dystrophy
    forceps
    heterochromia
    heterochromic cyclitis
    keratitis
    operation
    sign
    spot
    syndrome
fuchsin
    acid f.
    aldehyde f.
    aniline f.
    basic f.
    diamond f.
    new f.
fuchsinophil
fuchsinophilia
fuchsinophilic
fuchsinophilous
fucosan

fucose
α-L-fucosidase [alpha-]
fucoside
fucosidosis
fucoxanthin
fugacity
fugitive
fugue
    dissociative f.
    epileptic f.
    psychogenic f.
    f. state
fuguism
fuguismus
fugutoxin
Fukala operation
fulcrum full width at half-maximum
fulgurant
fulgurate
fulguration
    direct f.
    indirect f.
fulgurize
fuliginous
Fuller operation
full-lumen esophagoscope
fulminant
fulminate
Fulpit forceps
fumagillin
fumarase
fumarate
fumarate hydratase
fumaric acid
fumaroylacetoacetate hydrolase
fumarylacetoacetase
fume
fumigant
fumigation
fuming
functio laesa
function
    arousal f.
    Carnot f.
    carnotic f.
    cumulative distribution f.
    discriminant f.
    distribution f.
    ego f.
    frequency f.
    group f.
    isometric f.
    life table f.
    linear f.

F

function *(continued)*
    line-spread f.
    liver f.
    probability density f.
functional
    f. anastomosis
    f. image
    f. imaging
    f. status
functionalis
functionating
funda
fundal
fundament
fundamental
fundectomy
fundi
fundic
fundiform
fundoplasty
fundoplication
    Nissen f.
fundus (fundus)
    albinotic f.
    f. albipunctatus
    f. of bladder
    f. camera
    f. diabeticus
    f. of eye
    f. flavimaculatus
    fluorescein f. photography
    f. of gallbladder
    gastric f.
    f. gastricus
    f. of internal acoustic meatus
    leopard f.
    f. meatus acustici interni
    f. microscopy
    f. oculi
    salt and pepper f.
    f. of stomach
    tessellated f.
    f. tigroid
    f. tympani
    f. of urinary bladder
    f. uteri
    f. of uterus
    f. of vagina
    f. vaginae
    f. ventricularis
    f. ventriculi
    f. vesicae biliaris
    f. vesicae felleae
    f. vesicae urinariae
funduscope
funduscopic

funduscopy
fundusectomy
fungal
fungate
fungating growth
fungemia
fungi (plural of fungus)
fungicidal
fungicide
fungicidin
fungiform
fungistasis
fungistat
fungistatic
fungisterol
fungitoxic
fungitoxicity
fungoid
fungosity
fungous
funguria
fungus (fungi)
    f. balls
    beefsteak f.
    biphasic f.
    cerebral f.
    f. cerebri
    club fungi
    cutaneous f.
    dimorphic f.
    foot f.
    imperfect f.
    mosaic f.
    mycelial f.
    opportunistic f.
    pathogenic f.
    perfect f.
    proper fungi
    ray f.
    sac fungi
    slime f.
    subcutaneous f.
    systemic f.
    f. testis
    thread f.
    thrush f.
    true fungi
    umbilical f.
funic
funicular
funiculate
funiculi (genitive and plural of
    funiculus)
funiculitis
    endemic f.
    filarial f.

funiculoepididymitis
funiculopexy
funiculus (funiculi)
 f. amnii
 f. anterior medullae spinalis
 anterior f. of spinal cord
 cuneate f.
 f. cuneatus
 f. cuneatus lateralis
 f. cuneatus medullae
  oblongatae
 dorsal f. of spinal cord
 f. dorsalis medullae spinalis
 funiculi medullae spinalis
 funiculi of spinal cord
 f. gracilis medullae oblongatae
 hepatic f.
 hepatic f. of Rauber
 f. lateralis medullae
  oblongatae
 f. lateralis medullae spinalis
 lateral f. of medulla oblongata
 ligamentous f.
 f. medullae spinalis
 f. posterior medullae spinalis
 posterior f. of spinal cord
 f. of Rolando
 f. separans
 f. solitarius
 f. spermaticus
 funiculi of spinal cord
 f. of spinal cord, anterior
 f. of spinal cord, lateral
 f. of spinal cord, posterior
 f. teres
 f. umbilicalis
 f. ventralis
 f. ventralis medullae spinalis
 ventral f. of spinal cord
funiform
funis
 accessory müllerian f.
 f. brachii
 f. hippocratis
 mitral f.
 muscular f.
 pial f.
 vascular f.
funisitis
funnel
 accessory müllerian f.
 mitral f.
 muscular f.
 pial f.
 vascular f.
funnel chest

FUO—
 fever of undetermined origin
 fever of unknown origin
FUR—fluorouracil riboside
furan
furanose
furanoside
furazolidone
furcal
furcation
 denuded f.
 invaded f.
 f. invasion
 f. involvement
furcocercous
furcula
furfuraceous
furfural
furfuran
furfurol
Furniss
 anastomosis
 catheter
 clamp
 incision
Furniss-Clute clamp
Furniss-McClure-Hinton clamp
furor epilepticus
furrier's suture
furrow
 atrioventricular f.
 digital f.
 division f.
 genital f.
 gluteal f.
 Jadelot f's
 Liebermeister f's
 mentolabial f.
 nympholabial f.
 palpebral f.
 primitive f.
 Schmorl f.
 scleral f.
 Sibson f.
 skin f's
fursalan
Fürstner (Fuerstner) disease
furuncle
furuncular
furunculoid
furunculosis
 f. blastomycetica
 f. cryptococcica
furunculous
furunculus (furunculi)
 f. vulgaris

fury
  alcoholic f.
fusaridiosis
fusariotoxicosis
Fusarium
  F. graminearum
  F. moniliforme
  F. oxysporum
  F. poae
  F. roseum
  F. solani
  F. sporotrichiella
  F. sporotrichioides
  F. tricinctum
fuscin
fuse
fuseau
fusible
fusidate
fusidic acid
fusiform
fusimotor
fusion
  anterior cervical diskectomy
    and f. (ACDF)
  f. beats
  binocular f.
  cell f.
  centric f.
  Cloward back f.
  diaphyseal-epiphyseal f.
  flicker f.
  f. of joint
  protoplast f.
  renal f.
  spinal f.

fusion *(continued)*
  f. tubes
fusional
Fusobacterium
  F. gonidiaformans
  F. mortiferum
  F. naviforme
  F. nucleatum
  F. russii
  F. varium
fusocellular
fusospirillary
fusospirillosis
fusospirochetal
fusospirochetosis
fustigation
fusus (fusi)
  cortical fusi
  fracture fusi
  f. neuromuscularis
  f. neurotendineus
Futura splint
FV—fluid volume
FVC—forced vital capacity
FVL—femoral vein
    ligation
FW—
    Felix-Weil (reaction)
    Folin and Wu (method)
    fragment wound
FWHM—full width at half-
    maximum
FWR—Felix-Weil reaction
fx—fracture
FYI—for your information
FZ—focal zone

G

γ—
  gamma (Greek letter)
  the heavy chain of IgG
  the γ chains of fetal
    hemoglobin
g—gram(s)
g—standard gravity
G—
  gauge
  gauss

G— *(continued)*
  giga-
  gingival
  glucose
  gonidial (colony)
  good
  gravida
  Greek
  guanine
  guanosine

G; Gly—glycine
Ga—gallium
GA—
    Gamblers Anonymous
    gastric analysis
    general anesthesia
    gestational age
    gingivoaxial
    glucuronic acid
    glutaric aciduria
    gut-associated
^{57}Ga citrate [gallium Ga 57 citrate]
GABA—γ-aminobutyric acid [gamma-]
Gabarro
    graft
    operation
Gabriel proctoscope
Gabriel Tucker tube
G-actin
gadfly
gadoleic acid
gadolinium (Gd)
Gaenslen
    sign
    test
GAF—Global Assessment of Functioning (scale)
Gaffky
    scale
    table
gag
    Davis g.
    Davis-Crowe mouth g.
    Doyen g.
    incisor g.
    Mason g.
    McIvor g.
    molar g.
    mouth g.
    g. reflex
GAG—glycosaminoglycan
Gaillard operation
Gaillard-Arlt suture
gain
    antigen g.
    end g.
    epinosic g.
    near g.
    paranosic g.
    primary g.
    secondary g.
    swept g.
Gairdner test

Gaisböck
    disease
    syndrome
gait
    antalgic g.
    ataxic g.
    calcaneus g.
    cerebellar g.
    Charcot g.
    cogwheel g.
    double-step g.
    drag-to g.
    drop-foot g.
    drunken g.
    duck g.
    equine g.
    festinating g.
    footdrop g.
    four-point g.
    glue-footed g.
    gluteal g.
    gluteus maximus g.
    gluteus medius g.
    heel-toe g.
    helicopod g.
    hemiplegic g.
    hysterical g.
    intermittent double-step g.
    listing g.
    myopathic g.
    Oppenheim g.
    paraparetic g.
    Petren g.
    reeling g.
    scissors g.
    skaters' g.
    spastic equinus g.
    staggering g.
    stamping g.
    star g.
    g. and station
    steppage g.
    swaying g.
    swing-through g.
    swing-to g.
    tabetic g.
    tandem g.
    three-point g.
    Todd g.
    Trendelenburg g.
    two-point g.
    waddling g.
gal.—gallon
galactacrasia
galactagogue

G

galactemia
galactic
galactischia
galactitol
galactoblast
galactocele
galactocerebroside
galactochloral
galactogen
galactogenous
galactography
galactokinase
galactolipin
galactoma
galactometastasis
galactometer
galactophlebitis
galactophlysis
galactophore
galactophoritis
galactophorous
galactophygous
galactoplania
galactopoiesis
galactopoietic
galactopyra
galactorrhea
galactosamine-6-sulfatase
galactoscope
galactose epimerase
galactose 1-phosphate
　　uridyltransferase
α-galactosidase A [alpha-]
β-galactosidase [beta-]
galactoside
　　g. acetylase
　　g. permease
galactosis
galactostasis
galactosuria
galactosyl
galactotoxism
galactotrophy
galacturia
galacturonic acid
galantamine hydrobromide
galanthamine hydrobromide
galea
　　g. aponeurotica
　　tendinous g.
Galeati glands
galeatus
Galeazzi
　　fracture
　　sign

Galen
　　anastomosis
　　foramen
　　nerve
　　veins
　　ventricle
galenic
galenicals
galeropia
galeropsia
gall
　　Aleppo g.
　　ox g.
　　Smyrna g.
gallacetophenone
gallate
gallbladder
　　Courvoisier g.
　　fish-scale g.
　　floating g.
　　folded fundus g.
　　hourglass g.
　　mobile g.
　　phrygian cap g.
　　sandpaper g.
　　stasis g.
　　strawberry g.
　　wandering g.
Gall craniology
gallein
gallic acid
Gallie
　　operation
　　transplant
Galli-Mainini test
galling
gallisin
gallium (Ga)
　　g. 67, g. 68
　　g. citrate Ga 67
　　radioactive g. (gallium Ga 67)
　　g. scan
　　g. scanning
　　g. titrate Ga 67
　　g. uptake
gallnut
gallocyanin
gallon (gal.)
gallop
　　atrial g.
　　apical g.
　　early diastolic g.
　　mid diastolic g.
　　murmur, rub, or g.
　　protodiastolic g.

gallop *(continued)*
- g. rhythm
- S_3 g. [S3]
- S_4 g. [S4]
- g. sounds
- summation g.
- systolic g.
- ventricular g.

gallotannic acid
gallsickness
gallstone
- silent g.

GalNAc—*N*-acetylgalactosamine
GALT—
- gastrointestinal-associated lymphoid tissue
- gut-associated lymphoid tissue

galvanic epilator
galvanism
- dental g.

galvanization
galvanocautery
galvanochemical
galvanocontractility
galvanogustometer
galvanolysis
galvanometer
- Einthoven g.
- string g.
- thread g.

galvanonervous
galvanopalpation
galvanosurgery
galvanotaxis
galvanotherapeutics
galvanotherapy
galvanotropism
Gambee suture
gambir
gamekeeper's thumb
gamete
gametic
gametocidal
gametocide
gametocyst
gametocyte
gametocytemia
gametoid
Gamgee tissue
gamic
gamma
- Greek letter (γ; alphabetized as g)
- g.-aminobutyrate
- g.-aminobutyric acid (GABA)

gamma *(continued)*
- g. benzene hexachloride
- g. camera
- g.-carboxyglutamate
- g.-carboxyglutamic acid
- g. cascade
- g. chain disease
- g.-cystathionase
- g. emitter
- g. encephalography
- g. film
- g.-guanidinobutyramide
- g. globulin
- g.-glutamylcysteine synthetase (deficiency)
- g.-glutamyltransferase (GGT)
- g.-glutamyl transpeptidase (GGTP)
- g.-glutamyl transpeptidase deficiency
- g. heating
- g. heavy chain disease
- g.-hydroxybutyricaciduria
- g. interferon
- g.-lactone
- g.-pipradol
- g. radiation
- g. radiography
- g. scanning
- g. streptococci
- g. well counter

gammacism
gammaglobulinopathy
gammagram
gammagraphic
gamma ray
- g.r. counter
- g.r. level indicator
- g.r. scanner
- g.r. spectra
- g.r. spectrometer

gammexane
gammography
- cerebral g.

gammopathy
- benign monoclonal g.
- biclonal g.
- monoclonal g.
- polyclonal g.

Gamna
- disease
- nodules

Gamna-Favre bodies
gamogenesis
gamogenetic

gamogony
gamone
gamont
gamophagia
gamophobia
gampsodactyly
Gamstorp disease
Gandhi knife
Gandy clamp
Gandy-Gamna
   disease
   nodules
   spleen
Gandy-Nanta disease
ganglia (plural of ganglion)
ganglial
gangliform
ganglioblast
gangliocyte
gangliocytoma
ganglioglioma
ganglioglioneuroma
gangliolytic
ganglioma
ganglion (ganglia, ganglions)
   accessory ganglia
   acoustic g.
   acousticofacial g.
   Acrel g.
   Andersch g.
   aorticorenal g.
   ganglia aorticorenalia
   Arnold g.
   auditory g.
   Auerbach g.
   auricular g.
   autonomic ganglia
   ganglia of autonomic
     plexuses
   g. autonomicum
   azygous g.
   basal ganglia
   Bezold g.
   Bidder ganglia
   Blandin g.
   Bochdalek g.
   Bock g.
   Böttcher (Boettcher) g.
   cardiac g.
   g. cardiaca
   carotid g.
   celiac ganglia
   ganglia celiaca
   cephalic g.
   cerebrospinal ganglia

ganglion (ganglia, ganglions)
   (continued)
   g. cervicale inferius
   g. cervicale medium
   g. cervicale superius
   cervical g., inferior
   cervical g., middle
   cervical ganglia of uterus
   cervical g., superior
   cervicothoracic g.
   g. cervicothoracicum
   cervicouterine g.
   g. ciliare
   Cloquet g.
   coccygeal g.
   cochlear g.
   g. cochleare
   ganglia coeliaca
   collateral ganglia
   compound g.
   Corti g.
   ganglia craniospinalia
   craniospinal sensory
     ganglia
   diaphragmatic g.
   diffuse g.
   dorsal root g.
   g. of duct of Botallo
   Ehrenritter g.
   encephalospinal g.
   g. encephalospinale
   g. extracraniale
   ganglia of facial nerve
   false g.
   Frankenhäuser
     (Frankenhaeuser) g.
   Froriep g.
   Ganser g.
   gasserian g.
   geniculate g.
   g. geniculatum nervi
     facialis
   g. geniculi nervi facialis
   g. of glossopharyngeal
     nerve
   g. of habenulae
   hepatic g.
   Huber g.
   hypoglossal g.
   g. impar
   inferior g. of glossopharyngeal
     nerve
   inferior thyroid g.
   g. inferius nervi
     glossopharyngei

ganglion (ganglia, ganglions)
(continued)
  g. inferius nervi vagi
  inhibitory g.
  intercrural g.
  ganglia intermedia
  intermediate ganglia
  interpeduncular g.
  g. intervertebrale
  intracranial g.
  g. jugulare nervi vagi
  jugular g. of glossopharyngeal
    nerve
  jugular g. of vagus nerve
  Küttner g.
  Langley g.
  Laumonier g.
  Lee g.
  lesser g. of Meckel
  Lobstein ganglion
  lower g. of glossopharyngeal
    nerve
  lower g. of vagus nerve
  Ludwig g.
  ganglia lumbalia
  ganglia lumbaria
  g. lymphaticum
  Meckel g.
  Meissner g.
  mesenteric g., inferior
  mesenteric g., superior
  g. mesentericum inferius
  g. mesentericum
    superius
  g. of Müller
  nasal g.
  nerve g.
  g. nervi splanchnici
  neural g.
  nodose g.
  g. nodosum
  nonpermanent g.
  olfactory g.
  ophthalmic g.
  optic g.
  orbital g.
  otic g.
  g. oticum
  parasympathetic g.
  g. parasympatheticum
  paravertebral g.
  pelvic ganglia
  ganglia pelvina
  periosteal g.
  permanent g.

ganglion (ganglia, ganglions)
(continued)
  petrosal g.
  petrous g.
  phrenic g.
  ganglia phrenica
  ganglia plexuum
    autonomicorum
  ganglia plexuum
    sympathicorum
  ganglia plexuum
    visceralium
  posterior root g.
  prevertebral ganglia
  primary g.
  prostatic g.
  pterygopalatine g.
  g. pterygopalatinum
  Remak g.
  renal ganglia
  ganglia renalia
  g. retinae
  Ribes g.
  g. rostralis nervi
    glossopharyngei
  g. rostralis nervi vagi
  sacral ganglia
  ganglia sacralia
  Scarpa g.
  Schacher g.
  Schmiedel g.
  semilunar g.
  g. semilunare
  g. sensoriale
  sensory g.
  simple g.
  sinoatrial g.
  sinus g.
  sphenomaxillary g.
  sphenopalatine g.
  g. sphenopalatinum
  spinal g.
  g. spinale
  spiral g.
  g. spirale cochleae
  splanchnic g.
  splanchnic g. of Arnold
  splanchnic thoracic g.
  g. splanchnicum
  stellate g.
  g. stellatum
  sublingual g.
  g. sublinguale
  submandibular g.
  g. submandibulare

ganglion (ganglia, ganglions)
(continued)
    superior g. of glossopharyngeal
      nerve
    g. superius nervi
      glossopharyngei
    g. superius nervi vagi
    suprarenal g.
    g. sympatheticum
    g. sympathicum
    synovial g.
    terminal g.
    g. terminale
    ganglia thoracalia
    thoracic ganglia
    ganglia thoracica
    trigeminal g.
    g. trigeminale
    g. of trigeminal nerve
    Troisier g.
    ganglia trunci sympathetici
    ganglia trunci sympathici
    tympanic g.
    tympanic g. of Valentin
    g. tympanicum
    vagal g., inferior
    vagal g., superior
    g. of vagus nerve
    Valentin g.
    ventricular g.
    vertebral g.
    g. vertebrale
    vestibular g.
    g. vestibulare
    vestibulocochlear g.
    visceral ganglia
    ganglia visceralia
    Walther g.
    Wrisberg g.
    wrist g.
ganglionated
ganglion cell layer
ganglionectomy
ganglioneure
ganglioneuroblastoma
ganglioneurofibroma
    melanotic g.
ganglioneuroma
    dumbbell g.
    hourglass g.
ganglioneuromatosis
ganglionic
ganglionitis
    acute posterior g.
    gasserian g.

ganglionostomy
ganglioplegic
ganglioside
    g. G_{M1}
    g. G_{M2}
    g. storage disease
gangliosidosis (gangliosidoses)
    generalized g.
    GM_1 g. [GM1]
    GM_1 g., adult
    GM_1 g., infantile
    GM_1 g., juvenile
    GM_2 g. [GM2]
    GM_2 g., adult
    GM_2 g., juvenile
    GM_2 g. (types I–III)
    GM_2 g., variant AB
    GM_2 g., variant B
    GM_2 g., variant O
gangliospore
gangliosympathectomy
gangliosympatheticoblastoma
Ganglophe sign
gangrene
    angiosclerotic g.
    atherosclerotic g.
    chemical g.
    circumscribed g.
    cold g.
    cutaneous g.
    decubital g.
    diabetic g.
    disseminated cutaneous g.
    dry g.
    embolic g.
    emphysematous g.
    epidemic g.
    Fournier g.
    gas g.
    gaseous g.
    glycemic g.
    g. of lung
    hospital g.
    hot g.
    humid g.
    inflammatory g.
    ischemic g.
    Meleney g.
    mephitic g.
    moist g.
    oral g.
    Pott g.
    presenile spontaneous g.
    pressure g.
    primary g.

gangrene *(continued)*
    progressive g.
    progressive bacterial
      synergistic g.
    progressive postoperative g.
    progressive synergistic g.
    pulp g.
    Raynaud g.
    secondary g.
    senile g.
    static g.
    symmetric g.
    sympathetic g.
    thrombotic g.
    traumatic g.
    trophic g.
    venous g.
    wet g.
gangrenosis
gangrenous
ganja
ganoblast
Ganser
    basal nucleus of G.
    commissure
    ganglion
    nucleus basalis of G.
    symptom
    syndrome
Gant
    clamp
    line
    operation
gantry
gap
    air g.
    air-bone g.
    anion g.
    auscultatory g.
    Bochdalek g.
    chromatid g.
    interocclusal g.
    silent g.
GAPD, GAPDH—glyceraldehyde-3-
  phosphate dehydrogenase
gapes
Garcin syndrome
Gardner
    chair
    needle
    operation
    syndrome
Gardnerella vaginalis
Garfield-Holinger laryngoscope
gargalanesthesia

gargalesthesia
gargalesthetic
gargle
gargoylism
    X-linked recessive g.
Gariel pessary
Garland
    curve
    triangle
garment
    elastic g.
    pneumatic antishock g.
garnet
Garré
    disease
    osteitis
    osteomyelitis
Garrigue
    forceps
    speculum
garrot
garrulous
Gartner
    bacillus
    canal
    cyst
    duct
    phenomenon
    tonometer
gas
    alveolar g.
    g. angiocardiography
    arterial blood g's (ABGs)
    blood g.
    carrier g.
    choking g.
    g. chromatography (GC)
    coal g.
    g. density line
    ethyl g.
    expired g.
    hemolytic g.
    inert g.
    lacrimator g.
    laughing g.
    g.-liquid chromatography (GLC)
    marsh g.
    g. mediastinography
    mustard g.
    nerve g.
    noble g.
    sewer g.
    sneezing g.
    g.-solid chromatography (GSC)
    suffocating g.

G

gas *(continued)*
    sweet g.
    tear g.
    vesicating g.
    war g.
gaseous
gasiform
gaskin
gasogenic
gasometer
gasometric
gasometry
gasp
gas-permeable lens
Gasser
    ganglion
    syndrome
gasserectomy
gasserian
Gass scleral punch
Gastaut
    disease
    syndrome
gaster
Gasterophilus
    G. haemorrhoidalis
    G. intestinalis
    G. nasalis
gastradenitis
gastralgia
    appendicular g.
gastralgokenosis
gastratrophia
gastrectomy
    antecolic g.
    Billroth g.
    physiologic g.
    Roux-en-Y g.
gastric
    g. acid
    g. actinomycosis
    g. adenocarcinoma
    g. anoxia
    g. atrophy
    g. balloon implantation
    g. bubble
    g. by-pass surgery
    g. carcinoma
    g. chromoscopy
    g. dilation
    g. duplication
    g. dysfunction
    g. dysrhythmia
    g. emptying
    g. fiberscope
    g. freezing

gastric *(continued)*
    g. hyperemia
    g. hypersecretion
    g. ileus
    g. inhibitory polypeptides
    g. lavage
    g. mucosal barrier
    g. neurectomy
    g. outlet obstruction
    g. parietography
    g. pseudolymphoma
    g. resection (GR)
    g. retention
    g. rupture
    g. stasis
    g. teratoma
    g. ulcer
    g. varices
    g. volvulus
gastricsin
gastrin
gastrinoma
gastritic
gastritis
    antral g.
    atrophic g.
    atrophic-hyperplastic g.
    catarrhal g.
    chemical g.
    chronic cystic g.
    chronic follicular g.
    cirrhotic g.
    corrosive g.
    emphysematous g.
    eosinophilic g.
    erosive g.
    exfoliative g.
    follicular g.
    giant hypertrophic g.
    g. granulomatosa
      fibroplastica
    granulomatous g.
    hemorrhagic g.
    hypertrophic g
    idiopathic g.
    interstitial g.
    mycotic g.
    nonerosive g.
    phlegmonous g.
    polypous g.
    pseudomembranous g.
    purulent g.
    radiation g.
    superficial g.
    suppurating g.
    suppurative g.

gastritis *(continued)*
    syphilitic g.
    toxic g.
    tuberculous g.
    uremic g.
    zonal g.
gastroacephalus
gastroadenitis
gastroadynamic
gastroamorphus
gastroanastomosis
gastrocamera
    Olympus model GTF-A g.
gastrocardiac
gastrocele
gastrocnemius
gastrocoele
gastrocolic
gastrocolitis
gastrocolostomy
gastrocolotomy
gastrocutaneous
gastrodermis
gastrodiaphane
gastrodiaphanoscopy
gastrodiaphany
gastrodidymus
gastrodisciasis
Gastrodiscoides
   hominis
gastrodisk
gastroduodenal
gastroduodenectomy
gastroduodenitis
gastroduodenoenterostomy
gastroduodenoscopy
    Billroth g.
gastroduodenostomy
gastrodynia
gastroenteralgia
gastroenteric
gastroenteritis
    acute infectious g.
    eosinophilic g.
    infantile g.
    Norwalk g.
gastroenteroanastomosis
gastroenterocolitis
gastroenterocolostomy
gastroenterologic
gastroenterologist
gastroenterology
gastroenteropathy
    allergic g.
gastroenteroplasty
gastroenteroptosis

gastroenterostomy (GE)
    Balfour g.
    Billroth g. (I, II, III) g.
    Braun and Jaboulay g.
    Courvoisier g.
    Heineke-Mikulicz g.
    Hofmeister g.
    Polya g.
    Roux g.
    Roux-en-Y g.
    Schoemaker g.
    von Haberer-Finney g.
    Wölfler (Woelfler) g.
gastroenterotomy
gastroepiploic
gastroesophageal reflux disease
  (GERD)
gastroesophagitis
gastroesophagoplasty
gastroesophagostomy
gastrofiberscope
gastrogastrostomy
gastrogavage
gastrogenic
Gastrografin
gastrograph
gastrohepatic
gastrohepatitis
gastrohydrorrhea
gastrohypertonic
gastroileac
gastroileitis
gastroileostomy
gastrointestinal (GI)
    g.-associated lymphoid tissue
    g. bypass
    g. fistula
    g. fungal balls
    g. immunodeficiency
      syndrome
    g. peptide hormone
    g. reflux
    g. smooth muscle
gastrojejunocolic
gastrojejunoesophagostomy
gastrojejunostomy
    Billroth g.
    Roux-en-Y g.
gastrokinesograph
gastrolavage
gastrolienal
gastrolith
gastrolithiasis
gastrologist
gastrology
gastrolysis

G

gastromalacia
gastromegaly
gastromelus
gastromenia
gastromycosis
gastromyotomy
gastromyxorrhea
gastrone
gastro-omental
gastropagus parasiticus
gastropancreatitis
gastroparalysis
gastroparesis
gastroparietal
gastropathic
gastropathy
gastroperiodynia
gastroperitonitis
gastropexy
    Hill posterior g.
gastrophore
gastrophotography
gastrophrenic
gastrophthisis
gastroplasty
    Eckhout vertical g.
    Mason g.
    vertical banded g.
gastroplegia
gastroplication
gastropneumonic
gastropod
gastroptosis
gastroptyxis
gastropulmonary
gastropylorectomy
gastropyloric
gastroradiculitis
gastrorrhagia
gastrorrhaphy
gastrorrhea continua
  chronica
gastrorrhexis
gastroschisis
gastroscope
    ACMI g.
    Benedict g.
    Bernstein g.
    Chevalier Jackson g.
    Eder g.
    Eder-Chamberlin g.
    Eder-Hufford g.
    Eder-Palmer g.
    Ellsner g.
    fiberoptic g.

gastroscope *(continued)*
    flexible g.
    Herman-Taylor g.
    Hirschowitz g.
    Housset-Debray g.
    Janeway g.
    Kelling g.
    Schindler g.
    Wolf-Schindler g.
gastroscopic
gastroscopy
gastroselective
gastrosia fungosa
gastrosis
gastrospasm
gastrosplenic
gastrostaxis
gastrostenosis
gastrostogavage
gastrostolavage
gastrostoma
gastrostomy
    Beck-Jianu g.
    Beck g. scoop
    feeding g.
    Glassman g.
    Janeway g.
    Kader g.
    laparoscopic g.
    Martin g.
    percutaneous endoscopic g.
     (PEG)
    percutaneously inserted g.
     tube
    plug g.
    regression of g. tube
    Ssabanejew-Frank g.
    Stamm g.
    g. tube placement
    g. tube feeding
    Witzel g.
gastrosuccorrhea
    digestive g.
    g. mucosa
gastrothoracopagus dipygus
gastrotome
gastrotomy
gastrotonometer
gastrotonometry
gastrotoxin
gastrotropic
gastrotympanites
gastrula
gastrulation
Gatch bed

gate
gated
    g. blood pool imaging
    g. CT scanner
    g. imaging
    g. system
Gatellier
    incision
    operation
gating
Gaucher
    cells
    disease
    histiocyte
    splenomegaly
gauge
    beta ray g.
    bite g. (bitegage,
      bite-gage)
    Boley g.
    catheter g.
    strain g.
    x-ray thickness g.
Gault test
gauntlet
gauss
gaussian
    g. curve
    g. distribution
Gauss sign
gauze
    absorbable g.
    absorbent g.
    antiseptic g.
    iodoform g.
    Kling g.
    petrolatum g.
    ribbon g.
    tulle gras g.
    Xeroform g.
    zinc gelatin impregnated
gavage feeding
Gavello operation
Gay glands
Gayet operation
Gaylor forceps
Gay-Lussac law
Gaynor-Hart position
gaze
    conjugate g.
    disconjugate g.
    g. movement
    g. palsy
    g. paretic nystagmus
GB—gallbladder

GBA—
    ganglionic-blocking agent
    gingivobuccoaxial
G-banding
GBG—
    glycine-rich β glycoprival
    glycine-rich β glycoprotein
GBGase—glycine-rich β
    glycoproteinase
GBH—graphite-benzalkonium-
    heparin
GBM—glomerular basement
    membrane
GBS—gallbladder series
GC—
    gas chromatography
    glucocorticoid
    gonococcus
    granular cast
    guanine cytosine
GCA—giant cell arteritis
g-cal—gram-calorie
g-cm—gram-centimeter
GCS—
    general clinical service
    Glasgow Coma Scale
G-CSF—granulocyte colony-
    stimulating factor
GDC—Guglielmi detachable coil
GDH—glycerophosphate
    dehydrogenase
GDS—gradual dosage schedule
GE—
    gastroenterology
    gastroenterostomy
    General Electric
G/E—granulocyte-erythroid ratio
GE scan
gear
    cervical g.
    head g.
Gee disease
Gee-Herter disease
Gee-Herter-Heubner
    disease
    syndrome
Gee-Thaysen disease
gefilte fish
Gegenbaur cell
gegenhalten
Gehrung pessary
Geiger counter
Geiger-Müller
    counter
    survey meter

Geiger-Müller *(continued)*
    tube
Geiger-Nuttall law
gel
    aluminum carbonate g., basic
    aluminum hydroxide g.
    aluminum hydroxide g.,
      dried
    betamethasone benzoate g.
    corticotropin g.
    fluocinonide g.
    polyacrylamide g.
    silica g.
    sodium fluoride and
      orthophosphoric acid g.
    sodium fluoride and
      phosphoric acid g.
    tolnaftate g.
    tretinoin g.
gelasmus
gelastic
gelate
gelatification
gelatigenous
gelatin
    g. compound phenolized
    g. compression boot
    formalin g.
    glycerinated g.
    medicated g.
    silk g.
    g. of Wharton
    zinc g.
gelatinase
gelatiniferous
gelatinize
gelatinoid
gelatinolytic
gelatinosa
gelatinous
gelatinum
gelation
gelatum
Gelfilm dressing
Gel Flex lens
Gelfoam
    cookie
    dressing
    packing
gelidusi
Gélineau syndrome
Gellé test
Gellhorn
    forceps
    pessary

Gelocast dressing
gelometer
gelose
gelosis
gelotripsy
Gelpi retractor
Gelpi-Lowrie forceps
gelsemine
gelsemism
Gély suture
Gemella haemolysans
gemellary
gemellipara
gemellology
geminate
gemination
    false g.
geminus (gemini)
    gemini aequales
gemistocytic
gemistocytoma
gemma
gemmangioma
gemmation
gemmule
gen.—general
gena
genal
gender
gene
    allelic g.
    amorphic g.
    antimutator g.
    autosomal g.
    g. bank
    cell interaction (CI) g's
    chimeric g.
    g. code
    codominant g.
    complementary g.
    g. complex
    control g.
    cumulative g.
    cytoplasmic g.
    derepressed g.
    dominant g.
    env g.
    gag g.
    H (histocompatibility) g.
    hemizygous g.
    holandric g.
    hologynic g's
    homeotic g.
    immune response (Ir) g's
    immune suppressor (Is) g's

gene *(continued)*
    immunoglobulin g's
    jumping g.
    leaky g.
    lethal g.
    major g.
    g. mapping
    marker g.
    mimic g.
    modifying g.
    mutant g.
    mutator g.
    nonstructural g's
    operator g.
    pleiotropic g.
    pol g.
    g. pool
    recessive g.
    reciprocal g.
    regulator g.
    regulatory g.
    repressed g.
    repressor g.
    resistance g.
    restorer g.
    Rh g.
    sex-conditioned g.
    sex-influenced g.
    sex-limited g.
    sex-linked g.
    silent g.
    split g.
    structural g.
    sublethal g.
    suicide g.
    supplementary g.
    suppressor g.
    switch g.
    syntenic g's
    taster g.
    tat g.
    transposable g.
    tRNA g.
    tumor-suppressor g.
    uninducible g.
    wild-type g.
    X-linked g.
    Y-linked g.
geneogenous
genera (plural of genus)
general
General Electric CT/T7 scanner
generalization
    stimulus g.
generalize

generation
    alternate g.
    asexual g.
    direct g.
    filial g.
    nonsexual g.
    parental g.
    second filial g.
    sexual g.
    spontaneous g.
    virgin g.
generation time
generative
generator
    asynchronous pulse g.
    atrial synchronous pulse g.
    demand pulse g.
    direct current g.
    electric g.
    electrostatic g.
    fixed-rate pulse g.
    molybdenum-technetium g.
    polyphase g.
    pulse g.
    12-pulse 3-phase g.
    radionuclide g.
    resonance g.
    standby pulse g.
    supervoltage g.
    technetium-99m g.
    three-phase g.
    Van de Graaff g.
    ventricular-inhibited pulse g.
    ventricular-triggered pulse g.
    x-ray g.
generic
genesial
genesic
genesiology
genesis
genesistasis
gene-splicing
genestatic
genetic code
geneticist
genetics
    bacterial g.
    behavioral g.
    biochemical g.
    clinical g.
    developmental g.
    human g.
    mathematical g.
    medical g.
    microbial g.

G

genetics *(continued)*
    molecular g.
    population g.
    reverse g.
    statistical g.
genetotrophic disease
genetous
Geneva Convention
Gengou phenomenon
genial
genian
genic
genicula (plural of
    geniculum)
genicular
geniculate body
geniculocalcarine tract
geniculotemporal
geniculum (genicula)
    g. canalis facialis
    g. of facial nerve
    g. nervi facialis
genin
geniocheiloplasty
genioglossus
geniohyoglossus
geniohyoid
geniohyoideus
genioplasty
genital
    g. ridge
    g. tract
genitalia
    ambiguous external g.
    external female g.
    external male g.
    indifferent g.
    internal g.
genitaloid
genitocrural
genitofemoral
genitography
genitoinfectious
genitoplasty
genitourinary
genius
Gennari
    band
    line
    stria
    stripe
genoblast
genocopy
genodermatology
genodermatosis

genome
    mitochondrial g.
genomic
genotoxic
genotype
genotypic
gentianophil
gentianophilic
gentianophobic
gentianose
gentian violet
gentisate
gentisic acid
gentle curettage
genu
    g. capsulae internae
    g. corporis callosi
    g. extrorsum
    g. of facial canal
    g. of facial nerve
    g. impressum
    g. of internal capsule
    g. internum radicis nervi
        facialis
    g. introrsum
    g. nervi facialis
    g. radicis nervi facialis
    g. recurvatum
    g. valgum
    g. varum
genua
genual
genucubital
genufacial
Genupak tampon
genupectoral
genus (genera)
genyplasty
geobiology
geochemistry
geode
geogen
geographic, geographical
geographic tongue
geomedicine
Geomedic prosthesis
geometric
    g. axis
    g. equator
    g. perspective
    g. prosthesis
geometrical efficiency
geometry
geometry factor
geopathology

geophagia
geophilic
George Lewis technique
geotactic
geotaxis
geotrichosis
Geotrichum candidum
geotropic
geotropism
gephyrophobia
GER—gastroesophageal
    reflux
Gerald forceps
geraniol
geranyl pyrophosphate
geratic
geratology
gerbil
GERD—gastroesophageal reflux
    disease
Gerdy
    fibers
    fontanelle
    ligament
    loop
gereology
Gerhardt
    change of sound
    disease
    phenomenon
    reaction
    sign
    test for acetoacetic acid
    test for urobilin in urine
Gerhardt-Semon law
geriatric
geriatrician
geriatrics
    dental g.
GERL—Golgi endoplasmic
    reticulum lysosomes
Gerlach
    network
    valve
Gerlier disease
germ
    dental g.
    enamel g.
    hair g.
    tooth g.
    wheat g.
germanium (Ge)
germerine
germ-free
germicidal

germicide
germicides
germinal
germination
germinative
germinoblast
germinocyte
germinoma
    pineal g.
germitrine
germline, germ line
geroderma osteodysplastica
gerodermia
gerodontic
gerodontics
gerodontist
gerodontology
geromarasmus
geromorphism
    cutaneous g.
gerontal
gerontin
gerontologist
gerontology
gerontophilia
gerontopia
gerontotherapeutics
gerontotherapy
gerontotoxon
gerontoxon
geropsychiatry
Gerota
    capsule
    fascia
    method
Gerson diet
Gerson-Herrmannsdorfer
    diet
Gerstmann syndrome
Gerzog speculum
Gesell developmental schedule
gestaclone
gestagen
gestalt, Gestalt
    Bender G. test
    g. psychology
    g. theory
    g. therapy
gestaltism
gestation
    abdominal g.
    exterior g.
    interior g.
gestational
    g. age

G

gestational *(continued)*
    g. sac
    g. trophoblastic neoplasia
gestodene
gestosis
gestrinone
GET—
    gastric emptying time
    general endotracheal
GET½—gastric emptying half-time
GET anesthesia
GeV, Gev—giga electron volt
GF—
    germ-free
    gluten-free
    grandfather
GFAP—glial fibrillary acidic
  protein
GFD—gluten-free diet
GFR—glomerular filtration rate
GG—gamma globulin
GGA—general gonadotropic
  activity
GGT— gamma-glutamyl
  transferase
GGTP—gamma-glutamyl
  transpeptidase
GH—growth hormone
GHB—γ-hydroxybutyric acid
  [gamma-]
GHD—growth hormone deficiency
GH-IH—growth hormone–
  inhibiting hormone
Ghon
    complex
    focus
    lesion
    tubercle
Ghon-Sachs bacillus
Ghormley operation
ghost
    erythrocyte g.
    g. ophthalmoscope
    red cell g.
    g. vessels in cornea
GH-RF—growth hormone–
  releasing factor
GH-RH—growth hormone–
  releasing hormone
GH-RIH—growth hormone
  release–inhibiting hormone
GHz—gigahertz
GI—
    gastrointestinal
    globin insulin

Gianelli sign
Giannuzzi
    bodies
    cells
    crescents
    demilunes
Gianotti-Crosti syndrome
giant cell
    g.c. arteritis
    g.c. epulis
    g.c. granuloma
giantism
Giardia
    G. intestinalis
    G. lamblia
giardiasis
    intestinal g.
gibberish
Gibbon
    hernia
    hydrocele
    stent
Gibbon and Landis test
gibbosity
gibbous
Gibbs-Donnan equilibrium
Gibbs free energy theory
gibbus
Gibert
    disease
    pityriasis
Gibney
    bandage
    boot
    disease
    perispondylitis
    strapping
Gibson
    incision
    irrigator
    murmur
    operation
    rule
    suture
    vestibule
Gibson-Balfour retractor
giddiness
Giemsa
    method
    stain
Giemsa-Wright stain
Gierke (von Gierke)
    cells
    corpuscles
    disease

Giertz-Shoemaker rib shears
Gifford
    applicator
    curet
    forceps
    operation
    reflex
    retractor
    sign
Gifford-Galassi reflex
gigabecquerel (GBq)
gigahertz (GHz)
gigantism
    acromegalic g.
    cerebral g.
    constitutional g.
    digital g.
    eunuchoid g.
    fetal g.
    hyperpituitary g.
    hypothalamic g.
    normal g.
    pituitary g.
    primordial g.
    total lipodystrophy and
      acromegaloid g.
gigantoblast
gigantomastia
gigantosoma
Gigli
    operation
    wire saw
GIK—glucose, insulin, and
    potassium
Gilbert
    cholemia
    disease
    sign
    syndrome
Gilbert-Behçet syndrome
Gilbert-Dreyfus syndrome
Gilbert-Lereboullet syndrome
Gilchrist
    disease
    mycosis
gildable
gilding
Giliberty prosthesis
Gill
    knife
    operation
Gilles de la Tourette
    disease
    syndrome
Gillespie operation

Gilliam operation
Gilliam-Doleris operation
Gillies
    flap
    graft
    hook
    operation
    up-and-down flap
Gillies-Dingman hook
Gillies-Fry operation
Gilmer
    splint
    wiring
Gimbernat
    ligament
    reflex ligament
ginger
gingiva (gingivae)
    alveolar g.
    areolar g.
    attached g.
    buccal g.
    cemental g.
    cemented g.
    cleft g.
    free g.
    interdental g.
    interproximal g.
    labial g.
    lingual g.
    marginal g.
    papillary g.
    septal g.
    unattached g.
gingival periodontal index (GPI)
gingivalgia
gingivally
gingivectomy
    Ochsenbein g.
gingivitis
    acute necrotizing ulcerative g.
      (ANUG)
    acute ulcerative g.
    acute ulceromembranous g.
    atrophic senile g.
    bismuth g.
    catarrhal g.
    cotton roll g.
    desquamative g.
    Dilantin g.
    diphenylhydantoin g.
    eruptive g.
    fusospirochetal g.
    gonococcal g.
    g. gravidarum

G

gingivitis *(continued)*
 hemorrhagic g.
 herpetic g.
 hormonal g.
 hyperplastic g.
 marginal g., generalized
 marginal g., simple
 g. marginalis suppurativa
 necrotizing ulcerative g.
 papillary g.
 phagedenic g.
 pregnancy g.
 puberty g.
 scorbutic g.
 streptococcal g.
 suppurative marginal g.
 tuberculous g.
 ulceromembranous g.
 Vincent g.
gingivoaxial
gingivobuccoaxial
gingivoglossitis
gingivolabial
gingivolinguoaxial
gingivoperiodontitis
 necrotizing ulcerative g.
gingivoplasty
gingivosis
gingivostomatitis
 herpetic g.
 necrotizing ulcerative g.
 white folded g.
gingivostomatosis
 white folded g.
ginglyform
ginglymoarthrodial
ginglymoid
ginglymus
 helicoid g.
 lateral g.
ginseng
Giordano operation
GIP—
 gastric inhibitory polypeptide
 gastrointestinal polyposis
Girard
 method
 operation
 procedure
 treatment
Giraud-Teulon law
girdle
 hip g.
 Hitzig g.
 limbus g.

girdle *(continued)*
 Neptune g.
 pectoral g.
 pelvic g.
 shoulder g.
 thoracic g.
 upper limb g.
 white limbal g. of Vogt
Girdlestone
 operation
 resection
Girdner electric probe
GIS—
 gas in stomach
 gastrointestinal system
GIT—gastrointestinal tract
githagism
gitogenin
gitoxigenin
gitoxin
GITT—glucose-insulin tolerance
 test
Giuffrida-Ruggieri stigma
Givens method
gizzard
Gjessing syndrome
GK—glycerol kinase
Gl—glucinium
GL—greatest length
GLA—gingivolinguoaxial
glabella
glabellad
glabellar
 g. frown line
 g. rotation flap
 g. tap reflex
 g. tap sign
 g. wrinkle
glabellum
glabrous
glacial
γ-lactone [gamma-]
gladiate
gladiolic acid
gladiolus
gladiomanubrial
glairin
glairy
gland
 absorbent g.
 accessory g.
 acid g's
 acinar g.
 acinotubular g.
 acinous g.

gland *(continued)*
 admaxillary g.
 adrenal g.
 adrenal g's, accessory
 aggregate g's
 aggregated g's
 Albarran g.
 albuminous g.
 alveolar g.
 anal g's
 anteprostatic g.
 aortic g's
 apical g's of tongue
 apocrine g.
 aporic g.
 areolar g's
 arterial g.
 arteriococcygeal g.
 arytenoid g's
 Aselli g's
 axillary g's
 Bartholin g.
 Bauhin g's
 Baumgarten g.
 Blandin g's
 Blandin and Nuhn g's
 blood g's
 blood vessel g's
 Boerhaave g's
 Bonnot g.
 Bowman g's
 brachial g's
 bronchial g's
 Bruch g's
 Brunner g.
 buccal g's
 bulbocavernous g.
 bulbourethral g.
 BUS (Bartholin, urethral, and
  Skene) g's
 cardiac g's
 carotid g.
 g's of the caruncle
 celiac g's
 ceruminous g's
 cervical g's of uterus
 cheek g's
 Ciaccio g's
 ciliary g's
 circumanal g's
 Cloquet g.
 closed g's
 Cobelli g's
 coccygeal g.
 coil g.

gland *(continued)*
 compound g.
 conglobate g.
 conjunctival g's
 convoluted g.
 Cowper g.
 cutaneous g's
 cytogenic g.
 ductless g.
 duodenal g's
 Duverney g.
 Ebner g's
 eccrine g.
 Eglis g's
 endocrine g.
 endoepithelial g.
 endometrial g's
 epithelial g.
 esophageal g's
 excretory g.
 exocrine g.
 follicular g's of tongue
 fundic g's
 fundus g's
 Galeati g.
 gastric g's
 gastroepiploic g's
 Gay g's
 genal g's
 genital g.
 gingival g's
 Gley g's
 globate g.
 glomerate g's
 glomiform g.
 glossopalatine g's
 gustatory g's
 guttural g.
 Haller g's
 Harder g's
 harderian g's
 haversian g's
 hedonic g's
 hemal g's
 hemal lymph g's
 hemolymph g's
 Henle g's
 heterocrine g.
 hibernating g.
 holocrine g.
 Home g.
 incretory g's
 inferior lacrimal g.
 inguinal g.
 intercarotid g.

G

gland *(continued)*
- intermediate g's
- interscapular g.
- interstitial g.
- intestinal g's
- intraepithelial g.
- intramuscular g's of tongue
- jugular g.
- Krause g.
- labial g's of mouth
- lacrimal g.
- lacrimal g's, accessory
- lactiferous g.
- g's of large intestine
- large sweat g.
- laryngeal g's
- lateral nasal g. of Stensen
- lenticular g's of stomach
- Lieberkühn g.
- lingual g.
- Littre g.
- Luschka g.
- lymph g.
- lymphatic g.
- lymph g's, extraparotid
- malar g's
- malpighian g's
- mammary g.
- mammary g., accessory
- mandibular g.
- Manz g.
- marrow-lymph g.
- master g.
- Mehlis g.
- meibomian g.
- merocrine g.
- mesenteric g's
- mesocolic g's
- metrial g.
- mixed g's
- molar g's
- Moll g.
- monoptychial g.
- Montgomery g.
- Morgagni g's
- g's of mouth
- mucilaginous g's
- muciparous g.
- mucous g.
- mucous g. of urethra
- multicellular g.
- myometrial g.
- Naboth g.
- nabothian g's
- nasal g's

gland *(continued)*
- g. of neck
- Nuhn g's
- odoriferous g's of prepuce
- oil g.
- olfactory g's
- oxyntic g's
- palatine g.
- palpebral g's
- pancreaticosplenic g's
- parafrenal g's
- parathyroid g.
- paraurethral g.
- parotid g.
- parotid g., accessory
- pectoral g's
- peptic g's
- Peyer g's
- pharyngeal g's
- Philip g's
- pineal g.
- pituitary g.
- Poirier g's
- polyptychic g.
- pregnancy g's
- prehyoid g's
- preputial g.
- prostate g.
- puberty g's
- pyloric g's
- racemose g's
- retrolingual g.
- retromolar g's
- Rivinus g.
- Rosenmüller g.
- saccular g.
- salivary g.
- Sandström g's
- Schuller g.
- sebaceous g.
- seminal g.
- sentinel g.
- seromucous g.
- serous g.
- Serres g's
- sex g.
- sexual g.
- g's of Shambaugh
- Sigmund g's
- simple g.
- Skene g.
- solitary g's
- splenoid g.
- splenolymph g.
- Stahr g.

gland *(continued)*
   staphyline g's
   subauricular g's
   sublingual g.
   submandibular g.
   submandibular salivary g.
   submaxillary g.
   subtrigonal g.
   sudoriferous g.
   sudoriparous g.
   superior lacrimal g.
   suprahyoid accessory thyroid g.
   suprarenal g.
   Suzanne g.
   sweat g.
   synovial g's
   target g.
   tarsal g.
   tarsoconjunctival g's
   Theile g.
   thymus g.
   thyroid g.
   thyroid g's, accessory
   g's of tongue
   tracheal g's
   trachoma g's
   tubular g.
   tubuloacinar g.
   tympanic g's
   Tyson g's
   ultimobranchial g's
   unicellular g.
   urethral g.
   urethral g's of male urethra
   uropygial g.
   uterine g's
   utricular g's
   vaginal g.
   vascular g.
   vesical g's
   vestibular g.
   vestibular g., greater
   vestibular g's, lesser
   Virchow g.
   vitelline g.
   vulvovaginal g.
   Waldeyer g's
   Weber g's
   Willis g.
   Wolfring g.
   g's of Zeis
   zeisian g.
   Zuckerkandl g.
glanderous
glanders

glandes
glandilemma
glandula (glandulae)
   g. adrenalis
   glandulae areolares
   g. arytenoidea
   g. atrabiliaris
   g. basilaris
   glandulae bronchiales
   glandulae buccales
   g. bulbo-urethralis
   g. cardiaca esophagi
   g. cardiaca gastrica
   glandulae ceruminosae
   glandulae cervicales uteri
   glandulae ciliares
   g. ciliares palpebrarum
   glandulae circumanales
   glandulae conjunctivales
   glandulae cutis
   glandulae duodenales
   glandulae endocrinae
   g. epiglottica
   glandulae esophageae
   glandulae gastricae
   glandulae gastricae propriae
   g. glomiformis
   g. gustatoria
   glandulae hepaticae
   g. incisiva
   g. intercarotica
   glandulae intestinales
   glandulae labiales
   g. lacrimalis
   glandulae laryngeae
   glandulae linguales
   g. mammaria
   glandulae molares
   g. mucosa
   glandulae nasales
   glandulae oesophageae
   glandulae olfactoriae
   glandulae oris
   glandulae palatinae
   glandulae parathyroideae
   g. parotidea
   glandulae pharyngeae
   glandulae pharyngeales
   g. pinealis
   g. pituitaria
   g. prostata
   g. prostatica
   glandulae pyloricae
   g. sacculi laryngis
   glandulae salivariae majores

G

glandula (glandulae) *(continued)*
>glandulae salivariae minores
>g. sebacea
>g. sebaceae palpebrarum
>g. seminalis
>g. seromucosa
>g. serosa
>glandulae sine ductibus
>g. sublingualis
>g. submandibularis
>g. sudorifera
>g. suprarenalis
>glandulae tarsales
>g. thyroidea
>glandulae tracheales
>g. trigoni vesicae
>glandulae tubariae
>g. tympanicae
>glandulae urethrales
>g. uropygialis
>glandulae uterinae
>g. ventriculi laryngis
>glandulae vestibulares minores
>g. vestibularis major

glandular
>g. cystitis
>g. metaplasia

glandule
glandulous
glans
>g. clitoridis
>g. of clitoris
>g. penis

glanular
Glanzmann
>disease
>thrombasthenia

glare
>direct g.
>indirect g.

glarometer
glaserian fissure
Glasgow
>Coma Scale (GCS)
>score
>sign

glass
>cover g.
>crown g.
>cupping g.
>flint g.
>lithium g.
>object g.
>optical g.
>quartz g.

glass *(continued)*
>test g.
>vita g.
>watch g.
>Wood g.

glass blower's emphysema
glasses
>bifocal g.
>contact g.
>crutch g.
>Franklin g.
>Frenzel g.
>Hallauer g
>hyperbolic g.
>safety g.
>trifocal g.

Glassman
>clamp
>forceps

Glassman-Allis forceps
glassy
glaucoma
>absolute g.
>acute angle-closure g.
>acute congestive g.
>air block g.
>angle-closure g.
>angle-recession g.
>aphakic g.
>apoplectic g.
>auricular g.
>capsular g.
>g. capsulare
>chronic narrow-angle g.
>chronic open-angle g.
>chymotrypsin-induced g.
>closed angle g.
>congenital g.
>congestive g.
>g. consummatum
>contusion g.
>Donders g.
>enzyme g.
>fulminant g.
>ghost cell g.
>hemolytic g.
>hemorrhagic g.
>incompensated g.
>infantile g.
>inflammatory g.
>inverse g.
>juvenile g.
>lenticular g.
>low-tension g.
>malignant g.

glaucoma *(continued)*
    melanomalytic g.
    narrow-angle g.
    neovascular g.
    noncongestive g.
    obstructive g.
    open-angle g.
    phacogenic g.
    phacolytic g.
    pigmentary g.
    postinflammatory g.
    primary g.
    primary open-angle g.
    prodromal g.
    pseudoexfoliative capsular g.
    pupillary block g.
    secondary g.
    simple g.
    g. simplex
    steroid g.
    traumatic g.
    vitreous-block g.
    wide-angle g.
glaucomatous
glaucosis
glaucosuria
glaukomflecken
glaze
GLC—gas-liquid chromatography
GlcNAc—*N*-acetylglucosamine
gleaned
Gleason
    grading score
    score on prostate carcinoma
Glénard disease
Glenn
    operation
    procedure
    shunt
    technique
Glenner
    forceps
    retractor
glenohumeral
glenoid
Gley
    cells
    glands
GLI—glucagon-like
  immunoreactivity
glia
    ameboid g.
    cytoplasmic g.
    g. of Fañanás
    fibrillary g.

gliacyte
gliadin
glial
gliamilide
gliarase
glicentin
glide
    mandibular g.
    occlusal g.
gliobacteria
glioblast
glioblastoma
    giant cell g.
    magnocellular g.
    g. multiforme
gliococcus
gliocyte
    retinal g's
gliocytoma
gliofibrillary
gliofibrosarcoma
gliogenous
glioma
    astrocytic g.
    g. endophytum
    ependymal g.
    g. exophytum
    extramedullary g.
    ganglionic g.
    heterotopic g.
    malignant peripheral g.
    mixed g.
    g. multiforme
    nasal g.
    optic g.
    peripheral g.
    pontine g.
    g. retinae
    g. sarcomatosum
    telangiectatic g.
gliomatosis
    cerebral g.
    g. cerebri
    peritoneal g.
    g. peritonei
gliomatous
glioneuroma
gliophagia
gliopil
gliosa
gliosarcoma retinae
gliosis
    basilar g.
    cerebellar g.
    diffuse g.

G

gliosis *(continued)*
 g. endometrii
 hemispheric g.
 hypertrophic nodular g.
 isomorphic g.
 lobar g.
 perivascular g.
 progressive subcortical g.
 spinal g.
 unilateral g.
 g. uteri
gliosome
γ-lipotropin [gamma-]
glischrin
glischruria
glissade
glissadic
Glisson
 capsule
 cirrhosis
 disease
 sling
glissonitis
glitter cell
global
globe
globefish
globi (plural of globus)
globidiosis
globin
globinometer
globoid
globose
globoside
globular
globulariacitrin
globule
 dentin g's
 Dobie g.
 Marchi g's
 milk g's
 Morgagni g's
 myelin g's
 polar g's
globulin
 AC g.
 accelerator g.
 alpha$_2$ g.
 antihemophilic g. (AHG)
 anti–human g. serum
 antilymphocyte g. (ALG)
 antithymocyte g. (ATG)
 antitoxic g.
 Bence Jones g.

globulin *(continued)*
 beta g.
 corticosteroid-binding g.
 cortisol-binding g.
 D antigen immune g.
 gamma g.
 hepatitis B immune g.
 human gamma g.
 immune g.
 immune human serum g.
 immune serum g.
 measles immune g.
 pertussis immune g.
 rabies immune g. (HRIG)
 Rh$_0$(D) immune g.
 T g.
 testosterone-estradiol–binding g. (TEBG)
 tetanus immune g.
 thyroxine-binding g.
 vaccinia immune g. (VIG)
 varicella-zoster immune g. (VZIG)
 vitamin D–binding g.
 g. X
 zoster immune g. (ZIG)
globulinuria
globulose
globulus (globuli)
 globuli ossei
globus (globi)
 g. abdominalis
 esophageal g.
 g. of the heel
 g. hystericus
 g. major epididymidis
 g. minor epididymidis
 g. pallidus; globi pallidi
glomangioma
glomangiosis
 pulmonary g.
glomectomy
glomera (plural of glomus)
glomerate
glomerular
 g. filtration rate
 g. insufficiency
 g. proteinuria
 g. sclerosis
glomeruli (plural of glomerulus)
glomerulitis
 focal g.
 segmental g.
glomerulonephritis
 acute g.

glomerulonephritis *(continued)*
    acute benign hemorrhagic g.
    acute diffuse g.
    acute non-poststreptococcal g.
    acute post-streptococcal g.
    anti–glomerular basement
      membrane (anti-GBM)
      antibody g.
    autoimmune g.
    chronic hypocomplementemic g.
    circulating immune-complex g.
    congenital chronic g.
    crescentic g.
    diffuse g.
    diffuse lupus g.
    diffuse proliferative g.
    extracapillary g.
    focal g.
    focal embolic g.
    focal necrotizing g.
    focal proliferative g.
    focal sclerosing g.
    IgA g.
    immune complex g.
    lobular g.
    lobulonodular g.
    lupus g.
    malignant g.
    membranoproliferative g.
    membranous g.
    mesangial IgA/IgG g.
    mesangiocapillary g.
    nodular g.
    postinfectious acute g.
    rapidly progressive g.
    segmental g.
    subacute g.
glomerulonephropathy
glomerulopathy
    diabetic g.
    membranous g.
    minimum change g.
glomerulosclerosis
    congenital g.
    diabetic g.
    diffuse g.
    focal segmental g.
    intercapillary g.
    nodular g.
glomerulose
glomerulotropin
glomerulotubular
glomerulus (glomeruli)
    caudal arterial g.
    glomeruli arteriosi cochleae

glomerulus (glomeruli) *(continued)*
    g. of kidney
    malpighian glomeruli
    g. of mesonephros
    nonencapsulated nerve g.
    olfactory g.
    g. of pronephros
    renal glomeruli
    glomeruli renis
    Ruysch glomeruli
glomic
glomoid
glomus (glomera)
    glomera aortica
    g. body
    g. caroticum
    carotid g.
    g. cell
    choroid g.
    g. choroideum
    coccygeal g.
    g. coccygeum
    cutaneous g.
    digital g.
    g. intravagale
    jugular g.
    g. jugulare
    neuromyoarterial g.
    g. tumor
    g. tympanicum
glossa
glossagra
glossal
glossalgia
glossanthrax
glossectomy
Glossina
    G. fuscipes
    G. morsitans
    G. pallidipes
    G. palpalis
    G. swynnertoni
    G. tachinoides
glossitis
    g. areata exfoliativa
    atrophic g.
    benign migratory g.
    chronic superficial g.
    Clarke-Fournier g.
    cortical superficial
      sclerotic g.
    g. dissecans
    exfoliative g.
    Fournier g.
    gummatous g.

G

glossitis *(continued)*
    Hunter g.
    idiopathic g.
    interstitial sclerous g.
    median rhomboid g.
    g. migrans
    Moeller g.
    monilial g.
    g. parasitica
    parenchymatous g.
    rhomboid g.
    g. rhomboidea mediana
    syphilitic g.
    ulceromembranous g.
glossocele
glossocinesthetic
glossocoma
glossodesmus
glossodynamometer
glossodynia
    g. exfoliativa
    psychogenic g.
glossoepiglottic
glossoepiglottidean
glossograph
glossohyal
glossohyoidal
glossokinesthetic
glossolalia
glossology
glossolysis
glossomantia
glossoncus
glossopalatinus
glossopathy
glossopexy
glossopharyngeal
    g. breathing
    g. nerve
glossopharyngeum
glossopharyngeus
glossophobia
glossophytia
glossoplasty
glossoplegia
glossoptosis
glossopyrosis
glossorrhaphy
glossoscopy
glossospasm
glossosteresis
glossotilt
glossotomy
glossotrichia
glottal

glottic
glottis (glottides)
    false g.
    intercartilaginous g.
    respiratory g.
    true g.
glottogram
glottograph
glottography
glottology
glove
    Biobrane g.
Glover
    clamp
    drainage system
    forceps
glover's suture
glow
    cathode g.
    g. modular tube
GLP—group living program
glucagon
    gut g.
glucagonoma
glucal
glucan
glucan-1,4α-glucosidase
    [-alpha-]
α-glucan glycosyl [alpha-]
glucaric acid
glucatonia
glucemia
gluceptate
gluciphore
Gluck
    incision
    rib shears
glucoascorbic acid
glucocerebrosidase
glucocerebroside
glucocerebrosidosis
glucocinin
glucocorticoid
glucofuranose
glucogenesis
glucogenic
glucoglycinuria
glucohemia
glucokinase
glucokinetic
glucokinin
glucolactone
glucolysis
glucolytic
gluconate

gluconeogenesis
gluconeogenetic
gluconic acid
gluconolactone
glucopenia
glucophenetidin
glucophore
glucophylline
glucoprotein
glucopyranose
glucoregulation
glucosamine
    acetyl g.
    g. sulfate
glucosaminephosphate
  isomerase
glucosan
glucose
    Brun g.
    fasting plasma g. (FPG)
    gamma g.
    liquid g.
    g. oxidase
glucose-1-phosphate
glucose-1-phosphate
  phosphodismutase
glucose-1-phosphate
  uridylyltransferase
glucose-6-phosphatase
glucose-6-phosphatase deficiency
glucose-6-phosphate dehydrogenase
  (G6PD)
glucose-6-phosphate dehydrogenase
  (G6PD) deficiency
glucose-6-phosphate isomerase
α-glucosidase [alpha-]
α-1,4-glucosidase deficiency
  [alpha-]
glucoside
glucosidolytic
glucosin
glucosinolate progoitrin
glucosteroid
glucosum
glucosyl
glucosylceramidase
glucosyltransferase
glucoxylose
glucuronate
glucuronic acid
β-glucuronidase [beta-]
β-glucuronidase deficiency [beta-]
glucuronide
glucuronide transferase
glucuronoside

glucuronosyltransferase
glucuronyl transferase
glue
    plasma g.
Gluge corpuscles
glutamate
glutamate decarboxylase
glutamate dehydrogenase
glutamate formiminotransferase
glutamate oxaloacetate
  transaminase
glutamate pyruvate transaminase
glutamic acid
glutamic-oxaloacetic transaminase
  (GOT)
glutamic-pyruvic transaminase
  (GPT)
glutamic semialdehyde
glutaminase
glutamine synthase
glutaminyl
glutaminyl-peptide-γ-
  glutamyltransferase
glutamyl
glutaral concentrate
glutaraldehyde
    g.-tanned bovine collagen
      tubes
    g.-tanned porcine heart valve
glutaredoxin
glutargin
glutaric acid
glutaryl-CoA synthetase
glutathione
glutathionemia
glutathione peroxidase
glutathione reductase
glutathione synthetase deficiency
glutathionuria
gluteal bonnet
gluten
    g. enteropathy
    g.-free diet
    g. sensitivity
glutenin
gluteofemoral
gluteoinguinal
glutethimide
gluteus
    g. maximus
    g. medius
    g. minimus
glutinous
glutitis
glutose

G

Gly—glycine
glycal
glycan
glycate
glycated
glycation
glycemin
glycentin
glyceraldehyde
glyceraldehyde-3-phosphate
glyceraldehyde-3-phosphate
  dehydrogenase (GAPD)
glycerate
glyceric acid
glyceridase
glyceride
glycerin
    g. of alum
    g. of boric acid
    compound g. of thymol
    g. of ichthammol
    g. of lead subacetate
    g. of pepsin
    phenol g.
    starch g.
glycerinated
glycerinum
glycerite
    starch g.
    tannic acid g.
glycerogel
glycerogelatin
glycerol
    iodinated g.
    g. kinase
    g. phosphate
glycerol-3-phosphate
  dehydrogenase
glycerolize
glycerone phosphate
glycerophilic
glycerophosphatase
glycerophosphate
    ferric g.
glycerose
glyceryl
    g. guaiacolate
    g. monostearate
    g. triacetate
    g. trinitrate
glycinamide ribonucleotide
glycinate
glycine (G; Gly)
    g. amidinotransferase
glycinemia

glycinin
glycinol
glycinuria
    de Vries-type renal g.
    hereditary g.
glycobiarsol
glycocalix, glycocalyx
glycochenodeoxycholate
glycochenodeoxycholic acid
glycocholate
glycocholic acid
glycoclastic
glycocyamine
glycogelatin
    hepatic g.
    tissue g.
glycogen
    hepatic g.
    tissue g.
glycogenase
glycogenesis
glycogenetic
glycogenic
glycogenolysis
glycogenolytic
glycogenosis
    brancher deficiency g.
    generalized g.
    hepatophosphorylase
      deficiency g.
    hepatorenal g.
    myophosphorylase
      deficiency g.
glycogenous
glycogen phosphorylase
glycogen phosphorylase
  kinase
glycogen storage disease
glycogen synthase
glycogen synthetase
glycogeusia
glycohemia
glycohemoglobin
glycol
    g. methacrylate
    polyethylene g.
glycolate
glycolic acid
glycolipid
glycoluric acid
glycolyl
glycolysis
glycolytic
glycometabolic
glycometabolism

glycone
glyconucleoprotein
glycopenia
glycopeptide
glycopexia
glycopexic
glycopexis
glycophilia
glycophorin
glycopolyuria
glycoprival
glycoprotein
    g. IIb/IIIa
    α_1-acid g.
    glycine-rich β g. (GBG)
    g. Mac-1
    g. p150,95
    P-g. (Pgp)
    variable surface g. (VSG)
glycoptyalism
glycopyrrolate
glycopyrronium bromide
glycoregulation
glycoregulatory
glycorrhachia
glycorrhea
glycosamine
glycosaminoglycan
glycosaminolipid
glycosecretory
glycosemia
glycosene
glycosialia
glycosialorrhea
glycosidase
glycoside
    N-g.
    cardiac g.
    cyanophoric g.
    sterol g.
glycosometer
glycosphingolipid
glycosphingolipidosis
glycostasis
glycostatic
glycosuria
    alimentary g.
    artificial g.
    benign g.
    diabetic g.
    digestive g.
    emotional g.
    epinephrine g.
    factitious g.
    hyperglycemic g.

glycosuria *(continued)*
    magnesium g.
    nervous g.
    nondiabetic g.
    nonhyperglycemic g.
    normoglycemic g.
    orthoglycemic g.
    pathologic g.
    phlorhizin g.
    pituitary g.
    renal g.
    toxic g.
glycosuric acid
glycosyl
glycosylated
    g. hemoglobin
glycosylation
glycosyltransferase
glycotaxis
glycotropic
glycuresis
glycuronic acid
glycuronide
glycuronuria
glycyl
glycylglycine
glycyltryptophan
Glycyphagus domesticus
glycyrrhiza
glycyrrhizic acid
glycyrrhizin
glykemia
glyoxal
glyoxalin
glyoxisome
glyoxosome
glyoxylate
glyoxylic acid
glyoxysome
g-m—gram-meter
GM—
    gastric mucosa
    general medicine
    geometric mean
    grandmother
    grand multiparity
GMA—glyceryl methacrylate
GMC—general medical council
GM-CSF—granulocyte-macrophage
  colony–stimulating factor
Gmelin test
GMK—green monkey kidney
GMP—
    guanochlor sulfate
    monophosphate

GMP— *(continued)*
    guanosine monophosphate
3′,5′-GMP, cGMP—cyclic guanosine
    monophosphate
GM&S—general medical and
    surgical
GMT—geometric mean titer
GMW—gram-molecular weight
GN—
    glomerulonephritis
    gram-negative
G/N—glucose-nitrogen ratio
gnat
    buffalo g.
    eye g.
    turkey g.
gnathalgia
gnathic
gnathion
gnathitis
gnathocephalus
gnathodynamics
gnathodynamometer
    bimeter g.
gnathodynia
gnathography
gnathologic
gnathology
gnathopalatoschisis
gnathoplasty
gnathoplegia
gnathoschisis
gnathosoma
gnathostat
gnathostatics
Gnathostoma spinigerum
gnathostomiasis
GNB—gram-negative bacilli
GNID—gram-negative
    intracellular diplococci
gnosia
gnosis
gnotobiology
gnotobiota
gnotobiote
gnotobiotic
gnotobiotics
gnotophoresis
gnotophoric
GnRF—gonadotropin-releasing
    factor
Gn-RH—gonadotropin-releasing
    hormone
Goa powder
GOE—gas, oxygen, and ether

Goebel-Stoeckel operation
Goeckerman treatment
Goelet retractor
Goffe operation
Goggia sign
Gohrbrand dilator
goiter
    aberrant g.
    adenomatous g.
    Basedow g.
    cabbage g.
    colloid g.
    congenital g.
    cystic g.
    diffuse g.
    diving g.
    endemic g.
    exophthalmic g.
    familial g.
    fibrous g.
    follicular g.
    intrathoracic g.
    iodide g.
    lingual g.
    lymphadenoid g.
    multinodular g.
    myxedematous g.
    nodular g.
    nontoxic g.
    papillomatous g.
    parenchymatous g.
    perivascular g.
    plunging g.
    retrovascular g.
    simple g.
    substernal g.
    suffocative g.
    thoracic g.
    toxic g.
    toxic multinodular g.
    vascular g.
    wandering g.
goitrin
goitrogen
goitrogenic
goitrogenicity
goitrogenous
goitrous
GOK—God only knows
gold (Au)
    g. Au 198
    g. aurothiosulfate
    cohesive g.
    colloidal g.
    fibrous g.

gold (Au) *(continued)*
  inlay g.
  mat g.
  radioactive g.
  g. sodium thiomalate
  g. sodium thiosulfate
  g. thioglucose
  g. toning
Goldbacher
  anoscope
  needle
  proctoscope
  speculum
Goldberg MPC
  mediastinoscope
Goldblatt
  clamp
  hypertension
  kidney
  phenomenon
Goldenhar syndrome
Golden sign
Goldflam disease
Goldflam-Erb disease
Goldman curet
Goldman-Kazanjian forceps
Goldmann applanation tonometer
Goldscheider
  percussion
  test
Goldstein
  cannula
  classification
  disease
  hematemesis
  hemoptysis
  rays
  retractor
  syndrome
  toe sign
Goldstein-Reichmann syndrome
Goldthwait
  brace
  operation
  sign
  symptom
Golgi
  apparatus
  cells
  complex
  corpuscle
  neuron
  organ
  stain
golgiosome

Goll
  column
  fasciculus
  fibers
  nucleus
  tract
Goltz
  experiment
  syndrome
  theory
Goltz-Gorlin syndrome
Gombault
  degeneration
  neuritis
Gombault-Philippe triangle
Gomco clamp
gomitoli
Gomori
  method
  stains
Gompertz
  formula
  law
gomphosis
gonad
  indifferent g.
  primitive g.
  streak g's
gonadal dysgenesis
gonadarche
gonadectomize
gonadectomy
gonadial
gonadoblastoma
gonadocentric
gonadogenesis
gonadoinhibitory
gonadokinetic
gonadoma
  dysgenetic g.
gonadopathy
gonadopause
gonadorelin
gonadotrope
gonadotroph
gonadotropic
gonadotropin
  chorionic g.
  equine g.
  human chorionic g.
    (HCG; hCG)
  human menopausal g. (hMG)
  pituitary g.
  pregnant mare serum g.
  g.-releasing hormone (Gn-RH)

G

gonaduct
gonagra
gonalgia
gonangiectomy
gonarthritis
gonarthrocace
gonarthromeningitis
gonarthrosis
gonarthrotomy
gonatocele
Gonda sign
gonecyst
gonecystis
gonecystitis
gonecystolith
gonecystopyosis
goneitis
gonepoiesis
gonepoietic
Gongylonema
    G. neoplasticum
    G. pulchrum
    G. scutatum
gongylonemiasis
gonia (plural of gonion)
gonial angle of mandible
Gonin operation
Gonin-Amsler marker
Goniobasis silicula
goniodysgenesis
goniolens
goniometer
    Carroll finger g.
    finger g.
    universal g.
goniometry
gonion (gonia)
gonion gradient
    g.g. coil
    g.g. magnetic field
goniophotography
gonioprism
    Allen g.
goniopuncture
gonioscope
gonioscopy
goniosynechia
goniotomy
gonitis
    fungous g.
    g. tuberculosa
gonoblennorrhea
gonocampsis
gonocele
gonochorism

gonococcal proctitis
gonococcemia
gonococci (plural of gonococcus)
gonococcic
gonococcide
gonococcocide
gonococcus
gonocyte
    primordial g.
gonocytoma
gonoduct
gonoducts
gonomery
gononephrotome
gonophage
gonophore
gonorrhea
    Neisseria g.
    oropharyngeal g.
    pharyngeal g.
    rectal g.
gonorrheal
gonoscheocele
gonotokont
gonotome
gonotoxemia
gonyalgia paresthetica
gonycampsis
gonycrotesis
gonyectyposis
gonyocele
gonyoncus
Gonzales blood group
Good rasp
Goodale-Lubin catheter
Goodall-Power operation
Goodell
    dilator
    law
    sign
Goodenough test
Goodfellow cannula
Goodhill forceps
Goodpasture
    stain
    syndrome
Goodsall rule
Good syndrome
Goodyear knife
Goormaghtigh
    apparatus
    cells
goose bump
gooseflesh, goose flesh
gooseneck deformity

Gopalan syndrome
Gordius
    G. aquaticus
    G. robustus
Gordon
    bodies
    forceps
    reflex
    sign
    splint
    symptom
    syndrome
    test
gorget
    Teale g.
Gorlin
    cyst
    formula
    sign
    syndrome
Gorlin-Chaudhry-Moss syndrome
Gorlin-Goltz syndrome
Gorlin-Psaume syndrome
Goslee tooth
Gosselin fracture
Gosset retractor
gossypol
GOT—glutamic-oxaloacetic
  transaminase
Gott prosthesis
Gottlieb
    cuticle
    epithelial attachment
Gottron
    papules
    sign
    syndrome
Gottschalk
    aspirator
    operation
    saw
Gottstein
    curet
    fibers
    process
gouge
    Alexander g.
    Andrews g.
    Cobb g.
    Derlacki g.
    Hibbs g.
    Holmes g.
    Kelley g.
    Meyerding g.
    Moore g.

gouge *(continued)*
    Todd g.
    Troutman g.
Gougerot triad
Gougerot-Blum
    disease
    syndrome
Gougerot-Carteaud syndrome
Goulard
    extract
    lotion
    water
Gould suture
Gouley catheter
Goulian mammaplasty
goundou
gout
    abarticular g.
    articular g.
    calcium g.
    chalky g.
    idiopathic g.
    irregular g.
    latent g.
    lead g.
    masked g.
    misplaced g.
    oxalic g.
    polyarticular g.
    primary g.
    regular g.
    renal g.
    retrocedent g.
    rheumatic g.
    saturnine g.
    secondary g.
    tophaceous g.
    visceral g.
gouty
Govons curet
Gowers
    attack
    column
    contraction
    disease
    fasciculus
    panatrophy
    phenomenon
    sign
    solution
    syndrome
    tract
Goyrand hernia
GP—
    general paresis

GP— *(continued)*
  general practice
  general practitioner
  glycoprotein
  guinea pig
  gutta-percha
GPA—grade-point average
GPAIS—guinea pig anti-insulin
  serum
GPC—giant papillary conjunctivitis
GPCR—G protein–coupled
  receptors
G6PD, G6PDH—glucose-6-
  phosphate dehydrogenase
GPI—
  general paralysis of the insane
  gingival periodontal index
  glucose phosphate isomerase
GPT—glutamic-pyruvic
  transaminase
GPUT—galactose phosphate uridyl
  transferase
gr.—grain(s)
GR—
  gastric resection
  glutathione reductase
GRA—gonadotropin-releasing
  agent
graafian
  g. follicle
  g. ovules
  g. vesicles
Graber-Duvernay operation
Gracey curet
gracile
gracilis muscle
gracilothalamic
g-rad—gram-rad
gradatim
Gradenigo syndrome
Gradenigo-Lannois syndrome
gradient
  g. of approach
  atrioventricular g.
  g. of avoidance
  axial g.
  concentration g.
  density g.
  magnetic g.
  mitral g.
  proton g.
  systolic g.
  ventricular g.
grading
  Karnofsky tumor g.

grading system
  Hyams g.s.
Gradle
  electrode
  operation
  retractor
graduate
graduated tenotomy
Graefe (von Graefe)
  cautery
  cystotome
  disease
  forceps
  hook
  knife
  needle
  operation
  sign
  syndrome
Graefenberg ring
graft
  accordion g.
  activated g.
  allogeneic g.
  alloplast g.
  animal g.
  anorganic bone g.
  aortofemoral bypass g.
  aortorenal bypass g.
  autochthonous g.
  autodermic g.
  autoepidermic g.
  autogenous g.
  autogenous vein g.
  autologous g.
  autologous fat g.
  autoplastic g.
  avascular g.
  axillofemoral bypass g.
  B g.
  B-B g.
  bifurcated vascular g.
  bifurcation g.
  Blair-Brown g.
  bolus tie-over g.
  bone g.
  Braun g.
  Braun-Wangensteen g.
  brephoplastic g.
  bridge g.
  B-W g.
  cable g.
  cantilever g.
  chessboard g.
  chondrocutaneous g.

graft *(continued)*
- chorioallantoic g.
- composite g.
- corneal g.
- coronary artery bypass g. (CABG)
- cross-leg g.
- crossover bypass g.
- cuffs g.
- cutis g.
- Dacron g.
- Dardik Bio g.
- Davis g.
- DeBakey g.
- delayed g.
- derma-fat-fascia g.
- dermal g.
- dermic g.
- dermis-fat g.
- diced cartilage g's
- Douglas g.
- Dragstedt g.
- epidermal g.
- Esser g.
- extracranial-intracranial bypass g.
- fascia g.
- fascial g.
- fascia lata g.
- fascicular g.
- fat g.
- femoral-femoral g.
- femoral-tibial bypass g.
- femoropopliteal bypass g.
- fiber glass g.
- filler g.
- free g.
- free gingival g.
- full-thickness g.
- full-thickness skin g.
- Gabarro g.
- Gillies g.
- glutaraldehyde-tanned bovine carotid artery g.
- Gore-Tex g.
- heterodermic g.
- heterogenous g.
- heterologous g.
- heteroplastic g.
- heterotopic g.
- homogenous g.
- homologous g.
- homoplastic g.
- hyperplastic g.
- ileal g.

graft *(continued)*
- iliac g.
- inlay g.
- interposition g.
- island g.
- isogeneic g.
- isologous g.
- isoplastic g.
- jump g.
- Kebab g.
- Kiel bone g.
- König (Koenig) g.
- Krause-Wolfe g.
- lamellar g.
- Marlex g.
- mesh g.
- mesocaval H g.
- microvascular free g.
- mucosal g.
- nerve g.
- Nicoll bone g.
- Ollier-Thiersch g.
- omental g.
- onlay g.
- onlay bone g.
- orthotopic g.
- osseous g.
- outlay g.
- Padgett g.
- panel g.
- parathyroid g.
- patch g.
- pedicle g.
- pedicled bone g.
- penetrating g.
- periosteal g.
- Phemister g.
- pigskin g.
- pinch g.
- polytetrafluoroethylene (PTFE) g.
- preserved bone g.
- prosthetic vascular g.
- razor g.
- g. rejection
- Reverdin g.
- Russe bone g.
- saphenous vein bypass g.
- Seddon nerve g.
- seed g.
- sequential g.
- sheet g.
- sieve g.
- skin g.
- sleeve g.

G

graft *(continued)*
    snake g.
    splenorenal bypass g.
    split-rib g.
    split-skin g.
    split-thickness g.
    split-thickness skin g.
    stent g.
    syngeneic g.
    tantalum mesh g.
    Teflon g.
    thick-split g.
    Thiersch g.
    thin-split g.
    tube g.
    tunnel g.
    Van Millingen g.
    vascular g.
    vein g.
    Weavenit patch g.
    white g.
    Wolfe g.
    Wolfe-Krause g.
    xenogeneic g.
grafting
    interfascicular nerve g.
    mesh g.
    skin g.
graft-versus-host disease
  (GVHD)
Graham
    hook
    law
    test
Graham Little syndrome
Graham Steell murmur
grainage
grain (gr.)
graininess
Gram
    method
    solution
    stain
Gram-amphophilic
gram-atom
gram-calorie
gram-equivalent
gramicidin
gramine
graminin
graminivorous
gram-ion
grammeter
grammole
gram-molecule

gram-negative
gram-positive
gram-rad (g-rad)
gram-roentgen
grana
grandiose
grandiosity
grand mal
    g.m. epilepsy
    g.m. seizure
Grandry corpuscle
Granger
    line
    sign
granoplasm
Grant operation
Grant-Ward operation
granula iridica
granular
granularis
granulate
granulatio (granulationes)
    granulationes arachnoideae
    granulationes arachnoideales
    granulationes cerebrales
    granulationes pacchioni
granulation
    arachnoid g's
    arachnoidal g's
    Bayle g's
    Bright g's
    cell g's
    exuberant g's
    hypertrophic g.
    pacchionian g's
    pyroninophilic g's
    Reilly g's
    Virchow g's
granulationes (plural of granulatio)
granule
    acidophil g's
    acrosomal g.
    albuminous g's
    aleuronoid g's
    alpha g's
    amphophil g's
    argentaffine g's
    atrial g's
    azurophil g.
    Babès-Ernst g.
    basal g.
    basophil g.
    Bensley specific g's
    beta g's
    Birbeck g.

granule *(continued)*
 Bollinger g's
 bull's eye g.
 Bütschli g's
 carbohydrate g's
 chromatic g's
 chromophilic g's
 chromophobe g's
 cone g's
 cortical g's
 cytoplasmic g.
 delta g's
 dense g.
 dense core g.
 Ehrlich g's
 Ehrlich-Heinz g's
 elementary g's
 eosinophil g.
 Fauvel g.
 Fordyce g.
 fuchsinophil g's
 gamma g's
 glycogen g's
 Heinz g's
 hyperchromatin g.
 interstitial g.
 iodophil g's
 Isaac g's
 juxtaglomerular g's
 kappa g.
 keratohyalin g's
 Kölliker interstitial g's
 Kretz g's
 Langerhans g's
 Langley g's
 lipofuscin g.
 mast cell g.
 melanin g.
 membrane-coating g.
 meningeal g's
 metachromatic g.
 Much g's
 mucinogen g's
 mucous g.
 neurosecretory g.
 neutrophil g's
 Nissl g's
 oxyphil g's
 Palade g.
 Paschen g's
 perichromatin g's
 pigment g's
 polar g's
 proacrosomal g.
 protein g's

granule *(continued)*
 rod g's
 Schrön (Schroen) g.
 Schrön-Much g's
 Schüffner g's
 secondary g.
 secretory g's
 seminal g's
 specific atrial g's
 sphere g.
 sulfur g's
 tannophil g's
 thread g.
 toxic g's
 trichohyalin g's
 vermiform g's
 volutin g's
 yolk g's
 zymogen g.
granuliform
granuloadipose
granuloblast
granuloblastosis
granulocorpuscle
granulocytapheresis
granulocyte
 band-form g.
 heterophil g.
 neutrophil g.
 polymorphonuclear g.
 segmented g.
granulocytic
granulocytopathy
granulocytopenia
granulocytopoiesis
granulocytopoietic
granulocytosis
granulofatty
granuloma
 adjuvant g.
 alum g.
 amebic g.
 g. annulare
 apical g.
 aquarium g.
 beryllium g.
 candida g.
 candidal g.
 cholesterol g.
 chronic g.
 coccidioidal g.
 g. contagiosum
 dental g.
 g. endemicum
 eosinophilic g.

G

granuloma *(continued)*
    favic g.
    fish tank g.
    g. fissuratum
    foreign body g.
    g. fungoides
    g. gangraenescens
    g. gluteale infantum
    Hodgkin g.
    infectious g.
    g. inguinale
    intubation g.
    iodide g.
    g. iridis
    laryngeal g.
    lethal midline g.
    lipoid g.
    lipophagic g.
    lycopodium g.
    Majocchi g.
    malarial g.
    malignant g. of face
    g. malignum
    midline g.
    Miescher actinic g.
    Mignon eosinophilic g.
    monilial g.
    g. multiforme
    necrotic g.
    paracoccidioidal g.
    periapical g.
    plasma cell g.
    g. of prostate
    pseudopyogenic g.
    g. pudendi
    g. pudens
      tropicum
    pyogenic g.
    g. pyogenicum
    reticulohistiocytic g.
    rheumatic g's
    g. sarcomatodes
    septic g.
    silicotic g.
    swimming pool g.
    telangiectatic g.
    g. telangiectaticum
    trichophytic g.
    g. trichophyticum
    umbilical g.
    g. venereum
    Wegener g.
    xanthomatous g.
    zirconium g.

granulomatosis
    allergic g.
    beryllium g.
    bronchocentric g.
    chronic familial g.
    chronic X-linked g.
    g. disciformis progressiva et
      chronica
    Langerhans cell g.
    lipid g.
    lipophagic intestinal g.
    lymphomatoid g.
    malignant g.
    Miescher-Leder g.
    necrotizing respiratory g.
    pulmonary g.
    reticuloendothelial g.
    sarcoid g.
    g. siderotica
    Wegener g.
granulomatous
    g. prostatitis
    g. reaction
    g. rosacea
    g. uveitis
    g. vasculitis
granulomere
granulopenia
granulopexy
granuloplasm
granuloplastic
granulopoiesis
granulopoietic
granulopoietin
granulopotent
granulosa
    g. lutein
    g.–theca cell tumor
granulose
granulosis rubra nasi
granulosity
granulovacuolar
granum
grape
    Carswell g's
graph
graphesthesia
graphic
graphite pneumoconiosis
graphitosis
graphoanalysis
graphokinesthetic
graphology
graphomotor

graphorrhea
graphospasm
GRAS—
    generally recognized
      as safe
    generally regarded as safe
Grashey
    aphasia
    position
grasping
    forced g.
grasp reflex
GRASS—gradient-recalled
  acquisition in a steady state
grass
    scurvy g.
Grasset
    law
    phenomenon
    sign
Grasset-Bychowski sign
Grasset-Gaussel-Hoover sign
Grasset-Gaussel phenomenon
GRASS pulse sequence
graticule
    eyepiece g.
gratification
grating
    diffraction g.
Gratiola officinalis
grattage
grave
    g. condition
    g. illness
gravedo
gravel
Graves
    disease
    ophthalmic disease
    scapula
    speculum
grave-wax
gravid
gravida
gravidarum
gravidic
gravidism
graviditas
    g. examnialis
    g. exochorialis
gravidity
gravidocardiac
gravidopuerperal
gravimeter

gravimetric
gravistatic
gravitation
gravitometer
gravity
    specific g.
    standard g.
gray
    central g.
    g. line
    g. matter
    periaqueductal g.
    perihypoglossal g.
    scale ultrasonography
    silver g.
    steel g.
Gray forceps
gray-out
grease
grease-heel
great vessels
green
    acid g.
    brilliant g.
    bromcresol g.
    diamond g.
    diazin g. S
    ethyl g.
    fast g. FCF
    fast acid g. N
    Hoffman g.
    indocyanine g.
    Janus g. B
    light g. 2 G
    light g. 2 GN
    light g. N
    light g. SF yellowish
    malachite g.
    malachite g. G
    methyl g.
    methylene g.
    new solid g.
    Paris g.
    Schweinfurt g.
    solid g.
    solid g. O
    Victoria g.
Green [eponym]
    calipers
    curet
    dissector
    forceps
    hook
    knife

G

Green [eponym] *(continued)*
    needle holder
    replacer
    retractor
Green-Armytage operation
Greene curet
Greenfield
    disease
    filter
    syndrome
Greenhow incision
Greenwood-Yule method
gregaloid
Gregg syndrome
Greig syndrome
Greiling tube
Greither syndrome
grenz ray
Greulich and Pyle bone age staging
Grey Turner sign
GRF—gonadotropin-releasing
    factor
GRF; GH-RF—growth hormone–
    releasing factor
GRH; GH-RH—growth hormone–
    releasing hormone
Grice-Green operation
grid
    Amsler g.
    baby g.
    Bucky g.
    crossed g.
    fixed g.
    focused g.
    moving g.
    oscillating g.
    parallel g.
    Potter-Bucky g.
    stationary g.
    Thoms g.
    Wetzel g.
gridiron incision
Gridley stain
grief
Grieshaber
    keratome
    needle
    needle holder
    retractor
    trephine
Griesinger
    disease
    sign
    symptom
Griffith classification

Grignard reagent
grinders' disease
grinding
    night g.
    selective g.
    spot g.
grinding-in
grip
    devil's g.
    hook g.
    power g.
    precision g.
grip, grippe
    g. aurique
grippal
grisein
Grisel disease
gristle
Gritti
    amputation
    operation
Gritti-Stokes amputation
Grocco
    sign
    triangle
    triangular dullness
Groenholm retractor
Groenouw corneal dystrophy
grog
groin
Grollman pigtail catheter
grommet
Grönblad-Strandberg (Groenblad-
    Strandberg) syndrome
Grondahl-Finney operation
groove
    alveolobuccal g.
    alveololabial g.
    alveololingual g.
    anterior auricular g.
    anterolateral g.
    anteromedian g.
    arterial g's
    atrioventricular g.
    auriculoventricular g.
    basilar g.
    bicipital g.
    Blessig g.
    branchial g.
    buccal g.
    buccal developmental g.
    carotid g. of sphenoid bone
    cavernous g. of sphenoid bone
    central g.
    central developmental g.

groove *(continued)*
  cerebral g.
  chiasmatic g.
  costal g.
  deltopectoral g.
  developmental g's
  digastric g.
  distobuccal g.
  distobuccal developmental g.
  distolingual g.
  distolingual developmental g.
  duodenopyloric g.
  enamel g's
  ethmoidal g.
  g. for eustachian tube
  g. for facial artery on mandible
  free gingival g.
  genital g.
  hamular g.
  g. of helix
  inferior dental g.
  infraorbital g. of maxilla
  interatrial g.
  interdental g.
  interosseous g. of calcaneus
  intersphincteric g.
  intertubercular g. of humerus
  interventricular g., anterior
  interventricular g. of heart
  interventricular g., inferior
  interventricular g., posterior
  labial g.
  lacrimal g.
  laryngotracheal g.
  lateral phallic g.
  Liebermeister g's
  lingual g.
  lingual developmental g.
  g. of Lucas
  mastoid g.
  medullary g.
  meningeal g's
  mesiobuccal g.
  mesiobuccal developmental g.
  mesiolingual g.
  mesiolingual developmental g.
  musculospiral g.
  mylohyoid g.
  nail g.
  nasal g.
  nasolabial g.
  nasolacrimal g.
  nasomaxillary g.
  naso-optic g.
  nasopalatine g.

groove *(continued)*
  nasopharyngeal g.
  neural g.
  nuchal g.
  nutrient artery g.
  obturator g.
  occipital g.
  occlusal g.
  olfactory g.
  optic g.
  palatine g.
  palatomaxillary g.
  palatovaginal g.
  paracolic g.
  paraglenoid g's of hip bone
  pharyngeal g.
  pharyngotympanic g.
  popliteal g.
  posterior auricular g.
  preauricular g's
  preputiolabial g.
  primitive g.
  primitive dental g.
  pterygopalatine g.
  radial g.
  rhombic g.
  sagittal g.
  secondary branchial g.
  Sibson g.
  sigmoid g. of temporal bone
  sinus g.
  sphenobasilar g.
  spiral g.
  subclavius g.
  g. of subclavius muscle
  subcostal g.
  supplemental g's
  supra-acetabular g.
  g. suture
  tracheobronchial g.
  trigeminal g.
  tympanic g.
  ulnar g.
  urethral g.
  urogenital g.
  venous g's
  Verga lacrimal g.
  vertebral g.
  visceral g.
  vomerine g.
Groshong catheter
Gross
  clamp
  curet
  disease

G

Gross *(continued)*
    leukemia
    retractor
    spoon
    spud
    test
Gross-Pomeranz-Watkins retractor
grotesque
grotesquely
ground-glass
    g-g appearance
    g-g attenuation
    g-g density
    g-g inclusions
    g-g infiltrates
    g-g opacification
    g-g opacities
    g-g pattern
ground state
group
    alcohol g.
    alkalescens-dispar g.
    amide g.
    Arizona g.
    azo ġ.
    blood g.
    California g.
    closed g.
    CMN g.
    coli-aerogenes g.
    colon-typhoid-dysentery g.
    compatibility g.
    continuous g.
    control g.
    coryneform g.
    Diagnosis-Related Groups
      (DRG)
    dorsal respiratory g.
    encounter g.
    experimental g.
    functional g.
    glucophore g.
    hemorrhagic-septicemia g.
    incompatibility g.
    Kell-Cellano blood g.
    Kidd blood g.
    Lancefield g.
    leukocyte g.
    linkage g.
    Lutheran blood g.
    marathon g.
    methyl g.
    open g.
    osmophore g.
    paratyphoid-enteritidis g.

group *(continued)*
    peptide g.
    platelet g.
    PLT g.
    prosthetic g.
    reporter g.
    Runyon g.
    saccharide g.
    sapophore g.
    sensitivity g.
    sensitivity training g.
    sulfonic g.
    T-g.
    training g.
    ventral respiratory g.
    ventral thalamic g.
grouping
    blood g.
    haptenic g.
group-specific
group-transfer
growth
    absolute g.
    accretionary g.
    allometric g.
    appositional g.
    auxetic g.
    balanced g.
    condylar g.
    confluent g.
    g. cycle
    differential g.
    g. fraction
    heterogonous g.
    histiotypic g.
    g. hormone
    interstitial g.
    intrauterine g. retardation
      (IUGR)
    intussusceptive g.
    isometric g.
    multiplicative g.
    organotypic g.
    relative g.
GRP—gastrin-releasing
   peptide
grübelsucht, gruebelsucht
Gruber
    bougie
    fossa
    hernia
    speculum
    suture
    test
Gruber-Landzert fossa

Gruber-Widal
    reaction
    test
gruel
Gruenwald forceps
Gruenwald-Bryant forceps
grumose
grumous
Grünbaum-Widal (Gruenbaum-Widal) test
Grünfelder (Gruenfelder) reflex
grunting respirations in newborn
Grüntzig (Gruentzig)
    balloon-tip catheter
    catheter
    technique
Grynfeltt
    hernia
    triangle
Grynfeltt-Lesgaft triangle
gryochrome
gryphosis
gryposis
    g. penis
    g. unguium
GS—general surgery
G/S—glucose and saline
GSA—guanidinosuccinic acid
GSC—
    gas-solid chromatography
    gravity-settling culture
GSD—genetically significant dose
GSE—gluten-sensitive enteropathy
GSH—growth-stimulating hormone
GSR—
    galvanic skin response
    generalized Shwartzman reaction
GSSR—generalized Sanarelli-Shwartzman reaction
G-suit
GSW—gunshot wound
gt., gtt.—drop, drops (L. gutta, guttae)
GT—
    gingiva, treatment of
    glucose tolerance
    glutamyl transpeptidase
G&T—gowns and towels
GTH—gonadotropic hormone
GTN—
    gestational trophoblastic neoplasia
    glyceryl trinitrate

GTP—
    glutamyl transpeptidase
    guanochlor sulfate triphosphate
    guanosine triphosphate
GTP cyclohydrolase I
GTT—glucose tolerance test
GU—
    genitourinary
    gonococcal urethritis
guaiac
guanase
guanazolo
guanethidine
guanidase
guanidine-acetic acid
guanidinemia
guanidino
guanidinoacetic acid
guanidinosuccinic acid
guanido-acetic acid
guanidylate nucleotide
guanine
    g. deaminase
    g. nucleotide
guanosine
    cyclic g. monophosphate (cGMP)
    g. diphosphate (GDP)
    g. monophosphate (GMP)
    g. triphosphate (GTP)
guanylate cyclase
guanylic acid
guanyloribonuclease
guanylyl methylene diphosphonate
guarana
guaranine
guard
    bite g.
    mouth g.
    night g.
    occlusal g.
    Sachs g.
guarded chisel
guardian ad litem
guarding
Guarnieri
    bodies
    corpuscles
gubernacular
gubernaculum (gubernacula)
    chorda g.
    g. dentis
    Hunter g.
    g. testis

G

Gubler
    hemiplegia
    icterus
    line
    paralysis
    sign
    tumor
Gubler-Millard paralysis
Gubler-Robin typhus
Gudden
    commissure
    law
Guedel
    laryngoscope
    stage
Guelpa treatment
Guéneau de Mussy point
Guenther stain
Guepar prosthesis
Guérin
    fold
    fracture
    glands
    sinus
    valve
Guggenheim forceps
guaiacum resin
guidance
    child g.
    condylar g.
    contact g.
    incisal g.
guide
    adjustable anterior g.
    anterior g.
    condylar g.
    incisal g.
    light g.
    mold g.
guideline
    clasp g.
guidewire, guide wire
Guidi canal
Guild-Pratt speculum
Guilford stapedectomy
Guilford-Zimmerman personality
    test
Guillain-Barré
    polyneuritis
    reflex
    syndrome
Guilland sign
guillotine
    g. incision
    Sluder g. tonsillectomy

guillotine *(continued)*
    Sluder-Sauer g.
    Sluder tonsillar g.
    tonsil g.
    g. tonsillectomy
Guinard
    method
    treatment
guinea pig
Guinon disease
Guisez tube
Guist implant
Guleke-Stookey
  operation
gulf
    Lecat g.
Gull
    disease
    renal epistaxis
gullet
Gullstrand
    law
    slit lamp
gulonic acid
L-gulonolactone
gulose
gum
    g. acacia
    animal g.
    g. arabic
    Australian g.
    g. benjamin
    g. benzoin
    blue g.
    g. camphor
    Cape g.
    g. dragon
    eucalyptus g.
    free g.
    ghatti g.
    g. guaiac
    guar g.
    Indian g.
    g. juniper
    karaya g.
    Kordofan g.
    mesquite g.
    g. opium
    red g.
    g. senegal
    sterculia g.
    g. thus
    g. tragacanth
    wattle g.
    xanthan g.

gumboil
Gumboro disease
gumma (gummas, gummata)
    tuberculous g.
gummate
gummatous meningitis
gummi
gummy
gum-resin
gun-barrel enterostomy
guncotton
Gunn
    dots
    law
    phenomenon
    pupillary phenomenon
    sign
    syndrome
Günzberg (Guenzberg) test
Günz (Guenz) ligament
gurney
GUS—genitourinary system
Gusberg curet
Gussenbauer
    operation
    suture
gustation
    colored g.
gustatism
gustatory
gustin
gustometer
gustometry
gut
    blind g.
    g. chromic suture
    postanal g.
    preoral g.
    primitive g.
    ribbon g.
    ribbon g. suture
    silkworm g.
    silkworm g. suture
    surgical g.
    tail g.
    tiger g. suture
Gutglass forceps
Guthrie
    formula
    muscle
    test
gutta (guttae)
    g. ophthalmicae
    g. rosacea
gutta-percha

guttata
guttate
    g. parapsoriasis
    g. psoriasis
guttation
gutter
    paracolic g.
    pleuroperitoneal g's
    synaptic g.
guttering
gut-tie
Guttmann
    retractor
    speculum
guttur
guttural
gutturophony
gutturotetany
Gutzeit operation
Guyon
    amputation
    canal
    clamp
    dilator
    operation
    sign
    sound
Guyon-Péan clamp
guy suture
Guyton operation
Guyton-Friedenwald suture
Guyton-Maumenee speculum
Guyton-Park speculum
GV—gentian violet
GVH—graft-versus-host
GVHD—graft-versus-host disease
GVHR—graft-versus-host
    reaction
GW—group work
Gwathmey oil-ether anesthesia
Gy—gray(s)
gymnastics
    ocular g.
    Swedish g.
    vocal g.
Gymnema
gymnocarpous
gymnocyte
gymnoplast
gymnosperm
gymnospore
gymnothecium
gyn, GYN—gynecology
gynander
gynandrism

G

gynandroblastoma
gynandroid
gynandromorph
gynandromorphism
   bilateral g.
gynandromorphous
gynatresia
gynecic
gynecium
gynecogen
gynecogenic
gynecography
gynecoid
gynecologic, gynecological
gynecologist
gynecology
gynecomania
gynecomastia
   nutritional g.
   refeeding g.
   rehabilitation g.
gynecopathy
gynecophoral
gynecophoric
gyneduct
gynephilia
gynephobia
gynesin
gynogamon
gynogamone
gynogenesis
gynomerogon
gynomerogony
gynopathic
gynopathy
gynoplastic
gynoplastics
gynoplasty
gypsum
gyral
gyrase
gyrate
gyrate atrophy
gyration
gyrectomy
   frontal g.
gyrencephalic
gyri (plural of gyrus)
gyrochrome
gyromagnetic
gyromagnetic ratio
gyromele
gyrometer
gyrose
gyrospasm

gyrotrope
gyrus (gyri)
   angular g.
   g. angularis
   annectant gyri
   annectent gyri
   Broca g.
   callosal g.
   g. callosus
   central g., anterior
   central g., posterior
   g. centralis anterior
   g. centralis posterior
   cingulate g.
   g. cingulatus
   g. cinguli
   g. cunei
   cuneolingual g.
   deep transitional g.
   dentate g.
   g. dentatus
   g. descendens
   g. epicallosus
   external orbital g.
   g. fasciolaris
   g. fornicatus
   frontal g., ascending
   frontal g., inferior
   frontal g., middle
   frontal g., superior
   g. frontalis inferior
   g. frontalis medialis
   g. frontalis superior
   fusiform g.
   g. fusiformis
   g. geniculi
   gyri annectentes
   gyri breves insulae
   gyri cerebelli
   gyri cerebri
   gyri of cerebrum
   gyri insulae
   gyri olfactorii medialis et
     lateralis
   gyri orbitales
   gyri profundi cerebri
   gyri temporales transversi
   gyri transitivi cerebri
   Heschl gyri
   hippocampal g.
   g. hippocampi
   infracalcarine g.
   g. infracalcarinus
   internal orbital g.
   g. intralimbicus

gyrus (gyri) *(continued)*
  g. limbicus
  lingual g.
  g. lingualis
  long g. of insula
  g. longus insulae
  marginal g.
  marginal g. of Turner
  g. marginalis
  occipital g., inferior
  occipital gyri, lateral
  occipital g., superior
  occipitotemporal g., lateral
  occipitotemporal g., medial
  g. occipitotemporalis lateralis
  g. occipitotemporalis medialis
  g. olfactorius
  g. olfactorius medialis
  olfactory g., lateral
  olfactory g., medial
  orbital gyri
  g. orbitalis lateralis
  g. orbitalis medialis
  paracentral g.
  g. paracentralis
  parahippocampal g.
  g. parahippocampalis
  parahippocaudal g.
  parasplenial g.
  paraterminal g.
  g. paraterminalis
  parietal g.
  parietal g., ascending
  postcentral g.

gyrus (gyri) *(continued)*
  g. postcentralis
  postrolandic g.
  precentral g.
  g. precentralis
  preinsular gyri
  prerolandic g.
  g. rectus
  retrosplenal g.
  g. of Retzius
  g. rolandicus
  short gyri of insula
  splenial g.
  straight g.
  subcalcarine g.
  subcallosal g.
  g. subcallosus
  supracallosal g.
  g. supracallosus
  supramarginal g.
  g. supramarginalis
  temporal g.
  temporal g., inferior
  temporal g., middle
  temporal g., superior
  temporal gyri, transverse
  g. temporalis
  g. temporalis inferior
  g. temporalis medius
  g. temporalis superior
  uncinate g.
  g. uncinatus
GZ—Guilford-Zimmerman
GZ personality test

H

η—
  eta (Greek letter)
  absolute viscosity
[H⁺]—hydrogen ion concentration
h—hecto-
h.—hour (L. hora)
H—
  height
  high
  horizontal
  hormone
  Hounsfield unit

H— *(continued)*
  hour
  hydrogen
  hydrogen ion
  hypermetropia
  hyperopia
  hyperphoria
H.—Haemophilus
HA—
  headache
  height age
  hemadsorbent

HA— *(continued)*
   hemagglutinating antibody
   high anxiety
   hospital admission
   hyaluronic acid
   hydroxyapatite
HA1—hemadsorption virus, type 1
HA2—hemadsorption virus, type 2
HAA—hepatitis-associated antigen
Haab
   magnet
   reflex
   striae
HAART—highly active
  antiretroviral therapy
Haas
   operation
   position
Haase rule
habena (habenae)
habenal
habenar
habenula (habenulae)
   h. arcuata
   h. conarii
   habenulae perforatae
   Haller h.
   h. pectinata
   h. urethralis
habenular
Haber syndrome
Habermann disease
habilitation
habit
   clamping h.
   clenching h.
   endothelioid h.
   glaucomatous h.
   oral h.
   position h.
   tongue h.
habitat
habitual
habituation
habitus
   Buddha-like h.
   h. phthisicus
habu
HAD—hemadsorption
Hadfield-Clarke syndrome
HAdV—human adenovirus
  (serotypes A–F)
HAE—hereditary angioneurotic
  edema
H-Ae interval

Haemadipsa
   H. ceylonica
   H. chiliani
   H. japonica
   H. zeylandica
Haemaphysalis
   H. concinna
   H. humerosa
   H. leachi
   H. leporispalustris
   H. longicornis
   H. punctata
   H. spinigera
Haematobia irritans
Haematosiphon indorus
Haementeria officinalis
Haemodipsus ventricosus
Haemonchus contortus
Haemophilus
   H. aegyptius
   H. aphrophilus
   H. bovis
   H. ducreyi
   H. duplex
   H. equigenitalis
   H. gallinarum
   H. haemolyticus
   H. influenzae (type a, type b)
   H. paragallinarum
   H. parahaemolyticus
   H. parainfluenzae
   H. paraphrophilus
   H. parasuis
   H. somnus
   H. suis
   H. vaginalis
haemozoin
Haff disease
Hafnia alvei
hafnium (Hf)
Hagedorn
   needle
   operation
Hageman coagulation factor
Hagerty operation
Hagie pin
Haglund
   deformity
   disease
Hagner
   bag
   operation
Hahn operation
hahnemannian
hahnemannism

hahnium
Hahn sign
HAI; HI—hemagglutination
  inhibition (assay, test)
Haidinger brushes
Haig Ferguson forceps
Haight retractor
HAI; HI—hemagglutinin inhibition
Hailey-Hailey disease
Haines
    coefficient
    formula
    reagent
    test
hair
    auditory h.
    bamboo h.
    bayonet h.
    beaded h.
    burrowing h.
    club h.
    exclamation point h.
    Frey h's
    gustatory h's
    ingrown h.
    knotted h.
    lanugo h.
    moniliform h.
    h's of nose
    olfactory h's
    pubic h.
    resting h.
    ringed h.
    sensory h's
    stellate h.
    stinging h's
    tactile h's
    taste h's
    terminal h.
    twisted h.
    vellus h.
hairball
hair-on-end appearance
hairworm
hairy
    h. cell leukemia
    h. nevus
    h. tongue
Hajek
    chisel
    operation
    retractor
Hajek-Ballenger elevator
Hajek-Koffler forceps
Hajek-Skillern punch

halation
Halban
    disease
    sign
Halberg clip
Halbrecht syndrome
Haldane's law
Haldane-Priestley sampling
Hale forceps
half-cycle
half-hitch knot
half-layer
half-life
    antibody h.
    biological h.
    effective h.
    physical h.
    radioactive h.
half-moon
    red h.
half-thickness
half-time
    h. of exchange
    plasma iron clearance h.
half-value layer
halfway house
halide
halisteresis cerea
halisteretic
halitosis
halituous
halitus
Hall
    air drill
    band
    bur
    dermatome
    drill
    method
    neurotome
    sign
hallachrome
Hallauer glasses
Hallberg effect
Halle
    curet
    speculum
Hallé point
Haller (von Haller)
    ansa
    arch
    channel
    circle
    cone
    crypt

H

Haller (von Haller) *(continued)*
    duct
    fretum
    habenula
    insula
    layer
    line
    membrane
    plexus
    rete
    ring
    tripod
Hallermann-Streiff syndrome
Hallervorden-Spatz syndrome
Halle-Tieck speculum
Hallgren syndrome
Hallopeau
    acrodermatitis
    disease
Hallopeau-Siemens
    syndrome
Hall-Pallister syndrome
Hallpike maneuver
hallucal
halluces (plural of hallux)
hallucination
    auditory h.
    autoscopic h.
    blank h.
    depressive h.
    epileptic h.
    gustatory h.
    haptic h.
    hypnagogic h.
    hypnopompic h.
    kinesthetic h.
    lilliputian h.
    microptic h.
    olfactory h.
    h. of perception
    psychomotor h.
    reflex h.
    somatic h.
    stump h.
    tactile h.
    visual h.
hallucinative
hallucinatory
hallucinogen
hallucinogenesis
hallucinogenetic
hallucinogenic
hallucinosis
    acute alcoholic h.
    drug-induced h.

hallucinosis *(continued)*
    ethanolic h.
    organic h.
hallucinotic
hallux (gen. hallucis; pl.
    halluces)
    h. flexus
    h. malleus
    h. rigidus
    h. valgus
    h. varus
Hallwachs effect
halo
    anemic h.
    Fick h.
    h. glaucomatosus
    glaucomatous h.
    h.-pelvic traction
    peripapillary senile h.
    h. saturninus
    senile h.
    h. traction
halobacteria
halodermia
haloduric
halofenate
halogen
halogenation
halogeton
haloid
halometer
halometry
halophil
halophilic
halothane
haloxon
halquinols
Halsey needle holder
Halstead-Reitan
    battery
    test
Halsted
    clamp
    forceps
    hemostat
    incision
    operation
    radical mastectomy
    suture
halzoun
hamarthritis
hamartia
hamartial
hamartoblastoma
hamartochondromatosis

hamartoma
    chondromatous h.
    fetal h.
    intrapulmonary h.
    leiomyomatous h.
    h. of lung
    neuromuscular h.
    renal h.
    temporal h.
hamartomatosis
hamartomatous
hamate
hamatum
Hamburger
    interchange
    phenomenon
    test
Hamby retractor
Hamilton
    bandage
    method
    pseudophlegmon
    test
Hamm electrode
Hamman
    disease
    murmur
    sign
    syndrome
Hamman-Rich
    disease
    syndrome
hammer
    h. finger
    h. palsy
    Quisling hammer
    h. toe
Hammerschlag
    method
    test
hammock
    h. effect
    pelvic h.
Hammond
    syndrome
    disease
    operation
Hampton
    hump
    line
    maneuver
    view
hamster
    Syrian
        cardiomyopathic h.

hamstring
    inner h's
    lateral h.
    medial h's
    outer h.
Ham test
hamular
hamulate
hamulus
    h. cochleae
    h. of ethmoid bone
    frontal h.
    h. frontalis
    h. of hamate bone
    lacrimal h.
    h. lacrimalis
    h. laminae spiralis
    h. ossis hamati
    pterygoid h.
    h. pterygoideus
    trochlear h.
Hancock
    amputation
    M.O. II bioprosthesis porcine
        valve
    operation
    II porcine bioprosthesis
    II tissue valve
hand
    accoucheur's h.
    ape h.
    apostolic h.
    benediction h.
    Charcot h.
    claw h.
    cleft h.
    dead h.
    drop h.
    flat h.
    flipper h.
    frozen h.
    ghoul h.
    griffin-claw h.
    Krukenberg h.
    lobster-claw h.
    Marinesco succulent h.
    mirror h's
    mitten h.
    obstetrician's h.
    opera-glass h.
    phantom h.
    preacher's h.
    skeleton h.
    spade h.
    split h.

H

hand *(continued)*
  succulent h.
  trench h.
  trident h.
  writing h.
Hand [eponym]
  disease
  syndrome
handedness
  left h.
  right h.
handicap
handicapped
  perceptually h.
handle
  Beaver h.
  h. of malleus
Handley
  incision
  lymphangioplasty
  operation
handpiece
handprint
Hand-Schüller-Christian
  disease
  syndrome
handshaking
HANE—hereditary angioneurotic
  edema
Hanfmann-Kasanin test
Hanger test
hanging
  h.-drop test
  h. panniculus
hangman's fracture
hangnail
Hanhart syndrome
Hank dilator
Hank-Bradley dilator
Hannon curet
Hannover canal
Hanot
  cirrhosis
  disease
  syndrome
Hanot-Chauffard
  syndrome
Hansen
  bacillus
  disease
hanseniasis
Hansen-Street
  nail
  pin
Hansenula anomala

HAP—
  heredopathia atactica
    polyneuritiformis
  histamine phosphate acid
HAPA—hemagglutinating
  antipenicillin antibody
haphalgesia
haphephobia
Haplochilus panchax
haplodiploidy
haplodont
haploidentical
haploidentity
haploidy
haplomycosis
haplont
haplopathy
haplopia
Haplorchis taichui
haploscope
  mirror h.
haploscopic
haplosporangin
haplotype
Hapsburg
  jaw
  lip
hapten
  group A h.
haptenic
haptic
haptics
haptoglobin
haptometer
Harada
  disease
  syndrome
harara
harassment
hardening of arteries
Harden-Young ester
harderian
hard metal disease
hardness
  diamond pyramid h.
  indentation h.
  permanent h.
  temporary h.
Hardy-Rand-Ritter plates
Hardy-Weinberg
  equilibrium
  formula
  law
harelip
  bilateral h.

harelip *(continued)*
    lateral h.
    median h.
    h. suture
    unilateral h.
Hare syndrome
Hark operation
Harken
    forceps
    prosthesis
    rib spreader
harlequin fetus
Harley disease
harmaline
harmine
Harmon operation
harmonia
harmonic
harmony
    occlusal h.
    occlusal h., functional
harm's way
harness
    Pavlik h.
    shoulder h.
harpoon
Harrington
    forceps
    instrumentation
    nail
    operation
    retractor
    rod
    solution
Harrington-Mayo forceps
Harrington-Pemberton retractor
Harris
    forceps
    hematoxylin
    hematoxylin stain
    line
    migrainous neuralgia
    segregator
    separator
    staining method
    suture
    syndrome
    tube
Harris and Benedict standard
Harris-Beath operation
Harrison
    curve
    groove
    knife
    method

Harrison *(continued)*
    scissors
    sulcus
harrowing
Hart
    splint
    syndrome
Hartley-Krause operation
Hartman solution
Hartmann
    curet
    dewaxer speculum
    forceps
    fossa
    operation
    point
    pouch
    procedure
    punch
    rongeur
    speculum
    tuning fork
Hartmann-Citelli forceps
Hartmannella hyalina
hartmannelliasis
Hartmann-Gruenwald forceps
Hartmann-Herzfeld rongeur
Hartnup
    disease
    syndrome
hartshorn
Hartstein retractor
harvest
    organ h.
    saphenous vein h.
    tissue h.
Häser (Haeser)
    coefficient
    formula
HASHD—hypertensive
    arteriosclerotic heart disease
Hashimoto
    disease
    struma
    thyroiditis
hashish
Haslinger
    bronchoscope
    esophagoscope
    laryngoscope
    retractor
Hasner
    fold
    operation
    valve

H

Hassall
  bodies
  corpuscles
Hassall-Henle warts
HAT—hypoxanthine-aminopterin-
  thymidine
Hatcher pin
hatchet
  enamel h.
Haudek
  niche
  sign
haunch
hauptganglion of Kuttner
Hauser operation
haustellum
haustorium
haustra
haustra coli
haustral
haustration
haustrum (haustra)
  cecal h.
  haustra coli
  haustra of colon
haustus niger
haut-mal epilepsy
HAV—hepatitis A virus
Haven syndrome
Haverhill
  fever
  operation
Haverhillia
  H. moniliformis
  H. multiformis
haversian
  h. canal
  h. glands
  h. lamella
  h. space
  h. spaces
  h. system
Hawes-Pallister-Landor syndrome
Hawkins cervical biopsy forceps
hawkinsin
hawkinsinuria
Hawks-Dennen forceps
Hawley
  appliance
  retainer
Hayden curet
Hayem
  corpuscles
  encephalitis
  icterus

Hayem *(continued)*
  jaundice
  solution
Hayes clamp
hay fever
Haynes
  cannula
  operation
hayrake splint
hazard
Hb, Hgb—hemoglobin
HB—
  heart block
  hepatitis B
  housebound
HBB—hydroxybenzyl
  benzimidazole
HB$_c$—hepatitis B core
HBcAg—hepatitis B core antigen
HbCO—carboxyhemoglobin
HbCV—*Haemophilus influenzae*
  b conjugate vaccine
HBD, HBDH—hydroxybutyrate
  dehydrogenase
HB$_e$—hepatitis B e
HBeAg—hepatitis B e antigen
HBGV—hepatitis GB virus
HBI—high-serum-bound iron
HBLV—human B lymphotropic
  virus
HbO$_2$ [HBO2]—oxyhemoglobin
HBO—hyperbaric oxygen
HBP—high blood pressure
HbPV—*Haemophilus influenzae* b.
  polysaccharide vaccine
HB$_s$—hepatitis B surface
HBsAg—hepatitis B surface antigen
HBV—hepatitis B virus
HBW—high birthweight
HC—
  head compression
  hepatic catalase
  hospital corps
  hospital course
  house call
  hyaline cast(s)
  hydroxycorticoid
HCA—hypothalamic chronic
  anovulation
HCC—
  hepatocellular carcinoma
  hydroxycholecalciferol
β-hCG [beta hCG]
hCG; HCG—human chorionic
  gonadotropin

HCH—hexachlorocyclohexane
HCl—hydrochloric acid
HCL—hard contact lenses
HCM—hypertrophic
    cardiomyopathy
HCO₃ [HCO3]—bicarbonate
HCP—
    hepatocatalase peroxidase
    hereditary coproporphyria
Hct, hct—hematocrit
HCT—homocytotrophic
HCTZ—hydrochlorothiazide
HCU—homocystinuria
HD—
    hearing distance
    high dosage
HDC—histidine decarboxylase
HDCV—human diploid cell (rabies)
    vaccine
HDL—high-density lipoprotein
HDL₁—Lp(a) lipoprotein
HDL-C—high-density–lipoprotein
    cholesterol
HDLW—distance at which a watch
    is heard by the left ear
HDN—hemolytic disease of the
    newborn
HDRW—distance at which a watch
    is heard by the right ear
HDV—hepatitis D virus
HE—
    hereditary elliptocytosis
    human enteric
H&E—hematoxylin and eosin
    (stain)
head
    articular h.
    h. of astragalus
    box h.
    h. of caudate nucleus
    drum h.
    engaged h.
    h. of epididymis
    h. of femur
    h. of fibula
    floating h.
    hourglass h.
    h. of humerus
    little h. of humerus
    little h. of mandible
    h. of malleus
    h. of mandible
    medusa h.
    h. of metacarpal
    h. of metatarsal

head *(continued)*
    h. of muscle
    h. of optic nerve
    overriding h.
    h. of pancreas
    h. of penis
    h. of phalanx of fingers
    h. of phalanx of foot
    h. of phalanx of hand
    h. of phalanx of toes
    radial h. of humerus
    h. of radius
    h. of rib
    saddle h.
    h. of spermatozoon
    h. of spleen
    h. of stapes
    steeple h.
    swelled h.
    h. of talus
    h. of thigh bone
    tower h.
    h. of ulna
    white h.
Head [eponym]
    classification
    reflex
    zones
headache
    anemic h.
    bilious h.
    blind h.
    cluster h.
    congestive h.
    cough h.
    drainage h.
    dynamite h.
    exertional h.
    fibrositic h.
    functional h.
    hat band h.
    helmet h.
    histamine h.
    Horton h.
    hyperemic h.
    jolt h.
    lumbar puncture h.
    meningeal h.
    migraine h.
    miners' h.
    Monday morning h.
    muscle contraction h.
    neuralgic h.
    nitroglycerin h.
    organic h.

H

headache *(continued)*
    orgasmic h.
    paraplegic h.
    postconcussional h.
    postspinal h.
    pressor h.
    puncture h.
    pyrexial h.
    reflex h.
    rhinogenous h.
    sick h.
    spinal h.
    spinal fluid loss h.
    symptomatic h.
    tension h.
    thunderclap h.
    toxic h.
    traction h.
    traumatic h.
    vacuum h.
    vascular h.
    vasomotor h.
headcap
headgear
    Kloehn h.
Head-Holmes syndrome
headhunter catheter
headlight
head nodding, head-nodding
headrest
    Shambaugh h.
head-tilt test
heal
healing
    h. by first intention
    h. by granulation
    h. by second intention
    h. by third intention
    faith h.
    mental h.
    h. per primam intentionem
      (L. by first intention)
    h. per secundam intentionem
      (L. by second intention)
health
    holistic h.
    occupational h.
    public h.
health maintenance organization
  (HMO)
healthy
Healy forceps
Heaney
    clamp
    curet

Heaney *(continued)*
    forceps
    needle holder
    retractor
    vaginal hysterectomy
Heaney-Ballantine forceps
Heaney-Kanter forceps
Heaney-Rezek forceps
Heaney-Simon retractor
hearing
    color h.
    double disharmonic h.
    monaural h.
    residual h.
    visual h.
hearing aid
hearing loss
    Alexander h.
    conductive h.
    pagetoid h.
    paradoxic h.
    sensorineural h.
    transmission h.
heart
    abdominal h.
    addisonian h.
    amyloid h.
    armored h.
    artificial h.
    athlete's h.
    athletic h.
    atrophic h.
    beer h.
    beriberi h.
    h. block
    boat-shaped h.
    bony h.
    booster h.
    bovine h.
    cervical h.
    chaotic h.
    crisscross h.
    drop h.
    dynamite h.
    encased h.
    extracorporeal h.
    h. failure
    fat h.
    fatty h.
    fibroid h.
    flask-shaped h.
    frosted h.
    goiter h.
    hairy h.
    hanging h.

heart *(continued)*
    horizontal h.
    hypertensive h.
    hyperthyroid h.
    hypoplastic h.
    icing h.
    intermediate h.
    intracorporeal h.
    irritable h.
    Jarvik h.
    kyphoscoliotic h.
    left h.
    luxus h.
    lymph h.
    mechanical h.
    h. murmur
    myxedema h.
    ox h.
    paracorporeal h.
    parchment h.
    pear-shaped h.
    pectoral h.
    pendulous h.
    pulmonary h.
    Quain fatty h.
    rheumatic h.
    right h.
    round h.
    sabot h.
    scleroderma h.
    semihorizontal h.
    semivertical h.
    soldier's h.
    stony h.
    suspended h.
    systemic h.
    tabby cat h.
    three-chambered h.
    thrush breast h.
    thyroid h.
    thyrotoxic h.
    tiger h.
    tiger lily h.
    tobacco h.
    Traube h.
    triatrial h.
    trilocular h.
    h. valve
    vertical h.
    wandering h.
    wooden-shoe h.
heartbeat
heart block
    arborization h.b.
    atrioventricular h.b.

heart block *(continued)*
    2:1 AV (atrioventricular) h.b.
    bifascicular h.b.
    bundle branch h.b.
    complete h.b.
    congenital h.b.
    divisional h.b.
    entrance h.b.
    exit h.b.
    fascicular h.b.
    first-degree h.b.
    incomplete h.b.
    interventricular h.b.
    intraventricular h.b.
    Mobitz h.b.
    partial h.b.
    peri-infarction h.b.
    sinoatrial h.b.
    sinoauricular h.b.
    subjunctional h.b.
    Wenckebach h.b.
heartburn
heart failure
    acute congestive h.f.
    backward h.f.
    congestive h.f.
    forward h.f.
    high-output h.f.
    left ventricular h.f.
    right ventricular h.f.
heart valve prosthesis
heartworm
HEAT—human erythrocyte
    agglutination test
heat
    atomic h.
    h. of compression
    conductive h.
    convective h.
    conversive h.
    dry h.
    h. of fusion
    latent h.
    latent h. of fusion
    latent h. of sublimation
    latent h. of vaporization
    molecular h.
    prickly h.
    radiant h.
    specific h.
    h. of sublimation
    h. of vaporization
Heath
    curet
    dilator

H

Heath *(continued)*
    expressor
    forceps
    operation
heating
    conductive h.
    convective h.
    conversive h.
    radiant h.
    reflex h.
    ultrasonic h.
heat-labile
heatstroke
heave
    parasternal h.
heaves
    dry h.
heavy chain disease
heavy-metal screening
heavy particle therapy
hebdomadal
hebephrenia
hebephrenic
Heberden
    angina
    arthropathy
    asthma
    disease
    nodes
    nodosities
    rheumatism
    sign
hebetic
hebetude
hebiatrics
heboid
Hebra
    disease
    ointment
    pityriasis
    prurigo
HEC—hydroxyergocalciferol
hecatomeral
hecatomeric
Hecht
    phenomenon
    pneumonia
hectic
Hector tendon
HED—Haut-Einheits-Dosis unit
    [of x-ray dosage]
Hedblom
    elevator
    retractor
Hedinger syndrome

hedonic
hedonism
hedonophobia
hedrocele
heel
    anterior h.
    basketball h.
    black h.
    contracted h.
    cracked h's
    gonorrheal h.
    painful h.
    policeman's h.
    prominent h.
    Thomas h.
heelstick hematocrit
heel-to-shin test
HEENT—head, eyes, ears, nose,
    and throat
Heerfordt
    disease
    syndrome
Heermann
    incision
    operation
Heffernan speculum
Hefke-Turner sign
Hegar
    dilator
    operation
    sign
Hegglin anomaly
Heiberg-Esmarch maneuver
Heidenhain
    cells
    law
    rods
    stain
Heifitz
    clip
    operation
height
    apex h.
    h. of contour
    h. of contour, surveyed
    cusp h.
    facial h.
    midparental h.
    sitting h.
    sitting suprasternal h.
    sitting vertex h.
    standing h.
Heilbronner
    sign
    thigh

Heim-Kreysig sign
Heimlich maneuver
Heine operation
Heine-Medin disease
Heineke operation
Heineke-Mikulicz
    gastroenterostomy
    operation
    pyloroplasty
Heintz method
Heinz
    bodies
    granules
Heinz-Ehrlich bodies
Heisrath operation
Heister
    diverticulum
    fold
    valve
Heitz-Boyer procedure
HEK—human embryo kidney (cell culture)
Hektoen phenomenon
HEL—human embryo lung (cell culture)
HeLa cells
Helbing sign
helcoid
helcology
helcoma
helcosis
Held
    end-bulb
    foot
    striae
helenine
helianthin
heliation
helical
helical suture
helicase
helicin
helicine
Helicobacter
    H. cinaedi
    H. fennelliae
    H. pylori
helicoid
helicopod gait
helicotrema
heliosin
heliosis
heliotherapy
heliotrope B
heliotropism

helium (He)
    h. dilution method
    h. equilibration time
    h. washout
helix (helices, helixes)
    α h. [alpha]
    double h.
    h. of ear
    h. multihead nuclear imaging system
    Watson-Crick h.
hellebore
    American h.
    black h.
    green h.
    white h.
Heller
    disease
    esophagomyotomy
    myotomy
    operation
    plexus
    test
Heller-Döhle disease
Heller-Nelson syndrome
HELLP syndrome (hemolysis, elevated liver enzymes, and low platelet count occurring in association with preeclampsia)
Helly
    fixative
    fluid
Helmholtz
    ligament
    theory
helminthagogue
helminthemesis
helminthiasis
    cutaneous h.
    h. elastica
helminthic disease
helminthicide
helminthism
helminthoid
helminthology
helminthoma
helminthous
Helmont speculum
heloma
    h. durum
    h. molle
helosis
helotomy
helper cell

H

helplessness
   learned h.
Helvetius ligaments
Helweg
   bundle
   tract
HEMA—hydroxyethyl
   methacrylate
hemachrome
hemachrosis
hemacytometry
hemadostenosis
hemadsorbent
hemadsorption
   mixed h.
hemadynamometry
hemafacient
hemagglutination
   indirect h.
   passive h.
   viral h.
hemagglutinative
hemagglutinin
   cold h.
   warm h.
hemagogic
hemagonium
hemal
hemalum
   Mayer h.
hemanalysis
hemangiectasia
hemangiectasis
hemangioameloblastoma
hemangioblast
hemangioblastoma
   cerebellar h.
   h. retinae
   retinal h.
   spinal h.
hemangioblastomatosis
hemangioendothelioblastoma
   benign h.
   malignant h.
hemangioendothelioma
   benign h.
   epithelioid h.
   infantile h.
   kaposiform h.
   malignant h.
   spindle cell h.
   h. tuberosum multiplex
   vertebral h.
hemangioendotheliosarcoma
hemangiofibroma

hemangiogliomatosis retinae
hemangiolymphangioma
hemangioma
   ameloblastic h.
   capillary h.
   h. cavernosum
   cavernous h.
   cirsoid h.
   h. congenitale
   h. hypertrophicum cutis
   h. of kidney
   macular h.
   multiple hemorrhagic h's
      of Kaposi
   h. planum extensum
   racemose h.
   renal h.
   sclerosing h.
   h. simplex
   strawberry h.
   h.-thrombocytopenia
      syndrome
   venous h.
   verrucous h.
   verrucous keratotic h.
hemangiomatosis
   h. retinae
   systemic h.
hemangiomyolipoma
hemangiopericyte
hemangiopericytoma
   h. of kidney
   renal h.
hemangiosarcoma
hemapheic
hemaphein
hemapheism
hemapheresis
hemapophysis
hemarthrosis
hemastrontium
hematal
hematapostema
hematein
hematemesis
   Goldstein h.
   h. puellaris
hematencephalon
hematic
hematid
hematidrosis
hematin
   acid h.
hematinemia
hematinic

hematinometer
hematinuria
hematite pneumoconiosis
hematobilia
hematobium (hematobia)
hematoblast
    Hayem h.
hematocele
    parametric h.
    pudendal h.
    rectouterine h.
    retrouterine h.
    scrotal h.
    vaginal h.
hematocephalus
hematochezia
hematochlorin
hematochromatosis
hematochylocele
hematochyluria
hematocoelia
hematocolpometra
hematocolpos
hematocrit (Hct, hct)
    heelstick h.
    large vessel h.
    mean circulatory h.
    total body h.
    whole body h.
    Wintrobe h.
hematocryal
hematocyanin
hematocyst
hematocytolysis
hematocytopenia
hematocytosis
hematocyturia
hematodialysis
hematodyscrasia
hematodystrophy
hematoencephalic
hematogenesis
hematogenic
hematogenous
hematogone
hematohyaloid
hematoid
hematoidin
hematologic, hematological
hematologist
hematology
hematolymphangioma
hematoma
    aneurysmal h.
    auricular h.

hematoma *(continued)*
    h. auris
    cystic h.
    dissecting h.
    epidural h.
    extradural h.
    intracerebral h.
    intramural h.
    nasal septum h.
    pelvic h.
    perianal h.
    perinephric h.
    puerperal h.
    retroperitoneal h.
    retrouterine h.
    subdural h.
    sublingual h.
    submental h.
    subungual h.
    tuberous subchorial h.
hematomanometer
hematomphalocele
hematomphalus
hematomyelia
hematomyelitis
hematomyelopore
hematonephrosis
hematonic
hematopenia
hematophage
hematophagia
hematophagous
hematophyte
hematophytic
hematopiesis
hematoplast
hematoplastic
hematopoiesis
    extramedullary h.
hematopoietic
hematopoietin
hematoporphyria
hematoporphyrin
hematoporphyrinemia
hematoporphyrinism
hematoporphyrinuria
hematorrhachis
    h. externa
    h. interna
hematorrhea
hematosalpinx
hematosarcoma
hematoscheocele
hematosepsis
hematospectroscope

H

hematospectroscopy
hematospermatocele
hematospermia
hematospherinemia
hematostatic
hematosteon
hematotoxic
hematotoxicosis
hematotoxin
hematotrachelos
hematotropic
hematotympanum
hematoxylin
    alum h.
    Delafield h.
    Ehrlich h.
    h. and eosin (H&E) stain
    Harris h.
    Heidenhain iron h.
    iron h.
    Mayer h.
    Weigert iron h.
hematozemia
hematozoa
hematozoan
hematuresis
hematuria
    angioneurotic h.
    benign recurrent h.
    Egyptian h.
    endemic h.
    essential h.
    false h.
    hereditary h.
    initial h.
    microscopic h.
    primary h.
    recurrent h.
    renal h.
    terminal h.
    total h.
    urethral h.
    vesical h.
heme
hemendothelioma
hemeralope
hemeralopia
Hemerocampa leukostigma
hemerythrin
heme synthase
heme synthetase
hemiacardius
hemiacephalus
hemiacetal
hemiachromatopsia
hemiacidrin

hemiagenesis
hemiageusia
hemiagnosia for pain
hemialbumose
hemialbumosuria
hemialgia
hemiamblyopia
hemiamyosthenia
hemianacusia
hemianalgesia
hemianencephaly
hemianesthesia
    alternate h.
    bulbar h.
    cerebral h.
    crossed h.
    h. cruciata
    mesocephalic h.
    peduncular h.
    pontile h.
    spinal h.
hemianopia
    absolute h.
    altitudinal h.
    bilateral h.
    binasal h.
    binocular h.
    bitemporal h.
    color h.
    complete h.
    congruous h.
    crossed h.
    equilateral h.
    heteronymous h.
    homonymous h.
    horizontal h.
    incomplete h.
    incongruous h.
    lateral h.
    nasal h.
    quadrant h.
    quadrantic h.
    relative h.
    temporal h.
    true h.
    unilateral h.
    uniocular h.
hemianopic
hemianopsia
hemianoptic
hemianosmia
hemiapraxia
hemiarthrosis
hemiasomatognosia
hemiasynergia
hemiataxia

hemiathetosis
hemiatonia
hemiatrophy
    facial h.
    progressive lingual h.
    Romberg progressive
     facial h.
hemiaxial
hemiballismus
hemibladder
hemiblock
hemibody
hemic
hemicanities
hemicardia
    h. dextra
    h. sinistra
hemicardius
hemicellulose
hemicentrum
hemicephalalgia
hemicephalia
hemicephalus
hemicephaly
hemicerebrum
hemichorea
    paralytic h.
    posthemiplegic h.
    preparalytic h.
hemichrome
hemicolectomy
    left h.
    right h.
hemicorporectomy
hemicorticectomy
hemicrania
hemicraniectomy
hemicraniosis
hemidecortication
hemidesmosome
hemidiaphoresis
hemidiaphragms
hemidysergia
hemidysesthesia
hemidystrophy
hemiectromelia
hemielastin
hemiencephalon
hemiencephalus
hemiepilepsy
hemifacial
hemifacial microsomia
hemigastrectomy
    h. and vagotomy (H&V)
hemigeusia
hemigigantism

hemiglossal
hemiglossectomy
hemiglossitis
hemiglossoplegia
hemignathia
hemihepatectomy
hemihidrosis
hemihydranencephaly
hemihypalgesia
hemihyperesthesia
hemihyperhidrosis
hemihypermetria
hemihyperplasia
hemihypertonia
hemihypertrophy
    facial h.
hemihypesthesia
hemihypogeusia
hemihypometria
hemihypoplasia
hemihypothermia
hemihypotonia
hemikaryon
hemiketal
hemilaminectomy
    Ballantine h. retractor
hemilaryngectomy
    horizontal h.
    vertical h.
hemilarynx
hemilateral
hemilesion
hemilingual
hemimacrocephaly
hemimacroglossia
hemimandible
hemimandibulectomy
hemimandibuloglossectomy
hemimaxillectomy
hemimelia
    axial h.
    fibular h.
    radial h.
    tibial h.
    transverse h.
    ulnar h.
hemimelus
hemimetabolous
hemin
heminephrectomy
heminephroureterectomy
hemiobesity
hemiopalgia
hemiopia
hemiopic
hemipagus

H

hemiparalysis
hemiparanesthesia
hemiparaplegia
hemiparesis
hemiparesthesia
hemiparetic
hemiparkinsonism
hemipelvectomy
hemipelvis
hemipeptone
hemiphalangectomy
hemiplacenta
hemiplegia
    h. alternans hypoglossica
    alternate h.
    alternating oculomotor h.
    ascending h.
    Avellis h.
    bulbar h.
    capsular h.
    cerebellar h.
    cerebral h.
    collateral h.
    congenital h.
    contralateral h.
    crossed h.
    h. cruciata
    facial h.
    faciobrachial h.
    faciolingual h.
    flaccid h.
    functional h.
    Gubler h.
    hysterical h.
    infantile h.
    organic h.
    peduncular h.
    pontine h.
    spastic h.
    spinal h.
    superior alternate h.
    Wernicke-Mann h.
hemiplegic
hemiprosoplegia
hemiprostatectomy
hemipterous
hemipylorectomy
hemipyocyanin
hemipyonephrosis
hemirachischisis
hemisacralization
hemiscotosis
hemisection of spinal cord
hemisectomy
hemiseptum cerebri

hemisomus
hemisotonic
hemispasm
    facial h.
    glossolabial h.
hemisphere
    cerebellar h.
    cerebral h.
    dominant h.
    nondominant h.
    talking h.
hemispherectomy
hemispherium
    (hemispheria)
    h. bulbi urethrae
    h. cerebelli
    h. cerebralis
    h. cerebri
hemisphincter
    pharyngeal h.
hemisphygmia
Hemispora stellata
hemispore
hemisyndrome
hemiterata
hemiteratic
hemiterpene
hemitetany
hemithermoanesthesia
hemithorax
hemithyroidectomy
hemitomias
hemitonia
hemitoxin
hemitransfixion incision
hemitremor
hemivagotony
hemivertebra
hemizygosity
hemizygote
hemizygous
hemlock
    poison h.
    water h.
hemoaccess
hemobilia
hemobilinuria
hemoblast
    lymphoid h. of Pappenheim
hemocatheresis
hemocatheretic
Hemoccult
hemocholecyst
hemocholecystitis
hemochorial

hemochromatosis
  exogenous h.
hemochromatotic
hemochrome
hemochromogen
  hemoglobin h.
hemochromometer
hemochromometry
hemoclasia
hemoclasis
hemoclastic
hemoclip
hemocoagulin
hemocoel
hemocoelom
hemocoeloma
hemoconcentration
hemoconia
hemoconiosis
hemocrine
hemocryoscopy
hemoculture
hemocuprein
hemocyanin
  keyhole limpet h. (KLH)
hemocyte
hemocytoblast
hemocytocatheresis
hemocytogenesis
hemocytolytic
hemocytoma
hemocytometer
hemocytometry
hemocytophagia
hemocytophagic
hemocytopoiesis
hemocytotripsis
hemodiafiltration
hemodiagnosis
hemodialysis
  sequential ultrafiltration h.
  simultaneous h. and
    hemofiltration
hemodialyzer
  ultrafiltration h.
hemodiapedesis
hemodilution
hemodromography
hemodynamic
hemodynamics
hemodynamometry
hemodyscrasia
hemodystrophy
hemoendothelial
hemofilter

hemofiltration
  continuous arteriovenous h.
  simultaneous hemodialysis
    and h.
hemoflagellate
hemofuscin
hemogenesis
hemoglobin (Hb, Hgb)
  h. A
  h. A_{1c}
  h. A_2
  Bart h.
  h. C
  h. carbamate
  h. Chesapeake
  h. Constant Spring
  h. D
  deoxygenated h.
  h. E
  h. F
  fast h's
  fetal h.
  glycosylated h.
  Gower h.
  h. Gun Hill
  h. H
  homozygous h. C, D, E
  h. I
  h. J
  h. K
  h. Köln (Koeln)
  h. Lepore
  h. M
  mean corpuscular h.
  muscle h.
  h. N
  h. O
  oxidized h.
  oxygenated h.
  pyridoxilated stroma-free h.
  h. Rainier
  reduced h.
  h. S
  h. Seattle
  sickle h.
  slow h's
  unstable h.
  h. Yakima
  h. Zurich
hemoglobinated
hemoglobin C-thalassemia disease
hemoglobinemia
hemoglobin E-thalassemia disease
hemoglobinocholia
hemoglobinolysis

H

hemoglobinometer
Hemoglobinometry
hemoglobinopathy
hemoglobinopepsia
hemoglobinous
hemoglobinuria
    bacillary h.
    bovine h.
    intermittent h.
    malarial h.
    march h.
    paroxysmal cold h.
    paroxysmal nocturnal h. (PNH)
    toxic h.
hemoglobinuric
Hemogram
hemokinesis
hemokinetic
hemolymph
hemolymphadenosis
hemolymphangioma
hemolymphocytotoxin
hemolysate
hemolysin
    acid h.
    alpha h.
    bacterial h.
    beta h.
    cold h.
    delta h.
    gamma h.
    heterophile h.
    hot-cold h.
    immune h.
    natural h.
    specific h.
hemolysis
    alpha h.
    beta h.
    contact h.
    gamma h.
    immune h.
    osmotic h.
    passive h.
    siderogenous h.
    venom h.
    viridans h.
hemolytic
    h. anemia
    h. disease
    h. disease of the newborn
hemolyzable
hemolyzation
hemolyze
hemomanometer

hemomanometry
hemomediastinum
hemometer
hemomyelosis
hemonormoblast
hemopathic
hemopathology
hemopathy
hemoperfusion
    charcoal h.
    resin h.
hemopericardium
hemoperitoneum
hemopexin
hemophage
hemophagocyte
hemophagocytosis
hemophilia
    h. A
    h. B
    h. C
    classical h.
    Leyden h. B
    h. neonatorum
    vascular h.
hemophiliac
hemophilic
hemophilioid
hemophilus
    h. of Koch-Weeks
    h. of Morax-Axenfeld
hemophobia
hemophoresis
hemophthalmia
hemophthalmos
hemophthisis
hemopiezometer
hemoplasmopathy
hemopleura
hemopneumothorax
hemopoietin
hemoposia
hemoprecipitin
hemoproctia
hemoprotein
hemoprotozoa
hemopsonin
hemoptic
hemoptoic
hemoptysic
hemoptysis
    cardiac h.
    endemic h.
    Goldstein h.
    Manson h.

hemoptysis *(continued)*
    Oriental h.
    parasitic h.
    vicarious h.
hemopyelectasis
hemorepellant
hemorheology
hemorrhachis
hemorrhage
    accidental antepartum h.
    alveolar h.
    arterial h.
    blot h.
    brain h.
    capillary h.
    capsular h.
    capsuloganglionic h.
    cerebellar h.
    cerebral h.
    concealed h.
    critical h.
    dot h.
    Duret h.
    epidural h.
    essential h.
    expulsive h.
    external h.
    extradural h.
    fetomaternal h.
    fibrinolytic h.
    flame-shaped h's
    glomerular h.
    gravitating h.
    internal h.
    intracerebral h.
    intracranial h.
    intradural h.
    intramedullary h.
    intraparenchymal h.
    intrapartum h.
    intraventricular h.
    massive h.
    meningeal h.
    nasal h.
    neonatal subdural h.
    parenchymatous h.
    h. per rhexin
    petechial h.
    pontine h.
    postpartum h.
    primary h.
    pulmonary h.
    punctate h.
    putaminal h.
    recurring h.

hemorrhage *(continued)*
    renal h.
    salmon-patch h.
    secondary h.
    slit h.
    splinter h.
    spontaneous h.
    sternocleidomastoid h.
    subarachnoid h.
    subconjunctival h.
    subdural h.
    subgaleal h.
    subhyaloid h.
    thalamic h.
    unavoidable h.
    uterine h., essential
    venous h.
hemorrhagenic
hemorrhagic
    h. cystitis
    h. disease of newborn
    h. fever
    h. shock
    h. telangiectasia
hemorrhagin
hemorrhagiparous
hemorrheology
hemorrhoid
    combined h.
    external h.
    internal h.
    lingual h.
    mixed h.
    mucocutaneous h.
    prolapsed h.
    strangulated h.
    thrombosed h.
hemorrhoidal
hemorrhoidectomy
hemorrhoidolysis
hemosiderin
hemosiderinuria
hemosiderosis
    hepatic h.
    idiopathic pulmonary h.
    nutritional h.
    pulmonary h.
    transfusional h.
hemospermia
hemosporian
hemosporine
hemostasis
hemostat
    Avitene microfibrillar
      collagen h.

H

hemostat *(continued)*
    Corwin h.
    Dandy h.
    Dunhill h.
    Halsted h.
    Kolodny h.
    Maingot h.
hemostatic
    capillary h.
    return flow h. catheter
    h. sutures
hemostyptic
hemotherapeutics
hemotherapy
hemothorax
hemotoxicity
hemotoxin
    cobra h.
hemotroph
hemotrophic
Hemovac drain
hemozoin
hemozoon
hemp
    American h.
    Indian h.
hemuresis
henbane
hence
henceforth
Hench-Aldrich
    index
    test
Henderson operation
Henderson-Hasselbalch equation
Henderson-Jones disease
hendersonulosis
Hendrickson lithotrite
Henke
    space
    triangle
    trigone
Henle
    ampulla
    ansa
    canal
    cell
    fiber
    fissure
    gland
    internal cremaster
    layer
    ligament
    loop
    membrane

Henle *(continued)*
    reaction
    sheath
    sphincter
    spine
    tubules
Henle-Coenen sign
henna
Henneberg disease
Hennebert
    sign
    test
Henner retractor
Hennings sign
Henoch
    chorea
    disease
    purpura
Henoch-Schönlein (Henoch-
    Schoenlein, Henoch-Schonlein)
    purpura
    syndrome
henogenesis
Henrotin
    forceps
    speculum
Henry
    classification
    incision
    melanin test
    operation
    splenectomy
    system
Henry-Geist operation
Hensen
    body
    canal
    cell
    disk
    duct
    knot
    line
    node
Henshaw test
Hensing
    fold
    ligament
HEP—hepatoerythropoietic
    porphyria
HEPA—high-efficiency particulate
    air (filter)
hepar
    h. adiposum
    h. lobatum
    h. siccatum

heparan-α-glucosaminide *N*-acetyltransferase [-alpha-]
heparan *N*-sulfatase
heparan sulfate
heparan sulfate sulfamidase
heparan sulfate sulfatase
heparin
    h. calcium
    h. lock
    h. lyase
    h. sodium
heparinate
heparinemia
heparinize
heparitin sulfate
heparitinuria
hepatalgia
hepatatrophia
hepatectomize
hepatectomy
hepatic
    h. coma
    h. encephalopathy
    h. flexure
    h. vein catheterization
hepaticocholangiojejunostomy
hepaticocholedochostomy
hepaticodochotomy
hepaticoduodenostomy
hepaticoenterostomy
hepaticogastrostomy
hepaticojejunostomy
hepaticoliasis
hepaticolithotomy
hepaticolithotripsy
hepaticopulmonary fistula
hepaticostomy
hepaticotomy
hepatism
hepatitic
hepatitis (hepatitides)
    h. A
    acute h.
    acute parenchymatous h.
    aggressive h.
    alcoholic h.
    amebic h.
    anicteric h.
    autoimmune h.
    h. B
    h. B antigen
    h. B virus
    h. C
    cholangiolitic h.
    cholangitic h.

hepatitis (hepatitides) *(continued)*
    cholestatic h.
    chronic h.
    chronic active h.
    chronic aggressive h.
    chronic interstitial h.
    chronic persisting h.
    h. contagiosa canis
    h. D
    delta h.
    drug-induced h.
    h. E
    enterically transmitted non-A, non-B h. (ET-NANB)
    epidemic h.
    h. externa
    familial h.
    fulminant h.
    h. G
    giant cell h.
    halothane h.
    homologous serum h.
    infectious h.
    inoculation h.
    ischemic h.
    long-incubation h.
    lupoid h.
    neonatal h.
    neonatal giant cell h.
    non-A h.
    non-B h.
    peliosis h.
    plasma cell h.
    posttransfusion h.
    serum h.
    short-incubation h.
    subacute h.
    syphilitic h.
    toxic h.
    transfusion h.
    viral h.
hepatization
    gray h.
    red h.
    yellow h.
hepatized
hepatobiliary
    percutaneous h. cholangiography
    h. tract disease
hepatoblast
hepatoblastoma
hepatobronchial
hepatocarcinogenesis
hepatocarcinogenic

H

hepatocarcinoma
hepatocele
hepatocellular
hepatocerebral
hepatocholangeitis
hepatocholangiocarcinoma
hepatocholangioduodenostomy
hepatocholangioenterostomy
hepatocholangiogastrostomy
hepatocholangiojejunostomy
hepatocholangiostomy
hepatocholangitis
hepatocirrhosis
hepatocolic
hepatocuprein
hepatocystic
hepatocyte
hepatoduodenal
hepatoduodenostomy
hepatodynia
hepatodystrophy
hepatoenteric
hepatoenterostomy
hepatoflavin
hepatofugal
hepatogastric
hepatogenic
hepatogenous
hepatogram
    emission h.
    radionuclide h.
hepatography
hepatohemia
hepatoid
hepatojugular
hepatolenticular
hepatolenticular degeneration
hepatolienal
hepatolienography
hepatolienomegaly
hepatolith
hepatolithectomy
hepatolithiasis
hepatologist
hepatology
hepatolysin
hepatolysis
hepatolytic
hepatoma
    malignant h.
hepatomalacia
hepatomegalia glycogenica
hepatomegaly
    glycogenic h.

hepatomelanosis
hepatometry
hepatomphalocele
hepatomphalos
hepatonephric
hepatonephritic
hepatonephritis
hepatonephromegaly
hepatopancreas
hepatopath
hepatopathic
hepatopathy
hepatoperitonitis
hepatopetal
hepatopexy
hepatophage
hepatophlebitis
hepatophlebography
hepatopleural
hepatopneumonic
hepatoportal
hepatoptosis
hepatopulmonary
hepatorenal
hepatorrhagia
hepatorrhaphy
hepatorrhea
hepatorrhexia
hepatorrhexis
hepatoscan
hepatoscopy
hepatosis
    serous h.
hepatosolenotropic
hepatosplenic
hepatosplenitis
hepatosplenography
hepatosplenomegaly
hepatosplenometry
hepatosplenopathy
hepatostomy
hepatotherapy
hepatotomy
    transthoracic h.
hepatotoxemia
hepatotoxic
hepatotoxicity
hepatotoxin
hepatotropic
hepatovesicular
hepatozoonosis
heptachlor
heptachromic
heptad

heptadactyly
heptaene
heptanal
heptapeptide
heptatomic
heptavalent
heptoglobin
heptoglobinemia
heptose
heptosuria
herald
    patch
    plaque
herb
    death h.
    vulnerary h.
herbaceous
herbal
herbalist
Herbert
    operation
    pits
Herbert-Adams clamp
herbicide
herbivore
herbivorous
Herbst corpuscles
hereditary disease
heredity
    autosomal h.
    dominant h.
    sex-linked h.
    X-linked h.
heredoataxia
heredobiologic
heredoconstitutional
  disease
heredodegeneration
    spinocerebellar h.
heredodegenerative disease
heredodiathesis
heredofamilial
heredoimmunity
heredoinfection
heredolues
heredoluetic
heredopathia atactica
  polyneuritiformis
heredoretinopathia congenita
heredosyphilis
heredosyphilitic
heredosyphilology
Herellea vaginicola
heretofore

Herff clamp
Hering
    law
    nerve
    test
    theory
Hering-Breuer reflex
heritability
    broad sense h.
    narrow sense h.
heritable
heritage
Herlitz
    disease
    syndrome
Hermann-Perutz
    reaction
    test
Hermansky-Pudlak
    syndrome
Herman-Taylor gastroscope
hermaphrodism
hermaphrodite
    pseudo-h.
    true h.
hermaphroditic
hermaphroditism
    bilateral h.
    h. with excess
    false h.
    lateral h.
    ovotesticular h.
    protandrous h.
    protogynous h.
    spurious h.
    synchronous h.
    transverse h.
    true h.
    unilateral h.
Hermetia illucens
hermetic
hermetically
hernia
    abdominal h.
    acquired h.
    h. adiposa
    amniotic h.
    annular h.
    axial hiatal h.
    Barth h.
    Béclard h.
    Birkett h.
    h. of bladder
    Bochdalek h.

H

hernia *(continued)*
    h. of brain
    h. of broad ligament of
      uterus
    cecal h.
    cerebral h.
    h. cerebri
    Cheatle-Henry h.
    Cloquet h.
    complete h.
    concealed h.
    congenital h.
    congenital diaphragmatic h.
    Cooper h.
    crural h.
    diaphragmatic h.
    direct h.
    diverticular h.
    dry h.
    duodenojejunal h.
    encysted h.
    epigastric h.
    exomphalos h.
    external h.
    extrasaccular h.
    fat h.
    femoral h.
    foraminal h.
    funicular h.
    gastroesophageal h.
    Gibbon h.
    gluteal h.
    Goyrand h.
    Gruber h.
    Grynfeltt h.
    Hesselbach h.
    Hey h.
    hiatal h.
    hiatus h.
    Holthouse h.
    incarcerated h.
    incisional h.
    incomplete h.
    indirect h.
    infantile h.
    inguinal h.
    inguinocrural h.
    inguinofemoral h.
    inguinoproperitoneal h.
    inguinosuperficial h.
    h. in recto
    intermuscular h.
    internal h.
    interparietal h.
    intersigmoid h.

hernia *(continued)*
    interstitial h.
    intra-abdominal h.
    intraperitoneal h.
    irreducible h.
    ischiatic h.
    ischiorectal h.
    Krönlein h.
    labial h.
    Laugier h.
    levator h.
    linea alba h.
    Littré h.
    Littré-Richter h.
    lumbar h.
    h. of lung
    Maydl h.
    mesenteric h.
    mesocolic h.
    Morgagni h.
    mucosal h.
    h. of nucleus pulposus
    oblique h.
    obturator h.
    omental h.
    ovarian h.
    pantaloon h.
    paraduodenal h.
    paraesophageal h.
    parahiatal h.
    paraperitoneal h.
    parasaccular h.
    parastomal h.
    paraumbilical h.
    parietal h.
    pectineal h.
    perineal h.
    peritoneopericardial h.
    Petit h.
    pleuroperitoneal h.
    posterior vaginal h.
    prevascular femoral h.
    properitoneal h.
    pudendal h.
    pulsion h.
    rectal h.
    rectovaginal h.
    reducible h.
    retrocecal h.
    retrograde h.
    retroperitoneal h.
    retrosternal h.
    retrovascular h.
    Richter h.
    Rieux h.

hernia *(continued)*
    Rokitansky h.
    rolling h.
    sciatic h.
    scrotal h.
    Serafini h.
    sliding h.
    sliding hiatal h.
    slip h.
    slipped h.
    spigelian h.
    strangulated h.
    subpubic h.
    synovial h.
    tentorial h.
    thyroidal h.
    tonsillar h.
    transmesenteric h.
    Treitz h.
    h. of tunica albuginea
    tunicary h.
    umbilical h.
    h. uteri inguinalis
    uterine h.
    vaginal h.
    vaginolabial h.
    Velpeau h.
    ventral h.
    vesical h.
    voluminous h.
    w h.
hernial
herniary
herniated
    painful fat h.
    tonsillar h.
    uncal h.
herniation
    ascending transtentorial h.
    caudal transtentorial h.
    central h.
    cingulate h.
    descending transtentorial h.
    disk h.
    foraminal h.
    h. of intervertebral disk
    h. of nucleus pulposus
    painful fat h.
    rostral transtentorial h.
    subfalcial h.
    tentorial h.
    tonsillar h.
    tonsillar h. of nucleus pulposus
    transtentorial h.
    uncal h.

hernioappendectomy
hernioenterotomy
hernioid
herniolaparotomy
herniology
hernioplasty
    Cooper ligament h.
herniopuncture
herniorrhaphy
    Shouldice h.
herniotome
herniotomy
heroic
heroin
herpangina
herpes
    anorectal h.
    buccal h.
    h. catarrhalis
    h. corneae
    h. digitalis
    h. disseminatus
    h. facialis
    h. farinosus
    h. febrilis
    h. generalisatus
    genital h.
    h. genitalis
    h. gestationis
    h. gladiatorum
    h. zoster
    h. iridis
    h. labialis
    lingual h.
    h. meningoencephalitis
    menstrual h.
    h. menstrualis
    h. mentalis
    nasal h.
    neuralgic h.
    ocular h.
    h. odeus
    h. ophthalmicus
    orofacial h. simplex
    h. oticus
    pharyngeal h.
    h. pharyngitis
    h. phlyctaenodes
    h. praepuffalis
    h. praeputialis
    h. progenitalis
    h. recurrens
    recurrent h.
    h. simplex
    h. simplex recurrens

H

herpes *(continued)*
  h. tonsurans
  h. tonsurans
    maculosus
  traumatic h.
  h. varicella-zoster
    virus
  h. vegetans
  h. virus
  wrestler's h.
  h. zoster
  h. zoster auricularis
  h. zoster ophthalmicus
  h. zoster oticus
  h. zoster varicellosus
herpesencephalitis
Herpesvirus
  H. hominis
  H. simiae
  H. suis
herpesvirus
  h. B
  herpes whitlow h.
  h. simian B
herpetic
  h. proctitis
  h. whitlow
herpetiform
herpetiformis
  dermatitis h.
herpetologist
herpetology
herpetophobia
Herrick
  anemia
  clamp
Herring bodies
Herrmannsdorfer diet
hersage
Hers disease
Hertel exophthalmometer
Herter
  disease
  infantilism
  test
Herter-Heubner disease
Hertig-Rock ova
Hertwig sheath
Hertwig-Magendie
  phenomenon
  sign
  syndrome
hertz (Hz)
hertzian
  h. rays
  h. waves

Herxheimer
  fever
  fibers
  reaction
  spirals
Heryng sign
HES—hydroxyethyl starch
Heschl
  convolutions
  gyrus
hesperidin
Hess
  capillary test
  forceps
  operation
  spoon
Hess-Barraquer forceps
Hesselbach
  hernia
  ligament
  triangle
Hess-Horwitz forceps
Hess-Lees screen
HET—helium equilibration time
hetastarch
heteradelphia
heteradelphus
heteradenic
heteralius
heterauxesis
heteraxial
heterecious
heterecism
heterergic
heteresthesia
heterinoculation
heteroagglutination
heteroagglutinin
heteroalbumose
heteroalbumosuria
heteroallele
heteroallelic
heteroantibody
heteroantigen
heteroatom
heteroauxin
Heterobilharzi americana
heteroblastic
heterocellular
heterocentric
heterocephalus
heterochiral
heterochromatin
  constitutive h.
  facultative h.
  paracentric h.

heterochromatinization
heterochromatization
heterochromatosis
heterochromia
    binocular h.
    Fuchs h.
    h. iridis
    monocular h.
heterochromic
heterochromosome
heterochromous
heterochron
heterochronia
heterochronic
heterochthonous
heterochylia
heterocladic
heterocrine
heterocrisis
heterocycle
heterocyclic
heterocytotropic
heterodermic
heterodesmotic
heterodimer
heterodont
heterodromous
heteroduplex
heterodymus
heteroecious
heteroeroticism
heterofermentation
heterofermentative
heterofermenter
heterogamete
heterogametic
heterogamety
heterogamous
heterogamy
heteroganglionic
heterogeneity
    genetic h.
heterogeneous
heterogenesis
heterogenetic
heterogenic
heterogenote
heterogenous
heterogeusia
heteroglobulose
heterogonic
heterogony
heterograft
    bovine h.
    porcine h.
heterography

heterohemagglutination
heterohemagglutinin
heterohemolysin
heterohexosan
heteroimmune
heteroimmunity
heterointoxication
heterokaryon
heterokaryosis
heterokeratoplasty
heterokinesia
heterokinesis
heterolactic
heterolalia
heterolateral
heterolecithal
heteroliteral
heterolith
heterologous
heterology
heterolysin
heterolysis
heterolysosome
heterolytic
heteromastigote
heteromeric
heterometaplasia
heterometric
heterometropia
heteromorphosis
heteromorphous
heteronomous
heteronymous
hetero-osteoplasty
hetero-ovular
heteropagus
heteropancreatism
heteropathy
heteropentosan
heterophagosome
heterophagy
heterophany
heterophasia
heterophemia
heterophil
heterophile
heterophilic
heterophonia
heterophoralgia
heterophoria
heterophoric
heterophthalmia
heterophthalmos
Heterophyes
    H. brevicaeca
    H. heterophyes

H

Heterophyes (continued)
    H. katsuradai
heterophyiasis
heteroplasia
heteroplasm
heteroplastic
heteroplastid
heteroplasty
heteroploid
heteroploidy
Heteropoda venatoria
heteropodal
heteropolymeric
heteropolysaccharide
heteroprosopus
heteroproteose
heteropsia
heteropsychology
heteroptics
heteropyknosis
    negative h.
    positive h.
heteropyknotic
    negatively h.
    positively h.
heterosaccharide
heteroscedasticity
heteroscope
heteroscopy
heterosexual
heterosexuality
heterosis
heterosmia
heterosome
heterospecific
heterospore
heterosporous
heterosuggestion
heterotaxia
heterotaxic
heterothallic
heterothallism
heterotherapy
heterotherm
heterothermic
heterothermy
heterotonia
heterotonic
heterotopia
    nasal glial h.
    neuronal h.
heterotopic
heterotoxic
heterotoxin
heterotoxis

heterotransplant
heterotransplantation
heterotrichosis superciliorum
heterotroph
heterotrophia
heterotrophic
heterotrophy
heterotropia
heterotype
heterotypic
heterotypical
heterovaccine
heteroxenous
heteroxeny
heterozoic
heterozygosis
heterozygosity
heterozygote
    compound h.
    double h.
    inversion h.
    manifesting h.
heterozygous
HETP—hexaethyltetraphosphate
Heublein method
Heubner
    artery
    disease
    endarteritis
Heubner-Herter disease
heuristic
Heuter operation
hexabasic
hexabiose
hexacanth
hexachlorane
hexachlorobenzene
hexachlorocyclohexane
hexachloroethane
hexachlorophene
hexachromic
hexacosane
hexad
hexadactyly
hexadecanoate
hexadimethrine bromide
hexaene
hexafluorenium bromide
Hexagenia bilineata
hexahydric
hexamer
hexamethonium
    h. bromide
    h. chloride
hexamethylated

hexamethylenamine
hexamethylenaminesalicylsulfonic
  acid
hexamethylendiamine
hexamethyl violet
hexamitiasis
hexamylose
hexane
hexanoic acid
hexatomic
hexavaccine
hexavalent
hexavitamin
hexaxial
hexedine
hexenmilch
hexestrol
hexethal sodium
hexetidine
hexhydric sodium
hexobarbitone
hexobendine
hexocyclium methylsulfate
hexokinase
hexonate
hexone
hexonic acid
hexosamine
hexosaminidase
    h. A
    h. B
hexosan
hexosazone
hexose
hexose 1-phosphate
  uridylyltransferase
hexose
    h. diphosphate
    h. monophosphate
hexosediphosphoric acid
hexosephosphatase
hexosephosphate
hexosephosphate isomerase
hexose-1-phosphate
  uridylyltransferase
hexose phosphoric esters
hexosyltransferase
hexuronic acid
hexyl
Hey
    amputation
    derangement
    hernia
    internal derangement
    ligament

Hey *(continued)*
    operation
    skull saw
Heyer valve
Heyer-Schulte prosthesis
Hey Groves
    clamp
    operation
Heyman
    operation
    technique
Heymans law
Heynsius test
HF—
    Hageman factor
    heart failure
    high flow
    high frequency
HFI—hereditary fructose intolerance
HFP—hexafluoropropylene
Hg—mercury
Hgb, Hb—hemoglobin
HGBV—hepatitis GB virus
HGF—hyperglycemic-
  glycogenolytic factor
hGG—human gamma globulin
hGH; HGH—human growth
  hormone
Hg meralluride
HGPRT—hypoxanthine-guanine
  phosphoribosyl transferase
HGV—hepatitis G virus
HH—hydroxyhexamide
HHT—
    hereditary hemorrhagic
      telangiectasia
    hydroxyheptadecatrienoic acid
HI—
    hemagglutination inhibition
    high impulsiveness
    hydroxyindole
HIA—hemagglutination-inhibition
  antibody
5-HIAA—hydroxyindoleacetic acid
hiatal hernia
hiation
hiatopexy
hiatus
    adductor h.
    h. adductorius
    aortic h.
    h. aorticus
    Breschet h.
    buccal h.
    esophageal h.

hiatus *(continued)*
    h. esophageus
    h. of fallopian canal
    h. fallopii
    h. of Fallopius
    false h. of fallopian canal
    h. femoralis
    h. finalis sacralis
    h. hernia
    h. interosseus
    leukemic h.
    h. leukemicus
    h. lumbosacralis
    h. maxillaris
    neural h.
    h. oesophageus
    pleuropericardial h.
    h. pleuroperitonealis
    sacral h.
    h. sacralis
    saphenous h.
    h. saphenus
    Scarpa h.
    h. of Schwalbe
    semilunar h.
    h. semilunaris
    subarcuate h.
    h. tendineus
    tentorial h.
    h. totalis sacralis
    vena caval h.
    h. of Winslow
HIB—*Haemophilus influenzae*
  type b
HIB disease
HIB polysaccharide vaccine
Hibbs
    curet
    elevator
    forceps
    frame
    gouge
    operation
    osteotome
    retractor
hibernation
    artificial h.
hiccup
    epidemic h.
Hickey position
Hickman catheter
Hicks
    contractions
    sign
    version

HIDA—hepato-iminodiacetic acid
HIDA scan
hidebound
hidradenitis
    h. axillaris
    h. suppurativa
    suppurative h.
hidradenoid
hidradenoma
    clear cell h.
    eruptive h.
    papillary h.
    h. papilliferum
hidroa
hidroadenoma
    clear cell h.
    eruptive h.
    h. eruptivum
    papillary h.
hidrocystoma
hidropoiesis
hidropoietic
hidrorrhea
hidrosadenitis
    h. axillaris
    h. destruens suppurativa
hidroschesis
hidrosis
hidrotic
hiemal
hierarchy
    anxiety h.
hieric
hierolisthesis
high
    h. hyperopia
    h. lithotomy
high-density
high-density lipoprotein (HDL)
high-energy
highly selective vagotomy
Highmore
    antrum
    body
    corpus
highmori
    sinus maxillaris h.
high-risk
high-spin
high-spinal
HIHA—high impulsiveness, high
  anxiety
HI; HAI—hemagglutination
  inhibition (test)
hila

HILA—high impulsiveness,
  low anxiety
hilar
Hildebrandt test
Hildenbrand
    disease
    typhus
Hilgenreiner line
Hilger operation
hili
hilifuge
hilitis
Hill
    coefficient
    equation
    posterior gastropexy
    reaction
    sign
Hill-Ferguson retractor
Hillis retractor
Hillis-Müller maneuver
hillock
    anal h.
    auricular h's
    axon h.
    Doyère h.
    ear h's
    facial h.
    germ h.
    germ-bearing h.
    nerve h.
    seminal h.
Hilton
    law
    line
    muscle
    sac
hilum (hila)
    h. of adrenal gland
    h. of caudal olivary nucleus
    h. of dentate nucleus
    h. glandulae suprarenalis
    h. hepatis
    h. of inferior olivary nucleus
    h. of kidney
    h. lienale
    h. of lung
    h. of lymph node
    h. lymphoglandulae
    h. nodi lymphatici
    h. nodi lymphoidei
    h. nuclei dentati
    h. nuclei olivaris caudalis
    h. nuclei olivaris inferioris
    h. ovarii

hilum (hila) *(continued)*
    h. of ovary
    h. pulmonis
    renal h.
    h. renale
    h. renalis
    h. of spleen
    h. splenicum
    h. of suprarenal gland
hilus (hili)
    h. hepatis
    h. of kidney
    h. of lung
    h. of lymph node
    h. lymphoglandulae
    h. nodi lymphatici
    h. ovarii
    h. pulmonis
    h. renale
himantosis
Himmelstein valvulotome
hinchazon
hindbrain
hindfoot
hindgut
hind-kidney
hindwater
Hines-Brown
    rotating test
    test
hinge-bow
hinge osteotomy
Hinkle-James rectal speculum
Hinman reflux
Hinton test
hip
    h. pointer
    snapping h.
    total h. arthroplasty
hipped
Hippelates
    H. flavipes
    H. pallipes
    H. pusio
Hippel-Lindau disease
Hippeutis cantori
hippo
Hippobosca rufipes
hippocampal
hippocampus
    h. major
    h. minor
hippocoprosterol
hippocratic
    h. oath

H

hippocratic *(continued)*
    h. wreath
hippocratism
hippocratist
hippolite
hippolith
hippomane
hippomelanin
hippostercorin
hippulin
hippurate
hippuria
hippuric acid
hippuricase
hippus
hircismus
hircus (hirci)
Hirschberg
    magnet
    method
    reflex
    sign
Hirschfeld
    canals
    disease
    method
Hirschman
    anoscope
    forceps
    proctoscope
Hirschman-Martin
  proctoscope
Hirschowitz
    gastroduodenal fiberscope
    gastroscope
Hirschsprung disease
Hirst operation
Hirst-Emmett forceps
hirsute
hirsuties papillaris penis
hirsutism
    Apert h.
    constitutional h.
    idiopathic h.
Hirtz rales
hirudicidal
hirudicide
hirudin
hirudiniasis
    external h.
    internal h.
hirudinization
hirudinize
Hirudo
    H. aegyptiaca

Hirudo (continued)
    H. japonica
    H. javanica
    H. medicinalis
    H. quinquestriata
    H. sanguisorba
    H. troctina
His [eponym]
    band
    bundle of H.
    bursa
    canal
    disease
    duct
    isthmus
    rule
    space
    spindle
    tubercle
    zones
His-Held space
His-Purkinje
    conduction
    system
    tissue
Hiss capsule stain
histaminase
histamine
    $h._1$
    $h._2$
    h. acid phosphate
    h. challenge
    h. diphosphate
    h. phosphate
histamine-fast
histaminemia
histaminergic
histanoxia
His-Tawara node
histic
histidase
histidinase
histidine
    ammonia-lyase
histidine decarboxylase
histidinuria
histioblast
histiocyte
    cardiac h.
    sea-blue h.
    wandering h.
histiocytic
    h. lymphoma
    h. panniculitis
    h. reticulosis

histiocytoma
    benign fibrous h.
    h. cuffs
    h. cutis
    eruptive h.
    fibrous h.
    generalized eruptive h.
    juvenile h.
    lipoid h.
    malignant fibrous h.
histiocytomatosis
histiocytosis
    atypical h.
    cephalic h.
    malignant h.
    nonlipid h.
    pulmonary h.
    sinus h.
    h. X
histioid
histio-irritative
histionic
histoautoradiography
histoblast
histochemical
histochemistry
histochemotherapy
histochromatosis
histoclastic
histoclinical
histocompatibility complex
histocompatible
histodiagnosis
histodialysis
histodifferentiation
histofluorescence
histogenesis
histogenetic
histogenous
histogram
histography
histohematogenous
histohydria
histohypoxia
histoid
histoincompatibility
histoincompatible
histokinesis
histologic
histological
histologist
histology
    normal h.
    pathologic h.
    topographic h.

histolysate
histolysis
histolytic
histoma
histometaplastic
histomorphology
histomorphometric
histomorphometry
histone nucleinate
histoneurology
histonomy
histonuria
histopathogenesis
histopathology
histophagous
histophysiology
Histoplasma
    H. capsulatum
    H. capsulatum var.
      duboisii
    H. capsulatum var.
      farciminosum
    H. duboisii
    H. farciminosum
    H. pyriforme
histoplasmoma
histoplasmosis
    African h.
    disseminated h.
    ocular h.
historadiography
historetention
historrhexis
history
    case h.
    family h. (FH)
    incongruous h.
    marital h. (MH)
    medical h. (MH)
    occupational h. (OH)
    past h. (PH)
    past medical h. (PMH)
    past surgical h. (PSH)
    h. and physical examination
      (HPE)
    h. of present illness (HPI)
    social h. (SH)
    surgical h. (SH)
histospectroscopy
histo spots
histoteliosis
histotherapy
histothrombin
histotome
histotomy

H

histotoxic
histotroph
histotrophic
histotropic
histozoic
histrionic
histrionism
His-Werner disease
HIT—
  hemagglutination-inhibition
    test
  hypertrophic infiltrative
    tendinitis
Hitzenberg test
Hitzig
  girdle
  syndrome
  test
HIV—human immunodeficiency
  virus
hive
hives
HJ—Howell-Jolly
HJB—Howell-Jolly bodies
HK—
  heat-killed
  heel-to-knee
  hexokinase
HKAFO—hip-knee-ankle-foot
  orthosis
HKLM—heat-killed *Listeria
  monocytogenes*
Hl—latent hyperopia
HL—
  hearing level
  hearing loss
  histocompatibility locus
  hypermetropia, latent
H&L—heart and lungs
HLA—human leukocyte antigen
HLDH—heat-stable lactate
  dehydrogenase
hLH—human luteinizing hormone
HLHS—hypoplastic left heart
  syndrome
H-L-K—heart, liver, kidney
hLT—human lymphocyte
  transformation
HLV—herpes-like virus
Hm—manifest hyperopia
HM—
  human milk
  hydatidiform mole
HME—heat and moisture
  exchanger

HMF—hydroxymethylfurfural
HMG—hydroxymethylglutaryl
hMG—human menopausal
  gonadotropin
HML—human milk lysozyme
HMO—health maintenance
  organization
HMP—
  hexose monophosphate
  hexose monophosphate
    pathway
  hot moist pack
HMPS—hexose monophosphate
  shunt
HMSAS—hypertrophic muscular
  subaortic stenosis
HMSN—hereditary motor and
  sensory neuropathy
HMW-NC; HMW-NCF—high-
  molecular-weight neutrophil
  chemotactic factor
HN—
  hereditary nephritis
  hilar node
  nitrogen mustard
    (mechlorethamine)
HNP—herniated nucleus pulposus
HNPCC—hereditary nonpolyposis
  colorectal cancer
hnRNA—heterogeneous nuclear
  RNA
h/o, H/O—history of
HO—high oxygen
H_2O_2 [H2O2]—hydrogen peroxide
hoarse
hoarseness
Hoboken
  nodules
  valves
HOC—hydroxycorticoid
Hochenegg operation
hock
hockey-stick incision
HOCM—hypertrophic obstructive
  cardiomyopathy
Hodge
  forceps
  maneuver
  pessary
  plane
Hodgen
  apparatus
  splint
Hodgkin
  cells

Hodgkin *(continued)*
    cycle
    disease
    granuloma
    lymphoma
    Rye classification of H. disease
    sarcoma
Hodgson disease
hodograph
hodology
hodoneuromere
hoe
    Hough h.
Hoehne sign
Hoen
    plate
    skull plate
hof
    nuclear h.
Hofbauer cells
Hoffa
    disease
    operation
Hoffa-Kastert disease
Hoffa-Lorenz operation
Hoffmann
    anodyne
    atrophy
    drops
    duct
    forceps
    phenomenon
    punch
    reflex
    rongeur
    sign
Hoffmann-Werdnig syndrome
Hofmann
    bacillus
    violet
Hofmeister
    gastroenterostomy
    operation
    test
Hogan operation
Hoguet
    maneuver
    operation
Hohmann
    operation
    retractor
Hoke
    operation
    osteotome
holagogue

holandric
holarthritis
Holden curet
holder
    broach h.
    Castroviejo h.
    clamp h.
    needle h.
    rubber dam clamp h.
    sponge h.
holdfast
holergasia
Holger Nielsen method
holiday
    drug h.
Holinger
    applicator
    bronchoscope
    dissector
    esophagoscope
    forceps
    laryngoscope
    telescope
    tube
Holinger-Jackson bronchoscope
holism
holistic
Hollenhorst
    bodies
    plaque
hollow
    Sébileau h.
hollow-back
Holman-Mathieu cannula
Holmes
    ataxia
    degeneration
    gouge
    nasopharyngoscope
    operation
    phenomenon
    sign
Holmes-Adie syndrome
Holmes-Stewart phenomenon
Holmgren-Golgi canals
Holmgren test
holmium (Ho)
holoacardius
    h. acephalus
    h. acormus
    h. amorphus
holoanencephaly
holoantigen
holoblast
holoblastic

holocarboxylase synthetase
   deficiency
holocephalic
holocephaly
holocortex
holocrine
holodiastolic
holoendemic
holoenzyme
hologamy
hologastroschisis
hologenesis
hologram
holography
   acoustical h.
hologynic
holomastigote
holometabolous
holomorphosis
holonephros
holophytic
holoplexia
holoprosencephaly
    familial alobar h.
holorachischisis
holosaccharide
holoschisis
holosymphysis
holosystolic
holotelencephaly
holothurin
holotonia
holotonic
holotopy
holotrichous
holotype
holoxenic
holozoic
Holter shunt
Holth
   forceps
   operation
   punch
Holthouse hernia
Holt-Oram syndrome
Holtz curet
homalocephalus
homalography
homaluria
Homans
   operation
   sign
homarine
homatropine
   h. hydrobromide
   h. methylbromide

homaxial
Home
   gland
   lobe
Homén syndrome
homeochrome
homeograft
homeokinesis
homeometric
homeomorphous
homeo-osteoplasty
homeopathic
homeopathist
homeopathy
homeoplasia
homeoplastic
homeorrhesis
homeosis
homeostasis
   genetic h.
   immunologic h.
homeostatic
homeotherapy
homeotherm
homeothermal
homeothermic
homeothermy
homeotoxic
homeotoxin
homeotransplant
homeotransplantation
homeotypic
homeotypical
Homer
   law
   muscle
   ptosis
   pupil
   syndrome
homergic
Homer-Trantas spots
Homer-Wright rosette
homicidal
homicide
homicidomania
homidium
homilophobia
hominal
hominid
homininoxious
hominoid
homme rouge
Homo sapiens
homobiotin
homoblastic
homobody

homocarnosinase
homocarnosine
homocarnosinosis
homocentric
homochronous
homocinchonine
homocladic
homocyclic
homocysteine
homocysteine
  methyltransferase
homocysteine–tetrahydrofolate
  methyltransferase
homocystine
homocystinemia
homocytotropic
homodesmotic
homodont
homodromous
homodynamic
homodynamy
homoecious
homoerotic
homoeroticism
homofermentation
homofermenter
homogamete
homogametic
homogamous
homogamy
homogenate
homogeneity
homogeneous
homogeneously
homogenesis
homogenetic
homogenic
homogenization
homogenize
homogenote
homogenous
homogentisate
homogentisate
  1,2-dioxygenase
homogentisate oxidase
homogentisic acid
homogentisic acid oxidase
  deficiency
homogentisuria
homoglandular
homogonic
homograft
    isogenic h.
homoiopodal
homoiosmotic
homoiotoxin

homokaryon
homokeratoplasty
homolactic
homolateral
homologen
homologous
homologue
homology
    metameric h.
    serial h.
homolysin
homolysis
homomorphic
homomorphosis
homonomous
homonymous
    h. diplopia
    h. hemianopia
    h. hemianopsia
homophene
homophil
homophilic
homoplastic
homoplasty
homopolymer
homopolysaccharide
homorganic
homosalate
homoscedasticity
homoserine lactone
homosexual
homosexuality
    ego-dystonic h.
    latent h.
    unconscious h.
homospore
homosporous
homostimulant
homostimulation
homothallic
homothallism
homotonic
homotopic
homotransplant
homotransplantation
homotropism
homotype
homotypic
homovanillic acid
homoxenous
homozoic
homozygosis
homozygosity
homozygote
homozygous
homunculus

H

Honan cuff
honey
honeycomb lung
honk
    precordial h.
hood
    Rock-Mulligan h.
    tooth h.
HOOD—hereditary osteo-
  onychodysplasia
Hood dermatome
Hood and Kirklin incision
hook
    Adson h.
    Barr crypt h.
    Barr fistula h.
    Barr rectal h.
    Blair palate h.
    blunt h.
    Boettcher h.
    Bose h's
    Bose tracheostomy h.
    Boyes-Goodfellow h.
    Braun h.
    Buck h.
    Carroll bone h.
    Carroll h. curet
    Dandy h.
    Dudley h.
    Duplay h.
    dural h.
    Edwards h.
    Emmet h.
    fixation h.
    Frazier h. retractor
    Gillies h.
    Gillies-Dingman h.
    Graefe (von Graefe) h.
    Graham h.
    Green h.
    h. of hamate bone
    House h.
    Jameson h.
    Kelly h.
    Kimball h.
    Kirby h.
    Lillie h.
    Linton h.
    Loughnane h.
    Mayo h.
    muscle h.
    New h.
    Newman h.
    Nugent h.
    O'Connor h.

hook *(continued)*
    Pajot
    palate h.
    Pratt h.
    Rosser h.
    Schuknecht h.
    Schwartz h.
    Shambaugh h.
    Shea h.
    Smith h.
    squint h.
    Stevens h.
    Stewart h.
    tracheostomy h.
    Tyrrell h.
    Welch-Allyn h.
    Wiener h.
hooklet
hook-on bronchoscope
hook-up
hookworm
    American h.
    European h.
    New World h.
    Old World h.
hoolamite
Hoover sign
HOP—
    high oxygen pressure
    hydroxydaunomycin
      (doxorubicin), Oncovin
      (vincristine), and
      prednisone
Hope sign
Hopkins
    clamp
    operation
Hopkins-Cole test
Hoplopsyllus anomalus
Hopmann
    papilloma
    polyp
Hoppe-Goldflam syndrome
Hoppe-Seyler test
hordein
hordenine
hordeolum
    external h.
    internal h.
horehound
Horgan operation
horizon
    Streeter h's
horizontal
    h. gaze

horizontal *(continued)*
    h. hemilaryngectomy
    h. incision
    h. mattress suture
    h. meridian
    h. nystagmus
    h. raphe
    h. tube
horizontalis
hormesis
hormion
Hormodendrum
    H. carrionii
    H. compactum
    H. pedrosoi
hormonagogue
hormonal
hormone
    adaptive h.
    adenohypophysial
        (adenohypophyseal) h.
    adipokinetic h.
    adrenocortical h.
    adrenocorticotropic h.
    adrenomedullary h's
    androgenic h's
    anterior pituitary h.
    antidiuretic h.
    Aschheim-Zondek h.
    chondrotropic h.
    chorionic growth h.-prolactin
    chromaffin h.
    chromatophorotropic h.
    circulatory h.
    conjugated estrogen h's
    corpus luteum h.
    cortical h.
    corticotropin-releasing h. (CRH)
    diabetogenic h.
    estrogenic h's
    fat-mobilizing h's
    female h.
    follicle-stimulating h. (FSH)
    follicular h.
    galactopoietic h.
    gametogenic h.
    gametokinetic h.
    gastrointestinal h's
    glycoprotein h.
    gonadotropic h.
    gonadotropic h's, pituitary
    growth h. (GH)
    growth h. release–inhibiting h.
        (GH-RIH)
    gut h.

hormone *(continued)*
    human growth h. (hGH)
    human pituitary growth h.
    hypophysial (hypophyseal) h.
    hypophysiotropic h's
    hypothalamic inhibitory h.
    hypothalamic-releasing h.
    inhibiting h's
    inhibitory h.
    interstitial cell–stimulating h.
    intestinal h.
    intracellular h.
    juvenile h.
    ketogenic h.
    lactation h.
    lactogenic h.
    lipolytic h's
    lipotropic h.
    local h.
    luteal h.
    luteinizing h.
    luteinizing h.–releasing h.
        (LH-RH)
    luteotropic h.
    mammary-stimulating h.
    mammogenic h.
    melanocyte-stimulating h.
    melanocyte-stimulating
        h.–inhibiting h.
        (MIF, MSH-IF)
    melanocyte-stimulating
        h.–releasing h.
    melanophore-stimulating h.
    morphogenetic h.
    morphogenic h.
    N h.
    neurohypophysial
        (neurohypophyseal) h's
    orchitic h.
    ovarian h.
    oxytocic h.
    parathyroid h.
    placental h's
    placental growth h.
    plant h.
    posterior pituitary h's
    preproparathyroid h.
    progestational h.
    prolactin inhibitory h.
    prolactin-releasing h.
    proparathyroid h.
    prothoracicotropic h.
    releasing h's
    S h.
    sex h's

H

hormone *(continued)*
    somatotrophic h.
    somatotropic h.
    somatotropin release–
      inhibiting h.
    somatotropin-releasing h.
      (SRH)
    steroid h's
    sympathetic h.
    testicular h.
    testis h.
    thymic h.
    thyroid h's
    thyroid-stimulating h. (TSH)
    thyrotropic h.
    thyrotropin-releasing h. (TRH)
    tropic h's
hormonogen
hormonogenesis
hormonogenic
hormonology
hormonopoiesis
hormonopoietic
hormonoprivia
hormonosis
hormonotherapy
horn
    Ammon h.
    anterior h. of lateral ventricle
    anterior h. of spinal cord
    cicatricial h.
    h. of clitoris
    coccygeal h.
    cutaneous h.
    dorsal h. of spinal cord
    frontal h. of lateral ventricle
    gray h's of spinal cord
    greater h. of hyoid bone
    iliac h.
    inferior h. of cerebrum
    inferior h. of falciform margin
    inferior h. of lateral ventricle
    inferior h. of saphenous opening
    inferior h. of thyroid cartilage
    inferior h. of saphenous opening
    lateral h. of coccyx
    lateral h. of hyoid bone
    lateral h. of spinal cord
    lateral h. of uterus
    lesser h. of hyoid bone
    motor h.
    occipital h. of lateral ventricle
    posterior h. of lateral ventricle
    posterior h. of spinal cord
    h. of pulp

horn *(continued)*
    sacral h.
    sebaceous h.
    superior h. of falciform margin
    superior h. of hyoid bone
    superior h. of saphenous
      opening
    superior h. of thymus
    superior h. of thyroid cartilage
    temporal h. of lateral ventricle
    uterine h.
    h. of uterus
    ventral h. of spinal cord
    warty h.
Horn sign
Horner
    law
    muscle
    ptosis
    pupil
    syndrome
    teeth
Horner-Bernard syndrome
hornification
horny
horopter
    Vieth-Muller h.
horopteric
horripilation
horror
    h. autotoxicus
    h. fusionis
horsefly
horsehair suture
horse-race effect
horseshoe kidney
Horsley
    anastomosis
    bone-cutting forceps
    gastropexy
    pyloroplasty
    suture
    wax
Hortega
    cell
    method
hortobezoar
Horton
    arteritis
    cephalalgia
    disease
    headache
    syndrome
Horton-Devine operation
Horwitz-Adams operation

hose
    TED h.
    thromboembolic disease h.
Hosford spud
hosp—hospital
hospice
hospital
    base h.
    camp h.
    closed h.
    closed staff h.
    cottage h.
    day h.
    evacuation h.
    field h.
    for-profit h.
    geriatric day h.
    government h.
    lying-in h.
    maternity h.
    mental h.
    mobile army surgical h.
      (MASH)
    night h.
    open h.
    private h.
    proprietary h.
    psychogeriatric h.
    public h.
    teaching h.
    voluntary h.
    weekend h.
hospitalism
hospitalist
hospitalization
    partial h.
hospitalize
host
    accidental h.
    alternate h.
    dead-end h.
    definitive h.
    final h.
    incidental h.
    intermediate h.
    maintenance h.
    mechanical intermediate h.
    overwintering h.
    paratenic h.
    h. of predilection
    primary h.
    reservoir h.
    secondary h.
    transfer h.
    transport h.

hostility
hot
    h. appendix
    h. area
    h. caudate lobe
    h. contrast material
    h. lesion on scan
    h. nose sign
    h. spot artifact
    h. spot imaging
    h. spot on scan
    h. thyroid nodule
HOT—human old tuberculin
hot-box
Hotchkiss operation
hot-cross-bun
    h. appearance
    h. skull
hot line, hotline
hottentotism
hot-tip, hot-tipped
    h.-t. laser probe
    h.-t. probe
Hough
    hoe
    stapedectomy
Hounsfield unit
hourglass chest
house
    halfway h.
House
    adaptor
    chisel
    curet
    elevator
    forceps
    hook
    irrigator
    knife
    needle
    prosthesis
    rod
    scissors
    separator
    stapedectomy
    tube
House-Barbara needle
housefly
House-Rosen needle
House-Urban retractor
Houssay
    animal
    phenomenon
Houssay-Biasotti syndrome
Housset-Debray gastroscope

Houston
  muscle
  operation
  valve
hoven
Hovius
  canal
  circle
  membrane
  plexus
Howard
  abrader
  basket
  forceps
  method
  test
Howard-Dolman apparatus
Howel-Evans syndrome
Howell bodies
Howell-Jolly bodies
Howe silver nitrate
Howorth
  operation
  osteotome
Howship lacuna
Howship-Romberg sign
Hoxworth forceps
Hoyne sign
HP—history of present illness
H&P—history and physical
HPAA—hydroxyphenylacetic acid
HPA axis
HPE—history and physical
  examination
HPETE—
  hydroperoxyeicosatetraenoic
  acid
HPF—heparin-precipitable fraction
hpf—high-power field
HPFH—hereditary persistence of
  fetal hemoglobin
hPFSH—human pituitary follicle-
  stimulating hormone
hPG—human pituitary
  gonadotropin
HPI—history of present illness
HPL, hPL—human placental
  lactogen
HPLC—
  high-performance liquid
    chromatography
  high-pressure liquid
    chromatography
HPNS—high-pressure neurologic
  syndrome
HPO—high-pressure oxygen

HPP—hereditary
  pyropoikilocytosis
HPPA—hydroxyphenylpyruvic acid
HPRT—hypoxanthine
  phosphoribosyltransferase
HPS—
  hematoxylin-phloxine-saffron
  hypertrophic pyloric stenosis
HPT—hyperparathyroidism
HPV—
  Haemophilus pertussis vaccine
  human papillomavirus
HPVG—hepatic portal venous gas
hr—hour
Hr—blood type factor
HR—
  heart rate
  hospital record
  hospital report
H&R—hysterectomy and radiation
  therapy
HRA—health risk appraisal
H-reflex
HRF—histamine-releasing factor
HRIG—human rabies immune
  globulin
HRR—Hardy-Rand-Ritter (plates)
HRS—Hamilton Rating Scale
HRT—heart rate
Hruby lens
h.s.—at bedtime (L. hora somni)
HS—
  heat stable
  heme synthetase
  hereditary spherocytosis
  herpes simplex
  horse serum
  house surgeon
HSA—human serum albumin
HSAN—hereditary sensory and
  autonomic neuropathy
HSF—hydrazine-sensitive factor
HSG—hysterosalpingogram
H-shaped vertebra
HSR—homogeneously staining
  regions
HSV—herpes simplex virus
HSV encephalopathy
ht.—
  heart
  height
Ht—total hyperopia
HT—
  hypodermic tablet
  hypothalamus
HT, htn—hypertension

HTA—hydroxytryptamine
HTACS—human thyroid adenylate cyclase stimulators
HTC—homozygous typing cell(s)
³H-TdR
HTLV—
    human T-cell leukemia/ lymphoma virus
HTLV-1—human T-lymphotropic virus 1
HTLV-2—human T-lymphotropic virus 2
HTP—
    house-tree-person (test)
    hydroxytryptophan
HTV—herpes-type virus
HU—
    hemagglutinating unit
    Hounsfield unit
    hydroxyurea
    hyperemia unit
Hua
    H. ningpoensis
    H. toucheana
Hubbard tank
Huchard
    disease
    sign
    symptom
Hudson
    brace
    bur
    clamp
    drill
    forceps
    line
Hudson-Stähli (Staehli) line
Hueck ligament
Hueston spiral flap
Hueter
    bandage
    fracture sign
    line
    maneuver
Huët-Pelger nuclear anomaly
Huffman-Graves speculum
Hufnagel
    clamp
    knife
    operation
    prosthesis
Huggins operation
Hughes
    reflex
    implant
    operation

Huguenin edema
Huguier
    canal
    circle
    sinus
Huhner test
HuIFN—human interferon
Hulka clip
hum
    venous h.
human immunodeficiency virus (HIV)
human papillomavirus (HPV)
humatrope
Hume clamp
humectant
humectation
humeral
humeri (genitive and plural of humerus)
humeroradial
humeroscapular
humeroulnar
humerus (humeri)
    h. varus
humidifier
humidity
    absolute h.
    relative h.
Hummelsheim procedure
humor
    aqueous h.
    h. aquosus
    h. cristallinus
    crystalline h.
    ocular h.
    plasmoid h.
    vitreous h.
    h. vitreus
humoral
    h. immune response
    h. immunity
humoralism
hump
    buffalo h.
    Hampton h.
humpback
Humphries clamp
Humphry ligament
hummus
hunchback
hunchbacked
Hünermann disease
hunger
    affect h.

H

hunger *(continued)*
    air h.
    calcium h.
Hunner
    stricture
    ulcer
Hunt
    atrophy
    clamp
    disease
    forceps
    method
    neuralgia
    operation
    paradoxical phenomenon
    paralysis
    phenomenon
    striatal syndrome
    syndrome
    tremor
Hunter
    canal
    curet
    glossitis
    gubernaculum
    ligament
    line
    syndrome
hunterian chancre
Hunter-Schreger
  band
Huntington
    chorea
    disease
    operation
    sign
Hurd
    dissector
    elevator
    forceps
Hurler
    disease
    polydystrophy
    syndrome
Hurler-Scheie
    compound
    syndrome
Hurst
    bougie
    disease
Hürthle
    cell
    cell adenoma
    cell carcinoma
    cell tumor

Hurwitz
    clamp
    trocar
HUS—hyaluronidase unit for
  semen
Huschke
    auditory teeth
    canal
    foramen
    ligaments
    teeth
    valve
    vomerian cartilage
husk
Husks rongeur
Hutchins needle
Hutchinson
    disease
    facies
    freckle
    lentigo
    mask
    patch
    pupil
    sign
    syndrome
    teeth
    triad
Hutchinson-Boeck
    disease
    syndrome
Hutchinson-Gilford
    disease
    syndrome
hutchinsonian
Hutchison
    syndrome
    type
Hutinel disease
Huxley
    layer
    membrane
huygenian
Huygens (Huyghens)
    eyepiece
    ocular
    principle
HV—
    hepatic vein
    herpesvirus
    hospital visit
    hyperventilation
H&V—hemigastrectomy and
  vagotomy
HVA—homovanillic acid

HVE—high-voltage electrophoresis
HVH—herpesvirus hominis
HVL—half-value layer
HVM—high-velocity missile
HVSD—hydrogen-detected
  ventricular septal defect
Hx—history
hyalin
    hematogenous h.
hyaline
    h. membrane disease
    h. arteriosclerosis
    h. cartilage
    h. membrane disease
hyalinization
    tympanic h.
hyalinosis
    h. cutis et mucosae
    tympanic h.
hyalinuria
hyalitis
    asteroid h.
    h. punctata
    punctate h.
    h. suppurativa
    suppurative h.
hyalogen
hyaloid
    h. canal
    h. membrane
hyaloidin
hyaloidopathy
    asteroid h.
hyalomere
hyalomitome
Hyalomma
    H. marginatum
    H. truncatum
hyalomucoid
hyalonyxis
hyalophagia
hyaloplasm
    nuclear h.
hyaloserositis
    progressive
      multiple h.
hyalosis
    asteroid h.
    punctate h.
hyalosome
hyalotome
hyaluronate
hyaluronate lyase
hyaluronic acid
hyaluronidase

hyaluronoglucosaminidase
hyaluronoglucuronidase
Hyams
    clamp
    criteria
    grading system
    operation
    scleral knife
hybaroxia
hybenzate
hybrid
    F_1h. [F1]
    false h.
    somatic h.
hybridism
hybridity
hybridization
    cell h.
    cross h.
    DNA h.
    in situ h.
    molecular h.
hybridoma
    B lymphocyte h.
    T lymphocyte h.
hycanthone
hycanthone mesylate
hyclate
hydantoic acid
hydantoin
hydantoinate
hydatid
    alveolar h's
    h. disease
    h. of Morgagni
    nonpedunculated h.
    pedunculated h.
    sessile h.
hydatidiform
hydatidocele
hydatidosis
hydatidostomy
hydatiduria
hydatism
hydatoid
Hyde disease
hydracetin
hydraeroperitoneum
hydragogue
hydramine
hydramnios
hydranencephaly
hydrangiology
hydrargyria
hydrargyrism

hydrargyromania
hydrargyrorelapsing
hydrargyrosis
hydrarthrodial
hydrarthrosis
    intermittent h.
hydratase
hydrate
hydrated
hydration
hydraulics
hydrazine
hydrazinolysis
hydrazone
hydremia
hydrepigastrium
hydriatric
hydriatrics
hydric
hydride
hydrindicuria
hydriodic acid
hydrion
hydroa
    h. aestivale
    h. estivale
    h. febrile
    h. gestationis
    h. gravidarum
    h. puerorum
    h. vacciniforme
    h. vesiculosum
hydroadipsia
hydroappendix
hydrobilirubin
hydroblepharon
hydrobromic acid
hydrobromide
hydrocalycosis
hydrocalyx
hydrocarbarism
hydrocarbon
    alicyclic h.
    aliphatic h.
    aromatic h.
    carcinogenic h.
    chlorinated h.
    cyclic h.
    fluorinated h.
    halogenated h.
    saturated h.
    unsaturated h.
hydrocarbonism
hydrocardia

hydrocele
    bilocular h.
    cervical h.
    chylous h.
    h. colli
    communicating h.
    congenital h.
    diffused h.
    Dupuytren h.
    encysted h.
    h. feminae
    filarial h.
    funicular h.
    Gibbon h.
    hernial h.
    inguinal h.
    Maunoir h.
    h. muliebris
    h. of neck
    noncommunicating h.
    Nuck h.
    h. renalis
    scrotal h.
    spermatic h.
    h. spinalis
    h. of testis
hydrocelectomy
hydrocenosis
hydrocephalic
hydrocephalocele
hydrocephaloid
hydrocephaloid disease
hydrocephalus
    communicating h.
    compensating h.
    congenital h.
    external h.
    h. ex vacuo
    hypertonic h.
    internal h.
    low-pressure h.
    noncommunicating h.
    normal-pressure h.
    normal-pressure occult h.
    obstructive h.
    occult normal-pressure h.
    otitic h.
    postmeningitic h.
    post-traumatic h.
    primary h.
    thrombotic h.
    toxic h.
hydrochloric acid (HCl)
hydrochlorothiazide (HCT, HCTZ)

hydrocholecystis
hydrocholeresis
hydrocholeretic
hydrocholesterol
hydrocinchonidine
hydrocirsocele
hydrocodone bitartrate
hydrocodone resin complex
hydrocollidine
hydrocolloid
    irreversible h.
    reversible h.
hydrocolpocele
hydrocolpos
hydroconion
hydrocortisone
    h. acetate
    h. butyrate
    h. cyclopentylpropionate
    h. cypionate
    h. hemisuccinate
    h. probutate
    h. sodium phosphate
    h. sodium succinate
    h. valerate
hydrocrania
hydrocyanic acid
hydrocyanism
hydrocyst
hydrocystadenoma
hydrocytosis
hydrodiascope
hydrodiffusion
hydrodipsia
hydrodipsomania
hydrodiuresis
hydrodynamics
hydroelectric
hydroencephalocele
Hydroflex penile
    prosthesis
hydrofluoric acid
hydrogel
hydrogen (H)
    h. arsenide
    arseniuretted h.
    h. atom
    h. bromide
    h. chloride
    h. cyanide
    h. disulfide
    heavy h.
    h. ion [H+]
    light h.

hydrogen (H) *(continued)*
    ordinary h.
    h. peroxide
    radioactive h.
    h. selenide
    h. sulfate
    h. sulfide
    sulfuretted h.
hydrogenase
hydrogenate
hydrogenation
hydrogenize
hydrogenoid
hydrogenolysis
hydrogymnastic
hydrogymnastics
hydrohemarthrosis
hydrohematonephrosis
hydrohematosalpinx
hydrohepatosis
hydrohymenitis
hydrohystera
hydrokinesitherapy
hydrokinetic
hydrokinetics
hydrolabile
hydrolability
hydrolase
    murein h.
hydrology
hydro-lyase
hydrolymph
hydrolysate
    protein h.
hydrolysis
    papain h.
hydrolyst
hydrolyte
hydrolytic
hydrolyze
hydromassage
hydromeningitis
hydromeningocele
hydrometer
hydrometra
hydrometric
hydrometrocolpos
hydrometry
hydromicrocephaly
hydromorphone
hydromphalus
hydromyelia
hydromyelocele
hydromyelomeningocele

H

hydromyoma
hydronephrosis
    closed h.
    congenital h.
    external h.
    infected h.
    intermittent h.
    open h.
    perirenal h.
    subcapsular h.
hydronephrotic
hydronium
hydropancreatosis
hydroparasalpinx
hydroparotitis
hydropedesis
hydropenia
hydropenic
hydropericarditic
hydropericarditis
hydropericardium
hydroperinephrosis
hydroperion
hydroperitoneum
hydroperitonia
hydroperoxyeicosatetraenoic acid
hydropexic
hydropexis
hydrophagocytosis
hydrophilia
hydrophilic
hydrophilic lens
hydrophobia
    paralytic h.
hydrophobic
hydrophorograph
hydrophthalmia
hydrophthalmos
    h. anterior
    h. posterior
    h. totalis
hydrophthalmus
hydrophysometra
hydrophyte
hydropic
hydropigenous
hydroplasma
hydroplasmia
hydropleura
hydropneumatosis
hydropneumogony
hydropneumoperitoneum
hydropneumothorax
hydrops
    h. abdominis

hydrops *(continued)*
    h. ad matulam
    h. amnii
    h. antri
    h. articuli
    Bart hemoglobin h. fetalis
    h. of cornea
    endolymphatic h.
    fetal h.
    h. fetalis
    h. folliculi
    hypertensive meningeal h.
    immune h. fetalis
    h. labyrinthi
    labyrinthine h.
    nonimmune h. fetalis
    h. pericardii
    h. of pleura
    h. spurius
    h. tubae
    h. tubae profluens
    tympanic h.
hydropyonephrosis
hydroquinone
hydrorachis
hydrorachitis
hydrorchis
hydrorrhea
    h. gravidarum
    nasal h.
hydrosalpinx
    h. follicularis
    intermittent h.
    h. simplex
hydrosarcocele
hydroscheocele
hydrosol
hydrosoluble
hydrospermatocele
hydrosphygmograph
hydrospirometer
hydrostabile
hydrostat
hydrostatic
hydrostatics
hydrostomia
hydrosulfuric acid
hydrosynthesis
hydrosyringomyelia
Hydrotaea
    H. irritans
    H. meteorica
hydrotaxis
hydrotherapeutic
hydrotherapy

hydrothermic
hydrothioammonemia
hydrothionemia
hydrothionuria
hydrothorax
    chylous h.
hydrotomy
hydrotoxicity
hydrotropism
hydrotubation
hydrotympanum
hydroureter
hydroureteronephrosis
hydroureterosis
hydrouria
hydrous
hydrovarium
hydroxamic acids
hydroxide
11-hydroxy-17-ketosteroid
3-hydroxy-3-methylglutaryl CoA
    (HMG CoA) lyase deficiency
hydroxyacetanilide
3-hydroxyacyl-CoA
    dehydrogenase
hydroxyacylglutathione
    hydrolase
hydroxyamphetamine
    hydrobromide
hydroxybenzene
3-hydroxybutyrate dehydrogenase
hydroxybutyric acid
    β-h.
    γ-h. (GHB)
    3-h.
4-hydroxybutyricaciduria
25-hydroxycholecalciferol
25-hydroxydihydrotachysterol
hydroxydione sodium succinate
hydroxyeicosatetraenoic acid
25-hydroxyergocalciferol
hydroxyestradiols
hydroxyestrin benzoate
hydroxyformobenzoylic acid
hydroxyheptadecatrienoic acid
5-hydroxyindoleacetic acid
5-hydroxyindoleacetic acid
    (5-HIAA)
3-hydroxyisobutyryl-CoA hydrolase
11-hydroxy-17-ketosteroid
hydroxyl
hydroxylamine
hydroxylapatite
hydroxylase
    17α-h. [17-alpha-]

hydroxylase *(continued)*
    11β-h. [11-beta-]
    21-h.
hydroxylation
4-hydroxy-L-proline oxidase
    deficiency
hydroxylysine
5-hydroxymethyl cytosine
3-hydroxy-3-methylglutaryl CoA
    (HMG CoA) lyase deficiency
hydroxymethylglutaryl-CoA lyase
hydroxymethylglutaryl-CoA
    reductase
hydroxymethylglutaryl-CoA
    synthase
hydroxymethyltransferase
hydroxynervone
hydroxyphenamate
hydroxyphenylethylamine
4-hydroxyphenylpyruvate
    dioxygenase
p-hydroxyphenylpyruvate oxidase
    [p-, para-]
p-hydroxyphenylpyruvic acid
    (PHPPA) [p-, para-]
hydroxyphenyluria
17 α-hydroxyprogesterone aldolase
    [17-alpha-]
hydroxyprogesterone caproate
hydroxyproline oxidase
4-hydroxy-L-proline oxidase
    deficiency
hydroxyprolinuria
hydroxypropyl methylcellulose
8-hydroxyquinoline sulfate
hydroxystearin sulfate
hydroxysteroid
    3β-h. [3-beta-]
    17-h.
3β-hydroxy-δ5-steroid
    dehydrogenase [3-beta-, delta-5-]
hydroxystilbamidine isethionate
hydroxytetracycline
5-hydroxytryptamine (5-HT)
5-hydroxytryptophan
hydroxyvaline
hydrozoan
hydruria
hydruric
hyenanchin
hygieist
hygiene
    dental h.
    industrial h.
    mouth h.

H

hygiene *(continued)*
    occupational h.
    oral h.
    radiation h.
hygienic
hygienics
hygienist
    dental h.
hygienization
hygieology
hygiogenesis
hygiology
hygrechema
hygric
hygroblepharic
hygroma
    h. colli
    cystic h.
    h. cysticum
    Fleischmann h.
    h. praepatellare
    subdural h.
hygromatous
hygrometer
    dew point h.
    hair h.
    Saussure h.
hygrometric
hygrometry
hygroscopic
hyla
hylotropic
hylotropy
hymecromone
hymen
    annular h.
    h. bifenestratus
    h. biforis
    circular h.
    cribriform h.
    denticular h.
    falciform h.
    fenestrated h.
    imperforate h.
    infundibuliform h.
    lunar h.
    persistent h.
    septate h.
    h. septus
    subseptate h.
    h. subseptus
hymenal
    h. band
    h. ring
hymenectomy

hymenitis
hymenium
hymenolepiasis
Hymenolepis
    H. diminuta
    H. fraterna
    H. lanceolata
    H. nana
    H. nana var. *fraterna*
hymenology
Hymenoptera
hymenopteran
hymenopterism
hymenorrhaphy
hymenotomy
Hynes pharyngoplasty
hyobasioglossus
hyodeoxycholic acid
hyoepiglottic
hyoepiglottidean
hyoglossal
hyoid
hyolaryngeal
hyomandibular
hyomental
hyoscine
hyoscyamine
    h. hydrobromide
    h. sulfate
hyoscyamus
hyosternal
hyothyroid
hypacidemia
hypacusia
hypacusis
hypalgesia
hypalgesic
hypamnios
hypaphorine
hypaphrodisia
hyparterial bronchi
hypasthenia
hypaxial
hypazoturia
hypenchyme
hyperabsorption
hyperacanthosis
hyperacid
hyperacidaminuria
hyperacidity
    gastric h.
hyperactive
hyperactivity
hyperacuity
hyperacusis

hyperacute
hyperadenosis
hyperadiposis
hyperadrenal
hyperadrenalemia
hyperadrenalism
hyperadrenocortical
hyperadrenocorticism
hyperalbuminemia
hyperalbuminosis
hyperalcoholemia
hyperaldosteronemia
hyperaldosteronism
hyperaldosteronuria
hyperalgesia
    auditory h.
    muscular h.
hyperalgesic
hyperalimentation
    parenteral h.
    total parenteral h.
hyperalimented
hyperalimentosis
hyperalkalescence
hyperalkalinity
hyperallantoinuria
hyperalonemia
hyperalphalipoproteinemia
hyperaminoacidemia
hyperaminoaciduria
hyperammonemia
    cerebroatrophic h.
    congenital h., type I
    congenital h., type II
hyperammonuria
hyperamylasemia
hyperandrogenism
hyperaphia
hyperaphic
hyperarousal
hyperazotemia
hyperazoturia
hyperbaric
    h. chamber
    h. oxygen
hyperbarism
hyperbasophilic
hyper-beta-alaninemia
hyperbetalipoproteinemia
    familial h.
hyperbicarbonatemia
hyperbilirubinemia
    congenital h.
    conjugated h.
    constitutional h.

hyperbilirubinemia *(continued)*
    hereditary
      nonhemolytic h.
    h. I
    neonatal h.
    unconjugated h.
hyperbilirubinemic
hyperblastosis
hyperbrachycephalic
hyperbrachycephaly
hyperbradykininemia
hyperbradykininism
hypercalcemia
    familial hypocalciuric h.
    idiopathic h.
hypercalcipexy
hypercalcitoninemia
hypercalciuria
    absorptive h.
    idiopathic h.
    renal h.
    resorptive h.
    secondary h.
hypercapnia
    permissive h.
hypercapnic
hypercarbia
hypercarotenemia
hypercatabolic
hypercatabolism
hypercatharsis
hypercathartic
hypercellular
hypercellularity
    glomerular h.
hypercementosis
hyperchloremia
hyperchloremic
hyperchlorhydria
hyperchloridation
hyperchloriduria
hyperchloruration
hyperchloruria
hypercholesterolemia
    essential h.
    familial h.
    polygenic h.
hypercholesterolemic
hypercholesterolia
hypercholia
hyperchondroplasia
hyperchromaffinism
hyperchromasia
hyperchromatic
hyperchromatin

H

hyperchromatism
  macrocytic h.
hyperchromatopsia
hyperchromatosis
hyperchromemia
hyperchromia
  macrocytic h.
hyperchromic
hyperchromicity
hyperchylia
hyperchylomicronemia
  familial h.
hypercitruria
hypercoagulability
hypercoagulable
hypercorticalism
hypercorticism
hypercortisolism
hypercreatinemia
hypercryalgesia
hypercryesthesia
hypercupremia
hypercupriuria
hypercyanotic
hypercyesis
hypercythemia
hypercytochromia
hyperdactyly
hyperdiastole
hyperdicrotic
hyperdicrotism
hyperdiploid
hyperdipsia
hyperdistention
hyperdiuresis
hyperdontia
hyperdynamia uteri
hyperdynamic
hypereccrisia
hypereccritic
hyperechema
hyperechoic
hyperelastic
hyperelectrolytemia
hyperemesis
  h. gravidarum
  h. lactentium
hyperemetic
hyperemia
  active h.
  arterial h.
  Bier passive h.
  collateral h.
  conjunctival h.
  constriction h.

hyperemia *(continued)*
  fluxionary h.
  leptomeningeal h.
  passive h.
  reactive h.
  venous h.
hyperemic
hyperemization
hyperencephalus
hyperendemic
hyperendocrinism
hyperenergia
hypereosinophilia
  filarial h.
hyperepinephrinemia
hyperequilibrium
hypererethism
hypererergasia
hyperergia
hypererythrocythemia
hyperesophoria
  cerebral h.
  gustatory h.
  muscular h.
  olfactory h.
  oneiric h.
  optic h.
  tactile h.
hyperesthesia
  acoustic h.
  auditory h.
  cerebral h.
  gustatory h.
  muscular h.
  olfactory h.
  oneiric h.
  optic h.
  tactile h.
hyperesthetic
hyperestrinism
hyperestrogenemia
hyperestrogenism
hyperestrogenosis
hypereuryopia
hyperevolutism
hyperexcretory
hyperexophoria
hyperexplexia
hyperextension
hyperferremia
hyperferremic
hyperfibrinogenemia
hyperfibrinolysis
  systemic h.
hyperfiltration

hyperflexion
hyperfluorescence
hyperfolliculinism
hyperfractionation
hyperfunction
hyperfunctioning
hypergalactia
hypergalactous
hypergammaglobulinemia
  M-component h.
  monoclonal h.
  polyclonal h.
hypergastrinemia
hypergenesis
hypergenetic
hypergenitalism
hypergeusesthesia
hypergeusia
hypergia
hypergigantosoma
hyperglandular
hyperglobulia
hyperglobulinemia
hyperglobulism
hyperglucagonemia
hypergluconeogenesis
hyperglycemia
hyperglycemic
hyperglyceridemia
hyperglyceridemic
hyperglycerolemia
  infantile-type h.
  juvenile-type h.
  microdeletion-type h.
hyperglycinemia
  ketotic h.
  nonketotic h.
hyperglycinuria
hyperglycistia
hyperglycogenolysis
hyperglycorrhachia
hyperglycosuria
hyperglyoxylemia
hypergnosis
hypergonadism
hypergonadotropic
hypergonia
hypergranulation
  juxtaglomerular
    cell h.
hyperguanidinemia
hyperhedonia
hyperhemoglobinemia
hyperhemolytic
hyperheparinemia

hyperhepatia
hyperhidrosis
  axillary h.
  emotional h.
  gustatory h.
  h. lateralis
  unilateral h.
  h. unilateralis
  volar h.
hyperhidrotic
hyperhistaminemia
hyperhormonism
hyperhydration
hyperhydrochloria
hyperhydrochloridia
hyperhydroxyprolinemia
hyperhypnosis
hyperhypophysism
Hypericum perforatum
hyperimidodipeptiduria
hyperimmune globulin
hyperimmunity
hyperimmunization
  maternal h.
hyperimmunoglobulin E
hyperimmunoglobulinemia E
hyperindicanemia
hyperinflation
hyperingestion
hyperinnervation
hyperinsulinar
hyperinsulinemia
hyperinsulinism
  alimentary h.
  functional h.
  iatrogenic h.
hyperinvolution
hyperiodemia
hyperirritability
hyperisotonia
hyperisotonic
hyperisotonicity
hyperkalemia
hyperkaluria
hyperkeratinization
hyperkeratosis
  bullous ichthyosiform h.
  h. congenitalis palmaris et
    plantaris
  diffuse congenital h.
  epidermolytic h.
  h. excentrica
  h. figurata centrifuga
    atrophica
  follicular h.

hyperkeratosis *(continued)*
   h. follicularis et
     parafollicularis in cutem
     penetrans
   h. follicularis in cutem
     penetrans
   h. follicularis vegetans
   h. lacunaris
   h. lacunaris pharyngis
   h. lenticularis perstans
   h. linguae
   palmoplantar h.
   h. of palms and soles
   h. penetrans
   progressive dystrophic h.
   h. subungualis
   h. universalis congenita
hyperketonemia
hyperketonuria
hyperketosis
hyperkinemia
hyperkinemic
hyperkinesia
hyperkinesis
hyperkinetic
hyperkoria
hyperlactacidemia
hyperlactation
hyperlacticacidemia
hyperlecithinemia
hyperlethal
hyperleukocytosis
hyperleydigism
hyperlipemia
   carbohydrate-induced h.
   combined fat- and
     carbohydrate-induced h.
   endogenous h.
   essential familial h.
   familial h., essential
   familial fat-induced h.
   fat-induced h.
   idiopathic h.
   mixed h.
hyperlipidemia
   combined h.
   mixed h.
   multiple lipoprotein–type h.
hyperlipidemic
hyperlipoproteinemia
   acquired h.
   broad-beta h., familial
   combined h., familial
   familial h.
   familial h. (types I–V, IIa, IIb)

hyperlipoproteinemia *(continued)*
   Lp(a) h.
   mixed h.
hyperliposis
hyperlithemia
hyperlithic
hyperlithuria
hyperlordosis
hyperlucency
hyperlucent
hyperluteinization
hyperlutemia
hyperlysinuria
hypermagnesemia
hypermania
hypermastia
hypermature cataract
hypermedication
hypermelanosis
hypermelanotic
hypermenorrhea
hypermetabolic
hypermetabolism
     extrathyroidal h.
hypermetamorphosis
hypermetaplasia
hypermetria
hypermetrope
hypermetropia
hypermetropic
hypermicrosoma
hypermimia
hypermineralization
hypermnesia
hypermnesic
hypermodal
hypermorph
hypermotility
hypermyotonia
hypermyotrophy
hypernasal
hypernasality
hypernatremia
     hypodipsic h.
hypernatremic
hyperneocytosis
hypernephroid
hypernephroma
hypernidation
hypernitremia
hypernomic
hypernormal
hypernutrition
hyperocclusion
hyperoncotic

hyperonychia
hyperope
hyperopia
    absolute h.
    axial h.
    curvature h.
    facultative h.
    index h.
    latent h.
    manifest h.
    relative h.
    total h.
hyperopic
hyperorchidism
hyperorexia
hyperornithemia
hyperorthocytosis
hyperosmia
hyperosmolality
hyperosmolar coma
hyperosmolarity
hyperosmotic
hyperosphresia
hyperosteogenesis
hyperosteogeny
hyperostosis
    calvarial h.
    h. corticalis deformans
       juvenilis
    h. corticalis generalisata
    h. cranii
    flowing h.
    h. frontalis interna
    infantile conical h.
    infantile cortical h.
    Morgagni h.
    senile ankylosing h.
       of spine
hyperostotic
hyperovarianism
hyperovarism
hyperoxaluria
    enteric h.
    primary h.
       (type I, type II)
    secondary h.
hyperoxemia
hyperoxia
hyperoxic
hyperoxidation
hyperpallesthesia
hyperpancreorrhea
hyperparasite
    second-degree h.
hyperparasitoidism

hyperparathyroidism
    nutritional secondary h.
    primary h.
    secondary h.
    tertiary h.
hyperpathia
    thalamic h.
hyperpepsia
hyperpepsinemia
hyperpepsinia
hyperpepsinuria
hyperperistalsis
hyperpermeability
hyperpexia
hyperphagia
hyperphagic
hyperphalangia
hyperphenylalaninemia
    malignant h.
    maternal h.
    persistent h.
    transient h.
hyperphonesis
hyperphonia
hyperphoria
hyperphosphatasemia
    chronic congenital idiopathic h.
    h. tarda
hyperphosphatemia
hyperphosphaturia
hyperphosphoremia
hyperphrasia
hyperphrenia
hyperpiesia
hyperpiesis
hyperpietic
hyperpigmentation
hyperpinealism
hyperpipecolatemia
hyperpituitarism
    basophilic h.
    eosinophilic h.
hyperplasia
    adenomatous h.
    adrenal h.
    adrenal cortical h.
    adrenocortical h.
    angiofollicular mediastinal
       lymph node h.
    angiolymphoid h.
    angiolymphoid h. with
       eosinophilia
    basal cell h.
    benign mediastinal lymph
       node h.

H

hyperplasia *(continued)*
  benign prostatic h. (BPH)
  C-cell h.
  cementum h.
  chronic perforating pulp h.
  congenital adrenal h. (CAH)
  congenital adrenocortical h.
  congenital sebaceous gland h.
  congenital virilizing adrenal h.
  cutaneous lymphoid h.
  cystic-glandular h. of
    endometrium
  cystic h. of breasts
  cystic prostatic h.
  denture h.
  Dilantin h.
  endometrial h.
  h. endometrii
  epiphyseal h.
  fibromuscular h.
  fibrous inflammatory h.
  focal adenomyomatous h. of
    gallbladder
  focal nodular h. (FNH)
  focal nodular h. of liver
  follicular h.
  giant follicular h.
  giant lymph node h.
  gingival h.
  hilus cell h.
  inflammatory h.
  intimal h.
  islet cell h.
  juxtaglomerular cell h.
  Leydig cell h.
  lipoid h.
  lipoid adrenal h.
  lymphoid h.
  mesangial h.
  neoplastic h.
  nodular adrenocortical h.
  nodular lymphoid h.
  ovarian stromal h.
  polar h.
  polypoid h.
  postmenopausal h.
  proliferative h.
  pseudoepitheliomatous h.
  Schwann h.
  sebaceous h.
  stromal h.
  Swiss-cheese h.
  thymic medullary h.
  verrucous h.
hyperplasmia

hyperplasminemia
hyperplastic
    h. endometrium
    h. polyp
hyperploid
hyperploidy
hyperpnea
hyperpneic
hyperpolarization
hyperpolypeptidemia
hyperponesis
hyperponetic
hyperposia
hyperpotassemia
hyperpragic
hyperpraxia
hyperprebetalipoproteinemia
    familial h.
hyperpresbyopia
hyperprogesteronemia
hyperproinsulinemia
hyperprolactinemia
hyperprolactinemic
hyperprolactinism
hyperprolinemia
    familial h.
    h., type I
    h., type II
hyperprosessis
hyperprosexia
hyperprosody
hyperproteinemia
hyperproteosis
hyperpselaphesia
hyperptyalism
hyperpyremia
hyperpyretic
hyperpyrexia
    fulminant h.
    heat h.
    malignant h.
hyperpyrexial
hyperreactive airways
hyperreflexia
    autonomic h.
    detrusor h.
hyperreninemia
hyperreninemic
hyperresonance
hyperresonant
hyperresponsive
hyperresponsiveness
    airway h.
hypersalemia
hypersaline

hypersalivation
hypersarcosinemia
hypersecretion
    gastric h.
hypersegmentation
    hereditary h. of neutrophils
hypersensibility
hypersensitive
hypersensitivity
    atopic h.
    carotid sinus h.
    contact h.
    cutaneous basophil h.
    delayed h. (DH)
    delayed-type h. (DTH)
    immediate h.
    tuberculin-type h.
    type I–IV h.
hypersensitization
hyperserotonemia
hypersexuality
hypersomatotropism
hypersomia
hypersomnia
    continuous h.
    paroxysmal h.
    periodic h.
    primary h.
hypersomnolence
hypersphyxia
hypersplenism
hyperspongiosis
hypersteatosis
hyperstereoradiography
hypersthenia
hypersthenic
hypersthenuria
hyperstimulation
hypersuprarenalism
hypersusceptibility
hypersympathicotonus
hypertarachia
hypertaurodontism
hypertelorism
    canthal h.
    ocular h.
    orbital h.
hypertensin
hypertensinase
hypertensinogen
hypertension
    accelerated h.
    adrenal h.
    arterial h.
    benign intracranial h.

hypertension *(continued)*
    borderline h.
    diastolic h.
    endolymphatic h.
    episodic h.
    essential h.
    gestational h.
    Goldblatt h.
    idiopathic h.
    intracranial h.
    labile h.
    low-renin h.
    malignant h.
    neuromuscular h.
    ocular h.
    pale h.
    paroxysmal h.
    pituitary h.
    portal h.
    primary h.
    pulmonary h.
    red h.
    renal h.
    renin-dependent h.
    renoprival h.
    renovascular h.
    secondary h.
    splenoportal h.
    suprarenal h.
    symptomatic h.
    systemic venous h.
    systolic h.
    transient h.
    vascular h.
    venous h.
hypertensive
    h. crisis
    h. encephalopathy
    h. heart disease
    h. pulmonary vascular disease
    h. renal disease
    h. retinopathy
    h. vascular disease
hypertensor
hypertestosteronism
hyperthecosis
    testoid h.
hyperthelia
hyperthermal
hyperthermalgesia
hyperthermesthesia
hyperthermia
    h. of anesthesia
    malignant h.
    whole-body h.

H

hyperthrombinemia
hyperthymia
hyperthymic
hyperthymism
hyperthyroid
hyperthyroidism
    apathetic h.
    factitious h.
    iatrogenic h.
    iodine-induced h.
    masked h.
    primary h.
    secondary h.
hyperthyroxinemia
    familial dysalbuminemic h.
hypertonia
    h. oculi
    h. polycythaemica
hypertonicity
hypertonic saline
hypertoxic
hypertoxicity
hypertransfusion
hypertrichosis
    h. lanuginosa
    h. pinnae auris
    h. universalis
hypertriglyceridemia
    alimentary h.
    carbohydrate-induced h.
    endogenous h.
    exogenous h.
    familial h.
    familial fat-induced h.
hypertrophia musculorum vera
hypertrophic
hypertrophy
    adaptive h.
    adenoid h.
    adult h. of pylorus
    benign h. of pons
    benign prostatic h. (BPH)
    bilateral h. of masseters
    Billroth h.
    biventricular h.
    breast h. of newborn
    cardiac concentric h.
    cicatricial h.
    compensatory h.
    compensatory h. of heart
    complementary h.
    concentric h.
    congenital h. of bladder neck
    denture h.
    eccentric h.

hypertrophy *(continued)*
    false h.
    fibromuscular h.
    functional h.
    hemangiectatic h.
    hemifacial h.
    juxtaglomerular cell h.
    mammary h.
    Marie h.
    mulberry h.
    numeric h.
    physiologic h.
    prostatic h.
    pseudomuscular h.
    renal h.
    septal h.
    simple h.
    true h.
    unilateral h.
    ventricular h.
    vicarious h.
hypertropia
hypertyrosinemia
hyperuresis
hyperuricemia
    X-linked h.
hyperuricemic
hyperuricuria
hypervaccination
hypervascular
hyperventilation
    central neurogenic h.
    hysterical h.
hypervigilance
hyperviscosity
hypervitaminosis
    h. A
    h. D
hypervitaminotic
hypervolemia
hypervolemic
hypervolia
hypesthesia
hypha (hyphae)
hyphal
hyphedonia
hyphema
hyphidrosis
hyphomycete
hyphomycosis
hyphylline
hypisotonic
hypnagogic
hypnagogue
hypnalgia

hypnic
hypnoanalysis
hypnoanesthesia
hypnocinematograph
hypnocyst
hypnodontics
hypnogenic
hypnoid
hypnoidal
hypnology
hypnonarcosis
hypnopedia
hypnopompic
hypnosis
hypnosophy
hypnotherapy
hypnotic
hypnotism
hypnotist
hypnotization
hypnotize
hypnotoxin
hypnozoite
hypoacidity
hypoactive
    h. bowel sounds
    h. deep tendon reflexes
hypoactivity
hypoacusis
hypoadenia
hypoadrenalemia
hypoadrenalism
hypoadrenocortical
hypoadrenocorticism
    pituitary h.
    secondary h.
hypoaeration
hypoagnathus
hypoalbuminemia
hypoalbuminosis
hypoaldosteronemia
hypoaldosteronism
    hyporeninemic h.
    isolated h.
hypoaldosteronuria
hypoalimentation
hypoalkaline
hypoalkalinity
hypoallergenic
hypoalonemia
hypoalphalipoproteinemia
hypoaminoacidemia
hypoandrogenism
hypoazoturia
hypobaric

hypobarism
hypobaropathy
hypobetalipoproteinemia
    familial h.
hypobilirubinemia
hypoblast
hypoblastic
hypobranchial
hypobromite
hypobromous acid
hypocalcemia
    neonatal h.
hypocalcemic
hypocalcia
hypocalcification
    enamel h.
hypocalcipectic
hypocalcipexy
hypocalcitoninemia
hypocalciuria
hypocapnia
hypocapnic
hypocarbia
hypocatalasemia
hypocellular
hypocellularity
hypocenter
hypoceruloplasminemia
hypochloremia
hypochloremic
hypochlorhydria
hypochloridation
hypochlorite
    sodium h.
hypochlorization
hypochlorous acid
hypochloruria
hypocholesterolemia
hypocholesterolemic
hypocholia
hypocholuria
hypochondria (plural of
    hypochondrium)
hypochondriac
hypochondriacal
hypochondriasis
hypochondrium (hypochondria)
hypochondroplasia
hypochordal
hypochromasia
hypochromatic
hypochromatism
hypochromatosis
hypochromemia
    idiopathic h.

H

hypochromia
    idiopathic h.
hypochromic
hypochromicity
hypochromotrichia
hypochrosis
hypochylia
hypocistis
hypocitremia
hypocitruria
hypocoagulability
hypocoagulable
hypocomplementemia
hypocomplementemic
hypocondylar
hypocone
hypoconid
hypoconulid
hypocorticalism
hypocorticism
hypocrisy
hypocupremia
hypocyclosis
hypocythemia
hypocytosis
hypodactyly
hypoderm
Hypoderma
    H. bovis
    H. lineatum
hypodermatomy
hypodermiasis
hypodermic
    h. microscope
    h. needle
hypodermis
hypodermoclysis
hypodermolithiasis
hypodermomycosis
hypodiaphragmatic
hypodiploid
hypodiploidy
hypodipsia
hypodipsic
hypodontia
hypodynamia
    h. cordis
hypodynamic
hypoeccrisia
hypoeccritic
hypoechoic
hypoelectrolytemia
hypoeosinophilia
hypoepinephrinemia
hypoequilibrium

hypoergasia
hypoergia
hypoergic
hypoesophoria
hypoesthesia
    acoustic h.
    auditory h.
    gustatory h.
    olfactory h.
    tactile h.
hypoesthetic
hypoestrogenemia
hypoestrogenemism
hypoevolutism
hypoexcitability
hypoexcitable
hypoexophoria
hypoferremia
hypoferrism
hypofertile
hypofertility
hypofibrinogenemia
hypofluorescence
hypofunction
    convergence h.
    divergence h.
hypogalactia
hypogalactous
hypogammaglobulinemia
    acquired h.
    common variable h.
    congenital h.
    lymphopenic h.
    physiologic h.
    primary h.
    secondary h.
    Swiss-type h.
    transient h.
    transient h. of
      infancy
    X-linked h.
    X-linked infantile h.
hypoganglionosis
hypogastric
hypogastrium
hypogastropagus
hypogastroschisis
hypogenesis
    polar h.
hypogenetic
hypogenitalism
hypogeusia
hypoglandular
hypoglobulia
hypoglossal

hypoglossus
hypoglottis
hypoglucagonemia
hypoglycemia
    factitial h.
    factitious h.
    fasting h.
    functional h.
    ketotic h.
    leucine-induced h.
    mixed h.
    reactive h.
hypoglycemic
hypoglycemosis
hypoglycin (A or B)
hypoglycine
hypoglycogenolysis
hypoglycorrhachia
hypognathous
hypognathus
hypogonadal
hypogonadism
    eugonadotropic h.
    familial hypogonadotropic h.
    hypergonadotropic h.
    hypogonadotropic h.
    pituitary h.
    primary h.
    secondary h.
    h. with anosmia
hypogonadotropic
hypogonadotropism
hypogranulocytosis
hypohepatia
hypohidrosis
hypohidrotic
hypohormonal
hypohyal
hypohydration
hypohydrochloria
hypohypnotic
hypohypophysism
hypoinsulinemia
hypoinsulinism
hypointense
hypoiodidism
hypoisotonic
hypokalemia
hypokalemic
hypokinemia
hypokinesia
hypokinesis
hypokinetic
hypolactasia
hypolarynx

hypolemmal
hypolethal
hypoleukocytic
hypoleydigism
hypolipemia
hypolipidemic
hypolipoproteinemia
hypoliposis
hypoliquorrhea
hypolutemia
hypolymphemia
hypomagnesemia
hypomania
hypomanic
hypomastia
hypomelancholia
hypomelanism
    dominant oculocutaneous h.
hypomelanosis
    hereditary h.
    idiopathic guttate h.
    h. of Ito
hypomenorrhea
hypomere
hypomery
hypomesosoma
hypometabolic
hypometabolism
    euthyroid h.
hypometria
hypometropia
hypomicron
hypomicrosoma
hypomineralization
hypomnesia
hypomnesis
hypomorph
hypomotility
hypomyotonia
hypomyxia
hyponanosoma
hyponasality
hyponatremia
    depletional h.
    dilutional h.
    hyperlipemic h.
hyponatremic
hyponatruria
hyponeocytosis
hyponitremia
hyponoia
hyponychial
hyponychium
hyponychon
hypo-oncotic

hypo-orchidism
hypo-orthocytosis
hypo-osmolality
hypo-osmosis
hypo-osmotic
hypo-ovaria
hypo-ovarianism
hypopallesthesia
hypopancreatism
hypopancreorrhea
hypoparathyroid
hypoparathyroidism
　　familial h.
hypopepsia
hypopepsinia
hypoperfusion
hypoperistalsis
hypoperistaltic
hypopexia
hypophalangism
hypophamine
hypopharyngeal
hypopharyngoscope
hypopharyngoscopy
hypopharynx
hypophonesis
hypophonia
hypophoria
hypophosphatasia
hypophosphatemia
　　familial h.
　　hereditary h.
　　renal h.
　　X-linked h.
hypophosphatemic
hypophosphaturia
hypophosphite
　　ferric h.
hypophosphorous acid
hypophrenia
hypophrenic
hypophrenium
hypophrenosis
hypophyseal, hypophysial
hypophysectomize
hypophysectomy
　　transsphenoidal h.
hypophysial, hypophyseal
hypophysin
hypophysioportal
hypophysioprivic
hypophysiotropic
hypophysis
　　accessory h.
　　h. cerebri

hypophysis *(continued)*
　　pharyngeal h.
hypophysitis
hypopiesia
hypopiesis
hypopietic
hypopigmentation
hypopigmenter
hypopinealism
hypopituitarism
　　postpartum hemorrhagic h.
hypopituitary
hypoplasia
　　h. of aortic tract complexes
　　cartilage-hair h.
　　congenital generalized
　　　muscular h.
　　craniofacial h.
　　h. cutis congenita
　　enamel h.
　　focal dermal h.
　　granulocytic h.
　　hereditary brown h. of enamel
　　lobular h.
　　nasomaxillary h.
　　oligomeganephronic renal h.
　　oligonephronic h.
　　pluricystic h.
　　thymic h.
　　h. of tooth
　　Turner h.
hypoplastic
hypoploid
hypopnea
hypopneic
hypoponesis
hypoporosis
hypoposia
hypopotassemia
hypopotassemic
hypopotentia
hypopraxia
hypoproaccelerinemia
hypoproconvertinemia
　　hereditary h.
hypoprogesterone hexanoate
hypoprosody
hypoproteinemia
　　chronic idiopathic h. in child
　　prehepatic h.
hypoproteinemic
hypoproteinia
hypoproteinic
hypoproteinosis
hypoprothrombinemia

hypopselaphesia
hypopteronosis cystica
hypoptyalism
hypopyon
hyporeactive
hyporeflexia
hyporeninemia
hyporeninemic
hyporiboflavinosis
hyporrhea
hyposalemia
hyposalivation
hyposarca
hyposcheotomy
hyposcleral
hyposecretion
hyposegmentation
hyposensitive
hyposensitivity
hyposensitization
hyposensitize
hyposexuality
hyposialosis
hyposkeocytosis
hyposmia
hyposmolarity
hyposmosis
hyposomatotropism
hyposomia
hyposomnia
hypospadiac
hypospadias
    balanic h.
    balanitic h.
    female h.
    glandular h.
    penile h.
    penoscrotal h.
    perineal h.
    pseudovaginal h.
hyposphresia
hyposplenism
hypostasis
hypostatic
hyposteatolysis
hyposteatosis
hyposthenia
hypostheniant
hyposthenic
hyposthenuria
    tubular h.
hypostomia
hypostomial
hypostosis
hypostypsis

hypostyptic
hyposulfite
hyposuprarenalism
hyposympathicotonus
hyposynergia
hypotaxia
hypotelorism
    ocular h.
    orbital h.
hypotension
    arterial h.
    chronic idiopathic orthostatic h.
    chronic orthostatic h.
    controlled h.
    familial orthostatic h.
    idiopathic orthostatic h.
    induced h.
    intracranial h.
    orthostatic h.
    postural h.
    spinal h.
    vascular h.
    ventricular h.
hypotensive
hypotensor
hypothalamic
    h. suppression
hypothalamotomy
hypothalamus
hypothenar
    h. eminence
hypothermal
hypothermia
    endogenous h.
    induced h.
    moderate h.
    profound h.
    regional h.
hypothermic
hypothesis (hypotheses)
    alternative h.
    biogenic amine h.
    Buergi h.
    cardionector h.
    cascade h. of coagulation
    Dreyer and Bennett h.
    Gad h.
    gate h.
    Harrower h.
    insular h.
    jelly roll h.
    Keller h.
    lattice h.
    Lyon h.
    Makeham h.

H

hypothesis (hypotheses) *(continued)*
    null h.
    one gene–one enzyme h.
    one gene–one polypeptide
      chain h.
    Orgel h.
    permissive h. of affective
      disorders
    sliding filament h.
    Starling h.
    unitarian h.
    wobble h.
hypothrepsia
hypothrombinemia
hypothromboplastinemia
hypothymia
hypothymic
hypothymism
hypothyroid
hypothyroidism
    familial goitrous h.
    hypothalamic h.
    infantile h.
    postoperative h.
    primary h.
    tertiary h.
    thyroprivic h.
hypotonia
    benign congenital h.
    infantile h.
    ocular h.
    h. oculi
hypotonic
    h. duodenography
hypotonicity
hypotony
hypotoxicity
hypotransferrinemia
hypotrichiasis
hypotrichosis
hypotrichous
hypotrophy
hypotropia
hypotryptophanic
hypotympanic
hypotympanotomy
hypotympanum
hypouremia
hypouresis
hypouricemia
hypouricuria
hypourocrinia
hypovarianism
hypovasopressinemia
hypovenosity

hypoventilation
    alveolar h.
    central h.
    chronic alveolar h.
    primary alveolar h.
hypovigility
hypovitaminosis
hypovolemia
hypovolemic
hypovolia
hypoxanthine guanine
    phosphoribosyltransferase
    (HGPRT, HPRT)
hypoxanthine oxidase
hypoxanthine
    phosphoribosyltransferase
    (HPRT)
hypoxemia
hypoxemic
hypoxia
    anemic h.
    circulatory h.
    diffusion h.
    histotoxic h.
    hypoxic h.
    stagnant h.
hypoxic
    h. insult
hypoxidosis
hypsarrhythmia
hypsibrachycephalic
hypsicephalic
hypsicephaly
hypsiconchous
hypsiloid
hypsistaphylia
hypsistenocephalic
hypsocephalous
hypsochrome
hypsochromy
hypsodont
hypsokinesis
hypsonosus
hypsotherapy
hypurgia
Hyrtl
    anastomosis
    loop
    recess
    sphincter
hysteralgia
hysteratresia
hysterectomy
    abdominal h.
    abdominovaginal h.

hysterectomy *(continued)*
    Ballantine h. forceps
    Bonney h.
    Carmalt h. forceps
    cesarean h.
    chemical h.
    complete h.
    Doyen vaginal h.
    extrafascial h.
    Heaney vaginal h.
    intrafascial h.
    Lash h.
    Latzko radical h.
    Mayo-Ward vaginal h.
    paravaginal h.
    partial h.
    Porro h.
    radical h.
    Schauta radical vaginal h.
    Schauta-Amreich
      vaginal h.
    Spalding-Richardson h.
    subtotal h.
    supracervical h.
    supravaginal h.
    total h.
    total abdominal h.
      (TAH)
    total vaginal h.
      (TVH)
    vaginal h. (VH)
    Ward-Mayo vaginal h.
    Wertheim radical h.
hysteremphysema
hysteresis
    protoplasmic h.
hystereurynter
hystereurysis
    major h.
hysteria
    anxiety h.
    canine h.
    combat h.
    conversion h.
    degenerative h.
    dissociative h.
    epidemic h.
    fixation h.
    major h.
    h.-malingering
    masked h.
    monosymptomatic h.
    reflex h.
    retention h.
    traumatic h.

hysteric
hysterical
    h. amblyopia
    h. field
hystericism
hysterics
hysteriform
hysterobubonocele
hysterocarcinoma
hysterocele
hysterocleisis
hysterocolpectomy
hysterocolposcope
hysterocystic
hysterocystocleisis
hysterocystopexy
hysterodynia
hysteroedema
hysteroepilepsy
hysterogenic
hysterogram
hysterograph
hysterography
hysteroid
hysterolith
hysterology
hysterolysis
hysterometer
hysterometry
hysteromyoma
hysteromyomectomy
hysteromyotomy
hysteroneurosis
hystero-oophorectomy
hystero-ovariotomy
hysteropathy
hysteropexy
hysteropia
hysteroplasty
hysteropsychosis
hysteroptosia
hysteroptosis
hysterorrhaphy
hysterorrhexis
hysterosalpingectomy
hysterosalpingogram
hysterosalpingography
hysterosalpingo-
    oophorectomy
hysterosalpingostomy
hysterosalpinx
hysteroscope
    Baggish h.
    Baloser h.
    Storz h.

H

hysteroscopic
hysteroscopy
    laparoscopic-assisted vaginal
      h. (LAVH)
hysterospasm
hysterostat
hysterostomatomy
hysterothermometry
hysterotome
hysterotomy
    abdominal h.

hysterotomy *(continued)*
    vaginal h.
hysterotrachelectasia
hysterotrachelectomy
hysterotracheloplasty
hysterotrachelorrhaphy
hysterotrachelotomy
hysterotubography
Hz—hertz
HZ—herpes zoster
HZV—herpes zoster virus

I

ι—iota (Greek letter)
I—
    iodine
    incisor
    inosine
^{131}I—radioactive iodine [iodine
  I 131]
IA—
    internal auditory
    intra-aortic
    intra-arterial
IABP—intra-aortic balloon pump
IAC—internal auditory canal
IADH—inappropriate antidiuretic
  hormone
IADL—instrumental activities of
  daily living
IAEA—International Atomic
  Energy Agency
IAHA—immune adherence
  hemagglutination assay
IAM—internal auditory meatus
iamatology
IAS—
    interatrial septum
    intra-amniotic saline
IASD—interatrial septal defect
IAS infusion
IASP—International Association
  for the Study of Pain
IAT—
    invasive activity test
    iodine-azide test
iatraliptic
iatric
iatrochemical

iatrochemistry
iatrogenesis
iatrogenic
iatrology
iatromathematical
iatromechanical
iatrophysical
iatrophysics
IB—
    immune body
    inclusion body
IBB—intestinal brush border
IBC—iron-binding capacity
I-beam
IBF—immunoglobulin-binding factor
IBU—international benzoate unit
IC—
    immune complex
    inspiratory capacity
    intensive care
    intercostal
    intermediate care
    intermittent claudication
    internal conversion
    intracavitary
    intracellular
    intracerebral
    intracranial
    intracutaneous
    irritable colon
    isovolumic contraction
ICA—
    internal carotid artery
    intracranial aneurysm
ICAM-1—intercellular adhesion
  molecule-1

ICAO—internal carotid artery occlusion
ICC—intensive coronary care
ICCU—intensive coronary care unit
ICD—
    International Classification of Diseases
    intrauterine contraceptive device
    ischemic coronary disease
ice
    dry i.
ICE—iridocorneal-endothelial (syndrome)
Iceland disease
I-cell disease
ICF—intermediate care facility
ICG—indocyanine green
ichnogram
ichthammol
ichthyism
ichthyismus exanthematicus
ichthyoacanthotoxin
ichthyoacanthotoxism
ichthyocolla
ichthyohemotoxin
ichthyohemotoxism
ichthyoid
ichthyootoxin
ichthyootoxism
ichthyophagia
ichthyophagous
ichthyophthiriasis
ichthyosarcotoxin
ichthyosarcotoxism
ichthyosiform erythroderma
ichthyosis
    acquired i.
    i. congenita
    congenital i.
    i. cornea
    i. fetalis
    follicular i.
    i. follicularis
    i. hystrix
    i. intrauterina
    lamellar i.
    linear i.
    i. linearis circumflexa
    i. linguae
    nacreous i.
    i. palmaris
    i. palmaris et plantaris
    i. plantaris
    i. sauroderma

ichthyosis *(continued)*
    i. scutulata
    i. sebacea cornea
    senile i.
    i. serpentina
    sex-linked recessive i.
    i. simplex
    i. spinosa
    i. uteri
    i. vulgaris
    X-linked i.
ichthyotic
ichthyotoxic
ichthyotoxicology
ichthyotoxin
ichthyotoxism
ICM—intercostal margin
ICN—International Council of Nurses
icosanoic acid
icosanoid
icosapentaenoic acid
icosatrienoic acid
ICP—intracranial pressure
ICRP—International Commission on Radiological Protection
ICS—
    intercostal space
    International College of Surgeons
ICT—
    inflammation of connective tissue
    insulin coma therapy
    isovolumic contraction time
ictal
icteric
icteritious
icteroanemia
icterogenic
icterogenicity
icterohematuria
icterohematuric
icterohemoglobinuria
icterohepatitis
icteroid
icterus
    bilirubin i.
    i. catarrhalis
    choluric hemolytic i. with splenomegaly
    chronic familial i.
    congenital familial i.
    congenital hemolytic i.
    epidemic catarrhal i.
    i. gravis

I

icterus *(continued)*
    i. gravis neonatorum
    i. hemolyticus
    i. infectiosus
    i. melas
    i. neonatorum
    nuclear i.
    i. praecox
    i. simplex
    spirochetal i.
    i. typhoides
    urobilin i.
    i. viridans
ictus
    i. cordis
    i. epilepticus
    i. paralyticus
    i. sanguinis
    i. solis
ICU—intensive care unit
ICW—intracellular water
ID—
    identification
    immunodeficiency
    infant death(s)
    infectious disease(s)
    infective dose
    inside diameter
    internal diameter
    intradermal
I&D—
    incision and drainage
    irrigation and débridement
IDA—image display and analysis
IDD—insulin-dependent
  diabetes
IDDM—insulin-dependent diabetes
  mellitus
idea
    autochthonous i.
    complex of i's
    compulsive i.
    concatenated i's
    dominant i.
    fixed i.
    flight of i's
    imperative i.
    overproductive i's
    overvalued i.
    i's of reference
    referential i.
    ruminative i.
ideal
    ego i.
idealization

ideation
    homicidal i.
    incoherent i.
    paranoid i.
    suicidal i.
ideational
idée fixe
identification
    cosmic i.
    projective i.
identity
    body i.
    core gender i.
    i. crisis
    i. diffusion
    ego i.
    family i.
    gender i.
    i. integration
    sense of personal i.
    sexual i.
identity disorder
    i.d. of childhood
    dissociative i.d.
    psychosexual i.d.
    sexual and gender i.d.
ideogenetic
ideokinetic
ideology
ideomotion
ideomotor
IDI—induction-delivery
  interval
idioagglutinin
idiogenesis
idioglossia
idioglottic
idiogram
idiographic
idioheteroagglutinin
idioheterolysin
idiohypnotism
idioisoagglutinin
idioisolysin
idiolalia
idiologism
idiolysin
idiomuscular
idiopathic
    i. abortion
    i. amyloidosis
    i. atrophoderma of Pasini and
      Pierini
    i. cardiomyopathy
    i. cervical dystonia

idiopathic *(continued)*
    i. dilatation
    i. disease
    i. edema
    i. epilepsy
    i. glossitis
    i. gout
    i. guttate hypomelanosis
    i. hypercalcemia
    i. hypercalciuria
    i. hypertension
    i. hypertrophic
      osteoarthropathy
    i. hypertrophic subaortic
      stenosis (IHSS)
    i. intracranial hypertension
    i. livedo reticularis
    i. megacolon
    i. multiple pigmented
      hemorrhagic sarcoma
    i. muscular atrophy
    i. myocarditis
    i. neutropenia
    i. nodular panniculitis
    i. pericarditis
    i. photodermatosis
    i. postprandial syndrome
    i. proctitis
    i. pulmonary fibrosis
    i. purpura
    i. resorption
    i. respiratory distress of
      newborn
    i. retroperitoneal fibrosis
    i. steatorrhea
    i. thrombocythemia
    i. thrombocytopenic purpura
    i. unilobar emphysema
    i. urticaria
idiopathy
idiophrenic
idioreflex
idioretinal
idiosome
idiospasm
idiosyncrasy
idiosyncratic
idiotope
idiotopy
idiotrophic
idiotropic
idiotype
idiotypic
idiovariation
idioventricular rhythm

L-iditol 2-dehydrogenase
IDL—intermediate-density
  lipoprotein
IDM—infant of diabetic mother
L-idose
IDP—initial dose period
IDR—intradermal reaction
id reaction
IDS—
    immunity deficiency state
    inhibitor of DNA synthesis
IDU—
    idoxuridine
    iododeoxyuridine
iduronate-2-sulfatase
iduronic acid
iduronic sulfatase
α-L-iduronidase [alpha-]
IDVC—indwelling venous catheter
I/E—inspiratory-expiratory ratio
IEF—isoelectric focusing
IEL—intraepithelial lymphocytes
IEM—
    immune electron microscopy
    inborn error of metabolism
IEMG—integrated electromyogram
IEP—
    immunoelectrophoresis
    isoelectric point
    isoelectric precipitation
IF—
    immunofluorescence
    initiation factor
    interferon
    interstitial fluid
    intrinsic factor
IFA—
    immunofluorescence assay
    indirect fluorescent antibody
IFC—intrinsic factor
  concentrate
IFN—interferon
IFN-α—interferon-α
IFN-β—interferon-β
IFN-γ—interferon-γ
IFR—inspiratory flow rate
IFRA—indirect fluorescent rabies
  antibody
Ig—immunoglobulin
IG—
    immune globulin
    intragastric
IgA, IgD, IgE, IgG, IgM—
  immunoglobulin A, etc.
IgA deficiency

I

IGDM—infant of gestational
diabetic mother
IGF-1—insulin-like growth factor-1
Iglesias resectoscope
IgM deficiency
ignipuncture
ignis
ignisation
ignotine
IGT—impaired glucose tolerance
IGV—intrathoracic gas volume
IH—
    idiopathic hyperprolactinemia
    infectious hepatitis
    inner half
IHA—indirect hemagglutination
IHC—
    idiopathic hypercalciuria
    immunohistochemistry
IHD—ischemic heart disease
IHO—idiopathic hypertrophic
    osteoarthropathy
IHR—intrinsic heart rate
IHSA—iodinated human serum
    albumin
IHSS—idiopathic hypertrophic
    subaortic stenosis
IIF—indirect immunofluorescence
IJP—internal jugular pressure
IJV—internal jugular vein
IL—interleukin (IL-1 through
    IL-15)
ILA—
    insulin-like activity
    International Leprosy
        Association
ILB, ILBW—infant of low
    birthweight
ILD—
    interstitial lung disease
    ischemic leg disease
    ischemic limb disease
ileac
ileadelphus
ileal conduit diversion
ileectomy
ileitis
    backwash i.
    distal i.
    prestomal i.
    regional i.
    terminal i.
ileocecal cutaneous diversion
ileocecostomy
ileocecum

ileocolic
ileocolitis
    tuberculous i.
    i. ulcerosa chronica
ileocolostomy
ileocolotomy
ileocystoplasty
    Camey i.
    LeDuc-Camey i.
ileocystostomy
ileoileostomy
ileojejunitis
    granulomatous i.
    nongranulomatous i.
ileopexy
ileoproctostomy
ileorectal
ileorectostomy
ileorrhaphy
ileosigmoid
ileosigmoidostomy
ileostomy
    end i.
    Kock i.
ileotomy
ileotransverse
    i. colostomy
    end-to-side i. colostomy
ileotransversostomy
ileum
    duplex i.
    terminal i.
ileus
    adynamic i.
    angiomesenteric i.
    dynamic i.
    gallstone i.
    gastric i.
    hyperdynamic i.
    mechanical i.
    meconium i.
    occlusive i.
    paralytic i.
    i. paralyticus
    spastic i.
    i. subparta
    terminal i.
Ilfeld-Holder deformity
ilia (plural of ilium)
iliac
iliadelphus
Iliff operation
iliococcygeal
iliococcygeus
iliocolotomy

iliocostal
iliodorsal
iliofemoral
iliofemoroplasty
iliohypogastric
ilioinguinal
iliolumbar
iliolumbocostoabdominal
iliopagus
iliopectineal
iliopelvic
ilioperoneal
iliopsoas
iliopubic
iliosacral
iliosciatic
ilioscrotal
iliospinal
iliothoracopagus
iliotibial
iliotrochanteric
ilioxiphopagus
ilium (ilia)
Ilizarov leg-lengthening procedure
ill
    föhn i.
illacrimation
illaqueation
ill-defined
illicit
illinition
illness
    acute on chronic i.
    compressed-air i.
    debilitating i.
    emotional i.
    functional i.
    grave i.
    high-altitude i.
    mental i.
    psychosomatic i.
    radiation i.
    refractory i.
    terminal i.
illumination
    axial i.
    central i.
    contact i.
    critical i.
    darkfield i.
    dark-ground i.
    direct i.
    focal i.
    Köhler i.
    lateral i.

illumination *(continued)*
    oblique i.
    orthogonal i.
    surface i.
    through i.
illuminator
    Abbe i.
illuminism
illusion
    autokinetic i.
    i. or delusions
    epileptic i.
    Fregoli i.
    Kuhnt i.
    optical i.
illusional
illutation
IM—
    infectious mononucleosis
    internal medicine
    intramuscular
    intramuscularly
IMA—internal mammary artery
IMAA—iodinated macroaggregated
  albumin
image
    accidental i.
    acoustic i.
    i. aliasing
    i. amplifier
    i. analysis
    auditory i.
    body i.
    calculated i.
    i. chains
    conceptual i.
    i. contrast
    i. converter
    direct i.
    i. displacement
    double i.
    eidetic i., visual
    erect i.
    false i.
    fluoroscopic i.
    i.-forming system
    gamma i.
    gated i.
    heteronymous i.
    homonymous i.
    idealized i.
    incidental i.
    i. intensification
    i. intensifier system
    i. intensifier tube

I

image *(continued)*
- inversion recovery i.
- inverted i.
- i. jump
- memory i.
- mental i.
- mirror i.
- motor i.
- negative i.
- i. noise
- nuclear magnetic
  resonance i.
- optical i.
- parametric i.
- percept i.
- personal i.
- phantom i.
- i. point
- primary memory i.
- primary mental i.
- pulse echo i.
- Purkinje i's
- Purkinje-Sanson mirror i's
- i. quality
- radiographic i.
- radioisotope i.
- real i.
- i. reconstruction
- i. reformation
- renal i.
- i. resolution
- retinal i.
- Sanson i.
- saturation recovery i.
- scout i.
- sensory i.
- i. sharpness
- i. slice thickness
- specular i.
- spin echo i.
- static renal i.
- tactile i.
- true i.
- unconscious i.
- virtual i.
- x-ray i.

image-amplified fluoroscopy

imagery
- eidetic i.
- guided i.
- guided affective i.
- hypnagogic i.
- hypnopompic i.
- spontaneous i.

imagines (plural of imago)

imaging
- acoustic i.
- adrenal i.
- blood pool i.
- cardiac blood pool i.
- coded-aperture i.
- color flow Doppler i.
- diagnostic i.
- digital vascular i. (DVI)
- direct Fourier transformation i.
- dynamic i.
- dynamic volume i.
- echo-planar i.
- electrostatic i.
- flow i.
- Fourier i.
- gated blood pool i.
- gated cardiac blood pool i.
- gated magnetic resonance i.
- gray-scale i.
- heavy ion i.
- hot spot i.
- infarct-avid i.
- isotope colloid i.
- isotope hepatobiliary i.
- line i.
- longitudinal section i.
- lymph node i.
- magnetic resonance i. (MRI)
- microwave i.
- multigated i.
- multiplanar i.
- multiple-gated blood pool i.
- multiple line scan i.
- multiple spin echo total
  volume i.
- myocardial infarct i.
- myocardial perfusion i.
- nuclear i.
- nuclear magnetic resonance i.
- perfusion i.
- planar i.
- planar spin i.
- projection reconstruction i.
- pulse echo i.
- pyrophosphate i.
- quantitative brain i.
- radionuclide i.
- reconstructive i.
- reticuloendothelial i.
- rotating-frame i.
- selective excitation projection
  reconstruction i.
- sensitive plane projection
  reconstruction i.

imaging (continued)
  sequential first pass i.
  sequential plane i.
  sonographic i.
  spin-echo i.
  spin-warp i.
  static i.
  stop-action i.
  technetium Tc 99m
    pyrophosphate i.
  thallium-201 i.
  three-dimensional i.
  three-dimensional
    echo planar i.
  three-dimensional Fourier i.
  three-dimensional projection
    reconstruction i.
  through-transmission i.
  transverse section i.
  two-dimensional i.
  two-dimensional Fourier i.
  two-dimensional Fourier
    transformation i.
  ultrasound i.
  ventilation perfusion i.
  volume i.
imago (imagoes, imagines)
imagocide
IMB—intermenstrual bleeding
imbalance
  autonomic i.
  binocular i.
  electrolyte i.
  gene i.
  hormonal i.
  sex chromosome i.
  sympathetic i.
  vasomotor i.
IMBC—indirect maximum
  breathing capacity
imbibition
  hemoglobin i.
imbricate
imbricated suture
imbrication
IMC—irregular menstrual cycle
IM cocktail—intramuscular
  cocktail
ImD$_{50}$—median immunizing dose
Imerslund syndrome
Imerslund-Graesbeck syndrome
Imerslund-Najman-Graesbeck
  syndrome
IMH—idiopathic myocardial
  hypertrophy

Imhoff tank
IMHP—1-iodomercuri-
  2-hydroxypropane
IMI—intramuscular
  injection
imidogen
iminoglycinuria
  familial renal i.
iminourea
imitate
Imlach
  fat pad
  fat plug
  ring
immature cataract
immediate
immediately
immedicable
Immergut tube
immersion
  cold i.
  homogeneous i.
  oil i.
  water i.
immigration
imminent
immiscible
immobility
immobilization
immobilization device
immobilize
immune
  i. adherence
  i. complex
  i. deviation
  i. elimination
  i. globulin (IG)
  i. hemolysis
  i. interferon
  i. neutropenia
  i. paralysis
  i. response
  i. serum
  i. serum globulin
  i. suppression
  i. surveillance
  i. system
immunity
  acquired i.
  active i.
  adoptive i.
  antibacterial i.
  antitoxic i.
  antiviral i.
  artificial i.

I

immunity *(continued)*
- cell-mediated i.
- cellular i.
- community i.
- concomitant i.
- congenital i.
- cross i.
- familial i.
- functional i.
- genetic i.
- herd i.
- humoral i.
- induced i.
- infection i.
- inherent i.
- inherited i.
- innate i.
- intrauterine i.
- local i.
- maternal i.
- native i.
- natural i.
- nonspecific i.
- passive i.
- phagocytic i.
- placental i.
- preemptive i.
- protective i.
- residual i.
- species i.
- specific i.
- superinfection i.
- T cell–mediated i. (TCMI)
- tissue i.
- toxin-antitoxin i.
- transplantation i.

immunization
- active i.
- occult i.
- passive i.
- prophylactic i.

immunize
immunoadjuvant
immunoadsorbent
immunoadsorption
immunoagglutination
immunoassay
- enzyme i.
- enzyme-multiplied i. technique (EMIT)
- fluorescence polarization immunoassay (FPIA)
- label-based electrochemical i.
- multiplex i.
- nonradioisotopic i.

immunoassay *(continued)*
- radioisotopic i.
- sandwich enzyme i.
- solid-phase i.

immunobiology
immunoblast
immunoblastic
immunochemical
immunochemistry
immunochemotherapy
immunocompetence
immunocompetent
immunocompromised
immunoconglutinin
immunocyte
immunocytoadherence
immunocytochemistry
immunocytology
immunodeficiency
- acquired i. syndrome (AIDS)
- acquired primary i.
- cellular i.
- combined i.
- common variable i.
- common variable unclassifiable i.
- i. disease
- human i.
- i. with hyper-IgM
- primary i.
- severe combined i.
- i. with short-limbed dwarfism
- Swiss-type i.
- i. with thymoma
- thymus-dependent i.
- X-linked i.
- X-linked hyper-IgM i.

immunodeficient
immunodepression
immunodermatology
immunodetection
immunodeviation
immunodiagnosis
immunodiffusion
- radial i. (RID)

immunodominance
immunodominant
immunoelectrophoresis
- counter i.
- countercurrent i.
- crossed i.
- rocket i.
- two-dimensional i.

immunoferritin

immunofiltration
    analytical i.
immunofluorescence
    direct i.
    indirect i.
    i. microscopy
immunogen
immunogenetic
immunogenetics
immunogenic
immunogenicity
immunoglobulin (Ig)
    i. A (IgA)
    i. alpha chain
    Bence Jones monoclonal i.
    i. class
    i. class switching
    i. D (IgD)
    i. delta chain
    i. domain
    i. E (IgE)
    i. epsilon chain
    i. fold
    i. G (IgG)
    i. gamma chain
    i. gene rearrangement
    i. genes
    i. heavy chain
    i. kappa chain
    i. lambda chain
    i. light chain
    i. M (IgM)
    membrane i.
    monoclonal i.
    i. mu chain
    secretory i. A
    i. subclass
    i. superfamily
    surface i.
    thyroid-binding inhibitory i.
      (TBII)
    thyroid-stimulating i. (TSI)
    thyrotropin-binding inhibitory
      i. (TBII)
    TSH-binding inhibitory i. (TBII)
immunoglobulinopathy
immunohematology
immunohistochemical
immunohistochemistry
immunohistofluorescence
immunoincompetent
immunologic, immunological
    i. imbalance
    i. memory
    i. surveillance

immunologist
immunology
immunolymphoscintigraphy
immunomodulation
immunomodulator
immunoparasitology
immunopathogenesis
immunopathologic
immunopathology
immunoperoxidase
immunophoresis
immunophysiology
immunopotency
immunopotentiation
immunopotentiator
immunoprecipitation
immunoprecipitin
immunoproliferative
immunoprophylaxis
immunoprotein
immunoradiometric
immunoradiometry
immunoreactant
    glucagon i's
immunoreaction
immunoreactive
immunoreactivity
    glucagon-like i.
immunoregulation
immunoresponsiveness
immunoscintigraphy
immunoselection
immunosenescence
immunosmoelectrophoresis
immunosorbent
    enzyme-linked i. assay (ELISA)
immunostimulant
immunostimulation
immunosuppressant
immunosuppression
immunosuppressive
immunosurveillance
immunotherapy
    adoptive i.
immunotolerance
immunotolerant
immunotoxicology
immunotoxin
immunotransfusion
imp.—
    impression
    improved
IMP—inosine monophosphate
IMPA—incisal mandibular plane
    angle

I

impact
impacted
impaction
    ceruminal i.
    dental i.
    fecal i.
    food i.
    mucoid i.
impactor
impaired
impairment
    conductive hearing i.
    hearing i.
    percentage of i.
impalpable
impar
imparidigitate
impatency
impatent
impedance
    acoustic i.
    ear i.
    electrical i. plethysmography
    i. plethysmography
    i. venography
Imperatori forceps
imperception
imperforate
imperforation
imperialine
impermeable
impersistence
    motor i.
impervious
impetiginization
impetiginous
impetigo
    Bockhart i.
    i. bullosa
    bullous i.
    chronic symmetric i.
    circinate i.
    i. contagiosa
    i. contagiosa bullosa
    i. eczematodes
    follicular i.
    Fox i.
    furfuraceous i.
    i. herpetiformis
    miliary i.
    i. neonatorum
    i. pityroides
    i. simplex
    staphylococcal i.
    i. staphylogenes

impetigo *(continued)*
    streptococcal i.
    i. syphilitica
    i. variolosa
    i. vulgaris
impilation
impinge
impingement
implant
    acorn-shaped i.
    acrylic i.
    Allen i.
    Alpar i.
    Arruga i.
    Berens i.
    Berens-Rosa i.
    Binkhorst i.
    Boyd i.
    Brown-Dohlman i.
    build-up i.
    Bunker i.
    carcinomatous i's
    cartilaginous i.
    Choyce i.
    Choyce Mark VIII i.
    cochlear i.
    conical i.
    Copeland i.
    corneal i.
    Cutler i.
    dental i.
    deoxycortone acetate i.
    diodontic i.
    Doherty i.
    Dow-Corning i.
    dynamic i.
    endodontic i.
    endometrial i's
    endosseous i.
    endosteal i.
    Fox i.
    Frey i.
    glass sphere i.
    gold sphere i.
    Guist i.
    hemisphere i.
    hormone i.
    Hughes i.
    intraocular lens i. (IOL i.)
    intraosseous i.
    intraperiosteal i.
    Ivalon i.
    Little intraocular lens i.
    Lucite i.
    magnet i.

implant *(continued)*
    magnetic i.
    McGhan i.
    Mules i.
    needle endosteal i.
    oral i.
    osseointegrated i.
    penile i.
    pin endosteal i.
    plastic sphere i.
    Plexiglas i.
    polyethylene i.
    reverse-shape i.
    scleral i.
    scleral buckler i.
    semishell i.
    shelf-type i.
    shell i.
    Silastic i.
    silicone i.
    Snellen i.
    sphere i.
    spherical i.
    sponge i.
    Stone i.
    subperiosteal i.
    surface i.
    tantalum i.
    Teflon i.
    tire i.
    transmandibular i.
    Troutman i.
    tunneled i.
    Vitallium i.
    Wheeler i.
    wire mesh i.
implantation
    central i.
    circumferential i.
    delayed i.
    eccentric i.
    endometrial i.
    hypodermic i.
    interstitial i.
    intrafollicular i.
    juxtafollicular i.
    LeDuc i.
    nerve i.
    periosteal i.
    radioactive isotope i.
    superficial i.
    teratic i.
    tooth i.
implanted suture
implantodontics

implantodontist
implantodontology
implantologist
implantology
    dental i.
    oral i.
implosion
impotence
    functional i.
    organic i.
    orgastic i.
    paretic i.
    psychic i.
    secondary i.
    symptomatic i.
impotentia
    i. coeundi
    i. erigendi
    i. generandi
impoverishment
    personality i.
    i. in thinking
impregnate
impregnated dressing
impregnation
    artificial i.
impressio (impressiones)
    i. cardiaca hepatis
    i. cardiaca pulmonis
    i. colica hepatis
    impressiones digitatae
    i. duodenales hepatis
    i. esophagea hepatis
    i. esophagealis hepatis
    i. gastrica hepatis
    i. gastrica renis
    impressiones gyrorum
    i. ligamenti
        costoclavicularis
    i. meningealis
    i. muscularis renis
    i. oesophagea hepatis
    i. petrosa pallii
    i. renalis hepatis
    i. suprarenalis hepatis
impression
    anatomic i.
    basilar i.
    bridge i.
    cardiac i.
    cleft palate i.
    colic i. of liver
    colic i. of spleen
    complete denture i.
    composite i.

I

impression *(continued)*
    copper-ring i.
    costal i's
    i. of costoclavicular ligament
    deltoid i. of humerus
    dental i.
    digastric i.
    digital i's
    digitate i's
    direct bone i.
    duodenal i. of liver
    elastic i.
    esophageal i. of liver
    final i.
    fluid wax i.
    functional i.
    gastric i.
    gastric i. of liver
    gastric i. of spleen
    gyrate i's
    hydrocolloid i.
    lower i.
    mandibular i.
    maxillary i.
    meningeal i.
    mucodisplacement i.
    mucostatic i.
    partial denture i.
    petrous i.
    preliminary i.
    primary i.
    renal i. of liver
    rhomboid i. of clavicle
    secondary i.
    sectional i.
    suprarenal i. of liver
    trigeminal i. for gasserian
      ganglion
    trigeminal i. of temporal bone
    upper i.
impressiones (plural of impressio)
imprinting
impulse
    apex i.
    apical i.
    i. conduction
    i. control disorder
    ectopic i.
    episternal i.
    exteroceptive i's
    interoceptive i's
    involuntary i.
    irresistible i.
    left parasternal i.
    nerve i.

impulse *(continued)*
    neural i.
    point of maximal i. (PMI)
    proprioceptive i's
    right parasternal i.
impulsion
    wandering i.
IMR—infant mortality rate
IMS—incurred in military
   service
IMV—intermittent mandatory
   ventilation
IMViC, imvic—indole, methyl red,
   Voges-Proskauer, citrate
in.—inch
In—indium
IN—intranasal
INA—International Neurological
   Association
inacidity
inaction
inactivate
inactivation
    complement i.
    heat i.
    paternal-X i.
    random-X i.
    X-i.
    X-chromosome i.
inactivator
    anaphylatoxin i. (AI)
    C3b i.
inactivity
    electrocerebral i.
inadequacy
inadequate
inagglutinable
inalimental
inanimate
inanition
inappetence
inarticulate
in articulo mortis
inassimilable
inattention
    sensory i.
inborn
inbred
inbreeding
inc.—
    increase
    incurred
incandescent
incarcerated
incarceration

incarnatio unguis
incarnative
incasement
incendiarism
incentive spirometry
incertae sedis
incest
inch
^{111}In chloride [indium In 111 chloride]
incidence
incident
incineration
incipient
 i. heart attack
 i. tumor
incisal
incised
incision
 abdominal i.
 abdominothoracic i.
 ab externo i.
 Agnew-Verhoeff i.
 alar i.
 Alexander i.
 angular i.
 aortotomy i.
 arcuate i.
 areolar i.
 arteriotomy i.
 Auvray i.
 backcut i.
 Bar i.
 Bardenheuer i.
 Battle i.
 Battle-Jalaguier-Kammerer i.
 bayonet i.
 Bergmann i.
 Bergmann-Israel i.
 Bevan i.
 bivalve i., bivalved i.
 Brackin i.
 Brock i.
 bur-hole i.
 buttonhole i.
 celiotomy i.
 cervical i.
 Cherney i.
 Chernez i.
 chevron i.
 Chiene i.
 circular i.
 circumareolar i.
 circumcisional i.
 circumferential i.

incision *(continued)*
 circumlimbal i.
 circumscribing i.
 Clute i.
 Codman i.
 Coffey i.
 collar i.
 confirmatory i.
 conjunctival i.
 corneoscleral i.
 cortical i.
 Courvoisier i.
 crescent i.
 crosshatch i.
 crucial i.
 cruciate i.
 curved i.
 curvilinear i.
 Deaver i.
 decompression i.
 deltopectoral i.
 dorsolateral i.
 double-Y i.
 Dührssen (Duehrssen) i.
 dural i.
 Edebohls i.
 elliptical i.
 Elsberg i.
 endaural i.
 enterotomy i.
 epigastric i.
 exploratory i.
 Fergusson i.
 fishmouth i.
 flank i.
 flexed i.
 Fowler i.
 Fowler-Weir i.
 Furniss i.
 Gatellier i.
 Gibson i.
 Gluck i.
 Greenhow i.
 gridiron i.
 guillotine i.
 Halsted i.
 Handley i.
 Hayes Martin i.
 Heermann i.
 hemitransfixion i.
 Henry i.
 hockey-stick i.
 Hood and Kirklin i.
 horizontal i.
 inframammary i.

I

incision *(continued)*
    infraumbilical i.
    inguinal i.
    intercartilaginous i.
    intracapsular i.
    Jackson i.
    J-shaped i.
    Kammerer i.
    Kammerer-Battle i.
    Kehr i.
    Kocher i.
    Küstner i.
    lamellar i.
    Langenbeck (von Langenbeck) i.
    LaRoque herniorrhaphy i.
    lateral flank i.
    lateral rectus i.
    lazy H i.
    lazy S i.
    lazy Z i.
    Lempert i.
    Lilienthal i.
    limbal i.
    linear i.
    Linton i.
    longitudinal i.
    low transverse abdominal i.
    Lynch i.
    MacFee i.
    Mackenrodt i.
    Mason i.
    mastoid i.
    Maylard i.
    Mayo-Robson i.
    McBurney i.
    McLaughlin i.
    McVay i.
    meatal i.
    median i.
    Meyer hockey-stick i.
    midline i.
    Mikulicz i.
    Morison i.
    Munro Kerr i.
    muscle-splitting i.
    myringotomy i.
    Nagamatsu i.
    oblique i.
    Ollier i.
    Orr i.
    paracostal i.
    parainguinal i.
    paramedian i.
    paramuscular i.
    parapatellar i.

incision *(continued)*
    pararectus i.
    parasagittal i.
    parascapular i.
    paraumbilical i.
    paravaginal i.
    Parker i.
    Péan i.
    perianal i.
    periareolar i.
    perilimbal i.
    periscapular i.
    peritoneal i.
    Perthes i.
    Pfannenstiel i.
    Phemister i.
    popliteal i.
    postauricular i.
    posterior i.
    posterolateral i.
    proximal i.
    pyelotomy i.
    racquet i.
    radial i.
    rectus muscle–splitting i.
    recumbent i.
    relaxing i.
    relief i.
    retroauricular i.
    rim i.
    Risdon extraoral i.
    Robertson i.
    Rockey-Davis i.
    Rollet i.
    Rosen i.
    Roux-en-Y jejunal loop i.
    Ruddy i.
    saber-cut i.
    salmon backcut i.
    Sanders i.
    Schuchardt i.
    scratch-type i.
    semicircular i.
    semiflexed i.
    semilunar i.
    serpentine i.
    Shambaugh i.
    shelving i.
    shoulder-strap i.
    Simon i.
    Singleton i.
    Sloan i.
    smile i.
    smiling i.
    Smith-Peterson i.

incision *(continued)*
 Sorensen i.
 spiral i.
 stab wound i.
 stellate i.
 sternal-splitting i.
 Stewart i.
 Strömbeck i.
 subcostal i.
 subinguinal i.
 submammary i.
 subtrochanteric i.
 subumbilical i.
 supracervical i.
 suprapubic i.
 supraumbilical i.
 temporal i.
 Thomas-Warren i.
 thoracoabdominal i.
 thoracotomy i.
 transection i.
 transmeatal i.
 transrectus i.
 transverse i.
 trap-door i.
 T-shaped i.
 U-shaped i.
 vertical i.
 V-shaped i.
 Warren i.
 Watson-Jones i.
 Weber-Fergusson i.
 wedge i.
 Whipple i.
 Wilde i.
 W-shaped i.
 Yorke-Mason i.
 Z-flap i.
 Z-plasty i.
 Z-shaped i.
incisional
incisive suture
incisolabial
incisolingual
incisoproximal
incisor
 central i.
 first i.
 hawk-bill i's
 Hutchinson i's
 lateral i.
 medial i.
 second i.
 shovel-shaped i's
 winged i.

incisura (incisurae)
 i. acetabuli
 i. angularis
 i. angularis ventriculi
 i. anterior auriculae
 i. anterior auris
 i. apicis cordis
 i. cardiaca
 i. cardiaca ventriculi
 i. cerebelli
 i. cerebelli anterior
 i. clavicularis sterni
 incisurae costales sterni
 i. fastigii
 i. fibularis tibiae
 i. frontalis
 i. interarytenoidea
 i. interarytenoidea laryngis
 i. interlobaris hepatis
 i. interlobaris pulmonis
 i. intertragica
 i. ischiadica major
 i. ischiadica minor
 i. ischialis major
 i. ischialis minor
 i. jugularis sterni
 i. lacrimalis maxillae
 i. ligamenti teretis
 i. mandibulae
 i. mastoidea
 i. mastoidea ossis temporalis
 i. nasalis maxillae
 i. pancreatis
 i. parietalis
 i. peronea tibiae
 i. preoccipitalis
 i. pterygoidea
 i. radialis ulnae
 i. Rivini
 Santorini i.
 i. scapulae
 i. semilunaris tibiae
 i. semilunaris ulnae
 i. sphenopalatina
 i. supraorbitalis
 i. temporalis
 i. tentorii cerebelli
 i. terminalis auricularis
 i. terminalis auris
 i. thyroidea inferior
 i. thyroidea superior
 i. tragica
 i. trochlearis ulnae
 i. tympanica
 i. ulnaris radii

I

incisura (incisurae) *(continued)*
    i. umbilicalis
    i. vertebralis inferior
    i. vertebralis superior
incisural
incisure
    i. of acetabulum
    angular i.
    i. of apex of heart
    i. of calcaneus
    cardiac i. of left lung
    cardiac i. of stomach
    i. of cerebellum
    clavicular i. of sternum
    costal i's of sternum
    cotyloid i.
    digastric i. of temporal bone
    i's of Duverney
    i. of ear, anterior
    i. of ear, terminal
    ethmoidal i. of frontal bone
    falciform i. of fascia lata
    fibular i. of tibia
    frontal i.
    humeral i. of ulna
    iliac i., lesser
    interarytenoid i.
    interclavicular i.
    intertragic i.
    ischial i., greater
    ischial i., lesser
    i. of ischium, greater
    i. of ischium, lesser
    jugular i. of occipital bone
    jugular i. of sternum
    jugular i. of temporal bone
    lacrimal i. of maxilla
    i's of Lanterman
    i's of Lanterman-Schmidt
    lateral i. of sternum
    i. of mandible
    mastoid i. of temporal bone
    maxillary i., inferior
    nasal i. of frontal bone
    nasal i. of maxilla
    obturator i. of pubic bone
    palatine i.
    palatine i. of Henle
    parietal i. of temporal bone
    patellar i. of femur
    peroneal i. of tibia
    popliteal i.
    preoccipital i.
    pterygoid i.
    radial i. of ulna

incisure *(continued)*
    Rivinus i.
    i. of scapula
    Schmidt-Lanterman i's
    semilunar i.
    sigmoid i. of mandible
    sigmoid i. of ulna
    sphenopalatine i. of palatine bone
    sternal i.
    supraorbital i.
    suprascapular i.
    i. of talus
    temporal i.
    i. of tentorium of cerebellum
    thoracic i.
    thyroid i., inferior
    thyroid i., superior
    trochlear i. of ulna
    tympanic i.
    ulnar i. of radius
    umbilical i.
    vertebral i., greater
    vertebral i., inferior
    vertebral i., lesser
    vertebral i., superior
incitant
incitogram
inclinatio (inclinationes)
    i. pelvis
inclination
    axial i.
    condylar guidance i.
    condylar guide i.
    lateral condylar i.
    lingual i.
    pelvic i.
    i. of pelvis
    i. of tooth
inclinationes (plural of inclinatio)
incline
inclinometer
inclusion
    i. bodies
    cell i.
    Dawson i.
    dental i.
    fetal i.
    Guarnieri i's
    intranuclear i's
    leukocyte i's
    Walthard i's
incoagulability
incoagulable
incoherent

incomitant strabismus
incompatibility
    ABO i.
    chemical i.
    physiologic i.
    Rh i.
    therapeutic i.
incompatible
incompetence
    gastroesophageal i.
    ileocecal i.
    ileocolic i.
    relative i.
    i. of the cardiac valves
    valvular i.
    velopharyngeal i.
incompetent
incompressible
incongruence
incongruent
incongruous
    i. findings
    i. history
incontinence
    active i.
    fecal i.
    intermittent i.
    overflow i.
    paradoxical i.
    paralytic i.
    passive i.
    rectal i.
    sphincteric i.
    stress i.
    urge i.
    urgency i.
    urinary i.
    i. of urine
incontinent
incontinentia
    i. alvi
    Bloch-Sulzberger i. pigmenti
    Naegeli i. pigmenti
    i. pigmenti
    i. pigmenti achromians
    i. alvi
incoordination
    first-degree uterine i.
    second-degree uterine i.
    uterine i.
incorporation
incorrigible
incostapedial
increment
incretin

incretion
incross
incrustation
incubate
incubation
incubator
incubus
incudal
incudectomy
incudiform
incudius (plural of incus)
incudomalleal
incudostapedial
incumbent
incuneation
incurable
incurvation
incus (gen. of incudius)
incyclodeviation
incycloduction
incyclophoria
incyclotropia
incyclovergence
indacrinic acid
indanedione
indemnity
indenization
indentation
    aortic i. of esophagus
    i. of Hahn
    i. of tongue
    i. tonometry
independence
    statistical i.
independent
indeterminate
index (indexes, indices)
    absolute refractive i.
    absorbancy i.
    ACH i.
    acidophilic i.
    alpha i.
    altitudinal i.
    alveolar i.
    ankle-brachial i. (ABI)
    antitryptic i.
    arm-ankle i. (AAI)
    Arneth i.
    auricular i.
    auriculoparietal i.
    auriculovertical i.
    baric i.
    basilar i.
    Becker-Lennhoff i.
    body build i.

I

index (indexes, indices) *(continued)*
Boedecker i.
Bouchard i.
brachial i.
breadth-height i.
Broders i. (1–4)
Brugsch i.
calcium i.
cardiothoracic i.
I.-Catalogue
centromeric i.
cephalic i.
cephalic height i.
cephalo-orbital i.
cephalorhachidian i.
cephalospinal i.
cerebral i.
cerebrospinal i.
chemotherapeutic i.
coliform i.
Colour I.
combined thyroid hormone i.
community periodontal i. of
  treatment needs
coronofrontal i.
cranial i.
Cumulated I. Medicus
decayed, extracted, filled
  (DEF) caries i.
def i.
degenerative i.
dental i.
DMF (decayed, missing,
  or filled) i.
dyspnea i.
effective temperature i.
endemic i.
erythrocyte indices
facial i.
fatigue i.
femorohumeral i.
Flower i.
forearm-hand i.
Fourmentin thoracic i.
free thyroxin i. (FTI)
free triiodothyronine i.
gingival periodontal i. (GPI)
gnathic i.
habitus i.
hair i.
hand i.
height i.
hematopneic i.
hemolytic i.
hemophagocytic i.

index (indexes, indices) *(continued)*
hemorenal i.
hemorenal salt i.
Hench-Aldrich i.
high lateral myocardial i.
icteric i.
intermembral i.
juxtaglomerular i.
Kaup i.
Krebs leukocyte i.
length-breadth i.
length-height i.
Lennhoff i.
lower leg–foot i.
Macdonald i.
maturation i.
maxilloalveolar i.
I. Medicus
Mengert i.
i. of mental deterioration
metacarpal i.
mitotic i.
morphological i.
morphologic face i.
nasal i.
nucleoplasmic i.
obesity i.
opsonic i.
orbital i.
palatal i.
palatal height i.
palatine i.
palatomaxillary i.
parasite i.
pelvic i.
penile brachial i.
periodontal i.
phagocytic i.
physiognomonic upper face i.
Pignet i.
Pirquet i.
PMA (papilla, gingival margin,
  and attached gingiva) i.
ponderal i.
Pont i.
profunda-popliteal collateral i.
pulsatile i.
pyknotic i.
Quarterly Cumulative I.
  Medicus
radiohumeral i.
red blood cell i's, red cell i's
refractive i.
Röhrer (Roehrer) i.
Russell i.

index (indexes, indices) *(continued)*
    sacral i.
    salivary urea i.
    sedimentation i.
    short increment sensitivity i.
      (SISI)
    spleen i.
    splenic i.
    splenometric i.
    stimulation i. (SI)
    tension-time i.
    therapeutic i.
    thoracic i.
    tibiofemoral i.
    tibioradial i.
    trunk i.
    urea i.
    uricolytic i.
    vertical i.
    vital i.
    xanthoproteic i.
    Youden i.
    zygomaticoauricular i.
Indian
    method
    operation
    rhinoplasty
    rotation flap
indican
indicanemia
indicanmeter
indicanorachia
indicant
indicanuria
indicarmine
indicatio
    i. causalis
    i. curativa
    i. morbi
    i. symptomatica
indication
indicator
    anaerobic i.
    Andrade i.
    dew point i.
    fluorescent i.
    oxidation-reduction i.
    pH i.
    proportional mortality i.
    radioactive i.
    redox i.
    Schneider i.
    universal i.
    xylol pulse i.
indicophose

indifférence
    belle i., la belle i.
indifference
    i. reaction
    sexual i.
indifferent
indigenous
indigent
indigestible
indigestion
    acid i.
    fat i.
    gastric i.
    intestinal i.
    sugar i.
indigitation
indiglucin
indigo
indigo carmine
indigo carmine dye
indigogen
indigopurpurine
indigotin
indirect
    binocular i. ophthalmoscopy
    i. laryngoscopy
    i. ophthalmoscope
    i. ophthalmoscopy
    i. placentography
indirubin
indirubinuria
indiscernible
indiscrete
indiscriminate
indisposition
indistinct
indium (In)
    i. In 111
    i. In 111 DTPA
    i. In 111 oxyquinoline
    i. In 111 pentetate
    i. In 111 pentetreotide
    i. In 113m
individualization
individuation
INDM—infant of nondiabetic
  mother
indolaceturia
indolamine
indole
indole-3-acetic acid
indolent
    i. lesion
    i. tumor
indologenous

indoluria
indophenol
indoramin
indoxyl
indoxylemia
indoxyluria
induced
inducer cell
inductance
induction
    autonomous i.
    complementary i.
    enzyme i.
    induction of labor
    magnetic i.
    medical i. of labor
    ovulation i.
    Spemann i.
    spinal i.
    surgical i. of labor
inductive plethysmography
inductor
    gene i.
inductorium
inductotherm
inductothermy
indulin black
indulinophil
indulinophilic
indurated
    i. cellulitis
    i. lymphangitis
induration
    black i.
    brawny i.
    brown i.
    cyanotic i.
    fibroid i.
    fibrous i.
    Froriep i.
    granular i.
    gray i.
    laminate i.
    parchment i.
    penile i.
    phlebitic i.
    plastic i.
    red i.
    rigid i. of bladder neck
indurative
indusium griseum
industrial monitoring
indwelling catheter
INE—infantile necrotizing
  encephalomyelopathy

inebriant
inebriation
inebriety
inelastic
inert
inertia
    colonic i.
    immunological i.
    primary uterine i.
    psychic i.
    secondary uterine i.
    i. uteri
    uterine i.
inexcitable
inexorable
in extremis
inf.—
    inferior
    infusion
infancy
infant
    floppy i.
    i. Hercules
    immature i.
    liveborn i.
    low birth weight i. (LBW i.)
    mature i.
    moderately low birth weight i.
      (MLBW i.)
    newborn i.
    postmature i.
    postterm i.
    premature i.
    preterm i.
    stillborn i.
    term i.
    very low birth weight i.
      (VLBW i.)
infanticide
infantile celiac disease
infantilism
    Brissaud i.
    cachectic i.
    celiac i.
    dysthyroidal i.
    hepatic i.
    Herter i.
    hypophysial (hypophyseal) i.
    idiopathic i.
    intestinal i.
    Levi-Lorain i.
    Lorain i.
    lymphatic i.
    myxedematous i.
    pancreatic i.

infantilism *(continued)*
> partial i.
> pituitary i.
> proportionate i.
> regressive i.
> renal i.
> sexual i.
> symptomatic i.
> thyroid i.
> universal i.

infarct
> anemic i.
> aseptic i.
> bilirubin i
> bland i.
> bone i.
> Brewer i.
> calcareous i.
> cerebral i.
> cystic i.
> embolic i.
> hemorrhagic i.
> infected i.
> kidney i.
> mesenteric i.
> pale i.
> placental i.
> pulmonary i.
> red i.
> renal i.
> septic i.
> thrombotic i.
> uric acid i.
> white i.

infarctectomy

infarction
> anterior myocardial i.
> anteroinferior myocardial i.
> anterolateral myocardial i.
> anteroseptal myocardial i.
> apical myocardial i.
> atrial i.
> brain stem i.
> cardiac i.
> cerebral i.
> diaphragmatic i.
> diaphragmatic myocardial i.
> high-lateral myocardial i.
> inferior myocardial i.
> inferolateral myocardial i
> intestinal i.
> lacunar i.
> lateral myocardial i.
> mesenteric i.
> myocardial i. (MI)

infarction *(continued)*
> pituitary i.
> posterior myocardial i.
> posterolateral myocardial i.
> pulmonary i.
> renal i.
> right ventricular i.
> right ventricular myocardial i.
> Roesler-Dressler i.
> septal myocardial i.
> silent myocardial i.
> subendocardial i.
> through-and-through
>   myocardial i.
> transmural myocardial i.
> watershed i.

infaust
> i. case
> i. disease
> i. evolution
> predictable i. outcome
> i. prognosis
> i. prognostic sign

infect

infectible

infection
> abortive i.
> acute productive/lyric i.
> airborne i.
> apical i.
> ascending i.
> autochthonous i.
> bacterial i.
> colonization i.
> concurrent i.
> contact i.
> covert i.
> cross i.
> cryptogenic i.
> cryptosporidial i.
> cysticercosis i.
> defective i.
> diaplacental i.
> direct i.
> dormant i.
> droplet i.
> dust-borne i.
> ectogenous i.
> endogenous i.
> Epstein-Barr virus i.
> exogenous i.
> focal i.
> fungal i.
> germinal i.
> hepatitis B virus i.

I

infection *(continued)*
    herpes simplex i.
    herpes zoster i.
    iatrogenic i.
    inapparent i.
    indirect i.
    intercurrent i.
    invasive burn i.
    latent i.
    local i.
    lower respiratory tract i.
      (LRTI)
    mass i.
    metastatic i.
    metazoan i.
    mixed i.
    nonspecific i.
    nosocomial i.
    opportunistic i.
    parasitic i.
    perinatal i.
    phycomycotic i.
    protozoan i.
    puerperal i.
    pyogenic i.
    retrograde i.
    secondary i.
    silent i.
    slow i.
    subclinical i.
    toxoplasmosis, other
      agents, rubella,
      cytomegalovirus, herpes
      simplex (TORCH) i.
    transcervical i.
    transforming i.
    transplacental i.
    tunnel i.
    upper respiratory i.
      (URI)
    upper respiratory tract i.
      (URTI)
    urinary tract i. (UTI)
    vector-borne i.
    Vincent i.
    viral i.
    water-borne i.
    zoogenic i.
infectiosity
infectious mononucleosis
infectiousness
infective
infectivity
infecundity

inferior
    i. laryngotomy
    i. tracheotomy
inferiority
inferior vena cava (IVC)
inferofrontal
inferolateral
inferomedial
inferomedian
inferonasal
inferoparietal
inferoposterior
inferotemporal
infertile
infertility
    primary i.
    secondary i.
infest
infestation
infestive
infibulation
infiltrate
    Assmann tuberculous i.
    leukemic i.
infiltrating
infiltration
    adipose i.
    calcareous i.
    calcium i.
    cellular i.
    epituberculous i.
    fatty i.
    gelatinous i.
    glycogen i.
    gray i.
    inflammatory i.
    lymphocytic i.
    lymphocytic i. of skin
    mesentery i.
    paraneural i.
    parenchymal i.
    perineural i.
    pulmonary i. with
      eosinophilia
    round cell i.
    sanguineous i.
    serous i.
    tuberculous i.
    urinous i.
infirm
infirmary
infirmity
inflamed
inflammagen

inflammation
- acute i.
- adhesive i.
- allergic i.
- atrophic i.
- bacterial i.
- catarrhal i.
- chemical i.
- chronic i.
- cirrhotic i.
- croupous i.
- diffuse i.
- disseminated i.
- exudative i.
- fibrinopurulent i.
- fibrinous i.
- fibrosing i.
- focal i.
- granulomatous i.
- hyperplastic i.
- hypertrophic i.
- interstitial i.
- metastatic i.
- necrotic i.
- obliterative i.
- parenchymatous i.
- plastic i.
- productive i.
- proliferative i.
- pseudomembranous i.
- purulent i.
- sclerosing i.
- serofibrinous i.
- seroplastic i.
- serous i.
- simple i.
- specific i.
- subacute i.
- suppurative i.
- toxic i.
- traumatic i.
- ulcerative i.

inflammatory
inflation
inflator
inflection
inflexed
inflexion
inflorescence
inflow
influenza
- Asian i.
- avian i.
- endemic i.

influenza (continued)
- equine i.
- feline i.
- goose i.
- Hong Kong i.
- laryngeal i.
- Russian i.
- Spanish i.
- swine i.
- i. virus (A–C)

influenzal
info—information
infold
infolding
information
- genetic i.
- sensory i.

informosome
infra-alveolar
infra-auricular
infra-axillary
infrabulge
infracardiac
infracerebral
infraciliature
infraclass
infraclavicular
infraclinoid
infraclusion
infraconstrictor
infracortical
infracostal
infracotyloid
infraction
- Freiberg i.

infracture
infradentale
infradian
infradiaphragmatic
infraduction
infrageniculate
infragenual
infraglenoid
infraglottic
infrahyoid pharyngotomy
infrainguinal
inframammary incision
inframammillary
inframandibular
inframarginal
inframaxillary
infranatant
infranuclear
infraorbital suture

I

infrapatellar
infrapsychic
infrapulmonic
infrared
    far i.
    i. microscope
    near i.
    i. spectroscopy
infrarenal
infrascapular
infrasonic
infrasound
infraspecific
infraspinous
infrasternal
infrastructure
    implant i.
infratemporal
infratentorial
infrathoracic
infratonsillar
infratracheal
infratrochlear
infratubal
infraturbinal
infraumbilical incision
infravergence
infraversion
infravesical
infrazygomatic
infriction
infundibula (plural of
  infundibulum)
infundibular
infundibulectomy
    Brock i.
infundibuliform
infundibuloma
infundibulo-ovarian
infundibulopelvic
infundibulum
  (infundibula)
    cardiac i.
    crural i.
    i. crurale
    ethmoidal i.
    i. ethmoidale
    i. of fallopian tube
    i. of frontal sinus
    i. of heart
    i. of hypophysis
    i. hypothalami
    i. of hypothalamus
    i. of kidney

infundibulum (infundibula)
    (continued)
    i. nasi
    i. of nose
    i. pulmonis
    i. pulmonum
    infundibula renum
    i. tubae uterinae
    i. of urinary bladder
    i. of uterine tube
Infuse-a-Cath
Infuse-a-Port
infused
infusible
infusion
    amniotic fluid i.
    cold i.
    drip i. pyelography
    meat i.
    i. nephrotomography
    i. pyelography
    saline i.
infusodecoction
infusum
Ingals
    cannula
    speculum
ingenious
Ingersoll curet
ingestant
ingestion
ingestive
ingluvies
Ingram trocar catheter
Ingrassia
    apophysis
    process
    wings
ingravescent
ingress
ingrowth
    epithelial i.
inguen (inguina)
inguinal incision
inguinoabdominal
inguinocele
inguinocrural
inguinodynia
inguinolabial
inguinoscrotal
INH—
    isonicotine hydrazine inhibitor
    isonicotinic acid hydrazide
    (isoniazid)

inhalant
    antifoaming i.
inhalation
    isoproterenol sulfate i.
    naphtha i.
    smoke i.
inhale
inhaler
    Allis i.
    ether i.
    H. H. i.
    Junker i.
inherent
inheritance
    alternative i.
    autosomal i.
    biparental i.
    blending i.
    codominant i.
    complemental i.
    cytoplasmic i.
    dominant i.
    extrachromosomal i.
    extranuclear i.
    galtonian i.
    holandric i.
    hologynic i.
    homochronous i.
    homotropic i.
    intermediate i.
    maternal i.
    matrilinear i.
    mendelian i.
    mitochondrial i.
    monofactorial i.
    monogenic i.
    mosaic i.
    multifactorial i.
    particulate i.
    polygenic i.
    quantitative i.
    quasidominant i.
    recessive i.
    sex-linked i.
    unit i.
    X-linked i.
inherited
inhibin
inhibit
inhibition
    allogenic i.
    allosteric i.
    antidromic i.
    autogenous i.

inhibition *(continued)*
    central i.
    competitive i.
    contact i.
    endproduct i.
    enzyme i.
    feedback i.
    fertility i.
    hemagglutination i. (HI; HAI)
    mixed i.
    motor i.
    noncompetitive i.
    potassium i.
    proactive i.
    reciprocal i.
    recurrent i.
    reflex i.
    Renshaw i.
    retroactive i.
    selective i.
    substrate i.
    uncompetitive i.
    Wedensky i.
inhibitor
    α_2-plasmin i.
    active-site-directed
      irreversible i.
    aldosterone i.
    angiotensin-converting
      enzyme i's
    C1 i. (C1 INH)
    C1 esterase i.
    cholesterol i.
    competitive i.
    factor VIII i.
    inter-alpha-trypsin i.
    irreversible i.
    lupus i.
    membrane attack complex i.
      (MAC INH)
    mitotic i.
    monoamine oxidase i. (MAOI)
    noncompetitive i.
    plasminogen activator i. (PAI)
    reversible i.
    trypsin i.
inhibitory
inhomogeneity
inhomogeneous
iniac
iniad
iniencephalus
iniencephaly
iniodymus

I

inion
iniopagus
iniops
initial
initiation
initis
inj.—inject
inject
injectable
injected
injection

    anatomical i.
    circumcorneal i.
    coarse i.
    depot i.
    dextrose i.
    endermic i.
    epifascial i.
    ethiodized oil i.
    fine i.
    fructose i.
    gaseous i.
    gelatin i.
    hypodermic i.
    insulin i.
    intracutaneous i.
    intradermal i.
    intradermic i.
    intramuscular (IM) i.
    intrathecal i.
    intravascular i.
    intravenous (IV) i.
    iodinated I 125 albumin i.
    iodinated I 131 albumin i.
    iron dextran i.
    iron sorbitex i.
    jet i.
    lactated Ringer i.
    nasopalatine i.
    opacifying i.
    oxytocin i.
    paraperiosteal i.
    parathyroid i.
    parenchymatous i.
    perinephric air i.
    posterior pituitary i.
    preservative i.
    protamine sulfate i.
    protein hydrolysate i.
    repository i.
    Ringer i.
    sclerosing i.
    Silastic i.
    sodium chloride i.
    sodium pertechnetate Tc 99m i.

injection (continued)
    sodium radiochromate i.
    subcutaneous i.
    technetium Tc 99m albumin
        aggregated i.
    Teflon i. of vocal cord
    transduodenal fiberscopic
        duct i.
    trigger point i.
    vasopressin i.
injector
    jet i.
injure
injury
    air-blast i.
    atmospheric blast i.
    birth i.
    blast i.
    blunt i.
    bucket-handle i.
    bumper i.
    closed head i.
    compression i.
    contrecoup i.
    coup i. of brain
    coup-contrecoup i.
    crush i.
    deceleration i.
    egg-white i.
    Goyrand i.
    high-explosive i.
    hyperextension-hyperflexion i.
    immersion blast i.
    internal i.
    neonatal cold i.
    occupational i.
    open head i.
    patterned i.
    shell i.
    soft tissue i.
    steering wheel i.
    straddle i.
    unintentional i.
    vital i.
    whiplash i.
    wringer i.
[111]In-labeled IgG [Indium I 111 IgG]
inlay
    bone i.
    epithelial i.
    i. myringoplasty
    skin graft i.
inlet
    pelvic i.
    thoracic i.

innate
innervate
innervated
innervation
    double i.
    multiple i.
    plurisegmental i.
    polyneuronal i.
    reciprocal i.
innidiation
innocent
innocuous
innominatal
innominate
    i. artery
    i. osteotomy
    i. vein
innominatum
innoxious
innutrition
INO—internuclear
  ophthalmoplegia
inoblast
inoccipitia
inochondritis
inocula (plural of
  inoculum)
inoculability
inoculable
inoculate
inoculation
    protective i.
inoculative
inoculum (inocula)
inocyte
inogenesis
inogenous
inoglia
inohymenitis
inolith
inomyositis
inoperable
inopexia
inophragma
inorganic
    i. pyrophosphatase
inosclerosis
inoscopy
inosculate
inosculation
inosemia
inosinate
inosinic acid
inositide
inositis

inositol
    i. niacinate
    i. 1,4,5-triphosphate
inosituria
inostosis
inosuria
inotagma
inotrope
inotropic
    negatively i.
    positively i.
inotropism
in ovo
inpatient
input
INPV—intermittent negative-
  pressure assisted ventilation
inquest
    coroner's i.
inquiline
inquisition
insaccation
insalivation
insalubrious
insane
    criminally i.
insanitary
insanity
    adolescent i.
    affective i.
    alcoholic i.
    alternating i.
    anticipatory i.
    choreic i.
    circular i.
    collective i.
    communicated i.
    compound i.
    compulsive i.
    consecutive i.
    criminal i.
    cyclic i.
    double i.
    doubting i.
    emotional i.
    hereditary i.
    homicidal i.
    homochronous i.
    hysterical i.
    idiophrenic i.
    imposed i.
    impulsive i.
    induced i.
    manic-depressive i.
    moral i.

I

insanity *(continued)*
 partial i.
 perceptional i.
 periodic i.
 polyneuritic i.
 primary i.
 puerperal i.
 recurrent i.
 senile i.
 simultaneous i.
 toxic i.
inscriptio (inscriptiones)
 i. tendinea
 inscriptiones tendineae
  musculi recti abdominis
inscription
 tendinous i.
 tendinous i's of rectus
  abdominis muscle
inscriptiones (plural of inscriptio)
insect
insectarium
insecticide
insectifuge
insectivore
insectivorous
insemination
 artificial i.
 artificial i. donor
 donor i.
 heterologous i.
 homologous i.
insenescence
insensible
 i. fluid output
insert
 intramucosal i.
 mucosal i.
insertio
 i. velamentosa
insertion
 parasol i.
 thought i.
 velamentous i.
insheathed
insidious
insight
 i. fair
 i. and judgment
insipidus
 diabetes i.
in situ hybridization
insolation
 asphyxial i.
 hyperpyrexial i.

insoluble
insomnia
 fatal familial i.
 initial i.
 middle i.
 primary i.
 terminal i.
insomniac
insomnic
insonate
insorption
InsP$_3$—inositol 1,4,5-triphosphate
inspection
inspersion
inspirate
inspiration
 crowing i.
inspiratory
 i. dyspnea
 i.-expiratory (I/E)
  phase ratio
 i. flow
 i. flow rate (IFR)
 i.-inhibitory reflex
 maximum i. flow (MIF)
 maximum i. pressure (MIP)
 i. murmur
 i. pause time
 peak i. flow (PIF)
 post-tussive i. rhonchi
 i. pressure
 i. rales
 i. reserve capacity (IRC)
 i. reserve volume (IRV)
 i. rhonchi
 i. spasm
 i. stridor
 i. triggering pressure
 i. triggering volume
inspirometer
inspissant
inspissate
inspissated
inspissation
inspissator
instability
 lumbosacral i.
instar
instep
instill
instillation
instillator
instinct
 aggressive i.
 death i.

instinct *(continued)*
  ego i.
  herd i.
  life i.
  mother i.
  sexual i.
instinctive
institutionalization
institutionalize
instruction
instrument
  Acufex i.
  hand i.
  plugging i.
  stereotaxic i.
instrumental
instrumentarium
instrumentation
  Cotrel-Dubousset
    spinal i.
  Harrington i.
  Luque i.
insuccation
insudation
insufficiency
  active i.
  acute adrenocortical i.
  adrenal i.
  adrenocortical i.
  anterior pituitary i.
  aortic i.
  basilar i.
  capsular i.
  cardiac i.
  chronic adrenocortical i.
  coronary i.
  i. of the externi
  i. of the eyelids
  gastric i.
  gastromotor i.
  hepatic i.
  ileocecal i.
  i. of the interni
  mitral i.
  muscular i.
  myocardial i.
  myovascular i.
  pancreatic i.
  parathyroid i.
  placental i.
  post-traumatic pulmonary i.
  pseudoaortic i.
  pulmonary i.
  pyloric i.
  renal i.

insufficiency *(continued)*
  thyroid i.
  tricuspid i.
  uterine i.
  uteroplacental i.
  valvular i.
  vascular i.
  velopharyngeal i.
  venous i.
  vertebral i.
  vertebrobasilar i.
insufflate
insufflation
  cranial i.
  endotracheal i.
  i. of the lungs
  methylene blue i.
  perirenal i.
  presacral i.
  retroperitoneal gas i.
  tubal i.
insufflator
  Buckstein i.
  Kidde tubal i.
  Weber i.
insula (insulae)
  i. pancreaticae
  insulae of Peyer
  i. of Reil
insular
insularine
insulate
insulation
insulator
insulin
  beef i.
  beef-pork i.
  dealinated i.
  depot i.
  extended i. zinc
    suspension
  globin i.
  globin zinc i.
  hexamine i.
  human i.
  immunoreactive i.
  i. injection
  isophane i. suspension
  i. lispro
  neutral i.
  NPH (neutral protamine
    Hagedorn) i.
  pectin i.
  plant i.
  pork i.

I

insulin *(continued)*
    prompt i. zinc suspension
    protamine zinc i. suspension
    regular i.
    synalbumin i.
    three-to-one i.
    vegetable i.
    i. zinc suspension
insulinase
insulinemia
insulin-iodine
insulinlipodystrophy
insulinogenesis
insulinogenic
insulinoid
insulinoma
insulinopenia
insulinopenic
insulinoprivic
insulinotardic
insulism
insulitis
insuloma
insult
    cerebellar i.
    cerebral i.
    hemorrhagic i.
    hypoxic i.
    myocardial i.
    respiratory i.
insurance
    catastrophic health i.
    disability income i.
    health i.
    malpractice i.
    professional liability i.
    supplemental health i.
    Workers' Compensation i.
insusceptibility
int.—
    intermittent
    internal
intake
    acceptable daily i. (ADI)
    caloric i.
    conditional daily i.
    fluid i.
    provisional total weekly i.
    unconditional daily i.
integrating microscope
integration
    biological i.
    nervous i.
    structural i.
integrator

integument
    common i.
    spore i.
integumentary
integumentum
    i. commune
in tela
intellect
intellectualization
intelligence
    artificial i.
    i. quotient (IQ)
intemperance
intensification
    image i.
intensification factor
intensimeter
intensionometer
intensity
    electric i.
    intrauterine i.
    luminous i.
    pulse average i.
    spatial average i.
    spatial average temporal
      average i.
    spatial peak i.
    spatial peak temporal
      average i.
    temporal average i.
    temporal peak i.
    threshold i.
intensive
intensivist
intent
    criminal i.
intention
    first i.
    paradoxical i.
    primary i.
    secondary i.
intentional
interaccessory
interacinar
interaction
    complementary i.
    drug i.
    heme-heme i.
    ion-dipole i.
    primary i.
interalveolar
interamnios
interangular
interannular
interapophyseal

interarticular
interarytenoid
interatrial
interauricular
interaxonal
interbands
interbiopsy
interbrain
intercalary
intercalate
intercanalicular
intercanthal
intercapillary
intercarotic
intercarpal
intercartilaginous
    i. rim
    i. incision
intercavernous
intercede
intercellular
intercentral
intercerebral
interchange
    Hamburger i.
interchondral
intercilium
interclavicular
interclinoid
intercoccygeal
intercolumnar
intercondylar
intercornual
intercostal
intercostohumeral
intercourse
intercoxal
intercricothyrotomy
intercristal
intercritical
intercross
intercrural
intercurrent
intercuspal
intercuspation
intercusping
interdeferential
interdental
interdentale
interdentium
interdigit
interdigital
interdigitate
interdigitation
interectopic

interendognathic
    i. suture
interface
    dermoepidermal i.
    dineric i.
    gamma camera i.
interfacial
interfascicular
interfemoral
interference
    chiasma i.
    cuspal i.
    initial i.
    interceptive occlusal i.
    interchromosomal i.
    i. microscope
    occlusal i's
    premature i.
    proactive i.
    retroactive i.
    RNA i.
interfering
interferometer
interferometry
interferon (IFN)
    i.-α (IFN-α) [-alpha]
    antigenic i.
    i.-β (IFN-β) [-beta]
    epithelial i.
    fibroblast i.
    fibroepithelial i.
    i.-γ (IFN-γ), γ-i. [gamma]
    immune i.
    immunoreactive i.
    leukocyte i.
    lymphoblastoid cell i.
    type I i.
    type II i.
interfibrillar
interfibrous
interfilamentous
interfilar
interfrontal
interfurca (interfurcae)
interganglionic
intergemmal
intergenic
interglobular
intergluteal
intergonial
intergradation
intergrade
intergranular
intergyral
interhemicerebral

I

interhemispheric
interictal
interim
interior
interischiadic
interjugal
interkinesis
interlabial
interlamellar
interleukin (IL-1 through
    IL-15)
interligamentary
interligamentous
interlobar
interlobitis
interlobular
interlocking sutures
intermalar
intermalleolar
intermammary
intermammillary
intermarginal
intermarriage
intermaxillary suture
intermediary
intermediate
intermedin
intermediolateral
intermediomedial
intermedius
intermembranous
intermeningeal
intermenstrual
intermenstruum
intermetacarpal
intermetameric
intermetatarsal
intermission
intermitotic
intermittence
intermittency
intermittent
    i. claudication
    i. porphyria
intermolecular
intermural
intermuscular
intern
internal
    i. pharyngotomy
    i. proctotomy
    i. sphincterotomy
    i. urethrotomy
internal conversion
internalization

internal os
internarial
internasal suture
internatal
internation
International Classification of
    Diseases (ICD)
International Commission on
    Radiation Units and
    Measurements (ICRU)
International Commission on
    Radiological Protection (ICRP)
International Nonproprietary
    Names (INN)
international unit(s) (IU)
interneural
interneuron
    inhibitory i.
interneuronal
internist
internodal
internode of Ranvier
internodular
internship
internuclear
internuncial
internus
interobserver
interocclusal
interoception
interoceptive
interoceptor
interofection
interofective
interoinferiorly
interolivary
interorbital
interosseal
interosseous
interpalatine suture
interpalpebral
interparietal suture
interparoxysmal
interpediculate
interpeduncular
interphalangeal
interphase
interphyletic
interpial
interplant
interpleural
interpleuricostal
interpolar
interpolated
interpolation

interposition operation
interpositum
interpretation
interpreter
interprotometamere
interproximal
interpterygoid
interpubic
interpulse
interpulse time
interpupillary
interpyramidal
interradial
interradicular alveoloplasty
interrenal
interrogation
    Doppler i.
interrupted suture
interrupter
    ground fault circuit i.
interscapilium
interscapular
interscapulum
intersciatic
intersectio (intersectiones)
    i. tendinea
    intersectiones tendineae
      musculi recti
      abdominis
intersection
    aponeurotic i.
    tendinous i.
intersectiones (plural of
  intersectio)
intersegment
intersegmental
interseptal
interseptum
intersex
    female i.
    male i.
    true i.
intersexual
intersexuality
    female genital i.
    gonadal i.
    male genital i.
intersigmoid
interspace
    dineric i.
interspinal
interspinous
intersternal
interstice
interstimulus

interstitial
    i. disease (ID)
    i. markings
interstitium
intertarsal
intertendinous
intertragic
intertransversalis
intertransverse
intertrial
intertriginous candidosis
intertrigo
    i. labialis
    i. saccharomycetica
intertrochanteric osteotomy
intertubercular
intertubular
interureteral
interureteric
interuteroplacental
intervaginal
interval
    a–c i.
    Ae–H i.
    A–H i.
    atriocarotid i.
    atrioventricular (AV) i.
    auriculocarotid i.
    auriculoventricular i.
    a.–v. i.
    B–H i.
    c.–a. i.
    cardioarterial i.
    confidence i.
    coupling i.
    escape i.
    focal i.
    H–Ae i.
    H–V i.
    induction-delivery i.
    interectopic i.
    interstimulus i.
    intertrial i.
    isovolumetric i.
    lucid i.
    i. operation
    P–A i.
    P–J i.
    postmortem i.
    postsphygmic i.
    P–P i.
    PQ i.
    P–R i.
    presphygmic i.
    Q–M i.

I

interval *(continued)*
    Q–R i.
    QRS i.
    QRST i.
    Q–T i.
    Q–U i.
    reference i.
    RS–T i.
    S_2–OS [S2–OS] i.
    Sturm i.
    tolerance i.
    T–P i.
intervalvular
intervascular
intervention
    crisis i.
    percutaneous coronary i. (PCI)
interventricular
intervertebral
interview
    stress i.
intervillous
interzonal
intestinal
    i. atresia
    i. lymphangiectasia
    i. metaplasia
    i. obstruction
    i. peptides
    i. perfusion
    i. tube
intestine
    blind i.
    empty i.
    iced i.
    jejunoileal i.
    large i.
    mesenterial i.
    preoral i.
    segmented i.
    small i.
    straight i.
intestino-intestinal
intestinum
    i. crassum
    i. tenue
intima
intimal
intimectomy
intimitis
    proliferative i.
intoe
in-toeing
intolerance
    disaccharide i.

intolerance *(continued)*
    drug i.
    hereditary fructose i.
    hereditary galactose i.
    lactose i.
    leucine i.
    lysine i.
    lysinuric protein i.
    milk i.
    sucrose i.
intonation
    nasal i.
intorsion
intortor
in toto
intoxicant
intoxication
    acid i.
    alcohol i.
    alcohol idiosyncratic i.
    alkaline i.
    anaphylactic i.
    bongkrek i.
    citrate i.
    digitalis i.
    manganese i.
    pathological i.
    roentgen i.
    serum i.
    substance i.
    water i.
intra-abdominal
intra-acinous
intra-aortic balloon pump
intra-appendicular
intra-arachnoid
intra-arterial
intra-articular
intra-atrial baffle
intra-aural
intrabiopsy
intrabronchial electrocardiography
intrabuccal
intracaliceal
intracanalicular
intracapsular incision
intracardiac
    i. catheter
    i. phonocardiography
intracarpal
intracartilaginous
Intracath catheter
intracatheter
intracavernous
intracavitary electrocardiography

intracelial
intracellular
intracellular-like
intracephalic
intracerebellar
intracerebral
intracervical
intrachange
intrachondral
intrachondrial
intrachordal
intrachorionic
intracisternal
intracolic
intracordal
intracoronal
intracorporeal
intracorpuscular
intracostal
intracranial pressure (IP)
intracrureus
intractable
intracutaneous
intracystic
intracytoplasmic
intracytoplasmic inclusion cell
intrad
intradermal
    i. mattress suture
    i. suture
intradermic suture
intradermoreaction
intraduct
intraductal
intraduodenal
intradural
intraembryonic
intraepidermal
intraepiphyseal
intraepithelial
intraerythrocytic
intrafascial hysterectomy
intrafascicular
intrafat
intrafebrile
intrafetation
intrafilar
intrafissural
intrafistular
intrafollicular
intrafusal
intragalvanization
intragastric
intragemmal
intragenic

intraglandular
intraglobular
intragluteal
intragyral
intrahepatic cholangiojejunostomy
intrahyoid
intraictal
intraintestinal
intrajugular
intralamellar
intralaryngeal
intralesional
intraleukocytic
intraligamentous
intralingual
intralobar
intralobular
intralocular
intraluminal
    i. catheter
    i. stripper
intramammary
intramarginal sulcus
intramastoiditis
intramatrical
intramedullary
    i. drill
    i. tractotomy
intramembranous
intrameningeal
intrameniscal
intramenstrual
intramolecular
intramucosal
intramural
intramuscular (IM)
intramyocardial
intranarial
intranasal antrostomy
intranatal
intraneural
^{113m}In transferrin [indium In 113m
    transferrin]
intranuclear
intraocular
intraoperative cholangiography
intraoral
intraorbital
intraosseous venography
intraosteal
intraovarian
intraovular
intrapancreatic
intraparenchymatous
intraparietal

I

intrapartum
intrapelvic
intrapericardial
intraperineal
intraperitoneal catheter
intrapial
intraplacental
intrapleural
intrapontine
intraprostatic
intraprotoplasmic
intrapsychic
intrapulmonary
intrapulpal
intrapyretic
intrarachidian
intrarectal
intrarenal
intraretinal
intrascleral
intrascrotal
intrasegmental
intrasellar
intraseptal alveoloplasty
intrasheath tenotomy
intraspinal
intraspinous
intrasplenic
intrasternal
intrastitial
intrastromal
intrasynovial
intratarsal
intratendinous
intratesticular
intrathecal
intrathenar
intrathoracic
intratonsillar
intratrabecular
intratracheal
intratubal
intratubular
intratympanic
intraureteral
intraurethral
intrauterine
    endometrial laser i.
      thermotherapy (ELITT)
    i. fetal death
    i. growth retardation
      (IUGR)
intrauterine device (IUD)
    coil
    copper-7

intrauterine device (IUD)
    (continued)
    Lippes loop
    Mirena
    Progestasert
    Tatum-T
intravaginal
intravasation
intravascular coagulation
intravenation
intravenous
    i. angiocardiography
    i. aortography
    i. cholangiography (IVC)
    i. cholecystography
    i. pyelography (IVP)
    i. urography (IVU)
intraventricular
intraversion
intravertebral
intravesical
intravillous
intravitelline
intravitreal
intravitreous
intrinsic
    i. affinity
    i. association constant
introducer
    Carter i.
    Littleford-Spector i.
introfier
introflexion
introgastric
introgression
introitus
    marital i.
    i. oesophagi
    parous i.
    i. pelvis
    i. vaginae
    vaginal i.
introjection
intromission
intron
intropunitive
introrsus
introspection
introspective
introversion
introversion-extroversion
introvert
intrude
intrusion
intubate

intubation
  aqueductal i.
  blind nasal i.
  blind nasotracheal i.
  endotracheal i.
  nasal i.
  nasotracheal i.
  oral i.
  orotracheal i.
  i. tube
intubationist
intubator
intuition
intumesce
intumescence
intumescent
intumescentia
  i. cervicalis
  i. ganglioformis
  i. lumbalis
  i. lumbosacralis
  i. tympanica
intussusception
  agonic i.
  appendicular i.
  cecocolic i.
  colic i.
  colocolic i.
  double i.
  enteric i.
  enterocolic i.
  ileal i.
  ileocecal i.
  ileocolic i.
  ileoileal i.
  jejunogastric i.
  postmortem i.
  retrograde i.
intussusceptum
intussuscipiens
inulase
inulin
inuloid
inunction
inunctum mentholis compositum
in utero
in vacuo
invade
invaginate
invaginating suture
invagination
  basilar i.
  i. of enamel
  mammary i.
invaginator

invalid
invalidism
invariant
  i. chain
  I i.
invasin
invasion
invasive
invasiveness
inventory
  Maudsley Personality I.
  Millon Clinical Multiaxial
    Inventory
  Minnesota Multiphasic
    Personality Inventory
invermination
inverse square law
inversion
  i. of bladder
  carbohydrate i.
  chromosome i.
  forced i.
  i. of gradient
  lateral i.
  paracentric i.
  pericentric i.
  sexual i.
  sound i.
  spontaneous i.
  thermic i.
  T-wave i.
  i. of uterus
  visceral i.
inversion-recovery technique
inversus
invert
invertase
invertebrate
inverted suture
inverting suture
invertor
invertose
invest
investing
  i. the pattern
  vacuum i.
investment
  emotional i.
  fibrous i.
  hygroscopic i.
  myelin i.
inveterate
inviscation
in vitro
in vivo

I

involucre
involucrum
involuntary
involuntomotory
involute
involution
    buccal i.
    pituitary i.
    senile i.
    i. of uterus
involutional
involvement
    bifurcation i.
    trifurcation i.
I&O—
    in and out (surgery)
    intake and output
IO—
    internal os
    intestinal obstruction
    intraocular
iobenguane
    i. I 123
    i. I 123 sulfate
    i. I 131
iobenzamic acid
iocarmic acid
iocetamic acid
iodalbumin
iodamide
Iodamoeba buetschlii
iodate
iodemia
iodic acid
iodide
    ferrous i.
iodide peroxidase
iodimetry
iodinate
iodinated
    i. contrast media
    i. I 125 fibrinogen
    i. I 125 serum albumin
    i. I 131 aggregated albumin
        (human)
    i. I 131 serum albumin
        (human)
iodination
iodine (I)
    butanol-extractable i.
    i. green
    i. I 123
    i. I 125
    i. I 131
    imidecyl i.

iodine (I) *(continued)*
    Lugol i.
    povidone-i.
    protein-bound i.
    i. PVP bond
    radioactive i. (i. I 123, i. I 125,
        i. I 131)
iodine-fast
iodinin
iodinophil
iodinophilous
iodipamide
    i. meglumine
    i. sodium
iodism
iodixanol
iodize
iodoacetamide
iodoacetic acid
iodoantipyrine
iodobrassid
iodocasein
iodocholesterol
iodocholesterol I 131
5-iododeoxyuridine
iododerma
iodoform
    i. dressing
    i. gauze
    i. gauze packing
iodoformism
iodogenic
iodoglobulin
iodogorgonine
iodogorgoric acid
iodohippurate sodium
    i. I 123
    i. I 131
iodolography
iodomethamate
iodomethylnorcholesterol
iodometric
iodometry
iodopanoic acid
iodophenol
iodophilia
iodophor
iodoprotein
iodopsin
iodopyracet
iodostick
iodosulfate
iodotherapy
iodothyroglobulin
iodothyronine

iodotyrosine
iodotyrosine dehalogenase
iodotyrosine deiodinase
iodoventriculography
iodovolatilization
iodoxamic acid
iodoxyquinolinesulfonic
    acid
ioduria
ioglicic acid
ioglycamic acid
IOL—intraocular lens
ion
    amphoteric dipolar i.
    dipolar i.
    gram i.
    hydrogen i.
    hydronium i.
    i. microscope
Ionescu-Shiley
    prosthesis
    valve
ionic
ionium
ionization
    avalanche i.
    Townsend i.
ionize
ionocolorimeter
ionogen
ionogenic
ionometer
ionometry
ionone
ionophore
ionophose
ionoscope
ionotherapy
ion-protein
ions
iontherapy
iontophoresis
iontophoretic
iontotherapy
IOP—intraocular pressure
iopamidol
iopanoic acid
iophendylate
iophenoxic acid
iopromide
iopydol
iopydone
ioseric acid
iosulamide meglumine
iosumetic acid

iota —Greek letter (ι; alphabetized
    as i)
iotacism
iotetric acid
iothalamate
    i. meglumine
    i. sodium
iothalamic acid
iotroxic acid
IOU—intensive therapy
    observation unit
Iowa forceps
IP—
    incisoproximal
    incubation period
    instantaneous pressure
    interphalangeal
    intraperitoneal
    intraperitoneally
    isoelectric point
IP₃—inositol 1,4,5-triphosphate
IPA—International
    Psychoanalytical Association
I-para—primipara
IPC—isopropyl chlorophenyl
IPD—intermittent peritoneal
    dialysis
ipecac
    powdered i.
IPG—impedance
    plethysmography
IPH—idiopathic pulmonary
    hemosiderosis
IPL—intrapleural
ipomea
Ipomoea
    I. calobra
    I. muelleri
    I. orizabensis Ledenois
    I. violacea L.
IPP—intermittent positive
    pressure
IPPB—intermittent positive-
    pressure breathing
IPPI—interruption of pregnancy
    for psychiatric indication
IPPO—intermittent positive-
    pressure inflation with oxygen
IPPR—intermittent positive-
    pressure respiration
IPPV—intermittent positive-
    pressure ventilation
IPRT—interpersonal reaction test
IPS—initial prognostic score
ipsilateral

IPSP—inhibitory postsynaptic potential
IPU—inpatient unit
IPV—inactivated poliovirus vaccine
IQ—intelligence quotient
IR—
    immunoreactive
    internal resistance
IRA-400 resin
irascibility
IRC—inspiratory reserve capacity
IRG—immunoreactive glucagon
Ir genes—immune response genes
IRHCS—immunoradioassayable human chorionic somatomammotropin
IRhGH—immunoreactive human growth hormone
IRI—immunoreactive insulin
iridal
iridalgia
iridauxesis
iridavulsion
iridectasis
iridectome
iridectomesodialysis
iridectomize
iridectomy
    basal i.
    buttonhole i.
    complete i. (CI)
    laser i.
    optic i.
    optical i.
    peripheral i. (PI)
    preliminary i.
    preparatory i.
    sector i.
    stenopeic i.
    therapeutic i.
    total i.
iridectropium
iridemia
iridencleisis
iridentropium
irideremia
iridescence
iridescent
iridesis
iridiagnosis
iridial
iridian
iridic
iridis
    rubeosis i.

iridium (Ir)
iridization
iridoavulsion
iridocapsulitis
iridocapsulotomy
iridocele
iridochoroiditis
iridocoloboma
iridoconstrictor
iridocorneal-endothelial (ICE) syndrome
iridocorneosclerectomy
iridocyclectomy
iridocyclitis
    heterochromic i.
iridocyclochoroiditis
iridocystectomy
iridocyte
iridodesis
iridodiagnosis
iridodialysis
iridodiastasis
iridodilator
iridodonesis
iridokeratitis
iridokinesia
iridokinesis
iridokinetic
iridoleptynsis
iridology
iridolysis
iridomalacia
iridomesodialysis
iridomotor
iridoncus
iridoparalysis
iridopathy
iridoperiphakitis
iridoplegia
    accommodation i.
    complete i.
    reflex i.
    sympathetic i.
iridoptosis
iridopupillary
iridorhexis
iridoschisis
iridosclerotomy
iridosteresis
iridotasis
iridotome
iridotomy
iridovirus
iris (irides)
    bombé i.

iris (irides) *(continued)*
    i. coloboma
    i. crypts
    detached i.
    Florentine i.
    i. inclusion operation
    i. pigment dispersion
    i. prolapse
    i. scissors
    i. sphincter
    i. stroma
    tremulous i.
    umbrella i.
IRIS—International Research
  Information Service
irisin
irisopsia
iritic
iritis
    i. catamenialis
    diabetic i.
    Doyne i.
    follicular i.
    gouty i.
    i. papulosa
    plastic i.
    purulent i.
    serous i.
    spongy i.
    sympathetic i.
    tuberculous i.
    uratic i.
iritoectomy
iritomy
irium
IRMA—intraretinal microvascular
  abnormalities
iron (Fe)
    i. 55 (or 59)
    i. acetate
    i. adenylate
    i. and ammonium sulfate
    i. ascorbate
    available i.
    i. chloride
    i. choline citrate
    i. citrate
    i. dextrin
    i. gluconate
    i. hematoxylin
    i. hydroxide
    i. hypophosphate
    i. lactate
    i. malate
    nonheme i.

iron (Fe) *(continued)*
    i. oleate
    i. phosphate
    i. protosulfate
    i. pyrophosphate
    Quevenne i.
    i. and quinine citrate
    radioactive i.
    reduced i.
    i. sorbitex
    i. sulfate
    i. valerianate
irradiate
irradiated
irradiation
    interstitial i.
    intracavitary i.
    painful i.
    ultraviolet blood i.
    whole-body i.
irreducible
    i. dislocation
    i. fracture
    i. hernia
    i. umbilical mass
irregular
irregularity
    luminal i.
    i. of pulse
irremedial
irrespirable
irresponsibility
    criminal i.
irresuscitable
irreversibility of conduction
irreversible
irrigant
irrigate
irrigation
    acetic acid i.
    aminoacetic acid i.
    antral i.
    continuous i.
    Ringer i.
    sodium chloride i.
irrigator
    Buie i.
    DeVilbiss i.
    Fox i.
    Gibson i.
    House i.
    Rollet i.
    Shambaugh i.
    Shea i.
irrigoradioscopy

I

irritability
  chemical i.
  electric i.
  faradic i.
  galvanic i.
  mechanical i.
  muscular i.
  myotatic i.
  nervous i.
  specific i.
  tactile i.
  i. of the bladder
  i. of the stomach
  uterine i.
  ventricular i.
irritable bowel disease (IBD)
irritant
  primary i.
irritation
  cerebral i.
  direct i.
  functional i.
  meningeal i.
  spinal i.
  sympathetic i.
irritative
IRS—infrared spectrophotometry
Irukandji sting
IRV—inspiratory reserve
  volume
Irvine
  scissors
  syndrome
Irvine-Gass syndrome
Irving operation
IS—
  immune serum
  intercostal space
  interspace
  intraspinal
  insertion sequence
ISA—intrinsic sympathomimetic
  activity
Isaac differential distortion
  divergent method
Isaacs-Ludwig arteriole
Isambert disease
isatin
isauxesis
ischemia
  brachiocephalic i.
  brain stem i.
  i. cordis intermittens
  fascicular i.

ischemia *(continued)*
  mesenteric i.
  midgut i.
  myocardial i.
  postural i.
  renal i.
  i. retinae
  subendocardial i.
  subepicardial i.
  transient carotid i.
  transient cerebral i.
  vasospastic cerebral i.
ischemic
  transient i. attack (TIA)
ischesis
ischia
ischiadelphus
ischiadic
ischial weightbearing (weight-
  bearing) brace
ischialgia
ischiatic
ischidrosis
ischiectomy
ischioanal
ischiobulbar
ischiocapsular
ischiocavernous
ischiocele
ischiococcygeal
ischiococcygeus
ischiodidymus
ischiodymia
ischiodynia
ischiofemoral
ischiofibular
ischiohebotomy
ischiomelus
ischionitis
ischiopagia
ischiopagus
  i. parasiticus
  i. tetrapus
  i. tripus
ischiopubic
ischiopubiotomy
ischiopubis
ischiorectal
ischiosacral
ischiothoracopagus
ischiovaginal
ischiovertebral
ischium
ischogyria

ischospermia
ischuretic
ischuria
    i. paradoxa
    i. spastica
ISD, ISDN—isosorbide dinitrate
isethionate
isethionic acid
ISG—immune serum globulin
Is genes—immune suppressor
    genes
ISH—
    icteric serum hepatitis
    International Society of
       Hematology
Isherwood position
Ishihara
    plate
    test
isinglass
    Japanese i.
island
    blood i's
    bone i.
    i's of Calleja
    cartilage i's
    i's of Langerhans
    olfactory i's
    i's of pancreas
    Pander i's
    i. of Reil
    Wolff i.
islet
    blood i's
    Calleja i's
    i. cell
    Langerhans i.
    pancreatic i's
    Walthard i's
ISO—International Organization
    for Standardization
isoadrenocorticism
isoagglutination
isoagglutinin
isoallele
isoallelism
isoalloxazine
    mononucleotide
isoamylamine
isoamylethylbarbituric acid
isoamyl nitrite
isoantibody
isoantigen
isobar

isobaric
isobaric transition
isobolism
isobornyl thiocyanoacetate
isobutamben
isobutylallylbarbituric acid
isocaloric
isocarboxazid
isocellobiose
isocellular
isocenter
isocholesterol
isochromatic
isochromatophil
isochromosome
isochronia
isochronism
isochronous
isocitrate
    i. dehydrogenase–NAD$^+$
    i. dehydrogenase–NADP$^+$
    i. lyase
isocitric acid
isocolloid
isocomplement
Isocon camera
isocoria
isocortex
isocyanate
isocyanide
isocyclic
isocytolysin
isocytosis
isodactylism
isodesmosine
isodiagnosis
isodiametric
isodispersoid
isodontic
isodose
isodulcite
isodynamic
isodynamogenic
isoechoic
isoeffect
isoelectric
    i. focusing
    i. point
isoelectronic
isoenergetic
isoenzyme
    Regan i.
isoerythrolysis
    neonatal i.

I

isoetharine
isoflupredone acetate
isoflurane
isoflurophate
isoflurophosphate
isogamete
isogametic
isogamety
isogamous
isogamy
isogeneic
isogeneric
isogenesis
isogenic
isogenous
isograft
isohemagglutination
isohemagglutinin
isohemolysin
isohemolysis
isohemolytic
isohydric
isohydruria
isoiconia
isoiconic lens
isoimmunization
    Rh i.
    rhesus i.
isoindicial
isolabeling
isolactose
isolate
isolateral
isolation
    ethologic i.
    pulmonary i.
    sensory i.
isolator
    surgical i.
isolecithal
Isolette
isoleucine
isoleucyl
isoleukoagglutinin
isologous
isolysergic acid
isolysin
isolysis
isolytic
isomaltase
isomaltose
isomastigote
isomer
    cis-trans i.
    conformational i.

isomer *(continued)*
    geometric i.
    optical i.
isomerase
    phosphoribose i.
isomeric
    i. decay
    i. transition
isomeride
isomerism
    chain i.
    cis-trans i.
    configurational i.
    conformational i.
    constitutional i.
    functional group i.
    geometric i.
    optical i.
    position i.
    spatial i.
    stereochemical i.
    structural i.
    substitution i.
isomerization
isomethadone
isometheptene mucate
isometrics
isometropia
isometry
isomicrogamete
isomorphic
isomorphism
isomorphous
isomuscarine
isonaphthol
isonephrotoxin
isonicotinic acid
    i.a. hydrazide
isonicotinoylhydrazine
isonicotinylhydrazine
isonipecaine
isonormocytosis
iso-oncotic
Isopaque
Isoparorchis trisimilitubis
isopathy
isopentenyl diphosphate
isopentenyl-diphosphate
    δ-isomerase
    [delta-]
isopentenyl pyrophosphate
isophagy
isophan
isophene
isophoria

isophotometer
isopia
isoplastic
isopotential
isoprecipitin
isopregnenone
isoprenaline
isoprene
isoprenoid
isopropanol
isopropyl
    i. alcohol
    i. meprobamate
    i. myristate
    i. rubbing alcohol
    i. thiogalactoside
isopropylarterenol
isopropyl-benzanthracene
isopropylepinephrine
isoproterenol sulfate
isopter
isopyknic
isopyknosis
isopyknotic
isorhodeose
isorhythmic
isoriboflavin
isorrhea
isorrheic
isorrhopic
isorubin
isoscope
isosensitization
isosensitize
isoserine
isoserotherapy
isoserum
isosexual
isosmotic
isosmoticity
isosorbide dinitrate
Isospora
    I. belli
    I. bigemina
    I. felis
    I. hominis
    I. lacazei
    I. rivolta
    I. suis
isospore
isosporiasis
isosporous
isostere
isosthenuria
isosulfan blue

isotel
isothebaine
isotherapy
isothermic
isothermognosia
isothermognosis
isothiocyanate
isothiocyanic acid
isothipendyl
isothromboagglutinin
isotone
isotonia
isotonic
isotonicity
isotope
    i. bone scan
    i. colloid imaging
    i. effect
    heavy i.
    hepatobiliary imaging
      radioactive i.
    i. nephrography
    radioactive i.
    stable i.
    i. study
    i. ventriculography
    i. voiding cystourethrography
      (IVCU)
isotopic
isotopology
isotoxic
isotoxin
isotransplant
isotransplantation
isotretinoin
isotrimorphism
isotrimorphous
isotron
isotropic
isotropy
isotype
isotypic
isotypical
isouretin
isovaleric acid
isovaleric acid CoA dehydrogenase
    deficiency
isovalericacidemia
isovaleryl-CoA
    dehydrogenase
isovolume pressure
isoxepac
isoxicam
isozyme
ISP—interspace

Israel
    operation
    retractor
issue
IST—
    insulin sensitivity
      test
    insulin shock therapy
isthmectomy
isthmi (plural of isthmus)
isthmic
isthmica nodosa
isthmic-cornual
isthmitis
isthmoparalysis
isthmoplegia
isthmospasm
isthmus (isthmi)
    anterior i. of fauces
    i. of aorta
    i. aortae
    i. of auditory tube
    i. of cartilage of auricle
    i. cartilaginis auris
    i. of cingulate gyrus
    i. of eustachian tube
    i. of external auditory
      meatus
    i. of fallopian tube
    i. of fauces
    i. faucium
    i. glandulae thyroideae
    gyral i.
    i. gyri cingulatus
    i. gyri cinguli
    i. gyri fornicati
    Haller i.
    i. hippocampi
    i. of His
    Krönig (Kronig, Kroenig) i.
    i. of limbic lobe
    oropharyngeal i.
    i. prostatae
    i. rhombencephali
    i. of thyroid gland
    i. tubae auditoriae
    i. tubae uterinae
    tubal i.
    i. urethrae
    i. uteri
    i. of uterus
    i. of Vieussens
ISU—International Society of
  Urology
isuria

ISW—interstitial water
IT—
    implantation test
    inhalation test
    inhalation therapy
    intradermal test
    intrathecal
    intratracheal
    intratracheal tube
    intratumoral
    isomeric transition
Italian
    distant flap
    method
    operation
    rhinoplasty
Itard catheter
Itard-Cholewa sign
ITC—imidazolyl-thioguanine
  chemotherapy
itch
    Aujeszky i.
    bakers' i.
    barbers' i.
    bath i.
    Boeck i.
    chorioptic i.
    clam digger's i.
    copra i.
    Cuban i.
    dew i.
    dhobie i.
    dhobie mark i.
    filarial i.
    grain i.
    grocer's i.
    ground i.
    gym i.
    jock i.
    kabure i.
    mad i.
    Moeller i.
    Norway i.
    prairie i.
    sarcoptic i.
    Sawah i.
    seven-year i.
    straw i.
    summer i.
    swamp i.
    swimmer's i.
    water i.
    winter i.
itching
ITE—in-the-ear (hearing aid)

iter
    i. chordae anterius
    i. chordae posterius
    i. dentium
    i. of Sylvius
iteral
iterative
iteroparity
iteroparous
ithylordosis
ithyokyphosis
ITLC—instant thin-layer
   chromatography
Ito nevus
Ito-Reenstierna test
ITP—
    idiopathic thrombocytopenic
      purpura
    inosine triphosphate
ITPA—Illinois Test of
   Psycholinguistic Abilities
Itsenko disease
ITT—insulin tolerance test
ITU—intensive therapy unit
IU—
    immunizing unit
    international unit(s)
    intrauterine
IUCD—intrauterine
   contraceptive device
IUD—
    intrauterine contraceptive
      device
    intrauterine death
    intrauterine device
IUGR—
    intrauterine growth
      rate
    intrauterine growth
      restriction
    intrauterine growth
      retardation
IUM—intrauterine fetally
   malnourished
IUT—intrauterine
   transfusion
IV cocktail
IV—
    interventricular
    intervertebral
    intravascular
    intravenous
    intravenously
    intraventricular
    invasive

Ivalon
   implant
   suture
IVAP—in vivo adhesive platelet
IVC—
   inferior vena cava
   intravenous cholangiogram
IVCC—intravascular consumption
   coagulopathy
IVCD—intraventricular conduction
   defect
IVCP—inferior vena cava pressure
IVCU—isotope voiding
   cystourethrography
IVCV—inferior venacavography
IVD—intervertebral disk
Ivemark syndrome
Iverson dermabrader
Ives anoscope
IVGTT—intravenous glucose
   tolerance test
IVH—intraventricular hemorrhage
IVM—intravascular mass
ivory
IVP—
   intravenous pyelogram
   intravenous pyelography
   intraventricular pressure
IVRT—isovolumic relaxation time
IVS—interventricular septum
IVSD—interventricular septal
   defect
IVT—intravenous transfusion
IVTTT—intravenous tolbutamide
   tolerance test
IVU—intravenous urography
Ivy
   bleeding time test
   loop wiring
   method
   rongeur
   wire
   wiring
Iwanoff (Iwanow)
   cysts
   retinal edema
IWL—insensible water loss
IWMI—inferior wall myocardial
   infarction
Ixodes
   I. bicornis
   I. canisuga
   I. cavipalpus
   I. cookei
   I. dammini

I

Ixodes (continued)
   I. frequens
   I. hexagonus
   I. holocyclus
   I. pacificus
   I. persulcatus
   I. pilosus
   I. rasus
   I. ricinus

Ixodes (continued)
   I. rubicundus
   I. scapularis
   I. spinipalpus
ixodiasis
ixodic
ixodid
Ixodiphagus caucurtei
Izar reagent

J

J—
   joule
   journal
JA—juvenile arthritis
Jaboulay
   amputation
   button
   method
   operation
   pyloroplasty
Jaccoud
   arthritis
   arthropathy
   fever
   sign
   syndrome
jacket
   Kydex body j.
   Minerva j.
   orthoplast j.
   plaster-of-Paris j.
   porcelain j.
   Risser j.
   Sayre j.
   strait j.
jackscrew
Jackson
   appliance
   bougie
   bronchoscope
   clamp
   crib
   dilator
   elevator
   epilepsy
   esophagoscope
   forceps

Jackson *(continued)*
   incision
   laryngoscope
   law
   membrane
   operation
   paralysis
   retractor
   rule
   safety triangle
   scalpel
   scissors
   sign
   syndrome
   tenaculum
   theory
   tube
   veil
jacksonian
   j. epilepsy
   j. march
jacksonism
Jackson-Mosher dilator
Jackson-Pratt
   catheter
   tube
Jackson-Trousseau dilator
Jacob
   membrane
   ulcer
jacobine
Jacobs
   forceps
   uterine tenaculum
Jacobson
   anastomosis
   canal

Jacobson *(continued)*
 cartilage
 clamp
 forceps
 nerve
 organ
 plexus
 ramus
 retinitis
 retractor
 scissors
 spatula
 sulcus
Jacobs-Palmer laparoscope
Jacod syndrome
Jacod-Negri syndrome
Jacquemier sign
Jacques plexus
Jacquet
 dermatitis
 erythema
jactatio capitis nocturna
jactitation
 periodic j.
jaculiferous
Jadassohn
 anetoderma
 disease
 macular atrophy
 sebaceous nevus
 test
Jadassohn-Lewandowsky
 law
 syndrome
Jadassohn-Pellizari
 anetoderma
Jadelot
 furrows
 lines
Jaeger
 keratome
 lid plate
 test types
Jaesche operation
Jaesche-Arlt operation
Jaffe
 reaction
 test
Jako laryngoscope
Jakob
 disease
 pseudosclerosis
Jakob-Creutzfeldt
 disease
 syndrome

Jaksch (von Jaksch)
 anemia
 test
jalap resin
jamais vu
James fibers
James-Lange-Sutherland
 theory
Jameson
 calipers
 forceps
 hook
 operation
Jamshidi needle
Janet
 disease
 test
Janeway
 gastroscope
 gastrostomy
 lesion
 sphygmomanometer
 spots
janiceps
 j. asymmetros
 j. parasiticus
Janošík embryo
Jansen
 disease
 forceps
 operation
 retractor
 syndrome
 test
Jansen-Middleton forceps
Jansky-Bielschowsky
 disease
 syndrome
Jansky classification
Janthinosoma
 J. lutzi
 J. posticata
Japanese B encephalitis
Jaquet apparatus
jar
 anaerobic j.
 bell j.
 candle j.
 Coplin j.
 Leyden
jararaca
Jarcho
 cannula
 forceps
 pressometer

J

jargon
    j. agraphia
    j. aphasia, jargonaphasia
Jarisch-Herxheimer reaction
Jarjavay
    ligament
    muscle
Jarvik heart
Jarvis
    clamp
    operation
jaundice
    acholuric j.
    acholuric familial j.
    anhepatic j.
    anhepatogenous j.
    black j.
    breast milk j.
    cholestatic j.
    chronic acholuric j.
    congenital familial
      nonhemolytic j.
    congenital nonhemolytic j.
    congenital obliterative j.
    constitutional j.
    Crigler-Najjar j.
    epidemic j.
    familial acholuric j.
    familial nonhemolytic j.
    hemolytic j.
    hemorrhagic j.
    hepatocanalicular j.
    hepatocellular j.
    hepatogenic j.
    hepatogenous j.
    homologous serum j.
    human serum j.
    infectious j.
    infective j.
    latent j.
    leptospiral j.
    malignant j.
    mechanical j.
    nonhemolytic j., congenital
    nonhemolytic j., congenital
      familial
    nonobstructive j.
    nuclear j.
    obstructive j.
    parenchymatous j.
    physiologic j.
    picric acid j.
    regurgitation j.
    retention j.
    Schmorl j.

jaundice *(continued)*
    spirochetal j.
    syringe j.
    j. of the newborn
    toxemic j.
    toxic j.
    transfusion j.
Javal ophthalmometer
Javid
    bypass clamp
    shunt
jaw
    bird-beak j.
    cleft j.
    crackling j.
    Hapsburg j.
    inferior j.
    j.-limb
    locked j.
    lower j.
    phossy j.
    pipe j.
    snapping j.
    upper j.
    j.-winking phenomenon
    j.-winking syndrome
    j. wiring
jawbone
Jaworski
    bodies
    corpuscles
    test
JCA—juvenile chronic arthritis
JCAHO; JC—Joint Commission
    on Accreditation of Healthcare
    Organizations [now: The Joint
    Commission]
Jeanselme nodules
Jefferson
    fracture
    syndrome
jejunal cutaneous urinary
    diversion
jejunectomy
jejunitis
jejunocecostomy
jejunocolostomy
jejunogastric
jejunoileal
jejunoileitis
jejunoileostomy
jejunoileum
jejunojejunostomy
jejunoplasty
jejunorrhaphy

jejunostomy
    Baker j. tube
    needle catheter j.
jejunotomy
jejunum
Jelanko arch bar
Jellinek
    sign
    symptom
jelly
    cardiac j.
    contraceptive j.
    electrode j.
    enamel j.
    glycerin j.
    mineral j.
    petroleum j.
    Wharton j.
Jenckel method
Jendrassik
    maneuver
    sign
Jenner
    emphysema
    method
    stain
jennerian vaccine
jennerization
Jensen
    choroiditis
    disease
    procedure
    retinitis
jerk
    Achilles j.
    ankle j.
    biceps j.
    crossed j.
    elbow j.
    epileptic j.
    finger j.
    jaw j.
    knee j.
    massive myoclonic j.
    nystagmoid j's
    j. nystagmus
    pendular knee j.
    quadriceps j.
    supinator j.
    tendon j.
    triceps surae j.
Jervell and Lange-Nielsen syndrome
Jesberg
    bronchoscope
    clamp

Jesberg *(continued)*
    esophagoscope
Jesionek lamp
jessur
Jeune syndrome
Jewett
    bladder carcinoma classification
    extractor
    nail
    operation
    plate
    sound
Jewett-Strong system
JG—juxtaglomerular
jigger
jitter
jitteriness
jittery
JND—just noticeable difference
Jobert
    fossa
    suture
Jobst
    boot
    stockings
Job syndrome
Jodbasedow disease
Joest bodies
Joffroy
    reflex
    sign
Johanson-Blizzard syndrome
Johne disease
Johns Hopkins
    clamp
    forceps
Johnson
    basket
    calculation
    forceps
    needle holder
    operation
    position
    stone dislodger
    syndrome
    tube
Johnson-Stevens disease
joint
    acromioclavicular (AC) j.
    amphidiarthrodial j.
    ankle j.
    apophyseal j.
    arthrodial j.
    arycorniculate j.
    atlantoaxial j.

J

joint *(continued)*

  atlanto-occipital j.
  ball-and-socket j.
  biaxial j.
  bicondylar j.
  bilocular j.
  bleeder's j.
  Budin j.
  calcaneocuboid j.
  capitular j.
  carpal j's
  carpometacarpal j's
  cartilaginous j.
  Charcot j.
  Chopart j.
  Clutton j.
  coccygeal j.
  cochlear j.
  composite j.
  compound j.
  condylar j.
  condyloid j.
  costochondral j's
  costotransverse j.
  costovertebral j's
  cotyloid j.
  cricoarytenoid j.
  cricothyroid j.
  Cruveilhier j.
  cubital j.
  cuboideonavicular j.
  cuneocuboid j.
  cuneometatarsal j.
  cuneonavicular j.
  diarthrodial j.
  dry j.
  elbow j.
  ellipsoidal j.
  enarthrodial j.
  facet j's
  false j.
  femoropatellar j.
  femorotibial j.
  fibrocartilaginous j.
  fibrous j.
  flail j.
  freely movable j.
  fringe j.
  ginglymoid j.
  glenohumeral j.
  gliding j.
  hemophilic j.
  hinge j.
  hip j.

joint *(continued)*

  humeroradial j.
  humeroulnar j.
  immovable j.
  incudomalleolar j.
  incudostapedial j.
  inferior radioulnar j.
  inferior tibiofibular j.
  inferior sternal j.
  inferior tibiofibular j.
  interarticular j's
  intercarpal j.
  interchondral j's
  intercuneiform j's
  intermetacarpal j's
  interphalangeal j's
  irritable j.
  jaw j.
  knee j.
  ligamentous j.
  Lisfranc j.
  lumbosacral j.
  Luschka j.
  mandibular j.
  manubriosternal j.
  mediocarpal j.
  metacarpophalangeal (MCP) j's
  metatarsophalangeal (MTP) j's
  j. mice
  midcarpal j.
  midtarsal j.
  mixed j.
  mortise j.
  movable j.
  multiaxial j.
  open j.
  peg-and-socket j.
  pisotriquetral j.
  pivot j.
  plane j.
  polyaxial j.
  j. position sense
  radiocarpal j.
  rotary j.
  sacrococcygeal j.
  sacroiliac j.
  saddle j.
  saddle-shaped j.
  scapuloclavicular j.
  sellar j.
  shoulder j.
  simple j.
  skin j.
  slip j.

joint *(continued)*
    socket j. of tooth
    spheno-occipital j.
    spheroidal j.
    spiral j.
    sternoclavicular j.
    sternocostal j's
    stifle j.
    subtalar j.
    superior radioulnar j.
    superior tibiofibular j.
    suture j.
    synarthrodial j.
    synovial j.
    talocalcaneonavicular j.
    talocrural j.
    talonavicular j.
    talotibiofibular j.
    tarsal j.
    tarsal j., transverse
    tarsometatarsal j's
    temporomandibular j. (TMJ)
    thoracic j's
    through j.
    tibiofibular j.
    transverse tarsal j.
    trochoid j.
    uncovertebral j.
    uniaxial j.
    unilocular j.
    j's of vertebral column
    von Gies j.
    wrist j.
    xiphisternal j.
    zygapophyseal j's
joker elevator
Jolles test
Jolly
    bodies
    dilator
    reaction
    sign
    test
Jonas-Graves speculum
Jonas symptom
Jones
    criteria
    curet
    dilator
    forceps
    fracture
    operation
    position
    scissors

Jones *(continued)*
    splint
Jonnesco
    fold
    fossa
    operation
Joplin operation
Jordan-Day
    bur
    drill
Jorgenson scissors
Joseph
    clamp
    knife
    operation
    periosteotome
    rhinoplasty
    saw
    scissors
    syndrome
Joseph-Maltz saw
Josephs-Diamond-Blackfan
  syndrome
joule (J)
JRA—juvenile rheumatoid
  arthritis
J-shaped incision
Judd
    forceps
    pyloroplasty
    retractor
Judd-Allis forceps
Judd-DeMartel forceps
Judd-Masson retractor
Judet prosthesis
judgment
judicious
Judkins technique
Juers-Lempert forceps
Juevenelle clamp
juga (plural of jugum)
jugal suture
jugale
jugate
jugomaxillary
jugular
    j. pulse sphygmography
    j. venous distention
      (JVD)
    j. venous pressure (JVP)
    j. venous pulse (JVP)
jugulation
jugulodigastric nodes
jugulum

J

jugum (juga)
- juga alveolaria mandibulae
- juga alveolaria maxillae
- juga cerebralia ossium cranii
- j. sphenoidale

juice
- cancer j.
- cherry j.
- gastric j.
- intestinal j.
- pancreatic j.
- press j.
- raspberry j.

Jukes family

Julian forceps

jumper

jumping
- j. disease
- j. Frenchmen of Maine
- j. pain

jumping-the-bite
- j.b. appliance
- j.b. plate

junction
- adherens j.
- amelodentinal j.
- anorectal j.
- cardioesophageal j.
- cell j.
- cementodentinal j.
- cementoenamel j.
- cervicomedullary j.
- choledochoduodenal j.
- corneoscleral j.
- dentinocemental j.
- dentinoenamel j.
- dentogingival j.
- dermoepidermal j.
- esophagogastric j.
- fibromuscular j.
- gap j.
- gastroesophageal j.
- ileocecal j.
- intermediate j.
- intermembrane j.
- iridociliary j.
- j. of lips
- lumbosacral j.
- manubriogladiolar j.
- mucocutaneous j.
- mucogingival j.
- myoneural j.
- myotendinal j.
- neuromuscular j.
- occluding j.

junction *(continued)*
- osseous j.
- pentilaminar j.
- rectosigmoid j.
- root-cord j.
- sclerocorneal j.
- j. scotoma
- ST j.
- tendinous j's
- tight j.
- tympanostapedial j.
- ureteropelvic j.
- ureterovesical j.

junctional
- j. epidermolysis bullosa
- j. escape rhythm
- j. nevus

junctura
- juncturae cartilagineae
- j. fibrosa
- juncturae lumbosacralis
- juncturae ossium
- j. sacrococcygea
- juncturae synovialis
- juncturae tendinum
- juncturae zygapophyseales

juncture
- saphenofemoral j.

Jung
- method
- muscle

Jungbluth
- vasa propria
- vessels

jungian

juniper

Juniperus
- *J. communis*
- *J. oxycedrus*
- *J. sabina*
- *J. virginiana*

Junker
- apparatus
- bottle
- inhaler

Jurasz forceps

jurisprudence
- dental j.
- medical j.

justo major

justo minor

Jutte tube

juvenile
- j. gangliosidosis
- j. hyaline fibromatosis

juvenile *(continued)*
        j. lentigo melanoma
        j.-onset diabetes
        j. polyposis
        j. retinoschisis
        j. rheumatoid arthritis
        j. xanthogranuloma
juxta-articular
juxtacortical
juxtaductal coarctation
juxtaepiphyseal
juxtaglomerular
juxtallocortex
juxtamedullary

juxtangina
juxtapapillary
juxtaposition
juxtapyloric
juxtaspinal
juxtavesical
JV—
        jugular vein
        jugular venous
JVP—
        jugular venous pressure
        jugular venous pulse
JXG—juvenile xanthogranuloma

K

κ—
        kappa (Greek letter)
        one of the two types of
            immunoglobulin light chains
k—kilo-
k—Boltzmann constant
K—
        absolute zero
        cathode
        electrostatic capacity
        Kell blood system
        Kelvin
        potassium
K—equilibrium constant
*K*_a—acid dissociation constantf
KA—
        ketoacidosis
        King-Armstrong (units)
kabure
Kader
        gastrostomy
        operation
Kader-Senn operation
Kaes
        feltwork
        line
Kaes-Bekhterev
        band
        layer
        stripe
KAF—conglutinogen activating
    factor
KAFO—knee-ankle-foot orthosis

Kahlbaum
        catatonic stupor
        syndrome
Kahlbaum-Wernicke syndrome
Kahler
        disease
        forceps
        law
Kahn
        cannula
        tenaculum
Kahn-Graves speculum
kahweol
Kaiserling
        fixative
        method
        solution
Kaiserstuhl disease
kala-azar
        Mediterranean k.
kaladana
kalagua
kalemia
kaligenous
kalimeter
Kalischer disease
kaliuresis
kaliuretic
kallidin
Kallikak family
kallikrein
        plasma k.
        tissue k.

kallikreinogen
Kallmann syndrome
Kalt
    forceps
    needle holder
    suture
Kammerer incision
Kammerer-Battle incision
Kanavel
    apparatus
    brain-exploring cannula
    canal
    conductor
    line
    sign
    splint
    triangle
Kandori flock retina
Kane clamp
kangaroo tendon suture
Kanner syndrome
Kantor
    clamp
    sign
Kantrowitz clamp
kaolinosis
kaolin pneumoconiosis
Kapel operation
Kapeller-Adler test
Kaplan
    needle
    test
Kaplan-Meier
    method
    survival curve
Kaposi
    disease
    sarcoma
    varicelliform eruption
    xeroderma
kappa
    Greek letter (κ; alphabetized
        as k)
    k. angle
Kapp-Beck clamp
kara-kurt
karaya gum
Karell
    diet
    treatment
Karman catheter
Karnofsky
    rating scale
    status
    tumor grading

Karplus sign
Karroo syndrome
Kartagener
    disease
    syndrome
    triad
karyapsis
karyochrome
karyogamic
karyogamy
karyogenesis
karyogenic
karyokinesis
    asymmetrical k.
    hyperchromatic k.
    hypochromatic k.
karyokinetic
karyoklasis
karyoklastic
karyolobic
karyolobism
karyology
karyolymph
karyolysis
karyolytic
karyomastigont
karyomegaly
karyomere
karyometry
karyomicrosome
karyomitosis
karyomitotic
karyomorphism
karyon
karyonide
karyophage
karyoplasm
karyoplasmic
karyoplast
karyoplastin
karyopyknosis
karyopyknotic
karyoreticulum
karyorrhectic
karyorrhexis
karyosome
karyostasis
karyotheca
karyotype
karyotypic
karyozoic
Kasabach-Merritt syndrome
Kasai operation
kasal
Kashin-Bek (Kaschin-Beck) disease

Kast syndrome
kat—katal
katachromasis
katadidymus
katal per liter (kat/L)
katathermometer
Katayama
    disease
    fever
    syndrome
    test
katharometer
kathisophobia
katine
Katz formula
katzenjammer
Katzin scissors
Katzin-Barraquer forceps
Katz-Wachtel phenomenon
KAU—King-Armstrong
    units
Kaufman
    pneumonia
    vitrector
kava
kavaism
Kawasaki
    disease
    syndrome
Kay annuloplasty
Kay-Shiley prosthesis
Kazanjian
    forceps
    line
    operation
    splint
Kazanjian and Converse line
Kaznelson syndrome
kb—kilobase
KB—ketone body
K_b—base dissociation
    constant
KBr—potassium bromide
kc—kilocycle
Kcal, kcal, Cal—kilocalorie
K-capture
KCG—kinetocardiogram
kCi—kilocurie(s)
KCl—potassium chloride
kcps—kilocycles per second
KCT—kathodal closure
    tetanus
K_d—dissociation constant
KE—kinetic energy
Kearns-Sayre syndrome

keel
    McNaught k.
    k. operation
Keeley stripper
Keen
    operation
    sign
Kegel exercises
Kehr
    incision
    sign
Kehrer reflex
Kehrer-Adie syndrome
Keith
    bundle
    low-ionic diet
    needle
    node
Keith-Flack node
Keith-Wagener (K-W) classification
    (1–4)
Keith-Wagener-Barker
    classification (groups 1–4)
kelectome
Kell
    blood antibody type
    blood group
Keller
    arthroplasty
    bunionectomy
    hypothesis
    operation
    ultraviolet test
Keller-Blake splint
Kelling gastroscope
Kellogg-Speed operation
Kelly
    clamp
    curet
    cystoscope
    dilator
    endoscope
    forceps
    hook
    operation
    proctoscope
    retractor
    scissors
    sigmoidoscope
    sign
    speculum
    sphincteroscope
    suture
    tube
Kelly-Gray curet

K

Kelly-Stoeckel operation
Kelman
    forceps
    lens
    operation
keloid
    acne k's
    Addison k.
    Alibert k.
    k. of gums
kelosomus
kelotomy
kelp
Kelvin
    scale
    thermometer
Kempner diet
Kendall
    method
    rank correlation coefficient
    tau
Kennedy
    bar
    classification
    disease
    forceps
    operation
    syndrome
Kenny-Caffey syndrome
kenophobia
kenotoxin
Kent bundle
Kent-His bundle
K_{eq}—equilibrium constant
Kerandel
    sign
    symptom
kerasin
keratalgia
keratansulfaturia
keratectasia
keratectomy
keratic precipitates
keratin
    α-k. [alpha-]
    false k.
    hard k.
    soft k.
keratinase
keratinization
keratinize
keratinized
keratinocyte
keratinoid

keratinosome
keratinous
keratitic
keratitis
    Acanthamoeba k.
    acne rosacea k.
    actinic k.
    aerosol k.
    alphabet k.
    amebic k.
    anaphylactic k.
    annular k.
    arborescens k.
    artificial silk k.
    aspergillus k.
    band k.
    k. bandelette
    band-shaped k.
    k. bullosa
    catarrhal ulcerative k.
    deep k.
    deep pustular k.
    dendriform k.
    dendritic k.
    desiccation k.
    Dimmer k.
    disciform k.
    k. disciformis
    epithelial k.
    epithelial diffuse k.
    epithelial punctate k.
    exfoliative k.
    exposure k.
    fascicular k.
    k. filamentosa
    Fuchs k.
    furrow k.
    herpetic k.
    hypopyon k.
    infectious bovine k.
    interstitial k.
    lagophthalmic k.
    lattice k.
    marginal k.
    metaherpetic k.
    microbial k.
    mycotic k.
    necrogranulomatous k.
    neuroparalytic k.
    neurotrophic k.
    k. nummularis
    oyster shucker's k.
    parenchymatous k.
    k. petrificans

keratitis *(continued)*
  phlyctenular k.
  k. profunda
  k. punctata
  k. punctata leprosa
  k. punctata profunda
  k. punctata subepithelialis
  punctate k., deep
  punctate k., superficial
  purulent k.
  k. pustuliformis profunda
  k. ramificata
    superficialis
  reapers' k.
  reticular k.
  ribbon-like k.
  rosacea k.
  Schmidt k.
  sclerosing k.
  scrofulous k.
  secondary k.
  senile guttate k.
  serpiginous k.
  k. sicca
  striate k.
  stromal k.
  superficial punctate k.
  suppurative k.
  syphilitic k.
  Thygeson k.
  trachomatous k.
  trophic k.
  vascular k.
  vesicular k.
  xerotic k.
  zonular k.
keratoangioma
keratocele
keratocentesis
keratoconjunctivitis
  epidemic k.
  epizootic k.
  flash k.
  limbic k.
  phlyctenular k.
  shipyard k.
  k. sicca
  superior limbic k.
  vernal k.
  viral k.
  welder's k.
keratoconus
keratocyst
keratocyte

keratoderma
  k. blennorrhagica
  k. blennorrhagicum
  k. climactericum
  diffuse palmoplantar k.
  k. palmare et
    plantare
  palmoplantar k.
  plantar k.
  punctate k.
  symmetric k.
keratoectasia
keratogenesis
keratogenetic
keratogenous
keratoglobus
keratohelcosis
keratohemia
keratohyalin
keratohyaline
keratoid
keratoiridocyclitis
keratoiridoscope
keratoiritis
  hypopyon k.
keratoleptynsis
keratoleukoma
keratolysis
  k. exfoliativa
  k. neonatorum
  pitted k.
  k. plantare sulcatum
keratolytic
keratoma
  k. diffusum
  k. hereditaria mutilans
  k. hereditarium mutilans
  k. malignum congenitale
  k. palmare et plantare
  k. plantare sulcatum
  k. senile
keratomalacia
keratomata
keratome
  Agnew k.
  Beaver k.
  Berens k.
  Castroviejo k.
  Grieshaber k.
  Jaeger k.
  Kirby k.
keratometer
keratometric
keratometry

K

keratomileusis
  laser-assisted in situ k. (LASIK)
  laser-assisted intrastromal k. (LASIK)
keratomycosis linguae
keratonosus
keratonyxis
keratopathy
  band k.
  band-shaped k.
  bullous k.
  climatic k.
  exposure k.
  filamentary k.
  Labrador k.
  lipid k.
  striate k.
  vesicular k.
keratophakia
keratoplasty
  autogenous k.
  Barraquer k. knife
  Hippel (von Hippel) k.
  lamellar k. (LKP)
  optic k.
  penetrating k. (PKP)
  refractive k.
  tectonic k.
keratoprecipitates
keratoprotein
keratorrhexis
keratoscleritis
keratoscope
keratoscopy
keratosis (keratoses)
  actinic k.
  arsenic k.
  arsenical k.
  aural k.
  k. blennorrhagica
  k. diffusa fetalis
  k. follicularis
  k. follicularis contagiosa
  k. follicularis decalvans
  gonorrheal k.
  inverted follicular k.
  k. labialis
  lichenoid k.
  lichen planus–like k.
  k. linguae
  nevoid k.
  k. nigricans
  k. obliterans
  k. obturans

keratosis (keratoses) *(continued)*
  k. palmaris et plantaris
  k. pharyngea
  k. pilaris
  k. pilaris atrophicans
  k. pilaris atrophicans faciei
  k. pilaris rubra
  k. punctata
  roentgen k.
  k. rubra figurata
  seborrheic k.
  k. seborrheica
  senile k.
  k. senilis
  solar k.
  stucco k.
  k. suprafollicularis
  tar k.
  k. universalis congenita
  k. vegetans
  wax k.
keratosulfate
keratosulfaturia
keratotic
keratotomy
  delimiting k.
  radial k. (RK)
keratotorus
Kerckring (Kerkring)
  center
  folds
  ossicle
kerectasis
kerectomy
Kergaradec sign
kerion
  k. celsi
  Celsus k.
Kerley
  A lines
  B lines
kerma
Kern forceps
kernicterus
Kernig sign
keroid
kerosene
Kerr
  cesarean section
  sign
Kerrison
  forceps
  punch
  retractor
  rongeur

Keshan disease
Kesling
    appliance
    spring
Kessel plate
Kessler operation
Kestenbach-Anderson procedure
Kestenbaum
    procedure
    role
ketene
kethoxal
ketimine
keto acid
keto acid decarboxylase
keto acid decarboxylase deficiency
ketoacidemia
    branched-chain k.
ketoacidosis
    diabetic k.
ketoaciduria
    branched-chain k.
3-ketoacyl-CoA thiolase
keto-aldehyde
ketoaminoacidemia
ketodeoxyoctonate
Keto-Diastix
ketogenesis
ketogenetic
ketogenic
2-ketogluconate
α-ketoglutaric acid [alpha-]
ketoheptose
ketohexokinase
ketohexose
ketohydroxyestrin
ketol
ketol-isomerase
ketolysis
ketolytic
ketone
    dimethyl k.
ketone bodies
ketonemia
ketonic
ketonization
ketonuria
ketoplasia
ketoplastic
ketose
ketoside
ketosis
17-ketosteroid
ketosuria
keto-tetrahydrophenanthrene

ketotetrose
3-ketothiolase
3-ketothiolase deficiency
ketotic
ketotifen
ketotransferase
ketourine
ketoxime
keV, kev—kilo electron volts
Kevorkian curet
key
    determinative k.
    torquing k.
Key operation
Keyes
    biopsy punch
    dermal punch
    lithotrite
keynote
Key-Retzius
    connective tissue sheath
    foramen
keyway
Kezerian osteotome
KFAB—kidney-fixing antibody
kg—kilogram(s)
kg-cal—kilogram-calorie
KGS—ketogenic steroid
khellin
kHz—kilohertz
kick
    atrial k.
    k. counts
Kidd
    blood antibody type
    blood group
Kidde tubal insufflator
Kidner operation
kidney
    abdominal k.
    amyloid k.
    arteriosclerotic k.
    artificial k.
    atrophic k.
    cake k.
    cicatricial k.
    cirrhotic k.
    clump k.
    coarsely granular k.
    congenital double k.
    congested k.
    contracted k.
    crush k.
    cyanotic k.
    cystic k.

K

kidney *(continued)*
    definite k.
    definitive k.
    disk k.
    doughnut k.
    dump k.
    dystopic k.
    ectopic k.
    fatty k.
    finely granular k.
    flea-bitten k.
    floating k.
    Formad k.
    fused k.
    Goldblatt k.
    gouty k.
    granular k.
    head k.
    hind k.
    horseshoe k.
    hypermobile k.
    hypoplastic k.
    infarcted k.
    k. internal splint/stent (KISS)
      catheter
    lardaceous k.
    large red k.
    large white k.
    lumbar k.
    lump k.
    medullary sponge k.
    middle k.
    monopyramidal k.
    mortar k.
    movable k.
    multilobar k.
    mural k.
    myelin k.
    myeloma k.
    palpable k.
    pelvic k.
    polycystic k.
    primitive k.
    primordial k.
    k. punch
    putty k.
    Rokitansky k.
    Rose-Bradford k.
    sacciform k.
    sclerotic k.
    sigmoid k.
    single k.
    soapy k.
    solitary k.
    sponge k.

kidney *(continued)*
    k. stone
    sulfa k.
    supernumerary k.
    thoracic k.
    unilateral fused k.
    unilobar k.
    wandering k.
    washout k.
    waxy k.
Kiel classification
Kielland (Kjelland) forceps
Kielland-Luikart forceps
Kienböck
    disease
    dislocation
    phenomenon
    unit
Kienböck-Adamson points
kieselguhr
Kiesselbach
    area
    plexus
    space
Kilian line
killeen
Killian
    chisel
    elevator
    forceps
    knife
    nasal speculum
    operation
    rectal speculum
    triangle
    tube
Killian-Freer operation
Killian-King retractor
Kilner operation
kilobase
kilobecquerel (kBq)
kilocalorie (kcal, Cal)
kilocurie(s) (kCi)
kilocycle
kilogram (kg)
kilogram-calorie
kilogram-force (kgf)
kilohertz (kHz)
kilohm
Kiloh-Nevin
    myopathy
    syndrome
kilometer
kilopascal (kPa)
kilopond (kp)

kilounit
kilovolt (kV)
kilovoltage
kilovolts peak (kVp)
Kimball hook
Kimmelstiel-Wilson
    disease
    lesion
    nodule
    syndrome
kinanesthesia
kindling
kinematics
kinemia
kinemic
kineplasty
kinesalgia
kinescope
kinesia
    paradoxical k.
kinesiatrics
kinesics
kinesigenic
kinesimeter
kinesiology
kinesioneurosis
kinesis
kinesitherapy
kinesodic
kinesthesia
kinesthesiometer
kinesthetic
kinetia
kinetic
    k. energy
    k. perimetry
kinetics
    cell population k.
    chemical k.
    first-order k.
    Michaelis k.
    pre–steady-state k.
kinetin
kinetism
kinetocardiogram (KCG)
kinetocardiography
kinetochore
kinetodesma
kinetodesmata
kinetodesmos
kinetofragment
kinetogenic
kinetographic
kinetography
kinetonucleus

kinetoplasm
kinetoplast
kinetoplastid
kinetoscope
kinetoscopy
kinetosis
kinetosome
King
    operation
    retractor
    unit
King-Armstrong unit
kingdom
Kingella
    K. denitrificans
    K. indologenes
    K. kingae
King-Richards operation
Kingsley
    appliance
    plate
    splint
kinic acid
kinin
    C2 k.
    venom k.
    wasp k.
kininase
    k. I
    k. II
kininogen
kininogenase
kink
kinky hair disease
Kinnier Wilson disease
kinocentrum
kinocilia
kinohapt
kinomere
kinomometer
Kinsbourne syndrome
Kinsella-Buie clamp
kinship
Kinyoun stain
kiotome
kiotomy
Kirby
    forceps
    hook
    keratome
    knife
    operation
    retractor
    scissors
    spoon

K

Kirby *(continued)*
  suture
Kirk amputation
Kirkland
  disease
  knife
Kirschner
  apparatus
  splint
  suture
  wire
  wire splint
KISS—kidney internal splint/stent
  (catheter)
kissing-balloon technique
kissing choroidals
Kistner tube
kiting
Kitlowski operation
Kittner forceps
KIU—kallikrein-inhibiting unit
kj—
  knee jerk
Kjeldahl
  method; macro-Kjeldahl
    method
  test
Kjelland forceps
kL—kiloliter(s)
Klatskin needle
Klauder syndrome
Klebs disease
Klebsiella
  K. granulomatis
  K. mobilis
  K. oxytoca
  K. ozaenae
  K. planticola
  K. pneumoniae
  K. pneumoniae subsp.
    ozaenae
  K. pneumoniae subsp.
    rhinoscleromatis
  K. rhinoscleromatis
  K. terrigena
Klebs-Löffler bacillus
kleeblattschädel
KleenSpec sigmoidoscope
Kleihauer-Betke test
Kleihauer test
Kleine-Levin syndrome
Kleist
  classification
  phenomenon
  sign

Klemm
  sign
  tetanus
Klemme retractor
Klemperer disease
kleptolagnia
kleptomania
kleptomaniac
kleptophobia
Klestadt cyst
KLH—keyhole limpet hemocyanin
Klieg eye
Kligler agar
Klinefelter syndrome
Kline flocculation test
Klippel disease
Klippel-Feil
  malformation
  sign
  syndrome
Klippel-Feldstein syndrome
Klippel-Trénaunay syndrome
Klippel-Trénaunay-Weber
  syndrome
klismaphilia
Kloehn headgear
Kloepfer syndrome
Klotz syndrome
KLS—kidneys, liver, spleen
Kluge
  method
  sign
Klumpke
  palsy
  paralysis
Klumpke-Dejerine
  paralysis
  syndrome
KM—kanamycin
km—kilometer(s)
K_M—Michaelis constant
KMnO—potassium permanganate
KMV—killed measles virus vaccine
Knapp
  forceps
  knife
  needle
  operation
  procedure
  retractor
  rule
  scissors
  scoop
  spatula
  speculum

Knapp *(continued)*
    spoon
    streaks
    striae
    test
Knaus rule
kneading
knee
    back k.
    beat k.
    Brodie k.
    conventional single-axis k.
      prosthesis
    football k.
    housemaid's k.
    hydraulic k.
    k. of internal capsule
    knock k.
    little k. of fascial canal
    locked k.
    rugby k.
    septic k.
    total k. arthroplasty
    trick k.
    von Willebrandt k.
kneecap
kneippism
Knies sign
Kniest dysplasia
knife
    Adson k.
    Austin k.
    Ayerst k.
    Bailey-Glover-O'Neill k.
    Bailey-Morse k.
    Ballenger swivel k.
    Bard-Parker k.
    Barkan k.
    Barraquer keratoplasty k.
    Beaver k.
    Beck k.
    bladebreaker k.
    Blair-Brown k.
    Blair cleft palate k.
    Blair k.
    Bosher k.
    Brock k.
    Brophy k.
    Brown k.
    Buck k.
    Bucy k.
    button k.
    Caltagirone k.
    Canfield k.
    Carpenter k.

knife *(continued)*
    Castroviejo k.
    cataract k.
    cautery k.
    Colver k.
    Cottle k.
    Crile k.
    Dean k.
    Derlacki k.
    Derra k.
    Desmarres k.
    Douglas k.
    Downing k.
    electric k.
    Elschnig k.
    Ferris-Robb k.
    Fisher k.
    Fleming k.
    Fletcher k.
    Fomon k.
    Freer k.
    Freiberg k.
    Gandhi k.
    Gill k.
    gold k.
    Goldman-Fox k.
    Goodyear k.
    Graefe (von Graefe) k.
    Green k.
    Harrison k.
    House k.
    Hufnagel k.
    Humby k.
    Hyams scleral k.
    Joseph k.
    Killian k.
    Kirby k.
    Kirkland k.
    Knapp k.
    Lancaster k.
    Lebsche k.
    Leland k.
    Lempert k.
    lenticular k.
    Liston k.
    Lothrop k.
    Lynch k.
    MacKenty k.
    Maltz k.
    McHugh k.
    McPherson-Wheeler k.
    McPherson-Ziegler k.
    McReynolds k.
    meniscectomy k.
    Merrifield k.

K

knife *(continued)*
- Niedner k.
- Nunez-Nunez k.
- Pace k.
- Parker k.
- photon k.
- Ramsbotham sickle k.
- Robertson k.
- Rochester k.
- Rosen k.
- Scheie k.
- Schuknecht k.
- Seiler k.
- Sellor k.
- Sexton k.
- Shambaugh-Lempert k.
- Shea k.
- Sheehy k.
- Smillie k.
- Smith-Green k.
- Thiersch k.
- Tobold k.
- Tooke k.
- Tydings k.
- Virchow k.
- Weber k.
- Wheeler k.
- Wullstein k.
- Ziegler k.

knife needle
- Davis k.n.

Knight
- brace
- forceps
- scissors

Knight-Sluder
- forceps

Knight-Taylor brace
knismogenic
knitted vascular
- prosthesis

knitting
knob
- aortic k.
- basal k.
- embryonic k.
- surfers' k's
- synaptic k.

knock
- pericardial k.

knock-knee, knock-kneed
knot
- clove-hitch k.
- double k.
- enamel k.

knot *(continued)*
- false k.
- friction k.
- granny k.
- half-hitch k.
- Hensen k.
- primitive k.
- protochordal k.
- reef k.
- square k.
- stay k.
- surfers' k's
- surgeons' k.
- surgical k.
- syncytial k's
- true k.

Knowles
- pin
- scissors

knuckle
- aortic k.
- cervical aortic k.

knuckling
Kobelt
- tubes
- tubules

Köbner (Koebner)
- disease
- effect
- phenomenon

Koby cataract
KOC—kathodal
  (cathodal) opening
  contraction

Koch
- bacillus
- law
- lymph node
- node
- phenomenon
- postulate
- reaction
- reservoir
- triangle
- tuberculin

Kocher
- clamp
- dissector
- forceps
- incision
- line
- maneuver
- operation
- reflex
- retractor

Kocher *(continued)*
   sign
   ulcer
Kocher-Crotti retractor
Kocher-Debré-Sémélaigne
   syndrome
kocherization
kocherized
Koch-Weeks
   bacillus
   conjunctivitis
   hemophilus
Kock
   ileostomy
   pouch
   reservoir
Koeberlé forceps
Koebner phenomenon
Koenecke
   reaction
   test
Koeppe
   disease
   nodule
Koerber-Salus-Elschnig
   syndrome
Koffler forceps
Koffler-Lillie forceps
Kogoj spongiform pustule
Köhler bone disease
Köhler-Pellegrini-Stieda disease
Kohlmeier-Degos disease
Kohlrausch
   folds
   valves
Kohn pores
Kohnstamm phenomenon
koilocytosis
koilocytotic
koilonychia
koilorrhachic
koilosternia
koinonia
kojic acid
koktigen
Kolb forceps
Kölliker
   column
   granule
   membrane
   nucleus
Kollmann dilator
Kolmer test
Kolmogorov-Smirnov test
Kolodny hemostat

Kondoleon operation
König (Koenig)
   disease
   graft
   operation
   rods
   syndrome
koniocortex
koniology (coniology)
konometer
kophemia
Koplik
   sign
   spots
   stigma
koprosterin
Koranyi
   auscultation
   percussion
   sign
   treatment
Koranyi-Grocco triangle
Korean hemorrhagic
   nephrosonephritis
koro
koroscopy
Korotkoff
   method
   sounds
   test
Korsakoff (Korsakov)
   amnesia
   disease
   psychosis
   syndrome
Kos cannula
kosam
Koshevnikoff
   disease
   epilepsy
Kossel test
Kostmann
   disease
   syndrome
koumiss
Kovalevsky canal
Kozlowski degeneration
KP—
   keratitic precipitates
   keratitis punctata
KPTT—kaolin partial
   thromboplastin time
Krabbe
   disease
   hypoplasia

K

Krabbe *(continued)*
    leukodystrophy
    sclerosis
    syndrome
K radiation
Kraepelin classification
krait
Kramer speculum
Kraske
    operation
    position
kratom
kratometer
Kratz lens
kraurosis
    penile k.
    k. penis
    k. vulvae
    vulvar k.
Krause
    end bulbs
    cannula
    corpuscle
    forceps
    glands
    graft
    ligament
    line
    membrane
    operation
    snare
    suture
    syndrome
    valve
    ventricle
Krause-Wolfe
    graft
    operation
KRB—Krebs-Ringer bicarbonate
  buffer
krebiozen
Krebs
    cycle
    leukocyte index
kreotoxin
kreotoxism
kresofuchsin
Kretschmer types
Krimer operation
Krimsky method
Krishaber disease
Kristeller
    expression
    method
    technique
Kristiansen screw

Krogh
    apparatus
    spirometer
Kromayer
    burn
    lamp
Krompecher
    carcinoma
    tumor
Kron
    bile duct probe
    dilator
Kronecker
    center
    needle
    puncture
Kronfeld
    electrode
    forceps
    retractor
Krönig (Kronig, Kroenig)
    isthmus
    steps
    technique
Krönlein
    hernia
    operation
Krönlein-Berke operation
KRP—Krebs-Ringer
  phosphate
Krukenberg
    arm
    hand
    spindle
    tumor
    veins
Krumwiede agar
Krupin valve
Kruse brush
krypton Kr 85
KS—
    ketosteroid
    Kveim-Siltzbach (test)
KSC—kathodal (cathodal) closing
  contraction
K-shell
K_{sp}—solubility product constant
KST—kathodal closing tetanus
KU—Karmen units
KUB—kidney, ureter, bladder (x-ray)
kubisagari
Kufs disease
Kugelberg-Welander disease
Kuhn tube
Kuhne
    methylene blue

Kuhne *(continued)*
  muscular phenomenon
  spindle
  terminal plates
Kuhnt
  forceps
  illusion
  operation
Kuhnt-Szymanowski
  operation
  procedure
Kulchitsky carcinoid
Kulenkampff anesthesia
Kulvin-Kalt forceps
Külz
  cast
  cylinder
  test
Kümmell
  disease
  spondylitis
Kümmell-Verneuil disease
Kunkel syndrome
Küntscher
  driver
  nail
  reamer
Kupperman test
kupramite
Kurie plot
Kurten stripper
Kurthia zopfii
kurtosis
Kurtzke score
kuru
Kurzbauer position
Kushner-Tandatnick curet
Küss experiment
Kussmaul
  aphasia
  breathing
  disease
  paralysis
  pulse
  respiration
  sign
  symptom
Kussmaul-Kien respiration
Kussmaul-Landry paralysis
Kussmaul-Maier disease
Küstner
  incision
  law
  operation
  sign
kuttarosome

KV—
  kanamycin and
    vancomycin
  killed vaccine
  kilovolt
Kveim
  antigen
  reaction
  test
KVO—keep vein open (IV line)
kVp—kilovolts peak
kW—kilowatt(s)
KW—
  Keith-Wagener (classification,
    retinopathy)
  Kimmelstiel-Wilson (disease,
    syndrome)
  Kugelberg-Welander
    (syndrome)
K_W—the ion product of water
kwashiorkor
  marasmic k.
KWB—Keith, Wagener, Barker
  (classification, groups 1–4)
kW-hr—kilowatt-hour
Kyasanur Forest
  disease
  virus
Kydex body jacket
Kyle speculum
kymogram
kymograph
  x-ray k.
kymography
  roentgen k. (RKY)
kynocephalus
kynureninase
kynurenine
kynurenic acid
  k. 3-hydroxylase
  k. 3-monooxygenase
kyphectomy
kyphorachitis
kyphos
kyphoscoliosis
kyphosis
  angular k.
  dorsal k.
  k. dorsalis juvenilis
  juvenile k.
  post-traumatic k.
  Scheuermann k.
  Scheuermann juvenile k.
kyphotic
Kyrle disease
kyrtorrhachic

K

L

λ—lambda (Greek letter)
l-—levorotatory
L—
    lambert
    Latin
    left
    length
    leucine
    ligament
    light chain
    light sense
    liter(s)
    low
    lower
    lumbar vertebra
    lung
L.—
    Lactobacillus
    Leishmania
L1 through L5—lumbar
  vertebrae 1–5
LA—
    lactic acid
    latex agglutination (test)
    left arm
    left atrial
    left atrium
    linguoaxial
    local anesthesia
    low anxiety
L&A—light and accommodation
lab—laboratory
Labbé
    neurocirculatory syndrome
    syndrome
    triangle
    vein
label
    radioactive l.
labeling
    affinity l.
    ferritin l.
    isotope l.
    peroxidase l.
    pulse l.
    spin l.
la belle indifférence
labia (plural of labium)
labial
labialism
labially
labile
    l. affect
    l. blood pressure
    l. mood

lability
    affective l.
    autonomic l.
    cardiac repolarization l.
    emotional l.
    increased l.
    marked l.
    mood l.
labioalveolar
labioaxiogingival
labiocervical
labiochorea
labioclination
labiodental
labiogingival
labioglossolaryngeal
labioglossopharyngeal
labioincisal
labiolingual
labiomental
labiomycosis
labionasal
labiopalatine
labioplacement
labiotenaculum
labioversion
labium (labia)
    l. anterius ostii uteri
    l. cerebri
    l. externum cristae iliacae
    l. inferius oris
    l. internum cristae iliacae
    l. laterale lineae asperae
      femoris
    l. laterale sulci
      intertubercularis
    l. limbi tympanicum
    l. limbi vestibulare
    labia majora
    l. majus pudendi
    l. mandibulare
    l. maxillare
    l. medialis lineae asperae
      femoris
    labia minora
    l. minus pudendi
    labia oris
    l. posterius ostii uteri
    l. superius oris
    l. urethrae
    l. vestibulare laminae spiralis
    l. vocale
labor
    active l.
    arrested l.

labor *(continued)*
    artificial l.
    atonic l.
    complicated l.
    delayed l.
    desultory l.
    dry l.
    dyskinetic l.
    false l.
    habitual l.
    habitual premature l.
    immature l.
    induced l.
    inert l.
    instrumental l.
    mimetic l.
    missed l.
    multiple l.
    obstructed l.
    postmature l.
    postponed l.
    precipitate l.
    premature l.
    prodromal l.
    prolonged l.
    protracted l.
    spontaneous l.
    spurious l.
    stages of l.
    trial of l.
laboratory
    clinical l.
Laborde
    dilator
    forceps
    method
    sign
    test
labored breathing
laborious
    l. detail
    l. workup
labrale
    l. inferius
    l. superius
labrum (labra)
    l. acetabulare
    l. articulare
    l. glenoidale articulationis
      coxae
    l. glenoidale articulationis
      humeri
    l. ileocaecalis ostii ilealis
    l. ileocolicum ostii ilealis
    l. inferius ostii ilealis
    l. superius ostii ilealis

labyrinth
    acoustic l.
    bony l.
    cochlear l.
    cortical l.
    endolymphatic l.
    l. of ethmoid
    ethmoidal l.
    Ludwig l's
    membranous l.
    nonacoustic l.
    olfactory l.
    osseous l.
    perilymphatic l.
    posterior l.
    vestibular l.
    l. of vestibule
    vestibulocochlear l.
labyrinthectomy
    membranous l.
    transtympanic l.
    ultrasonic l.
labyrinthi (genitive and plural of
    labyrinthus)
labyrinthine nystagmus
labyrinthitis
    circumscribed l.
    serous l.
    suppurative l.
    traumatic l.
labyrinthotomy
labyrinthus (labyrinthi)
    l. cochlearis
    l. corticis
    l. ethmoidalis
    l. membranaceus
    l. osseus
    l. vestibularis
lac.—laceration
lac (lacta)
    l. femininum
lacelike
lacerable
lacerate, lacerated
laceration
    brain l.
    dicing l.
    fishmouth l.
    perianal l.
    l. of the perineum
lacertus
    l. cordis
    l. fibrosus musculi bicipitis
      brachii
    l. medius Weitbrechtii
    l. medius Wrisbergii

L

lacertus *(continued)*
    l. musculi recti lateralis bulbi
lace suture
Lacey rotating-hinge arthroplasty
Lachman test
lacquer cracks
lacrimal
    l. apparatus
    l. artery
    l. bone
    l. canaliculi
    l. duct
    l. gland
    l. lake
    l. nerve
    l. papilla
    l. probe
    l. sac
lacrimation
lacrimator
lacrimatory
lacrimoconchal suture
lacrimoethmoidal suture
lacrimomaxillary suture
lacrimonasal duct
lacrimotome
lacrimotomy
lacrimoturbinal suture
lacta (plural of lac)
lactacidemia
lactaciduria
lactalbumin
β-lactam antibiotic
    [beta-]
β-lactamase [beta-]
lactamide
lactase deficiency
lactate
L-lactate dehydrogenase (LDH)
lactation
lactational
lacteal
    central l.
    l. vessel
lactenin
lactescence
lactescent
lactic
    l. acid
    l. acidosis
    l. acidemia
lactiferous
lactim
lactinated
lactivorous

Lactobacillus (lactobacilli)
    L. acidophilus
    L. bifidus
    L. bulgaricus
    L. salivarius
lactobezoar
lactoferrin
lactogen
    human placental l. (hPL)
lactoglobulin
γ-lactone [gamma-]
lactone
lactoprotein
lactose
    anhydrous l.
    β-lactose [beta-]
    l. intolerance
    l. synthase
lactoside
lactosuria
lactosylceramide
lactotoxin
lactotroph
lactotrophin, lactotropin
lactovegetarian
lactovegetarianism
lactoylglutathione lyase
lactulose
lacuna (lacunae)
    absorption l.
    bone l.
    cartilage l.
    cerebral lacunae
    great l. of urethra
    Howship l.
    intervillous l.
    lacunae laterales
    l. magna
    l. of muscles, l. musculorum
    osseous l.
    parasinusoidal lacunae
    l. pharyngis
    resorption l.
    tonsillar l.
    lacunae of urethra, urethral
        lacunae
    lacunae urethrales
    vascular l.
    l. of vessels
lacunar infarct
lacunule
lacus lacrimalis
LAD—
    left anterior descending
        (coronary artery)

LAD— *(continued)*
 leukocyte adhesion deficiency
LADA—left anterior descending
 artery
Ladd calipers
Ladd-Franklin theory
laden
Ladendorff test
Ladin sign
LAE—left atrial enlargement
Laënnec
 catarrh
 cirrhosis
 disease
 pearls
 sign
laeve
 chorion l.
LAF—
 laminar air flow
 lymphocyte-activating factor
Lafora
 bodies
 disease
 epilepsy
 sign
LaForce
 adenotome
 spud
 tonsillectome
LaForce-Grieshaber adenotome
lag
 anaphase l.
 eyelid l.
 globe l.
 lid l.
 nitrogen l.
 phenomic l.
 phenotypic l.
LAG—
 labiogingival
 lymphangiogram
lageniform
lagophthalmos
Lagrange
 operation
 scissors
LAH—
 left anterior hemiblock
 left atrial hypertrophy
Lahey
 carrier
 clamp
 forceps
 operation

Lahey *(continued)*
 retractor
 tenaculum
Lahey-Péan forceps
LAI—labioincisal
Laing plate
laiose
Laird-McMahon anorectoplasty
LAIT—latex agglutination-
 inhibition test
lake
 capillary l.
 lacrimal l.
 marginal l's
 subchorial l.
 venous l.
Laki-Lorand factor
LAL—limulus amebocyte lysate
lallation
Lallemand bodies
Lallemand-Trousseau bodies
lalognosis
lalopathy
lalophobia
Lalouette pyramid
Lamaze method
lambda
 Greek letter (λ; alphabetized
  as l)
 l. bacteriophage
lambdacism
lambdoid, lambdoidal
 l. suture
Lambert forceps
Lambert-Eaton myasthenic
 syndrome
Lambotte
 clamp
 forceps
 osteotome
Lambotte-Henderson osteotome
Lambrinudi operation
lame
lame foliacée
lamella (lamellae)
 annulate lamellae
 articular l.
 basic l.
 circumferential l.
 concentric l.
 cornoid l.
 elastic l.
 enamel lamellae
 endosteal l.
 ground l.

L

lamella (lamellae) *(continued)*
    haversian l.
    intermediate l.
    interstitial l.
    osseous l.
    periosteal l.
    peripheral l.
    posterior border l. of Fuchs
    triangular l.
    vitreous l.
lamellar
    l. exfoliation
    l. granules
    l. ichthyosis
    l. incision
    l. keratoplasty (LKP)
lamelliform
lamina (laminae)
    l. affixa
    alar l.
    l. alaris
    laminae albae cerebelli
    anterior limiting l.
    l. anterior vaginae musculi
      recti abdominis
    l. arcus vertebrae
    basal l.
    basal l. of ciliary body
    basal l. of choroid
    l. basalis
    l. basalis choroideae
    l. basalis corporis ciliaris
    basement l.
    l. basilaris ductus cochlearis
    bony spiral l.
    Bowman l.
    l. cartilaginis cricoideae
    l. cartilaginis lateralis tubae
      auditivae
    l. cartilaginis medialis tubae
      auditivae
    l. cartilaginis thyroideae
      dextra/sinistra
    l. choroidocapillaris
    cribriform l. of ethmoid bone
    cribriform l. of transverse
      fascia
    l. cribrosa ossis ethmoidalis
    l. cribrosa sclerae
    l. of cricoid cartilage
    l. densa
    dental l., l. dentalis
    l. dentata
    dentogingival l.
    l. dots

lamina (laminae) *(continued)*
    l. dura
    l. elastica anterior (Bowmani)
    l. elastica posterior (Demoursi)
    elastic l., external
    elastic l., internal
    episcleral l., l. episcleralis
    epithelial l., l. epithelialis
    l. externa calvariae
    l. externa cranii, l. externa
      ossium cranii
    external l. of peritoneum
    external l. of pterygoid process
    l. fibrocartilaginea interpubica
    l. fibroreticularis
    fibrous nuclear l.
    l. fusca sclerae
    l. granularis externa
    l. granularis interna
    l. horizontalis ossis palatini
    inferior l. of sphenoid bone
    l. interna calvariae
    l. interna cranii, l. interna
      ossium cranii
    internal l. of pterygoid process
    interpubic l., fibrocartilaginous
    labial l.
    labiodental l.
    labiogingival l.
    lateral l. of cartilage of
      auditory tube
    l. lateralis cartilaginis tubae
      auditivae
    l. lateralis processus pterygoidei
    lateral l. of pterygoid process
    l. limitans anterior corneae
    l. limitans posterior corneae
    limiting l., anterior
    limiting l., posterior
    l. lucida
    medial l. of cartilage of
      auditory tube
    l. medialis cartilaginis tubae
      auditivae
    l. medialis processus
      pterygoidei
    medial l. of pterygoid process
    l. medullaris lateralis corporis
      striati
    l. medullaris medialis corporis
      striati
    l. medullaris transversa
      corporis quadrigemini
    medullary l. of corpus
      striatum, external

lamina (laminae) *(continued)*
    medullary l., external
    medullary l., internal
    medullary l. of lentiform
      nucleus
    medullary laminae of thalamus
    l. membranacea tubae
      auditivae
    membranous l. of auditory tube
    l. mesenterii propria
    l. modioli
    l. molecularis
    l. multiformis
    l. muscularis mucosae
    l. muscularis mucosae esophagi
    l. muscularis mucosae gastris
    l. muscularis mucosae
      intestini crassi
    l. muscularis mucosae
      ventriculi
    nuclear l.
    orbital l.
    l. orbitalis ossis ethmoidalis
    palatine l. of maxilla
    l. papyracea
    l. parietalis pericardii serosi
    l. parietalis tunicae vaginalis
      testis
    periclaustral l.
    l. perpendicularis ossis
      ethmoidalis
    l. perpendicularis ossis
      palatini
    l. plexiformis corticis cerebri
    posterior limiting l.
    l. posterior vaginae musculi
      recti abdominis
    l. pretrachealis fasciae
      cervicalis
    l. prevertebralis fasciae
      cervicalis
    l. profunda fasciae temporalis
    l. profunda musculi levatoris
      palpebrae superioris
    proper l. of mesentery
    l. propria membranae
      tympanicae
    l. propria mucosae
    l. pyramidalis
    l. pyramidalis externa
    l. pyramidalis interna
    l. quadrigemina
    l. rara externa
    l. rara interna
    reticular l., l. reticularis

lamina (laminae) *(continued)*
    reticular l. of the cochlea
    reticular l. of the spiral organ
    Rexed laminae
    rostral l., l. rostralis
    l. septi pellucidi
    l. of septum pellucidum
    spinal l., l. spinalis X
    spiral l., bony
    l. spiralis ossea
    l. spiralis secundaria
    spiral l., osseous
    spiral l., secondary
    l. superficialis fasciae cervicalis
    l. superficialis fasciae
      temporalis
    l. superficialis musculi
      levatoris palpebrae
      superioris
    suprachoroid l., l.
      suprachoroidea
    l. supraneuroporica
    l. tectalis mesencephali
    tectal l. of mesencephalon
    l. tecti mesencephali
    l. of tectum of mesencephalon
    terminal l. of hypothalamus
    l. terminalis hypothalami
    l. of thyroid cartilage, right
      and left
    l. tragi, l. tragica
    vascular l. of choroid
    vascular l. of stomach
    l. vasculosa choroideae
    l. of vertebra
    l. of vertebral arch
    l. visceralis pericardii serosi
    l. visceralis tunicae vaginalis
      testis
    l. vitrea, vitreal l., vitreous l.
    white laminae of cerebellum
    zonal l.
    l. zonalis of cerebellum
laminaplasty
laminar
    l. air flow chamber
    l. breach
    l. cortical infarcts
    l. drusen
    l. screws
    l. sheet
Laminaria
laminaria
    l. for cervical ripening
    l. insertion

L

laminaria *(continued)*
    l. tent
laminated
lamination
laminectomy
    Beckman-Adson l. retractor
    cervical l.
    decompressive l.
    lumbar l.
    thoracic l.
L-amino-acid oxidase
laminotomy
Lamont
    elevator
    saw
lamp
    black light fluorescent l.
    diagnostic l.
    Duke-Elder l.
    fluorescent sun l.
    Gullstrand slit l.
    slit l.
    sun l.
    ultraviolet (UV) l.
    Wood l.
lana (lanae)
Lancaster
    knife
    magnet
    operation
    red-green test
    speculum
Lancaster Regan dial
Lancefield classification
lanceolate
Lancereaux-Mathieu disease
Lancereaux nephritis
lancet
    abscess l.
    acne l.
    gingival l.
    gum l.
    spring l.
    thumb l.
Lancet coefficient
lancinating pain
Lancisi
    nerves
    stria
Landau
    reflex
    test
landmark
Landolt
    bodies

Landolt *(continued)*
    chart
    eyelid reconstruction
    operation
Landouzy
    disease
    dystrophy
    purpura
    type
Landouzy-Dejerine
    atrophy
    dystrophy
    type
Landry
    disease
    palsy
    paralysis
    syndrome
Landry-Guillain-Barré
    syndrome
Landsteiner classification
Landzert fossa
Lane
    band
    catheter
    clamp
    disease
    elevator
    forceps
    kink
    mouth gag
    operation
    plate
Langdon Down disease
Lange
    operation
    reaction
    skinfold calipers
    solution
    speculum
    test
Langenbeck (von Langenbeck)
    amputation
    elevator
    flap
    incision
    operation
    saw
    triangle
Langendorff preparation
Langer
    axillary arch
    lines
    muscle
Langer-Giedion syndrome

Langerhans
   cells
   granules
   islands
   islets
Langer-Saldino syndrome
Langhans
   cells
   layer
   stria
Langley
   ganglion
   granules
   nerves
Langmuir trough
Langoria sign
language
Lannelongue foramina
lanolin
Lanterman
   clefts
   incisures
Lanterman-Schmidt incisures
lanthanic
lanthanum (La)
lanthopine
lanuginous
lanugo
Lanz tube
LAO—left anterior oblique
  (projection)
LAP—
   left atrial pressure
   leucine aminopeptidase (test)
   leukocyte alkaline
     phosphatase
lapactic
laparocholecystotomy
laparocolectomy
laparocolostomy
laparocolotomy
laparocystectomy
laparocystotomy
laparoenterostomy
laparoenterotomy
laparogastroscopy
laparogastrostomy
laparogastrotomy
laparohepatotomy
laparohysterectomy
laparohystero-oophorectomy
laparohysterosalpingo-
  oophorectomy
laparohysterotomy
laparoileotomy

laparomonodidymus
laparomyitis
laparomyomectomy
laparomyomyotomy
laparorrhaphy
laparosalpingectomy
laparosalpingo-oophorectomy
laparosalpingostomy
laparosalpingotomy
laparoscope
   ACMI l.
   Eder l.
   Jacobs-Palmer l.
   Lent l.
   Wolf l.
laparoscopic-assisted vaginal
  hysteroscopy (LAVH)
laparoscopy
laparosplenectomy
laparosplenotomy
laparotome
laparotomy
   exploratory l.
   second-look l.
   staging l.
Lapides
   needle holder
   urethropexy
Lapidus
   operation
   osteotomy
lapsus
   l. calami
   l. linguae
   l. memoriae
Laquerriére-Pierquin position
LAR—left arm recumbent
lardaceous
lariat-like
lariat loop knot
larkspur
Larmor
   equation
   frequency
LaRocca tube
Laron
   dwarf
   syndrome
LaRoque
   herniorrhaphy incision
   technique
Larrey
   amputation
   cleft
   ligation

L

Larrey *(continued)*
    operation
    spaces
Larrey-Weil disease
Larry
    rectal director
    rectal probe
Larsen
    disease
    syndrome
Larsen-Johansson disease
larva (larvae)
    l. currens
    cutaneous l. migrans
    ocular l. migrans
    visceral l. migrans
larvaceous
larval
larvate
larvicide
larviparous
laryngalgia
laryngeal
    l. catheterization
    l. stridor
    l. web
laryngectomee
laryngectomy (LG)
    frontolateral partial l.
    lateral partial l.
    supraglottic l.
    total l.
larynges (plural of larynx)
laryngismus
    l. paralyticus
    l. stridulus
laryngitic
laryngitis
    acute spasmodic l.
    atrophic l.
    catarrhal l.
    chronic catarrhal l.
    chronic hyperplastic l.
    chronic nonspecific l.
    croupous l.
    diphtheritic l.
    edematous l.
    membranous l.
    necrotic l.
    phlegmonous l.
    reflux l.
    l. sicca
    simple l.
    l. stridulosa
    subglottic l.

laryngitis *(continued)*
    supraglottic l.
    syphilitic l.
    tuberculous l.
    vestibular l.
laryngocele
    external l.
    internal l.
    ventricular l.
    l. ventricularis
laryngocentesis
laryngofissure
laryngogram
laryngography
    contrast l.
laryngohypopharynx
laryngologist
laryngology
laryngomalacia
laryngometry
laryngoparalysis
laryngopathy
laryngopharyngeal
laryngopharyngectomy
laryngopharyngeus
laryngopharyngitis
laryngopharynx
laryngophony
laryngophthisis
laryngoplasty
laryngoplegia
laryngoptosis
laryngopyocele
laryngorrhagia
laryngorrhaphy
laryngorrhea
laryngoscleroma
laryngoscope
    Albert-Andrews l.
    Atkins-Tucker l.
    Bizzarri-Giuffrida l.
    Broyles l.
    Chevalier Jackson l.
    Clerf l.
    commissure l.
    Dedo l.
    Dedo-Pilling l.
    fiberoptic l.
    Fink l.
    Foregger l.
    Garfield-Holinger l.
    Guedel l.
    Haslinger l.
    Holinger l.
    Jackson l.

laryngoscope *(continued)*
    Jako l.
    Lewy l.
    Lynch l.
    MacIntosh l.
    Magill l.
    Miller l.
    reverse-bevel l.
    Roberts l.
    rotating l.
    Rusch l.
    Sanders l.
    self-retaining l.
    slotted l.
    suspension l.
    Tucker l.
    Welch-Allyn l.
    Wis-Hipple l.
    Yankauer l.
laryngoscopic
laryngoscopist
laryngoscopy
    direct l.
    endoscopic l.
    fiberoptic l.
    indirect l.
    mirror l.
    suspension l.
    video l.
laryngospasm
laryngostat
laryngostenosis
laryngostomy tube
laryngostroboscope
laryngotome
laryngotomy
    inferior l.
    lateral l.
    median l.
    subhyoid l.
    superior l.
    thyrohyoid l.
    l. tube
laryngotracheal
laryngotracheitis
laryngotracheobronchitis
laryngotracheobronchoscopy
laryngotracheoesophageal cleft
  (type I–IV)
laryngotracheoscopy
laryngotracheotomy
larynx
    artificial l.
    supraglottic l.
    l. transplantation

Larzel anemia
Lasègue
    maneuver
    sign
    test
laser
    l. angioplasty
    argon l.
    l. beam
    carbon dioxide (CO_2) l.
    endometrial l. intrauterine
      thermotherapy (ELITT)
    helium-neon (He-Ne) l.
    Hruby l.
    ion l.
    l. iridectomy
    krypton l.
    l. microscope
    Nd:YAG (neodymium:yttrium-
      aluminum-garnet) l.
    l. photocoagulation
    ruby l.
    Sharplan 733 CO_2 [CO2] l.
    l. speckle
    l. trabeculoplasty
    Visulas Nd:YAG l.
    xenon arc l.
Lash
    hysterectomy
    operation
    technique
LASIK—
    laser-assisted in situ
      keratomileusis
    laser-assisted intrastromal
      keratomileusis
Lassa
    fever
    virus
lassitude
Latarjet
    nerve
    vein
latency
    absolute l.
    distal l.
    motor l.
    proximal l.
    reducible l.
    REM (rapid eye movement) l.
    residual l.
    sensory l.
    sleep l.
    terminal l.
    total reflex l.

L

latent
- l. diabetes mellitus
- l. infection
- l. phase
- l.-phase endometrium
- l. phase of labor

laterad
lateral
lateralis
laterality
- crossed l.
- dominant l.
- mixed l.

lateralization
- sound l.

lateritious sediment
lateroabdominal
laterodeviation
lateroduction
lateroflexion
lateroposition
lateropulsion
lateroretrusive
laterotorsion
laterotrusion
lateroversion
latex
- l. allergy
- l. catheter
- l. drain

lathyrism
lathyritic
lathyrogen
lathyrogenic
latissimus dorsi
latitude
Latrobe retractor
latrodectism
Latrodectus mactans
LATS—long-acting thyroid
    stimulator
LATS-p—LATS protector
latter
lattice
- l. degeneration
- space l.

Latzko
- cesarean section
- closure
- operation
- radical hysterectomy

Lauber disease
laudable
laudanosine
laudanine

laudanum
Lauenstein and Hickey projection
Laufe forceps
Laufe-Barton-Kielland forceps
Laufe-Piper forceps
laugh
- canine l.
- sardonic l.

laughter
- compulsive l.
- forced l.
- obsessive l.

Laugier
- hernia
- sign

Laumonier ganglion
Launois syndrome
Launois-Cléret syndrome
Laurence-Biedl syndrome
Laurence-Moon syndrome
Laurence-Moon-Biedl
- law
- syndrome

Laurens operation
laureth 9
lauric acid
Lauth
- canal
- ligament
- sinus
- violet

Lautier test
LAV—lymphadenopathy-associated
    virus
lavage
- bronchoalveolar l. (BAL)
- gastric l.
- intestinal l.
- peritoneal l.
- pleural l.

lavation
Laveran
- bodies
- corpuscles

laveur
law
- Allen's paradoxical l.
- all-or-none l.
- Aran's l.
- Arndt's l., Arndt-Schulz l.
- l's of articulation
- Avogadro's l.
- Bastian's l., Bastian-Bruns l.
- Boyle's l.
- l. of conservation of energy

law *(continued)*
    l. of conservation of mass
    Courvoisier's l.
    Coutard's l.
    Dalton's l.
    Desmarres' l.
    Donders' l.
    Einthoven's l.
    Ewald's l.
    Flatau's l.
    Flourens' l.
    Gerhardt-Semon l.
    Giraud-Teulon l.
    Gullstrand's l.
    Gull-Toynbee l.
    Hanau's l's of articulation
    Hellin-Zeleny l.
    Hering's l.
    l. of inertia
    Jackson's l.
    Kahler's l.
    Knapp's l.
    Küstner's l.
    Laplace's l.
    Listing's l.
    Marey's l.
    Mendel's l's, mendelian l.
    Meyer's l.
    Minot's l.
    l. of multiple proportions
    l. of multiple variants
    Nernst's l.
    Nysten's l.
    Ohm's l.
    Ollier's l.
    Pajot's l.
    Pitres' law
    Pflüger's (Pflueger's) l.
    l. of reciprocity
    l. of referred pain
    l. of refraction
    Rubner's l.
    Sherrington's l.
    l. of similars
    Starling's l., Starling's l. of the
        heart
    Stokes' l.
    Teevan's l.
    Virchow's l.
    Wolff's l.
    Wundt-Lamansky l.
    Yerkes-Dodson l.
Law [eponym]
    position
    views
lawn
    bacterial l.
Lawrence position
Lawrence-Seip syndrome
lawrencium (Lw)
lawsone
Lawson Tait
laxation
laxative
    bulk l.
    bulk-forming l.
laxity
    congenital l. of ligaments
layer
    l. I–VI
    adamantine l.
    anterior elastic l.
    anterior limiting l. of iris
    anterior l. of rectus abdominis
        sheath
    bacillary l.
    basal l. of endometrium
    basal l. of epidermis
    basement l.
    Bowman l.
    Bruch l.
    buffy l.
    cambium l.
    Chievitz l.
    choriocapillary l.
    circular l. of drumhead
    circular l. of eardrum
    circular l. of muscular coat of
        colon
    circular l. of muscular coat of
        rectum
    circular l. of muscular coat of
        small intestine
    circular l. of muscular coat of
        stomach
    circular l. of tympanic
        membrane
    clear l. of epidermis
    columnar l.
    compact l.
    compact l. of endometrium
    cortical l.
    cutaneous l. of tympanic
        membrane
    cuticular l.
    deep l's of cervical fascia, l's of
        deep cervical fascia
    deep l. of triangular ligament
    deep l. of urogenital diaphragm
    dense l.

L

layer *(continued)*
  dermic l.
  Dobie l.
  enamel l., inner and outer
  ependymal l.
  epitrichial l.
  fibrous l. of articular capsule
  Floegel l.
  functional l. of endometrium
  fusiform l. of cerebral cortex
  ganglion cell l.
  ganglionic l. of cerebellum
  ganglionic l. of cerebral cortex
  ganglionic l. of optic nerve
  ganglionic l. of retina
  germinative l. of epidermis
  germinative l. of nail
  granular l. of cerebellum
  granular l. of cerebral cortex,
    external
  granular l. of epidermis
  granular l. of follicle of ovary
  granular l. of Tomes
  gray l. of superior colliculus
  half-value l.
  Haller l.
  Henle fiber l.
  horny l.
  horny l. of epidermis
  horny l. of nail
  Huxley l.
  inferior l. of pelvic diaphragm
  inferior l. of urogenital
    diaphragm
  inner muscular l. of stomach
  investing l. of cervical fascia
  Kaes-Bekhterev l.
  Langhans l.
  lateral cartilaginous l.
  limiting l., internal
  longitudinal l. of muscular
    coat of colon
  longitudinal l. of muscular
    coat of rectum
  longitudinal l. of muscular
    coat of small intestine
  longitudinal l. of muscular
    coat of stomach
  malpighian l.
  mantle l.
  marginal l.
  matching l.
  medial cartilaginous l.
  medullary l's of thalamus,
    internal and external

layer *(continued)*
  membranous l. of perineum
  Meynert l.
  molecular l. of cerebellar
    cortex
  molecular l. of cerebellum
  molecular l. of cerebral cortex
  molecular l., external and
    internal
  molecular l., inner and outer
  molecular l. of olfactory bulb
  mucous l. of epidermis
  mucous l. of tympanic
    membrane
  multiform l. of cerebral cortex
  muscular l.
  nerve fiber l.
  neural l. of retina
  neuroepidermal l.
  Nitabuch l.
  nuclear l. of cerebellum
  nuclear l., external and internal
  nuclear l., inner and outer
  odontoblastic l.
  Ollier l.
  osteogenetic l.
  palisade l.
  Pander l.
  papillary l. of dermis
  parietal l. of pelvic fascia
  parietal l. of tunica vaginalis
    of testis
  perforated l. of sclera
  peripheral l.
  pigmented l. of ciliary body
  pigmented l. of eyeball
  pigmented l. of iris
  pigmented l. of retina
  piriform neuronal l.
  plexiform l. of cerebellum
  plexiform l. of cerebral cortex
  plexiform l., external and
    internal
  plexiform l., inner and outer
  polymorphic l. of cerebral
    cortex
  posterior l. of rectus sheath
  pretracheal l.
  prickle cell l.
  Purkinje cell l.
  pyramidal l. of cerebral cortex,
    external and internal
  radiate l. of tympanic
    membrane
  Rauber l.

layer *(continued)*

    reticular l. of dermis
    l. of rods and cones
    Rohr l.
    Sattler l.
    sclerotogenous l.
    second half-value l.
    somatic l.
    spinous l.
    splanchnic l.
    spongy l.
    spongy l. of endometrium
    subcallosal l.
    subcutaneous l.
    subendocardial l.
    subendothelial l.
    subepicardial l.
    submantle l.
    submucous l. of bladder
    submucous l. of colon
    submucous l. of pharynx
    submucous l. of small intestine
    submucous l. of stomach
    subodontoblastic l.
    subpapillary l.
    subserous l.
    subserous l. of peritoneum
    superficial l. of fascia of
        perineum
    superficial l. of triangular
        ligament
    superficial l. of urogenital
        diaphragm
    superior l. of pelvic diaphragm
    suprachoroid l.
    supragranular l.
    synovial l. of articular capsule
    Tomes granular l.
    trophic l.
    vascular l. of choroid
    vascular l. of testis
    vegetative l.
    vertical l. of ethmoid bone
    vessel l. of iris
    visceral l. of pelvic fascia
    visceral l. of pericardium
    visceral l. of tunica vaginalis
        of testis
    Waldeyer l.
    Weil basal l.
    white l's
    yellow l.
    Zeissel l.
    zonal l. of cerebellum
    zonal l. of cerebral cortex

layer *(continued)*

    zonal l. of quadrigeminal body
    zonal l. of thalamus
lazy
    l. eye
    l. H incision
    l. leukocyte syndrome (LLS)
    l. S incision
    l. Z incision
lb.—pound (L. libra)
LB—
    laboratory data
    live birth(s)
LBB—left bundle branch
LBBB—left bundle branch block
LBCD—left border of cardiac
    dullness
LBI—low serum-bound iron
LBM—lean body mass
LBNP—lower-body negative
    pressure
LBW—low birthweight
LBWI—low-birthweight infant
LBWR—lung-body weight ratio
LC—
    lethal concentration
    living children
LCA—
    left circumflex coronary artery
    left coronary artery
    leukocyte common antigens
LCAT—lecithin–cholesterol
    acyltransferase
LCD—liquor carbonis detergens
LCF, LCx—left circumflex
    (coronary artery)
LCFA—long-chain fatty acid
LCL—
    Levinthal-Coles-Lillie (bodies)
    lymphocytic lymphosarcoma
LCM—
    left costal margin
    lymphocytic choriomeningitis
LCT—long-chain triglyceride
LD—
    left deltoid
    lethal dose
    linguodistal
    living donor
    low dosage
    lymphocyte-defined (antigens)
L-D—Leishman-Donovan (bodies)
LDA—
    left descending artery
    left dorsoanterior (position)

LDD—light-dark discrimination
LDH—lactate dehydrogenase
  (ʟ-lactate dehydrogenase)
LDL—
    loudness discomfort level
    low-density lipoprotein
LDL-C—low-density–lipoprotein
  cholesterol
LDP—left dorsoposterior
LE—
    left eye
    lower extremity
    lupus erythematosus
leaching
lead (Pb)
    black l.
    radioactive l.
lead
    l's I–III
    Accufix l.
    active fixation l.
    anterior precordial l.
    anterolateral l.
    anteroseptal l.
    atrial l.
    augmented bipolar limb l's
    augmented limb l's
      (aV$_F$, aV$_L$, aV$_R$)
    bipolar l.
    bipolar limb l.
    bipolar precordial l.
    chest l.
    deep limb l.
    direct l.
    dual electrode l.
    ECG (electrocardiogram) l.
    EEG (electroencephalogram) l.
    EKG (electrocardiogram) l.
    electroencephalographic l.
    esophageal l.
    Frank XYZ orthogonal l.
    grid l.
    indirect l.
    inferior l.
    inferior precordial l.
    inferolateral l.
    intracardiac l.
    lateral l.
    lateral precordial l.
    left precordial l.
    left-sided l.
    limb l's
    line l.
    multi-electrode l.
    orthogonal Frank XYZ l.

lead (continued)
    pacemaker l., pacing l.
    precordial l's (V$_1$–V$_6$)
    reversed arm l.
    right precordial l. (V$_{3r}$, V$_{4r}$, etc.)
    right-sided chest l.
    right-sided EEG l.
    semidirect l.
    sphenoid fossa l.
    standard (bipolar) l's (I, II, III)
    sternal l.
    unipolar l.
    unipolar limb l.
    unipolar precordial l.
    V l's (V$_1$–V$_6$)
    ventricular l.
    white EEG l.
    Wilson l's
    XYZ Frank ECG l.
Leadbetter
    ileal loop diversion
    maneuver
Leadbetter-Politano
    ureterovesicoplasty
Leader-Kollmann dilator
leaflet
    aortic valve l.
    mitral valve l.
Leahey operation
Leão spreading depression
learning disability
learning-disabled
leash
Leber
    amaurosis congenita
    atrophy
    congenital amaurosis
    corpuscle
    disease
    hereditary optic atrophy
    idiopathic stellar neuroretinitis
    plexus
Leboyer
    method
    technique
Lebsche
    forceps
    knife
    shears
lecithal
lecithid
    cobra l.
lecithin
lecithin–cholesterol acyltransferase
  (LCAT)

lecithoprotein
lecithovitellin
Leclanché cell
lectin
LED—lupus erythematosus
  disseminatus
Ledbänder
Le Dentu suture
Lederer anemia
Leder stain
ledging
LeDuc
    implantation
    technique
LeDuc-Camey ileocystoplasty
Lee
    bronchus clamp
    wedge resection clamp
leech
    artificial l.
    medicinal l.
leeching
Leede-Rumpel phenomenon
Leff stethoscope
Le Fort
    amputation
    apertognathia repair (I)
    bougie
    catheter
    fracture (I–III)
    operation
    osteotomy (I–III)
    sound
    suture
Le Fort-Neugebauer operation
left-handed
leg
    badger l.
    baker l.
    bandy l.
    bayonet l.
    bow l.
    milk l.
    restless l's
    rider's l.
    scissor l.
    tennis l.
    white l.
Legal [eponym]
    disease
    test
Le Gendre (Legendre) sign
Legg
    disease
    osteotome

Legg-Calvé-Perthes
    disease
    syndrome
Legg-Calvé-Waldenström disease
legionella (legionellae)
    l. pneumonia
legionellosis
legionnaires'
    l. disease
    l. pneumonia
Legroux remission
Legueu retractor
legume
legumelin
legumin
Lehman catheter
leiasthenia
Leichtenstern
    encephalitis
    phenomenon
    sign
    type
Leifson flagella stain
Leigh
    disease
    encephalopathy
    syndrome
Leinbach
    osteotome
    screw
Leiner
    dermatitis
    disease
leiodermia
leiodystonia
leiomyoblastoma
leiomyofibroma
leiomyoma (leiomyomas,
  leiomyomata)
    bizarre l.
    l. cutis
    epithelioid l.
    parasitic l.
    l. of seminal vesicles
    l. uteri
    Zenker l.
leiomyomatosis
    intracardiac l.
leiomyomatous
leiomyosarcoma
Leishman
    anemia
    cells
    stain
Leishman-Donovan bodies

L

Leishmania
- *L. aethiopica*
- *L. amazonensis*
- *L. arabica*
- *L. brasiliensis*
- *L. chagasi*
- *L. colombiensis*
- *L. donovani*
- *L. garnhami*
- *L. guyanensis*
- *L. infantum*
- *L. killicki*
- *L. lainsoni*
- *L. major*
- *L. mexicana*
- *L. naiffi*
- *L. panamensis*
- *L. peruviana*
- *L. pifanoi*
- *L. shawi*
- *L. tropica*
- *L. venezuelensis*

leishmanial
leishmaniasis
- American l.
- anergic l.
- anergic cutaneous l.
- canine l.
- cutaneous l.
- diffuse cutaneous l.
- Indian mucosal l.
- lupoid l.
- mucocutaneous l.
- New World cutaneous l.
- l. recidivans
- rural cutaneous l.
- urban cutaneous l.
- visceral l.

leishmanicidal
leishmanid
leishmanin
leishmanoid
- dermal l.
- post–kala-azar dermal l.

Leitner syndrome
Lejeune
- applicator
- scissors
- syndrome

Leksell
- apparatus
- forceps
- rongeur
- technique

Leland knife

Leland-Jones forceps
Lell esophagoscope
Leloir disease
lema
Lembert suture
lemmocyte
lemniscus (lemnisci)
- l. lateralis
- l. medialis
- l. spinalis
- l. trigeminalis

Lempert
- bur
- curet
- elevator
- fenestration operation
- forceps
- incision
- knife
- perforator
- retractor
- rugine

Lempert-Colver endaural speculum
Lenard rays
Lendrum inclusion body stain
Lenègre
- disease
- syndrome

length
- arch l.
- basialveolar l.
- basinasal l.
- cranial l.
- crown-heel l. (CHL)
- crown-rump l. (CRL)
- dental l.
- focal l.
- foot l.
- l. of gestation
- greatest l.
- mean l. of life
- sitting l.
- stem l.
- wave l.

lenitive
Lennarson tube
Lennert classification
Lennhoff
- index
- sign

Lennox syndrome
Lennox-Gastaut syndrome
Lenoir facet
lens
- absorptive l.

lens *(continued)*
    achromatic l.
    acoustic l.
    acrylic l.
    adherent l.
    anastigmatic l.
    aniseikonic l.
    anterior chamber intraocular
      l. (IOL)
    AO soft l.
    aplanatic l.
    apochromatic l.
    Aquaflex l.
    aspheric l.
    astigmatic l.
    Bagolini l.
    bandage l.
    baseball l.
    biconcave l.
    biconvex l.
    bicylindrical l.
    bifocal l.
    Binkhorst l.
    bispherical l.
    bitoric contact l.
    Brücke l.
    cataract l.
    Comberg l.
    compound l.
    concave l.
    concavoconcave l.
    concavoconvex l.
    condensing l.
    contact l., gas-permeable
    converging l.
    convex l.
    convexoconcave l.
    Coquille plano l.
    corneal l.
    Crookes l.
    crossed l.
    l. crystallina
    crystalline l.
    cylindrical l.
    decentered l.
    dispersing l.
    diverging l.
    electron l.
    flat l.
    Fresnel l.
    gas-permeable l.
    Gel Flex l.
    hard contact l.
    honey bee l.
    Hruby l.

lens *(continued)*
    hydrophilic l.
    hydrophobic l.
    immersion l.
    intraocular l. (IOL)
    iridocapsular l.
    iridocapsular/iris fixation l.
    iris plane l.
    iseikonic l.
    isoiconic l.
    Lieb and Guerry cataract
      implant l.
    meniscus l., converging
    meniscus l., diverging
    meniscus l., negative
    meniscus l., positive
    meter l.
    minus l.
    multifocal intraocular l.
    non–gas permeable hard
      contact l.
    omnifocal l.
    orthoscopic l.
    periscopic l.
    periscopic concave l.
    periscopic convex l.
    photochromic l.
    photosensitive l.
    piggyback l.
    plane l.
    plano l.
    planoconcave l.
    planoconvex l.
    plus l.
    PMMA contact l.
    posterior chamber intraocular
      l. (IOL)
    progressive l.
    prosthetic l.
    punctal l.
    punktal l.
    retinal laser l.
    rigid contact l.
    safety l.
    scleral contact l.
    Shearing l.
    Sheets l.
    silicone l.
    Simcoe l.
    Sinskey l.
    soft contact l.
    spherical l.
    spherocylindrical l.
    stigmatic l.
    Stokes l.

L

lens *(continued)*
    l. sutures
    Thorpe plastic l.
    toric l.
    trial l.
    trifocal l.
Lent laparoscope
lenticel
lenticonus
lenticula
lenticular nuclear sclerosis
lenticulo-optic
lenticulostriate
lenticulothalamic
lentiform
lentigines (plural of lentigo)
lentiginosis
    progressive cardiomyopathic l.
lentiginous
lentiglobus
lentigo (lentigines)
    l. maligna
    l. maligna melanoma
    nevoid lentigines
    senile lentigines
    l. senilis
    l. simplex
    solar lentigines
lentivirus
Lentulo spiral drill
Leonard-George position
leontiasis
    l. ossea
    l. ossium
Leopold
    maneuver
    operation
leotropic
lepidic
Lépine-Froin syndrome
L'Episcopo operation
Lepley-Ernst tube
lepocyte
lepra
leprechaunism
leproma
lepromatous
lepromin
leprosarium
leprostatic
leprosy
    borderline l.
    cutaneous l.
    diffuse l. of Lucio and
      Latapí

leprosy *(continued)*
    indeterminate l.
    lazarine l.
    lepromatous l.
    multibacillary l.
    neuritic l.
    nodular l.
    ocular l.
    paucibacillary l.
    pure neuritic l.
    spotted l.
leprotic
leprous
leptocephalic
leptocephalous
leptocephaly
leptochromatic
leptocyte
leptocytosis
leptodactylous
leptodactyly
leptodontous
leptomeningeal
leptomeninges (plural of
  leptomeninx)
leptomeningitis
    sarcomatous l.
leptomeninx (leptomeninges)
leptopellic
leptoprosope
leptoprosopia
leptoprosopic
leptorrhine
leptosomatic
Leptospira
    L. interrogans
    L. interrogans serovar
      australis
    L. interrogans serovar
      autumnalis
    L. interrogans serovar *bataviae*
    L. interrogans serovar *canicola*
    L. interrogans serovar
      grippotyphosa
    L. interrogans serovar *hardjo*
    L. interrogans serovar
      hebdomadis
    L. interrogans serovar
      icterohaemorrhagiae
    L. interrogans serovar *pomona*
    L. interrogans serovar
      pyrogenes
    L. interrogans serovar *tarassovi*
leptospiral
leptospire

leptospirosis
  anicteric l.
  benign l.
  icteric l.
  l. icterohaemorrhagica
leptospiruria
leptostaphyline
Leptotrichia buccalis
Leredde syndrome
Léri
  disease
  pleonosteosis
  sign
  syndrome
Leriche
  disease
  forceps
  operation
  syndrome
Léri-Weill syndrome
Lermoyez
  punch
  syndrome
les—local excitatory state
lesbian
lesbianism
Lesch-Nyhan syndrome
Leser-Trelat sign
lesion
  annular l.
  Antopol-Goldman l.
  apple core l.
  Armanni-Ebstein l.
  Baehr-Löhlein l.
  Bankart
  benign lymphoepithelial l.
  birds' nest l.
  blueberry muffin l.
  Blumenthal l.
  Bracht-Wächter l.
  Brown-Séquard l.
  bull's-eye l.
  butterfly l.
  capsular drop l.
  caviar l.
  cavitary pulmonary l.
  central l.
  circumscribed l.
  coin l.
  cold l.
  Cole herpetiform l.
  complement l.
  compressive l. of lumbosacral
    region
  congenital l.

lesion *(continued)*
  coronary artery bifurcation l.
  Councilman l.
  cutaneous l.
  cystic l.
  dendritic l.
  de novo l.
  desmoid l.
  destructive l.
  diffuse l.
  discharging l.
  disseminated l.
  doughnut l.
  DREZ (dorsal root entry zone) l.
  dumbbell l.
  Duret l.
  Ebstein l.
  ellipsoid l.
  focal l.
  frondy l.
  functional l.
  Ghon primary l.
  gross l.
  hepatic veno-occlusive l.
  herpetiform l. of Cole
  Hill-Sachs l.
  histologic l.
  hot l.
  hyaline l.
  impaction l.
  indiscriminate l.
  initial syphilitic l.
  irritative l.
  Janeway l.
  jet l.
  Kimmelstiel-Wilson l.
  local l.
  local glomerular l.
  Löhlein-Baehr l.
  lower motor neuron l.
  macroscopic l.
  mass l.
  metastatic l.
  molecular l.
  napkin-ring l.
  nodular l.
  onion scale l.
  onionskin l.
  organic l.
  partial l.
  peripheral l.
  phlyctenule l.
  pinguecula l.
  precancerous l.
  primary l.

L

lesion *(continued)*
 retrocochlear l.
 ring-like l.
 ring-wall l.
 satellite l.
 Scheibe l.
 sessile l.
 shagreen l.
 solitary l.
 space-occupying l.
 space-occupying
  intracranial l.
 spherical l.
 structural l.
 suspicious l.
 swan-neck tubular l.
 systemic l.
 target l.
 total l.
 trophic l.
 tumor-like l.
 wedge-shaped l.
 wire-loop l.
Lesshaft
 space
 triangle
Lester Martin procedure
LET—linear energy transfer
let-down
lethal
lethality
lethargic
lethargy
 progressive l.
 unexplained l.
lethologica
Letterer-Siwe disease
leucine
leucine amino-peptidase (LAP)
[4-leucine] oxytocin
leucinimide
leucinosis
leucinuria
leucitis
leucosin
leucovorin rescue
Leudet
 bruit
 sign
 tinnitus
leukapheresis
leukemia
 acute lymphoblastic l. (ALL)
 acute monoblastic l. (AMOL)
 acute myeloblastic l. (AML)

leukemia *(continued)*
 acute myelomonoblastic l.
  (AMMOL)
 acute nonlymphocytic l. (ANLL)
 acute promyelocytic l.
 adult T-cell l.
 aleukemic l.
 aleukocythemic l.
 aplastic l.
 basophilic l.
 blast cell l.
 blastic l.
 Burkitt-like acute
  lymphoblastic l.
 chronic granulocytic l.
 chronic lymphocytic l. (CLL)
 chronic myelocytic l. (CML)
 l. cutis
 embryonal l.
 eosinophilic l.
 granulocytic l.
 Gross l.
 hairy cell l.
 hemoblastic l.
 hemocytoblastic l.
 histiocytic l.
 leukopenic l.
 lymphatic l.
 lymphoblastic l.
 lymphocytic l.
 lymphogenous l.
 lymphoid l.
 lymphosarcoma cell l.
 mast cell l.
 mature cell l.
 medullary l.
 megakaryocytic l.
 micromyeloblastic l.
 monoblastic l.
 monocytic l.
 myeloblastic l.
 myelocytic l.
 myelogenous l.
 myeloid l.
 myeloid granulocytic l.
 myelomonocytic l.
 Naegeli l.
 neutrophilic l.
 nonlymphocytic l.
 null cell lymphoblastic l.
 plasma cell l.
 plasmacytic l.
 polymorphocytic l.
 progranulocytic l.
 prolymphocytic l.

leukemia *(continued)*
    promyelocytic l.
    reticuloendothelial cell l.
    Rieder cell l.
    Schilling l.
    smoldering l.
    splenic l.
    splenomedullary l.
    splenomyelogenous l.
    stem cell l.
    subleukemic l.
    testicular l.
    undifferentiated cell l.
leukemic
leukemid
leukemogen
leukemogenic
leukemoid
leukencephalitis
leukin
leukoagglutinin
leukoblast
    granular l.
leukoblastosis
leukocidin
    Panton-Valentine (P-V) l.
leukocyte
    acidophilic l.
    agranular l's
    l. alkaline phosphatase (LAP)
    basophilic l.
    l. count
    differential peripheral l. count
    endothelial l.
    eosinophilic l.
    l. esterase-positive
    granular l's (granulocytes)
    heterophilic l's
    human l. antigen (HLA)
    hyaline l.
    l. inhibitory factor
    lymphoid l's
    mast l.
    mononuclear l.
    motile l.
    neutrophilic l.
    nonfilament
      polymorphonuclear l.
    nongranular l's
    nonmotile l.
    passenger l.
    peripheral l's
    polymorphonuclear (PMN) l.
    polynuclear neutrophilic l.
    l.-poor red blood cells

leukocyte *(continued)*
    Türk irritation l.
leukocytic
leukocytoid
leukocytolysin
leukocytolysis
    venom l.
leukocytolytic
leukocytoma
leukocytophagy
leukocytoplania
leukocytosis
    absolute l.
    agonal l.
    basophilic l.
    eosinophilic l.
    lymphocytic l.
    mononuclear l.
    neutrophilic l.
    l. of the newborn
    pathologic l.
    physiologic l.
    pure l.
    relative l.
    terminal l.
    toxic l.
leukocytotherapy
leukocytotoxicity
leukocytotropic
leukocyturia
leukoderma
    l. acquisitum centrifugum
    l. colli
    genital l.
    occupational l.
    postinflammatory l.
    syphilitic l.
leukodermatous
leukodextrin
leukodystrophy
    cerebral l.
    globoid cell l.
    hereditary adult-onset l.
    hereditary cerebral l.
    Krabbe l.
    metachromatic l.
    progressive cerebral l.
    spongiform l.
    sudanophilic l.
    vanishing white matter l.
leukoedema
leukoencephalitis
    acute hemorrhagic l.
    acute hemorrhagic l. of Weston
      Hurst

L

leukoencephalitis *(continued)*
    concentric periaxial l.
    l. periaxialis concentrica
    subacute sclerosing l.
    van Bogaert sclerosing l.
leukoencephalomalacia
leukoencephalopathy
    metachromatic l.
    multifocal progressive l.
    necrotizing l.
    progressive multifocal l.
    subacute sclerosing l.
leukoerythroblastosis
leukokeratosis
    congenital oral l.
leukokinesis
leukokinetic
leukokinin
leukokoria
leukokraurosis
leukoma (leukomata)
    adherent l.
leukomaine
leukomainic
leukomalacia
    cystic periventricular l.
    periventricular l. (PVL)
leukomatous
leukon
leukonecrosis
leukonychia
leukopedesis
leukopenia
    basophilic l.
    eosinophilic l.
    lymphocytic l.
    malignant l.
    monocytic l.
    neutrophilic l.
    pernicious l.
leukopenic
leukoplakia
    atrophic l.
    l. buccalis
    hairy l.
    l. of larynx
    l. lingualis
    oral l.
    oral hairy l.
    l. of penis
    speckled l.
    l. vulvae
leukopoiesis
leukopoietic
leukopoietin

leukoprecipitin
leukopsin
leukorrhagia
leukorrhea
    menstrual l.
    periodic l.
leukorrheal
leukosarcoma
leukotactic
leukotaxis
leukothrombin
leukotome
leukotoxic
leukotoxicity
leukotoxin
leukotrichia
leukotriene
leukourobilin
levan
levansucrase
Levant stone dislodger
levator (levatores)
    l. ani
    l. claviculae
    l. muscle
Lev disease
LeVeen
    peritoneal shunt
    valve
level
    α l. [alpha]
    air-fluid l.
    l. of anesthesia
    background l.
    barbiturate l.
    bone-conduction hearing l.
    l's of brightness
    butyrylcholinesterase l.
    complement l.
    l's of consciousness
    continuous noise l.
    developmental l.
    ethanol l.
    lead l.
    loudness discomfort l.
    lowest observed adverse effect
      l. (LOAEL)
    lowest observed effect l. (LOEL)
    no adverse effect l.
    no detectable effect l.
    no effect l.
    no observable effect l.
    no observed adverse effect l.
      (NOAEL)
    no observed effect l. (NOEL)

level *(continued)*
    sensation l.
    sensorineural acuity l.
    l's of brightness
    l's of consciousness
    sound pressure l.
    threshold l.
    tonal l.
leveling
levicellular
levigation
Lévi-Lorain
    dwarf
    dwarfism
    infantilism
    syndrome
    type
Levin tube
Levine
    agar
    clenched-fist sign
    EMB (eosin–methylene blue)
      agar
    operation
    sign
levitation
levocardia
    isolated l.
    mixed l.
levoclination
levoduction
levorotation
levorotatory
levotorsion
levoversion
Levret forceps
levulinate
levulinic acid
levulosan
Lévy-Roussy syndrome
Lewandowsky nevus elasticus
Lewandowsky-Lutz disease
Lewin
    dissector
    forceps
    splint
Lewin-Stern splint
Lewis
    acid
    base
    blood group
    cystometer
    forceps
    line
    rasp

Lewis *(continued)*
    scoop
    snare
    tube
Lewis and Pickering test
lewisite
Lewisohn method
Lewkowitz forceps
Lewy
    bodies
    laryngoscope
Lewy-Rubin needle
Lexer operation
Leyden
    ataxia
    crystals
    disease
    hemophilia B
Leyden-Möbius
    dystrophy
    syndrome
    type
Leydig
    cells
    cylinders
    duct
Leyro-Diaz forceps
LFA—
    left femoral artery
    left frontoanterior (position)
LFD—
    lactose-free diet
    least fatal dose
LFP—left frontoposterior (position)
LFT—
    latex flocculation test
    left frontotransverse (position)
    liver function test
LGB—lateral geniculate body
LGN—lateral geniculate nucleus
LGV—lymphogranuloma venereum
LH—
    lower half
    luteinizing hormone
Lhermitte sign
LHL—left hepatic lobe
LHRF; LH-RF—luteinizing
    hormone–releasing factor
LHRH; LH-RH—luteinizing
    hormone–releasing hormone
LI—
    linguoincisal
    low impulsiveness
LIA—leukemia-associated
    inhibitory activity

L

liability
  l. insurance
  medical l.
  professional l.
liaison
LIBC—latent iron-binding capacity
libidinal
libidinous
libido (libidines)
Libman-Sacks
  disease
  endocarditis
  syndrome
Libman sign
library
  gene l.
lice (plural of louse)
license
licentiate
licentious
lichen
  l. amyloidosus
  l. aureus
  bullous l. planus
  follicular l. planus
  hypertrophic l. planus
  l. myxedematosus
  l. nitidus
  l. planopilaris
  l. planus
  l. planus actinicus
  l. planus atrophicus
  l. planus follicularis
  l. planus hypertrophicus
  l. planus pilaris
  l. planus subtropicus
  l. planus tropicus
  l. ruber planus
  l. sclerosis
  l. sclerosus
  l. sclerosus et atrophicus
  l. scrofulosorum
  l. simplex chronicus
  l. spinulosus
  l. striatus
  vesiculobullous l. planus
lichenification
licheniformin
lichenoid
  l. dermatosis
  l. phase
Lich-Gregoire repair
Lichtenstein hernia repair
Lichtheim
  aphasia

Lichtheim (continued)
  disease
  plaques
  sign
  syndrome
  tests
licorice powder
lid
  granular l's
  l. lag
  l. retraction
  l. speculum
  tucked l. of Collier
Liddell and Sherrington
  reflex
Liddle aorta clamp
lid everter
  Walker l.e.
lidofenin
lidofilcon A
lid plate
  Jaeger l.p.
lie
  longitudinal l.
  oblique l.
  transverse l.
Lieb and Guerry cataract implant
  lens
Lieben
  reaction
  test
Lieberkühn
  ampulla
  crypts
  follicles
  glands
Lieberman
  proctoscope
  sigmoidoscope
Liebermann test
Liebermann-Burchard
  reaction
  test
Liebermeister
  furrows
  grooves
Liebig test
Liebreich symptom
lien
  l. accessorius
  l. mobilis
lienal
lienculus, lienunculus
lienorenal
lienteric

lientery
lienunculus, lienculus
Liepmann apraxia
Liesegang
    phenomenon
    striae
    waves
Lieutaud
    body
    triangle
    uvula
LIF—
    left iliac fossa
    leukocyte inhibitory factor
life
    antenatal l.
    fetal l.
    intrauterine l.
    mean l.
    mean effective l.
    potential years of l. lost
    uterine l.
lifetime
lift and heave
ligament
    accessory l. of Henle
    accessory l. of humerus
    accessory l's of
      metacarpophalangeal joints
    accessory patellar l.
    accessory l's, plantar
    accessory l's, volar
    acromioclavicular l.
    acromiocoracoid l.
    adipose l. of knee
      (of Cruveilhier)
    alar l's
    alar l's of knee
    alveolodental l.
    annular l.
    annular l. of ankle
    annular l. of base of stapes
    annular l. of carpus
    annular l's of digits of foot
    annular l's of digits of hand
    annular l. of femur
    annular l's of fingers
    annular l. of malleolus
    annular l. of radius
    annular l. of stapes
    annular l. of tarsus
    annular l's of tendon sheaths
      of fingers
    annular l's of toes
    annular l. of wrist

ligament *(continued)*
    anococcygeal l.
    l. of antebrachium of Weitbrecht
    anterior l. of ankle joint
    anterior l. of colon
    anterior cruciate l.
    anterior l. of head of fibula
    anterior l. of head of rib
    anterior l. of malleus
    anterior l. of neck of rib
    anterior l. of radiocarpal joint
    apical l. of dens
    apical dental l.
    apical odontoid l.
    appendiculo-ovarian l.
    Arantius l.
    arcuate l.
    arcuate l. of diaphragm
    arcuate l. of knee
    arcuate popliteal l.
    arcuate pubic l., arcuate l.
      of pubis
    articular l. of vertebrae
    arytenoepiglottic l.
    atlantooccipital l.
    auricular l.
    Barkow l.
    Bellini l.
    Bérard l.
    Berry l.
    Bertin l.
    Bichat l.
    bifurcate l., bifurcated l.
    bifurcate l's of Arnold
    Bigelow l.
    bigeminate l's of Arnold
    l. of Botallo
    Bourgery l.
    brachiocubital l.
    brachioradial l.
    broad l. of liver
    broad l. of uterus
    Brodie l.
    Burns l.
    calcaneocuboid l.
    calcaneofibular l.
    calcaneonavicular l.
    calcaneotibial l.
    Caldani l.
    Campbell l.
    Camper l.
    canthal l's
    capitular l.
    capsular l.
    capsular l. of hip joint

L

ligament *(continued)*
- cardinal l.
- caroticoclinoid l.
- carpal l.
- carpometacarpal l's
- Casser l., casserian l.
- ceratocricoid l.
- cervical l.
- cervical l. of sinus tarsi
- cervicobasilar l.
- check l's of axis
- chondrosternal l.
- chondroxiphoid l's
- l. of Civinini
- Clado l.
- clavicular l.
- Cloquet l.
- coccygeal l.
- collateral l. of carpus, radial
- collateral l. of carpus, ulnar
- collateral l., fibular
- collateral l's of interphalangeal articulations of foot
- collateral l's of metacarpophalangeal articulations
- collateral l's of metatarsophalangeal articulations
- collateral l's of midcarpal joint
- collateral l., radial
- collateral l., radial carpal
- collateral l., tibial
- collateral l., ulnar
- collateral l., ulnar carpal
- Colles l.
- l's of colon
- common l. of knee of Weber
- common l. of wrist joint
- conoid l.
- conus l.
- Cooper l.
- Cooper suspensory l's
- coracoacromial l.
- coracoclavicular l.
- coracohumeral l.
- coracoid l. of scapula
- cordiform l. of diaphragm
- coronary l. of liver
- coronary l. of radius
- costocentral l.
- costoclavicular l.
- costocolic l.
- costocoracoid l.
- costopericardiac l.

ligament *(continued)*
- costosternal l's, radiate
- costotransverse l.
- costotransverse l. of Krause
- costovertebral l.
- costoxiphoid l's
- cotyloid l.
- Cowper l.
- cricoarytenoid l.
- cricopharyngeal l. of Luschka
- cricothyroid l.
- cricotracheal l. of Luschka
- crucial l's of fingers
- crucial l. of foot
- cruciate l. of atlas
- cruciate l's of knee
- cruciate l. of leg
- cruciate l's of toes
- cruciform l. of atlas
- crural l.
- Cruveilhier l's
- cubitoradial l.
- cubitoulnar l.
- cuboideometatarsal l's
- cuboideonavicular l., dorsal
- cuboideonavicular l., oblique
- cuboideonavicular l., plantar
- cubonavicular l.
- cuboscaphoid l., plantar
- cuneocuboid l., dorsal
- cuneocuboid l., plantar
- cuneonavicular l's, dorsal
- cuneonavicular l's, plantar
- cutaneophalangeal l's
- cysticoduodenal l.
- deltoid l. of ankle
- deltoid l. of elbow
- deltoid l. of talocrural joint
- Denonvilliers l.
- dental l.
- dentate l. of spinal cord
- denticulate l.
- Denucé l.
- diaphragmatic l.
- dorsal l's of bases of metacarpal bones
- dorsal l's of bases of metatarsal bones
- dorsal l's, carpal
- dorsal l. of radiocarpal joint
- dorsal l., talonavicular
- dorsal l's of tarsus
- dorsal l. of wrist
- Douglas l.
- duodenohepatic l.

ligament *(continued)*
  duodenorenal l.
  epihyal l.
  external l's of Barkow, plantar
  external l. of mandibular
    articulation
  extracapsular accessory l's
  fabellofibular l.
  falciform l.
  falciform l. of liver
  fallopian l., l. of Fallopius
  false l.
  Ferrein l.
  fibrous l's
  fibrous l's of breast
  fibular collateral l.
  flaval l's
  Flood l.
  fundiform l. of clitoris
  fundiform l. of penis
  gastrocolic l.
  gastrohepatic l.
  gastrolienal l.
  gastropancreatic l's of Huschke
  gastrophrenic l.
  gastrosplenic l.
  genitoinguinal l.
  Gerdy l.
  Gillette suspensory l.
  Gimbernat l.
  gingivodental l.
  glenohumeral l's
  glenoid l's of Cruveilhier
  glenoid l. of humerus
  glenoid l. of Macalister
  glenoid l. of mandibular fossa
  Grayson l.
  Günz l.
  hamatometacarpal l.
  hammock l.
  l. of head of femoral bone
  l. of head of femur
  Helmholtz l.
  l's of Helvetius
  Henle l.
  Hensing l.
  hepatic l's
  hepatocolic l.
  hepatocystocolic l.
  hepatoduodenal l.
  hepatogastric l.
  hepatogastroduodenal l.
  hepatorenal l.
  hepatoumbilical l.
  Hesselbach l.

ligament *(continued)*
  Hey l.
  Hueck l.
  Humphry l.
  Hunter l.
  Huschke l's
  hyaloideocapsular l.
  hyoepiglottic l.
  iliocostal l.
  iliofemoral l.
  iliolumbar l.
  iliopectineal l.
  iliopubic l.
  iliosacral l's
  iliotibial l. of Maissiat
  iliotrochanteric l.
  inferior l. of epididymis
  inferior l. of neck of rib of Henle
  inferior l. of tubercle of rib
  infundibulo-ovarian l.
  infundibulopelvic l.
  inguinal l's
  inguinal l. of Blumberg
  inguinal l. of Cooper
  inguinal l., reflex
  interarticular l. of articulation
    of humerus
  interarticular l. of head of rib
  interarticular l. of hip joint
  interarticular sternocostal l.
  intercarpal l's
  interchondral l.
  interclavicular l.
  interclinoid l.
  intercornual l.
  intercostal l's
  intercuneiform l's
  interfoveolar l.
  interlaminar l's
  intermaxillary l.
  intermetacarpal l's
  intermetacarpal l's,
    transverse, dorsal
  intermetacarpal l's,
    transverse, volar
  intermetatarsal l's
  intermetatarsal l's, transverse,
    dorsal
  intermetatarsal l's, transverse,
    plantar
  intermuscular l's
  intermuscular l., fibular
  internal l. of neck of rib
  interosseous l's of Barkow,
    internal

L

ligament *(continued)*

> interosseous l's of bases of metacarpal bones
> interosseous l's of bases of metatarsal bones
> interosseous l. of Cruveilhier, costovertebral
> interosseous l. of Cruveilhier, transversocostal
> interosseous cuboideonavicular l.
> interosseous cuneometatarsal l's
> interosseous intercarpal l's
> interosseous intercuneiform l's
> interosseous intermetacarpal l's
> interosseous intermetatarsal l's
> interosseous l's of knee
> interosseous l. of leg
> interosseous metacarpal l's
> interosseous metatarsal l's
> interosseous l. of pubis of Winslow
> interosseous l., radioulnar
> interosseous sacroiliac l's
> interosseous talocalcaneal l.
> interosseous l's of tarsus
> interosseous l's, transverse metacarpal
> interprocess l.
> interpubic l.
> interspinal l's, interspinous l's
> intertarsal l's
> intertransverse l. of vertebral arch
> interureteral l.
> intervertebral l.
> intraarticular costovertebral l.
> intraarticular l. of head of rib
> intraarticular sternocostal l.
> intrinsic l. of auricle
> ischiocapsular l.
> ischiofemoral l.
> ischioprostatic l.
> ischiosacral l's
> Jarjavay l.
> keystone l.
> Krause l.
> laciniate l.
> lacunar l. of Gimbernat
> lambdoid l.
> Lannelongue l.
> lateral l. of ankle joint
> lateral l's of bladder
> lateral l. of carpus, radial

ligament *(continued)*

> lateral l. of carpus, ulnar
> lateral check l. of eyeball
> lateral l. of colon
> lateral l. of elbow
> lateral false l.
> lateral l's of joints of fingers
> lateral l's of joints of toes
> lateral l. of knee
> lateral l's of liver
> lateral l. of malleus
> lateral l's of metacarpophalangeal joints
> lateral l's of metatarsophalangeal joints
> lateral meniscofemoral l.
> lateral palpebral l.
> lateral puboprostatic l.
> lateral l. of rectum
> lateral l. of talocrural joint
> lateral l. of temporomandibular articulation
> lateral l. of temporomandibular joint
> lateral l's of wrist joint
> Lauth l.
> l. of left superior vena cava
> lienophrenic l.
> lienorenal l.
> Lisfranc l.
> l. of Lockwood
> longitudinal l's
> longitudinal l. of abdomen
> long posterior sacroiliac l.
> lumbocostal l. of Henle
> l's of Luschka
> Mackenrodt l.
> l. of Maissiat
> Mauchart l's
> maxillary l's
> l. of Mayer
> Meckel l.
> medial check l. of eyeball
> medial l. of elbow joint
> medial palpebral l.
> medial puboprostatic l.
> medial l. of temporomandibular articulation
> medial l. of temporomandibular joint
> medial l. of wrist
> meniscofemoral l's
> mesocolic l. of colon

ligament *(continued)*

metacarpal l's
metacarpophalangeal l's
metatarsal l's
metatarsal l's of Weitbrecht
metatarsal l's proper of Weber
metatarsophalangeal l's
middle glenohumeral l.
middle l. of neck of rib
middle umbilical l.
l. of nape
natatory l.
navicularicuneiform l's
nephrocolic l.
nuchal l.
oblique l. of Cooper
oblique l. of forearm
oblique l. of knee
oblique l. of scapula
oblique l. of superior
  radioulnar joint
obturator l., atlantooccipital
obturator l. of atlas
obturator l. of pelvis
occipitoaxial l.
occipitoodontoid l's
odontoid l.
odontoid l's of axis
olecranon l.
orbicular l. of radius
ovarian l.
palmar l. of carpus
palmar l. of radiocarpal joint
palmar l., transverse, deep
palpebral l's
pancreaticosplenic l.
patellar l's
pectinal l. of iris
pectinate l. of iridocorneal angle
pectineal l. of Cooper
pelvic l's
pelviprostatic l., basal
pericardiovertebral l.
perineal l. of Carcassone
perineal l., transverse
periodontal l.
peritoneal l.
Petit l.
Pétrequin l.
petrosphenoid l.
pharyngeal l.
phrenicocolic l.
phrenicolienal l.
phrenicosplenic l.
phrenocolic l.

ligament *(continued)*

pisimetacarpal l.
pisohamate l.
pisometacarpal l.
pisounciform l.
pisouncinate l.
plantar l's of bases of
  metatarsal bones
plantar l., long
plantar l. of second metatarsal
  bone
plantar l. of tarsus
popliteal l., arcuate
popliteal l., external
popliteal l., oblique
posterior annular l. of carpus
posterior cricoarytenoid l.
posterior false l. of bladder
posterior l. of head of fibula
posterior l. of incus
posterior meniscofemoral l.
  of Wrisberg
posterior l. of pinna
posterior l. of radiocarpal joint
Poupart l.
preurethral l. of Waldeyer
prismatic l. of Weitbrecht
proper l.
proper l's of costal cartilages
proper l. of ovary
pterygomandibular l.
pterygomaxillary l.
pterygospinal l.
pterygospinous l.
pubic arcuate l.
pubic l. of Cowper
pubic l. of Cruveilhier
pubocapsular l.
pubocervical l.
pubofemoral l.
puboischiadic l. of prostate
  gland
puboprostatic l.
puborectal l.
pubovesical l.
pulmonary l.
quadrate l.
quadrate l. of Denucé
radial collateral l. of elbow joint
radial collateral l. of wrist
radial l. of cubitocarpal
  articulation
radiate l. of carpus
radiate l. of head of rib
radiate l., lateral

L

ligament *(continued)*
    radiate l. of Mayer
    radiate sternocostal l.
    radiate l. of wrist
    radiocarpal l's
    rectouterine l.
    reflected l.
    reflex l. of Gimbernat
    reflex inguinal l.
    reinforcing l's
    Retzius l.
    rhomboid l. of clavicle
    rhomboid l. of wrist
    ring l. of hip joint
    Robert l.
    round l. of acetabulum
    round l. of Cloquet
    round l. of femur
    round l. of forearm
    round l. of liver
    round l. of uterus
    sacciform l.
    sacrococcygeal l's
    sacrogenital l.
    sacroiliac l's,
    sacrosciatic l's
    sacrospinal l., sacrospinous l.
    sacrotuberal l., sacrotuberous l.
    sacrouterine l.
    salpingopharyngeal l.
    Santorini l.
    Sappey l.
    scaphocuneiform l's, plantar
    l. of Scarpa
    Schlemm l's
    scrotal l. of testis
    Sebileau suspensory l's
    serous l.
    short lateral l.
    short plantar l.
    short posterior sacroiliac l.
    Soemmering l.
    sphenoidal l.
    sphenomandibular l.
    spinoglenoid l.
    spinosacral l.
    spiral l. of cochlea
    splenocolic l.
    splenogastric l.
    splenophrenic l.
    splenorenal l.
    spring l.
    Stanley cervical l.
    stapedial l.
    stellate l.

ligament *(continued)*
    sternoclavicular l's
    sternocostal l's
    sternopericardiac l's,
        sternopericardial l's
    l. of Struthers
    stylohyoid l.
    stylomandibular l.
    stylomaxillary l.
    stylomylohyoid l.
    subflaval l.
    subpubic l.
    superficial l. of carpus
    superior l. of epididymis
    superior glenohumeral l.
    superior l. of hip
    superior l. of incus
    superior l. of malleus
    superior l. of neck of rib
    superior l. of pinna
    suprascapular l.
    supraspinal l's
    supraspinous l's
    suspensory l. of axilla
    suspensory l. of axis
    suspensory l. of bladder
    suspensory l's of breast
    suspensory l. of clitoris
    suspensory l. of duodenum
    suspensory l. of eyeball
    suspensory l. of humerus
    suspensory l. of lens
    suspensory l. of liver
    suspensory l's of mammary
        gland
    suspensory l. of ovary
    suspensory l. of penis
    suspensory l. of spleen
    sutural l.
    synovial l.
    synovial l. of hip
    talocalcaneal l's
    l. of talocrural joint
    talofibular l's
    talonavicular l.
    talotibial l's
    tarsal l., anterior
    tarsometatarsal l's
    temporomandibular l.
    tendinotrochanteric l.
    tensor l.
    Teutleben l's
    Thompson l.
    thyroepiglottic l.
    thyrohyoid l's

ligament *(continued)*

    tibial collateral l.
    tibiocalcaneal l.,
      tibiocalcanean l.
    tibiofibular l's
    tibionavicular l.
    l. of Toldt
    Toynbee l.
    tracheal l's
    tracheal annular l's
    transverse l. of acetabulum
    transverse l. of atlas
    transverse l. of carpus
    transverse humeral l.
    transverse l. of knee
    transverse l. of leg
    transverse l. of little head of rib
    transverse l. of pelvis
    transverse l's of scapula
    transverse l. of tibia
    transverse l's of wrist
    transversocostal l.
    trapezoid l.
    Treitz l.
    triangular l. of abdomen
    triangular l. of Colles
    triangular l. of linea alba
    triangular l's of liver
    triangular l. of pubis
    triangular l. of scapula
    triangular l. of thigh
    triangular l. of urethra
    trigeminate l's of Arnold
    triquetral l. of foot
    triquetral l. of scapula
    trochlear l's of foot
    trochlear l's of hand
    trochlear l's of little heads of
      metacarpal bones
    true l. of bladder
    tuberososacral l.
    tubopharyngeal l. of Rauber
    Tuffier inferior l.
    ulnar l. of carpus
    ulnocarpal l's
    umbilical l's
    utero-ovarian l.
    uteropelvic l's
    uterosacral l.
    uterovesical l.
    vaginal l's of fingers
    vaginal l's of toes
    l's of Valsalva
    venous l. of liver
    ventricular l. of larynx

ligament *(continued)*

    vertebropelvic l.
    vertebropericardial l.
    vertebropleural l.
    l. of Vesalius
    vesical l.
    vesicopubic l.
    vesicoumbilical l.
    vesicouterine l.
    vestibular l.
    vocal l.
    volar l's of bases of metacarpal
      bones
    volar l. of carpus
    volar l. of wrist
    Walther oblique l.
    Weitbrecht l.
    Whitnall l.
    Winslow l.
    Wrisberg l.
    xiphicostal l's of Macalister
    xiphoid l's
    Y l.
    yellow l's
    l. of Zaglas
    Zinn l.
    zonal l. of thigh
    zonular l.

ligamentopexy

ligamentous

ligamentum (ligamenta)

    l. acromioclaviculare
    ligamenta alaria
    l. anococcygeum
    l. anulare radii
    l. anulare stapediale, l.
      anulare stapedis
    ligamenta anularia digitorum
      manus
    ligamenta anularia digitorum
      pedis
    ligamenta anularia tracheae
    l. apicis dentis
    l. apicis dentis epistrophei
    l. arcuatum laterale
    l. arcuatum mediale
    l. arcuatum medianum
    l. arteriosum
    l. atlantooccipitale anterius
    l. atlantooccipitale laterale
    l. auriculare anterius
    l. auriculare posterius
    l. auriculare superius
    ligamenta auricularia
    l. bifurcatum

L

ligamentum (ligamenta) *(continued)*
l. calcaneocuboideum
l. calcaneocuboideum plantare
l. calcaneofibulare
l. calcaneonaviculare
l. calcaneonaviculare dorsale
l. calcaneonaviculare plantare
l. calcaneotibiale
l. capitis costae
  intraarticulare
l. capitis costae radiatum
l. capitis femoris
l. capitis fibulae anterius
l. capitis fibulae posterius
l. capituli costae
  interarticulare
l. capituli costae radiatum
ligamenta capituli fibulae
ligamenta capsularia
l. cardinale
l. carpi dorsale
l. carpi radiatum
l. carpi transversum
l. carpi volare
ligamenta carpometacarpalia
  dorsalia
ligamenta carpometacarpalia
  palmaria
l. caudale integumenti
  communis
l. ceratocricoideum
l. collaterale carpi radiale
l. collaterale carpi ulnare
l. collaterale fibulare
l. collaterale laterale
  articulationis talocruralis
l. collaterale mediale
  articulationis talocruralis
l. collaterale radiale
l. collaterale tibiale
l. collaterale ulnare
ligamenta collateralia
  articulationum digitorum
  manus
ligamenta collateralia
  articulationum digitorum
  pedis
ligamenta collateralia
  articulationum
  interphalangealium
  manus
ligamenta collateralia
  articulationum
  interphalangealium pedis

ligamentum (ligamenta) *(continued)*
ligamenta collateralia
  articulationum
  interphalangearum manus
ligamenta collateralia
  articulationum
  interphalangearum pedis
ligamenta collateralia
  articulationum
  metacarpophalangealium
ligamenta collateralia
  articulationum
  metacarpophalangearum
ligamenta collateralia
  articulationum
  metatarsophalangealium
ligamenta collateralia
  articulationum
  metatarsophalangearum
l. colli costae
l. conoideum
l. coracoacromiale
l. coracoclaviculare
l. coracohumerale
l. coronarium hepatis
l. costoclaviculare
l. costotransversarium
l. costotransversarium laterale
l. costotransversarium superius
ligamenta costoxiphoidea
l. cricoarytenoideum posterius
l. cricopharyngeum
l. cricothyroideum medianum
l. cricotracheale
ligamenta cruciata digitorum
  manus
ligamenta cruciata digitorum
  pedis
ligamenta cruciata genualia,
  ligamenta cruciata genus
l. cruciatum anterius genus
l. cruciatum posterius genus
l. cruciforme atlantis
l. cuboideonaviculare dorsale
l. cuboideonaviculare plantare
l. cuneocuboideum dorsale
l. cuneocuboideum interosseum
l. cuneocuboideum plantare
ligamenta cuneometatarsalia
  interossea
ligamenta cuneonavicularia
  dorsalia
ligamenta cuneonavicularia
  plantaria

ligamentum (ligamenta) *(continued)*
- l. deltoideum articulationis talocruralis
- l. denticulatum (ligamenta denticulata)
- l. epididymidis inferius
- l. epididymidis superius
- ligamenta extracapsularia
- l. extraperitoneale
- l. falciforme hepatis
- l. flavum (ligamenta flava)
- l. fundiforme clitoridis
- l. fundiforme penis
- l. gastrocolicum
- l. gastrolienale
- l. gastrophrenicum
- l. gastrosplenicum
- l. genitoinguinale
- ligamenta glenohumeralia
- ligamenta hepatis
- l. hepatocolicum
- l. hepatoduodenale
- l. hepatogastricum
- l. hepatorenale
- l. hyoepiglotticum
- l. iliofemorale
- l. iliolumbale
- l. incudis posterius
- l. incudis superius
- l. inguinale
- l. inguinale reflexum
- ligamenta intercarpalia dorsalia
- ligamenta intercarpalia interossea
- ligamenta intercarpalia palmaria
- l. interclaviculare
- ligamenta intercuneiformia dorsalia
- ligamenta intercuneiformia interossea
- ligamenta intercuneiformia plantaria
- l. interfoveolare
- ligamenta interspinalia
- ligamenta intertransversaria
- ligamenta intracapsularia
- l. ischiocapsulare
- l. ischiofemorale
- l. laciniatum
- l. lacunare
- l. laterale articulationis talocruralis

ligamentum (ligamenta) *(continued)*
- l. laterale articulationis temporomandibularis
- l. laterale puboprostaticum
- l. laterale pubovesicale
- l. latum uteri
- l. lienorenale
- l. longitudinale anterius
- l. longitudinale posterius
- l. lumbocostale
- l. mallei anterius
- l. mallei laterale
- l. mallei superius
- l. malleoli lateralis anterius
- l. malleoli lateralis posterius
- l. mediale articulationis talocruralis
- l. mediale articulationis temporomandibularis
- l. mediale puboprostaticum
- l. mediale pubovesicale
- l. meniscofemorale anterius
- l. meniscofemorale posterius
- l. metacarpale transversum profundum
- l. metacarpale transversum superficiale
- ligamenta metacarpalia dorsalia
- ligamenta metacarpalia interossea
- ligamenta metacarpalia palmaria
- l. metatarsale transversum profundum
- l. metatarsale transversum superficiale
- ligamenta metatarsalia dorsalia
- ligamenta metatarsalia interossea
- ligamenta metatarsalia plantaria
- l. mucosum
- ligamenta navicularicuneiformia dorsalia
- ligamenta navicularicuneiformia plantaria
- l. nuchae

L

ligamentum (ligamenta) *(continued)*
    ligamenta ossiculorum auditoriorum
    ligamenta ossiculorum auditus
    ligamenta ovarii proprium
    ligamenta palmaria articulationum interphalangealium manus
    ligamenta palmaria articulationum interphalangearum manus
    ligamenta palmaria articulationum metacarpophalangealium
    ligamenta palmaria articulationum metacarpophalangearum
    l. palpebrale laterale
    l. palpebrale mediale
    l. patellae
    l. pectinatum anguli iridocornealis
    l. pectineale, l. pectineum
    l. phrenicocolicum
    l. phrenicolienale
    l. phrenicosplenicum
    l. pisohamatum
    l. pisometacarpeum
    l. plantare longum
    ligamenta plantaria articulationum interphalangealium pedis
    ligamenta plantaria articulationum interphalangearum pedis
    ligamenta plantaria articulationum metatarsophalangealium
    ligamenta plantaria articulationum metatarsophalangearum
    l. popliteum arcuatum
    l. popliteum obliquum
    l. pterygospinale
    l. pubicum inferius
    l. pubicum superius
    l. pubocapsulare
    l. pubofemorale
    l. puboprostaticum
    l. pubovesicale
    l. pubovesicale laterale
    l. pubovesicale mediale
    l. pulmonale
    l. quadratum

ligamentum (ligamenta) *(continued)*
    l. radiocarpale dorsale
    l. radiocarpale palmare
    l. recti laterale
    l. rectouterinum
    l. sacrococcygeum anterius
    l. sacrococcygeum dorsale profundum
    l. sacrococcygeum dorsale superficiale
    l. sacrococcygeum laterale
    l. sacrococcygeum posterius profundum
    l. sacrococcygeum posterius superficiale
    l. sacrococcygeum ventrale
    ligamenta sacroiliacum anterius
    ligamenta sacroiliacum dorsalis
    ligamenta sacroiliacum interosseum
    ligamenta sacroiliacum posterius
    ligamenta sacroiliacum ventralis
    l. sacrospinale
    l. sacrospinosum
    l. sacrotuberale
    l. sacrotuberosum
    l. serosum
    l. sphenomandibulare
    l. spirale cochleae, l. spirale ductus cochlearis
    l. splenorenale
    l. sternoclaviculare
    l. sternoclaviculare anterius
    l. sternoclaviculare posterius
    l. sternocostale interarticulare
    l. sternocostale intra-articulare
    ligamenta sternocostalia radiata
    ligamenta sternopericardiaca
    l. stylohyoideum
    l. stylomandibulare
    l. supraspinale
    l. suspensoria mammaria
    l. suspensorium clitoridis
    l. suspensorium duodeni
    l. suspensorium ovarii
    l. suspensorium penis
    l. talocalcaneare interosseum
    l. talocalcaneare laterale
    l. talocalcaneare mediale

ligamentum (ligamenta) *(continued)*
  l. talocalcaneum interosseum
  l. talocalcaneum laterale
  l. talocalcaneum mediale
  l. talofibulare anterius
  l. talofibulare posterius
  l. talonaviculare
  l. talotibiale anterius
  l. talotibiale posterius
  ligamenta tarsi
  ligamenta tarsi dorsalia
  ligamenta tarsi interossea
  ligamenta tarsi plantaria
  ligamenta tarsometatarsalia
    dorsalia
  ligamenta tarsometatarsalia
    plantaria
  l. temporomandibulare
  l. teres femoris
  l. teres hepatis
  l. teres uteri
  l. thyroepiglotticum
  l. thyrohyoideum laterale
  l. thyrohyoideum medianum
  l. tibiofibulare anterius
  l. tibiofibulare posterius
  l. tibionaviculare
  ligamenta trachealia
  l. transversum
  l. transversum acetabuli
  l. transversum atlantis
  l. transversum cervicis
  l. transversum cruris
  l. transversum genuale
  l. transversum genus
  . l. transversum pelvis
  l. transversum perinei
  l. transversum scapulae
    inferius
  l. transversum scapulae
    superius
  l. trapezoideum
  l. triangulare dextrum hepatis
  l. triangulare sinistrum hepatis
  l. tuberculi costae
  l. ulnocarpale palmare
  l. umbilicale medianum
  l. uteroovaricum
  ligamenta vaginalia digitorum
    manus
  ligamenta vaginalia digitorum
    pedis
  l. venae cavae sinistrae
  l. venosum
  l. ventriculare

ligamentum (ligamenta) *(continued)*
  l. vestibulare
  l. vocale
ligand
ligase
ligate
ligation
  Barron l.
  Desault l.
  high saphenous vein l.
  proximal l.
  quadruple l.
  rubber band l.
  saphenous vein l.
  surgical l.
  l. suture
  teeth l.
  tubal l.
ligator
ligature
  l. in continuity
  double l.
  elastic l.
  free l. suture
  grass-line l.
  interlacing l.
  interlocking l.
  lateral l.
  McGraw elastic l.
  occluding l.
  provisional l.
  soluble l.
  Stannius l.
  suboccluding l.
  suture l.
  terminal l.
  thread-elastic l.
  Woodbridge l.
light
  actinic l.
  cold l.
  diffused l.
  idioretinal l.
  infrared l.
  l. microscopy (LM)
  neon l.
  polarized l.
  reflected l.
  refracted l.
  ultraviolet (UV) l.
  white l.
  Wood l.
lightening
lightning
light reflex

L

Lightwood-Albright syndrome
Lightwood syndrome
Lignac
    disease
    syndrome
Lignac-Fanconi
    disease
    syndrome
ligneous
lignoceric acid
LIHA—low impulsiveness, high
  anxiety
LILA—low impulsiveness, low
  anxiety
Liley chart
Lilienfeld position
Lilienthal
    incision
    probe
Lillehei-Kaster
    prosthesis
    valve
Lillie
    forceps
    hook
    scissors
    speculum
limb
    anacrotic l.
    l's of anthelix
    ascending l.
    catacrotic l.
    descending l.
    l. of incus, long
    l. of incus, short
    inferior l.
    l. of internal capsule, anterior
    l. of internal capsule, posterior
    lower l.
    pectoral l.
    pelvic l.
    phantom l.
    l. of stapes, anterior
    l. of stapes, posterior
    superior l.
    thick ascending l.
    thick descending l.
    thick l. of loop of Henle
    thoracic l.
    upper l.
    l. venography
limbal
    l. groove
    l. incision
    l. suture

limbal *(continued)*
    l. vasculitis
Limberg flap
limbic
limbus (limbi)
    l. acetabuli
    l. alveolaris mandibulae
    l. alveolaris maxillae
    alveolar l. of mandible
    alveolar l. of maxilla
    l. angulosus
    l. anterior palpebrae
    l. chorioideus
    l. conjunctivae
    l. of cornea, l. corneae
    l. corticalis
    l. foraminis ovalis
    l. fossae ovalis
    l. fossae ovalis Vieussenii
    l. laminae spiralis osseae
    l. luteus retinae
    l. medullaris
    l. membranae tympani
    limbi palpebrales anteriores
    limbi palpebrales posteriores
    l. of sclera
    l. of sphenoid bone
    spiral l.
    l. of Vieussens
lime
    barium hydroxide l.
    chlorinated l.
    slaked l.
    soda l.
limen (limina)
    l. of insula
    l. insulae
    l. nasi
    l. of twoness
limes
liminal
limit
    assimilation l.
    audibility l.
    emergency exposure l.
    exposure l.
    l. of flocculation
    l. of perception
    saturation l.
limitans
limitation
    eccentric l.
limit dextrinase
limitrophic
limonene

limophthisis
limosis
limp
limulus lysate test
lindane
Lindau
    disease
    tumor
Lindau-von Hippel disease
Lindbergh pump
Lindblom position
Lindemann method
Lindeman-Silverstein tube
Linder sign
Lindner
    bodies
    operation
    spatula
line
    abdominal l.
    accretion l's
    acetabular l.
    adrenal l.
    ala-tragal l.
    Aldrich-Mees l's
    alveolobasilar l.
    Amberg lateral sinus l.
    l. of Amici
    angular l.
    anococcygeal l., white
    anocutaneous l.
    anorectal l.
    anterior axillary l.
    anterior humeral l.
    arcuate l. of ilium
    arcuate l. of innominate bone
    arcuate l. of occipital bone
    arcuate l. of pelvis
    arcuate l. of sheath of rectus
      abdominis muscle
    arterial l.
    atropic l.
    auricular l.
    auriculobregmatic l.
    axial l.
    axillary l.
    l's of Baillarger
    base l.
    base-apex l.
    basinasal l.
    basiobregmatic l.
    Baudelocque l.
    Beau l.
    biauricular l.
    biiliac l.

line *(continued)*
    bismuth l.
    blood l.
    blue l.
    Brödel (Broedel) bloodless l.
    Brödel (Broedel) white l.
    Brücke l's
    Bryant l.
    Burton l.
    calcification l's
    Camper l.
    canthomeatal l.
    cell l.
    cement l.
    cervical l.
    Chamberlain l.
    Clapton l.
    clavicular l.
    cleavage l's
    Conradi l.
    contour l.
    Converse l.
    copper l.
    Correra l.
    Corrigan l.
    costoarticular l.
    costoclavicular l.
    costophrenic septal l's
    Crampton l.
    crease l.
    cricoclavicular l.
    crinkle l.
    cruciate l.
    curved l. of ilium
    curved l. of occipital bone
    Czermak l's
    Daubenton l.
    l. of demarcation
    dentate l.
    dependency l.
    De Salle l.
    developmental l's
    division l.
    Dobie l.
    dominant l.
    l. of Douglas
    Duhot l.
    dynamic facial l.
    Eberth l's
    l's of Ebner
    ectental l.
    Egger l.
    elastic l.
    election l.
    epiphyseal l.

L

line *(continued)*

l's of expression
expression folds l.
external oblique l.
facial l.
Farre white l.
Feiss l.
finish l.
fissural l.
l. of fixation
Fleischner l.
flexion l.
flexure l.
focal l., anterior
focal l., posterior
force l.
Fränkel l.
Frommann l's
fulcrum l., retentive
fulcrum l., stabilizing
Futcher l.
Gant l.
gas density l.
genal l.
l. of Gennari
germ l.
gingival l.
gluteal l.
Gottinger l.
grain l.
Granger l.
gravitational l.
gray l.
growth arrest l.
Gubler l.
gum l.
Haller l.
Hampton l.
Harris l's
health l.
heave l.
Helmholtz l.
Hensen l.
Hilgenreiner l.
Hilton white l.
Holden l.
hot l.
Hudson l.
Hudson-Stähli (Staehli) l.
Hueter l.
Hunter l.
iliopectineal l.
l. imaging
imbrication l's of cementum
imbrication l's of Pickerill

line *(continued)*

increased tension l.
incremental l's
incremental l's of cementum
incremental l's of Ebner
inflating l.
infracostal l.
infraorbital l.
infrascapular l.
intercondylar l.
intercondyloid l.
intermediate l. of iliac crest
interorbital l.
interpupillary l.
interspinal l.
intertrochanteric l.
intertuberal l.
intertubercular l.
intraperiod l's
isoeffect l's
isoelectric l.
Jadelot l's
junction l.
l. of Kaes
Kanavel l.
Kazanjian l.
Kazanjian and Converse l.
Kerley A l's
Kerley B l's
Kilian l.
Kocher l.
Krause l.
labial l.
Lanz l.
lateral l.
lateral sinus l.
lateral sternal l.
lead l.
Lewis l.
lip l., high
lip l., low
Lorentzian l.
lower lung l.
magnetic l's of force
major dense l's
major period l's
mammary l.
mammillary l.
maximal tension l.
McGregor l.
McKee l.
median l.
median axillary l.
medioclavicular l.
Mees l's

line *(continued)*

 mercurial l.
 mesenteric l.
 Meyer l.
 midaxillary l.
 midclavicular l.
 middle l. of scrotum
 midspinal l.
 midsternal l.
 milk l.
 l's of minimal tension
 minimum extensibility l.
 Monro l.
 Monro-Richter l.
 Morgan l.
 Moyer l.
 mucogingival l.
 Muercke l's
 muscular l's of scapula
 mylohyoidean l.
 mylohyoid l. of mandible
 nasal l.
 nasobasal l.
 nasobasilar l.
 nasolabial l.
 nasosubnasal l.
 natural l.
 Nélaton l.
 neonatal l.
 nigra l.
 nipple l.
 nuchal l.
 Obersteiner-Redlich l.
 oblique l. of femur
 oblique l. of fibula
 oblique l. of mandible
 oblique l. of radius
 oblique l. of thyroid cartilage
 oblique l. of tibia
 obturator l.
 l. of occlusion
 oculozygomatic l.
 Ogston l.
 omphalospinous l.
 orthostatic l.
 Ouchterlony l.
 l's of Owen
 papillary l.
 pararectal l.
 parasternal l.
 paravertebral l.
 Pastia l's
 pectinate l.
 pectineal l.
 pelvic pain l.

line *(continued)*

 period l's
 Pickerill imbrication l's
 pigmented l. of the cornea
 pleuroesophageal l.
 Poirier l.
 popliteal l. of femur
 popliteal l. of tibia
 postaxillary l.
 posterior axillary l.
 Poupart l.
 preaxillary l.
 precentral l.
 primitive l.
 profile l.
 protrusive l.
 pubococcygeal l.
 pupillary l.
 pure l.
 quadrate l.
 radial longitudinal l.
 recessional l's
 regression l.
 Reid base l.
 relaxed skin tension l's
 Retzius l's
 Richter-Monro l.
 Robson l.
 Rolando l.
 Roser l.
 rough l.
 rough l. of femur
 Salter incremental l's
 scan l.
 l. scanning
 scapular l.
 Schoemaker l.
 l's of Schreger
 Schwalbe l.
 segmental l's
 semicircular l. of Douglas
 semicircular l. of frontal bone
 semicircular l. of occipital bone
 semicircular l. of parietal bone
 semicircular l's, supreme
 semilunar l. of Spieghel
 septal l.
 Sergent white adrenal l.
 Shenton l.
 l. of sight
 simian l.
 Skinner l.
 soleal l. of tibia
 Spieghel l.
 spigelian l., Spigelius l.

L

line *(continued)*
   spiral l. of femur
   Stähli (Staehli) pigment l.
   Stark l.
   sternal l.
   sternomastoid l.
   subcostal l.
   subscapular l's
   superficial l. of the cornea
   supracondylar l. of femur
   l. supracondylaris lateralis
     femoris
   l. supracondylaris medialis
     femoris
   supracrestal l.
   supraorbital l.
   survey l.
   suture l.
   Sydney l.
   sylvian l.
   temporal l.
   temporal l. of frontal bone
   temporal l. of parietal bone
   tension l.
   terminal l. of pelvis
   Terry l.
   Thompson l.
   thyroid red l.
   l. of Toldt, white l. of Toldt
   Topinard l.
   tram l's
   transverse l's of sacral bone
   transverse l. of sacrum
   trapezoid l.
   triradiate l's
   Trümmerfeld l.
   type l.
   Ullmann l.
   umbilicoiliac l.
   l. of Venus
   vertebral l.
   Veslingius l.
   vibrating l.
   Virchow l.
   visual l.
   Voigt l's
   Wagner l.
   Webster l.
   Weiger l.
   white l.
   white adrenal l.
   white l. of Brödel (Broedel)
   white l. of Fränkel
   white l. of ischiococcygeal
     muscle

line *(continued)*
   white l. of pelvic fascia
   white l. of pelvis
   white l. of pharynx
   white l. of Toldt
   l. width
   Wimberger l.
   working l.
   wrinkle l.
   Wrisberg l's
   Y l.
   Z l.
   l's of Zahn
   Zöllner l's.
linea (lineae)
   l. alba abdominis
   l. alba cervicalis
   lineae albicantes
   l. anocutanea
   l. anorectalis
   l. arcuata ossis ilii
   l. arcuata vaginae musculi
     recti abdominis
   l. aspera
   l. axillaris anterior
   l. axillaris media
   l. axillaris posterior
   l. epiphysialis
   l. glutea anterior
   l. glutea inferior
   l. glutea posterior
   l. iliopectinea
   l. innominata
   l. intercondylaris
   l. intercondyloidea
   l. intermedia cristae iliacae
   l. intertrochanterica posterior
   l. mammillaris
   l. mediana anterior
   l. mediana posterior
   l. medioaxillaris
   l. medioclavicularis
   lineae musculares scapulae
   l. musculi solei
   l. mylohyoidea mandibulae
   l. nigra
   l. nuchalis inferior
   l. nuchalis superior
   l. nuchalis suprema
   l. obliqua cartilaginis
     thyroideae
   l. obliqua fibulae
   l. obliqua mandibulae
   l. obliqua tibiae
   l. pararectalis

line *(continued)*
- l. parasternalis
- l. paravertebralis
- l. pectinata
- l. pectinea
- l. poplitea tibiae
- l. postaxillaris
- l. preaxillaris
- l. scapularis
- l. semicircularis Douglasi
- l. semilunaris (Spigeli)
- l. spiralis
- l. splendens
- l. sternalis
- l. supracondylaris lateralis
- l. supracondylaris medialis
- l. temporalis inferior ossis parietalis
- l. temporalis ossis frontalis
- l. temporalis superior ossis parietalis
- l. terminalis pelvis
- lineae transversae ossis sacri
- l. trapezoidea
- l. vertebralis

lineage
- cell l.
- sympathetic cell l.

lineal

linear
- l. attenuation
- l. focus
- l. incision
- l. osteotomy
- l. proctotomy
- l. tomography

liner
- cavity l.
- soft l.

Lineweaver-Burk
- equation
- plot

lingua (linguae)
- l. cerebelli
- l. dissecta
- l. fissurata
- l. frenata
- l. geographica
- l. nigra
- l. plicata
- l. villosa nigra

lingual

linguale

lingualis

lingually

linguiform

linguistic deficit

lingula (lingulae)
- l. cerebelli
- l. of cerebellum
- l. of left lung
- l. of lower jaw
- l. of mandible
- l. mandibulae
- l. pulmonis sinistri
- l. of sphenoid
- sphenoidal l.
- l. of sphenoidalis

lingular
- l. infiltrates

lingulate

lingulectomy

linguoaxial

linguoaxiogingival

linguocervical

linguodental

linguodistal

linguogingival

linguoincisal

linguomesial

linguo-occlusal

linguopapillitis

linguoplacement

linguoplate
- palatal l.

linguopulpal

linguoversion

liniment

linin

lining
- soft l.

linitis plastica

link

linkage
- sex l.
- Y l.

linked

linoleic acid

linolein

linolenic acid

linseed

Linser method

lint

lintin

Linton
- clamp
- hook
- incision
- lipectomy
- operation

L

Linton *(continued)*
>   retractor
>   tube
Linzenmeier test
lip
>   acetabular l.
>   anterior l. of cervix of uterus
>   anterior l. of ostium of uterus
>   anterior l. of pharyngeal
>   opening of auditory tube
>   articular l.
>   cleft l.
>   double l.
>   external l. of iliac crest
>   external l. of linea aspera of
>   femur
>   fibrocartilaginous l. of
>   acetabulum
>   glenoid l. of articulation of hip
>   glenoid l. of articulation of
>   humerus
>   greater l. of pudendum
>   Hapsburg l.
>   inferior l.
>   inferior l. of ileocecal valve
>   internal l. of iliac crest
>   lateral l. of linea aspera of
>   femur
>   lesser l. of pudendum
>   lower l.
>   medial l. of linea aspera of
>   femur
>   posterior l. of cervix of uterus
>   posterior l. of ostium of
>   uterus
>   posterior l. of pharyngeal
>   opening of auditory tube
>   rhombic l.
>   superior l. of ileocecal valve
>   tapir l's
>   tympanic l. of limb of spiral
>   lamina
>   upper l.
>   vestibular l. of limb of spiral
>   lamina
LIP—lymphocytic interstitial
>   pneumonitis
lipacidemia
lipaciduria
lipase
>   acid l.
>   hepatic l.
>   lingual l.
>   pancreatic l.
lipasuria

lipectomy
>   abdominal l.
>   aspiration l.
>   circumferential belt l.
>   Linton l.
>   submental l.
>   suction l., suction-assisted l.
>   total-block l.
lipedema
lipemia
>   alimentary l.
>   diabetic l.
>   postprandial l.
>   l. retinalis
lipemic
lipid
>   l. A
>   Gaucher l.
>   Niemann-Pick l.
>   skin surface l.
lipidemia
lipidic
lipidolysis
lipidolytic
lipidosis (lipidoses)
>   cerebral l.
>   cerebroside l.
>   galactosylceramide l.
>   ganglioside l.
>   glucosylceramide l.
>   hereditary dystopic l.
>   neurovisceral l.
>   sphingomyelin l.
>   sulfatide l.
lipiduria
lipoadenoma
lipoamide reductase
lipoarthritis
lipoatrophy
>   insulin l.
lipoblast
lipoblastoma
lipoblastomatosis
lipocardiac
lipocatabolic
lipochondroma
lipochrome
lipochromemia
lipochromogen
lipocyanine
lipocyte
lipodermatosclerosis
lipodystrophy
>   acquired generalized l.
>   acquired partial l.

lipodystrophy *(continued)*
  cephalothoracic l.
  congenital generalized l.
  congenital progressive l.
  familial l. of limbs and trunks
  generalized l.
  inferior l.
  insulin l.
  intestinal l.
  partial l.
  progressive l.
  progressive congenital l.
  progressive partial l.
  reverse partial l.
  total l.
  total l. and acromegaloid
    gigantism
lipoferous
lipofibroma
lipofuscin
lipofuscinosis
  infantile neuronal ceroid l.
  juvenile neuronal ceroid l.
lipogenesis
lipogenic
lipogenous
lipogranuloma
lipogranulomatosis
  Farber l.
  l. subcutanea
lipohemarthrosis
lipohistiodieresis
lipohyalin
lipohyalinosis
lipohypertrophy
  insulin l.
lipoic acid
lipoid
  anisotropic l.
  Forssman l.
  l. nephrosis
  l. proteinosis
lipoidosis
  arterial l.
  cerebroside l.
  cholesterol l.
  l. cutis et mucosae
  Erdheim-Chester l.
  pulmonary l.
  renal l.
lipolytic
lipoma
  l. annulare colli
  l. arborescens
  calcified l.

lipoma *(continued)*
  l. capsulare
  l. cavernosum
  chondroid l.
  l. of corpus callosum
  diffuse l.
  diffuse symmetrical l's of neck
  l. diffusum renis
  l. dolorosa
  epidural l.
  fat cell l., fetal
  l. fibrosum
  intermuscular l.
  intradural l.
  intramedullary l.
  intramuscular l.
  intraspinal l.
  l. myxomatodes
  nevoid l.
  l. ossificans
  ossifying l.
  pleomorphic l.
  renal l.
  l. sarcomatodes
  l. of spermatic cord
  spinal l.
  spindle cell l.
  telangiectatic l.
  l. telangiectodes
lipomatoid
lipomatosis
  l. atrophicans
  congenital l. of pancreas
  diffuse l.
  l. dolorosa
  l. gigantea
  medullary l.
  l. neurotica
  nodular circumscribed l.
  renal l.
  l. renis
  replacement l. of kidney
  symmetrical l.
lipomatous
lipomeningocele
lipomeria
lipometabolic
lipometabolism
lipopathy
lipopectic
lipopenia
lipopenic
lipopexia
lipophage
lipophagia granulomatosis

L

lipophanerosis
lipophil
lipophilia
lipophilic
lipophilin
lipophore
lipoplastic
lipoplasty
lipopolysaccharide
lipoprotein
    α-l., alpha l.
    l. (a), Lp(a)
    β-l., beta l.
    familial l. deficiency
    familial high-density l. (HDL)
      deficiency
    high-density l. (HDL)
    intermediate-density l. (IDL)
    l. lipase (LPL)
    l. lipase (LPL) deficiency,
      familial
    low-density l. (LDL)
    Lp(a) l.
    l. metabolism
    plasma l.
    very high-density l. (VHDL)
    very low-density l. (VLDL)
    l. X
lipoproteinemia
liposarcoma
    dedifferentiated l.
    myxoid l.
    pleomorphic l.
    round cell l.
    well-differentiated l.
liposoluble
liposome
liposuction
lipoteichoic acid
lipothymia
lipotroph
lipotrophic
lipotrophy
lipotropic
β-lipotropin [beta-]
γ-lipotropin [gamma-]
lipotropism
lipovaccine
lipovitellin
lipoxanthine
lipoxygenase
Lippes loop IUD
lipping
lippitude
Lippman prosthesis

lip-print
Lipschütz (Lipschuetz)
    bodies
    cell
    disease
    erythema
    ulcer
liquefacient
liquefaction
    gas l.
liquefactive
liquefy
liquescent
liquid
    Altmann l.
    l. crystal thermography
      (LCT)
    Fleming l.
    gas-l. chromatography (GLC)
    high-performance l.
      chromatography (HPLC)
    high-pressure l.
      chromatography (HPLC)
    Müller l.
    Thoma l.
liquiform
liquor (liquors, liquores)
    l. amnii
    l. carbonis detergens (LCD)
    l. cerebrospinalis
    l. chorii
    l. entericus
    l. folliculi
    l. gastricus
    mother l.
    l. pancreaticus
    l. puris
    l. of Scarpa
    l. seminis
liquorice
LIS—lobular in situ
Lisfranc
    amputation
    joint
    ligament
    operation
    tubercle
lisp
lisping
Lissauer
    column
    marginal zone
    paralysis
    tract
    zone

lissencephaly
lissive
list
listening
    dichotic l.
Lister
    dressing
    forceps
    scissors
Lister-Burch speculum
Listeria monocytogenes
listerial
listeriosis
Liston
    knife
    operation
    splint
Liston-Stille forceps
liter (L)
lithate
lithiasic
lithiasis
    appendicular l.
    biliary l.
    cholecystic l.
    l. conjunctivae
    l. conjunctivitis
    gallbladder l.
    pancreatic l.
    renal l.
    urinary l.
lithic
lithic acid
lithium (Li)
lithocholate
lithocholic acid
lithocholylglycine
lithocholyltaurine
lithoclast
lithogenesis
lithogenic
lithogenous
lithokelyphopedion
lithokelyphos
litholapaxy
litholysis
litholytic
lithonephritis
lithopedion
lithotomy
    bilateral l.
    dorsal l. position
    high l.
    lateral l.
    median l.

lithotomy *(continued)*
    mediolateral l.
    perineal l.
    l. position
    prerectal l.
    rectal l.
    rectovesical l.
    suprapubic l.
    vaginal l.
    vesicovaginal l.
lithotresis
    ultrasonic l.
lithotripsy
    electrohydraulic l.
    extracorporeal shock wave l.
     (ESWL)
    laser l.
    pneumatic l.
    ultrasonic l.
lithotriptic
lithotriptor
    Dornier gallstone l.
lithotrite
    Alcock l.
    Alcock-Hendrickson l.
    Bigelow l.
    cystoscopic l.
    electrohydraulic l.
    Hendrickson l.
    Keyes l.
    Lowsley l.
    Thompson l.
lithotrity
lithotroph
litmus
Littauer
    forceps
    scissors
Littauer-Liston forceps
Litten
    diaphragm
     phenomenon
    diaphragm sign
litter
Little [eponym]
    area
    disease
    intraocular lens (IOL)
     implant
    paralysis
    retractor
Littler operation
Littlewood operation
Littré (Littre)
    crypts

L

Littré (Littre) *(continued)*
  glands
  hernia
  suture
Littré-Richter hernia
littritis
Litwak scissors
Litzmann obliquity
Livaditis circular myotomy
live-born
livedo
  cutaneous l.
  generalized l.
  necrotic l.
  l. racemosa
  l. reticularis, idiopathic
  l. reticularis,
    symptomatic
livedoid
liver
  albuminoid l.
  amyloid l.
  biliary cirrhotic l.
  brimstone l.
  bronze l.
  cirrhotic l.
  degraded l.
  desiccated l.
  l. dysfunction
  fatty l.
  l. flap
  floating l.
  foamy l.
  frosted l.
  l. function test (LFT)
  hobnail l.
  icing l.
  infantile l.
  iron l.
  lardaceous l.
  nutmeg l.
  pigmented l.
  polycystic l.
  sago l.
  l. scan
  l. span
  stasis l.
  sugar-icing l.
  wandering l.
  waxy l.
livetin
livid
lividity
  cadaveric l.
  postmortem l.

Livierato
  reflex
  test
livor (livores)
  l. mortis
lixiviation
lixivium
LK—left kidney
LKP—lamellar keratoplasty
LL—
  left leg
  left lower
  left lung
  lower lobe
LLC—long leg cast
LLE—left lower extremity
LLL—left lower lobe
Lloyd
  catheter
  sign
  syndrome
LLQ—left lower quadrant
LLS—lazy leukocyte syndrome
LM—
  light microscopy
  linguomesial
LMA—left mentoanterior (position)
LMD—local medical doctor
LMP—
  last menstrual period
  left mentoposterior (position)
LMR—localized magnetic
  resonance
LMT—left mentotransverse
  (position)
LMWD—low-molecular-weight
  dextran
LN—
  lipoid nephrosis
  lupus nephritis
  lymph node
LNMP—last normal menstrual
  period
LNPF—lymph node permeability
  factor
LO—linguo-occlusal
Loa loa
LOA—
  leave of absence
  left occipitoanterior (position)
load
  filtered l.
  genetic l.
  mutational l.
  occlusal l.

loading
    carbohydrate l.
    l. dose
LOAEL—lowest observed adverse
  effect level
lobar
    l. atelectasis
    l. pneumonia
lobate
lobation
    renal l.
lobe
    ansiform l.
    anterior l. of hypophysis
    anterior l. of pituitary gland
    appendicular l.
    azygos l.
    caudate l. of cerebrum
    caudate l. of liver
    l's of cerebellum
    l's of cerebrum
    crescentic l. of cerebellum
    cuneate l.
    cuneiform l.
    flocculonodular l.
    frontal l.
    gracile l. of cerebellum
    grand l. limbique of Broca
    hepatic l's
    Home l.
    inferior crescentic l. of
      cerebellum
    inferior l. of left lung
    inferior l. of right lung
    lateral l's of prostate gland
    left lower l. (LLL)
    left upper l. (LUL)
    limbic l.
    linguiform l.
    l's of liver
    lower l. of lung
    l's of mammary gland
    median l. of prostate
    middle l. of right lung
    neural l. of hypophysis
    neural l. of neurohypophysis
    neural l. of pituitary gland
    occipital l.
    olfactory l.
    optic l's
    parietal l.
    piriform l.
    l's of placenta
    polyalveolar l.
    posterior l. of hypophysis

lobe *(continued)*
    posterior l. of pituitary gland
    l's of prostate
    pulmonary l's
    pyramidal l. of thyroid gland
    pyriform l.
    quadrangular l. of cerebellum
    quadrate l. of cerebral
      hemisphere
    quadrate l. of liver
    renal l's
    Riedel l.
    right lower l. (RLL)
    right upper l. (RUL)
    semilunar l's
    side l.
    spigelian l.
    superior crescentic l. of
      cerebellum
    superior l. of left lung
    superior l. of right lung
    temporal l.
    temporosphenoidal l. of
      cerebral hemisphere
    l's of thymus
    l's of thyroid gland
    upper l. of lung
    vagal l.
    vermiform l.
    visceral l.
lobectomy
    occipital l.
    sleeve l.
    temporal l.
    thoracoscopic l.
    thyroid l.
    VATS (video-assisted thoracic
      surgery) l.
α-lobeline [alpha-]
lobi (genitive and plural of lobus)
lobite
lobitis
Lobo disease
lobomycosis
lobotomy
    frontal l.
    prefrontal l.
    transorbital l.
    traumatic l.
Lobstein
    disease
    ganglion
    syndrome
lobular
lobulated

L

lobulation
  fetal l.
  portal l.
lobule
  ansiform l.
  anterior l. of pituitary gland
  anterior lunate l.
  l. of auricle
  l. of azygos vein
  biventral l.
  central l. of cerebellum
  cerebellar l.
  cortical l's of kidney
  digastric l.
  ear l.
  l's of epididymis
  floccular l.
  fusiform l.
  glandular l.
  glomerular l.
  gracile l.
  hepatic l's
  l's of liver
  l's of lung
  l's of mammary gland
  l. of pancreas
  paracentral l.
  paramedian l.
  parietal l., inferior
  parietal l., superior
  portal l.
  posteromedian l.
  primary l. of lung
  pulmonary l's
  quadrangular l. of
    cerebellum
  quadrate l.
  renal l.
  respiratory l.
  secondary l. of lung
  semilunar l., caudal
  semilunar l., cranial
  semilunar l., inferior
  semilunar l., superior
  spermatic l's
  l. of testis
  l's of thymus
  l's of thyroid gland
lobulette
lobulose
lobulus (lobuli)
  l. auriculae, l. auricularis
  l. biventer cerebelli
  l. centralis cerebelli
  lobuli corticales renis

lobulus (lobuli) *(continued)*
  lobuli epididymidis
  lobuli glandulae mammariae
  lobuli glandulae thyroideae
  l. gracilis cerebelli
  lobuli hepatis
  lobuli mammae
  l. paracentralis
  l. paramedianus cerebelli
  l. parietalis inferior
  l. parietalis superior
  l. quadrangularis anterior
    cerebelli
  l. quadrangularis posterior
    cerebelli
  l. semilunares
  l. semilunaris caudalis
  l. semilunaris inferior
  l. semilunaris rostralis
  l. semilunaris superior
  l. simplex cerebelli
  lobuli testis
  lobuli thymi
lobus (lobi)
  l. anterior cerebelli
  l. anterior hypophyseos
  l. caudalis cerebelli
  l. caudatus hepatis
  l. caudatus Spigeli
  l. cerebelli anterior
  lobi cerebrales
  lobi cerebri
  l. cranialis cerebelli
  l. flocculonodularis
  l. frontalis
  lobi glandulae mammariae
  l. glandulae thyroideae
  l. hepatis dexter
  l. hepatis sinister
  l. inferior pulmonis dextri
  l. inferior pulmonis sinistri
  l. insularis
  lobi mammae
  l. medius prostatae
  l. medius pulmonis dextri
  l. nervosus
    neurohypophyseos
  l. occipitalis
  l. olfactorius
  l. parietalis
  lobi placentae
  l. posterior cerebelli
  l. posterior hypophyseos
  l. posterior hypophysis
  lobi prostatae dexter et sinister

lobus (lobi) *(continued)*
 l. pyramidalis glandulae thyroideae
 l. quadratus hepatis
 lobi renales
 l. rostralis cerebelli
 l. spigelii
 l. superior pulmonis dextri
 l. superior pulmonis sinistri
 l. temporalis
 l. thymi dexter et sinister
 l. vagi
local
localization
 cerebral l.
 germinal l.
 pneumotaxic l.
 precise l.
 selective l.
 spatial l.
 tumor l.
localized
localizer
locator
 abutment l.
 apex l.
 Berman-Moorhead l.
 electroacoustic l.
 Moorehead foreign body l.
lochia
 l. alba
 l. cruenta
 l. rubra
 l. sanguinolenta
 l. serosa
lochial
lochiocolpos
lochiocyte
lochiometra
lochiometritis
lochiorrhea
lochioschesis
lochiostasis
lock
 bite l., bitelock, bite-lock
 friction l.
 transfer l.
Locke
 fluid
 solution
Locke-Ringer solution
locking
 head l.
 l. suture
lockjaw

lock-stitch suture
Lockwood
 clamp
 forceps
 ligament
 tendon
locomotion
 brachial l.
 fictive l.
locomotive
locomotor
locomotorial
locomotorium
locomotory
locular
loculate
loculated pleural effusion
loculation
loculus (loculi)
locum
 l. tenens
 l. tenent
locus (loci)
 l. caeruleus, l. ceruleus
 complex l.
 l. ferrugineus
 l. of HLA (human leukocyte antigen)
 minor histocompatibility l.
 l. minoris resistentiae
 l. niger
 operator l.
 l. perforatus anticus
 l. perforatus posticus
 PTC (phenylthiocarbamide) l.
 l. ruber
 T l.
LOD—line of duty
Loeb
 deciduoma
 reaction
LOEL—lowest observed effect level
Loenen sign
Loevit cell
Loewi
 reaction
 symptom
Löffler (Loeffler)
 agar
 blood serum
 culture medium
 disease
 endocarditis
 eosinophilia
 pneumonia

L

Löffler (Loeffler) *(continued)*
    stain
    suture
    syndrome
logadectomy
logamnesia
Logan bow
logaphasia
loge de Guyon
logic
logoclonia
logomania
logopathy
logoplegia
logorrhea
    jargon aphasic l.
logospasm
Löhlein
    operation
    diameter
    nephritis
loiasis
loin
LOM—
    limitation of motion
    loss of motion
Lombard test
Lombard-Boies rongeur
Long
    coefficient
    forceps
    formula
longevity
longilineal
longimanous
longipedate
Long Island forceps
longissimus
longitudinal
    l. incision
    l. magnetization
    l. relaxation
    l. section tomography
    l. suture
    l. suture of palate
longitudinalis
longitypical
long leg brace
long tract signs
longus
loop
    afferent l.
    Axenfeld nerve l.
    Bricker l.
    Cannon endarterectomy l.

loop *(continued)*
    capillary l's
    C l. of duodenum
    cervical l.
    closed l.
    Cordonnier ureteroileal l.
    cutting l.
    efferent l.
    gamma l.
    Gerdy interatrial l.
    Granit l.
    Henle l., l. of Henle
    l. of hypoglossal nerve
    Hyrtl l.
    intestinal l.
    jejunal l.
    lenticular l.
    Lippes l. IUD
    Meyer l.
    nephronic l.
    l.-on mucosa suture
    open l.
    P l.
    l. of the pectoral nerves
    peduncular l.
    platinum l.
    QRS l.
    l. of recurrent laryngeal nerve
    regulatory feedback l.
    Roux-en-Y l.
    sentinel l.
    Silastic l's
    l's of spinal nerves
    Stoerck l.
    subclavian l.
    l. suture
    terminal ileal l.
    ventricular l.
    l. of Vieussens
loopful
loopogram
loose bodies
loosening of associations
Looser transformation zones
Looser-Milkman syndrome
LOP—left occipitoposterior (position)
lophophorine
LOQ—lower outer quadrant
loquacious
Lorain
    disease
    infantilism
Lorain-Levi dwarf
Lord operation
lordoscoliosis

lordosis
    compensatory l.
    dorsal l.
lordotic
    anteroposterior l. projection
    apical l. projection
Lore-Lawrence tube
Lorentzian line
Lorenz
    operation
    osteotomy
    position
    sign
Lortat-Jacobs disease
loss
    autoimmune sensorineural
        hearing l.
    birth l.
    conductive hearing l.
    congenital hearing l.
    dissociated sensory l.
    hearing l.
    noise-induced hearing l.
    nonorganic hearing l.
    ototoxic hearing l.
    profound hearing l.
    saddle sensory l.
    sensorineural hearing l.
LOT—left occipitotransverse
    (position)
Lotheissen operation
Lotheissen-McVay technique
Lothrop
    knife
    retractor
lotion
    hydrocortisone l.
    lindane l.
    nystatin l.
    selenium sulfide l.
Lottes
    nail
    operation
loudness
Louis angle
Louis-Bar
    disease
    syndrome
Louisiana pneumonia
Lounsbury curet
loupe
    corneal l.
louse (lice)
    biting l.
    body l.

louse (lice) *(continued)*
    clothes l.
    crab l.
    head l.
    pubic l.
Love retractor
Love-Adson elevator
Love-Gruenwald
    forceps
    rongeur
Love-Kerrison forceps
Lovelace forceps
Loven reflex
Lovset maneuver
Low-Beers projection
LowBI—low-birthweight infant
low-cervical cesarean section
low-density lipoprotein (LDL)
Löwe
    disease
    ring
    syndrome
Löwenberg (Lowenberg)
    canal
    forceps
    scala
    sign
    test
Löwenstein (Lowenstein,
    Loewenstein)
    climbing pupil
    descending pupil
    low-intensity reaction
    medium
Löwenstein-Jensen agar
Lower [eponym]
    forceps
    rings
    tubercle
lowering
    vapor pressure l.
Lowman
    balance board
    clamp
Lown-Ganong-Levine syndrome
Lown and Woolf method
low-osmolar contrast media
    (LOCM)
Lowsley
    forceps
    lithotrite
    operation
    tractor
Lowsley-Peterson cystoscope
low-spin

L

loxarthron
loxia
Loxosceles reclusa
loxoscelism
    viscerocutaneous l.
loxotomy
lozenge
LP—
    latency period
    leukocyte-poor
    light perception
    linguopulpal
    lipoprotein
    lumbar puncture
LPA—left pulmonary artery
LPE—lipoprotein electrophoresis
LPF—
    localized plaque formation
    low-power field
LPL—lipoprotein lipase
lpm—liter(s) per minute
LPN—licensed practical nurse
LPO—
    left posterior oblique
      (projection)
    light perception only
LPS—lipopolysaccharide
LPV—left pulmonary vein
LR—
    lactated Ringer
    light reaction
L/R—left-to-right ratio
L&R—left and right
LRQ—lower right quadrant
LRS—lactated Ringer solution
LRT—lower respiratory tract
LS—
    left side
    legally separated
    liver and spleen
    lumbosacral
L/S—lecithin-sphingomyelin
    (ratio)
LSA—left sacroanterior (position)
LSB—left sternal border
LScA—left scapuloanterior (position)
LScP—left scapuloposterior
    (position)
LSCS—lower segment cesarean
    section
LSD—lysergic acid diethylamide
LSH—lutein-stimulating hormone
LSM—late systolic murmur
LSO—lumbosacral orthosis
LSP—left sacroposterior (position)

LST—left sacrotransverse (position)
LSV—left subclavian vein
lt—left
LT—
    left thigh
    leukotriene
    levothyroxine
    long-term
    lymphotoxin
LTB—laryngotracheobronchitis
LTB_4, LTC_4, etc.—symbols for
    various leukotrienes
LTF—lymphocyte-transforming
    factor
LTH—
    lactogenic hormone
    luteotropic hormone
LTPP—lipothiamide pyrophosphate
LU—left upper
L&U—lower and upper
lubb-dupp
lubricant
Luc
    forceps
    operation
Lucae
    forceps
    mallet
Lucas
    groove
    sign
Lucas-Championnière disease
Lucas-Cottrell operation
lucent defect
lucid
lucidity
luciferase
luciferin
lucifugal
Lucio
    leprosy
    phenomenon
lucipetal
Luck
    fasciatome
    operation
lückenschädel (lueckenschaedel)
Luckett operation
Luder-Sheldon syndrome
Ludloff
    operation
    sign
Ludwig
    angina
    angle

Ludwig *(continued)*
    ganglion
    theory
LUE—left upper extremity
Luer
    forceps
    retractor
    tube
Luer-Korte scoop
lues
Luft
    disease
    syndrome
lug
    occlusal l.
    retention l.
Lugol
    caustic
    solution
    stain
lugubrious
Luhr maxillofacial system
Luikart forceps
Luikart-Bill traction handle
Luikart-Simpson forceps
Lukens
    retractor
    trap
Lukes-Collins classification
LUL—left upper lobe (of lung)
luliberin
lumbar
    l. nephrectomy
    l. sympathectomy
lumbarization
lumboabdominal
lumbocolostomy
lumbocolotomy
lumbocostal
lumbocrural
lumbodorsal
    l. splanchnicectomy
    l. sympathectomy
lumbodynia
lumboiliac
lumboinguinal
lumbosacral
    l. kyphosis
    l. plexus
    l. radiculopathy
    l. spine
lumbrical
lumbus
lumen (lumina)
    arterial l., l. of artery

lumen (lumina) *(continued)*
    dark-l. MR colonography
    double-l. endotracheal tube
    gastric l.
    intestinal l.
    minimal l. diameter
    rectal l.
    residual l.
    uterine l.
    vaginal l.
    vessel l.
lumichrome
lumiflavin
luminal
luminance
luminescence
luminiferous
luminophor
luminous
lumirhodopsin
lumpectomy
lumps
lunar
lunare
lunate bone
lunatomalacia
Lund operation
Lund-Browder burn scale
Lundh meals
lung
    arc welder's l.
    artificial l.
    bird breeders' l.
    bird fanciers' l.
    black l.
    brown l.
    cardiac l.
    coal miners' l.
    l. collapse, collapsed l.
    colliers' l.
    drowned l.
    eosinophilic l.
    farmers' l.
    fibroid l.
    fluid l.
    harvesters' l.
    honeycomb l.
    hyperlucent l.
    iron l.
    l. transplantation
    l. markings
    masons' l.
    miners' l.
    mushroom workers' l.
    pigeon breeders' l.

L

lung *(continued)*
 polycystic l.
 postperfusion l.
 l. root
 shock l.
 silo fillers' l.
 threshers' l.
 traumatic wet l.
 uremic l.
 vanishing l.
 Vietnam l.
 welders' l.
 wet l.
 white l.
lung aggregate reagent
lunula (lunulae)
 lunulae of aortic valve
 lunulae of cusps of aortic valve
 lunulae of cusps of pulmonary
 valve
 l. of nail
 l. of scapula
 lunulae of semilunar valves
 of aorta
 l. unguis
 lunulae of valves of pulmonary
 trunk
 lunulae valvularum
 semilunarium valvae aortae
 lunulae valvularum
 semilunarium valvae trunci
 pulmonalis
Luongo retractor
lupiform
lupoid
lupus
 butterfly rash of l.
 chilblain l., chilblain l.
 erythematosus
 cutaneous l. erythematosus
 discoid l. erythematosus (DLE)
 disseminated follicular l.
 disseminated l. erythematosus
 drug-induced l.
 l. erythematosus (LE)
 l. erythematosus discoides
 l. erythematosus disseminatus
 l. erythematosus profundus
 l. erythematosus tumidus
 l. fibrosus
 hypertrophic l. erythematosus
 laryngeal l.
 l. miliaris disseminatus faciei
 neonatal l.
 l. nephritis

lupus *(continued)*
 l. pernio
 photosensitive l. erythematosus
 l. profundus
 l. sclerosus
 l. serpiginosus
 systemic l. erythematosus
 (SLE)
 transient neonatal systemic l.
 erythematosus
 l. tumidus
 l. vorax
 l. vulgaris
 l. vulgaris fibromatosus
LUQ—left upper quadrant
Luschka
 bursa
 cartilage
 crypts
 cystic gland
 duct
 foramen
 joints
 laryngeal cartilage
 muscle
 nerve
 tonsil
Lust
 phenomenon
 reflex
Lustig-Galeotti vaccine
luteal
luteectomy
lutein
 serum l.
luteinic
luteinization
luteinize
luteinizing hormone (LH)
Lutembacher
 complex
 disease
 syndrome
luteogenic
luteolysin
 uterine l.
luteolysis
luteoma
luteotropic
luteotropin
lutetium (Lu)
luteum
Lutheran blood group
Lutz forceps
Lutz-Miescher disease

Lutz-Splendore-Almeida disease
lux
luxatio
    l. coxae congenita
    l. erecta
    l. imperfecta
    l. perinealis
luxation
    Malgaigne l.
luxuriant
Luys
    body
    body syndrome
    nucleus
    segregator
    separator
LV—
    left ventricle
    leukemia virus
    live virus
LVAD—left ventricular assist device
LVDP—left ventricular diastolic pressure
LVE—left ventricular enlargement
LVEDP—left ventricular end-diastolic pressure
LVEDV—left ventricular end-diastolic volume
LVEF—left ventricular ejection fraction
LVET—left ventricular ejection time
LVF—left ventricular failure
LVH—left ventricular hypertrophy
LVN—licensed vocational nurse
LVP—left ventricular pressure
LVS—left ventricular strain
LVSP—left ventricular systolic pressure
LVSV—left ventricular stroke volume
LVSW—left ventricular stroke work
LVW—left ventricular work
LW—
    lacerating wound
    Lee-White (method)
L&W, L/W—living and well
lyase
Lyb antigens
lycanthropy
lycine
lycopene
lycopenemia

lycoperdonosis
lycorexia
lycorine
Lycosa tarentula
lye
Lyell
    disease
    syndrome
lying
    pathologic l.
lying-in
Lyle syndrome
Lyman-Smith brace
Lyme
    arthritis
    borreliosis
    disease
lymph
    aplastic l.
    corpuscular l.
    croupous l.
    euplastic l.
    fibrinous l.
    inflammatory l.
    intercellular l.
    intravascular l.
    l. node
    l. nodule
    thyroidal l. node scintigraphy
    tissue l.
lympha
lymphaden
lymphadenectasis
lymphadenectomy
lymphadenitis
    acute suppurative l.
    caseous l.
    mesenteric l.
    nonbacterial regional l.
    paratuberculous l.
    regional l.
    tuberculoid l.
    tuberculous l.
    venereal suppurative benign l.
lymphadenocele
lymphadenocyst
lymphadenography
lymphadenoid
lymphadenoleukopoiesis
lymphadenopathy
    angioimmunoblastic l.
    angioimmunoblastic l. with dysproteinemia (AILD)
    dermatopathic l.
    giant follicular l.

L

lymphadenopathy *(continued)*
    immunoblastic l.
    subcarinal l.
    tuberculous l.
lymphadenosis
    acute epidemic l.
    aleukemic l.
    benign l.
    leukemic l.
    malignant l.
lymphadenotomy
lymphadenovarix
lymphagogue
lymphangial
lymphangiectasia
    intestinal l.
lymphangiectasis
    congenital pulmonary l.
    cystic l.
    pericaliceal l.
    pulmonary l.
    l. of the scrotum
lymphangiectatic
lymphangiectodes
lymphangiectomy
lymphangioendothelioma
lymphangiofibroma
lymphangiogram
lymphangiography
    pedal l.
lymphangioma
    capillary l.
    l. cavernosum, cavernous l.
    l. circumscriptum
    cystic l., l. cysticum
    fissural l.
    simple l., l. simplex
lymphangiomatous
lymphangiomyoma
lymphangiomyomatosis
    pulmonary l.
lymphangion
lymphangiophlebitis
lymphangioplasty
    Handley l.
lymphangiosarcoma
lymphangiotomy
lymphangitic sporotrichosis
lymphangitis
    l. carcinomatosa
    carcinomatous l.
    gummatous l.
    nonvenereal sclerosing l.
lymphatic
lymphaticostomy
lymphatitis

lymphatogenous
lymphatolysis
lymphatolytic
lymphectasia
lymphedema
    congenital l.
    filarial l.
    hereditary l. (type I, type II)
    l. praecox
    secondary l.
    l. tarda
lymphenteritis
lymphepithelioma
lymphization
lymphoblast
lymphoblastic
lymphoblastoma
    giant follicular l.
lymphoblastosis
lymphocele
lymphocerastism
lymphocytapheresis
lymphocyte
    l.-activating factor (LAF)
    amplifier T l.
    atypical l.
    B l's
    cytotoxic T l's (CTL)
    Downey-type l.
    educated T l.
    helper T l.
    killer l.
    large granular l's
    plasmacytoid l.
    primed l.
    l. recirculation
    Rieder l.
    small l.
    suppressor T l.
    T l's
    thymus-dependent l's
    thymus-independent l's
    l. transformation
    variant thymus-independent l.
lymphocytic interstitial
  pneumonitis (LIP)
lymphocytoma
    benign cutaneous l.
    l. cutis
lymphocytopenia
lymphocytopoiesis
lymphocytopoietic
lymphocytorrhexis
lymphocytosis
    acute infectious l.
    neutrophilic l.

lymphocytosis *(continued)*
    l.-promoting factor
    relative l.
lymphocytotic
lymphocytotoxicity
lymphocytotoxin
lymphoduct
lymphoepithelioma
lymphogenesis
lymphogenous
lymphoglandula (lymphoglandulae)
lymphogram
lymphogranuloma
    l. benignum
    l. inguinale
    l. malignum
    Schaumann benign l.
    venereal l.
    l. venereum (LGV)
lymphogranulomatosis
    benign l.
    l. cutis
    l. inguinalis
    l. maligna
lymphography
lymphohistiocytic
lymphohistiocytosis
    erythrophagocytic l.
    hemophagocytic l.
lymphoid
lymphoidectomy
lymphokentric
lymphokine
lymphokinesis
lympholysis
    cell-mediated l. (CML)
lympholytic
lymphoma
    adult T-cell leukemia l.
    African l.
    B-cell l.
    Burkitt l.
    centroblastic l.
    centrocytic l.
    convoluted l.
    cutaneous T-cell l.
    l. cutis
    diffuse l.
    fascicular l.
    follicular l.
    follicular center cell l.
    giant follicle l.
    giant follicular l.
    granulomatous l.
    histiocytic l.
    Hodgkin l.

lymphoma *(continued)*
    immunoblastic l.
    intestinal l.
    large cell l.
    Lennert l.
    lymphoblastic l.
    lymphocytic l.
    lymphocytic l. of intermediate
      differentiation
    lymphocytic l., plasmacytoid
    lymphocytic l., poorly
      differentiated
    lymphocytic l., well-
      differentiated
    lymphoepithelioid cell l.
    lymphoplasmacytic l.
    malignant l.
    Mediterranean l.
    mixed lymphocytic-histiocytic l.
    nodular l.
    non-Hodgkin l.
    null cell–type non-Hodgkin l.
    plasmacytoid lymphocytic l.
    pleomorphic l.
    prolymphocytic l.
    sclerosing l.
    signet-ring cell l.
    small B-cell l.
    stem cell l.
    T-cell l., convoluted
    T-cell l., cutaneous
    T-cell l., small lymphocytic
    testicular l.
    U-cell (undefined) l.
    undifferentiated l.
    well-differentiated l.
lymphomatoid
    l. granulomatosis
    l. papulosis
    l. vasculitis
lymphomatosis
    neural l.
    ocular l.
    osteopetrotic l.
lymphomatosum
    papillary adenocystoma l.
lymphomatous
lymphomyxoma
lymphonodulus (lymphonoduli)
    lymphonoduli splenici
lymphonodus (lymphonodi)
lymphopathia
    l. venerea
    l. venereum
lymphopathy
    ataxic l.

L

lymphopenia
lymphoplasia
    cutaneous l.
lymphoplasm
lymphoplasmapheresis
lymphopoiesis
lymphopoietic
lymphopoietin
lymphoproliferative disorder
lymphoreticular disorder
lymphoreticulosis
    benign l.
lymphorrhage
lymphorrhea
lymphorrhoid
lymphosarcoleukemia
lymphosarcoma
    fascicular l.
    lymphocytic l.
    Murphy-Sturm l.
    poorly differentiated l.
    sclerosing l.
lymphosarcomatosis
lymphosarcomatous
lymphoscintigraphy
    radiocolloid l.
lymphostasis
lymphotaxis
lymphotism
lymphotoxic
lymphotoxin
lymphotrophy
lymphotropic
lymphous
lymphs—lymphocytes
Lynch
    dissector
    forceps
    incision
    knife
    laryngoscope
    operation
    scissors
lyochrome
Lyon-Horgan operation
Lyon hypothesis
lyonization
lyonized
Lyon-Russell hypothesis
lyophil
lyophilic
lyophilization
lyophilize
lyophobe
lyophobic

lyosorption
lyotropic
lysate
lyse
lysergic acid diethylamide
    (LSD)
lysin
    beta-l.
    sperm l.
lysine
    l. dehydrogenase
    l. ketoglutarate reductase
    l. ketoglutarate reductase
        deficiency
L-lysine:NAD oxidoreductase
    deficiency
lysinogen
lysinosis
lysis
    bone l.
    hot-cold l.
    immune l.
    osmotic l.
    reactive l.
lysocythin
lysogen
lysogenesis
lysogenic
lysogenicity
lysogenization
lysogeny
lysokinase
lysolecithin
lysophosphatidate
lysophosphatide
lysophosphatidic acid
lysophosphatidylcholine
lysophospholipase
lysophospholipid
lysosomal α-glucosidase deficiency
    [alpha-]
lysosomal storage disease
lysosome
    primary l.
    secondary l.
lysostaphin
lysozyme
lysozymuria
Lyssavirus
lysyl hydroxylase
lysyl oxidase
Lyt antigens
lyterian
lytic
lyxose

μ—
 mu (Greek letter)
 micro-
 micron
m—
 median
 meter
 molar, deciduous
 thousand (L. mil., milli)
M—
 male
 married
 mesial
 mix
 molar, permanent
 month
 mother
 multipara
 murmur
 muscle
 myopia
M.—
 Micrococcus
 Microsporum
 Mycobacterium
 Mycoplasma
M_1—mitral first sound
M_2—mitral second sound
mA—milliampere(s)
MA—
 medical audit
 mental age
 Miller-Abbott (tube)
 moderately advanced
MAA—macroaggregated albumin
MABP—mean arterial blood
  pressure
MAC—
 maximum allowable
   concentration
 minimum alveolar
   concentration
 Mycobacterium avium complex
MacAusland operation
MACC—methotrexate, Adriamycin,
 cyclophosphamide, CCNU
 (lomustine)
MacCallum patch
MacConkey agar
MacDonald clamp
Macdonald index
mace
macerate, macerated
maceration

macerative
Macewen
 operation
 osteotomy
 sign
 triangle
MacFee neck flap
Machado-Joseph disease
machine
 Cybex m.
 heart-lung m.
 panoramic rotating m.
 Stryker Surgilav m.
 Surgitron m.
 Van de Graaff m.
Machover test
MacIntosh
 fiberoptic laryngoscope blade
 laryngoscope
 prosthesis
Mack tonsillectome
MacKay-Marg electronic tonometer
Mackenrodt
 incision
 ligament
 operation
MacKenty
 choanal plug
 elevator
 knife
 tube
Mackenzie
 amputation
 disease
 syndrome
MacLean-Maxwell disease
Macleod
 capsular rheumatism
 syndrome
macradenous
macrencephaly
macroabrasion
macroadenoma
macroaggregate
macroaggregated albumin (MAA)
macroamylase
macroamylasemia
macroamylasemic
macroanalysis
macrobiotic diet
macroblepharia
macrobrachia
macrocardius
macrocephalic

macrocephaly
macrocheilia
macrocheiria
macrochylomicron
macroclitoris
macrocnemia
macrocolon
macrocornea
macrocrania
macrocyst
macrocyte
macrocythemia
    hyperchromatic m.
macrocytic
macrocytosis
macrodactyly
macrodontia
macrodystrophia lipomatosa
macroerythroblast
macroesthesia
macrogenia
macrogenitosomia praecox
macrogingivae
macroglia
macroglial
macroglobulin
    α_2-m. [alpha-2-m.]
macroglobulinemia
    Waldenström m.
macroglossia
macrognathia
macrography
macrogyria
macrolabia
macrolide antibiotic
macrolymphocyte
macromastia
macromelia
macromelus
macromethod
macromineral
macromolecular
macromolecules
macromonocyte
macromyeloblast
macronodular
macronormoblast
macronucleus
macronutrient
macronychia
macro-orchidism
macro-ovalocyte
macroparasite
macropathology
macropenis

macrophage
    activated m.
    alveolar m.
    armed m's
    fixed m.
    free m.
    inflammatory m.
    suppressor m.
    tingible-body m.
macrophagocyte
macrophagocytosis
macrophallus
macrophthalmia
macroplasia
macropolycyte
macroprolactinoma
macropromyelocyte
macroprosopia
macropsia
macrorhinia
macroscopic magnetization vector
macroscopy
macrosigmoid
macrosis
macrosmatic
macrosomatia adiposa congenita
macrosomia
macrospore
macrostereognosia
macrostomia
macrostructural
Macrotec (technetium TC-99m
    albumin aggregated)
macrotia
macrotome
macrotooth (macroteeth)
macula (maculae)
    acoustic maculae, maculae
      acusticae
    m. adherens
    maculae atrophicae
    cerebral m.
    maculae ceruleae
    m. communis
    maculae cribrosae
    m. cribrosa inferior
    m. cribrosa media
    m. cribrosa superior
    m. densa
    false m.
    m. flava laryngis
    m. flava retinae
    m. lutea, m. lutea retinae
    maculae of membranous
      labyrinth

macula (maculae) *(continued)*
    m. retinae
    m. sacculi
    m. utriculi
macular
    cystoid m. edema
    m. degeneration
    m. detachment
    m. displacement
    m. dystrophy
    m. edema
    m. holes
    m. pigmentation
    m. pucker
    m. schisis
    m. sparing
    m. splitting
    m. star
maculate
maculation
macule
    annular m.
    ash-leaf m.
    black m.
    blue-gray m.
    brown-to-black m.
    café au lait m.
    chalky white m.
    coal m.
    dark brown m.
    erythematous m.
    flat m.
    hypopigmented m.
    ivory m.
    lance-ovate m.
    melanotic m.
    pigmented m.
    purple m.
    reddish m.
    smooth m.
    telangiectatic m.
maculocerebral
maculopapular
maculopathy
    age-related m.
    bull's eye m.
    cellophane m.
    crystalline m.
    cystic m.
    diabetic m.
    ischemic m.
    oxalosis m.
    persistent placoid m.
    polymorphous vitelliform m.
madarosis

MADD—multiple acyl CoA
    dehydrogenation deficiency
Madden technique
Maddox
    prism
    rod
    wing
Madelung
    deformity
    disease
    lipoma
    neck
    subluxation
    syndrome
Madlener operation
madness
    myxedema m.
Madura foot
Madurella
    M. grisea
    M. mycetomi
maduromycosis
MAF—macrophage-activating
    factor
Maffucci syndrome
MAFH—macroaggregated ferrous
    hydroxide
mafilcon A hydrophilic contact lens
magenblase
Magendie
    foramen
    law
    sign
    solution
    space
    symptom
Magendie-Hertwig sign
magenstrasse
magenta
maggot
Magill laryngoscope
magistral
Magitot operation
magma
Magnan
    movement
    symptom
magnesemia
magnesia
    milk of m.
magnesium (Mg)
    m. carbonate
    m. chloride
    m. citrate
    m. gluconate

M

magnesium (Mg) *(continued)*
    m. hydroxide
    m. lactate
    m. sulfate
magnet
    denture m.
    Grüning (Gruening) m.
    Haab m.
    Hirschberg m.
magnetic
    m. field gradient
    m. gradient
    nuclear m. resonance (NMR)
    m. relaxation time
    m. resonance angiography
      (MRA)
    m. resonance imaging (MRI)
    m. resonance signal
    m. resonance spectroscopy
magnetocardiography
magnetoencephalography
magnetotherapy
magnetron
magnification
magnify
magnum
    os m.
Magnus operation
Magnus and de Kleijn neck reflexes
Magnuson operation
Magnuson-Stack
    arthroplasty
    operation
    shoulder arthrotomy
Magovern prosthesis
mAh, mA-h—milliampere-hour
Mahaim bundle
Mahoney speculum
Mahorner-Mead operation
ma huang
MAI—*Mycobacterium
   avium-intracellulare*
Maier
    forceps
    sinus, sinus of Maier
maim
main
    m. d'accoucheur
    m. de tranchées
    m. en crochet
    m. en griffe
    m. en lorgnette
    m. en pince
    m. en singe
    m. en squelette
    m. en succulente

main *(continued)*
    m. fourchée
main bronchi
Maingot hemostat
main stem bronchus
maintainer
    space m.
Mainz pouch urinary reservoir
Maisonneuve
    amputation
    bandage
    sign
    urethrotome
Maissiat
    band
    ligament
    tract
Majewski syndrome
Majocchi
    disease
    granuloma
    purpura
major
    m. operation
    m. surgery
Makeham hypothesis
Makkas operation
mal
    m. de mer
    grand m.
    haut m.
    m. de Meleda
    m. de mer
    m. morado
    m. perforant du pied
    petit m.
    m. rouge
malabsorption
    carbohydrate m.
    congenital glucose-galactose m.
    congenital lactose m.
    familial glucose-galactose m.
    fat m.
    hereditary familial folate m.
    intestinal m.
    lipid m.
    sucrose-isomaltose m.
Malacarne
    antrum
    pyramid
    space
malacia
    metaplastic m.
    porotic m.
malacic
malacoplakia

malacosteon
malacotic
maladie
    m. des jambes
    m. de plongeurs
    m. de Roger
    m. du sommeil
    m. des tics maladjustment
malady
malaise
malakoplakia
malalignment
malar
malaria
    acute m.
    airport m.
    algid m.
    benign tertian m.
    bilious remittent m.
    cerebral m.
    chronic m.
    congenital m.
    dysenteric m.
    falciparum m.
    hemorrhagic m.
    induced m.
    intermittent m.
    latent m.
    malignant tertian m.
    ovale m.
    pernicious m.
    Plasmodium falciparum m.
    Plasmodium malariae m.
    Plasmodium ovale m.
    Plasmodium vivax m.
    quartan m.
    quotidian m.
    recrudescent m.
    relapsing m.
    remittent m.
    tertian m.
    transfusion m.
    vivax m.
malariacidal
malarial
malaris
malarticulation
Malassez
    disease
    epithelial rests
    rests
Malassezia
    M. furfur
    M. ovalis
malassimilation
malathion

malaxate
malaxation
maldevelopment
maldigestion
male
    m. androgenetic alopecia
    m. castration
    m. erectile disorder
    m. factor infertility
    m. orgasmic disorder
    m. pattern baldness
    m. pseudohermaphrodite
    m. sex hormone
    m. sterility
Malecot
    catheter
    drain
maleic hydrazide
malemission
maleruption
maleylacetoacetate isomerase
malformation
    Abernathy m.
    anorectal m.
    Arnold-Chiari. m.
    arteriovenous m. (AVM)
    atrioventricular m. (AVM)
    cerebral cavernous m.
    Chiari-type m.
    congenital m.
    cystic adenomatoid m.
    Dandy-Walker m.
    Dieulafoy vascular m.
    Ebstein m.
    Ebstein-like m. of mitral valve
    fetal m.
    Klippel-Feil m.
    major m.
    minor m.
    Mondini m.
    Taussig-Bing m.
    vascular m.
    venous m.
malfunction
    cannula m.
    catheter m.
    dialysis access m.
    drain m.
    eustachian tube m.
    implantable cardioverter-
      defibrillator (ICD) m.
    insulin pump m.
    intrathecal pump m.
    lead m.
    mechanical shunt m.
    pacemaker m.

M

malfunction *(continued)*
 vascular access m.
 ventilator m.
Malgaigne
 amputation
 luxation
 triangle
Malherbe calcifying
 epithelioma
malic enzyme
malign
malignancy
malignant
malignin
malingerer
malingering
malinterdigitation
Malis coagulator
malleability
malleable
mallear
malleation
malleoincudal
malleolar
malleolus (malleoli)
 external m.
 m. externus
 m. fibulae
 fibular m.
 inner m.
 internal m.
 m. internus
 lateral m.
 lateral m. of fibula
 m. lateralis
 m. lateralis fibulae
 medial m.
 m. medialis
 m. medialis tibiae
 medial m. of tibia
 outer m.
 radial m.
 m. radialis
 m. tibiae
 tibial m.
 ulnar m.
 m. ulnaris
malleotomy
mallet
 Crane m.
 m. finger
 Lucae m.
 Meyerding m.
 Rush m.
 m. toe

malleus
 cog tooth of m.
Mallory
 acid fuchsin
 bodies
 stain
Mallory-Azan stain
Mallory-Weiss
 syndrome
 tear
malnutrition
 advanced m.
 extreme m.
 malignant m.
 protein m.
 protein-calorie m.
malnutrition-inflammation-
 atherosclerosis syndrome
malocclusion
 class I to III m.
 closed-bite m.
 deep-bite m.
 division 1 to 2 m.
 open-bite m.
 sub-clinical m.
Maloney dilator
malonic acid
Malpighi
 pyramids
 vesicles
malpighian
 m. bodies
 m. capsule
 m. cell
 m. corpuscle
 m. glomerulus
 m. layer
 m. rete
 m. stigma
 m. tubule
 m. tuft
malposed
malposition
malpractice
malpresentation
malrotation
MALT—mucosa-associated
 lymphoid tissue
maltase
maltitol
maltodextrin
MALToma, maltoma
maltose
maltoside
maltosuria

maltotriose
malturned
Maltz
    knife
    rasp
    saw
Maltz-Lipsett rasp
malum
    m. coxae senilis
    m. perforans
    m. perforans pedis
    m. vertebrale suboccipitale
malunion
malvaria
mAm, mA-m—milliampere-minute
MAM—methylazomethanol
M+Am—myopia plus astigmatism
mamelon
mamillary, mammillary
mamma (mammae)
    m. accessoria
    accessory mammae
    m. areolata
    m. masculina
    supernumerary mammae
    m. virilis
mammaplasty
    Aries-Pitanguy m.
    Ashford m.
    augmentation m.
    Biesenberger m.
    Conway m.
    Goulian m.
    reconstructive m.
    reduction m.
    reverse dual-plane m.
    Strömbeck m.
    Y-scar vertical m.
mammary Paget disease
mammary artery
    left internal m.a. (LIMA)
    right internal m.a. (RIMA)
mammiform
mammillary suture
mammillated
mammillopeduncular tract
mammogram
mammography
mammoplasia
    adolescent m.
mammose
mammotropic
Manchester
    operation
    ovoid

Mancini plates
mandate, mandated
mandelic acid
mandible
mandibula (mandibulae)
mandibular resection
mandibulectomy
mandibulofacial
mandibulopharyngeal
mandrel
mandrin
maneuver
    abdominal drawing-in m.
    Adson m.
    Allen m.
    Barlow m.
    Belghiti liver-hanging m.
    Bracht m.
    Brandt-Andrews m.
    Bruhat m.
    canalith repositioning m.
    Catell m.
    Chassard-Lapiné m.
    Cottle m.
    Credé m.
    cross-leg Patrick m.
    DeLee m.
    Dix-Hallpike vertigo-
      triggering m.
    doll's head m.
    Engel-Lysholm m.
    Epley m.
    forward-bending m.
    Fowler m.
    Gowers m.
    Halstead m.
    Hampton m.
    Heimlich m.
    Hodge m.
    Hoguet m.
    Hueter m.
    jaw thrust m.
    Jendrassik m.
    Jonnson m.
    key-in-lock m.
    Kocher m.
    Kristeller m.
    Lasègue m.
    Leadbetter m.
    Lecompte m.
    Leopold m.
    Levret m.
    life-saving m.
    liver-hanging m.
    Lovset m.

M

maneuver *(continued)*
    Massini m.
    Mattox m.
    Mauriceau m.
    Mauriceau-Smellie m.
    Mauriceau-Smellie-Veit m.
    McDonald m.
    McMurray circumduction m.
    McRoberts m.
    Müller (Mueller) m.
    Müller-Hillis m.
    Munro-Kerr m.
    Nagahara phaco-chop m.
    Neer m.
    Nylen-Bárány m.
    Ortolani m.
    Osler m.
    Pajot m.
    Phalen m.
    Phaneuf m.
    pharyngeal squeeze m.
    Pinard m.
    pivot-shift m.
    Politzer m.
    Ponseti m.
    Prague m.
    Pringle m.
    Proust-Lichtheim m.
    Queckenstedt m.
    Ritgen m.
    Roos m.
    Saxtorph m.
    Scanzoni m.
    Schatz m.
    Schreiber m.
    Sellick m.
    Smellie-Veit m.
    squeeze m.
    stent-in-stent m.
    Thorn m.
    Toynbee m.
    Valsalva m.
    Westphal m.
    Wigand m.
    Wigand-Martin m.
    Zavanelli m.
manganese (Mn)
    m. pneumonitis
    m. poisoning
manganic
manganism
manganous
mania
    acute hallucinatory m.
    akinetic m.

mania *(continued)*
    alcoholic m.
    antidepressant-associated m.
    Bell m.
    bipolar m.
    delirious m.
    full m.
    lamotrigine-induced m.
    new-onset m.
    poststroke m.
    posttraumatic m.
    psychotic m.
    puerperal m.
    pure m.
    religious m.
    secondary m.
    transitory m.
    unproductive m.
    ziprasidone-associated m.
maniac
maniacal
manic
manic-depressive
manifest
    m. content
    m. deviation
    m. hyperopia
    m. refraction
    m. strabismus
manifestation
    clinical m.
    ictal epileptic m's
    interictal epileptic m's
    postictal epileptic m's
    preictal epileptic m's
    somatic m.
manikin
manipulation
    chiropractic m.
    conjoined m.
    endocrine m.
    fracture m.
    hormonal m.
    object m.
    osteopathic m.
    pharmacologic m.
    spinal m.
    stone m.
Mann
    forceps
    sign
Mann-Bollman fistula
manner
    in a m. after Tom Jones
    m. of death

manner *(continued)*
    dose-dependent m.
    dose-response m.
    McLean m.
    systematic m.
mannerism
    hand-washing m.
mannitol
mannosidosis
Mann-Whitney test
Mann-Williamson ulcer
manometry
    Cartesian diver m.
manoptoscope
manslaughter
Manson
    disease
    hemoptysis
    pyosis
    schistosomiasis
Mansonella
    M. ozzardi
    M. perstans
    M. streptocerca
mansonelliasis
mansonellosis
mantle
    brain m.
    m. cell lymphoma
    cement m.
    cortical m.
Mantoux
    conversion
    reaction
    skin test
    test
manual
manubrial
manubriosternal
manubrium (manubria)
    m. mallei, m. of
        malleus
    m. sterni, m. of sternum
manuduction
manus
    m. cava
    m. extensa
    m. flexa
    m. plana
    m. superextensa
    m. valga
    m. vara
many-tailed dressing
manzanita
Manz glands

MAO—
    maximal acid output
    monoamine oxidase
map
    chromosome m.
    cognitive m.
    cytogenetic m.
    fate m.
    gene m.
    genetic m.
    linkage m.
MAP—
    mean aortic pressure
    mean arterial pressure
    muscle action potential
MAPF—microatomized protein
    food
maple syrup urine disease (MSUD)
maplike
mapping
    cytologic m.
    deletion m.
    fine structure genetic m.
Maquet technique
Maragliano tuberculin
Marañón
    sign
    syndrome (I, II, III)
marasmatic
marasmic
marasmoid
marasmus
    enzootic m.
    nutritional m.
marbleization
Marburg
    disease
    hemorrhagic fever
    triad
    virus
march
    jacksonian m.
Marchand
    adrenals
    organs
marche á petits pas
Marchesani syndrome
Marchetti test
Marchi
    balls
    globule
    method
    reaction
    tract
Marchiafava-Bignami disease

M

Marchiafava-Micheli
    disease
    syndrome
Marcus Gunn
    dots
    pupillary phenomenon
    pupillary syndrome
    sign
Marcy operation
Maréchal-Rosin test
Maréchal test
Marey reflex
Marfan
    sign
    syndrome
marfanoid
margarine
margin
    m. of acetabulum
    acute m. of heart
    alveolar m. of mandible
    alveolar m. of maxilla
    anterior m. of fibula
    anterior m. of lung
    anterior m. of scapula
    anterior m. of spleen
    anterior m. of tibia
    anterior m. of ulna
    axillary m. of scapula
    buccal m.
    cartilaginous m. of acetabulum
    cervical m.
    ciliary m. of iris
    convex m. of testis
    coronal m. of frontal bone
    coronal m. of parietal bone
    crenate m. of spleen
    cristate m. of spleen
    dentate m.
    dorsal m. of radius
    enamel m.
    external m. of scapula
    falciform m. of fascia lata
    falciform m. of saphenus
      hiatus
    falciform m. of white line of
      pelvic fascia
    free gingival m.
    free gum m.
    free m. of eyelid
    free m. of nail
    free m. of ovary
    frontal m. of greater wing of
      sphenoid bone
    frontal m. of parietal bone

margin *(continued)*
    gingival m.
    gum m.
    hidden m. of nail
    incisal m.
    inferior m. of liver
    inferior m. of lung
    inferior m. of suprarenal
      gland
    infraorbital m. of body of
      maxilla
    infraorbital m. of maxilla
    infraorbital m. of orbit
    interosseous m. of fibula
    interosseous m. of tibia
    interosseous m. of ulna
    lacrimal m. of maxilla
    lambdoid m. of occipital bone
    lambdoid m. of parietal bone
    lateral m. of humerus
    lateral m. of kidney
    lateral m. of nail
    lateral m. of orbit
    lateral m. of scapula
    lateral m. of uterus
    left m. of heart
    malar m. of greater wing
    mammillary m.
    mastoid m. of occipital bone
    mastoid m. of parietal bone
    medial m. of foot
    medial m. of humerus
    medial m. of kidney
    medial m. of orbit
    medial m. of suprarenal gland
    medial m. of tibia
    mesovarial m. of ovary
    nasal m. of frontal bone
    obtuse m. of heart
    obtuse m. of spleen
    occipital m. of parietal bone
    occipital m. of temporal bone
    orbital m.
    outer m.
    parietal m. of frontal bone
    parietal m. of great wing of
      sphenoid bone
    parietal m. of occipital bone
    parietal m. of parietal bone
    parietal m. of squamous part
      of temporal bone
    parietal m. of temporal bone
    parietofrontal m. of great wing
      of sphenoid bone
    posterior m. of fibula

margin *(continued)*

    pupillary m. of iris
    radial m. of forearm
    red m.
    m. of resection
    right m. of heart
    m. of safety
    sagittal m. of parietal bone
    sphenoidal m. of parietal bone
    sphenoidal m. of squamous
      part of temporal bone
    sphenoidal m. of temporal bone
    sphenotemporal m. of parietal
      bone
    squamous m. of great wing of
      sphenoid bone
    squamous m. of parietal bone
    straight m. of testis
    superior m. of pancreas
    superior m. of scapula
    superior m. of spleen
    superior m. of suprarenal gland
    supraorbital m. of frontal bone
    supraorbital m. of orbit
    surgical m.
    temporal m. of parietal bone
    tibial m. of foot
    m. of tongue
    tumor-free m.
    ulnar m's of fingers
    ulnar m. of forearm
    m. of uninvolved tissue
    m. of uterus, right and left
    vertebral m. of scapula
    volar m. of radius
    volar m. of ulna
    wound m.
    zygomatic m. of great wing of
      sphenoid bone

marginal

margination

marginoplasty

margo (margines)

    m. acetabuli, m. acetabularis
    m. alveolaris
    m. anterior corporis pancreatis
    m. anterior fibulae
    m. anterior hepatis
    m. anterior pulmonis
    m. anterior radii
    m. anterior splenis
    m. anterior testis
    m. anterior tibiae
    m. anterior ulnae
    m. arcuatus hiatus sapheni

margo (margines) *(continued)*

    m. axillaris scapulae
    m. ciliaris iridis
    m. dexter cordis
    m. dorsalis radii
    m. dorsalis ulnae
    m. falciformis fasciae latae
    m. falciformis hiatus sapheni
    m. fibularis pedis
    m. frontalis alae magnae,
      m. frontalis alae majoris
    m. frontalis ossis parietalis
    m. gingivalis
    m. incisalis
    m. inferior cerebri
    m. inferior corporis
      pancreatis
    m. inferior hepatis
    m. inferior lienis
    m. inferior pulmonis
    m. inferior splenis
    m. inferolateralis hemispherii
      cerebri
    m. inferomedialis hemispherii
      cerebri
    m. infraglenoidalis tibiae
    m. infraorbitalis corporis
      maxillae
    m. infraorbitalis orbitae
    m. interosseus fibulae
    m. interosseus radii
    m. interosseus tibiae
    m. interosseus ulnae
    m. lacrimalis maxillae
    m. lambdoideus ossis
      occipitalis
    margines laterales digitorum
      pedis
    m. lateralis antebrachii
    m. lateralis humeri
    m. lateralis linguae
    m. lateralis orbitae
    m. lateralis pedis
    m. lateralis renis
    m. lateralis scapulae
    m. lateralis unguis
    m. lateralis uteri
    m. liber ovarii
    m. liber unguis
    m. linguae
    m. mastoideus ossis occipitalis
    m. medialis antebrachii
    m. medialis cerebri
    margines medialis digitorum
      pedis

M

margo (margines) *(continued)*
 m. medialis glandulae
  suprarenalis
 m. medialis humeri
 m. medialis orbitae
 m. medialis pedis
 m. medialis renis
 m. medialis scapulae
 m. medialis tibiae
 m. mesovaricus ovarii
 m. nasalis ossis frontalis
 m. occipitalis ossis parietalis
 m. occipitalis ossis temporalis
 m. occultus unguis
 m. orbitalis
 m. palpebrae
 m. parietalis alae magnae, m.
  parietalis alae majoris
 m. parietalis ossis frontalis
 m. parietalis partis squamosae
  ossis temporalis
 m. parietalis squamae
  temporalis
 m. posterior corporis pancreatis
 m. posterior fibulae
 m. posterior partis petrosae
  ossis temporalis
 m. posterior radii
 m. posterior splenis
 m. posterior testis
 m. posterior ulnae
 m. pupillaris iridis
 m. radialis antebrachii
 m. radialis humeri
 m. sagittalis ossis parietalis
 m. sphenoidalis partis
  squamosae ossis temporalis
 m. sphenoidalis squamae
  temporalis
 m. squamosus alae magnae,
  m. squamosus alae majoris
 m. squamosus ossis parietalis
 m. superior corporis pancreatis
 m. superior glandulae
  suprarenalis
 m. superior hemispherii cerebri
 m. superior lienis
 m. superior partis petrosae
  ossis temporalis
 m. superior scapulae
 m. superior splenis
 m. superomedialis cerebri
 m. supraorbitalis orbitae
 m. supraorbitalis ossis frontalis
 m. tibialis pedis

margo (margines) *(continued)*
 m. ulnaris antebrachii
 m. ulnaris humeri
 m. uteri
 m. vertebralis scapulae
 m. volaris radii
 m. volaris ulnae
 m. zygomaticus alae magnae
 m. zygomaticus alae majoris
Margulies coil IUD
marian lithotomy
Marie
 ataxia
 disease
 hypertrophy
 sclerosis
 sign
 syndrome (I, II)
Marie-Bamberger disease
Marie-Foix sign
Marie-Strümpell
 disease
 spondylitis
 syndrome
Marie-Tooth disease
marihuana, marijuana
Marin Amat phenomenon
Marinesco
 sign
 succulent hand
Marinesco-Radovici reflex
Marinesco-Sjögren syndrome
Marinesco-Sjögren-Garland
 syndrome
marinobufagin
Marion disease
Mariotte spot
marital
 m. status
 m. therapy
maritonucleus
mark
 beauty m.
 birth m.
 hesitation m's
 lightning m.
 mulberry m.
 pock m.
 Pohl-Pinkus m.
 port-wine m.
 quillon m.
 raspberry m.
 strawberry m.
marker
 Amsler m.

marker *(continued)*
    cell-surface m.
    Crane-Kaplan pocket m.
    D'Assumpçao rhytidoplasty m.
    Freeman cookie-cutter
      areola m.
    genetic m.
    Gonin-Amsler m.
marking
    Fontana m's
    interstitial m.
    pulmonary vascular m.
Marlex
    atraumatic tenaculum
    bandage
    graft
    mesh
    suture
Marlow test
Marmo method
marmoration
marmoreal
Maroteaux-Lamy
    disease
    syndrome (I, II)
marrow
    bone m.
    depressed m.
    fat m.
    gelatinous m.
    red m.
    spinal m.
    yellow m.
Marshall
    fold
    surgical sucker
    syndrome
    test
    vein
Marshall Hall
    facies
    method
Marshall-Jewett-Strong
   classification
Marshall-Marchetti
    operation
    test
Marshall-Marchetti-Birch
   operation
Marshall-Marchetti-Krantz (MMK)
   operation
Marshall and Tanner pubertal
   staging
Marsh disease
Marshik forceps

marsupialization
marsupium (marsupia)
    marsupia patellaris
Martel clamp
martial arts
Martin
    bandage
    disease
    forceps
    gastrostomy
    needle
    operation
    pelvimeter
    retractor
    speculum
    syndrome
    tube
Martin and Davy speculum
Martinotti cells
Martius operation
Martius-Harris operation
Martorell
    syndrome
    ulcer
Maryan forceps
mAs, mA-s—milliampere-second
maschaladenitis
masculine
masculinity
masculinization
masculinize
masculinizing
maser
MASH—Mobile Army Surgical
   Hospital
mask
    BLB m.
    Boothby m.
    bulbulian m.
    death m.
    ecchymotic m.
    face m. (facemask)
    m. facies
    full-face m.
    Hutchinson m.
    laryngeal m. airway
    luetic m.
    meter m.
    nonrebreathing m.
    oxygen m.
    Parkinson m.
    partial rebreathing m.
    m. of pregnancy
    tabetic m.
    tracheostomy m.

M

mask *(continued)*
    Venturi m.
MASK—microkeratome-assisted
  additive stromal keratoplasty
masker
    central m.
    tinnitus m.
masking
    central m.
masochism
masochist
Mason
    gastroplasty
    incision
Mason-Allen splint
Mason-Auvard speculum
mass
    achromatic m.
    amorphous m.
    appendiceal m.
    atomic m.
    benign m. lesion
    biopsy-proven m.
    blue m.
    body cell m.
    body m. index (BMI)
    breast m.
    critical m.
    cystic m.
    m. effect
    encapsulated m.
    fat m.
    fibrillar m.
    fluctuant m., fluctuating m.
    m. fragmentography
    injection m.
    intraluminal m.
    irregular m.
    lateral m. of atlas
    lateral m. of ethmoid bone
    lateral m. of occipital bone
    lateral m. of sacrum
    lateral m. of vertebrae
    lean body m.
    lean tissue m.
    lobulated m.
    localized m.
    lung m.
    mediastinal m.
    molecular m.
    muscle m.
    ovarian m.
    painless m.
    palpable m.
    parahilar m.

mass *(continued)*
    pill m., pilular m.
    polypoid m.
    m. radiography
    m. roentgenography
    sarcoplasmic m's
    slow-growing m.
    solid m.
    soft tissue m.
    m. spectrometry
    tigroid m's
    total red cell m.
    translucent m.
    yellow-pink conjunctival m.
massa (massae)
    m. innominata
    m. intermedia
    m. lateralis atlantis
    m. lateralis ossis ethmoidalis
    m. lateralis ossis sacri
    m. lateralis vertebrae
massage
    adjuvant m. therapy
    cardiac m.
    carotid sinus m.
    closed-chest cardiac m.
    deep muscle m.
    deep tissue m.
    electrovibratory m.
    external cardiac m.
    gingival m.
    heart m.
    hydropneumatic m.
    lymphatic m.
    nerve-point m.
    open-chest cardiac m.
    prostatic m.
    spray m.
    Swedish m.
    m. therapist
    m. therapy
    trigger-point m.
    vapor m.
    vibratory m.
Masselon spectacles
masseter
masseur
masseuse
Massie nail
Massini maneuver
massive
Masson-Judd retractor
massotherapy
MAST—
    military anti-shock trousers

MAST— *(continued)*
 multiple antigen stimulation
  test
mastadenitis
mastadenoma
mastalgia
mastatrophy
mastauxe
mast cell
mastectomy
 bilateral m.
 extended radical m.
 Halsted radical m.
 modified m.
 modified radical m.
 nipple-sparing m.
 partial m.
 prophylactic m.
 radical m. (RM)
 secondary m.
 segmental m.
 simple m. (SM)
 skin-sparing m.
 subcutaneous m.
 total m.
Master 2-step exercise test
mastic
masticate
mastication
 muscles of m.
masticatory
Mastin clamp
mastitis
 brucella m.
 chronic cystic m.
 cystic m.
 eosinophilic m.
 glandular m.
 idiopathic granulomatous
  lobular m.
 infectious m.
 interstitial m.
 lupus m.
 m. neonatorum
 m. obliterans
 parenchymatous m.
 periductal m.
 phlegmonous m.
 plasma cell m.
 postpartum m.
 puerperal m.
 recurrent m.
 retromammary m.
 stagnation m.
 subclinical m.

mastitis *(continued)*
 suppurative m.
 tuberculous m.
mastocyte
mastocytoma
mastocytosis
 cutaneous m.
 diffuse cutaneous m.
 malignant m.
 systemic m.
mastodynia
mastoid
 m. abscess
 acellular m.
 m. angle of parietal bone
 m. antrum
 m. artery
 m. bone
 m. bowl
 m. canaliculus
 m. cavity
 m. cells
 m. cortex
 diploic m.
 m. empyema
 m. foramen
 m. fossa
 ivory m.
 m. lymph nodes
 m. margin of occipital bone
 m. margin of parietal bone
 m. notch of temporal bone
 m. obliteration operation
 pneumatized m.
 m. process
 m. region
 sclerotic m.
 m. sinuses
 m. suture
mastoidal
mastoidale
mastoidalgia
mastoidea
mastoidectomy
 Bondy m.
 canal wall down m.
 canal wall up m.
 combined approach m.
 conservative m.
 cortical m.
 Gülhane m.
 modified radical m.
 radical m.
 retrograde m.
 robotic m.

M

mastoidectomy *(continued)*
    Schwartze m.
    simple m.
    Tos m.
mastoiditis
    acute m.
    Bezold m.
    coalescent m.
    masked m.
    silent m.
    tuberculous m.
mastoidotomy
masto-occipital
mastoparietal
mastopathia
    benign m.
    m. chronica
    m. cystica
    m. fibrocystica
mastopathy
    cystic m.
    diabetic m.
    diabetic fibrous m.
    fibrocystic m.
    proliferative m.
mastopexy
    doughnut m.
    one-stage m.
    staged m.
mastoptosis
mastorrhagia
mastosquamous
mastostomy
mastotomy
masturbation
Masugi nephritis
MAT—multifocal atrial tachycardia
Matas
    band
    operation
    test
Matchett-Brown prosthesis
matching
    cross m.
    impedance m.
mater
    dura m.
    pia m.
materia
    m. alba
    m. dentica
    m. medica
material
    air-equivalent m.
    baseplate m.

material *(continued)*
    dental m.
    genetic m.
    impression m.
    target m.
    tissue equivalent m.
    trace m.
materialization
maternal
maternity
Mathews speculum
Mathieu forceps
matrical
matricectomy
matrilineal
matrix (matrices)
    amalgam m.
    m. band
    bone m.
    m. calculus
    capsular m.
    cartilage m.
    m. cells
    cytoplasmic m.
    extracellular m.
    functional m.
    hair m.
    intercellular m.
    m. metalloproteinase (MMP)
    nail m.
    resin m.
    m. retainer
    m. unguis
matroclinous
Matsner median episiotomy and
  repair
Matson
    elevator
    operation
matt, matte
matter
    gelatinous m.
    gray m. of nervous system
    gray m. of spinal cord
    medullary white m.
    radiant m.
    white m. of nervous system
Mattox
    clamp
    maneuver
mattress
    alternating pressure m.
    divided m.
    egg-crate m.
    end-on m. suture

mattress *(continued)*
    horizontal m. suture
    intradermal m. suture
    right-angle m. suture
    ripple m.
    m. suture
    vertical m. suture
maturate
maturation
    m. arrest
    m. index
    ovarian follicular m.
maturation-development
mature, matured
maturity-onset diabetes of the
  young (MODY)
matutinal
Mauchart ligament
Mauck operation
Maugeri syndrome
Maumenee-Park speculum
Maunoir hydrocele
Maunsell suture
Maurer
    clefts
    dots
    spots
    stippling
Mauriac syndrome
Mauriceau
    lance
    maneuver
Mauriceau-Smellie maneuver
Mauriceau-Smellie-Veit maneuver
Mauthner
    cell
    fiber
    membrane
    sheath
    test
MAVIS—mobile artery and vein
  imaging system
max.—maximum
maxilla (maxillae, maxillas)
    frontal processes of maxillae
    inferior m.
maxillary
    radical m. antrostomy
    m. resection
    total m. osteotomy
maxillectomy
maxillitis
maxillodental
maxilloethmoidectomy
maxillofacial prosthesis

maxillolabial
maxillomandibular
maxillotomy
maximal
Maximow
    method
    stain
maximum
Maxwell
    ring
    spot
Maydl
    hernia
    operation
Mayer
    glycerin-albumin
      mixture
    hemalum stain
    hematoxylin stain
    mucihematein stain
    pessary
    position
    reagent
    reflex
    speculum
    splint
    test
    view
    waves
Mayer-Rokitansky-Kustner
  syndrome
Mayfield
    clip
    osteotome
mayfly
May-Grünwald stain
May-Hegglin anomaly
Maylard incision
Mayo
    cannula
    carrier
    clamp
    forceps
    hook
    linen suture
    needle
    operation
    probe
    retractor
    scissors
    scoop
    sign
    stripper
Mayo-Blake forceps
Mayo-Collins retractor

M

Mayo-Harrington scissors
Mayo-Lovelace retractor
Mayo-Noble scissors
Mayo-Ochsner forceps
Mayor
    scarf
    sign
Mayo-Robson
    forceps
    incision
    line
    operation
    point
    position
    scoop
Mayo-Russian forceps
Mayo-Sims scissors
Mayo-Ward vaginal hysterectomy
Mays operation
maze
    m. atrial fibrillation ablation
        procedure
    Cox m. III procedure
    radiation m.
mazoplasia
Mazur operation
Mazzoni corpuscle
MB—
    mesiobuccal
    methylene blue
MBAS—methylene blue active
    substance
MB bands
MBC—
    maximal breathing capacity
    maximum breathing capacity
    minimal bactericidal
        concentration
MBD—
    methylene blue dye
    minimal brain damage
    minimal brain dysfunction
MBF—myocardial blood flow
MBL—minimal bactericidal level
MBO—mesiobucco-occlusal
MBP—
    mean blood pressure
    mesiobuccopulpal
    myelin basic protein
mbundu
Mc—megacycle(s)
MC—
    maximum concentration
    Medical Corps
    metacarpal

MC— *(continued)*
    mineralocorticoid
    myocarditis
MCA—middle cerebral artery
McArdle
    disease
    syndrome
McAtee screw
McAtee-Tharias-Blazina
    arthroplasty
MCBR—minimum concentration of
    bilirubin
McBride operation
McBurney
    incision
    operation
    point
    sign
McCall operation
McCarey-Kaufman (M-K) medium
McCarroll operation
McCarthy
    cystoscope
    electrode
    evacuator
    forceps
    Foroblique panendoscope
    reflex
    resectoscope
    telescope
McCarthy-Alcock forceps
McCarthy-Campbell cystoscope
McCarthy-Peterson cystoscope
McCash-Randall operation
McCaskey curet
McClintock sign
McClure scissors
McCort sign
MCCU—mobile coronary care unit
McCullough forceps
McCune-Albright syndrome
MCD—
    mean corpuscular diameter
    multiple carboxylase
        deficiency
McDonald, W. Dean
    clamp
    maneuver
    operation
    rule
MCF—macrophage chemotactic
    factor
MCFA—medium-chain fatty acid(s)
mcg, μg—microgram(s)
McGannon retractor

McGaw pump
McGee operation
McGhan implant
McGill operation
McGinn-White sign
McGoon technique
McGregor
    forehead flap
    line
McGuire
    operation
    scissors
MCH, MCHg—mean corpuscular
    hemoglobin
MCHC—mean corpuscular
    hemoglobin concentration
McHenry forceps
McHugh
    knife
    speculum
µCi [microCi]—microcurie(s)
mCi—millicurie(s)
MCi—megacurie(s)
µCi-hr [microCi-hr]—microcurie-
    hour
mCi-hr—millicurie-hour
McIndoe
    elevator
    operation
McIntire aspiration-irrigation
    system
McIvor mouth gag
McKay forceps
McKee line
McKee-Farrar
    acetabular cup
    arthroplasty
    prosthesis
McKeever
    operation
    prosthesis
McKenzie
    bur
    clip
    drill
    forceps
McKinnon test
McKissock operation
McKrae herpesvirus
MCL—
    midclavicular line
    midcostal line
    most comfortable loudness
        level
McLane forceps

McLane-Tucker forceps
McLane-Tucker-Luikart forceps
McLaughlin
    incision
    operation
    plate
    screw
McLean
    formula
    index
    manner
    scissors
    tonometer
McLean-Maxwell disease
McLeod blood phenotype
MCMI—Millon Clinical Multiaxial
    Inventory
McMurray
    sign
    test
McNealy-Glassman-Babcock
    forceps
McNealy-Glassman-Mixter forceps
McNemar test
MCP—metacarpophalangeal
McPheeters treatment
McPherson
    forceps
    needle holder
    scissors
    spatula
    speculum
McPherson-Castroviejo scissors
McPherson-Vannas scissors
McPherson-Wheeler
    blade
    knife
McPherson-Ziegler knife
Mcps—megacycles per second
MCQ—multiple choice question
MCR—metabolic clearance rate
McReynolds
    adapter
    knife
    operation
M-CSF—macrophage colony–
    stimulating factor
MCT—
    mean circulation time
    mean corpuscular thickness
    medium-chain triglyceride
    medullary carcinoma of
        thyroid
MCTD—mixed connective tissue
    disease

M

MCV—mean corpuscular volume
McVay
    incision
    operation
Md—mendelevium
MD—
    manic depressive
    movement disorder
    muscular dystrophy
    myocardial damage
MD; M.D.—medical doctor
    (L. Medicinae Doctor)
MDC—minimum detectable
    concentration
MDD—mean daily dose
MDF—
    mean dominant frequency
    myocardial depressant factor
MDH—malic dehydrogenase
MDMA—methylene
    dioxymethamphetamine
MDP—methylene diphosphonate
MDR—minimum daily
    requirement
MDTR—mean diameter-thickness
    ratio
MDY—month, date, year
ME—
    medical examiner
    middle ear
M/E—myeloid-erythroid [ratio]
MEA—
    multiple endocrine
        abnormalities
    multiple endocrine
        adenomatosis
    multiple endocrine
        adenopathies
Meadox vascular graft
meal
    barium m.
    fatty test m.
    opaque m.
    test m.
mean deviation
Mean sign
measles
    atypical m.
    confluent m.
    German m.
    three-day m.
    m. virus
    m. vaccine
measly
measure

measurement
    end-point m.
    kinetic m.
    OFC (occipitofrontal
        circumference) m.
    real-time m.
    skinfold m's
    SNA (sella, nasion, point A) m.
    SNB (sella, nasion, point B) m.
    torr m.
meatal incision
meatitis
    ulcerative m.
meatoplasty
    Stacke m.
meatorrhaphy
meatoscope
meatoscopy
    ureteral m.
meatotome
meatotomy
    ureteral m.
meatus (meatus)
    acoustic m.
    acoustic m., bony external
    acoustic m., bony internal
    acoustic m., external
        cartilaginous
    m. acusticus externus
        cartilagineus
    m. acusticus externus osseus
    m. acusticus internus osseus
    m. auditorius externus
        cartilagineus
    m. auditorius externus osseus
    m. auditorius internus osseus
    auditory m., bony external
    auditory m., bony internal
    auditory m., external
        cartilaginous
    external acoustic m.
    external urinary m.
    fish-mouth m.
    inferior m. of nose
    internal urinary m.
    middle m. of nose
    nasal m., bony common
    nasal m., bony inferior
    nasal m., bony middle
    nasal m., bony superior
    m. nasi inferior
    m. nasi medius
    m. nasi superior
    nasopharyngeal m.
    m. nasopharyngeus

meatus (meatus) *(continued)*
    m. of nose
    superior m. of nose
    ureteral m., ureteric m.
    m. of urethra, urethral m.
    m. urinarius, urinary m.
mecalil provocation test
mechanics
    body m.
    developmental m.
mechanism
    coping m.
    defense m.
    Duncan m.
    escape m.
    feedback m.
    Frank-Starling m.
    m. of labor
    mental m.
    neutralizing m.
    oculogyric m.
    pinchcock m.
    pressoreceptive m.
    reentrant m.
    scapegoat m.
    Schultze m.
    sliding filament m.
    Starling m.
    suspensory m.
mechanist
mechanoreceptor
mechanotherapy
mechanothermy
mecism
mecistocephalic
Meckel
    band
    cartilage
    cavity
    diverticulum
    ganglion
    ligament
    plane
    rod
    scan
    space
    syndrome
meckelectomy
mecobalamine
meconate
meconic acid
meconiorrhea
meconium
    m. aspiration
    m. ileus

meconium *(continued)*
    m. periorchitis
    m. peritonitis
    m. plug
    m. staining
mecrylate
mecystasis
med.—
    median
    medical
    medicine
MED—
    minimal effective dose
    minimal erythema dose
MEDAC—multiple endocrine
    deficiency–autoimmune
    candidiasis
medallion
media (plural of medium)
mediad
medial meniscectomy
medialis
    vastus m. muscle
median
    m. bar of prostate
    m. episiotomy
    m. incision
    m. laryngotomy
    m. lithotomy
    m. palatine suture
    m. pharyngotomy
    m. rhinoscopy
    m. sternotomy
    m. strumectomy
medianus
mediastina (plural of
    mediastinum)
mediastinal
    m. collagenosis
    m. crunch
    m. lymphadenitis
    m. teratoma
mediastinitis
    fibrous m.
    indurative m.
mediastinography
    gas m.
    opaque m.
mediastinopericarditis
mediastinoscope
    Carlens m.
    Goldberg MPC m.
mediastinoscopic
mediastinoscopy
mediastinotomy

M

mediastinum (mediastina)
 anterior m.
 m. anterius
 inferior m.
 m. inferius
 m. medium
 middle m.
 posterior m.
 m. posterius
 superior m.
 m. superius
 m. testis
mediation
 chemical m.
mediator
medicable
Medicaid
medical
 m. corps
 m. curettage
 m. diathermy
 m. discharge
 m. ethics
 m. ophthalmoscopy
 m. thyroidectomy
 m. vagotomy
medicament
medicamentous
Medicare
medicate, medicated
medication
 conservative m.
 conventional m.
 dialytic m.
 discharge m's
 m. errors
 hypodermic m.
 ionic m.
 over-the-counter (OTC) m.
 preanesthetic m.
 prescription m.
 prophylactic m.
 psychotropic m.
 sublingual m.
 substitutive m.
 transduodenal m.
medicator
medicinal
medicine
 adolescent m.
 aerospace m.
 alternative m.
 aviation m.
 behavioral m.
 Chinese herbal m.

medicine *(continued)*
 clinical m.
 community m.
 comparative m.
 complementary m.
 compound m.
 domestic m.
 emergency m.
 environmental m.
 evidence-based m.
 family m.
 fetal-maternal m.
 folk m.
 forensic m.
 general m.
 genomic m.
 geriatric m.
 group m.
 herbal m.
 holistic m.
 hyperbaric m.
 industrial m.
 internal m.
 ionic m.
 legal m.
 manipulative m.
 maternal-fetal m.
 mind-body m.
 naturopathic m.
 neonatal m.
 nuclear m.
 occupational m.
 oral m.
 osteopathic m.
 perinatal m.
 physical m.
 podiatric m.
 preclinical m.
 preventive m.
 prophylactic m.
 proprietary m.
 psychosomatic m.
 rehabilitation m.
 space m.
 sports m.
 state m.
 tropical m.
medicolegal
medifrontal
Medin
 disease
 poliomyelitis
mediocre
mediolateral
 m. approach

mediolateral *(continued)*
- m. diameter
- m. direction
- m. displacement
- m. distribution
- m. episiotomy
- m. laxity
- m. lithotomy
- m. oblique view

mediolysis

mediolytic

medionecrosis
- m. of aorta
- cystic m.
- Erdheim-Gsell cystic m.
- non-Marfan idiopathic m.

mediopatellar plica

mediotarsal amputation

mediotemporal

mediotrusion

MediPort vascular access device

mediscalenus

medisect

meditation
- mindful m., mindfulness m.
- transcendental m.

medium (media, mediums)
- brain-heart infusion m.
- Cary-Blair transport m.
- clearing m.
- contrast m.
- culture m.
- deoxycholate-citrate m.
- dioptric media
- disperse m., dispersion m., dispersive m.
- Dubos m.
- HAT m.
- Löwenstein (Lowenstein, Loewenstein) m.
- Löwenstein-Jensen m.
- marking m.
- McCarey-Kaufman (M-K) m.
- motility test m.
- mounting m.
- Novy, McNeal, and Nicolle (NNN) m.
- nutrient m.
- refracting media
- Sabouraud m.
- Stuart transport m.
- Thayer-Martin m.
- transparent m. of eye
- Wickersheimer m.

medius

Medrafil wire suture

medronate disodium

medronate scan

meds—
- medications
- medicines

Medtronic-Hall valve

medulla (medullae)
- adrenal m.
- m. of bone
- m. glandulae suprarenalis
- m. of hair shaft
- m. of kidney
- m. of lymph node
- m. nodi lymphatici, m. nodi lymphoidei
- m. oblongata
- m. ossium
- m. ossium flava
- m. ossium rubra
- m. ovarii
- m. of ovary
- renal m.
- m. renalis, m. renis
- spinal m.
- m. spinalis
- suprarenal m.
- m. of suprarenal gland
- m. thymi
- m. of thymus

medullaris
- cavitas m.
- conus m.

medullary
- m. artery
- m. canal
- m. cystic disease
- m. fold
- m. foramen
- m. groove
- m. lamina
- m. layer
- m. plate
- m. segment
- m. sheath
- m. sinuses
- m. space
- m. sponge kidney
- m. streak
- m. stria
- m. tractotomy
- m. tube

medullated
- m. fibers
- m. neuroma

M

medullation
medullectomy
medullitis
medullization
medulloadrenal
medulloarthritis
medulloblast
medulloblastoma
    Cushing m.
    desmoplastic m.
medulloepithelioma
medullopontine sulcus
medullospinal
medusa head
medusae
    caput m.
Medx
    M. camera
    M. scanner
Meek-Wall dermatome
Mees lines
Meesmann dystrophy
MEF—maximal expiratory flow
MEFR—maximum expiratory flow
    rate
MEFV—maximum expiratory flow
    volume
MEG—magnetoencephalograph
megabecquerel (MBq)
megabladder
megacalicosis
megacardia
megacecum
megacholedochus
megacolon
    acquired m.
    acquired functional m.
    acute m.
    aganglionic m.
    congenital m.
    idiopathic m.
    toxic m.
megacurie (MCi)
megacycle (Mc)
megacystis-megaureter syndrome
megaduodenum
megadyne
megaelectronvolt (MeV, Mev)
megaesophagus
megahertz (MHz)
megakaryoblast
megakaryocyte
    basophilic m.
    lymphoid m.
    stage II m.

megakaryocytic leukemia
megakaryocytopenia
megakaryocytopoiesis
megakaryocytosis
megalencephalon
megalencephaly
megaloblast
megaloblastic anemia
megaloblastoid
megaloblastosis
megalocheiria
megalocornea
megalocystis
megalocyte
megalocytic
    m. anemia
    m. degeneration
    m. interstitial nephritis
megalocytosis
megalodactyly
megalomania
megalophthalmos
    anterior m.
Megalopyge opercularis
megarectum
megaroentgen (MR)
Megaselia scalaris
megaseme
megasigmoid
megasoma
megasomia
megaunit
megavitamin
megavolt (MV)
Méglin point
meglumine
megrim
MEGX— monoethylglycinexylidide
meibomian
    m. cyst
    m. foramen
    m. froth
    m. gland
    m. stye
meibomianitis, meibomitis
Meige disease
Meigs
    capillaries
    suture
    syndrome
Meigs-Cass syndrome
Meinicke
    reaction
    test
meiosis

meiotic
Meirowsky phenomenon
Meissner
    corpuscles
    ganglion
    plexus
mel
melagra
melalgia
melancholia
    affective m.
    m. agitata, agitated m.
    m. with delirium
    m. hypochondriaca
    involution m., involutional m.
    m. simplex
    stuporous m.
melancholic
melanemesis
melanemia
melanicterus
melaniferous
melanin
    artificial m.
    factitious m.
    m.-laden macrophages
    m. pigment
melanoacanthoma
melanoameloblastoma
melanoblast
    amelanotic m.
melanoblastoma
melanoblastosis
melanocarcinoma
melanocyte
    dendritic m.
    m.-stimulating hormone
melanocytic
    congenital m. nevi
    m. lesion
    m. markers
    m. neoplasm
    m. nevus
    m. tumor
melanocytoma
    compound m.
    dermal m.
    extrapapillary m.
    iris m.
    meningeal m.
    optic disk m.
    optic nerve m.
    pigmented epithelioid m.
    uveal tract m.
    well-differentiated m.

melanocytosis
    acquired dermal m.
    dermal m.
    diffuse m.
    epidermal m.
    leptomeningeal m.
    metastatic peritoneal
     neurocutaneous m.
    ocular m.
    oculodermal m.
    pagetoid m.
melanoderma
    diffuse m.
    macular m.
    mosaic subclinical m.
    mottled m.
    parasitic m.
    postinflammatory m.
    senile m.
melanodermatitis
    lichenoid m.
melanogen
melanogenic
melanoid
melanoleukoderma
melanoma
    acral lentiginous m.
    amelanotic m.
    animal-type m.
    benign juvenile m.
    Cloudman S91 m. cell line
    cutaneous malignant m.
    desmoplastic m.
    juvenile m.
    lentiginous m.
    lentigo maligna m.
    malignant m.
    multiple m.
    nodular m.
    oral mucosal m.
    pagetoid m.
    spindle cell m.
    subungual m.
    superficial spreading m.
melanomatosis
melanomatous
melanonychia
melanophage
melanoplakia
melanoptysis
melanosis
    Becker m.
    m. bulbi
    circumscribed precancerous m.
     of Dubreuilh

M

melanosis *(continued)*
    m. coli
    Dubreuilh precancerous m.
    m. iridis, m. of iris
    linear m.
    mucocutaneous m.
    neurocutaneous m.
    m. oculi
    oculocutaneous m.
    periorbital m.
    primary acquired m.
    pustular m.
    Riehl m.
    m. sclerae
    tar m.
    transient neonatal
      pustular m.
    whorled m.
melanosome
    compound m.
melanotic
    m. ameloblastoma
    m. cancer
    m. carcinoma
    m. neuroectodermal tumor
    m. pigment
    m. sarcoma
    m. whitlow
melanotropic
melanotropin
melanuria
melanuric
melasma
    epidermal m.
    facial m.
    hormonally induced m.
    recalcitrant m.
    resistant m.
melatonin
Meleda disease
melena
    massive m.
    recurrent m.
    repeated episodes of m.
    unexplained m.
Meleney
    chronic undermining ulcer
      (types I and II)
    synergistic gangrene
melenic
melezitose
melibiose
melitis
Melkersson syndrome
Melkersson-Rosenthal syndrome

Meller
    operation
    retractor
Mellinger speculum
mellitus
    diabetes m.
Melnick-Needles
    disease
    osteodysplasty
    syndrome
melodidymus
meloplasty
melorheostosis
melosalgia
meloschisis
melotia
Meltzer
    anesthesia
    method
    nasopharyngoscope
    punch
Meltzer-Lyon test
MEM—minimum essential
  medium
membra (plural of membrum)
membrana (membranae)
    m. adamantina
    m. adventitia
    m. agnina
    m. atlanto-occipitalis anterior
    m. atlanto-occipitalis posterior
    m. basalis
    m. basalis ductus
      semicircularis
    m. capsularis
    m. choriocapillaris
    m. cricovocalis
    m. epipapillaris
    m. fibroelastica laryngis
    m. fibrosa capsulae articularis
    m. flaccida
    m. fusca
    m. germinativa
    m. granulosa
    m. granulosa externa
    m. granulosa interna
    m. hyaloidea
    m. intercostalis externa
    m. intercostalis interna
    m. interossea antebrachii
    m. interossea cruris
    m. limitans
    m. nictitans
    m. obturatoria
    m. perforata

membrana (membranae) *(continued)*
    m. perinei
    m. pituitosa
    m. propria
    m. propria ductus
        semicircularis
    m. pupillaris
    m. quadrangularis
    m. reticularis organi spiralis
    m. ruyschiana
    m. sacciformis
    m. serosa
    m. serotina
    m. spiralis ductus cochlearis
    m. stapedialis
    m. statoconiorum macularum
    m. sterni
    m. suprapleuralis
    m. synovialis capsulae
        articularis
    m. synovialis inferior
        articulationis
        temporomandibularis
    m. synovialis superior
        articulationis
        temporomandibularis
    m. tectoria
    m. tectoria ductus cochlearis
    m. tensa
    m. thyrohyoidea
    m. tympanica secundaria
    m. tympani secundaria
    m. vestibularis ductus
        cochlearis
    m. vibrans
    m. vitellina
    m. vitrea
membranate
membrane
    abdominal m.
    accidental m.
    adamantine m.
    allantoid m.
    alveolar-capillary m.
    alveolocapillary m.
    alveolodental m.
    anal m.
    antral m.
    apical m.
    aponeurotic m.
    arachnoid m.
    Ascherson m.
    asphyxial m.
    atlantooccipital m., anterior
    atlantooccipital m., posterior

membrane *(continued)*
    basal m. of semicircular duct
    basement m.
    basilar m. of cochlear duct
    basolateral m.
    Bichat m.
    Bowman m.
    Bruch m.
    Brunn m.
    bucconasal m.
    buccopharyngeal m.
    capsular m.
    capsulopupillary m.
    cell m.
    chorioallantoic m.
    cloacal m.
    complex m.
    compound m.
    Corti m.
    costocoracoid m.
    cribriform m.
    cricothyroid m.
    cricotracheal m.
    cricovocal m.
    croupous m.
    crural interosseous m.
    cyclitic m.
    cytoplasmic m.
    Debove m.
    decidual m's
    Descemet m.
    dialysis m.
    diphtheritic m.
    drum m.
    enamel m.
    endoneural m.
    endoral m.
    epiretinal m.
    external elastic m.
    extraembryonic m's
    false m.
    fenestrated m.
    fetal m's
    fibroelastic m. of larynx
    fibrous m. of articular capsule
    filtration slit m.
    germinal m.
    glassy m.
    glomerular basement m.
    glomerular capillary m.
    gradocol m's
    ground m.
    Haller m.
    Hannover intermediate m.
    hemodialyzer m.

M

membrane *(continued)*

    Henle m.
    Henle elastic m.
    Henle fenestrated m.
    Heuser m.
    homogeneous m.
    hyaline m.
    hyaloid m.
    hymenal m.
    hyoglossal m.
    hyothyroid m.
    intercostal m.
    internal elastic m.
    interosseous m. of forearm
    interosseous m. of leg
    interosseous m., radioulnar
    interspinal m's
    intersutural m.
    Jackson m.
    Jacob m.
    keratogenous m.
    Kölliker m.
    Krause m.
    ligamentous m.
    limiting m.
    limiting m., external
    limiting m., inner
    limiting m., internal
    limiting m., outer
    Mauthner m.
    medullary m.
    mucocutaneous m.
    mucous m.
    mucous m. of colon
    mucous m. of esophagus
    mucous m. of female urethra
    mucous m. of gallbladder
    mucous m. of large intestine
    mucous m. of male urethra
    mucous m. of mouth
    mucous m. of pharynx
    mucous m. of rectum
    mucous m. of small intestine
    mucous m. of stomach
    mucous m. of tongue
    mucous m. of ureter
    mucous m. of urinary bladder
    mucous m. of vagina
    Nasmyth m.
    nuclear m.
    oblique m. of forearm
    obturator m.
    obturator m. of atlas, anterior
    obturator m. of atlas, posterior
    occipitoaxial m., long

membrane *(continued)*

    olfactory m.
    oral m.
    oronasal m.
    oropharyngeal m.
    otolithic m.
    ovular m.
    palatine m.
    paroral m.
    pericolic m.
    peridental m.
    perineal m.
    m. of perineum
    periodontal m.
    periorbital m.
    pharyngeal m.
    pial-glial m.
    pituitary m. of nose
    placental m.
    plasma m.
    platelet demarcation m.
    pleuropericardial m.
    pleuroperitoneal m.
    postsynaptic m.
    presynaptic m.
    proligerous m.
    proper mucous m.
    proper m. of semicircular duct
    prophylactic m.
    pseudoserous m.
    PTFE
      (polytetrafluoroethylene) m.
    pulmonary hyaline m.
    pupillary m.
    pyophylactic m.
    quadrangular m.
    Reissner m.
    respiratory m.
    reticular m.
    reticular m. of organ of Corti
    reticulated m.
    Rivinus m.
    m. of round window
    Ruysch m., ruyschian m.
    Scarpa m.
    schneiderian m.
    Schwann m.
    semipermeable m.
    serous m.
    shell m.
    m. of Slavianski
    slit m.
    spiral m. of cochlear duct
    stapedial m.
    sternal m.

membrane *(continued)*
- striated m.
- subepithelial m.
- submucous m.
- suprapleural m.
- synaptic m.
- synovial m.
- synovial m. of articular capsule
- synovial m. of temporomandibular joint, inferior
- synovial m. of temporomandibular joint, superior
- tarsal m.
- tectorial m.
- tectorial m. of cochlear duct
- tendinous m.
- Tenon m.
- thyrohyoid m.
- Toldt m.
- tympanic m. (TM)
- tympanic m., secondary
- unit m.
- urogenital m.
- vascular m. of viscera
- vernix m.
- vestibular m. of cochlear duct
- virginal m.
- vitelline m.
- vitreous m.
- Volkmann m.
- Wachendorf m.
- yolk m.
- Zinn m.

membranectomy
membraniform
membranocartilaginous
membranoid
membranolysis
membranous
- m. adhesions
- m. glomerulonephritis
- m. glomerulopathy
- m. labyrinthectomy
- m. nephropathy
- m. urethra

membrum (membra)
- m. inferius
- m. superius
- m. virile

Memorial Sloan-Kettering protocol
memory
- anterograde m.
- echoic m.

memory *(continued)*
- eye m.
- iconic m.
- m. image
- immediate m.
- immunologic m.
- kinesthetic m.
- long-term m.
- motor m.
- m. probe
- random-access m.
- recent m.
- remote m.
- retrograde m.
- rote m.
- screen m.
- short-term m.
- virtual m.
- visual m.

MEN—multiple endocrine neoplasia
menacme
menalgia
menarche
- age at m., age of m.
- delayed m.
- early-onset m.

menarcheal
mendacity
Mendel
- reflex
- test

Mendel-Bekhterev
- reflex
- sign

mendelevium (Md)
Mendelson syndrome
Ménétrier disease
Menge
- operation
- pessary

Mengert index
Menghini needle
Ménière disease
meningeal
- m. anthrax
- m. artery
- m. carcinoma
- m. carcinomatosis
- m. filament
- m. irritation
- m. melanocytosis
- m. nerve
- m. plexus
- primary m. lymphoma

meningeal *(continued)*
  m. signs
meningeorrhaphy
meninges (plural of meninx)
meninghematoma
meningioma
  aggressive m.
  anaplastic m.
  angioblastic m.
  angiomatous m.
  atypical m.
  cerebellopontine angle m.
  clinically silent m.
  clival m.
  convexity m.
  cystic m.
  endotheliomatous m.
  falcine m.
  falx m.
  fibroblastic m.
  fibrous m.
  intracranial m.
  meningothelial m.
  meningotheliomatous m.
  mesodermal m.
  microcystic m.
  mixed m.
  myxomatous m.
  olfactory groove m.
  parasagittal m.
  petroclival m.
  posterior fossa m.
  progesterone
   receptor–positive m.
  psammomatous m.
  suprasellar m.
  syncytial m.
  tentorial m.
  transitional m.
  tuberculum sellae m.
meningiomatosis
meningism
meningismus
meningitic
meningitis (meningitides)
  acute aseptic m.
  acute septic m.
  anthrax m.
  aseptic m.
  bacterial m.
  m. of the base of the brain
  basilar m.
  benign lymphocytic m.
  cerebral m.
  cerebrospinal m.

meningitis (meningitides) *(continued)*
  chemical m.
  chronic m.
  community-acquired m.
  cryptococcal m.
  eosinophilic m.
  epidemic cerebrospinal m.
  external m.
  fungal m.
  gonococcal m.
  granulomatous m.
  gummatous m.
  herpetic m.
  Hib (*Haemophilus influenzae*
   type b) m.
  infectious m.
  internal m.
  lymphocytic m.
  meningococcal m.
  metastatic m.
  Mollaret m.
  mumps m.
  mycobacterial m.
  mycotic m.
  neonatal m.
  neoplastic m.
  occlusive m.
  otitic m.
  otogenic m.
  parameningococcus m.
  pneumococcal m.
  post-traumatic m.
  purulent m.
  pyogenic m.
  sarcoid m.
  septic m.
  m. serosa circumscripta
  serous m.
  spinal m.
  staphylococcal m.
  sterile m.
  streptococcal m.
  suppurative m.
  m. sympathica
  syphilitic m.
  tubercular m., tuberculous m.
  viral m.
meningoarteritis
meningocele
  anterior m.
  cranial m.
  extradural m.
  rudimentary m.
  sacral m.
  spinal m.

meningocele *(continued)*
    spurious m.
    temporal m.
    traumatic m.
meningococcal
    m. conjugate vaccine
    m. meningitis
    m. pneumonia
    m. polysaccharide vaccine
meningococcemia
    acute fulminating m.
    chronic m.
    disseminated m.
    fulminant m.
meningococcosis
meningococcus (meningococci)
meningocortical
meningocyte
meningoencephalitis
    amebic m.
    chronic m.
    cryptococcal m.
    eosinophilic m.
    granulomatous m.
    infective m.
    mumps m.
    primary amebic m.
    syphilitic m.
    thromboembolic m.
    toxoplasmic m.
meningoencephalocele
meningoencephalomyelitis
meningoencephalomyelopathy
meningoencephalopathy
meningofibroblastoma
meningogenic labyrinthitis
meningomalacia
meningomyelitis
    blastomycotic m.
    eosinophilic m.
    mycobacterial m.
    sporotrichotic m.
    syphilitic m.
    torular m.
meningomyelocele
meningomyeloencephalitis
meningomyeloradiculitis
meningo-osteophlebitis
meningopathy
meningopneumonitis
meningopolyneuritis
meningorachidian
meningoradicular
meningoradiculitis
meningoradiculomyelitis

meningorecurrence
meningorrhagia
meningorrhea
meningosis
meningothelioma
meningovascular
meninx (meninges)
    cerebellar m.
    cervical m.
    primary m.
    m. primitiva, primitive m.
    spinal m.
meniscal
    m. fragment
    m. injury
    m. lesion
    m. migration
    m. tear
meniscectomy
    arthroscopic m.
    m. knife
    lateral m.
    medial m.
    open m.
    partial m.
    total m.
menisci (plural of meniscus)
meniscitis
meniscocyte
meniscocytosis
meniscofemoral ligament
meniscosynovial
meniscotome
    Bircher m.
    Bowen-Grover m.
    Smillie m.
    V-shaped m.
meniscotomy
meniscus (menisci)
    m. of acromioclavicular joint
    articular m., m. articularis
    converging m.
    discoid m., discoid lateral m.
    diverging m.
    m. of inferior radioulnar joint
    intact m.
    joint m.
    Kuhnt m.
    m. lateralis articulationis genus
    lateral m. of knee joint
    m. lens
    m. medialis articulationis genus
    medial m. of knee joint
    m. tactus
    native m.

M

meniscus (menisci) *(continued)*
    negative m.
    positive m.
    m. sign
    tactile menisci
    m. of temporomandibular joint
    torn m.
Menkes syndrome
Mennell sign
menolipsis
menometrorrhagia
menopausal
menopause
    artificial m.
    early m.
    induced m.
    natural m.
    m. praecox
    premature m.
    surgical m.
menoplania
menorrhagia
    functional m.
    unexplained m.
menorrhea
menorrheal
menoschesis
menotropins
menouria
menses
mens rea
menstrual
    m. age
    m. cycle
    m. decidua
    m. epilepsy
    last m. period (LMP)
    m. period
    m. phase
menstruant
menstruate
menstruation
    anovular m.,
      anovulatory m.
    delayed m.
    difficult m.
    infrequent m.
    nonovulational m.
    ovulatory m.
    profuse m.
    regurgitant m.
    retained m.
    retrograde m.
    scanty m.
    supplementary m.

menstruation *(continued)*
    suppressed m.
    vicarious m.
menstruous
menstruum
mental
    m. aberration
    m. age
    m. agraphia
    m. artery
    m. blind spot
    m. block
    m. canal
    m. crest
    m. deficiency
    m. disease
    m. disorder
    m. fog
    m. foramen
    m. illness
    m. image
    m. nerve
    m. point
    m. process
    m. protuberance
    m. retardation
    m. scotoma
    m. spine
    m. tubercle
mentalis muscle
mentality
mentation
menthol
menthyl anthranilate
mentoanterior
mentolabial
menton
    m. deviation
    gonion-m. distance
    m.-nasion length
    m. point
mentoplasty
mentoposterior
mentotransverse
mentum
    m. anterior position
    hypoplastic m.
    m. osseum
    m. posterior position
    m. transverse position
MEP—
    motor evoked potential
    multimodality evoked
      potential
mephitic

mEq—milliequivalent(s)
MER—
    mean ejection rate
    methanol extraction residue
meralgia paresthetica
M/E (myeloid-erythroid) ratio
mercapturic acid
Mercier
    bar
    barrier
    valve
mercocresols
mercurial
    m. necrosis
    m. stomatitis
mercurialism
p-mercuribenzoate [p-, para-]
mercuric
    m. chloride
    m. oxide, yellow
    m. sulfide
mercurous
mercury (Hg)
    ammoniated m.
    m. bichloride
    m. bougies
    m. dilators
    methyl m.
    millimeters of m. (mm Hg, mmHg)
    m. nephropathy
    m. oleate
    m. perchloride
    m. pneumonitis
    m. poisoning
    m. test
    m. thermometer
Merendino technique
meridian
    m. of cornea
    m's of eyeball
    horizontal m.
    vertical m.
meridianus (meridiani)
    meridiani bulbi oculi
meridional
meritorious
Merkel
    cell carcinoma
    cells
    corpuscles
    disk
    filtrum
    fossa
    muscle

Merkel *(continued)*
    tactile cells
Merkel-Ranvier cells
meroacrania
meroanencephaly
Merocel packing
merocoxalgia
merocrine
merocyte
meromelia
meromicrosomia
meromyosin
meropia
merorachischisis
merosmia
merostotic
Merseburg triad
Mersilene
    gauze dressing
    suture
Merzbacher-Pelizaeus
    disease
    sclerosis
mesangial
    m. cells
    m. proliferative
        glomerulonephritis
mesangiocapillary
    glomerulonephritis
mesangiolysis
mesangium
    extraglomerular m.
    glomerular m.
    renal m.
mesarteritis
    Mönckeberg m.
mesatikerkic
mesatipellic
mescal
mescaline
mescalism
mesencephalic
    m. arteries
    m. flexure
    m. tract of trigeminal nerve
    m. tractotomy
    m. veins
mesencephalitis
mesencephalohypophysial,
    mesencephalohypophyseal
mesencephalon
mesencephalotomy
mesenchymal
    m. cells
    m. chondrosarcoma

M

mesenchymal *(continued)*
    m. epithelium
    m. tissue
mesenchyme
    interzonal m.
mesenchymoma
    benign m.
    malignant m.
mesenterectomy
mesenterial intestine
mesenteric
    m. adenitis
    m. arterial thrombosis
    m. arteriography
    m. artery
    m. axis
    m. cyst
    m. fibromatosis
    m. ganglion
    m. glands
    m. hernia
    m. infarction
    m. ischemia
    m. lipodystrophy
    m. lymphadenitis
    m. lymphadenopathy
    m. lymph nodes
    m. panniculitis
    m. pregnancy
    m. vein
    m. venous thrombosis
mesentericoparietal
    m. fossa
    m. hernia
mesenteriolum appendicis
    vermiformis
mesenteriopexy
mesenteriorrhaphy
mesenteriplication
mesenteritis
    retractile m.
    sclerosing m.
mesenterium commune
mesenteroaxial volvulus
mesentery
    m. of ascending part of colon
    m. of descending part of colon
    m. of rectum
    m. of sigmoid colon
    m. of transverse part of colon
    m. of vermiform appendix
mesh
    Dexon m.
    fine m. dressing
    Marlex m.

mesh *(continued)*
    steel m. suture
    tantalum m.
    Teflon m.
    Vitallium m.
    wire m.
meshwork
    trabecular m.
mesiad
mesial
mesially
mesien
mesiobuccal (MB)
mesiobucco-occlusal (MBO)
mesiobuccopulpal (MBP)
mesiocervical
mesioclination
mesioclusion
mesiodens (mesiodentes)
mesiodistal
mesiogingival (MG)
mesioincisodistal (MID)
mesiolabial (MLA)
mesiolabioincisal (MLAI)
mesiolingual (ML)
mesiolinguoincisal (MLI)
mesiolinguo-occlusal (MLO)
mesiolinguopulpal (MLP)
mesion
mesio-occlusal (MO)
mesio-occlusodistal (MOD)
mesiopulpal (MP)
mesiopulpolabial (MPLA)
mesiopulpolingual (MPL)
mesioversion
mesitylene
mesmerism
mesoaortitis
    rheumatic m.
    syphilitic m.
mesoappendicitis
mesoappendix
mesobilin
mesobilirubin
mesobilirubinogen
mesobiliverdin
mesoblast
mesoblastema
mesoblastic
    m. nephroma
    m. segment
mesoblastoma
    m. ovarii
    m. vitellinum
mesobranchial area

mesocardia
mesocardium
    dorsal m.
    lateral m.
    venous m.
    ventral m.
mesocarpal
mesocaval shunt
mesocecal
mesocecum
mesocephalic
    m. hemianesthesia
mesochondrium
mesochoroidea
mesocolic
    m. glands
    m. lymph nodes
mesocolon
    ascending m., m. ascendens
    descending m., m. descendens
    iliac m.
    left m.
    pelvic m.
    right m.
    sigmoid m., m. sigmoideum
    transverse m., m. transversum
mesocolopexy
mesocoloplication
mesocord
mesocornea
mesocortex
mesocranic
mesocuneiform bone
mesocyst
mesoderm
    cardiogenic m.
    extraembryonic m.
    gastral m.
    head m.
    lateral m.
    paraxial m.
    peristomal m.
    somatic m.
    splanchnic m.
mesodermal mixed tumor
mesodermic
mesodont
mesodontic
mesodontism
mesoduodenal
mesoduodenum
mesoepididymis
mesoesophagus
mesogastric
mesogastrium

mesoglea
mesogluteal
mesogluteus
mesognathous
mesoileum
mesojejunum
mesolateral fold
mesomelic
mesomere
mesomeric
mesometrium
mesomorph
mesomorphic
mesomorphy
meson
mesonasal
mesonephric
    m. duct
    m. fold
    m. ridge
    m. tubules
mesonephroma
mesonephron
mesonephros (mesonephroi)
    caudal m.
    cranial m.
    genital m.
mesoomentum
mesophilic bacterium
mesophlebitis
mesophryon
mesopia
mesopic
mesopneumon
mesoporphyrin
mesoprosopic
mesopulmonum
mesorachischisis
mesorchial
mesorchium
mesorectum
mesoropter
mesorrhine
mesosalpinx
mesoscapula
mesoseme
mesosigmoid
mesosigmoiditis
mesosigmoidopexy
mesosome
mesostaphyline
mesosternum
mesostroma
mesotaurodontism
mesotendineum

M

mesothelial cells
mesothelioma
  benign fibrous m.
  diffuse m.
  localized fibrous m.
  malignant m.
  mesenteric m.
  peritoneal m.
  pleural m.
  m. of testis
  m. of tunica vaginalis
  m. xenografts
mesothelium
mesothenar muscle
mesotropic
mesotympanum
mesouterine fold
mesovarial margin of
  ovary
mesovarian
mesovarium
messenger
  first m.
  m. RNA
  second m.
mesuranic
met—methionine
met, mets [unit]
metabasis
metabolic
  m. acidosis
  m. alkalosis
  m. antagonist
  m. block
  m. burst
  m. cataract
  m. cirrhosis
  m. coma
  m. craniopathy
  m. detoxification
  m. disease
  m. encephalopathy
  m. myopathy
  m. syndrome
metabolimetry
metabolism
  basal m.
  drug m.
  endogenous m.
  energy m.
  excess m. of exercise
  exogenous m.
  glucose m.
  inborn error of m.
  intermediary m.

metabolite
  essential m.
metabolizable
metabolize
metacarpal
  m. arteries
  m. bones
  m. index
  m. ligaments
  m. region
  m. veins
metacarpectomy
metacarpophalangeal (MCP) joints
metacarpus
metacercaria (metacercariae)
metachromasia
metachromatic
  m. dye
  m. stain
metachromatin
metachromatophil
metachromophil
metachronous
metachrosis
metacone
metaconid
metaconule
metacresol
  m. purple
  m. sulfonphthalein
metacyesis
metafemale
metagaster
metagastrula
metagelatin
metagenesis
metagonimiasis
Metagonimus
  M. ovatus
  M. yokogawai
metaherpetic
metaicteric
metainfective
metaiodobenzylguanidine (MIBG)
  I-123 m.
  m. scanning
  m. scintigraphy
metal
  alkali m.
  alkaline earth m's
  m. base
  m. ceramic
  colloidal m.
  m. fume fever
  fusible m.

metal *(continued)*
 hard m. disease
 heavy m.
 heavy m. stain
 m. insert tooth
 noble m.
metallic
 m. echo
 m. melanism
 m. rale
 m. sound
 m. tremor
metallized
metallizing
metallocyanide
metalloenzyme
metalloflavoprotein
metalloid
metallophil cells
metallophilic
metalloporphyrin
metalloprotein
metalloproteinase
metallotherapy
metallothionein
metamorphopsia
metamorphosis
 fatty m.
 ovulational m.
 platelet m.
 retrograde m.
 retrogressive m.
 revisionary m.
 skeletal m.
 structural m.
 tissue m.
 viscous m.
metamorphotic
metamyelocyte
metanephric
 m. blastema
 m. bud
 m. cap
 m. diverticulum
 m. duct
 m. mass
 m. tubules
 m. vesicles
metanephrine
metanephrogenic tissue
metanephron
metanephros (metanephroi)
metaneutrophil
metanil yellow, metaniline yellow
metaphase plate

metaphosphoric acid
metaphyseal
 m. chondrodysplasia
 m. dysostosis
 m. dysplasia
 m. fibrous defect
metaphysis (metaphyses)
 distal m.
 femoral m.
 proximal m.
 radial m.
 tibial m.
 ulnar m.
metaphysitis
metaplasia
 agnogenic myeloid m.
 apocrine m.
 Barrett m.
 chondroid m.
 florid squamous m.
 gastric m.
 intestinal m.
 myeloid m.
 nephrogenic m.
 osseous m.
 primary myeloid m.
 proliferative squamous m.
 pseudopyloric m.
 m. of pulp
 squamous m.
metaplastic
metapneumonic
metapneumovirus
metapodialia
metapsychology
metarteriole
metarubricyte
metastable state
metastasectomy
metastasis (metastases)
 biochemical m.
 calcareous m.
 cannonball m.
 contact m.
 crossed m.
 direct m.
 hematogenous m.
 implantation m.
 lymphangitic m.
 mediastinal m.
 nodular m.
 osteoblastic m.
 osteolytic m.
 pleural m.
 retrograde m.

M

metastasize
metastatic
metasternum
metasyncrisis
metatarsal
metatarsalgia
metatarsectomy
metatarsophalangeal
    (MTP) joint
metatarsus
    m. adductocavus
    m. adductovarus
    m. adductus
    m. atavicus
    m. brevis
    m. latus
    m. primus varus
    m. varus
metathalamus
metathetic
metathrombin
metatrophia
metatypical
metavanadate
    sodium m.
Metchnikoff theory
metencephalic
metencephalon
metencephalospinal
meteorism
meteoropathy
meteororesistant
meteorosensitive
meteorotropic
meteorotropism
meter
    dosage m.
    dose-rate m.
    integrating dose m.
    peak flow m.
    rate m.
    sound level m.
metergasis
methacholine
    m. chloride
    m. pulmonary challenge
        test
methacrylate
methacrylic acid
methane
methanesulfonic acid
methanol
metHb—methemoglobin
methemalbumin
methemalbuminemia
metheme

methemoglobin (metHb)
methemoglobinemia
    acquired m.
    benzocaine-induced m.
    congenital m.
    dapsone-induced m.
    hereditary m.
    medication-induced m.
    postoperative m.
    toxic m.
    transient m.
methemoglobinemic
methemoglobin reductase
methemoglobinuria
methenamine
    Gomori m. silver (GMS)
    m. silver staining method
methionine C 11
methionyl
method
    Abbott m.
    Altmann-Gersh m.
    autoclave m.
    back pressure–arm lift m.
    Barger m.
    Barraquer m.
    bench m.
    Bethea m.
    Bobath m.
    border detection m.
    Born m. of wax plate
        reconstruction
    Brandt-Andrews m.
    breath alcohol m.
    brine flotation m.
    broth dilution m.
    broth microdilution m.
    Brunnstrom m.
    buffy coat m.
    caliper m.
    Callahan m.
    Carrel m.
    Castaneda m.
    chest pressure–arm lift m.
    Chick-Martin m.
    chloropercha m.
    Ciaccio m.
    Clark-Collip m.
    Clauss m.
    closed-plaster m.
    Converse m.
    Couette m.
    Coutard m.
    Credé m. of expressing placenta
    Cronin m.
    Cuignet m.

method *(continued)*
    cup plate m.
    Dakin-Carrel m.
    definitive m.
    deletion m.
    Denis and Leche m.
    Denman m.
    Dickinson m.
    differential
      agglutination m.
    dilution m.
    direct m.
    direct aeration m.
    direct centrifugal flotation m.
    disk diffusion m.
    Domagk m.
    Duke m.
    dye dilution m.
    Eicken m.
    Ellinger m.
    Eskimo m.
    expired air m.
    external rotation m.
    Fahraeus m.
    falling drop m.
    Faust m.
    Fay m.
    Feldenkrais m.
    Fick m.
    Fishberg m.
    Fiske m.
    Fiske and Subbarow m.
    flash m.
    flotation m.
    flush m.
    Folin m.
    Folin and Wu m.
    Fülleborn (Fuelleborn) m.
    Gerota m.
    Giemsa m.
    Gomori m.
    Gram m.
    Hamilton m.
    Heublein m.
    hippocratic m.
    Hirschberg m.
    Hoffa tendon-shortening m.
    holding m.
    Holger Nielsen m.
    horizontal scrub m.
    impedance m.
    India ink m.
    indirect m.
    introspective m.
    Isaac differential distortion
      divergent m.

method *(continued)*
    Ivy m.
    Jenckel
      cholecystoduodenostomy m.
    Jendrassik-Grof m.
    Johnson m.
    Kaplan-Meier m.
    Kety-Schmidt m.
    Kirstein m.
    Kjeldahl m.
    Klüver-Barrera m.
    Kocher m.
    Korotkoff m.
    Laborde m.
    Lamaze m.
    Lane m.
    Lange tendon-lengthening m.
    lateral condensation m.
    Leboyer m.
    Mauriceau-Smellie-Veit m.
    Milch m.
    Monte Carlo m.
    Mosley anterior shoulder
      repair m.
    mouth-to-mouth m.
    multiple cone m.
    Nègre and Bretey m.
    Nielsen m.
    Nikiforoff m.
    no-touch m.
    nutritional table m.
    Ogino-Knaus m.
    optical density m.
    Orr m.
    Orsi-Grocco m.
    panoptic m.
    Pap silver m.
    parallax m.
    piggybacking m.
    point source m.
    Politzer m.
    Ponseti m.
    potassium hydroxide
      concentration m.
    product-limit m.
    projective m.
    proprioceptive neuromuscular
      facilitation m.
    psychometric m.
    psychophysical m.
    pulse reflection m.
    radioactive balloon m.
    recall m.
    recognition m.
    reference m.
    retrofilling m.

M

method *(continued)*
    reverse Giemsa m.
    rhythm m.
    Rideal-Walker m.
    Ritchie formalin–ethyl
      acetate m.
    Ritgen m.
    Romanovsky (Romanowsky) m.
    Rood m.
    Rosen m.
    Sahli m.
    Schafer m.
    sectional m.
    segmentation m.
    Sheather sugar flotation
      method, modified
    sib-pair m.
    silver point (cone) m.
    Silvester m.
    single cone m.
    Sluder m.
    Smellie-Veit m.
    Somogyi m.
    split-cast m.
    Stimson m.
    m. of successive approximations
    suction m.
    sulfosalicylic acid m. for
      proteinuria
    Sumner m.
    suspension m.
    syringe-capillary m.
    template m.
    Thane m.
    thermal dilution m.
    thick-film m.
    Torkildsen shunt m.
    traction-countertraction m.
    triangle m.
    Trueta m.
    turbidity m.
    van Gehuchten m.
    Van Slyke m.
    vertical condensation m.
    Wardill m., four-flap, two-flap
    Welcker m.
    Westergren m.
    Whipple m.
    Wintrobe m.
    Wynn m.
    Yuzpe m.
    Ziehl-Neelsen staining m.
    Zsigmondy gold number m.
methodology
methoxychlor

methoxyflurane
methyl
    m. alcohol
    m. aminolevulinate HCl
    m. benzene
    m. blue
    m. bromide
    m. chloride
    m. ethyl-pyrrole
    m. green-pyronin stain
    m. hydride
    m. hydroxy-furfural
    m. iodide
    m. isobutyl ketone
    m. mercury
    m. methacrylate
    m. orange
    m. red test
    m. red-Voges-Proskauer
      (MR-VP) broth
    m. salicylate
    m. violet
    m. yellow
α-methylacetoacetic acid [alpha-]
α-methylacetoaceticaciduria
    [alpha-]
α-methylacetoacetyl CoA thiolase
    [alpha-]
methylamine
methylated
methylation
methylazoxymethanol
methylcellulose
    m. gel
    hydroxypropyl m.
methylchloroformate
3-methylcholanthrene (MCA)
3-methylcrotonyl CoA carboxylase
    deficiency
β-methylcrotonylglycinuria
    [beta-]
methyldichlorarsin
methylene
    m. azure
    m. blue
    m. blue insufflation
    m. chloride
    m. green
    m. iodide
    polychrome m. blue
    m. violet
methylenetetrahydrofolate
    reductase (MTHFR) deficiency
methylenophil
methylenophilous

3-methylglutaconic acid
3-methylglutaconicaciduria
3-methylglutaric acid
methylguanidine
methylguanosine
3-methylhistidine
methylhydantoin
methylmalonic acid
methylmalonicacidemia
methylmalonicaciduria
methylmalonyl-CoA epimerase
methylmalonyl-CoA mutase
methylmalonyl-CoA racemase
methylmercaptan
methylpyridine
5-methyltetrahydrofolate
methyltheobromine
methylthionine chloride
methyltransferase
5-methyluracil
methylxanthine
metmyoglobin
metonymy
metopic suture
metopion
metopism
metopodynia
metopopagus
metopoplasty
metra
Metras catheter
metratonia
metratrophia
metrectopia
metreurynter
metric
    m. ophthalmoscopy
    m. system
metriocephalic
metritis
    m. dissecans
    puerperal m.
metrizamide
    m.-assisted computed
        tomography
    m. cisternography
metrizoate sodium contrast
    medium
metrocystosis
metrogenous
metroleukorrhea
metrolymphangitis
metromalacia
metromenorrhagia
metronoscope

metroparalysis
metroperitoneal
metroperitonitis
metrophlebitis
metroplasty
metroptosis
metrorrhagia myopathica
metrorrhea
metrorrhexis
metrosalpingitis
metrosalpingogram
metrosalpingography
metrosalpinx
metrostasis
metrostaxis
metrostenosis
mets—metastases
Mett (Mette)
    method
    test tubes
metyrapone tartrate
Metzenbaum
    forceps
    scissors
Metzenbaum-Lipsett scissors
Meulengracht
    diet
    method
Meunier sign
mevalonate kinase
mevalonic acid
mevalonicaciduria
Meyer
    disease
    hockey-stick incision
    line
    loop
    mastectomy
    operation
    organ
    retractor
    sinus
    stripper
    system
Meyer-Betz disease
Meyerding
    curet
    gouge
    mallet
    osteotome
    retractor
Meyer-Overton theory
Meyhoeffer curet
Meynert
    bundle

M

Meynert *(continued)*
    cells
    commissure
    decussation
    fasciculus
    fibers
    layer
    tract
MF—
    medium frequency
    microscopic factor
    mycosis fungoides
    myelin figures
M&F—mother and father
MFB—metallic foreign body
MFD—
    midforceps delivery
    minimum fatal dose
MFR—mucus flow rate
MFWs—multiple fragment wounds
μg; mcg—microgram(s)
mg—milligram(s)
mg%—milligrams percent
Mg—magnesium
MG—
    mesiogingival
    muscle group
    myasthenia gravis
MGF—macrophage growth factor
mg/L—milligrams per liter
MGN—membranous
  glomerulonephritis
MGP—marginal granulocyte pool
MGR—modified gain ratio
mGy—milligray(s)
MH—
    marital history
    medical history
    mental health
MHA—
    methemalbumin
    microhemagglutination assay
MHA-TP—microhemagglutination
  assay–*Treponema pallidum*
MHb—methemoglobin
MHB—maximum hospital benefit
MHC—major histocompatibility
  complex
MHN—massive hepatic necrosis
MHR—maximal heart rate
MHz—megahertz
MI—
    mitral incompetence
    mitral insufficiency
    myocardial infarction

Mibelli porokeratosis
MIBG—metaiodobenzylguanidine
MIC—
    Maternity and Infant Care
    minimal inhibitory
      concentration
mica pneumoconiosis
micaceous
mication
micatosis
mice
    joint m.
micelle
Michaelis
    rhomboid
    stain
Michaelis-Gutmann bodies
Michel
    clip
    deafness
    deformity
    trephine
micranatomy
micrencephalon
micrencephalous
micrencephaly
microabrasion
microabscess
    central stellate m.
    dense neutrophilic m.
    eosinophilic m.
    focal dermal m.
    m. formation
    intraepithelial m.
    Munro m.
    Pautrier m.
    sebaceous m.
microabsorption spectroscopy
microadenectomy
microadenoma
microadenopathy
microaerosol
microaggregate
microalbuminuria
microanalysis
microanastomosis
microanatomist
microanatomy
microaneurysm
microangiogram
microangiography
    fluorescence m.
    synchrotron radiation m.
    three-dimensional (3-D) m.
microangiopathic

microangiopathy
    diabetic m.
    inflammatory m.
    posttransplantation
        thrombotic m.
    small vessel obliterative m.
    thrombotic m.
    vasa nervorum m.
microangioscopy
micro-Astrup method
microbacteria
Microbacterium lacticum
microbe
microbial
microbian
microbicidal
microbicide
microbioassay
microbiological
microbiologist
microbiology
microbiotic
microblast
microblepharia
microbrachia
microbrachius
microbrenner
microbubbles
microcalcification
microcalculus (microcalculi)
microcalix
microcapsule
microcardia
microcephalic
microcephalus
microcephaly
    encephaloclastic m.
    schizencephalic m.
microcheilia
microcheiria
microchemical
microchimerism
microcirculation
microcirculatory
microcnemia
micrococcus (micrococci)
Micrococcus luteus
microcolon
microconcentration
microcoria
microcornea
microcrania
microcrystalline
microcurie(s) (μCi, microCi)
microcurie-hour (μCi-hr, microCi-hr)

microcyst
microcyte
microcythemia
microcytic
    m. anemia
    m. erythrocytes
    m. hypochromic anemia
    m. hypochromic indices
    m. hypochromic parameters
microcytosis
microcytotoxicity
microdactyly
microdeletion
microdermatome
microdetermination
microdilution
microdiscectomy, microdiskectomy
    arthroscopic m.
    cervical m.
    lumbar m.
    open m.
    percutaneous m.
microdissection
microdont
microdontia
microdontic
microdosage
microdose
microdrepanocytic
microdrepanocytosis
microelectrode
microelectrophoresis
microelectrophoretic
microembolization
microembolus (microemboli)
microerythrocyte
microfarad (μf)
microfibril
microfilaremia
microfilaria
    m. bancrofti
    m. diurna
    m. loa
    sheathed m.
    m. streptocerca
    m. volvulus
microfiliariasis
microfilter
microfollicular
microfracture
microgamete
microgamy
microgastria
microgenia
microgenitalism

M

microglia
microglial
microglobulin
β_2 microglobulin [beta-2-]
microglossia
micrognathia
micrognathia-glossoptosis syndrome
micrognathism
microgram(s) (µg, mcg)
micrographia
microgyrus (microgyri)
microhematocrit
microhematuria
microhepatia
microimmunofluorescent test
microincineration
microincision
microinfarct
microinjection
microinjector
microinvasion
microinvasive
microkeratome
microlaparoscopic
　　m. approach
　　m.-assisted lumboperitoneal
　　　shunt placement
microlaparoscopy
microlaryngoscopy
microleakage
microlesion
microliter (µL, microL)
microlith
microlithiasis
　　cholesterol m.
　　pulmonary alveolar m. (PAM)
　　testicular m.
micromandible
micromanipulation
micromanipulator
micromanometric
micromastia
micromaxilla
micromegalopsia
micromelia
　　rhizomelic m.
micromelus
micromere
micrometastasis
micrometer
　　caliper m.
　　slide m.
micromethod
micrometry
micromolar (µM, microM)

micromolecular
micromyelia
micromyeloblast
microneedle
microneurography
microneurosurgery
micronize, micronized
micronodular
micronormoblast
micronutrient
micronychia
micronystagmus
micro-orchidism
microorganism
micropathology
micropenis
microperfusion
microphage
microphagocyte
microphakia
microphallus
microphonic
　　cochlear m.
　　microphthalmic
microphthalmos
micropigmentation
micropinocytosis
micropipet
micropituicyte
microplasia
microplethysmography
micropodia
microprecipitation
microprobe
　　laser m.
microprolactinoma
microprosopus
microproteinuria
micropsia
microptic
micropuncture
micropus
micropyknometer
microquantity
microradiogram
microradiography
microrhinia
microroentgen (µR, microR)
microsaccades
microscelous
microscope
　　acoustic m.
　　beta ray m.
　　binocular m.
　　capillary m.

microscope *(continued)*
 centrifuge m.
 color-contrast m.
 comparison m.
 compound m.
 corneal m.
 darkfield m.
 dissecting m.
 electron m.
 fluorescence m.
 hypodermic m.
 infrared m.
 integrating m.
 interference m.
 ion m.
 laser m.
 light m.
 ocular m.
 Omni operating m.
 opaque m.
 operating m.
 optical m.
 phase m., phase-contrast m.
 polarizing m., rectified
 projection x-ray m.
 reflecting m.
 Rheinberg m.
 scanning electron m.
 schlieren m.
 simple m.
 slit lamp m.
 stereoscopic m.
 stroboscopic m.
 surgical m.
 trinocular m.
 ultra-m.
 ultrapaque m.
 ultrasonic m.
 ultraviolet m.
 Wild operating m.
 x-ray m.
 Zeiss m.
microscopic, microscopical
microscopy
 brightfield m.
 clinical m.
 darkfield m.
 electron m.
 epifluorescence m.
 epiluminescence m.
 fluorescence m.
 fundus m.
 immersion m.
 immune electron m. (IEM)
 immunofluorescence m.

microscopy *(continued)*
 light m. (LM)
 phase-contrast m.
 scanning electron m. (SEM)
 scanning transmission
  electron m.
 television m.
 transmission electron m. (TEM)
microsection
microseme
microshock
microslide
microsmatic
microsoma
microsomal
microsome
microsomia fetalis
microspectrophotometry
microsphere
microspherolith
microsphygmia
microsplenia
microsplenic
microsporosis capitis
Microsporum
 M. audouinii
 M. canis
 M. cookei
 M. felineum
 M. ferrugineum
 M. fulvum
 M. gypseum
 M. lanosum
 M. nanum
 M. persicolor
 M. vanbreuseghemii
microsteatosis
microstomia
microstrabismus
microsurgery
 laser m.
microsuture
microsyringe
microtechnic
microthelia
microthrombosis
microthrombus (microthrombi)
microtia
microtiter
microtome
 cryostat m.
 freezing m.
 hard tissue m.
 rocking m.
 rotary m.

M

microtome *(continued)*
    sliding m.
    Stadie-Riggs m.
microtomy
microtransfusion
microtrauma
microtropia
microtubule
    chromosomal m.
    kinetochore m.
    spindle m.
    subpellicular m.
microvascular
microvasculature
microvessel
microvillus (microvilli)
    placental m.
microvivisection
microvolt (µV, microV)
microwave
microxycyte
microxyphil
micrurgic
micrurgy
micturate
micturating cystourethrography
micturition cystourethrography
MICU—medical intensive care unit
MID—
    mesioincisodistal
    minimum infective dose
midaxilla
midbody
midbrain
midcarpal
midclavicular
mid-diastolic
middle palatine suture
middlepiece
Middleton curet
midepigastric
midfoot
midfrontal
midge
midget
midline
    m. incision
    m. myelotomy
    m. shift
midoccipital
midparental height
midperiphery
midphalangeal
midplane
midriff

midsection
midsegment
midsternum
midtarsal
midtegmentum
midthorax
midventral
midwife
Mierzejewski effect
Miescher
    actinic granuloma
    granulomatous cheilitis
    tube
    tubule
MIFR—maximal inspiratory flow rate
migraine
    abdominal m.
    acute confusional m.
    m. aura
    m. aura without headache
    basilar m., basilar artery m.
    Bickerstaff m.
    classic m.
    common m.
    complicated m.
    m. equivalent
    familial hemiplegic m.
    m. headache
    hemiplegic m.
    hormonal m.
    menstrual m.
    neurologic m.
    ocular m.
    ophthalmic m.
    ophthalmoplegic m.
    retinal m.
    m. variant
migraineur
migrainoid
migrainous
migrate, migrated
migration
    band m.
    catheter m.
    cuff m.
    m. defect
    electrode m.
    external m.
    filter m.
    foreign body m.
    graft m.
    implant m.
    internal m.
    m. of leukocytes

migration *(continued)*
    m. of ovum
    retrograde m.
    screw m.
    m. of stone
    tube m.
    tooth m., pathologic
    tooth m., physiologic
    transperitoneal m.
migratory
    m. azygos vein
    m. eruption
    m. erythema
    m. neuralgias
    m. ophthalmia
    m. pneumonia
    m. subcutaneous nodules
    m. tumor
MIH—migratory inhibitory hormone
mika operation
Mikulicz (von Mikulicz)
    angle
    aphthae
    cells
    clamp
    disease
    drain
    incision
    operation
    pad
    procedure
    pyloroplasty
    syndrome
Mikulicz-Radecki syndrome
Mikulicz-Sjögren syndrome
Milch operation
mildew
Miles operation
milestone
    developmental m's
milia (plural of milium)
Milian
    erythema
    sign
    syndrome
miliaria
    m. alba
    apocrine m.
    m. crystallina
    exercise-induced m.
    m. papulosa
    m. profunda
    m. propria
    pustular m.
    m. pustulosa

miliaria *(continued)*
    m. rubra
    m. vesiculosa
miliary
milieu
    cultural m.
    m. extérieur, external m.
    m. intérieur, internal m.
    social m.
    m. therapy
militate, militated
milium (milia)
    colloid m.
    multiple eruptive milia
    m. neonatorum
milk
    acidophilus m.
    m. anemia
    breast m.
    certified m.
    condensed m.
    cow's m. anemia
    m. culture medium
    m. cyst
    dried m.
    m. ducts
    m. ejection reflex
    evaporated m.
    m. fat
    fortified m.
    goat's m. anemia
    grade A m.
    grade B m.
    homogenized m.
    lactic acid m.
    lowfat m.
    m. of magnesia (MOM)
    modified m.
    nonfat m.
    pasteurized m.
    protein-enriched m.
    skim m.
    sour m.
    sterilized m.
    vegetable m.
    vitamin D m.
milking
Milkman syndrome
Millar asthma
Millard
    island flap
    operation
    test
Millard-Gubler
    paralysis

M

Millard-Gubler *(continued)*
    syndrome
millennium
Millen technique
Miller
    laryngoscope
    operation
    position
    scissors
    speculum
    syndrome
Miller-Abbott (MA) tube
mill-house murmur
milliampere(s) (mA)
    m.-hour (mAh, mA-h)
    m.-minute (mAm, mA-m)
    m.-second (mAs, mA-s)
millibar(s) (mbar)
millicoulomb(s) (mC)
millicurie(s) (mCi)
    m. destroyed (mCiδ) [mCi-delta]
    m.-hour (mCi-hr)
milliequivalent(s) (mEq)
milligram(s) (mg)
    m's percent (mg%)
    m's per liter (mg/L)
milligray(s) (mGy)
millihertz (mHz)
millijoule(s) (mJ)
Millikan rays
millikatal (mkat)
    m's per liter (mkat/L)
milliliter(s) (mL)
millimeter(s) (mm)
    cubic m. (c mm, cu mm, mm^3)
    m's of mercury (mm Hg)
    square m. (mm^2, sq mm)
    m's of water (mm H$_2$O)
millimolar (mM)
millimole(s) (mmol)
    m. per liter (mmol/L)
Millin
    forceps
    tube
Millin-Bacon
    retractor
    spreader
milling-in
Millin-Read operation
milliosmole(s) (mOsm)
millirad(s) (mrad)
millirem (mrem)
milliroentgen(s) (mR)
millisecond(s) (ms, msec)
milliunit(s) (mU)
millivolt(s) (mV)
Millon
    reaction
    reagent
    test
Mills
    disease
    test
Mills-Reincke phenomenon
milphosis
Milroy
    disease
    edema
Mils cautery
Milton
    disease
    edema
    urticaria
Milwaukee brace
mimesis
mimetic
mimic
    genetic m.
mimicry
    antigenic m.
    molecular m.
min.—
    minimal
    minute
Minamata
    disease
    syndrome
mind
Miner osteotome
mineral
    trace m's
mineralization
mineralocorticoid
miner's nystagmus
Minerva jacket
mini-arousals
minification
minify
minilaparoscopy
minilaparotomy
minim (m.)
minimal
minimum (minima)
    m. audibile, m. audible
    m. cognoscibile
    m. legibile
    light m.
    m. sensibile
    m. separabile
    m. visibile

Minin light
minipill
miniplate
Minkowski figure
Minkowski-Chauffard syndrome
Minnesota Multiphasic Personality
    Inventory (MMPI)
Minnesota tube
Minor
    disease
    sign
Minot-Murphy
    diet
    treatment
Minsky operation
minuscule
minute (M, min)
    m. gun cough
MIO—minimal identifiable odor
miodidymus
miopragia
miopus
miosis
    irritative m.
    paralytic m.
    spastic m.
    spinal m.
miotic effect
MIP—maximum inspiratory
    pressure
Mira
    photocoagulator
    unit
miraculin
Mirault operation
Mirault-Brown-Blair operation
mire
Mirena (IUD)
mirror
    dental m.
    Glatzel m.
    m. hands
    head m.
    m. image
    m.-image dextrocardia
    laryngeal m.
    m. laryngoscopy
    nasopharyngeal m.
    Purkinje-Sanson m.
        images
    m. speech
    m. writing
mirroring
MIRU—myocardial infarction
    research unit

misanthropy
miscarriage
misce
miscegenation
miscible
misclassification
misidentification
    delusional m.
mismatch
    acoustic m.
misogamy
misogyny
mist
    ultrasonic m.
mistletoe
Mitchell
    basket
    bunionectomy
    disease
    operation
    osteotomy
    treatment
Mitchell-Diamond forceps
mite
    chigger m.
    flour m.
    food m.
    grain m.
    grain itch m.
    hair follicle m.
    house dust m.
    itch m.
    louse m.
    meal m.
    onion m.
    red m.
mitella
mithridatism
miticidal
miticide
mitigate
mitis
mitochondria
mitochondrial
mitogen
    pokeweed m.
    T-cell m.
mitogen-activated protein kinase
    (MAPK, MAP kinase)
mitogenesis
mitogenetic
mitogenic
mitosin
mitosis (mitoses)
mitotane

M

mitotic
mitral
    m. annulus
    m. commissurotomy
    m. incompetence
    m. insufficiency
    m. opening snap
    percutaneous m.
      commissurotomy (PMC)
    percutaneous transluminal m.
      valvuloplasty (PTMV)
    m. prolapse
    m. prosthesis
    m. regurgitation
    m. stenosis
    m. valve
    m. valve prolapse
    m. valve prosthesis
    m. valvotomy
    m. valvulitis
    m. valvuloplasty
mitrale
    P m.
mitralization
Mitrofanoff procedure
Mitsuda
    antigen
    reaction
    test
mittelschmerz
Mittendorf dot
mixed connective tissue disease
mixed dust pneumoconiosis
mixoscopia
Mixter forceps
mixture
    Gunning m.
    Mayer glycerin-albumin m.
    racemic m.
    Ringer m.
mJ—millijoule(s)
M-K—McCarey-Kaufman
  (medium)
MKV—killed-measles vaccine
μL, microL—microliter(s)
mL, ml—milliliter(s)
ML—
    mesiolingual
    middle lobe
    midline
M/L—monocyte-lymphocyte ratio
MLA—
    left mentoanterior (L.
      mentolaeva anterior)
    Medical Library Association

Mladick
    abdominoplasty
    ear reconstruction
MLAI—mesiolabioincisal
MLAP—mean left atrial pressure
MLBW—moderately low birth
  weight
MLC—
    minimal lethal concentration
    mixed lymphocyte culture
MLD—
    median lethal dose
    minimum lethal dose
MLF—medial longitudinal
  fasciculus
MLI—mesiolinguoincisal
MLN—mesenteric lymph node
MLNS—mucocutaneous lymph
  node syndrome
MLO—mesiolinguo-occlusal
MLP—
    left mentoposterior
      (L. mentolaeva posterior)
    mesiolinguopulpal
MLR—mixed lymphocyte reaction
MLSI—multiple line scan
  imaging
MLT—left mentotransverse
  (L. mentolaeva transverse)
μm—micrometer
mμ—meson
mm—
    millimeter(s)
    muscles
mm^2 [mm2], sq mm—square
  millimeter(s)
mm^3 [mm3], cu mm—cubic
  millimeter(s)
mM—millimolar
MM—
    malignant melanoma
    Marshall-Marchetti
    medial malleolus
    mucous membrane
    multiple myeloma
    muscularis mucosae
    myeloid metaplasia
M&M—milk and molasses
MMC—minimum medullary
  concentration
MMEF, MMF—
    maximal midexpiratory flow
MMEFR, MMFR—maximal
  midexpiratory flow rate
mm Hg—millimeters of mercury

mm H₂O [mm H2O]—millimeters of water

MMIHS—megacystis-microcolon–intestinal hypoperistalsis syndrome

MMK—Marshall-Marchetti-Krantz (operation)

MMM—
    myeloid metaplasia with myelofibrosis

M-mode
    M-m. cardiography
    M-m. echocardiography
    M-m. scanning

mmol—millimole(s)

mmol/L—millimoles per liter

MMP—matrix metalloproteinase

MMPI—Minnesota Multiphasic Personality Inventory

mm pp—millimeters partial pressure

MMPR—methylmercaptopurine riboside

MMR—
    measles, mumps, rubella (vaccine)
    myocardial metabolic rate

MMTV—mouse mammary tumor virus

mN—millinormal

Mn—manganese

MN—
    midnight
    multinodular
    myoneural

M'Naghten
    rule
    test

MNCV—motor nerve conduction velocity

mnemonic

MNU—methylnitrosourea

mo—month

Mo—molybdenum

MO—
    medical officer
    mesio-occlusal
    mineral oil

Moberg arthrodesis

mobility
    electrophoretic m.

mobilization
    chromosome m.
    early m.
    stapes m.

mobilization (continued)
    stem cell m.

mobilizer
    Derlacki m.
    patient m.

Mobin-Uddin filter

Mobitz atrioventricular (AV) heart block (I, II)

Möbius
    disease
    sign
    syndrome (I, II)

moccasin
    cottonmouth water m.

mod.—moderate

MOD—mesio-occlusodistal

modality (modalities)
    primary m.
    salvage m.
    therapeutic m.
    treatment m.

mode
    A-m.
    assist m., assisted m.
    assist-control m.
    B-m.
    control m., controlled m.
    isocontour m.
    list m.
    M-m.
    pacing m.
    pressure control m.
    pressure support m.
    radial m.
    TM-m.

model
    animal m.
    Danielli-Davson m.
    figure-of-eight m.
    Hassell-Varley m.
    leading circle m.
    ring m.
    Watson-Crick m.

modeling

modification
    behavior m.
    effect m.
    Mason-Likar limb lead m.
    racemic m.

modified
    m. mastectomy
    m. radical mastectomy
    m. radical mastoidectomy

modifier

modioliform

M

modiolus
    cochlear m.
    hypoplastic m.
modular prosthesis
modulation
    amplitude m.
    antigenic m.
    biochemical m.
    frequency m.
    image m.
    intensity m.
    object m.
    m. transfer function
modulator
MODY—maturity-onset diabetes of
  the young
Moe
    brace
    plate
Moeller
    glossitis
    itch
    reaction
Moeller-Barlow disease
Moerner-Sjöqvist
    method
    test
Moersch
    bronchoscope
    esophagoscope
    forceps
Moersch-Woltman syndrome
mogiarthria
mogilalia
mogiphonia
Mohrenheim
    fossa
    triangle
Mohs
    chemosurgery
    procedure
    surgery
    technique
moiety
    antioxidant m.
    carbohydrate m.
    estradiol m.
mol—mole(s)
molal
molality
molar (M, *M*)
    m. volume
molar
    dome-shaped m.
    Moon m's

molar *(continued)*
    mulberry m.
    m. pregnancy
    sixth-year m.
    supernumerary m.
    third-year m.
    m. tooth
    twelfth-year m.
molariform
molaris tertius
molarity
molasses
mold
    m. growth
    slime m.
    white m.
molding
    border m.
    compression m.
    cranial m.
    injection m.
    nasoalveolar m.
    nuclear m.
    presurgical nasal m.
    tissue m.
mole (mol) [SI unit]
mole
    atypical m.
    blood m.
    Breus m.
    carneous m.
    cystic m.
    false m.
    fleshy m.
    gram m.
    grape m.
    hairy m.
    hemorrhagic m.
    hydatid m., hydatidiform m.
    invasive m.
    malignant m.
    maternal m.
    metastasizing m.
    pigmented m.
    placental m.
    stone m.
    true m.
    tubal m.
    tuberous m.
    vesicular m.
    warty m.
molecular
    m. hybridization probe
    m. mimicry
    m. vibrations

molecule
  adhesion m's
  cell adhesion m's (CAM)
  cell interaction (CI) m's
  diatomic m.
  effector m.
  hexatomic m.
  intercellular adhesion m. 1
    (ICAM-1)
  intercellular adhesion m. 2
    (ICAM-2)
  monatomic m.
  nonpolar m.
  polar m.
  tetratomic m.
  triatomic m.
molimen (molimina)
  menstrual m.
Molisch
  reaction
  test
Mollaret meningitis
Moll glands
mollities ossium
molluscous
molluscum
  m. bodies
  m. conjunctivitis
  m. contagiosum
  m. fibrosum
  m. pendulum
mollusk
Moloney
  reaction
  test
molting
mol. wt.—molecular weight
molybdate
molybdenosis
molybdenum (Mo)
  stainless steel with m. (SMo)
molybdic acid
molybdoenzyme
molybdoflavoprotein
molybdoprotein
molybdous
MOM—milk of magnesia
MOMA—methoxyhydroxymandelic
  acid
moment
  m. of death
  golden m.
  magnetic m.
momentum
  angular m.

Monakow (von Monakow)
  bundle
  fascia
  fasciculus aberrans
  fibers
  striae
  syndrome
  theory
  tract
Monaldi
  drainage system
  operation
monangle
monarthric
monarthritis
  m. deformans
  traumatic deforming m.
monathetosis
monauchenos
monaural
Mönckeberg
  arteriosclerosis
  calcification
  degeneration
  mesarteritis
  sclerosis
  syndrome
Moncrieff
  irrigating cannula
  operation
Mondini deafness
Mondonesi reflex
Mondor
  disease
  syndrome
monerula (monerulae)
monesthetic
Monge disease
monilated
monilethrix
monilial
  m. esophagitis
  m. infection
  m. intertrigo
  m. vaginitis
moniliform
Moniliformis moniliformis
monitor
  ambulatory ECG m.
  apnea m.
  blood glucose m.
  depth-of-anesthesia m.
  Doppler m.
  Holter m.
  ICP (intracranial pressure) m.

M

monitor *(continued)*
    radiation m.
    tumescence m.
monitoring
    biological m.
    cardiac m.
    drug m.
    electronic fetal m.
    fetal m.
    oxygen m.
    24-hour pH m.
    wound m.
monitory
monkey
    cynomolgus m.
    rhesus m.
Monks
    malar elevator
    operation
Monks-Esser island flap
Monneret pulse
monoamine oxidase (MAO)
  inhibitor
monoaminergic
monoamnionic
monoanesthesia
monoauricular
monobacterial
monobasic
monobenzone
monoblast
monoblastoma
monoblepsia
monobrachia
monobrachius
monobromated
monocalcic
monocarboxylic acid
monocephalus
    m. tetrapus dibrachius
    m. tripus dibrachius
monochorea
monochorionic
monochroic
monochromacy
monochromat
monochromatic
monochromatism
    cone m.
    rod m.
monochromatophil
monoclonal antibody (MAb)
monocontaminated
monocontamination
monocorditis

monocrotic
monocrotism
monocular
monoculus
monocyclic
monocyte
monocytic
monocytoid
monocytoma
monocytopenia
monocytopoiesis
monocytosis
monodactyly
monodermal
monodermoma
monodiplopia
monoesterase
monoethanolamine
monoethylglycinexylidide (MEGX)
monofactorial
monofilament
    absorbable m. suture
    m. mucosectomy snare
    nonabsorbable m. suture
    nylon m. suture
    m. polypropylene sling
    m. polypropylene suture
    Semmes-Weinstein m. test
    m. sensory test
    m. suture
    von Frey m.
    m. wire
monofilm
monofixation syndrome
monogamous
monogamy
monoganglial
monogastric
monogen
monogenesis
monogenetic
monogenic
monoglyceride
monograph
monohydrated
monohydric
monoinfection
monoiodotyrosine
monokine
monolayer
monolobular
    m. cirrhosis
    m. megakaryocytes
monolocular
monomania

monomaxillary
monomelic
monomer
    fibrin m.
monomeric
monometallic
monomethylhydrazine
monomicrobial
monomolecular
monomorphic
monomorphism
monomorphous
monomphalus
monomyoplegia
monomyositis
mononeural
mononeuralgia
mononeuritis
mononeuropathy
    cranial m.
    multifocal m.
    m. multiplex
mononuclear
mononucleate
mononucleosis
    acute m.
    chronic m.
    cytomegalovirus m.
    Epstein-Barr virus–associated
      m.
    infectious m.
    post-transfusion m.
mononucleotide
monooctanoin
mono-osteitic
monooxygenase
monoparesis
monoparesthesia
monopathy
monophagia
monophasia
monophasic
monophenol monooxygenase
monophosphate
monophthalmus
monoplasmatic
monoplast
monoplegia
monoplegic
monopodia
monopodial
monopolar
monoptychial
monopus
monorchid

monorhinic
monos—monocytes
monosaccharide
monosodium glutamate (MSG)
monosome
monosomic
monosomy
    m. 7 syndrome
monospasm
monospecific
monospermy
Monospot test
monostotic
monostratal
monostratified
monosubstituted
monosyllabic
monosymptom
monosymptomatic
monosynaptic
monotherapy
monothermia
monothioglycerol
monotic
monounsaturated fatty acid
monovalent
monovision
monovular
monovulatory
monoxenic
monoxide
monozygosity
monozygotic twins
Monro
    abscess
    bursa
    fissure
    foramen
    line
    sulcus
Monro-Richter line
mons (montes)
    m. pubis
    m. ureteris
    m. veneris
monster
    Gila m.
monstrosity
montage
Montague
    proctoscope
    sigmoidoscope
Monte Carlo method
Monteggia
    dislocation

M

Monteggia *(continued)*
 fracture
montes (plural of mons)
Montevideo units
Montgomery
 cups
 follicles
 glands
 strap
 tape
 T tube
 tubercles
monticulus cerebelli
mood
 m. alterations
 depressed m., depressive m.
 m. disorder
 dysphoric m.
 elevated m.
 euthymic m.
 expansive m.
 irritable m.
 negative m.
 organic m. syndrome
 seasonal m. disorder
 substance-induced m.
  disorder
mood-congruent delusion
mood-incongruent delusion
moon
 m. boot
 crescent m. shape
 m. face, m. facies
Moon
 molars
 teeth
Moore
 chisel
 extractor
 fracture
 gouge
 nail
 operation
 osteotome
 pin
 prosthesis
 reamer
 scoop
 syndrome
 template
 tracheostomy button
Mooren ulcer
moot
 m. point
 m. question

MOPP—nitrogen mustard, Oncovin,
 prednisone, procarbazine
MOPV—monovalent oral poliovirus
 vaccine
Morand
 foot
 foramen
 spur
Morawitz theory
Morax operation
Morax-Axenfeld
 bacillus
 conjunctivitis
 diplococcus
 hemophilus
Moraxella
 M. catarrhalis
 M. lacunata
 M. liquefaciens
morbid
morbidity
 puerperal m.
morbific
morbilli
morbilliform
Morbillivirus
morbillous
MORC—Medical Officers Reserve
 Corps
morcel
morcellated
morcellation
 electromechanical m.
 tumor m.
morcellement
Morch tube
mordant
Morel
 ear
 syndrome
Morel-Kraepelin disease
Morelli
 reaction
 test
Morel-Wildi syndrome
Moreno clamp
mores
Morestin operation
Morgagni
 appendix
 caruncle
 columns
 crypts
 foramen
 fossa

Morgagni *(continued)*
    fovea
    globules
    hernia
    hydatid
    lacunae
    nodules
    prolapse
    sinus
    tubercle
    valves
    ventricle
Morgagni-Adams-Stokes syndrome
morgagnian cyst
Morgan bacillus
Morganella morganii
morgan unit (M)
morgue
moria
moribund
Morison
    incision
    method
    pouch
Morita therapy
Moritz
    reaction
    test
Moritz-Schmidt forceps
Mörner (Moerner)
    reagent
    test
Moro
    embrace reflex
    reflex
    test
Moro-Heisler diet
morphallactic
morphallaxis
morphea
    deep m.
    generalized m.
    guttate m.
    linear m., m. linearis
    plaque m.
    m. profunda
    subcutaneous m.
morpheaform
morpheme
morphine
    dimethyl m.
    m. hydrochloride
    m. sulfate
morphinic
morphinism

morphinization
morphodifferentiation
morphogen
morphogenesis
morphogenetic
morphological
morphology
morpholysis
morphometry
morphosis
morphotic
morpion
Morquio
    sign
    syndrome
Morquio-Brailsford
  syndrome
Morquio-Ullrich disease
morrhua
morrhuate sodium
morrhuic acid
Morris
    cannula
    syndrome
mors thymica
morsal
Morse scissors
morselize
morsicatio
    m. buccarum
    m. linguarum
morsulus
morsus humanus
mortal
mortality
mortar
mortician
mortification
Mortimer
    disease
    malady
mortis
    rigor m.
mortise
    ankle m.
Morton
    cough
    current
    disease
    foot
    metatarsalgia
    neuralgia
    neuroma
    test
    toe

M

mortuary
morula
morular
morulation
moruloid
Morvan
    chorea
    syndrome
mOs—milliosmolal
mosaic
    de novo m.
    m. disorder
    human cone m.
    m. trisomy 20
    m. Turner syndrome
mosaicism
    confined placental m.
    erythrocyte m.
    gonadal m.
    haploid-diploid m.
    somatic m.
    somatic CHD7 m.
    trisomy 20 m.
    Turner m.
    XO/XY m.
mosaicplasty
Moschcowitz
    disease
    operation
    sign
    test
Mosetig-Moorhof
    bone wax
    filling
Mosher
    air cells
    curet
    esophagoscope
    punch
    speculum
    tube
Mosher-Toti operation
Mosler sign
Mosley method
mOsm—milliosmole(s)
mosquito
    m. clamp
    m. forceps
mosquitocidal
mosquitocide
Moss classification
Mossbauer spectrometer
Mosse syndrome
Mosso
    ergograph

Mosso *(continued)*
    sphygmomanometer
Motais operation
moth
    brown-tail m.
    flannel m.
    io m.
    meal m.
    peppered m.
    puss m.
    silkworm m.
    tussock m.
mother
    m. cell
    m. cyst
    expectant m.
    genetic m.
    gestational m.
    surrogate m.
    m. yaw
motile
motilin
motility
    altered sperm m.
    colon m.
    m. disorder
    esophageal m.
    gastrointestinal (GI) m.
    ineffective esophageal m. (IEM)
    reduced m.
    segmental m.
    voluntary m.
motion
    active range of m.
    continuous passive m. (CPM)
    range of m.
    systolic anterior m. (SAM)
motivation
motive
    achievement m.
    aroused m.
motoceptor
motofacient
motoneuron
    alpha m's
    beta m's
    gamma m's
    heteronymous m's
    homonymous m's
    lower m's
    peripheral m's
    upper m's
motor
    plastic m.
motoricity

motorius
    dorsalis m. nervi vagi
    m. nerve
    m. nucleus
motorogerminative
MOTT—mycobacteria other than
    tubercle bacilli
Mott law of anticipation
mottled
mottling
    dental m., enamel m.
    miliary m.
    pigment m., pigmentary m.
    retinal pigment epithelial
      (RPE) m.
Mouchet disease
moulage
Moult curet
mound
    anal m.
    breast m.
    malar m.
    pubic m.
mounding
    cortical m.
    Essix m.
    muscle m.
    m. phenomenon
Mounier-Kuhn syndrome
mount
    wet m.
Mount syndrome
mountant
mounting
    split-cast m.
Mount-Mayfield forceps
Mount-Reback syndrome
Moure esophagoscope
Moure-Coryllos rib shears
mourning
mouse (mice)
    joint m.
    peritoneal m.
    pleural m.
mouse-tooth forceps
mouse units (m.u.)
mouth
    m. breathing
    burning m. syndrome
    denture sore m.
    dry m.
    m. gag
    glass blowers' m.
    m. guard
    sore m.

mouth *(continued)*
    tapir m.
    trench m.
    white m.
mouth gag
    Crowe-Davis m.g., Davis-
      Crowe m.g.
    Denhardt m.g.
    Denhardt-Dingman m.g.
    Dott m.g.
    Lane m.g.
    McIvor m.g.
    Roser m.g.
    Sluder-Jansen m.g.
mouth prop
mouthwash
movement
    active m.
    adversive m.
    angular m.
    associated contralateral m.
    athetoid m's
    automatic m.
    Bennett m.
    border m.
    border tissue m's
    bowel m.
    cardinal m's
    choreic m's, choreiform m's
    circus m.
    circum m. tachycardia
    conjugate m's
    contralateral associated m.
    curtain m.
    m. disorder
    dystonic m.
    euglenoid m.
    excursive m's
    fetal m.
    forced m.
    free mandibular m.
    functional mandibular m's
    gliding m.
    hinge m.
    intermediary m's,
      intermediate m's
    involuntary m.
    jaw m.
    Magnan trombone m.
    mandibular m.
    masticatory m's
    mirror m.
    morphogenetic m.
    opening m.
    passive m.

M

movement *(continued)*
    pedal m.
    pendular m.
    percussion m's
    posterior opening m.
    rapid eye m. (REM)
    reflex m.
    resistive m.
    rolling m.
    running m.
    saccadic m.
    scissors m.
    segmentation m.
    m. sense
    spontaneous m.
    stepping m's
    stereotypic m. disorder
    streaming m.
    Swedish m.
    synkinetic m's
    m. therapy
    tipping m.
    vermicular m's
    voluntary m.
mover
    prime m.
moxa
moxibustion
Moynahan syndrome (I, II)
Moynihan
    clamp
    cream
    forceps
    needle
    operation
    pancreatitis
    position
    probe
    scoop
    test
    ulcer
Mozart ear
MP—
    mean pressure
    melting point
    menstrual period
    mercaptopurine
    mesiopulpal
    metacarpophalangeal
    monophosphate
    mucopolysaccharide
    multiparous
MPA—
    main pulmonary artery
    medroxyprogesterone acetate
    methylprednisolone acetate

MPAP—mean pulmonary arterial
    pressure
MPC—meperidine, promethazine,
    chlorpromazine
MPD—maximum permissible dose
M period
MPGN—membranoproliferative
    glomerulonephritis
MPH—Master of Public Health
MPHR—maximum predicted heart
    rate
MPJ—metacarpophalangeal joint
MPL—mesiopulpolingual
MPLA—mesiopulpolabial
MPS—mononuclear phagocyte
    system
MPS (I-VII)—
    mucopolysaccharidosis (I-VII)
MPS I-H—mucopolysaccharidosis
    I-H
MPS I-H/S—mucopolysaccharidosis
    I-H/S
MPS I-S—mucopolysaccharidosis
    I-S
MPSS—methylprednisolone
    sodium succinate
μR, microR—microroentgen(s)
mR—milliroentgen(s)
MR—
    megaroentgen(s)
    mental retardation
    metabolic rate
    methyl red
    mitral regurgitation
    muscle relaxant
M_r—relative molecular mass
MRA—magnetic resonance
    angiography
mrad—millirad(s)
MRAP—mean right atrial pressure
MRC—Medical Reserve Corps
MRD—minimum reacting dose
mrem—millirem(s)
MRF—mesencephalic reticular
    formation
MRFIT—Multiple-Risk Factor
    Intervention Trial
MRI—magnetic resonance imaging
mRNA—messenger RNA
MRSA—methicillin-resistant
    Staphylococcus aureus
MRT—
    median recognition threshold
    milk-ring test
MRVP—mean right ventricular
    pressure

μs—microsecond(s)
ms; msec—millisecond(s)
MS—
    Master of Science
    Master of Surgery
    mental status
    mitral stenosis
    morphine sulfate
    multiple sclerosis
    musculoskeletal
MSB—Martius yellow, scarlet, and
    blue (stain)
μsec, microsec—microsecond(s)
msec; ms—millisecond
MSER—mean systolic ejection rate
MSG—monosodium glutamate
MSH—melanocyte-stimulating
    hormone
MSK—medullary sponge kidney
MSL—midsternal line
MSLT—multiple sleep latency test
MSR—monosynaptic reflex
MSRPP—Multidimensional Scale
    for Rating Psychiatric Patients
MSU—monosodium urate
MSUD—maple syrup urine disease
MSV—
    maximal sustained
        ventilation
    Moloney sarcoma virus
    murine sarcoma virus
MSVC—maximal sustained
    ventilatory capacity
MT—
    malignant teratoma
    maximal therapy
    medical technologist
    medical transcriptionist
    membrana tympani
    metatarsal
MTC—mitomycin C
MTD—maximum tolerated dose
MTDT—modified tone decay test
MTF—maximum terminal flow
MTI—minimum time interval
MTP—metatarsophalangeal
MTR—Meinicke turbidity
    reaction
MTT—mean transit time
MTX—methotrexate
μU, microU—microunit(s)
mu—
    Greek letter (μ; alphabetized
        as m)
    mouse unit(s)
mU—milliunit(s)

MU—
    Mache unit
    Montevideo unit
MUAP—motor unit action
    potential
MUC—maximum urinary
    concentration
Mucha disease
Mucha-Habermann disease
mucicarmine
mucicarminophilic
muciferous
mucigen
mucigogue
mucihematein
    Mayer m.
mucilage
    acacia m.
    tragacanth m.
mucilaginous
mucilloid
    psyllium hydrophilic m.
mucin
mucinase
mucinoblast
mucinoid
mucinolytic
mucinosis
    acral persistent papular m.
    cutaneous lupus m.
    dermal m.
    focal m.
    follicular m.
    pandermal m.
    papular m.
    papulonodular m.
    plaquelike m.
    reticular erythematous m.
    self-healing juvenile
        cutaneous m.
mucinous
mucinuria
muciparous
Muckle-Wells syndrome
mucobuccal
    m. fold
    m. reflections
mucocartilage
mucocele
    ethmoid sinus m.
    frontal sinus m.
    frontoethmoid m.
    giant appendiceal m.
    lacrimal m.
    maxillary sinus m.
    nasolacrimal sac m.

M

mucocele *(continued)*
    paranasal sinus m.
    petrous apex m.
    superficial m.
    suppurating m.
mucociliary
mucoclasis
mucocolitis
mucocolpos
mucocutaneous
    m. candidiasis
    m. fistula
    m. hemorrhoid
    m. herpes simplex
    m. junction
    m. leishmaniasis
    m. lymph node syndrome
    m. membrane
    m. pemphigus vulgaris
    m. plasmacytosis
mucocyst
mucocyte
mucoderm
mucoepidermoid
mucofibrous
mucoflocculent
mucogingival
mucogingivitis
mucoid
mucolipidosis I-IV
mucolytic
mucomembranous
mucopeptide
mucoperichondrial
mucoperichondrium
mucoperiosteal
mucoperiosteum
mucopoiesis
mucopolysaccharide
mucopolysaccharidosis
  (mucopolysaccharidoses) (MPS)
    m. I–XIII (MPS I–XIII)
    m. I-H (MPS I-H)
    m. I-H/S (MPS I-H/S)
    m. I-S (MPS I-S)
mucopolysacchariduria
mucoprotein
    Tamm-Horsfall m.
mucopurulent
mucopus
Mucor
    M. circinelloides
    M. racemosissimus
mucoraceous
mucorin

mucormycosis
    auricular m.
    cerebral m.
    cutaneous m.
    gastrointestinal m.
    m. peritonitis
    pulmonary m.
    rhinocerebral m.
    rhino-orbital m.
    sino-orbital-cranial m.
mucosa
    alveolar m.
    antral m.
    buccal m.
    colonic m.
    duodenal m.
    endocervical m.
    esophageal m.
    gastric m.
    gastroduodenal m.
    jejunal m.
    labial m.
    laryngeal m.
    masticatory m.
    muscular m.
    olfactory m.
    oral m.
    pharyngeal m.
    redundant supraglottic m.
    respiratory m.
    retromolar m.
    retrotuberosity m.
    tracheal m.
mucosal
    m. disease
    m. fold
    gastric m. barrier
    m. graft
    m. melanoma
    m. neuroma syndrome
    m. prolapse
    m. relief radiography
mucosanguineous
mucosectomy
    circumferential transanal m.
    m. cap
    endogastric m.
    endorectal m.
    endoscopic m.
    monofilament m. snare
    transanal rectal m.
mucoserous
mucosin
mucositis
    modified oral m. index (MOMI)

mucositis *(continued)*
    oral m.
    radiation-induced m.
mucostatic
mucosulfatidosis
mucotome
mucous
    m. cells
    m. coat of tympanic cavity
    m. coat of urinary bladder
    m. colitis
    m. corpuscles
    m. crypts of duodenum
    m. cyst
    m. degeneration
    m. diarrhea
    m. edema
    m. enteritis
    m. fistula
    m. fold
    m. glands
    m. hypersecretion
    m. layer
    m. membrane
    m. patch
    m. rale
    m. sheaths
mucoviscidosis
mucro (mucrones)
    m. sterni
mucronate
mucroniform
mucus
    airway m. obstruction
    cervical m.
    clear m.
    m. clearance
    excessive m. production
    m. extravasation phenomenon
    m. hypersecretion
    m. layer
    nasal m.
    m. plug
    m. plugging
    m. retention cyst
    m. secretion
    m. strands
    thick m., thickened m.
Muehrcke lines
Mueller
    cautery
    clamp
    maneuver
    needle
    operation

Mueller *(continued)*
    prosthesis
    retractor
    speculum
Mueller-Frazier tube
muelleri
    ductus m.
Mueller-Pool tube
Mueller-Pynchon tube
Mueller-Yankauer tube
Muer anoscope
muffle
MUGA (multiple gated acquisition)
  scanning
mugwort
mu heavy chain disease
Muir-Torre syndrome
mulberry
    m. lesion
    m. nodules
    outside-in m. knot suture
      technique
    m. pattern
mulberry-like
    m-l. appearance
    m-l. granulomatous lesions
    m-l. tumor
    m-l. ulcerations
mulberry-type hydroxyapatite
  concretions
Mulder angle
Muldoon dilator
Mules
    implant
    operation
    scoop
muliebria
mull
    plaster m.
Müller
    canal
    capsule
    cells
    duct
    fibers
    fluid
    liquid
    maneuver
    muscle
    operation
    radial cells
    sign
    test
    trigone
    tubercle

M

Müller-Hillis maneuver
müllerian (muellerian)
    m. agenesis
    m. capsule
    m. duct
    m. mixed tumor
    m. tubercle
mulling
multangular
multiallelic
multiarticular
multiaxial
multicapsular
multicellular
multicellularity
multicentric
multicentricity
multicipital muscle
multiclonal
multicontaminated
multicore
multicrystal camera
multicuspid
multicuspidate
multicystic
multidentate
multidetermination
multidigitate
multifactorial
multifid
multifidus
multifilament suture
multifocal
multiform
multiganglionic
multigated
    m. angiography
    m. imaging
multigravida
    grand m.
multihallucalism
multi-infarct
    m. dementia
    m. encephalopathy
multi-infection
multilobar
    m. consolidation
    m. disease
    m. infiltrates
    m. involvement
    m. opacities
    m. pneumonia
multilobular
    m. aneurysm
    m. appearance

multilobular *(continued)*
    m. biliary cirrhosis
    m. mass lesion
    m. tumor
multilocular
    m. crypt
    m. cyst
    familial m. cystic nephroma
    m. infection
    m. lesion
    m. mass
    m. thymic cyst
    m. tumor
multilocularity
multiloculated
multimammae
multimer
multimodal
multinodal
multinodular
    m. hepatocellular carcinoma
    m. mass
    nontoxic m. goiter
    m. thyroid
    toxic m. goiter
    m. tumor
multinucleate
multipara
    grand m.
multiparity
multiparous
multipartite
multipennate
    m. appearance
    m. structure
multiphasic
multiplanar
    m. imaging
    m. scanning
multiple
    m. endocrine neoplasia
    m. lymphomatous polyposis
    m. myeloma
    m. organ failure
    m. risk factors
    m. sclerosis (MS)
multiplexer
multiplication
    countercurrent m.
multiplicitas cordis
multipolar
multipollicalism
multipollicism
multirooted
multiscalar

multisensitivity
multistrand suture
multisynaptic
multisystem disease
multiterminal
multitoothed forceps
multituberculate
multivalent
multivariate
multivisceral
multivitamin (MV)
Mumford-Gurd operation
Mummery pink tooth
mummification
    fetal m.
    m. of pulp
mumps
    iodine m.
    m. meningoencephalitis
    metastatic m.
mumu
Münchausen
    by proxy syndrome
    syndrome
Münchmeyer disease
Mundie forceps
Munk disease
Munro
    abscess
    microabscess
    point
Munro Kerr
    cesarean section
    incision
    maneuver
Munson sign
Munster prosthesis
MUP—motor unit potential
mural
muralium (muralia)
muramic acid
muramidase
Murat sign
Murchison-Pel-Ebstein fever
Murdock-Wiener speculum
murein hydrolase
murexide
murexine
muriatic acid
muriform
murine T-cell phenotype
murmur
    amphoric m.
    anemic m.
    aneurysmal m.

murmur *(continued)*
    aortic m.
    apex m.
    apical m.
    apical diastolic m.
    arterial m.
    attrition m.
    Austin Flint m.
    bellows m.
    blowing m.
    brain m.
    cardiac m.
    cardiopulmonary m.
    Carey Coombs m.
    continuous m.
    cooing m.
    crescendo m.
    crescendo-decrescendo m.
    Cruveilhier-Baumgarten m.
    decrescendo m.
    deglutition m.
    diamond-shaped m.
    diastolic m.
    Duroziez m.
    early diastolic m.
    early systolic m.
    ejection m.
    extracardiac m.
    Flint m.
    flow m.
    friction m.
    functional m.
    Gibson m.
    Graham Steell m.
    Hamman m.
    harsh m.
    heart m.
    hemic m.
    holodiastolic m.
    holosystolic m.
    hourglass m.
    humming-top m.
    incidental m.
    innocent m.
    late systolic m.
    machinery m.
    mid-diastolic m.
    midsystolic m.
    mill-house m.
    mill-wheel m.
    mitral m.
    musical m.
    organic m.
    outflow tract m.
    pansystolic m.

M

murmur *(continued)*
    pericardial m.
    physiologic m.
    pleuropericardial m.
    prediastolic m.
    presystolic m.
    pulmonary m.
    pulmonic m.
    regurgitant m.
    Roger m.
    seagull m.
    seesaw m.
    short systolic m.
    Steell m.
    stenosal m.
    Still m.
    systolic m.
    systolic ejection m.
    to-and-fro m.
    transmitted m.
    tricuspid m.
    vascular m.
    venous m.
    vesicular m.
    water-wheel m.
Murphy
    button
    dilator
    needle
    percussion
    retractor
    sign
    test
    treatment
Murphy-Sturm lymphosarcoma
Murray Valley
    disease
    encephalitis
    virus
Murri
    disease
    syndrome
musca (muscae)
    muscae hispanicae
    muscae volitantes
muscacide
muscardine
muscarine
muscarinic
muscarinism
muscegenetic
muscimol
muscle
    abductor m.
    abductor m. of great toe

muscle *(continued)*
    abductor m. of little finger
    abductor m. of little toe
    abductor m. of thumb
    accessory flexor m.
    accessory m.
    accessory m's of respiration
    adductor m.
    adductor m. of great toe
    adductor m. of thumb
    Aeby m.
    agonistic m.
    Albinus m.
    anconeus m.
    antagonistic m.
    antitragus m.
    appendicular m's
    arrector m's of hair
    articular m.
    articular m. of elbow
    articular m. of knee
    aryepiglottic m.
    arytenoid m., oblique
    arytenoid m., transverse
    m's of auditory ossicles
    auricular m.
    axial m.
    Bell m.
    biceps m. of arm
    bicipital m.
    bipennate m.
    bipenniform m.
    Bowman m.
    brachial m.
    brachioradial m.
    Braune m.
    bronchoesophageal m.
    Brücke m.
    buccinator m.
    buccopharyngeal m.
    bulbar m's
    bulbocavernous m.
    canine m.
    cardiac m.
    Casser m., Casser perforated
      m., casserian m.
    ceratocricoid m.
    ceratopharyngeal m.
    Chassaignac axillary m.
    chondroglossus m.
    chondropharyngeal m.
    ciliary m.
    circumpennate m.
    cleidohyoid m.
    coccygeal m's

muscle *(continued)*

- compound m. action potential
- compressor naris m.
- compressor urethrae m.
- constrictor m. of pharynx
- continuous m. activity syndrome
- coracobrachial m.
- corrugator m., superciliary
- Crampton m.
- cremaster m.
- cricoarytenoid m.
- cricopharyngeal m.
- cricothyroid m.
- cruciate m.
- cutaneous m.
- dartos m.
- deltoid m.
- depressor m. of angle of mouth
- depressor m. of lower lip
- depressor m. of septum of nose
- depressor m., superciliary
- dermal m.
- detrusor m. of bladder
- diaphragmatic m.
- digastric m.
- dilator m. of naris
- dilator m. of pupil
- dorsal m's
- epicranial m.
- epimeric m.
- epitrochleoanconeus m.
- erector m. of penis
- erector m. of spine
- eustachian m.
- extensor m. of digits
- external oblique m.
- extraocular m's (EOMs)
- extrinsic m.
- facial m's, m's of facial expression
- fast m.
- femoral m.
- fibular m.
- fixation m's, fixator m's
- fixator m. of base of stapes
- flexor m., accessory
- flexor m.'s of the digits
- flexor m. of wrist, radial
- flexor m. of wrist, ulnar
- Folius m.
- frontal m.
- fusiform m.
- gastrocnemius m.
- Gavard m.

muscle *(continued)*

- gemellus m.
- genioglossus m.
- geniohyoid m.
- glossopalatine m.
- glossopharyngeal m.
- gluteal m.
- gracilis m.
- great adductor m.
- greater trochanter m.
- Guthrie m.
- hamstring m's
- helicis m. (major, minor)
- m. of helix
- Hilton m.
- m. hook
- Horner m.
- Houston m.
- hyoglossal m., hyoglossus m.
- m's of hyoid bone
- hypomeric m.
- hypothenar m's
- iliac m.
- iliococcygeal m.
- iliocostal m's
- iliocostal m. of neck
- iliocostal m. of thorax
- iliopsoas m.
- incisive m's of lip
- inferior oblique m.
- inferior oblique m. of head
- inferior rectus m.
- infrahyoid m's
- infraspinatus m.
- infraspinous m.
- inspiratory m.'s
- interarytenoid m's
- intercostal m's
- interfoveolar m.
- internal oblique m.
- interosseous m.
- interosseous m's of foot
- interosseous m's of hand
- interosseous m's, palmar
- interosseous m's, plantar
- interosseous m's, volar
- interspinal m's
- interspinal m's of thorax
- intertransverse m's
- intrinsic m.
- involuntary m.
- ischiocavernous m.
- ischiococcygeal m.
- Jarjavay m.
- Jung m.

M

muscle *(continued)*
    Koyter m.
    Landström m.
    Langer m.
    m's of larynx
    lateral malleolus m.
    lateral rectus m.
    lateral rectus m. of bulb
    lateral straight m.
    levator m.
    levator m. of angle of mouth
    levator m. of palatine
      velum
    levator m. of prostate
    levator m's of ribs
    levator m. of scapula
    levator m. of thyroid gland
    levator m. of upper eyelid
    levator m. of upper lip
    levator m. of upper lip and ala
      of nose
    lingual m's
    long abductor m. of thumb
    long adductor m.
    long m. of head
    longitudinal m. of tongue
    long m. of neck
    lumbrical m's of foot
    lumbrical m's of hand
    masseter m.
    m's of mastication
    masticatory m.
    medial rectus m.
    medial straight m.
    Merkel m.
    mesothenar m.
    Müller m.
    multicipital m.
    multifidus m's
    multipennate m.
    mylohyoid m.
    mylopharyngeal m.
    nasal m.
    m's of neck
    nonstriated m.
    oblique m. of abdomen
    oblique m. of auricle
    oblique m. of eyeball
    oblique m. of head
    oblique m. of head, inferior
    obturator m.
    occipital m.
    occipitofrontal m.
    ocular m's, oculorotatory m's
    Oddi m.

muscle *(continued)*
    Oehl m.
    omohyoid m.
    opposing m. of little finger
    opposing m. of thumb
    orbicular m.
    orbicular m. of eye
    orbicular m. of mouth
    orbital m.
    organic m.
    m's of palate and fauces
    palatine m's
    palatoglossus m.
    palatopharyngeal m.
    palmar m.
    papillary m.
    papillary m. of left ventricle
    papillary m. of right ventricle
    paraspinal m.
    pectinate m's
    pectinate m's of right atrium
    pectineal m.
    pectoral m.
    m's of pelvic diaphragm
    pennate m., penniform m.
    perineal m's, m's of perineum
    peroneal m.
    pharyngeal constrictor m.
    pharyngopalatine m.
    Phillips m.
    m. phosphofructokinase
    m. phosphorylase
    piriform m.
    plantar m.
    m. plate
    platysma m.
    pleuroesophageal m.
    popliteal m.
    postaxial m.
    posterior intertransverse m's
      of neck
    postural m's
    preaxial m.
    procerus m.
    pronator m., quadrate
    pronator m., round
    psoas major m.
    psoas minor m.
    pterygoid m.
    pterygopharyngeal m.
    puboanal m.
    pubococcygeal m.
    puboperineal m.
    puboprostatic m.
    puborectal m.

muscle *(continued)*
  pubovaginal m.
  pubovesical m.
  pyloric sphincter m.
  pyramidal m.
  pyramidal m. of auricle
  quadrate m.
  quadrate m. of lower lip
  quadrate pronator m.
  quadrate m. of sole
  quadrate m. of thigh
  quadrate m. of upper lip
  quadriceps m. of thigh
  radial flexor m. of wrist
  rectococcygeal m.
  rectourethral m.
  rectouterine m.
  rectovesical m.
  rectus m.
  rectus abdominis m.
  rectus m. of eyeball
  rectus femoris m.
  red m.
  m. relaxant
  rhomboid m.
  ribbon m's
  rider's m's
  Riolan m.
  risorius m.
  rotator m's
  rotator m's of neck
  rotator m's of thorax
  Rouget m.
  Ruysch m.
  sacrococcygeal m.
  sacrospinal m.
  salpingopharyngeal m.
  Santorini m.
  sartorius m.
  scalene m
  Sebileau m.
  semimembranous m.
  semipennate m.
  semispinal m.
  semispinal m. of head
  semispinal m. of neck
  semispinal m. of thorax
  semitendinous m.
  serratus m.
  serratus anterior m.
  serratus inferior m.
  serratus posterior m.
  m.-setting exercise
  short abductor m. of thumb
  short adductor m.

muscle *(continued)*
  Sibson m.
  skeletal m's
  slow m.
  smallest adductor m.
  smooth m.
  soleus m.
  somatic m's
  sphincter m.'s
  sphincter m. of anus
  sphincter m. of bile duct
  sphincter m. of
    hepatopancreatic ampulla
  sphincter m. of membranous
    urethra
  sphincter m. of pancreatic duct
  sphincter m. of pupil
  sphincter m. of pylorus
  sphincter m. of urethra
  sphincter m. of urinary
    bladder
  spinal m.
  spinal m. of head
  spinal m. of neck
  spinal m. of thorax
  splenius m. of head
  splenius m. of neck
  spurt m's
  stapedius m.
  sternal m.
  sternocleidomastoid m.
  sternohyoid m.
  sternomastoid m.
  sternothyroid m.
  strap m's
  striated m.
  striped m.
  styloglossus m.
  stylohyoid m.
  stylopharyngeal m.
  subanconeus m.
  subclavius m.
  subcostal m's
  suboccipital m's
  subscapular m.
  subvertebral m's
  superciliary corrugator m.
  superciliary depressor m.
  superior constrictor m.
  superior oblique m.
  superior rectus m.
  supinator m.
  suprahyoid m's
  supraspinatus m.
  supraspinous m.

M

muscle *(continued)*

    suspensory m. of duodenum
    synergic m's, synergistic m's
    tarsal m.
    temporal m.
    temporoparietal m.
    tensor m. of fascia lata
    tensor tympani m.
    tensor m. of tympanic
      membrane
    tensor m. of tympanum
    tensor veli palatini m.
    tensor m. of velum palatinum
    teres major m.
    teres minor m.
    Theile m.
    thenar m's
    thyroarytenoid m.
    thyroepiglottic m.
    thyrohyoid m.
    thyropharyngeal m.
    tibial m.
    m's of tongue
    tracheal m.
    trachelomastoid m.
    m. of tragus, tragicus m.
    transverse m's
    transverse m. of abdomen
    transverse abdominal m.
    transverse m. of auricle
    transverse m. of chin
    transverse m. of nape
    transverse m. of neck
    transverse perineal m.
    transverse m. of perineum
    transverse m. of thorax
    transverse m. of tongue
    transversospinal m.
    transversus abdominis m.
    trapezius m.
    m. of Treitz
    triangular m.
    triceps m. of arm
    triceps m. of calf
    tricipital m.
    trigonal m.
    twitch m.
    ulnar flexor m. of wrist
    unipennate m.
    unstriated m.
    m's of urogenital diaphragm
    m. of uvula
    vastus lateralis m.
    vastus medialis m.
    vertical m. of tongue

muscle *(continued)*

    vestigial m.
    visceral m.
    vocal m.
    voluntary m.
    white m.
    white m. disease
    Wilson m.
    yoked m's
    zygomatic m.
muscle-splitting incision
muscle-trimming
musculamine
muscular
muscularis
    m. mucosae
    m. propria
muscularity
muscularize
musculature
musculi (plural of musculus)
musculoaponeurotic
musculocutaneous
musculodermic
musculoelastic
musculofascial
musculofibrous
musculointestinal
musculoligamentous
musculomembranous
musculophrenic
musculoplasty
musculorachidian
musculoskeletal
musculospiral
musculotegumentary
musculotendinous
musculotropic
musculus (musculi)
    musculi abdominis
    m. abductor digiti minimi
      manus
    m. abductor digiti minimi pedis
    m. abductor hallucis
    m. abductor pollicis brevis
    m. abductor pollicis longus
    m. adductor brevis
    m. adductor hallucis
    m. adductor longus
    m. adductor magnus
    m. adductor minimus
    m. adductor pollicis
    m. anconeus
    m. anorectoperineales
    m. antitragicus

musculus (musculi) *(continued)*
    musculi arrector pili
    m. articularis
    m. articularis cubiti
    m. articularis genus
    m. aryepiglotticus
    m. arytenoideus obliquus
    m. arytenoideus transversus
    musculi auriculares
    m. auricularis anterior
    m. auricularis posterior
    m. auricularis superior
    m. biceps brachii
    m. biceps femoris
    m. bipennatus
    m. brachialis
    m. brachioradialis
    m. bronchooesophageus
    m. buccinator
    m. buccopharyngeus
    musculi bulbi
    m. bulbocavernosus
    m. bulbospongiosus
    musculi capitis
    m. ceratocricoideus
    m. ceratopharyngeus
    m. cervicis
    m. chondroglossus
    m. chondropharyngeus
    m. ciliaris
    m. coccygeus
    musculi colli
    m. compressor naris
    m. compressor urethrae
    m. constrictor pharyngis
      inferior
    m. constrictor pharyngis
      medius
    m. constrictor pharyngis
      superior
    m. coracobrachialis
    m. corrugator supercilii
    m. cremaster
    m. cricoarytenoideus lateralis
    m. cricoarytenoideus posterior
    m. cricopharyngeus
    m. cricothyroideus
    m. cruciatus
    m. cutaneus
    m. dartos
    m. deltoideus
    m. depressor anguli oris
    m. depressor labii inferioris
    m. depressor septi nasi
    m. depressor supercilii

musculus (musculi) *(continued)*
    m. detrusor urinae, m.
      detrusor vesicae urinariae
    musculi diaphragmatis pelvis
    m. digastricus
    m. dilator
    m. dilator naris
    m. dilator pupillae
    musculi dorsi
    m. epicranius
    m. epitrochleoanconeus
    m. erector spinae
    m. extensor carpi radialis brevis
    m. extensor carpi radialis
      longus
    m. extensor carpi ulnaris
    m. extensor digiti minimi
    m. extensor digiti quinti
      proprius
    m. extensor digitorum
    m. extensor digitorum brevis
    m. extensor digitorum
      communis
    m. extensor digitorum longus
    m. extensor hallucis brevis
    m. extensor hallucis longus
    m. extensor indicis
    m. extensor indicis proprius
    m. extensor pollicis brevis
    m. extensor pollicis longus
    musculi externi bulbi oculi
    musculi extremitatis inferioris
    musculi extremitatis
      superioris
    musculi faciales, musculi faciei
    m. fibularis brevis
    m. fibularis longus
    m. fibularis tertius
    m. flexor accessorius
    m. flexor carpi radialis
    m. flexor carpi ulnaris
    m. flexor digiti minimi brevis
      manus
    m. flexor digiti minimi brevis
      pedis
    m. flexor digiti quinti brevis
      manus
    m. flexor digiti quinti brevis
      pedis
    m. flexor digitorum brevis
    m. flexor digitorum longus
    m. flexor digitorum profundus
    m. flexor digitorum sublimis
    m. flexor digitorum superficialis
    m. flexor hallucis brevis

M

musculus (musculi) *(continued)*

    m. flexor hallucis longus
    m. flexor pollicis brevis
    m. flexor pollicis longus
    m. frontalis
    m. fusiformis
    m. gastrocnemius
    m. gemellus inferior
    m. gemellus superior
    m. genioglossus
    m. geniohyoideus
    m. glossopalatinus
    m. glossopharyngeus
    m. gluteus maximus
    m. gluteus medius
    m. gluteus minimus
    m. gracilis
    m. helicis major
    m. helicis minor
    m. hyoglossus
    m. iliacus
    m. iliococcygeus
    m. iliocostalis
    m. iliocostalis cervicis
    m. iliocostalis colli
    m. iliocostalis dorsi
    m. iliocostalis lumborum
    m. iliocostalis thoracis
    m. iliopsoas
    musculi incisivi labii inferioris
    musculi incisivi labii superioris
    m. incisurae terminalis
    musculi infrahyoidei
    m. infraspinatus
    musculi intercostales externi
    musculi intercostales interni
    musculi intercostales intimi
    musculi interossei dorsales
      manus
    musculi interossei dorsales
      pedis
    musculi interossei palmares
    musculi interossei plantares
    musculi interossei volares
    musculi interspinales
    musculi interspinales cervicis
    musculi interspinales colli
    musculi interspinales
      lumborum
    musculi interspinales thoracis
    musculi intertransversarii
    musculi intertransversarii
      anteriores cervicis
    musculi intertransversarii
      anteriores colli

musculus (musculi) *(continued)*

    musculi intertransversarii
      laterales lumborum
    musculi intertransversarii
      mediales lumborum
    musculi intertransversarii
      posteriores laterales cervicis
    musculi intertransversarii
      posteriores laterales colli
    musculi intertransversarii
      posteriores mediales cervicis
    musculi intertransversarii
      posteriores mediales colli
    musculi intertransversarii
      thoracis
    m. ischiocavernosus
    m. ischiococcygeus
    musculi laryngis
    m. latissimus dorsi
    m. levator anguli oris
    m. levator ani
    musculi levatores costarum
    musculi levatores costarum
      breves
    musculi levatores costarum
      longi
    m. levator glandulae thyroideae
    m. levator labii superioris
    m. levator labii superioris
      alaeque nasi
    m. levator palpebrae superioris
    m. levator prostatae
    m. levator scapulae
    m. levator veli palatini
    musculi linguae, musculi
      linguales
    m. longissimus
    m. longissimus capitis
    m. longissimus cervicis
    m. longissimus colli
    m. longissimus dorsi
    m. longissimus thoracis
    m. longitudinalis inferior
      linguae
    m. longitudinalis superior
      linguae
    m. longus capitis
    m. longus cervicis
    m. longus colli
    musculi lumbricales manus
    musculi lumbricales pedis
    m. masseter
    musculi masticatorii
    musculi membri inferioris
    musculi membri superioris

musculus (musculi) *(continued)*
- m. mentalis
- musculi multifidi
- m. multipennatus
- m. mylohyoideus
- m. mylopharyngeus
- m. nasalis
- m. obliquus auriculae
- m. obliquus auricularis
- m. obliquus capitis inferior
- m. obliquus capitis superior
- m. obliquus externus abdominis
- m. obliquus inferior bulbi
- m. obliquus inferior oculi
- m. obliquus internus abdominis
- m. obliquus superior bulbi
- m. obliquus superior oculi
- m. obturator externus
- m. obturator internus
- m. obturatorius externus
- m. obturatorius internus
- m. occipitalis
- m. occipitofrontalis
- musculi oculi
- m. omohyoideus
- m. opponens digiti minimi
- m. opponens digiti quinti manus
- m. opponens pollicis
- m. orbicularis
- m. orbicularis oculi
- m. orbicularis oris
- m. orbitalis
- musculi ossiculorum auditoriorum
- musculi ossis hyoidei
- musculi palati
- musculi palati mollis et faucium
- m. palatoglossus
- m. palatopharyngeus
- m. palmaris brevis
- m. palmaris longus
- musculi papillares
- m. papillaris anterior ventriculi dextri
- m. papillaris anterior ventriculi sinistri
- m. papillaris posterior ventriculi dextri
- m. papillaris posterior ventriculi sinistri
- musculi pectinati atrii dextri
- musculi pectinati atrii sinistri
- m. pectineus
- m. pectoralis major

musculus (musculi) *(continued)*
- m. pectoralis minor
- m. pennatus
- musculi perineales, musculi perinei
- m. peroneus brevis
- m. peroneus longus
- m. peroneus tertius
- musculi pharyngis
- m. pharyngopalatinus
- m. piriformis
- m. plantaris
- m. pleurooesophageus
- m. popliteus
- m. procerus
- m. pronator quadratus
- m. pronator teres
- m. prostaticus
- m. psoas major
- m. psoas minor
- m. pterygoideus lateralis
- m. pterygoideus medialis
- m. pterygopharyngeus
- m. puboanalis
- m. pubococcygeus
- m. puboperinealis
- m. puboprostaticus
- m. puborectalis
- m. pubovaginalis
- m. pubovesicalis
- m. pyramidalis
- m. pyramidalis auriculae
- m. pyramidalis auricularis
- m. quadratus
- m. quadratus femoris
- m. quadratus lumborum
- m. quadratus plantae
- m. quadriceps femoris
- m. rectococcygeus
- m. rectourethrales
- m. rectouterinus
- m. rectovesicalis
- m. rectus abdominis
- m. rectus capitis anterior
- m. rectus capitis lateralis
- m. rectus capitis posterior major
- m. rectus capitis posterior minor
- m. rectus femoris
- m. rectus inferior bulbi
- m. rectus inferior oculi
- m. rectus lateralis bulbi
- m. rectus lateralis oculi
- m. rectus medialis bulbi

M

musculus (musculi) *(continued)*
  m. rectus medialis oculi
  m. rectus superior bulbi
  m. rectus superior oculi
  m. rhomboideus major
  m. rhomboideus minor
  m. risorius
  musculi rotatores
  musculi rotatores breves
  musculi rotatores cervicis
  musculi rotatores colli
  musculi rotatores longi
  musculi rotatores lumborum
  musculi rotatores thoracis
  m. sacrococcygeus anterior
  m. sacrococcygeus dorsalis
  m. sacrococcygeus posterior
  m. sacrococcygeus ventralis
  m. sacrospinalis
  m. salpingopharyngeus
  m. sartorius
  m. scalenus anterior
  m. scalenus medius
  m. scalenus minimus
  m. scalenus posterior
  m. semimembranosus
  m. semipennatus
  m. semispinalis
  m. semispinalis capitis
  m. semispinalis cervicis
  m. semispinalis dorsi
  m. semispinalis thoracis
  m. semitendinosus
  m. serratus anterior
  m. serratus posterior inferior
  m. serratus posterior superior
  m. soleus
  m. sphincter
  m. sphincter ampullae
    hepatopancreaticae
  m. sphincter ani externus
  m. sphincter ani internus
  m. sphincter ductus biliaris
  m. sphincter ductus choledochi
  m. sphincter ductus pancreatici
  m. sphincter pupillae
  m. sphincter pylori
  m. sphincter pyloricus
  m. sphincter supracollicularis
  m. sphincter urethrae
  m. sphincter urethrae
    externus urethrae femininae
  m. sphincter urethrae
    externus urethrae
    masculinae

musculus (musculi) *(continued)*
  m. sphincter urethrae
    internus
  m. sphincter urethrae
    membranaceae
  m. sphincter urethrovaginalis
  m. sphincter vesicae urinariae
  m. spinalis
  m. spinalis capitis
  m. spinalis cervicis
  m. spinalis dorsi
  m. spinalis thoracis
  m. splenius capitis
  m. splenius cervicis
  m. stapedius
  m. sternalis
  m. sternocleidomastoideus
  m. sternohyoideus
  m. sternothyroideus
  m. styloglossus
  m. stylohyoideus
  m. stylopharyngeus
  m. subclavius
  musculi subcostales
  musculi suboccipitales
  m. subscapularis
  m. supinator
  musculi suprahyoidei
  m. supraspinatus
  m. suspensorius duodeni
  m. tarsalis inferior
  m. tarsalis superior
  m. temporalis
  m. temporoparietalis
  m. tensor fasciae latae
  m. tensor tympani
  m. tensor veli palatini
  m. teres major
  m. teres minor
  musculi thoracis
  m. thyroarytenoideus
  m. thyroepiglotticus
  m. thyrohyoideus
  m. thyropharyngeus
  m. tibialis anterior
  m. tibialis posterior
  m. trachealis
  m. tragicus
  musculi transversospinales
  m. transversus abdominis
  m. transversus auriculae
  m. transversus auricularis
  m. transversus linguae
  m. transversus menti
  m. transversus nuchae

musculus (musculi) *(continued)*
    m. transversus perinei
      profundus
    m. transversus perinei
      superficialis
    m. transversus thoracis
    m. trapezius
    m. triangularis
    m. triceps brachii
    m. triceps surae
    musculi trigoni vesicae
      urinariae
    m. trigoni vesicae urinariae
      profundus
    m. trigoni vesicae urinariae
      superficialis
    m. unipennatus
    m. uvulae
    m. vastus intermedius
    m. vastus lateralis
    m. vastus medialis
    m. ventricularis
    m. verticalis linguae
    m. vocalis
    m. zygomaticus
    m. zygomaticus major
    m. zygomaticus minor
Museholdt forceps
mushroom
    m. catheter
    Silastic m. catheter
mushroom worker's disease
musicogenic epilepsy
music therapy
Musset sign
mussitation
MUST—medical unit, self-
  contained, transportable
mustache dressing
mustard
    nitrogen m.
    L-phenylalanine m. (L-PAM)
    uracil m.
Mustard vascular operation
Mustardé
    flap
    otoplasty
mutagen
mutagenesis
    directed m.
    insertional m.
mutagenic
mutagenicity
mutagenize
mutant

mutarotation
mutase
mutation
    allelic m's
    amber m.
    auxotrophic m.
    back m.
    biochemical m.
    chromosomal m.
    clear plaque m.
    cold-sensitive m.
    conditional m.
    conditional lethal m.
    constitutive m.
    dynamic m.
    forward m.
    frameshift m.
    genomic m.
    germinal m.
    heat-sensitive m.
    heterozygous m.
    induced m.
    leaky
    lethal m.
    missense m.
    natural m.
    neutral m.
    nonsense m.
    nutritional m.
    ochre m.
    opal m.
    point m.
    polar m.
    reading frameshift m.
    reverse m.
    silent m.
    somatic m.
    spontaneous genetic m.
    suppressor m.
    synonymous m.
    temperature-sensitive (t-s) m.
    umber m.
    visible m.
mutational
mute
    deaf-m.
mutein
mutilate
mutilation
mutism
    akinetic m.
    deaf-m.
    elective m.
    hysterical m.
    selective m.

M

µV, microV—microvolt(s)
mV—millivolt(s)
Mv—mendelevium
MV—
    megavolt(s)
    mitral valve
    mixed venous
    veterinary physician (L.
      Medicus Veterinarius)
MVP—mitral valve prolapse
MVR—massive vitreous retraction
MVV—maximum voluntary
  ventilation
mw—microwave
mW—milliwatt(s)
MW—
    megawatt(s)
    molecular weight
My—myopia
myalgia
    m. abdominis
    m. capitis
    m. cervicalis
    epidemic m.
    lumbar m.
    spastic m.
myasthenia
    m. gravis
    m. gravis, familial infantile
    m. gravis pseudoparalytica
    m. laryngis
    neonatal m.
myasthenic
myatrophy
mycete
mycetism
mycetismus
    m. cerebris
    m. choleriformis
    m. gastrointestinalis
    m. nervosus
    m. sanguinarius
mycetogenic
mycetogenous
mycetoma
    actinomycotic m.
    eumycotic m.
mycobacteriosis
mycobacterium (mycobacteria)
    anonymous mycobacteria
    atypical mycobacteria
    groups I–IV mycobacteria
    nontuberculous
Mycobacterium
    M. abscessus

Mycobacterium (continued)
    M. africanum
    M. avium
    M. avium-intracellulare (MAI)
    M. bovis
    M. chelonae
    M. fortuitum
    M. gordonae
    M. haemophilum
    M. intracellulare
    M. kansasii
    M. leprae
    M. malmoense
    M. marinum
    M. scrofulaceum
    M. simiae
    M. smegmatis
    M. szulgai
    M. tuberculosis
    M. ulcerans
    M. xenopi
mycobactin
mycoid
mycolic acids
mycophagy
mycoplasma (mycoplasmas,
  mycoplasmata)
    T-strain m.
Mycoplasma
    M. faucium
    M. fermentans
    M. hominis
    M. orale
    M. orale type 1
    M. pharyngis
    M. pneumoniae
mycoplasmal pneumonia
mycoplasmosis
mycoprecipitin
mycopus
mycose
mycoside
mycosis (mycoses)
    cutaneous m.
    m. fungoides
    m. fungoides d'emblée
    m. leptothrica
    splenic m.
mycosterol
mycotic
mycotoxicology
mycotoxicosis
mycotoxin
mycotoxinization
mycteroxerosis

mydaleine
mydriasis
    alternating m.
    bounding m.
    paralytic m.
    spasmodic m.
    spastic m.
    spinal m.
    springing m.
mydriatic effect
myectomy
myectopia
myelalgia
myelatelia
myelatrophy
myelauxe
myelemia
myelencephalon
myelencephalospinal
myelin
myelinated
myelinic
myelinization
myelinogenesis
    dystopic cortical m.
myelinogenetic
myelinolysis
    central pontine m.
myelinopathy
myelinosis
    pontine m.
myelinotoxic
myelinotoxicity
myelitic
myelitis
    acute m.
    ascending m.
    bulbar m.
    cavitary m.
    central m.
    chronic m.
    compression m.
    concussion m.
    cornual m.
    descending m.
    diffuse m.
    disseminated m.
    hemorrhagic m.
    neuro-optic m.
    periependymal m.
    postinfectious m.
    postvaccinal m.
    radiation m.
    subacute m.
    subacute necrotic m.

myelitis *(continued)*
    syphilitic m.
    systemic m.
    transverse m.
    m. vaccinia
    viral m.
myeloablation
myeloablative
myeloarchitecture
myeloblast
myeloblastemia
myeloblastic
myeloblastoma
myeloblastomatosis
myeloblastosis
myelocele
myeloclast
myelocyst
myelocystic
myelocystocele
myelocystography
myelocystomeningocele
myelocyte
myelocythemia
myelocytic
myelocytoma
myelocytomatosis
myelocytosis
myelodysplasia
myeloencephalitis
    eosinophilic m.
    epidemic m.
myelofibrosis
    m. with myeloid metaplasia
    osteosclerosis m.
myelogenesis
myelogenous
    acute m. leukemia (AML)
    chronic m. leukemia (CML)
myelogeny
myelogone
myelogonic
myelogram
myelography
    air m.
    computed m.
    computer-assisted m. (CAM)
    opaque m.
    oxygen m.
myeloid metaplasia
myeloidin
myeloidosis
myelokentric
myelolipoma
myelolysis

M

myeloma
    Bence Jones m.
    extramedullary m.
    giant cell m.
    indolent m.
    localized m.
    multiple m.
    plasma cell m.
    solitary m.
myelomalacia
myelomatoid
myelomatosis
myelomenia
myelomeningocele
myelomere
myelomonocyte
myelomonocytic
myelo-opticoneuropathy
    subacute m.
myelopathic
myelopathy
    anterior m.
    ascending m.
    carcinomatous m.
    cervical m.
    cervical spondylotic m.
    cervical stenotic m.
    cervical vertebral
        stenotic m.
    chronic progressive m.
    compression m.
    concussion m.
    cystic m.
    descending m.
    focal m.
    funicular m.
    hemorrhagic m.
    hereditary m.
    HTLV-1-associated m.
    necrotizing m.
    paracarcinomatous m.
    paraneoplastic m.
    radiation m.
    spondylotic cervical m.
    systemic m.
    transverse m.
    traumatic m.
    vascular m.
myeloperoxidase (MPO)
  deficiency
myelophage
myelophthisic
myelophthisis
myeloplast
myeloplegia

myelopoiesis
    ectopic m.
    extramedullary m.
myelopoietic
myelopore
myeloproliferative
myeloradiculitis
myeloradiculodysplasia
myeloradiculopathy
myelorrhagia
myelosarcoma
myelosarcomatosis
myeloschisis
myelosclerosis
myeloscope
myeloscopy
myelosis
    aleukemic m.
    chronic nonleukemic m.
    erythremic m.
    nonleukemic m.
myelospongium
myelosuppression
myelosuppressive
myelosyphilis
myelotherapy
myelotome
myelotomy
    Bischof m.
    commissural m.
myelotoxic
myelotoxicity
myenteric
myenteron
Myers method
Myerson
    forceps
    saw
    sign
myesthesia
MyG—myasthenia gravis
myiasis
    aural m.
    creeping m.
    cutaneous m.
    dermal m.
    intestinal m.
    nasal m.
    ocular m.
    subcutaneous m.
    traumatic m.
myiodesopsia
Myles
    curet
    forceps

Myles *(continued)*
    punch
    snare
    speculum
    tonsillectome
mylohyoid
mylopharyngeal
myoadenylate deaminase deficiency
myoalbumin
myoarchitectonic
myoblast
myoblastic
myoblastoma
    granular cell m.
myoblastomyoma
myobradia
myocardial
    m. bridging
    m. concussion
    m. contractility
    m. contractions
    m. depolarization
    m. disease
    m. edema
    m. failure
    m. fiber shortening
    m. function
    m. hibernation
    m. hypertrophy
    m. imaging
    m. infarction
    m. ischemia
    m. metabolism
    m. necrosis
    m. oxygen consumption
    m. perfusion imaging
    m. perfusion scintigraphy
    m. perfusion study
    m. rupture
    m. stiffness
    m. stunning
    m. tension
    m. tissue
myocardiogram
myocardiography
myocardiopathy
    alcoholic m.
    chagasic m.
    idiopathic m.
myocardiorrhaphy
myocarditic
myocarditis
    acute bacterial m.
    acute isolated m.
    chronic m.

myocarditis *(continued)*
    diphtheritic m.
    Fiedler m.
    fragmentation m.
    giant cell m.
    granulomatous m.
    hypersensitivity m.
    idiopathic m.
    indurative m.
    infectious m.
    interstitial m.
    parenchymatous m.
    protozoal m.
    rheumatic m.
    rickettsial m.
    syphilitic m.
    toxic m.
    tuberculous m.
    viral m.
myocardium
    hibernating m.
    stunned m.
myocele
myocelialgia
myocelitis
myocellulitis
myoclonia
    m. congenita
    m. epileptica
    m. fibrillaris multiplex
    fibrillary m.
    pseudoglottic m.
myoclonic
myoclonus
    action m.
    Baltic m.
    cortical m.
    cortical reflex m.
    epileptic m.
    essential m.
    intention m.
    jaw m.
    m. multiplex
    nocturnal m.
    ocular m.
    opsoclonus-m.
    palatal m.
    palatopharyngolaryngeal m.
    reflex m.
    startle m.
myocolpitis
myocomma
myoctonine
myoculator
myocutaneous

M

myocyte
    Anitschkow (Anichkov) m.
myocytolysis
    coagulative m.
    focal m. of heart
myocytoma
myodegeneration
myodiastasis
myodiopter
myodynamic
myodynamics
myodynia
myodystonia
myodystrophia fetalis
myoedema
myoelastic
myoelectric, myoelectrical
    m. prosthesis
myoendocarditis
myoepithelial
myoepithelioma
myoepithelium
myofascial
myofasciitis
myofiber
myofibril
myofibrilla (myofibrillae)
myofibrillar
myofibroblast
myofibroma
myofibromatosis
    infantile m.
myofibrosis cordis
myofibrositis
myofilament
myofunctional
myogelosis
myogen
myogenesis
myogenetic
myogenic
myogenous
myoglia
myoglobin (Mb)
myoglobinemia
myoglobinuria
    familial m.
    paralytic m.
    spontaneous m.
myoglobulin
myoglobulinuria
myognathus
myogram
myograph
myographic

myography
myohemoglobin
myohypertrophia kymoparalytica
myoid
    visual cell m.
myoideum
myoidism
myo-inositol
myoischemia
myokinase
myokinesimeter
myokinesiogram
myokinesis
myokinetic
myokymia
myolemma
myolipoma
myolysis cardiotoxica
myoma (myomas, myomata)
    m. striocellulare
    m. uteri, uterine m.
myomagenesis
myomalacia cordis
myomatosis
myomatous
myomectomy
    abdominal m.
    vaginal m.
myomelanosis
myomere
myometer
myometrial
myometritis
myometrium
myomotomy
myon
myonecrosis
    clostridial m.
myoneural
myopachynsis
myopalmus
myoparalysis
myoparesis
myopathia
    m. cordis
    m. infraspinata
myopathic
myopathy
    acromegalic m.
    ACTH m.
    acute thyrotoxic m.
    alcoholic m.
    capture m.
    carcinomatous m.
    central core m.

myopathy *(continued)*
    centronuclear m.
    corticosteroid-induced m.
    Cushing disease m.
    deep pectoral m.
    degenerative m.
    diabetic m.
    distal m.
    Duchenne m.
    endocrine m.
    fibrotic m.
    glucocorticoid-induced m.
    glycolytic m.
    granulomatous m.
    hyperparathyroid m.
    hypertrophic branchial m.
    hypothyroid m.
    infiltrative m.
    inflammatory m.
    Kiloh-Nevin m.
    Landouzy-Dejerine m.
    late distal hereditary m.
    lipid m.
    metabolic m.
    mitochondrial m.
    myogranular m.
    myotonic m.
    myotubular m.
    myxedematous m.
    nemaline m.
    nutritional m.
    ocular m.
    ossifying m.
    primary progressive m.
    progressive atrophic m.
    rod m.
    sarcoid m.
    scapuloperoneal m.
    slow hereditary distal m.
    steroid m.
    thyrotoxic m.
    uremic m.
    Welander m., Welander
      distal m.
myope
myopectineal
myopericarditis
myophage
myophagism
myophosphorylase deficiency
myopia (M)
    axial m.
    curvature m.
    index m.
    malignant m.

myopia (M) *(continued)*
    primary m.
    prodromal m.
    progressive m.
    simple m.
myopic
    m. crescent
    m. degeneration
myoplasm
myoplastic
myoplasty
myoprotein
myorrhaphy
myorrhythmia
    oculofacioskeletal m.
    oculomasticatory m.
myosalpingitis
myosalpinx
myosarcoma
myoschwannoma
myosclerosis
myoscope
myoseptum
myosin ATPase
myosinuria
myositic
myositis
    acute disseminated m.
    acute progressive m.
    m. a frigore
    eosinophilic m.
    m. fibrosa
    generalized m. ossificans
    inclusion body m.
    infectious m.
    interstitial m.
    multiple m.
    orbital m.
    m. ossificans
    m. ossificans
      circumscripta
    m. ossificans progressiva
    m. ossificans traumatica
    parenchymatous m.
    primary multiple m.
    progressive ossifying m.
    proliferative m.
    m. purulenta
    rheumatoid m.
    m. serosa
    spontaneous bacterial m.
    tropical m.
myospasm
myospherulosis
myostatin

M

myosteoma
myosthenic
myostroma
myostromin
myosynizesis
myotactic
myotasis
myotatic
myotendinosis
myotendinous
myotenositis
myotenotomy
myotherapy
myothermic
myotilin
myotome
myotomic
myotomy
    cricopharyngeal m.
    Heller m.
    laparoscopic m.
    Livaidatis circular m.
    supracoronary m.
myotonia
    m. atrophica
    chondrodystrophic m.
    m. congenita
    congenital m.
    m. dystrophica
    m. hereditaria
    m. tarda
myotonic
myotonoid
myotonometer
myotonus
myotrophic
myotrophy
myotropic
myotubular
myotubule
myovascular
myricyl
myringa
myringectomy
myringitis
    m. bullosa
    bullous m.
myringodermatitis
myringoplasty
    bilateral m.
    cartilage graft m.
    chemical m.
    fat graft m.
    inlay m.

myringoplasty *(continued)*
    onlay graft m.
    perichondrium m.
    transcanal m.
    transtympanic m.
    underlay m.
myringostapediopexy
myringotome
myringotomy
    bilateral m.
    m. incision
    m. with ventilation tube
      insertion
    Venturi m. tube
myrinx
myristate
    isopropyl m.
myristic acid
myrrh
myrtenol
myrtiform
mysophilia
mysophobia
mysophobic
mytacism
mythophobia
myxadenitis labialis
myxangitis
myxasthenia
myxedema
    circumscribed m.
    congenital m.
    nodular m.
    operative m.
    papular m.
    pituitary m.
    pretibial m.
    primary m.
    secondary m.
myxedematoid
myxedematous
myxiosis
myxochondrofibrosarcoma
myxochondroma
myxochondrosarcoma
myxocystitis
myxocystoma
myxocyte
myxoenchondroma
myxoendothelioma
myxofibroma
myxofibrosarcoma
myxoglioma
myxoglobulosis

myxoid
myxolipoma
myxoma (myxomas,
  myxomata)
    atrial m.
    cystic m.
    enchondromatous m.
    m. fibrosum
    m. of heart
    infectious m.
    lipomatous m.
    nerve sheath m.
    odontogenic m.
    m. sarcomatosum

myxoma (myxomas, myxomata)
    (continued)
      vascular m.
myxomatosis
    m. cuniculi
    infectious m.
myxomatous
myxomyoma
myxopapilloma
myxopoiesis
myxosarcoma
myxosarcomatous
myxovirus
MZ—monozygotic

N

ν—
    nu (Greek letter)
n—
    refractive index
    sample size
n.—nerve (L. nervus)
N—
    nasal
    neurology
    nitrogen
    normal
    size of sample
    unit of neutron dosage
N—
    Avogadro number
    neutron number
    number
    population size
N.—
    Neisseria
    Nocardia
Na—sodium
NA—
    neutralizing antibody
    not admitted
N/A, NA—
    not applicable
    not available
N_A—refractive index
NAA—no apparent abnormalities
Nabatoff stripper
nabothian cyst

NaBr—sodium bromide
Nachlas tube
NaCl—sodium chloride
nacreous
NAD—
    nicotinamide adenine
      dinucleotide
    no acute distress
    no apparent distress
    no appreciable disease
Nadbath akinesia
nadir
NADP—nicotinamide adenine
    dinucleotide phosphate
NADPH—nicotinamide adenine
    dinucleotide phosphate, reduced
Naegeli
    leukemia
    syndrome
Naegleria fowleri
naegleriasis
Naffziger
    decompression
    operation
    syndrome
    test
Nagamatsu incision
Nagel anomaloscope
Nägele (Naegele)
    obliquity
    pelvis
    rule

Nageotte
    bracelets
    cell
Nager
    acrofacial dysostosis
    syndrome
Nager-De Reynier syndrome
Nagler
    effect
    reaction
    test
nail
    Augustine n.
    cloverleaf n.
    double-edge n.
    eggshell n.
    n. en raquette
    fracture n.
    hang n., hangnail
    Hansen-Street n.
    Harrington n.
    hippocratic n.
    ingrown n.
    Jewett n.
    Kuntscher n.
    Lottes n.
    Massie n.
    Moore n.
    Neufeld n.
    parrot beak n.
    pitted n.
    Pugh n.
    racket n.
    reedy n.
    Schneider n.
    Smillie n.
    Smith-Petersen n.
    spoon n.
    Thornton n.
    turtle-back n.
    Venable-Stuck n.
    watch-crystal n.
    Zickel n. fixation
nail bed
nailing
    intramedullary n.
    marrow n.
    medullary n.
nail nipper
    Amico n.n.
Nairobi eye
Nakayama
    reagent
    test

naked
    n. DNA
    n. eye
    n. fat sign
name
    British Approved N. (BAN)
    generic n.
    International Nonproprietary
      N. (INN)
    nonproprietary n.
    proprietary n.
    scientific n.
    semisystematic n.
    semitrivial n.
    systematic n.
    trivial n.
    United States Adopted N.
      (USAN)
    vernacular n.
NAMI—National Alliance for the
    Mentally Ill
naming
nanism
    mulibrey n.
    pituitary n.
    senile n.
nanocormia
nanocurie (nCi)
nanogram (ng)
nanoid
nanoliter (nl)
nanometer (nm)
nanosecond (ns, nsec)
nanounit (nU)
NAP—nasion, point A,
    pogonion
nape
napex
naphtha
naphthalene
    chlorinated n.
naphthol
    α-n. [alpha-], 1-n.
    β-n. [beta-n.], 2-n.
naphthylamine
napiform
napkin-ring
    n.r. annular stenosis
    n.r. annular tumor
    n.r. carcinoma
    n.r. defect
    n.r. lesion
    n.r. trachea
naprapathy

narcissism
  healthy n.
  pathological n.
  primary n.
  secondary n.
narcissistic
  n. features
  n. personality disorder
  n. traits
narcolepsy
narcoleptic
narcoma
narcomania
narcosis
  basal n.
  carbon dioxide n.
  nitrogen n.
  prolonged n.
narcostimulant
narcotic
  n. analgesic
  n. antagonist
  n. blockade
  n. poisons
narcotine
narcotize
Nardi test
naris (nares)
  anterior n.
  external n.
  internal nares
  posterior nares
narrow-beam half-thickness
narrowing
  diffuse n.
  irregular n.
  joint space n.
  luminal n.
  nonostial n.
  pharyngeal n.
  post-exercise airway n.
  proximal n.
  significant n.
nasal
  n. allergy
  n. aperture
  n. arch
  n. asthma
  n. bone
  bony n. septum
  n. calculus
  n. canal
  n. cannula
  n. cartilages

nasal *(continued)*
  cartilaginous n. septum
  n. cavity
  n. concha
  n. congestion
  n. crest
  n. deformity
  n. diphtheria
  n. dome
  n. drip
  n. duct
  n. eczema
  n. filtration
  n. fin
  n. flaring
  n. foramina
  n. fossa
  n. glioma
  n. groove
  n. hemianopia
  n. hemorrhage
  n. index
  n. intubation
  n. line
  n. margin of frontal bone
  n. meatus
  membranous n. septum
  n. notch of frontal bone
  n. notch of maxilla
  n. mastocytosis
  n. obstruction
  osseous n. septum
  n. packing
  n. plane
  n. polyposis
  n. polyps
  n. process
  n. prominence
  n. prongs
  n. reflex
  Rönne n. step
  n. septal defect
  n. septum
  n. solar dermatitis
  n. speculum
  n. spine
  n. sulcus
  n. suture
  n. tampon
  n. turbinate
  n. valve
  n. vestibule
  n. vestibulitis
nasalis

N

nasality
nascent
nasioiniac
nasion
Nasmyth membrane
nasoantral
nasoantritis
nasoantrostomy
nasobasal line, nasobasilar line
nasobregmatic arc
nasobronchial
nasobuccal
nasociliary
　　n. nerve
　　n. neuralgia
　　n. root
nasoendoscope
nasoendoscopy
naso-ethmoidal
nasofacial
nasofrontal
　　n. duct
　　n. suture
　　n. vein
nasogastric
　　n. catheter
　　n. intubation
　　n. suction
　　n. tube
nasojejunal
nasolabial
　　n. line
　　n. lymph node
　　n. reflex
　　n. sulcus
nasolacrimal
　　n. duct
　　n. groove
nasomandibular fixation
nasomaxillary suture
nasomental reflex
naso-occipital
naso-oral
nasopalatine
　　n. artery
　　n. canals
　　n. duct cyst
　　n. groove
　　n. nerve
　　n. plexus
nasopharyngeal
　　n. airway
　　n. carcinoma
　　n. diphtheria
　　n. fibroangioma

nasopharyngeal *(continued)*
　　n. fold
　　n. groove
　　n. roof
　　n. speculum
　　n. tube
nasopharyngitis
nasopharyngolaryngoscope
　　fiberoptic n.
　　flexible n.
　　Olympus ENP-P n.
nasopharyngoscope
　　Broyles n.
　　fiberoptic n.
　　flexible n.
　　Holmes n.
　　Meltzer n.
　　Olympus ENF-P2
　　pediatric n.
　　URA-1 n.
nasopharyngoscopy
　　dynamic n.
　　endoscopic n.
　　video n.
nasopharynx
nasoscope
nasoseptal
nasoseptitis
nasosinusitis
nasospinale
nasotracheal
　　n. catheter
　　n. intubation
　　n. tube
nasoturbinal concha
natal
　　n. cleft
　　n. tooth
natality
natatory ligament
nates (plural of natis)
Nathan test
National cystoscope
National Academy of Sciences
　　(NAS)
National Cancer Institute (NCI)
National Formulary (NF)
National Institute of Allergy and
　　Infectious Diseases (NIAID)
natis (nates)
native
　　n. coronary arteries
　　n. organ
　　n. tissue
natremia

natriuresis
    pressure n.
natriuretic
natural
    n. antibodies
    n. dentition
    n. family planning
    n. immunity
    n. killer (NK) cells
    n. ventilation
naturopath
naturopathic medicine
naturopathy
Nauheim
    bath
    treatment
Naunyn-Minkowski method
nausea
    epidemic n.
    n. gravidarum
    n. marina
nauseant
nauseated
nauseous
navel
    blue n.
    enamel n.
    n. piercing
    n. reinsertion
    n. transposition
navicula
navicular
    n. abdomen
    n. arthritis
    n. bone
    n. disease
    n. fossa of Cruveilhier
    n. fossa of male urethra
    n. fossa of sphenoid bone
naviculocuneiform
Nb—niobium
NB—newborn
NBM—nothing by mouth
NBS—normal blood serum
NBT—nitroblue tetrazolium
NBTE—nonbacterial thrombotic
  endocarditis
NBW—normal birthweight
NC—
    no change
    noncontributory
    not cultured
N/C—no complaints
NCA—
    neurocirculatory asthenia

NCA—*(continued)*
    nonspecific cross-reacting
    antigen
NCD—not considered disabling
NCF—neutrophil chemotactic
  factor
nCi—nanocurie(s)
NCI—National Cancer Institute
NCV—nerve conduction velocity
nD—refractive index
Nd—neodymium
ND—
    neonatal death
    neurotic depression
    no data
    no disease
    nondisabling
    normal delivery
    not detectable
    not detected
    not determined
    not done
NDA—
    no data available
    no demonstrable antibodies
NDMA—*p*-nitrosodimethylaniline
NDP—net dietary protein
NDV—Newcastle disease virus
Nd:YAG—neodymium:yttrium-
  aluminum-garnet (laser)
Ne—neon
NE—
    nerve ending
    neurologic examination
    no effect
    norepinephrine
    not evaluated
    not examined
Neal cannula
near-and-far suture
nearsighted
nearsightedness
nearthrosis
nebula (nebulae)
    n. formation
    n. frontalis
    proud n.
nebulization
nebulizer
    Aeroneb Micropump n.
    DeVilbiss n.
    eFlow electronic n.
    jet n.
    MistyNeb n.
    Pari LC Plus n.

N

nebulizer *(continued)*
    ultrasonic n.
    vibrating mesh n.
nebulous
NEC—
    necrotizing enterocolitis
    not elsewhere classifiable
Necator americanus
necatoriasis
necessary
necessity
    pharmaceutic n.,
      pharmaceutical n.
neck
    anatomical n. of humerus
    n. of ankle bone
    bladder n.
    n. brace
    bull n.
    n. of condyloid process of
      mandible
    dental n.
    n. of dorsal head of spinal cord
    false n. of humerus
    femoral n.
    n. of fibula
    n. of gallbladder
    n. of glans penis
    n. of head of posterior horn of
      spinal cord
    n. of humerus
    Madelung n.
    n. of malleus
    n. of mandible
    n. of pancreas
    n. of posterior horn of spinal
      cord
    radical n. dissection
    n. of radius
    n. of rib
    n. of scapula
    n. sign
    stiff n.
    surgical n.
    n. of talus
    n. of tooth
    true n. of humerus
    turkey gobbler n.
    n. of urinary bladder
    uterine n.
    n. of vertebra
    webbed n.
    wry n.
neck flap
    hair-bearing bipedicle n.f.
    MacFee n.f.

necklace
    n. arteriovenous hemodialysis
      graft
    n. bypass graft
    Casal n.
    n. distribution
    pearl n. sign
    n. sign
    stone n.
    n. of vessels
necrectomy
necrencephalus
necrobacillosis
necrobiosis
    n. lipoidica
    n. lipoidica diabeticorum
necrobiotic xanthogranuloma
necrocytosis
necrogenic wart
necrogenous
necrologic
necrolysis
    toxic epidermal n.
necrolytic migratory erythema
necromania
necromimesis
necrophagous
necrophilia
necrophilic
necrophilism
necrophilous
necrophobia
necropsy
necrosadism
necroscopy
necrose, necrosed
necrosis (necroses)
    acute tubular n.
    arteriolar n.
    aseptic n.
    avascular n.
    bacillary n.
    Balser fatty n.
    bilateral renal cortical n.
    bland n.
    bridging n.
    caseous n.
    central n.
    cerebrocortical n.
    cheesy n.
    chemical n.
    coagulation n.
    coagulative n.
    cold-induced n.
    colliquative n.
    contraction band n.

necrosis (necroses) *(continued)*
    cortical n.
    coumarin n.
    cystic medial n.
    decubital n.
    diphtheritic n.
    dry n.
    embolic n.
    enzymatic fat n.
    epiphyseal ischemic n.
    Erdheim cystic medial n.
    exanthematous n.
    fat n.
    fibrinoid n.
    focal n.
    gangrenous pulp n.
    glomerular n.
    gummatous n.
    hyaline n.
    icteric n.
    infectious bulbar n.
    infectious pancreatic n.
    ischemic n.
    laminar cortical n.
    liquefaction n.
    liquefactive n.
    mandibular n.
    massive hepatic n.
    medial n.
    mercurial n.
    moist n.
    mummification n.
    nephrotoxic tubule n.
    Paget quiet n.
    papillary n.
    peripheral n.
    phosphorus n.
    physical n.
    piecemeal n.
    pituitary n.
    postpartum n.
    pressure n.
    progressive emphysematous n.
    quiet n.
    radiation n.
    renal coagulation n.
    septic n.
    simple n.
    spontaneous n.
    subacute hepatic n.
    subcutaneous fat n.
    subendocardial n.
    submassive hepatic n.
    superficial n.
    syphilitic n.
    total n.

necrosis (necroses) *(continued)*
    transmural n.
    tubular n.
    n. ustilaginea
    Zenker n.
necrospermia
necrospermic
necrotic
    n. arachnidism
    n. caries
    n. cyst
    n. dermatitis
    n. enteritis
    n. infectious conjunctivitis
    n. inflammation
    n. laryngitis
    n. osteitis
    n. pump
    n. rhinitis
    n. stomatitis
necrotizing
    n. amebic colitis
    n. amebic pancolitis
    n. angiitis
    n. arteriolitis
    n. arteritis
    n. cellulitis
    n. enterocolitis (NEC)
    n. fasciitis
    n. funisitis
    n. gingivitis
    n. leukoencephalopathy
    n. myelopathy
    n. nephrosis
    n. otitis externa
    n. papillitis
    n. pneumonia
    n. sarcoid granulomatosis
    n. scleritis
    n. sialometaplasia
    n. ulcerative gingivitis
    n. ulcerative
        gingivoperiodontitis
    n. ulcerative gingivostomatitis
    n. vasculitis
necrotomy
    contusion n.
    osteoplastic n.
    radical n.
necrotoxin
necrozoospermia
NED—no evidence of
    disease
needle
    Abrams n.
    Adson n.

N

needle *(continued)*
    Amsler n.
    aneurysm n.
    aspirating n.
    atraumatic n.
    Babcock n.
    biopsy n.
    Bowman iris n.
    Brown n.
    Bunnell n.
    butterfly n.
    cataract n.
    n. catheter jejunostomy
    Chiba n.
    Child-Phillips n.
    Cibis ski n.
    Cone n.
    Cope n.
    Cournand n.
    Craig n.
    Curry n.
    Cushing n.
    cutting n.
    Davis n.
    Davis knife n.
    Dees n.
    Denis Browne n.
    Deschamps n.
    discission n.
    docking n.
    n. electromyography
    electrosurgical n.
    fascia n.
    fine n.
    Fischer n.
    Floyd n.
    Flynt n.
    Frankfeldt n.
    Franklin-Silverman n.
    Frederick n.
    Gardner n.
    Goldbacher n.
    Graefe (von Graefe) n.
    Grieshaber n.
    Hagedorn n.
    House n.
    House-Barbara n.
    House-Rosen n.
    Hutchins n.
    hypodermic n.
    Jamshidi n.
    Kaplan n.
    Keith n.
    Klatskin n.
    Knapp n.

needle *(continued)*
    knife n.
    Kronecker n.
    Lewy-Rubin n.
    ligature n.
    lumbar puncture n.
    Martin n.
    Mayo n.
    Menghini n.
    Mueller n.
    Murphy n.
    New n.
    Parhad-Poppen n.
    Pereyra n.
    pop-off n.
    radium n.
    Retter n.
    Reverdin n.
    Rochester n.
    Rosen n.
    Sachs n.
    Sanders-Brown-Shaw n.
    Seldinger n.
    Shambaugh n.
    Sheldon-Spatz n.
    Shirodkar n.
    side-cutting spatulated n.
    Silverman n.
    skinny n.
    Smiley-Williams
      arteriography n.
    spinal n.
    Stocker n.
    stop n.
    swaged n.
    Travenol n.
    Tru-Cut n.
    Tuohy n.
    Turkel n.
    Veenema-Gusberg n.
    ventriculopuncture n.
    Veress n.
    Vicat n.
    Vim-Silverman n.
    Voorhees n.
    Ward-French n.
    Weeks n.
    Wood n.
needle holder
    Barraquer n.h.
    Boynton n.h.
    Castroviejo n.h.
    Castroviejo-Kalt n.h.
    Derf n.h.
    Ellis n.h.

needle holder *(continued)*
    Green n.h.
    Grieshaber n.h.
    Halsey n.h.
    Heaney n.h.
    Johnson n.h.
    Kalt n.h.
    Lapides n.h.
    McPherson n.h.
    Paton n.h.
    Stratte n.h.
    Young n.h.
    Young-Millin n.h.
needling
NEEP—negative end-expiratory
    pressure
Neer prosthesis
NEFA—nonesterified fatty
    acid(s)
negation
negative
    false n.
    n. G
negativism
neglect
    benign n.
    dental n.
    emotional n.
    hemispatial n.
    medical n.
    senile n.
    sensory n.
    spatial n.
    unilateral n.
    visual n.
negligence
    comparative n.
    contributory n.
    medical n.
Negri bodies
Negro [eponym]
    phenomenon
    sign
Negus
    bronchoscope
    dilator
    esophagoscope
    tube
Neill-Mooser
    bodies
    reaction
Neil-Moore electrode
Neisser
    diplococcus
    syringe

Neisseria
    N. flavescens
    N. gonorrhoeae
    N. lactamica
    N. meningitidis
    N. mucosa
    N. sicca
    N. subflava
neisserial
Neisser-Wechsberg
    phenomenon
Neivert retractor
Nélaton
    catheter
    dislocation
    line
    operation
    probe
    sphincter
Nelson
    forceps
    scissors
    syndrome
nemaline
    n. bodies
    n. myopathy
    n. rods
nemathelminth
nematocide
nematocyst
nematode
nematodiasis
    intestinal n.
    nonpatent n.
nematoid
neoadjuvant
    n. chemohormonal therapy
    n. chemoradiotherapy
    n. chemotherapy
    n. hormonal therapy
    n. radiotherapy
    n. therapy
neobladder
neocortex
neocystostomy
    ureteral n.
    ureteroileal n.
neocytosis
neodymium:yttrium-aluminum-
    garnet (Nd:YAG) laser
neoendorphin
neoformation
    fibrous connective tissue n.
    tendon n.
    vascular n.

N

neoglottic
  n. closure
  n. vibrations
neoglottis
  phonatory n.
neointima
neologism
neomembrane
neon (Ne)
  n. light
  n. particle protocol
neonatal
  n. conjunctivitis
  n. diarrhea
  n. hemochromatosis
  n. hepatitis
  n. herpes
  n. hyperbilirubinemia
  n. hypoglycemia
  n. hypothermia
  n. icterus
  n. intensive care unit
    (NICU)
  n. jaundice
  n. myasthenia
  n. neutropenia
  n. respiratory distress
    syndrome
  n. tetanus
  n. tetany
  n. thrombocytopenia
  n. tooth
  n. TSH screening
  n. tyrosinemia
neonate
neonatologist
neonatology
neophobia
  food n.
neoplasia
  cervical intraepithelial n.,
    grade 1-3 (CIN-1 to CIN-3)
  colorectal n.
  gestational trophoblastic n.
    (GTN)
  intraepithelial n.
  keratinocytic intraepithelial
    n. (KIN)
  lobular n.
  multiple endocrine n. (MEN
    1-3, MEN 2A, and MEN 2B)
  nonpolypoid colorectal n.
  polypoid colorectal n.
  vaginal intraepithelial n.
    (VIN)

neoplasm
  adrenal n.
  benign n.
  clear cell mesenchymal n.
  colorectal n.
  histoid n.
  intraductal papillary
    mucinous n. (IPMN)
  malignant n.
  mesenchymal n.
  metastatic n.
  organoid n.
  papillary bladder n.
  stromal cell n.
  stromal-epithelial n.
  trophoblastic n.
  urothelial papillary n.
  vascular n.
neoplastic
neoplastigenic
neorectum
neosalpingostomy
neosphincter
neostomy
neostriatum
neovagina
neovascular
neovascularization
nephelometry
nephrectomy
  abdominal n.
  anterior n.
  cytoreductive n.
  laparoscopic n.
  laser-supported partial n.
  live donor n.
  lumbar n.
  paraperitoneal n.
  partial n.
  posterior n.
  radical n.
  simple n.
  total n.
nephric
nephritic
  n. calculus
  C3 n. factor
  n. retinitis
  n. sediment
  n. syndrome
nephritis (nephrides)
  acute n.
  acute focal bacterial n.
  acute interstitial n.
  acute serum sickness n.

nephritis (nephritides) *(continued)*
    acute tubulointerstitial n.
    allergic interstitial n.
    anaphylactoid purpura n.
    anti-GBM antibody n.
    anti–glomerular basement
      membrane (anti-GBM) n.
    antitubular basement
      membrane n.
    arteriosclerotic n.
    bacterial n.
    Balkan n.
    chronic n.
    chronic interstitial n.
    chronic tubulointerstitial n.
    congenital n.
    diffuse n.
    epidemic n.
    exudative n.
    fibrous n.
    focal n.
    glomerular n.
    granulomatous n.
    granulomatous interstitial n.
    n. gravidarum
    hemorrhagic n.
    Henoch-Schönlein purpura n.
    hereditary n.
    hereditary tubulointerstitial n.
    Heymann n.
    interstitial n.
    interstitial granulomatous n.
    latent n.
    lupus n.
    megalocytic interstitial n.
    nephrotoxic serum n.
    parenchymatous n.
    pneumococcal n.
    post-streptococcal n.
    potassium-losing n.
    n. of pregnancy
    radiation n.
    salt-losing n.
    saturnine n.
    Schönlein-Henoch (Schoenlein-
      Henoch) purpura n.
    shunt n.
    suppurative n.
    syphilitic n.
    transfusion n.
    tuberculous n.
    tubular n.
    tubulointerstitial n.
nephritogenic
nephroabdominal

nephroangiosclerosis
nephroblastoma
nephroblastomatosis
nephrobronchial fistula
nephrocalcinosis
nephrocapsulectomy
nephrocele
nephrocolic
    n. fistula
    n. ligament
nephrocolonic fistula
nephrocutaneous
    n. bypass
    n. fistula
    n. sinus
    n. tract
nephrocystitis
nephrocystosis
nephrogastric
nephrogenic
    n. adenoma
    n. diabetes insipidus
    n. fibrosing dermopathy
    gadolinium-induced n.
      systemic fibrosis
    n. metaplasia
    n. rests
    n. systemic fibrosis
    n. tissue
nephrogenous cyclic adenosine
    monophosphate (cAMP)
nephrogram
nephrography
    diuretic n.
    captopril-enhanced n.
    contrast-enhanced n.
    dynamic magnetic resonance n.
    furosemide isotope n.
    isotope n.
    radionuclide n.
nephroid
nephrolith
nephrolithiasis
    calcium oxalate n.
    uric acid n.
nephrolithotomy
nephrologic
nephrologist
nephrolysis
nephrolytic
nephroma
    embryonal n.
    malignant n.
    mesoblastic n.
    multilocular cystic n.

N

nephromalacia
nephromegaly
nephron
    n. loop
    lower n.
nephronophthisis
nephropathia epidemica
nephropathic
    n. amyloidosis
    n. cystinosis
nephropathy
    acute hypokalemic n.
    acute urate n.
    acute uric acid n.
    amyloid n.
    analgesic n.
    Balkan endemic n.
    BK virus n.
    cadmium n.
    cast m.
    contrast-induced n.
    contrast medium–induced n.
    C1q n.
    diabetic n.
    familial n.
    gouty n.
    heavy metal n.
    human immunodeficiency
      virus–associated n. [HIV-]
    hypercalcemic n.
    hypokalemic n.
    IgA n., immunoglobulin A n.
    IgM n., immunoglobulin M n.
    ischemic n.
    lead n.
    light chain n.
    malarial n.
    membranous n.
    mercury n.
    mesangial n.
    minimal change n.
    mycotoxic n.
    myeloma cast n.
    obstructive n.
    oxalate n.
    polyomavirus type BK n.
    n. of potassium depletion
    potassium-losing n.
    radiocontrast n.
    reflux n.
    salt-losing n.
    saturnine n.
    sickle cell n.
    thin basement membrane n.
    toxic n.

nephropathy *(continued)*
    tubular n.
    urate n., uric acid n.
    vasomotor n.
nephropexy
    laparoscopic n.
    retroperitoneoscopic n.
nephroptosis
nephropyelitis
nephropyelography
nephropyelolithotomy
nephrorrhagia
nephrorrhaphy
nephrosclerosis
    arterial n.
    arteriolar n.
    benign n.
    congenital n.
    hyaline arteriolar n.
    hyperplastic arteriolar n.
    intercapillary n.
    malignant n.
    senile n.
nephrosclerotic
nephroscope
nephroscopy
nephrosis (nephroses)
    congenital n.
    lipoid n.
    osmotic n.
    toxic n.
nephrostogram
nephrostolithotomy
    percutaneous n. (PCNL)
nephrostomy
    n. catheter
    percutaneous n.
    n. tract
    n. tube
nephrotic
    n. edema
    n. syndrome
nephrotomography
    infusion n.
    linear n.
nephrotomy
    abdominal n.
    anatrophic n.
    lumbar n.
    percutaneous n.
    radial n.
nephrotoxic
    n. acute tubular necrosis
    n. agents
    n. compounds

nephrotoxic *(continued)*
    n. drugs
    n. effects
    n. insult
    n. medications
    n. serum nephritis
nephrotoxicity
    contrast media–induced n.
    drug-associated n.
    salicylate n.
nephrotoxin
nephroureterectomy
nephroureterocystectomy
nephroureteroscopy
neptunium (Np)
NER—no evidence of recurrence
NERD—no evidence of recurrent
  disease
Neri sign
nerve
    abducens n., abducent n.
    accelerator n's
    accessory n., spinal
    accessory n., vagal
    acoustic n.
    afferent n.
    alveolar n's
    ampullary n's
    anal n's, inferior
    Andersch n.
    anococcygeal n.
    antebrachial cutaneous n's
    Arnold n.
    articular n.
    auditory n.
    auricular n's
    auricular n. of vagus n.
    auriculotemporal n.
    autonomic n.
    axillary n.
    Bell n.
    Bock n.
    brachial cutaneous n's
    buccal n.
    buccinator n.
    cardiac n's
    cardiac n's, supreme
    cardiac n's, thoracic
    caroticotympanic n's
    carotid n's
    cavernosal n's
    cavernous n's of clitoris
    cavernous n's of penis
    celiac n's
    centrifugal n.

nerve *(continued)*
    centripetal n.
    cerebral n's
    cervical cardiac n's
    cervical n., descending
    cervical n., transverse
    chorda tympani n.
    ciliary n's, long
    ciliary n's, short
    circumflex n.
    clunial n's
    coccygeal n.
    cochlear n.
    n. conduction study
    n. of Cotunnius
    cranial n's (I–XII, 1–12, 1st
      through 12th)
    crural interosseous n.
    cubital n.
    cutaneous n's
    cutaneous n. of abdomen,
      anterior
    cutaneous n. of arm, lateral,
      inferior
    cutaneous n. of arm, lateral,
      superior
    cutaneous n. of arm, medial
    cutaneous n. of arm, posterior
    cutaneous n. of calf, lateral
    cutaneous n. of calf, medial
    cutaneous n. of foot, dorsal,
      intermediate
    cutaneous n. of foot, dorsal,
      lateral
    cutaneous n. of foot, dorsal,
      medial
    cutaneous n. of forearm, dorsal
    cutaneous n. of forearm, lateral
    cutaneous n. of forearm, medial
    cutaneous n. of forearm,
      posterior
    cutaneous n. of neck, anterior
    cutaneous n. of neck,
      transverse
    cutaneous n. of thigh,
      intermediate
    cutaneous n. of thigh, lateral
    cutaneous n. of thigh, medial
    cutaneous n. of thigh,
      posterior
    dental n., inferior
    depressor n.
    diaphragmatic n.
    digastric n.
    digital n's of foot, dorsal

N

nerve *(continued)*

digital n's of lateral plantar nerve, common plantar
digital n's of lateral plantar nerve, proper plantar
digital n's, radial dorsal
digital n's, ulnar dorsal
dorsal n. of clitoris
dorsal n. of penis
dorsal scapular n.
efferent n.
encephalic n's
ethmoidal n's
excitor n.
excitoreflex n.
n. of external acoustic meatus
facial n.
facial n., temporal
femoral n.
femoral cutaneous n's
fibular n., common
fibular n., deep
fibular n., superficial
frontal n.
furcal n.
fusimotor n's
Galen n.
gangliated n.
gastric n's
genitofemoral n.
glossopharyngeal n.
gluteal n's
greater cavernous n. of penis
great sciatic n.
gustatory n's
hemorrhoidal n's, inferior
Hering n.
hypogastric n.
hypoglossal n.
iliohypogastric n.
ilioinguinal n.
iliopubic n.
infraorbital n.
infratrochlear n.
inhibitory n.
intercostal n's
intercostobrachial n's
intermediary n., intermediate n.
interosseous n. of forearm
interosseous n. of leg
ischiadic n.
Jacobson n.
jugular n.
labial n's
lacrimal n.

nerve *(continued)*

n's of Lancisi
Langley n's
laryngeal n's
laryngeal n., recurrent
Latarjet n.
n. to lateral pterygoid
lesser cavernous n. of penis
n. to levator ani muscle
lingual n.
longitudinal n's of Lancisi
lumbar n's
lumboinguinal n.
n. of Luschka
mandibular n.
masseteric n.
maxillary n.
n. to medial pterygoid
median n.
meningeal n.
mental n.
mixed n., n. of mixed fibers
motor n.
motor n. of tongue
musculocutaneous n.
musculocutaneous n. of leg
musculospiral n.
myelinated n.
mylohyoid n., n. to mylohyoid
nasociliary n.
nasopalatine n.
obturator n.
obturator n., accessory
n. to obturator internus
n. to obturator internus and gemellus superior
occipital n., greater
occipital n., least
occipital n., lesser; occipital n., smaller
occipital n., third
oculomotor n.
olfactory n's
ophthalmic n.
optic n.
pain n.
palatine n's
palatine n., greater
palatine n., posterior
parasympathetic n.
parotid n's
n. to pectineus muscle
pectoral n's
perforating cutaneous n.
perineal n's

nerve *(continued)*
    peripheral n.
    peroneal n., accessory deep
    peroneal n., common
    peroneal n., deep
    peroneal n., superficial
    petrosal n., deep
    petrosal n., greater
    petrosal n., greater superficial
    petrosal n., lesser
    petrosal n., lesser superficial
    pharyngeal n.
    phrenic n.
    phrenic n's, accessory
    phrenicoabdominal n's
    pilomotor n's
    piriform n., n. to piriformis
    plantar n's
    pneumogastric n.
    popliteal n's
    presacral n.
    pressor n.
    pterygoid n's
    n. of pterygoid canal
    pterygopalatine n's
    pudendal n.
    n. to quadratus femoris and
      gemellus inferior
    n. to quadratus femoris muscle
    radial n.
    radial n., deep
    radial n., superficial
    rectal n's, inferior
    recurrent n.
    recurrent n., ophthalmic
    saccular n.
    sacral n's
    saphenous n.
    n. to sartorius
    scapular n., dorsal
    Scarpa n.
    sciatic n., small
    scrotal n's
    secretomotor n.
    secretory n.
    sensory n.
    sinus n.
    sinu-vertebral n.
    somatic n's
    spermatic n., external
    sphenopalatine n's
    n. to sphincter ani
    spinal n's
    splanchnic n's
    splanchnic n., greater

nerve *(continued)*
    splanchnic n., least
    splanchnic n., lesser
    splanchnic n., lowest
    splanchnic n's, lumbar
    splanchnic n's, pelvic
    splanchnic n's, sacral
    stapedial n., stapedius n.
    stylohyoid n.
    stylopharyngeal n.
    subclavian n.
    n. to subclavius muscle
    subcostal n.
    sublingual n.
    suboccipital n.
    subscapular n's
    sudomotor n's
    supraclavicular n's
    supraorbital n.
    suprascapular n.
    supratrochlear n.
    sural n.
    sural cutaneous n's
    n. suture
    sympathetic n.
    temporal n's, deep
    temporal n's, subcutaneous
    n. to tensor tympani
    n. to tensor veli palatini
    tentorial n.
    terminal n.
    thoracic n., long
    thoracic splanchnic n., greater
    thoracic splanchnic n., lesser
    thoracic splanchnic n., lowest
    thoracodorsal n.
    tibial n.
    Tiedemann n.
    tonsillar n's
    transverse n. of neck
    trigeminal n.
    trochlear n.
    tympanic n.
    ulnar n.
    unmyelinated n.
    utricular n.
    utriculoampullary n.
    vaginal n's
    vagus n.
    Valentin n.
    vascular n's
    vasoconstrictor n.
    vasodilator n.
    vasomotor n.
    vasosensory n.

N

nerve *(continued)*
vertebral n.
vestibular n.
vestibulocochlear n.
vidian n.
visceral n.
n. of Willis
Wrisberg n.
zygomatic n.
zygomaticofacial n.
zygomaticotemporal n.
nerve block
ambulatory continuous
femoral n.b.
dorsal penile n.b. (DPNB)
peripheral n.b.
sacral plexus n.b.
sciatic n.b.
nervi (plural of nervus)
nervimotor
nervine
nervonic acid
nervous
autonomic n. system
n. breakdown
central n. system
n. dyspepsia
n. irritability
parasympathetic n. system
peripheral n. system
n. plexus
n. prostration
n. stimulation
nervousness
nervus (nervi)
n. abducens
n. accessorius
n. acusticus
nervi alveolares superiores
n. alveolaris inferior
n. ampullaris anterior
n. ampullaris lateralis
n. ampullaris posterior
nervi anales inferiores
n. anococcygeus
n. articularis
nervi auriculares anteriores
n. auricularis magnus
n. auricularis posterior
n. auriculotemporalis
n. autonomicus
n. axillaris
n. buccalis
n. canalis pterygoidei
nervi cardiaci thoracici

nervus (nervi) *(continued)*
n. cardiacus cervicalis inferior
n. cardiacus cervicalis medius
n. cardiacus cervicalis superior
nervi carotici externi
nervi caroticotympanici
n. caroticus internus
nervi cavernosi clitoridis
nervi cavernosi penis
nervi cervicales
nervi ciliares breves
nervi ciliares longi
nervi clunium inferiores
nervi clunium medii
nervi clunium superiores
n. coccygeus
n. cochlearis
nervi craniales
n. cutaneus
n. cutaneus antebrachii
lateralis
n. cutaneus antebrachii medialis
n. cutaneus antebrachii
posterior
n. cutaneus brachii lateralis
inferior
n. cutaneus brachii lateralis
superior
n. cutaneus brachii medialis
n. cutaneus brachii posterior
n. cutaneus dorsalis
intermedius
n. cutaneus dorsalis lateralis
n. cutaneus dorsalis medialis
n. cutaneus femoralis lateralis
n. cutaneus femoralis posterior
n. cutaneus femoris lateralis
n. cutaneus femoris posterior
n. cutaneus perforans
n. cutaneus surae lateralis
n. cutaneus surae medialis
nervi digitales dorsales
hallucis lateralis et digiti
secundi medialis
nervi digitales dorsales nervi
radialis
nervi digitales dorsales nervi
ulnaris
nervi digitales dorsales pedis
nervi digitales palmares
communes nervi mediani
nervi digitales palmares
communes nervi ulnaris
nervi digitales palmares
proprii nervi mediani

nervus (nervi) *(continued)*
   nervi digitales palmares
      proprii nervi ulnaris
   nervi digitales plantares
      communes nervi plantaris
      lateralis
   nervi digitales plantares
      communes nervi plantaris
      medialis
   nervi digitales plantares proprii
      nervi plantaris lateralis
   nervi digitales plantares proprii
      nervi plantaris medialis
   n. dorsalis clitoridis
   n. dorsalis penis
   n. dorsalis scapulae
   nervi encephalici
   nervi erigentes
   n. ethmoidalis anterior
   n. ethmoidalis posterior
   n. facialis
   n. femoralis
   n. fibularis communis
   n. fibularis profundus
   n. fibularis superficialis
   n. frontalis
   n. genitofemoralis
   n. glossopharyngeus
   n. gluteus inferior
   n. gluteus superior
   n. hypogastricus
   n. hypoglossus
   n. iliohypogastricus
   n. ilioinguinalis
   n. iliopubicus
   n. infraorbitalis
   n. infratrochlearis
   nervi intercostales
   nervi intercostobrachiales
   n. intermediofacialis
   n. intermedius
   n. interosseus antebrachii
      anterior
   n. interosseus antebrachii
      posterior
   n. interosseus cruris
   n. ischiadicus
   n. jugularis
   nervi labiales anteriores
   nervi labiales posteriores
   n. lacrimalis
   n. laryngealis recurrens
   n. laryngealis superior
   n. laryngeus recurrens
   n. laryngeus superior

nervus (nervi) *(continued)*
   n. lingualis
   nervi lumbales, nervi lumbares
   n. lumboinguinalis
   n. mandibularis
   n. massetericus
   n. maxillaris
   n. meatus acustici externi
   n. medianus
   n. meningeus medius
   n. mentalis
   n. mixtus
   n. motorius
   n. musculi obturatorii interni
   n. musculi piriformis
   n. musculi quadrati femoris
   n. musculi tensoris tympani
   n. musculi tensoris veli palatini
   n. musculocutaneus
   n. mylohyoideus
   n. nasociliaris
   n. nasopalatinus
   n. nervorum
   n. obturatorius accessorius
   n. obturatorius internus
   n. occipitalis major
   n. occipitalis minor
   n. occipitalis tertius
   n. octavus
   n. oculomotorius
   n. olfactorius
   n. ophthalmicus
   n. opticus
   nervi palatini
   nervi palatini minores
   n. palatinus major
   n. pectoralis lateralis
   n. pectoralis medialis
   nervi perineales
   n. peroneus communis
   n. peroneus profundus
   n. peroneus profundus
      accessorius
   n. peroneus superficialis
   n. petrosus major
   n. petrosus minor
   n. petrosus profundus
   n. pharyngeus
   n. phrenicus
   nervi phrenici accessorii
   n. piriformis
   n. plantaris lateralis
   n. plantaris medialis
   n. presacralis
   n. pterygoideus lateralis

N

nervus (nervi) *(continued)*
n. pterygoideus medialis
n. pudendus
n. quadratus femoris
n. radialis
nervi rectales inferiores
n. saccularis
nervi sacrales
nervi sacrales n. coccygeus
n. saphenus
n. sciaticus
nervi scrotales anteriores
nervi scrotales posteriores
n. sensorius
n. spermaticus externus
nervi spinales
nervus spinosus
nervi splanchnici lumbales
n. splanchnici lumbares
nervi splanchnici pelvici
nervi splanchnici sacrales
n. splanchnicus imus
n. splanchnicus major
n. splanchnicus minor
n. splanchnicus thoracicus imus
n. splanchnicus thoracicus
    major
n. splanchnicus thoracicus
    minor
n. statoacusticus
n. subclavius
n. subcostalis
n. sublingualis
n. suboccipitalis
nervi subscapulares
nervi supraclaviculares
nervi supraclaviculares
    intermedii
nervi supraclaviculares
    laterales
nervi supraclaviculares
    mediales
nervi supraclaviculares
    posteriores
n. supraorbitalis
n. suprascapularis
n. supratrochlearis
n. suralis
nervi temporales profundi
n. tensoris veli palatini
n. terminalis
nervi thoracici
n. thoracicus longus
n. thoracodorsalis
n. tibialis

nervus (nervi) *(continued)*
n. transversus cervicalis
n. transversus colli
n. trigeminalis
n. trigeminus
n. trochlearis
n. tympanicus
n. ulnaris
n. utricularis
n. utriculoampullaris
nervi vaginales
n. vagus
nervi vasorum
n. vertebralis
n. vestibularis
n. vestibulocochlearis
n. visceralis
n. zygomaticus
nesidiectomy
nesidioblast
nesidioblastoma
    malignant n.
nesidioblastosis
Nessler
    reagent
    solution
    test
nesslerization
nesslerize
nest
    bird's n. filter
    bird's n. lesions
    Brunn epithelial n's
    cancer n's
    cell n.
    junctional n.
    von Brunn n.
    Walthard cell n's
Netherton syndrome
nettle
Nettleship syndrome
Nettleship-Falls–type ocular
    albinism
Nettleship-Wilder dilator
network
    acromial n.
    arterial n.
    articular n. of knee
    articular vascular n.
    calcaneal n.
    cell n.
    Chiari n.
    cis-Golgi n.
    idiotype–anti-idiotype n.
    lateral malleolar n.

network *(continued)*
 lymphocapillary n.
 medial malleolar n.
 neurofibrillar n.
 patellar n.
 peritarsal n.
 Purkinje n.
 subpapillary n.
 trabecular n.
 trans-Golgi n.
 venous n.
Neubauer-Fischer test
Neuberg ester
Neufeld
 nail
 reaction
 test
Neumann
 cells
 disease
 law
 sheath
 syndrome
neural
 n. arc, n. arch
 n. atrophy
 n. canal
 n. crest
 n. cyst
 n. fold
 n. foramen
 n. ganglion
 n. groove
 n. hiatus
 n. lymphomatosis
 n. muscular dystrophy
 n. nevus
 n. plate
 n. pathway
 n. segment
 n. septum
 n. spine
 n. tube
 n. tube defect
neuralgia
 atypical facial n.
 brachial n.
 cervicobrachial n.
 cervico-occipital n.
 cranial n.
 femoral n.
 Fothergill n.
 geniculate n.
 glossopharyngeal n.
 hallucinatory n.

neuralgia *(continued)*
 Harris migrainous n.
 herpetic n.
 Hunt n.
 idiopathic n.
 intercostal n.
 mandibular joint n.
 migrainous n.
 Morton n.
 nasociliary n.
 obturator n.
 occipital n.
 Parsonage and Turner
  amyotrophic n.
 peripheral n.
 postherpetic n.
 pudendal plexus n.
 red n.
 reminiscent n.
 retrobulbar n.
 sciatic n.
 Sluder n.
 sphenopalatine n.
 stump n.
 supraorbital n.
 symptomatic
 trigeminal n.
 trifacial n.
 trigeminal n.
 Vail n.
neuralgic
 n. amyotrophy
 focal n. deficit
 hereditary n. amyotrophy
 n. syndrome
neuralgiform
neuraminic acid
neurapraxia
neurasthenia
neurasthenic
neuratrophic
neuraxial
 n. anesthesia
 n. block
 n. edema
neurectomy
 gastric n.
 ilioinguinal n.
 presacral n.
 tympanic n.
 vestibular n.
neurenteric
 n. canal
 n. cyst
neurilemma

N

neurilemmal
neurilemmoma
    acoustic n.
    base-of-tongue n.
    glossal n.
    malignant n.
    retroperitoneal n.
    solitary n.
    trigeminal n.
neurinoma
    acoustic n.
    malignant n.
neuritic
    n. muscular atrophy
    n. plaques
neuritis
    alcoholic n.
    ascending n.
    brachial n.
    compression n.
    descending n.
    diabetic n.
    femoral n.
    hereditary optic n.
    interstitial n.
    ischemic n.
    leprous n.
    multiple n.
    optic n.
    paralytic brachial n.
    peripheral n.
    pressure n.
    radiation n.
    radicular n.
    retrobulbar n.
    sciatic n.
    serum n.
    traumatic n.
neuro—neurologic
neuroacanthocytosis
neuroactive
neuroanastomosis
neuroanatomy
neuroarthropathy
neurobehavioral
neurobiology
neuroblast
    n. migration
    n. proliferation
    sympathetic n.
neuroblastoma
    localized n.
    olfactory n.
    Pepper-type n.
neuroborreliosis

neurobrucellosis
neurocardiac
neurochemistry
neurochorioretinitis
neurochoroiditis
neurocirculatory
    n. asthenia
    n. reflex
    sympathetic n. failure
neurocranial
neurocranium
neurocrine
neurocristopathy
neurocutaneous
    n. melanosis
    n. syndrome
neurocysticercosis
neurocytology
neurocytoma
    central n.
    intraventricular n.
    olfactory n.
neurodegeneration
neurodegenerative
neurodermatitis
    circumscribed n.
    n. disseminata
    disseminated n.
    exudative n.
    localized n.
    nummular n.
neurodevelopmental
neurodiagnosis
neurodynamic
neuroectodermal
    n. tumor of infancy
    n. tumor of the kidney
    n. tumor of the ovary
neuroendocrine
    n. cells
    n. tumor
neuroendoscope
neuroendoscopy
neuroenteric
    congenital n. cyst
    n. fistula
    intradural n. cyst
neuroepidermal
neuroepithelial
    n. cells
    n. tumor
neuroepithelioma
neuroepithelium
    n. of ampullary crest
    n. cristae ampullaris

neuroepithelium *(continued)*
   n. of maculae
   n. macularum
neurofiber
   afferent n's
   association n's
   commissural n's
   efferent n's
   postganglionic n's
   preganglionic n's
   projection n's
   somatic n's
   tangential n's
   visceral n's
neurofiberscope
neurofiberscopic biopsy
neurofibra (neurofibrae)
   neurofibrae afferentes
   n. associationis
   neurofibrae autonomicae
   n. commissuralis
   neurofibrae efferentes
   neurofibrae
     postganglionares
   neurofibrae preganglionares
   neurofibrae preganglionicae
   n. projectionis
   neurofibrae somaticae
   neurofibrae tangentiales
   neurofibrae viscerales
neurofibril
neurofibrilla (neurofibrillae)
neurofibrillar
   n. bundles
   n. degeneration
   n. network
   n. senile plaques
neurofibrillary
   Alzheimer n. degeneration
   n. changes
   n. lesions
   n. tangles
neurofibroma
   acoustic n.
   dumbbell n.
   n. gangliocellulare
   n. ganglionare
   granular cell n.
   malignant n.
   symmetrical bundle n's
neurofibromatosis
neurofibrosarcoma
neuroganglioma
neuroganglion
neurogastric

neurogenic
   n. arthropathy
   n. bladder
   n. claudication
   n. fracture
   n. impotence
   n. pain
   n. precocious puberty
   n. shock
   n. torticollis
   n. tumor
   n. ulcer
neurogenous
neuroglia
   fascicular n.
   interfascicular n.
   peripheral n.
   protoplasmic n.
neuroglial
   n. choristoma
   n. heterotopia
   mixed n. tumor
   n. stem cell
neurogliocytoma
neuroglioma
neuroglycopenia
neurogram
neurography
neurohistology
neurohormonal
neurohormone
neurohypophysectomy
neurohypophysial, neurohypophyseal
   n. diverticulum
   n. hormones
neurohypophysis
neuroid
neuroimaging
neuroimmunologic
neuroimmunomodulation
neuroimmunomodulatory
neuroinflammation
neurointensivist
neuroinvasive
neurokinin
neurolabyrinthitis
   unilateral n.
   vestibular n.
   vestibulocochlear n.
   viral n.
neurolathyrism
neuroleptanalgesia
neuroleptanalgesic
neuroleptanesthesia
neuroleptanesthetic

N

neuroleptic
    n. drugs
    n. malignant syndrome
neuroleukin
neurolinguistic programming (NLP)
neurolinguistics
neurologic, neurological
neurologist
neurology
neurolues
neurolymphomatosis
    n. gallinarum
    peripheral n.
neurolysin
neurolysis
    alcohol n.
    chemical n.
    endoscopic ultrasound–guided
      n. [EUS-]
    intramuscular n.
    intrathecal n.
    lumbar sympathetic n.
    phenol n.
    trigeminal n.
neurolytic block
neuroma
    acoustic n.
    amputation n.
    amyelinic n.
    appendiceal n.
    n. cutis
    cystic n.
    false n.
    fascicular n.
    ganglionated n.
    ganglionic n.
    malignant n.
    medullated n.
    Morton n.
    multiple n's
    myelinic n.
    nevoid n.
    plexiform n.
    post-traumatic n.
    stump n.
    n. telangiectodes
    traumatic n.
    true n.
    Verneuil n.
    n. verum
neuromalacia
neuromatosis
neuromatous
neuromediator
neuromelanin

neuromeningeal
neuromere
neurometrics
neuromimetic
neuromodulation
neuromodulator
neuromotor
neuromuscular
    n. blockade
    n. blocking agent
    n. contractility
    n. junction
    n. spindle
neuromyasthenia
    epidemic n.
neuromyelitis optica
neuromyopathic
neuromyopathy
    carcinomatous n.
    colchicine-induced n.
    critical illness n.
    cyclosporin-induced toxic n.
    drug-induced n.
neuromyositis
neuromyotonia
neuron
    afferent n.
    alpha motor n.
    bipolar n.
    central n.
    connector n.
    effector n.
    efferent n.
    exciter n.
    first-order n.
    gamma motor n.
    Golgi n's (types I and II)
    horizontal n's
    long n.
    motor n.
    multipolar n.
    peripheral motor n.
    peripheral sensory n.
    phasic motor n.
    postganglionic n's
    preganglionic n's
    premotor n.
    primary n.
    primary sensory n.
    pyramidal n.
    second-order n.
    sensory n.
    short n.
    superior motor n.
    n. threshold

neuron *(continued)*
 tonic motor n.
 unipolar n.
 upper motor n.
neuronal
 n. colonic dysplasia
 n. lesion
neuronitis
 myoclonic spinal n.
 vestibular n.
neuronography
neuronopathy
neuronophagia
neuronotrophic
neuron-specific enolase
neuro-ophthalmology
neuropacemaker
neuropapillitis
neuroparalysis
neuroparalytic
 n. keratitis
 n. ophthalmia
neuropathic
 n. arthritis
 n. arthropathy
 n. atrophy
 n. joint disease
neuropathogenesis
neuropathogenicity
neuropathology
neuropathy
 acute autonomic n.
 alcoholic n.
 amyloid n.
 Andrade-type amyloid n.
 angiopathic n.
 arsenic n., arsenical n.
 ascending n.
 autonomic n.
 axonal n.
 brachial plexus n.
 carcinomatous n.
 compression n.
 compression-entrapment n.
 Dejerine-Sottas n.
 Denny-Brown sensory
  radicular n.
 descending n.
 diabetic n.
 dying-back n.
 entrapment n.
 femoral n.
 focal n.
 giant axonal n.
 hepatic n.

neuropathy *(continued)*
 hereditary hypertrophic n.
 hereditary hypertrophic
  interstitial n.
 hereditary motor and sensory n.
  (HMSN)
 hereditary optic n.
 hereditary sensorimotor n.
  (types I–III)
 hereditary sensory n.
 hereditary sensory and
  autonomic n. (HSAN)
 hereditary sensory radicular n.
 hypertrophic n.
 hypertrophic interstitial n.
 infectious n.
 intercostal n.
 ischemic n.
 isoniazid n.
 lead n.
 Leber hereditary optic n.
 Leber optic n.
 lumbar plexus n.
 lumbosacral plexus n.
 motor n.
 multifocal n.
 multiple n.
 nitrofurantoin n.
 nutritional n.
 optic n.
 paraneoplastic n.
 peripheral n.
 plexus n.
 porphyric n.
 pressure n.
 progressive hypertrophic n.
 progressive hypertrophic
  interstitial n.
 radiation n.
 sacral plexus n.
 sarcoid n.
 selective autonomic n.
 sensorimotor n.
 sensory n.
 suprascapular n.
 tomaculous n.
 toxic n.
 traumatic n.
 trigeminal n.
 uremic n.
 vasculitic n.
neuropeptide Y
neuropharmacological
neuropharmacology
neurophilic

N

neurophysin
neurophysiology
neuropil
neuroplasm
neuroplasmic
neuroplasty
neuroplexus
neuroprosthesis
neuroprotectant
neuroprotection
neuroprotective
neuropsychiatrist
neuropsychiatry
neuropsychic
neuropsychologic,
   neuropsychological
    n. disorder
    n. evaluation
    n. function
    n. test, n. testing
neuropsychology
neuropsychometric
neuropsychopharmacology
neuropsychosis (neuropsychoses)
neuroradiology
neuroregulation
neuroretinal
neuroretinitis
neuroretinopathy
   hypertensive n.
neurorrhaphy
neurosarcoma
neuroschistosomiasis
neuroscience
neuroscientist
neurosecretion
neurosecretory
neurosegmental
neurosensory
neurosis (neuroses)
    association n.
    character n.
    compensation n.
    prison n.
    transference n.
    true n.
neuroskeletal
neurospasm
neurostimulator
neurosurgeon
neurosurgery
   functional n.
   microvascular n.
   stereotactic n., stereotaxic n.
neurosuture

neurosyphilis
   asymptomatic n.
   meningovascular n.
   parenchymatous n.
   paretic n.
   tabetic n.
neurotendinous
   n. organ
   n. spindle
neurotensin
neurothekeoma
neurotherapy
neurotic
   n. depression
   n. disorder
   n. excoriation
neuroticism
neurotization
neurotmesis
neurotome
   Hall n.
neurotomography
neurotomy
   opticociliary n.
   radio frequency n.,
    radiofrequency n.
   retrogasserian n.
neurotonic
   n. congestion
   n. reaction
neurotony
neurotoxic
neurotoxicity
neurotoxin
neurotransducer
neurotransmission
neurotransmitter
   false n.
neurotrauma
neurotrophic
   n. atrophy
   n. keratitis
neurotrophin
neurotrophy
neurotropic virus
neurotubule
neurovascular
neurovegetative
neurovirulence
neurovirulent
neurovirus
neurovisceral
neutral
   n. fat
   n. flux

neutral *(continued)*
- n. occlusion
- n. reaction
- n. red
- n. salt
- n. stain
- n. zone of His

neutralism

neutrality

neutralization
- n. equivalent
- n. test
- viral n.

neutralize

neutralizing antibody

neutron
- n. radiography
- n. therapy

neutropenia
- alloimmune neonatal n.
- autoimmune n.
- chronic benign n.
- chronic benign n. of childhood
- chronic familial n.
- chronic hypoplastic n.
- congenital n.
- cyclic n.
- drug-induced n.
- familial benign chronic n.
- hypersplenic n.
- idiopathic n.
- isoimmune neonatal n.
- Kostmann n.
- malignant n.
- neonatal n.
- periodic n.
- peripheral n.
- primary splenic n.
- severe congenital n.
- toxic n.

neutropenic
- n. fever of unknown origin
- n. typhlitis

neutrophil
- band n.
- n. chemotactic factor
- giant n.
- immature n.
- mature n.
- nonfilamented n.
- polymorphonuclear n. (PMN)
- rod n.
- segmented n.
- stab n.

neutrophilia

neutrophilic
- n. abscess
- n. cell
- n. dermatoses
- n. eccrine hidradenitis
- n. figurate erythema
- n. leukemoid reaction
- n. leukocyte
- n. leukocytosis
- polynuclear n. leukocyte
- rheumatoid n. dermatitis

nevertheless

nevi (plural of nevus)

Neviaser operation

Neville prosthesis

nevocellular

nevocytic

nevoid
- n. cyst
- n. hypertrichosis
- n. lentigo
- n. neuroma
- n. telangiectasia

nevolipoma

nevus (nevi)
- achromic n.
- acquired n.
- amelanotic n.
- n. anemicus
- n. angiectodes
- n. araneus
- balloon cell n.
- basal cell n.
- bathing trunk n.
- Becker n.
- blue n.
- blue rubber bleb n.
- n. cavernosus
- cellular n.
- cellular blue n.
- n. cerebelliformis
- CHILD n.
- choroidal n.
- Clark n.
- comedo n.
- compound n.
- congenital n.
- congenital hairy n.
- connective tissue n.
- n. depigmentosus
- dermal n.
- dysplastic n.
- n. elasticus
- n. elasticus of Lewandowsky

N

nevus (nevi) *(continued)*
    epidermal n.
    epithelial nevi
    fatty n.
    n. fibrosus
    n. flammeus
    n. fuscoceruleus
      acromiodeltoideus
    n. fuscoceruleus
      ophthalmomaxillaris
    giant congenital hairy n.
    giant congenital pigmented n.
    giant pigmented n.
    hair follicle n.
    hairy n.
    halo n.
    ichthyosiform n.
    inflammatory linear verrucous
      epidermal n.
    intradermal n.
    Ito n.
    Jadassohn n.
    Jadassohn-Tièche n.
    junction n., junctional n.
    kissing n.
    Lewandowsky n. elasticus
    linear epidermal n.
    n. lipomatosus
    n. lipomatosus cutaneus
      superficialis
    lipomatous n.
    malignant blue n.
    melanocytic n.
    Miescher n.
    nape n.
    neural n., neuroid n.
    nevocellular n.
    nevocytic n.
    nevus cell n.
    nonpigmented n.
    organoid n.
    Ota n.
    pigmented hairy epidermal n.
    pigmented n.
    n. pigmentosus
    port-wine n.
    sebaceous n.
    sebaceous n. of Jadassohn
    sebaceous n. syndrome
    n. sebaceus syndrome
    n. simplex
    speckled lentiginous n.
    spider n.
    n. spilus
    n. spilus tardus

nevus (nevi) *(continued)*
    spindle cell n.
    spindle and epithelioid cell n.
    Spitz n.
    n. spongiosus albus mucosae
    stellar n.
    straight hair n.
    strawberry n.
    Sutton n.
    n. unius lateralis
    n. unius lateris
    Unna n.
    uveal n.
    vascular n.
    n. verrucosus
    verrucous n.
    white sponge n.
New [eponym]
    forceps
    hook
    needle
    scissors
    sickle flap
    tube
newborn
Newcastle disease
Newcastle-Manchester bacillus
New England Baptist arthroplasty
New-Lambotte osteotome
Newman
    forceps
    hook
    proctoscope
newton (N)
Newton
    alloy
    disks
    law
    rings
newtonian gravitational constant
nexin
nexus
Nezelof syndrome
NF—
    National Formulary
    none found
    normal flow
    not found
NFLPN—National Federation of
    Licensed Practical Nurses
NFTD—normal full-term delivery
ng—nanogram(s)
NG—nasogastric
NGF—nerve growth factor
NGU—nongonococcal urethritis

NHA—nonspecific hepatocellular abnormality
NHC—neonatal hypocalcemia
NHL—non-Hodgkin lymphoma
NHLI—National Heart and Lung Institute
NHS—normal human serum
Ni—nickel
NI—
    no information
    not identified
    not isolated
NIA—no information available
niacinamide
niacinamidosis
NIAID—National Institute of Allergy and Infectious Diseases
NIAMD—National Institute of Arthritis and Metabolic Diseases
nib
niche
    Barclay n.
    enamel n.
    Haudek n.
    n. of round window
    n. sign
NICHHD—National Institute of Child Health and Human Development
Nichol procedure
Nichols clamp
nick, nicked
nickel (Ni)
    n. carbonyl
nicking
    arteriovenous (AV) n.
Nicola operation
Nicolas-Favre disease
Nicoll bone graft
Nicol prism
nicotinate
nicotine
    n. poisoning
    n. sulfate poisoning
nicotinic acid
nicotinism
nicotinolytic
β-nicotyrine [beta-]
nictitate
nictitation
NICU—
    neonatal intensive care unit
    neurological intensive care unit
Nida operation

NIDA—National Institute on Drug Abuse
nidal
    n. border
    n. embolization
    n. filling
    n. inflow
    n. obliteration
    n. outflow
    n. volume
nidation
NIDD—noninsulin-dependent diabetes
NIDDM—noninsulin-dependent diabetes mellitus
NIDR—National Institute of Dental Research
nidus (nidi)
    n. avis
Niebauer prosthesis
Niedner knife
Nielsen method
Niemann
    disease
    splenomegaly
Niemann-Pick
    cells
    disease
    lipid
nightmare
nightshade
    deadly n.
nigra
    n. line
    substantia n.
nigral
nigricans
    acanthosis n.
    hyperkeratosis n.
    ichthyosis n.
    onychomycosis n.
nigrities linguae
nigropallidal encephalomalacia
nigrosin
nigrostriatal
    n. fibers
    n. tract
NIH—National Institutes of Health
NIH catheter
nihilism
    therapeutic n.
Nikolsky sign
nil disease
NIMH—National Institute of Mental Health

N

NINDB—National Institute of Neurological Diseases and Blindness
niobium (Nb)
NIOSH—National Institute of Occupational Safety and Health
nipple
    n. adenoma
    n.-areolar complex
    n.-areolar reconstruction
    crackled n.
    crater n.
    erosive adenomatosis of n.
    florid papillomatosis of n.
    free n. graft
    n. grafting
    herniated n.
    insensate n.
    invaginated n.
    inverted n.
    n. line
    pacifier n.
    n. pedicle
    n. repositioning
    retracted n.
    n. retraction
    n. shield
    n.-sparing mastectomy
    n. transfer
Nisbet chancre
nisin
Nissen
    fundoplication
    operation
Nissl
    bodies
    degeneration
    granules
    method of staining
    substance
nisus
nit
Nitabuch
    layer
    stria
    zone
nitrate reductase
nitrates
nitremia
nitric acid
nitridation
nitride
nitrification
nitrifier
nitrifying
nitrile

nitrites
nitritoid
nitrituria
nitrobacteria
nitroblue tetrazolium assay
nitrogen (N)
    n. 13
    n. 15
    amide n.
    n. balance
    blood urea n. (BUN)
    n. dioxide
    n. equilibrium
    n. fixation
    n. mustard
    n. narcosis
    nomadic n.
    nonprotein n. (NPN)
    n. pentoxide
    n. peroxide
    rest n.
    n. tetroxide
    urea n.
nitrogenase
nitrogen-fixing bacteria
nitrogenous
nitronaphthalene
nitrophenol
nitrosamine
nitrosification
nitrosifying
nitrosourea
nitrosyl
nitrous oxide
nitryl
NK—
    natural killer (cells)
    not known
NKA—no known allergies
NKDA—no known drug allergies
NKH—nonketotic hyperosmotic
nl—nanoliter(s)
NLA—neuroleptanalgesia
NLP—
    Neurolinguistic Programming
    no light perception
NLT—normal lymphocyte transfer (test)
nm—nanometer(s)
NM—
    neuromuscular
    not measurable
    not measured
    not mentioned
    nuclear medicine

NMG—no Marcus Gunn (phenomenon)

NMP—normal menstrual period

NMR—nuclear magnetic resonance

NMRI—Naval Medical Research Institute

NND—neonatal death

NNM—Nicolle-Novy-MacNeal (medium)

No—nobelium

No.; no.—number (L. numero)

NO—nitric oxide

N/O—none obtained

NOAEL—no observed adverse effect level

nobelium (No)

Noble forceps

Nocardia
  N. asteroides
  N. brasiliensis
  N. farcinica
  N. otitidis-caviarum

nocardial

nocardin

Nocardiopsis dassonvillei

nocardiosis
  cerebral n.
  disseminated n.
  granulomatous n.
  ocular n.
  pulmonary n.
  systemic n.

nociception
  peripheral n.
  polymodal n.

nociceptive pain

nocturia

nocturnal
  n. enuresis
  n. penile tumescence (NPT)
  n. polysomnography

nocuous
  n. agent
  n. effects
  n. stimulation
  n. stimuli

nod
  bishop's n.

nodal
  n. arrhythmia
  n. artery
  atrioventricular (AV) n. reentrant tachycardia
  atrioventricular n. artery
  atrioventricular n. bigeminy
  n. beat

nodal *(continued)*
  n. bigeminy
  n. bradycardia
  n. escape
  n. extrasystole
  n. rhythm
  sinoatrial n. artery
  sinus n. reentry
  n. tachycardia
  n. tissue

node
  abdominal lymph n's, parietal
  abdominal lymph n's, visceral
  accessory lymph n's
  anorectal lymph n's
  anterior axillary lymph n's
  n. of anterior border of epiploic foramen
  anterior cervical lymph n's
  anterior jugular lymph n's
  anterior mediastinal lymph n's
  anterior superficial cervical lymph n's
  anterior tibial lymph n.
  anterior vesical lymph n's
  aortic lymph n's
  apical axillary lymph n's
  apical lymph n's
  appendicular lymph n's
  Aschoff n.
  Aschoff–Tawara n.
  atrioventricular (AV) n.
  axillary lymph n's
  axillary lymph n's, apical
  axillary lymph n's, central
  axillary lymph n's, pectoral
  axillary lymph n's, subscapular
  Babès n's
  Bouchard n.
  brachial lymph n's
  bronchopulmonary lymph n's
  buccal lymph n.
  buccinator lymph n.
  caval lymph n's
  celiac lymph n's
  central lymph n's
  cervical lymph n's
  cervical lymph n's, deep
  cervical lymph n's, prelaryngeal
  cervical lymph n's, superficial
  Cloquet n.
  colic lymph n's
  colic lymph n's, terminal
  coronary n.
  cubital lymph n's
  cystic n.

node *(continued)*
   cystic lymph n.
   deep anterior cervical lymph n's
   deep inguinal lymph n's
   deep lateral cervical lymph n's
   deep lymph n's of upper limb
   deep parotid lymph n's
   deep popliteal lymph n's
   Delphian n.
   deltoideopectoral lymph n's
   deltopectoral lymph n's
   diaphragmatic lymph n's
   epicolic lymph n's
   epigastric lymph n's, inferior
   n. of epiploic foramen
   epitrochlear lymph n's
   Ewald n.
   facial lymph n's
   fibular lymph n.
   Flack n.
   foraminal n.
   foraminal lymph n.
   gastric lymph n's
   gastroepiploic lymph n's
   gastro-omental lymph n's
   gluteal lymph n's
   gouty n.
   Haygarth n's
   Hensen n.
   hepatic lymph n's
   hilar lymph n's
   ileocolic lymph n's
   iliac n.
   iliac lymph n's, circumflex
   iliac lymph n's, common
   iliac lymph n's, external
   iliac lymph n's, intermediate
      common
   iliac lymph n's, intermediate
      external
   iliac lymph n's, internal
   iliac lymph n's, lateral common
   iliac lymph n's, lateral external
   iliac lymph n's, medial common
   iliac lymph n's, medial external
   iliac lymph n's, promontory
      common
   iliac lymph n's, subaortic
      common
   inferior deep cervical lymph n's
   inferior epigastric lymph n's
   inferior gluteal lymph n's
   inferior inguinal lymph n's
   inferior mesenteric lymph n's
   inferior pancreatic lymph n's

node *(continued)*
   inferior pancreaticoduodenal
      lymph n's
   inferior phrenic lymph n's
   inferior superficial inguinal
      lymph n's
   inferior tracheobronchial
      lymph n's
   infra-auricular deep parotid
      lymph n's
   infraclavicular n's
   infrahyoid lymph n's
   inguinal lymph n's, deep
   inguinal lymph n's, inferior
      superficial
   inguinal lymph n's, superficial
   inguinal lymph n's,
      superolateral superficial
   inguinal lymph n's,
      superomedial superficial
   intercostal lymph n's
   interiliac lymph n's
   intermediate colic lymph n's
   intermediate common iliac
      lymph n's
   intermediate external iliac
      lymph n's
   intermediate lacunar lymph n.
   intermediate lumbar lymph n's
   internal iliac lymph n's
   internal thoracic n's
   interpectoral lymph n's
   intraglandular deep parotid
      lymph n's
   intrapulmonary lymph n's
   jugular lymph n's
   jugulodigastric lymph n.
   jugulo-omohyoid lymph n.
   juxta-articular n.
   juxtaintestinal lymph n's
   juxtaintestinal mesenteric
      lymph n's
   Keith n., Keith-Flack n.
   lacunar lymph n.,
      intermediate
   lacunar lymph n., lateral
   lacunar lymph n., medial
   lateral aortic lymph n's
   lateral axillary lymph n's
   lateral caval lymph n's
   lateral common iliac lymph n's
   lateral external iliac lymph n's
   lateral jugular lymph n's
   lateral lacunar lymph n.
   lateral pericardial lymph n's

node *(continued)*

lateral vesicular lymph n's
left colic lymph n.
left gastric lymph n.
left gastroepiploic lymph n.
left gastro-omental lymph n.
left lumbar lymph n's
lingual lymph n's
lumbar lymph n's
lumbar lymph n's, intermediate
lymph n.
lymph n. of arch of azygos vein
lymph n. of ligamentum
  arteriosum
malar lymph n.
mandibular lymph n.
mastoid lymph n's
medial common iliac lymph n's
medial external iliac lymph n's
medial lacunar lymph n.
mediastinal lymph n's, posterior
mesenteric lymph n's
mesenteric lymph n's, central
  superior
mesenteric lymph n's,
  juxtaintestinal
mesocolic lymph n's
milker's n's
nasolabial lymph n.
n. of neck of gallbladder
obturator lymph n's
occipital lymph n's
Osler n's
pancreatic lymph n's
pancreaticoduodenal lymph n's
para-aortic lymph n.
paracardial lymph n's
paracolic lymph n's
paramammary lymph n's
pararectal lymph n's
parasternal lymph n's
paratracheal lymph n's
parauterine lymph n's
paravaginal lymph n's
paravesicular lymph n's
parietal abdominal lymph n's
parietal lymph n's
parietal pelvic lymph n's
parotid lymph n's, deep
parotid lymph n's,
  infra-auricular deep
parotid lymph n's,
  intraglandular deep
parotid lymph n's,
  preauricular deep

node *(continued)*

parotid lymph n's, superficial
Parrot n's
pectoral axillary lymph n's
pectoral lymph n's
pelvic lymph n's, parietal
pelvic lymph n's, visceral
pericardial lymph n's
peroneal lymph n's
phrenic lymph n's
popliteal lymph n's
postaortic lymph n's
postcaval lymph n's
posterior axillary lymph n's
posterior mediastinal lymph n's
posterior tibial lymph n.
postvesicular lymph n's
preaortic lymph n's
preauricular deep parotid
  lymph n's
preauricular lymph n's
precaval lymph n's
prececal lymph n's
prelaryngeal cervical lymph n's
prelaryngeal lymph n.
prepericardial lymph n's
pretracheal n.
pretracheal lymph n's
prevertebral lymph n's
prevesicular lymph n's
primitive n.
promontory common iliac
  lymph n's
pulmonary juxtaesophageal
  lymph n's
pulmonary lymph n.
pyloric lymph n's
n's of Ranvier
retroaortic lymph n's
retroauricular lymph n's
retrocaval lymph n's
retrocecal lymph n's
retropharyngeal lymph n's
retropyloric n's
retrovesicular lymph n's
right colic lymph n.
right gastric lymph n.
right gastroepiploic lymph n.
right gastro-omental lymph n.
right lumbar lymph n's
Rosenmüller n.
Rotter n's
n. of Rouvière
SA (sinoatrial) n.
sacral lymph n's

N

node *(continued)*

Schmorl n.
sentinel n.
shotty n.
sigmoid lymph n's
signal n.
singer's n.
sinoatrial n., sinuatrial n., sinus n.
Sister Mary Joseph n.
splenic lymph n's
sternal lymph n's
subaortic common iliac lymph n's
submandibular lymph n's
submental lymph n's
subpyloric n's
subscapular axillary lymph n's
subscapular lymph n's
superficial inguinal lymph n's
superficial lateral cervical lymph n's
superficial lymph n's of upper limb
superficial parotid lymph n's
superficial popliteal lymph n's
superior deep cervical lymph n's
superior gluteal lymph n's
superior mesenteric lymph n's
superior pancreatic lymph n's
superior pancreaticoduodenal lymph n's
superior phrenic lymph n's
superior rectal lymph n's
superior tracheobronchial lymph n's
superolateral superficial inguinal lymph n's
superomedial superficial inguinal lymph n's
supraclavicular lymph n's
suprapyloric lymph n.
supratrochlear lymph n's
syphilitic n.
n. of Tawara
teacher's n.
terminal colic lymph n's
thyroid lymph n's
tibial lymph n., anterior
tibial lymph n., posterior
tracheal lymph n's
tracheobronchial lymph n.
triticeous n.
Troisier n.

node *(continued)*

vesicular lymph n's
Virchow n.
visceral abdominal lymph n's
visceral lymph n's
visceral pelvic lymph n's
vital n.
vocal n's
nodi (plural of nodus)
nodosa
periarteritis n.
nodose ganglion
nodosity
nodular
nodularity
nodulated
nodulation
nodule
aggregated lymphatic n's of small intestine
Albini n's
n's of Arantius
Aschoff n's
Babès n's
Bianchi n's
Bohn n's
Bouchard n's
Busacca n's
Caplan n's
n. of cerebellum
cirrhotic n.
cold n.
Cruveilhier n's
Dalen-Fuchs n's
discrete n.
dysplastic n.
enamel n.
Gamna n's
Gandy-Gamna n's
glial n.
Hoboken n's
hot n.
Jeanselme n's
n's of Kerckring
Koeppe n's
Koester n.
Leishman n's
lumbar-sacral n's
lymphatic n's
lymphoid n's of stomach
macroregenerative n.
malpighian n.
milker's n's
Morgagni n's
pearly n.

nodule *(continued)*
- periosteal n's
- primary n.
- pulmonary n's
- pulp n.
- rabic n's
- regenerative n.
- regenerative n., monoacinar
- regenerative n., multiacinar
- rheumatic n's
- Schmorl n.
- secondary n.
- siderotic n's
- subcutaneous n.
- surfers' n's
- triticeous n.
- typhoid n.
- typhus n's
- n. of vermis
- vestigial n.
- vocal cord n's
- warm n.

nodulous

nodulus (noduli)
- noduli aggregati processus vermiformis
- n. cerebelli
- n. lymphatici aggregati cavitatis laryngis
- noduli lymphatici aggregati Peyeri
- n. lymphatici aggregati tubae auditivae
- noduli lymphatici bronchiales
- noduli lymphatici conjunctivales
- noduli lymphatici gastrici
- noduli lymphatici laryngei
- noduli lymphatici recti
- noduli lymphatici solitarii intestini crassi
- noduli lymphatici tubarii tubae auditivae
- noduli lymphatici vaginales
- noduli lymphatici vesicales
- n. lymphaticus
- n. primarius
- noduli thymici accessorii
- noduli valvularum aortae
- n. valvularum semilunarium valvae aortae
- noduli valvularum semilunarium ventriculi dextri
- n. vermis

nodus (nodi)
- n. arcus venae azygos
- n. atrioventricularis
- n. buccinatorius
- n. cursorius
- n. cysticus
- n. fibularis
- n. foraminalis
- n. jugulodigastricus
- n. jugulo-omohyoideus
- nodi juxta-intestinales
- n. lacunaris intermedius
- n. lacunaris lateralis
- n. lacunaris medialis
- n. ligamentis arteriosi
- nodi lymphatici abdominis parietales
- nodi lymphatici abdominis viscerales
- nodi lymphatici anorectales
- nodi lymphatici aortici laterales
- nodi lymphatici apicales
- nodi lymphatici appendiculares
- nodi lymphatici axillares
- nodi lymphatici brachialis
- nodi lymphatici bronchopulmonales
- nodi lymphatici cavales laterales
- n. lymphatici centrales
- nodi lymphatici cervicales anteriores
- nodi lymphatici cervicales laterales profundi
- nodi lymphatici coeliaci
- nodi lymphatici colici
- n. lymphatici colici dextri
- n. lymphatici colici medii
- n. lymphatici colici sinistri
- nodi lymphatici cubitales
- nodi lymphatici epigastrici inferiores
- nodi lymphatici faciales
- nodi lymphatici gastrici dextri
- nodi lymphatici gastrici sinistri
- nodi lymphatici gastroepiploici dextri
- nodi lymphatici gastroepiploici sinistri
- nodi lymphatici gastro-omentales dextri
- nodi lymphatici gastro-omentales sinistri

N

nodus (nodi) *(continued)*

nodi lymphatici gluteales
inferiores
nodi lymphatici gluteales
superiores
nodi lymphatici hepatici
nodi lymphatici hilares
nodi lymphatici ileocolici
nodi lymphatici iliaci
communes
nodi lymphatici iliaci
communes intermedii
nodi lymphatici iliaci
communes laterales
nodi lymphatici iliaci
communes mediales
nodi lymphatici iliaci
communes promontorii
nodi lymphatici iliaci
communes subaortici
nodi lymphatici iliaci externi
nodi lymphatici iliaci externi
intermedii
nodi lymphatici iliaci externi
laterales
nodi lymphatici iliaci externi
mediales
nodi lymphatici iliaci interni
n. lymphatici infra-auriculares
nodi lymphatici inguinales
inferiores
nodi lymphatici inguinales
profundi
nodi lymphatici inguinales
superficiales
nodi lymphatici inguinales
superolaterales
nodi lymphatici intercostales
nodi lymphatici interiliaci
nodi lymphatici
interpectorales
nodi lymphatici jugulares
anteriores
nodi lymphatici jugulares
laterales
nodi lymphatici juxta-
esophageales pulmonales
n. lymphatici laterales
nodi lymphatici lienales
nodi lymphatici linguales
nodi lymphatici lumbales
nodi lymphatici lumbales
dextri
nodi lymphatici lumbales
intermedii

nodus (nodi) *(continued)*

nodi lymphatici lumbales
sinistri
nodi lymphatici lumbares dextri
nodi lymphatici lumbares
intermedii
nodi lymphatici lumbares
sinistri
nodi lymphatici mastoidei
nodi lymphatici mediastinales
anteriores
nodi lymphatici mediastinales
posteriores
nodi lymphatici membri
superioris profundi
nodi lymphatici mesenterici
nodi lymphatici mesenterici
inferiores
nodi lymphatici mesenterici
superiores
n. lymphatici mesocolici
nodi lymphatici obturatorii
nodi lymphatici occipitales
nodi lymphatici pancreatici
nodi lymphatici pancreatici
inferiores
nodi lymphatici pancreatici
superiores
nodi lymphatici
pancreaticoduodenales
inferiores
nodi lymphatici paracolici
nodi lymphatici paramammarii
nodi lymphatici pararectales
nodi lymphatici parasternales
nodi lymphatici paratracheales
nodi lymphatici para-uterini
nodi lymphatici paravaginales
nodi lymphatici paravesiculares
nodi lymphatici parotidei
profundi
nodi lymphatici parotidei
superficiales
nodi lymphatici pectorales
nodi lymphatici pelvis
parietales
nodi lymphatici pelvis
viscerales
nodi lymphatici pericardiales
laterales
nodi lymphatici phrenici
inferiores
nodi lymphatici phrenici
superiores
nodi lymphatici popliteales

nodus (nodi) *(continued)*
    nodi lymphatici popliteales
      profundi
    nodi lymphatici popliteales
      superficiales
    nodi lymphatici postaortici
    nodi lymphatici postcavales
    nodi lymphatici postvesiculares
    nodi lymphatici pre-aortici
    n. lymphatici preauriculares
    nodi lymphatici precaecales,
      nodi lymphatici prececales
    nodi lymphatici precavales
    nodi lymphatici prelaryngeales
    nodi lymphatici
      prepericardiales
    nodi lymphatici pretracheales
    nodi lymphatici prevertebrales
    nodi lymphatici prevesiculares
    nodi lymphatici pulmonales
    nodi lymphatici pylorici
    nodi lymphatici rectales
      superiores
    nodi lymphatici
      retroauriculares
    nodi lymphatici retrocaecales,
      nodi lymphatici retrocecales
    nodi lymphatici
      retropharyngeales
    nodi lymphatici sacrales
    nodi lymphatici splenici
    nodi lymphatici
      submandibulares
    nodi lymphatici submentales
    nodi lymphatici subscapulares
    nodi lymphatici
      supraclaviculares
    nodi lymphatici thyroidei
    nodi lymphatici tracheales
    nodi lymphatici
      tracheobronchiales inferiores
    n. lymphatici vesicales laterales
    nodi lymphatici vesiculares
      laterales
    n. lymphaticus
    n. lymphaticus buccalis
    n. lymphaticus buccinatorius
    n. lymphaticus
      jugulodigastricus
    n. lymphaticus
      jugulo-omohyoideus
    n. lymphaticus malaris
    n. lymphaticus mandibularis
    n. lymphaticus nasolabialis
    n. lymphoideus

nodus (nodi) *(continued)*
    n. malaris
    n. mandibularis
    nodi mesocolici
    n. nasolabialis
    nodi retropylorici
    nodi sigmoidei
    n. sinuatrialis
    nodi subpylorici
    nodi superiores centrales
    n. suprapyloricus
    n. tibialis anterior
    n. tibialis posterior
    n. viscerales abdominis
NOEL—no observed effect level
Noguchi
    reagent
    test
noise
    transient n.
    white n.
Nölke position
noma
    n. pudendi
    n. vulvae
nomadic
nomenclature
    Systematized N. of Medicine
      Clinical Terms
      (SNOWMED CT) n.
    Terminologia Anatomica (TA) n.
nomogram
    blood volume n.
nonabsorbable
    n. hydrogel polymer
    n. Prolene mesh
    n. surgical suture
nonadherent
non–anion gap acidosis
nonantigenic
nonarticular
noncompliance
noncompliant
non compos mentis
nondisjunction
    primary n.
    secondary n.
    somatic n.
nonencapsulated
nonendocrine
    n. autoimmune disorder
    n. malignancy
    n. origin
    n. pancreatic disease
nonetheless

N

nonfunctioning
  n. gallbladder
  n. heart valve
  n. kidney
nonhomogeneity
nonhomogeneous
nonigravida
noninfectious
noninvasive
nonionic
nonipara
nonlinearity
nonmedullated
Nonne
  syndrome
  test
Nonne-Apelt
  phase
  reaction
  test
Nonne-Milroy-Meige syndrome
nonneurogenic
non-neuronal
non-nucleated
nonocclusion
nonocclusive intestinal infarction
nonoliguric
nononcogenic
nonopaque
nonparametric
nonpenetrant
nonperforating
  n. Crohn disease
  n. trauma
  n. ulcer
nonpermissive
nonplussed
nonpolar
nonprotein nitrogen (NPN)
non-REM—non–rapid eye movement
nonrotation of the intestine
nonsecretor
nonself
nonseminomatous
nonseptate
non sequitur
nonspecific
nonsurgical
nontaster
nonunion
  established n.
nonvalent
nonviable
  n. fetus
  n. tissue

nonvisualization
nonweightbearing,
  non-weightbearing
Noonan syndrome
Noorden treatment
noose suture
nootropic
noradrenergic
norethindrone test
norethynodrel test
Norland-Cameron photon
  densitometry
norleucine
norm
norma
  n. anterior
  n. basalis
  n. basilaris
  n. facialis
  n. frontalis
  n. inferior
  n. lateralis
  n. occipitalis
  n. posterior
  n. sagittalis
  n. superior
  n. temporalis
  n. ventralis
  n. verticalis
normal
  n.-pressure hydrocephalus
    (NPH)
  n. saline (NS)
  n. spontaneous vaginal
    delivery (NSVD)
normality
normalization
normalize
normalized plateau slope
Norman-Wood syndrome
normative
normoactive
normoblast
  acidophilic n.
  basophilic n.
  early n.
  eosinophilic n.
  intermediate n.
  late n.
  orthochromatic n.
  oxyphilic n.
  polychromatic n.
  polychromatophilic n.
normoblastic
normoblastosis

normocalcemia
normocalcemic
normocapnic
normocephalic
normocholesterolemic
normochromatic
normochromia
normochromic
normocrinic
normocyte
normocytic
normocytosis
normoglycemic
normokalemic
normoreflexic
normospermic
normosthenuric
normotensive
normothermic
normotonic
normotrophic
normouricemic
normouricuric
normovolemic
nornicotine
Norovirus
norovirus
    n. infection
    n. gastroenteritis
Norrie
    disease
    syndrome
Norris corpuscles
Northbent scissors
NOS—not otherwise specified
nose
    cleft n.
    copper n.
    external n.
    familial hump n.
    potato n.
    rabbit n.
    saddle n.
    saddle-back n.
    strawberry n.
    swayback n.
    Swedish n.
    telescope n.
    whiskey n.
nosebleed
nosegay
    Riolan n.
Nosema
    N. connori
    N. ocularum

nosematosis
nosencephalus
nosepiece
    quick-change n.
    rotating n.
nosocomial
nosogenic
nosography
nosologic
nosophobia
nosopoietic
nostril
nostrum
notalgia paresthetica
notanencephalia
notch
    acetabular n.
    angular n.
    antegonial n.
    anterior n. of auricle (ear)
    aortic n.
    n. of apex of heart
    auricular n.
    n. of cardiac apex
    cardiac n. of left lung
    cardiac n. of stomach
    Carhart n.
    cerebellar n., anterior
    cerebellar n., posterior
    clavicular n.
    clavicular n. of sternum
    coracoid n.
    costal n's of sternum
    cotyloid n.
    craniofacial n.
    dicrotic n.
    digastric n. of temporal bone
    n. of ethmoid
    ethmoidal n. of frontal bone
    fibular n.
    fibular n. of tibia
    frontal n.
    n. of gallbladder
    gastric n.
    greater n. of ischium
    hamular n.
    inferior n. of neck of pancreas
    interarytenoid n.
    interclavicular n.
    interclavicular n. of occipital bone
    interclavicular n. of temporal bone
    intercondylar n.
    intercondylar n. of femur

N

notch *(continued)*
    interlobar n.
    intertragic n.
    intervertebral n.
    ischiadic n., greater
    ischiadic n., lesser
    ischial n., greater
    ischial n., lesser
    jugular n. of manubrium of
      sternum
    jugular n. of occipital bone
    jugular n. of sternum
    jugular n. of temporal bone
    Kernohan n.
    lacrimal n. of maxilla
    lesser n. of ischium
    n. of ligamentum teres
    mandibular n.
    mastoid n.
    mastoid n. of temporal bone
    median prostatic n.
    nasal n. of frontal bone
    nasal n. of maxilla
    obturator n. of pubic bone
    palatine n.
    pancreatic n.
    parietal n. of temporal bone
    parotid n.
    popliteal n.
    preoccipital n.
    presternal n.
    n. projection
    pterygoid n.
    radial n.
    radial n. of ulna
    rivinian n.
    n. of Rivinus
    sacrosciatic n., greater
    sacrosciatic n., lesser
    scapular n.
    sciatic n., greater
    sciatic n., lesser
    semilunar n.
    semilunar n. of mandible
    semilunar n. of scapula
    Sibson n.
    sigmoid n.
    sigmoid n. of ulna
    sphenopalatine n. of palatine
      bone
    spinoglenoid n.
    sternal n.
    Stryker n. projection
    supraorbital n.
    suprascapular n.

notch *(continued)*
    suprasternal n.
    tentorial n.
    terminal n. of auricle
    thyroid n., inferior
    thyroid n., superior
    trigeminal n.
    trochlear n.
    trochlear n. of ulna
    tympanic n.
    ulnar n.
    ulnar n. of radius
    umbilical n.
    vertebral n.
    vertebral n., inferior
    vertebral n., superior
notching
    n. of alae, alar n.
    n. deformity
    femoral neck n.
    inferior glenoid n.
    optic disk n.
    rib n.
    n. of R wave
    n. of S wave
    T-wave n.
note
    bell n.
    cracked-pot n.
    percussion n.
Nothnagel
    acroparesthesia
    bodies
    sign
    syndrome
noticeable improvement
notifiable
notification of birth
Nott speculum
noumenal
Novak curet
novel
Novy, McNeal, and Nicolle culture
    medium
noxa (noxae)
noxious
    n. exposure
    n. event
    n. stimulation
    n. stimuli
Noyes forceps
Noyes-Shambaugh scissors
Np—neptunium
NP—
    nasopharyngeal

NP— *(continued)*
    nasopharynx
    neuropathology
    neuropsychiatric
    normal plasma
    not performed
    nurse practitioner
NPB—nodal premature beat
NPC—near point of convergence
NPCTG—National Prostatic
  Cancer Treatment Group
NPDL—nodular, poorly
  differentiated lymphocytes
NPH—
    neutral protamine Hagedorn
      (insulin)
    normal-pressure hydrocephalus
n.p.o., NPO—nothing by mouth
  (L. nil per os)
NPT—nocturnal penile tumescence
NRC—
    National Research Council
    normal retinal correspondence
    Nuclear Regulatory
      Commission
NREM—non–rapid eye movement
nRNA—nuclear RNA
NS—
    nervous system
    neurologic survey
    neurosurgery
    nonspecific
    nonsymptomatic
    normal saline
    no sample
    no specimen
    not significant
    not sufficient
NSA—no significant abnormality
NSAIA—nonsteroidal anti-
  inflammatory agent
NSC—
    no significant change
    not service-connected
NSCD—nonservice-connected
  disability
NSD—
    normal spontaneous delivery
    no significant defect
    no significant difference
    no significant disease
NSE—neuron-specific enolase
nsec—nanosecond
NSHD—nodular sclerosing
  Hodgkin disease

NSILA—nonsuppressible
  insulin-like activity
NSND—nonsymptomatic,
  nondisabling
NSQ—not sufficient quantity
NSR—normal sinus rhythm
NSS—normal saline solution
NST—nonstress test
NSU—nonspecific urethritis
NSVD—normal spontaneous
  vaginal delivery
NT—
    nasotracheal
    not tested
NTG—nontoxic goiter
NTN—nephrotoxic nephritis
NTP—normal temperature and
  pressure
nu—Greek letter
  (ν; alphabetized as n)
nucha
nuchal
    n. cord
    n. edema
    n. ligament
    n. ridge
    n. rigidity
    n. translucency sonography
Nuck
    canal
    diverticulum
    hydrocele
nuclear
    n. aggregate
    n. angiography
    n. cardiology
    n. cytoplasmic ratio alteration
    n. decay
    n. disintegration
    n. emulsion
    n. energy
    n. fission
    n. force
    n. fusion
    n. imaging
    n. inclusion body
    n. magnetic moment
    n. magnetic resonance
      imaging (NMRI)
    n. medicine
    n. particle
    n. pore alteration
    n. probe
    n. radiation
    n. reaction

N

nuclear *(continued)*
    n. reactor
    n. relaxation
    n. scanner
    n. scanning
    n. scintigraphy
    n. sclerosis
    n. signal
    n. spin
    n. structure
    n. vacuolization
nuclear magnetic resonance (NMR)
    n.m.r. Fourier transformation
    n.m.r. image
    n.m.r. imaging (NMRI)
    n.m.r. phantom
    pulsed n.m.r.
    n.m.r. relaxation rate
      enhancement
    n.m.r. scanning sequence
    n.m.r. signal intensity
    n.m.r. spectra
    n.m.r. spectral parameters
    n.m.r. spectroscopy
    n.m.r. spin warp method
    n.m.r. tomography
nuclease
nucleated
nucleation
nuclei (genitive and plural of nucleus)
nucleic acid
nucleiform
nucleinic acid
nucleocytoplasmic
nucleoid
nucleolar
nucleoli (plural of nucleolus)
nucleoliform
nucleonics
nucleophagocytosis
nucleophile
nucleophilic
nucleorrhexis
nucleosidase
nucleoside
    n. analogue
    n. phosphorylase
nucleosis
nucleotide
    cyclic n's
nucleotoxin
nucleotropic
nucleus (nuclei)
    n. abducens
    n. of abducens nerve

nucleus (nuclei) *(continued)*
    accessory n.
    accessory n. of auditory
      nerve
    accessory oculomotor n.
    accessory n. of ventral column
      of spinal cord
    acetabular n.
    nuclei of acoustic nerve
    n. alae cinereae
    ambiguous n.
    n. ambiguus
    n. amygdalae
    amygdaloid n.
    n. angularis
    n. ansae lenticularis
    n. of ansa lenticularis
    nuclei anteriores thalami
    anterior thalamic nuclei
    anterior nuclei of thalamus
    n. anterodorsalis thalami
    n. anteromedialis thalami
    n. anteroventralis thalami
    n. arciformes
    arcuate nuclei of medulla
      oblongata
    n. arcuati, n. arcuatus
    n. arcuatus hypothalami
    nuclei areae H, H_1, H_2
    n. of atom, atomic n.
    nuclei of auditory nerve
    auditory n., large cell
    autonomic n. of oculomotor
      nerve
    n. autonomicus
    Balbiani n.
    basal nuclei
    nuclei basales
    n. basalis of Meynert
    basal olfactory n.
    Béclard n.
    Bekhterev (Bechterew) n.
    Blumenau n.
    n. of Burdach column
    n. caeruleus
    n. of caudal colliculus
    n. caudalis centralis
    caudal olivary nuclei
    caudal salivatory n.
    caudal vestibular n.
    caudate n.
    cell n., cellular n.
    central caudal n.
    n. centralis lateralis thalami
    n. centralis medialis thalami

nucleus (nuclei) *(continued)*
    central n. of ventral column of spinal cord
    centrodorsal n.
    n. centromedianus thalami
    nuclei cerebelli
    n. of cerebellum, dentate
    n. of cerebellum, medullary
    cervical n., lateral
    cholane n.
    n. of circumolivary bundle of the pyramid
    Clarke n.
    cleavage n.
    cochlear n., anterior
    cochlear n., dorsal
    cochlear n., posterior
    cochlear nuclei
    cochlear n., ventral
    nuclei cochleares
    n. cochlearis anterior
    n. cochlearis dorsalis
    n. cochlearis posterior
    n. cochlearis ventralis
    n. colliculi caudalis
    n. colliculi inferioris
    commissural n.
    n. commissuralis
    compact n.
    conjugation n.
    n. corporis geniculati lateralis
    n. corporis geniculati medialis
    n. corporis trapezoidei
    n. of corpus striatum, intraventricular
    cortical n. of amygdala
    nuclei of cranial nerves
    cranial salivatory n.
    cuneate n., accessory
    cuneate n., lateral
    n. cuneatus accessorius
    Darkschewitsch (Darkshevich) n.
    daughter n.
    Deiters n.
    dental n.
    dentate n. of cerebellum
    n. dentatus cerebelli
    n. of descending fifth nerve
    descending vestibular n.
    diploid n.
    dorsal n. (of Clarke)
    n. dorsalis corporis trapezoidei
    n. dorsalis nervi glossopharyngei

nucleus (nuclei) *(continued)*
    n. dorsalis nervi vagi
    dorsal paramedian n.
    dorsal n. of trapezoid body
    dorsal vagal n.
    dorsal n. of vagus nerve
    dorsolateral n. of ventral column of spinal cord
    n. dorsomedialis hypothalami
    dorsomedial n. of thalamus
    dorsomedial n. of ventral column of spinal cord
    droplet nuclei
    drumstick n.
    Edinger n.
    Edinger-Westphal n.
    n. of eleventh cranial nerve
    emboliform n.
    n. emboliformis
    enamel n.
    entopeduncular n.
    n. entopeduncularis
    external cuneate n.
    n. facialis
    n. of facial nerve
    fastigial n.
    n. fastigiatus
    n. fastigii
    fertilization n.
    fibrous n. of tongue
    free n.
    n. funiculi cuneati
    n. funiculi gracilis
    gametic n.
    n. gelatinosus
    geniculate n., lateral
    geniculate n., medial
    n. geniculatus lateralis
    n. geniculatus medialis
    germ n., germinal n.
    gingival n.
    globose n.
    n. globosus cerebelli
    n. of glossopharyngeal nerve, dorsal
    Goll n.
    gonad n.
    n. gracilis
    gray n.
    nuclei of habenula
    habenular nuclei
    haploid n.
    hypoglossal n.
    n. hypoglossalis
    n. of hypoglossal nerve

N

nucleus (nuclei) *(continued)*
 hypothalamic n., anterior
 hypothalamic n., dorsal
 hypothalamic n., dorsomedial
 hypothalamic n., posterior
 hypothalamic n., ventromedial
 n. hypothalamicus anterior
 n. hypothalamicus dorsalis
 n. hypothalamicus
  dorsomedialis
 n. hypothalamicus posterior
 n. hypothalamicus
  ventromedialis
 n. of hypothalamus, arcuate
 n. of inferior colliculus
 n. inferior nervi trigemini
 inferior olivary nuclei
 inferior salivatory n.
 infundibular n.
 n. infundibularis hypothalami
 n. intercalatus
 intermediate ventral n. of
  thalamus
 intermediolateral n.
 n. intermediolateralis
 intermediomedial n.
 n. intermediomedialis
 n. of internal geniculate body
 interpeduncular n.
 n. interpeduncularis
 interstitial n. of Cajal
 n. interstitialis
 intracerebellar nuclei
 nuclei intralaminares thalami
 intralaminar thalamic nuclei
 Kölliker-Fuse n.
 large cell auditory n.
 laryngeal n.
 nuclei laterales thalami
 lateral geniculate n.
 n. of lateral geniculate body
 n. lateralis cervicalis
 n. lateralis dorsalis thalami
 n. lateralis medullae oblongatae
 n. lateralis posterior thalami
 n. of lateral lemniscus
 lateral reticular nuclei
 lateral thalamic nuclei
 lateral tuberal n.
 laterodorsal tegmental n.
 n. lemnisci lateralis
 n. of lens
 lenticular n.
 n. lenticularis
 n. lentiformis

nucleus (nuclei) *(continued)*
 n. lentis
 n. of Luys
 magnus raphe n.
 n. mammillaris lateralis
 n. mammillaris medialis
 masticatory n.
 medial accessory olivary n.
 nuclei mediales thalami
 n. mediales ventralis
 medial geniculate n.
 n. of medial geniculate body
 n. medialis centralis thalami
 n. medialis dorsalis thalami
 medial thalamic nuclei
 nuclei mediani thalami
 median raphe n.
 median thalamic nuclei
 n. mediodorsalis
 n. medullaris cerebelli
 medullary n. of cerebellum
 n. of mesencephalic tract of
  trigeminal nerve
 mesencephalic n. of trigeminal
  nerve
 metastable n.
 n. of Meynert
 Monakow n.
 motor n.
 motor n. of spinal cord
 motor n. of trigeminal nerve
 n. nervi abducentis
 n. nervi accessorii
 nuclei nervi acustici
 nuclei nervi cochlearis
 nuclei nervi cranialis
 n. nervi facialis
 n. nervi facialis of Arnold
 n. nervi glossopharyngei
 n. nervi hypoglossi
 n. nervi oculomotorii
 n. nervi olfactorii
 n. nervi phrenici
 nuclei nervi trigemini
 n. nervi trochlearis
 n. nervi vagi
 nuclei nervi vestibularis
 nuclei nervi vestibulocochlearis
 oculomotor n.
 n. of oculomotor nerve
 n. oculomotorii accessorii
 n. oculomotorii autonomici
 n. oculomotorius
 n. of olfactory tract
 n. oliva cerebellaris

nucleus (nuclei) *(continued)*
   nuclei olivares caudales
   n. olivaris accessorius dorsalis
   n. olivaris accessorius medialis
   n. olivaris accessorius posterior
   n. olivaris caudalis
   n. olivaris cranialis
   n. olivaris inferior
   n. olivaris rostralis
   n. olivaris superior
   n. olivaris superioris
   olivary n., accessory
   olivary n., caudal
   olivary n., inferior
   olivary n., medial accessory
   olivary n., posterior accessory
   olivary n., rostral
   olivary n., superior
   Onuf n., n. of Onufrowicz
   n. originis
   parabducent n.
   parabigeminal n.
   n. paracentralis thalami
   paracentral n. of thalamus
   parafascicular n.
   n. parafascicularis thalami
   parafascicular n. of thalamus
   paramedian n., dorsal
   paramedian n., posterior
   paramedian reticular n.
   n. paramedianus dorsalis
   n. paramedianus posterior
   n. parasolitarius, parasolitary n.
   nuclei parasympathici sacrales
   paraventricular nuclei
   n. paraventricularis
     hypothalami
   perihypoglossal n.
   n. periventricularis posterior
   Perlia n.
   phenanthrene n.
   n. of phrenic nerve
   phrenic n. of ventral column of
     spinal cord
   n. pigmentosus pontis
   polymorphic n.
   nuclei of pons
   pontine nuclei
   pontine n. of trigeminal nerve
   n. pontinus nervi trigemini
   n. pontinus nervi trigeminalis
   nuclei pontis
   pontobulbar n.
   posterior accessory olivary n.
   nuclei posteriores thalami

nucleus (nuclei) *(continued)*
   n. posterior hypothalami
   posterior paramedian n.
   n. posterior thalami
   posterior nuclei of thalamus
   posterior ventral n. of thalamus
   posterolateral ventral n. of
     thalamus
   posteromarginal n.
   premammillary n.
   preolivary n.
   nuclei preoptici medialis et
     lateralis
   preoptic nuclei, lateral and
     medial
   n. prepositus
   n. of prerubral field
   pretectal n.
   n. pretectalis
   principal sensory n. of
     trigeminal nerve
   n. proprius of posterior horn
   n. pulposus disci
     intervertebralis
   pulpy n.
   nuclei pulvinares thalami
   pyknotic n.
   pyramidal n.
   n. radicis descendentis nervi
     trigemini
   nuclei raphae medullae
     oblongatae
   nuclei of raphe
   raphe nuclei
   rapheal nuclei
   red n.
   reproductive n.
   reticular nuclei
   n. reticularis tegmenti
   n. reticularis thalami
   reticular n., lateral
   reticular n. of subthalamus
   reticular n. of thalamus
   reticular thalamic n.
   reticulotegmental n.
   n. reuniens thalami
   n. rhomboidalis thalami
   rhomboid thalamic n.
   Roller n.
   roof nuclei
   n. of roof of cerebellum
   n. of Rose
   rostral olivary n.
   n. ruber
   sacral parasympathetic nuclei

N

nucleus (nuclei) *(continued)*

n. salivatorius caudalis
n. salivatorius cranialis
n. salivatorius inferior
n. salivatorius rostralis
n. salivatorius superior
salivatory n., caudal
salivatory n., cranial
salivatory n., inferior
salivatory n., rostral
salivatory n., superior
n. of Sappey
Schwalbe n.
Schwann n.
secondary n.
segmentation n.
semilunar n.
sensory n. of trigeminal nerve, lower
sensory n. of trigeminal nerve, principal
septal n.
shadow n.
Siemerling n.
n. of sixth cranial nerve
nuclei solitarii
n. solitarius
solitary n.
n. of solitary tract
somatic n.
sperm n.
spherical n.
spinal n.
spinal n. of accessory nerve
n. spinalis
n. of spinal tract of trigeminal nerve
spinal n. of trigeminal nerve
spinocerebellar n.
Spitzka n.
Staderini n.
steroid n.
Stilling n.
striate n.
n. subcaeruleus
n. subceruleus
subependymal n.
sublingual n.
submedial n. of thalamus
subthalamic n.
n. subthalamicus
superior n.
superior olivary n.
n. of superior olive
suprachiasmatic n.

nucleus (nuclei) *(continued)*

suprageniculate n.
supramammillary n.
n. supraopticus hypothalami
supraspinal n.
n. sympathicus lateralis
n. tecti
tectoral n.
tegmental nuclei
nuclei tegmentales anteriores
n. of tegmental field
n. tegmentalis pedunculopontinus
nuclei tegmenti
n. tegmenti mesencephalici
terminal n.
nuclei terminationis
n. of thalamus
thoracic n.
n. thoracicus
n. of tongue, fibrous
n. tractus solitarii
n. of trapezoid body, dorsal
n. of trapezoid body, ventral
triangular n.
n. triangularis
trigeminal mesencephalic n.
n. trochlearis
n. of trochlear nerve
trophic n.
nuclei tuberales
tuberal nuclei, lateral
nuclei tuberis lateralis
n. vagalis dorsalis
vagoglossopharyngeal n.
vegetative n.
n. ventrales thalami
n. ventralis anterior thalami
n. ventralis anterolateralis thalami
n. ventralis corporis trapezoidei
n. ventralis intermedius thalami
n. ventralis lateralis thalami
n. ventralis medialis thalami
n. ventralis posterolateralis thalami
n. ventralis posteromedialis thalami
ventral n. of thalamus
ventral n. of trapezoid body
n. ventrobasolateralis
nuclei ventrolaterales thalami
ventrolateral nuclei of thalamus

nucleus (nuclei) *(continued)*
    ventrolateral n. of ventral
      column of spinal cord
    ventromedial n. of
      hypothalamus
    n. ventromedialis
    n. ventromedialis hypothalami
    ventromedial n. of ventral
      column of spinal cord
    vesicular n.
    vestibular n.
    vestibular n., caudal
    vestibular n., cranial
    nuclei vestibulares
    vestibular n., inferior
    n. vestibularis caudalis
    n. vestibularis cranialis
    n. vestibularis inferior
    n. vestibularis lateralis
    n. vestibularis medialis
    n. vestibularis rostralis
    n. vestibularis superior
    vestibular n., lateral
    vestibular n., rostral
    vestibular n., superior
    vestibulocochlear nuclei
    Voit n.
    Westphal nuclei
    yolk n.
    zygote n.
nuclide
    radioactive n.
Nuel spaces
NUG—necrotizing ulcerative
  gingivitis
Nu-gauze dressing
Nugent
    forceps
    hook
Nugent-Gradle scissors
Nuhn glands
nuisance
null
    n. cell lymphoblastic
      leukemia
    n.-type non-Hodgkin
      lymphoma
nulligravid
nulligravida
nullipara
nulliparity
nulliparous
numb
number
    atomic n.

number *(continued)*
    mass n.
    Mohs hardness n.
    random n.
numbering
numbness
nummular
Nunez-Nunez knife
nunnation
Nurolon suture
nurse
    charge n.
    clinical n. specialist
    n. clinician
    community n.
    community health n.
    district n.
    general duty n.
    graduate n.
    head n.
    hospital n.
    licensed practical n. (LPN)
    licensed vocational n.
    monthly n.
    occupational health n.
    operating room n.
    practical n.
    n. practitioner (NP)
    private duty n.
    probationer n.
    public health n.
    registered n. (RN)
    school n.
    scrub n.
    special n.
    n. specialist
    student n.
    theater n.
    trained n.
    visiting n.
    wet n.
nurse-anesthetist
nurse-midwife
nursery
    day care n.
nursing
Nussbaum
    clamp
    experiment
    narcosis
nut
    betel n.
nutation
nutatory
nutmeg

N

nutrient
    essential n's
    secondary n.
    trace n.
nutriment
nutrition
    adequate n.
    high n.
    total enteral n.
    total parenteral n. (TPN)
nutritional
nutritionist
nutritious
nutritive
Nuttall operation
nux
    n. moschata
    n. vomica
Nv—naked vision
NV—negative variation
N&V—nausea and vomiting
NVA—near visual acuity
nvCJD—new variant Creutzfeldt-
  Jakob disease
NVD—
    nausea, vomiting, diarrhea
    Newcastle virus disease
NWB—
    nonweightbearing,
      non-weightbearing,
      non–weight-bearing
    no weightbearing
Nycore pigtail catheter
nyctalopia
nyctophobia
NYD—not yet diagnosed
NYHA (New York Heart
  Association) classification
  (I–IV)
Nylen-Bárány maneuver
nylon monofilament suture
nymphectomy
nymphitis
nymphocaruncular
nymphohymeneal
nymphoid
nymphomania
nymphoncus
nymphotomy
nystagmic
nystagmiform
nystagmoid
nystagmus
    amaurotic n.
    amblyopic n.

nystagmus *(continued)*
    ataxic n.
    aural n.
    Baer n.
    Bekhterev (Bechterew) n.
    benign positional n.
    caloric n.
    central n.
    cervical torsion n.
    Cheyne n.
    Cheyne-Stokes n.
    congenital n., congenital
      hereditary n.
    convergence n.
    deviational n.
    disjunctive n.
    dissociated n.
    downbeat n.
    electrical n.
    end-point n.
    end position n.
    fixation n.
    galvanic n.
    gaze n.
    gaze paretic n.
    incongruent n.
    jerk n., jerky n.
    labyrinthine n.
    latent n.
    lateral n.
    miner's n.
    monocular n.
    n.-myoclonus
    occupational n.
    ocular n.
    opticokinetic n., optokinetic n.
      (OKN)
    oscillating n.
    palatal n.
    paretic n.
    pendular n.
    periodic alternating n.
    phasic n.
    positional n.
    postrotational n.
    postural n.
    provocation n.
    railroad n.
    rebound n.
    resilient n.
    retraction n., n.
      retractorius
    rhythmical n.
    rotary n.
    rotatory n.

nystagmus *(continued)*
   secondary n.
   see-saw n.
   spontaneous n.
   train-dispatcher's n.
   undulatory n.
   unilateral n.
   upbeat n.

nystagmus *(continued)*
   vertical n.
   vestibular n.
   vibratory n.
   visual n.
   voluntary n.
nystaxis
nyxis

O

θ—theta (Greek letter; alphabetized as th)
o—omicron (Greek letter)
ω—omega (Greek letter)
O.—eye (L. oculus)
O_2 (O2)—oxygen (molecular)
O_2 cap (O2 cap)—oxygen capacity
OA—
   occipital artery
   occiput anterior
   ocular albinism
   osteoarthritis
   oxalic acid
OA1—ocular albinism type 1
OA2—ocular albinism type 2
OAAD—ovarian ascorbic acid depletion
OAF—osteoclast-activating factor
oak
   poison o.
OAP—osteoarthropathy
OAR—other administrative reasons
oasis (oases)
Oasis wound matrix
OAT—ornithine aminotransferase
oatmeal
   colloidal o.
OAV—oculoauriculovertebral (dysplasia)
OB—
   objective benefit
   obstetrics
obedience
   automatic o.

O'Beirne
   sphincter
   tube
obeliac
obeliad
obelion
Ober
   operation
   sign
   test
Ober-Barr procedure
Obermayer test
Obermüller test
Oberst operation
Obersteiner-Redlich
   area
   zone
obese
obesity
   adrenocortical o.
   adult-onset o.
   alimentary o.
   centripetal o.
   endocrine o.
   endogenous o.
   exogenous o.
   hyperinsulinar o.
   o. of hyperinsulinism
   hyperinterrenal o.
   hyperplasmic o.
   hyperplastic-hypertrophic o.
   hypertrophic o.
   hypogonad o.
   hypoplasmic o.
   hypothalamic o.
   hypothyroid o.
   lifelong o.
   morbid o.

obesity *(continued)*
    plethoric o.
    simple o.
obesogenous
obex
obfuscation
OBG, OB-GYN—obstetrics and
  gynecology
object
    transitional o.
objective
    achromatic o.
    apochromatic o.
    binocular o's
    dry o.
    flat field o.
    fluorite o.
    immersion o.
    oil-immersion o.
    semiapochromatic o.
obligate
oblique
    external o. muscle
    o. incision
    internal o. muscle
obliquity
    biparietal o.
    Litzmann o.
    Nägele (Naegele) o.
    o. of pelvis
    Roederer o.
obliquus
    o. capitis inferior muscle
    o. capitis superior muscle
    o. reflex
obliteration
    complete o.
    cortical o.
    frontal sinus o.
    nidus o.
    percutaneous transhepatic o.
      of varices
oblongata
    medulla o.
oblongatal
obnubilation
    morning o.
    postictal o.
O'Brien
    akinesia
    block
    cataract
    forceps
OBS—organic brain
  syndrome

observation
    direct o.
    o. tube
obsession
    bowel o. syndrome
    death o.
obsessive-compulsive
    o-c. disorder
    o-c. neurosis
    o-c. personality disorder
    o-c. reaction
obsessive personality
obsolescence
    glomerular o.
obsolete
obstetric, obstetrical
    o. cholestasis
    o. forceps
obstetrician
obstetrics
obstipation
obstruction
    airway o.
    benign prostatic o.
    bladder outlet o.
    chronic airflow o.
    closed loop o.
    biliary tract o.
    false colonic o.
    gastric outlet o.
    idiopathic ureteropelvic
      junction o.
    intestinal o.
    left ventricular outflow o.
    pyloric outlet o.
    renal pelvic o.
    small-bowel o.
    subaortic o.
    tracheobronchial o.
    ureteral o.
    ureterovesical o.
    urinary tract o.
    uteropelvic junction o.
    vena cava o.
obstructive
    o. anuria
    o. apnea
    o. appendicitis
    o. atelectasis
    o. azoospermia
    o. cardiomyopathy
    chronic o. pancreatitis
    chronic o. pulmonary disease
      (COPD)
    o. coronary artery disease

obstructive *(continued)*
    o. dysmenorrhea
    o. emphysema
    o. glaucoma
    o. hydrocephalus
    hypertrophic o.
      cardiomyopathy
    o. jaundice
    localized o. emphysema
    o. megaureter
    o. nephropathy
    o. pneumonia
    o. pulmonary overinflation
    reversible o. airway disease
    o. sleep apnea (OSA)
    o. small airways disease
    o. thrombus
    o. uropathy
    o. vomiting
obstruent
obtund
obtundation
obtundent
obtundity
obturation
    canal o.
    mechanical o.
    prosthetic o.
obturator
    Alcock-Timberlake o.
    buccofacial o.
    Cripps o.
    o. foramen
    Timberlake o.
obtuse
    o. marginal branch
    o. marginal (OM) coronary
      artery
    o. margin of the heart
    o. margin of the spleen
obtusion
OC—
    occlusocervical
    office call
    on call
    oral contraceptive
OCA—
    oculocutaneous albinism
    oral contraceptive agent
occasion
occipital
    o. lobectomy
    o. suture
occipitalis
occipitalization

occipitoanterior
occipitoatloid
occipitoaxoid
occipitobasilar
occipitobregmatic
occipitocalcarine
occipitocervical
occipitofacial
occipitofrontal circumference (OFC)
occipitofrontalis
occipitomastoid suture
occipitomental
occipitoparietal suture
occipitopontine
occipitoposterior
occipitosphenoidal suture
occipitotemporal
occipitothalamic
occiput
occludable
occlude
occludens
    zonula o.
occluder
occlusal
occlusion
    abnormal o.
    acentric o.
    acquired eccentric o.
    afunctional o.
    anatomic o.
    anterior o.
    balanced o.
    branch retinal vein o.
    buccal o.
    centric o.
    o. clamp
    convenience o.
    coronary o.
    distal o.
    dynamic o.
    eccentric o.
    edge-to-edge o.
    enteromesenteric o.
    equilibrated o.
    fimbrial o.
    functional o.
    gliding o.
    habitual o.
    hepatic vein o.
    hyperfunctional o.
    ideal o.
    isthmic cornual o.
    labial o.
    lateral o.

O

occlusion *(continued)*
    lingual o.
    locked o.
    mechanically balanced o.
    mesenteric artery o.
    mesial o.
    midsegment o.
    neutral o.
    normal o.
    pathogenic o.
    physiologically balanced o.
    posterior o.
    postnormal o.
    prenormal o.
    protrusive o.
    o. of renal artery
    retrusive o.
    skeletal o.
    spherical form of o.
    terminal o.
    thrombotic o.
    traumatic o.
    traumatogenic o.
    tubal o.
    venous o. plethysmography
    working o.
occlusive
    o. dressing
    o. ileus
    o. meningitis
    o. mesenteric infarction
    o. mesenteric ischemia
occlusocervical
occult
    o. bleeding
    o. blood
    o. blood test
    o. border of nail
    o. cancer
    o. filariasis
    o. malignancy
    o. normal-pressure
      hydrocephalus
    o. tail
occupancy
occurrence
OCD—obsessive-compulsive disorder
OCG—oral cholecystogram
ochronosis
    exogenous o.
    ocular o.
ochronotic
Ochsenbein gingivectomy
Ochsner
    clamp

Ochsner *(continued)*
    forceps
    muscle
    probe
    ring
    scissors
    treatment
    trocar
    tube
Ochsner-Dixon forceps
Ockerblad clamp
OCL—Ortho Casting Lab
OCL splint
O'Connor
    hook
    operation
O'Connor-Peter operation
OCP—oral contraceptive pills
OCR—optical character recognition
OCT—oxytocin challenge test
octadecanoate
octahedral
octahedron
octamethyl
    o. derivatives
    o. ethers
    o. pyrophosphoramide
octane
octanoic acid breath test
octavalent pneumococcal
  polysaccharide vaccine
octet
octigravida
octipara
Octopus automatic perimeter
Octopus suction stabilizer
ocufilcon A hydrophilic contact lens
  material
ocular
    o. adnexa
    o. albinism
    o. aspergillosis
    o. bobbing
    o. density
    o. dysmetria
    o. flutter
    o. histoplasmosis
    o. hypertelorism
    o. hypertension
    o. hypotony
    o. microscope
    o. motility
    o. myoclonus
    o. myopathy
    o. pemphigus

ocular *(continued)*
    o. prosthesis
    o. torticollis
oculi (genitive and plural of oculus)
oculoauricular
    o. dysplasia
    o. reflex
oculocardiac reflex
oculocephalic reflex
oculocerebral hypopigmentation
  syndrome
oculocerebrorenal
    o. dystrophy
    o. syndrome of Lowe
oculocutaneous
    o. albinism
    o. melanosis
    o. oncocytic tumor
    o. sarcoid
    o. telangiectasia
    o. tyrosinemia, type II
oculodentodigital
    o. dysplasia
    o. syndrome
oculodermal melanocytosis
oculofacial-skeletal myorrhythmia
oculoglandular
    Parinaud o. syndrome
    o. tularemia
oculogyric
    o. crisis
    o. mechanism
oculomotor
    o. nerve
    o. nuclear complex
    o. nucleus
    o. paralysis
    o. sulcus
oculomycosis
oculonasal
oculopathy
    pituitarigenic o.
oculopharyngeal
    o. dystrophy
    o. reflex
    o. syndrome
oculopupillary reflex
oculosensory reflex
oculospinal
oculovagal reflex
oculozygomatic
oculus (oculi)
    o. dexter (OD) [L. right eye]
    orbicularis oculi muscle
    o. sinister (OS) [L. left eye]

oculus (oculi) *(continued)*
    o. uterque (OU) [L. each eye]
OCV—ordinary conversational voice
OD—
    optical density
    outside diameter
    overdose
    right eye (L. oculus dexter)
OD, O.D.—Doctor of Optometry
ODD—oculodentodigital
ODD dysplasia
odditis
ODN—ophthalmodynamometry
odontalgia
    phantom o.
odontalgic
odontectomy
odontic
odontoameloblastoma
odontoblastoma
odontodysplasia
odontogenesis imperfecta
odontogenic
    adenomatoid o. tumor
    benign epithelial o. tumor
    calcifying o. cyst
    central o. fibroma
    clear-cell o. tumor
    o. cyst
    o. fibers
    o. fibroma
    o. fibrosarcoma
    o. myxoma
    o. myxosarcoma
    peripheral o. fibroma
    squamous o. tumor
    o. tumor
odontogenous
odontogram
odontography
odontoid
odontolith
odontolithiasis
odontologist
odontology
    forensic o.
odontolysis
odontoma
    ameloblastic o.
    calcified o.
    complex o.
    composite o.
    compound o.
    coronal o.
    cystic o.

O

odontoma (continued)
  dilated o.
  dilated composite o.
  embryoplastic o.
  epithelial o.
  fibrous o.
  mixed o.
  radicular o.
odontopathic
odontopathy
odontoperiosteum
odontoplasty
odontosarcoma
  ameloblastic o.
odontoschism
odontosis
odontotomy
odontotripsis
odor
  ammonia-like o.
  fish o. syndrome
  fishy o.
  rotten cabbage o.
  sickeningly sweet o.
  sweetish o.
odorant
odoriferous
odorous
odynophagia
O&E—observation and
  examination
oedipism
Oedipus complex
Oehler symptom
OER—oxygen enhancement ratio
Oertel treatment
oesophagostomiasis
OFC—occipitofrontal circumference
OFD—
  oral-facial-digital
  orofaciodigital
OFD dysplasia
OFD syndrome (I, II)
off-loading splint
Ogilvie
  operation
  syndrome
Ogino-Knaus method
Ogston
  line
  operation
Ogston-Luc operation
OGTT—oral glucose tolerance test
Oguchi disease
OH—occupational history

O'Hanlon forceps
Ohara disease
Ohlmacher solution
ohm(s) (Ω)
OHP—oxygen under high
  pressure
OI—osteogenesis imperfecta
OIC—osteogenesis imperfecta
  congenita
oil
  cod liver o.
  flaxseed o.
  krill o.
  mineral o.
  olive o.
  peanut o.
  safflower o.
  volatile o.
ointment
  bacitracin o.
  bacitracin ophthalmic o.
  benzocaine o.
  betamethasone valerate o.
  boric acid o.
  calamine o.
  coal tar o.
  compound o. of capsicum
  Credé o.
  erythromycin o.
  erythromycin ophthalmic o.
  hydrocortisone o.
  hydrocortisone acetate o.
  hydrocortisone acetate
    ophthalmic o.
  ichthammol o.
  Jarisch o.
  lanolin o.
  lidocaine o.
  neomycin sulfate o.
  Nitrol o.
  nystatin o.
  Pagenstecher o.
  paraffin o.
  pine tar o.
  polyethylene glycol o.
  polymyxin B sulfate o.
  triamcinolone acetonide o.
  Whitfield o.
  zinc o.
  zinc oxide o.
OJ—orange juice
Oken
  body
  canal
  corpus

OKN—opticokinetic nystagmus
Oldberg
    dissector
    forceps
    retractor
oleaginous
oleander
olecranal
olecranoid
olecranon (olecrana)
    o. bursitis
    o. process
    o. spur
    o. tip
olein
oleogranuloma
oleoma
oleoresin
    capsicum o.
oleothorax
olfactant
olfaction
olfactism
olfactive
olfactory
    o. anesthesia
    o. angle
    o. area
    o. bulb
    o. canal
    o. cilia
    o. cortex
    o. epithelium
    o. foramina
    o. fossa
    o. ganglion
    o. glands
    o. glomerulus
    o. groove
    o. gyrus
    o. hairs
    o. hallucination
    o. hyperesthesia
    o. islands
    o. knob
    o. labyrinth
    o. lobe
Oligella
    O. ureolytica
    O. urethralis
oligemia
oligemic shock
oligo-1,6-glucosidase
oligoamnios
oligoanalgesia

oligoanuria
oligoarthritis
oligoasthenospermia
oligoastrocytoma
oligoblast
oligochromasia
oligoclonal
    o. bands, o. banding
    o. gammopathy
    o. immune response
    o. T cells
oligoclonality
oligocystic
oligodactyly
oligodendroblastoma
oligodendrocyte
oligodendroglia
oligodendroglioma
oligodendrogliomatosis
oligodipsia
oligodontia
oligodynamic
oligoencephalon
oligogalactia
oligogenic
oligohidrosis
oligohydramnios
oligohydruria
oligohypermenorrhea
oligohypomenorrhea
oligomeganephronia
oligomeganephronic renal
  hyperplasia
oligomenorrhea
oligonucleotide probe
oligo-ovulation
oligophrenia
oligophrenic
oligopnea
oligosaccharide
oligospermatic
oligospermatism
oligospermia
oligosymptomatic
oligosynaptic
oligotrophic
oliguria
oliguric
olisthy
oliva (olivae)
    o. cerebellaris
olivary
    o. body
    o. complex
    o. nuclei

O

olive
  inferior o.
  medullary o.
  pyloric o.
  o. ring
  spurge o.
  superior o.
  o. wire
Olivecrona clip
Oliver-Rosalki method
Oliver sign
olive-tip, olive-tipped
  o.t. bougie
  o.t. catheter
olivocerebellar
  o. fibers
  o. tract
olivocochlear
  o. bundle of Rasmussen
  o. fasciculus
olivocortical tract
olivopontocerebellar
  o. atrophy
  o. degeneration
olivospinal tract
Ollier
  disease
  dyschondroplasia
  incision
  law
  layer
  operation
  osteochondromatosis
  syndrome
Ollier-Thiersch
  graft
  operation
Olshausen
  operation
  sign
Olshevsky tube
Olympus
  BML-4Q lithotripsy
  EM30 radial
    echoendoscope
  fiberscope
  flexible endoscope
  GIF-N230 endoscope
  GIF-2T240M multibending
    scope
  GTF-A gastrocamera
  V-Scope
OM—
  obtuse marginal (coronary
    artery)

OM— *(continued)*
  otitis media
  outer membrane
Ombrédanne operation
omega—Greek letter
  (ω; alphabetized as o)
omenta (plural of omentum)
omental
omentectomy
omentitis
omentopexy
omentoplasty
omentorrhaphy
omentum (omenta)
  colic o.
  gastric o.
  gastrocolic o.
  gastrohepatic o.
  gastrosplenic o.
  greater o.
  lesser o.
  o. majus
  o. minus
  splenogastric o.
OMI—old myocardial
  infarction
omicron—Greek letter
  (o; alphabetized as o)
Ommaya reservoir
Omni operating microscope
Omnicarbon valve
Omnipen
omnipotence of thought
Omniscience valve
omnivorous
omoclavicular
  o. triangle
  o. trigone
omohyoid
omosternum
omothyroid
OMPA—otitis media, purulent,
  acute
omphalectomy
omphalic
omphalitis
omphaloangiopagous
omphaloangiopagus
omphalocele
omphalochorion
omphalodidymus
omphaloenteric duct
omphalogenesis
omphaloischiopagus
omphaloma

omphalomesenteric
    o. canal
    o. circulation
    o. duct
    o. duct cyst
    o. fistula
    o. veins
omphaloncus
omphalopagus
omphalophlebitis
omphalorrhagia
omphalorrhea
omphalorrhexis
omphalosite
omphalotomy
omphalus
OMT—osteopathic manipulative
  therapy
onanism
Onchocerca volvulus
onchocerciasis
    ocular o.
onchocercoma
onchodermatitis
oncocyte
oncocytic adenoma
oncocytoma
    renal o.
oncocytosis
oncofetal antigen
oncogene
    viral o.
oncogenetic
oncogenic
    o. osteomalacia
    o. virus
oncogenicity
oncogenous
oncoides
oncologic
oncologist
oncology
    radiation o.
oncolysate
oncolysis
oncolytic
oncoma
oncornavirus
oncosis
oncosphere
oncotherapy
oncothlipsis
oncotic pressure
oncotomy
oncotropic

oncovirus
Ondine curse
oneiric hyperesthesia
oneirism
oneiroid
oneirophrenia
onlay
    epithelial o.
    o. graft
    o. graft myringoplasty
onomatopoiesis
onychauxis
onychectomy
onychia
onychocryptosis
onychodystrophy
onychogenic
onychogryphosis
onychogryposis
onychoheterotopia
onycholysis
onychomadesis
onychomalacia
onychomatricoma
onychomycosis
    dermatophytic o.
onycho-osteodysplasia
onychopathic
onychopathology
onychopathy
onychophagia
onychophosis
onychoptosis
onychorrhexis
onychoschizia
onychosis
onychotillomania
onychotomy
O'nyong-nyong
onyx
onyxis
OOB—out of bed
oocyesis
oocyst
oocyte
    o. donation
    primary o.
    secondary o.
oogenic
oophoralgia
oophorectomize
oophorectomy
oophoritis parotidea
oophorocystectomy
oophorocystosis

O

oophorohysterectomy
oophoroma folliculare
oophoropathy
oophoropexy
oophoroplasty
oophorosalpingectomy
oophorosalpingitis
oophorostomy
oophorotomy
oophorrhagia
OP—
    opening pressure
    operation
    osmotic pressure
OP; OPT—outpatient
O&P—ova and parasites
opacification
opacified
opacify
opacity
    Caspar ring o.
    snowball o's
opalescent
opaline
Opalski cell
opaque
    o. arthrography
    o. catheter
    o. mediastinography
    o. microscope
    o. myelography
OPC—outpatient clinic
OPD—outpatient department
open
    o. operation
    o. reduction and internal
      fixation (ORIF)
    o. tenotomy
open-angle glaucoma
opening
    o. in adductor magnus muscle
    anterior o. of aqueduct of
      Sylvius
    aortic o.
    aortic o. in diaphragm
    o. of aqueduct of cochlea,
      external
    bite o.
    o. of bladder
    cardiac o.
    o. of coronary sinus
    cutaneous o. of male urethra
    duodenal o. of stomach
    esophageal o. in diaphragm
    o. of Hunter's canal, inferior

opening *(continued)*
    ileocecal o.
    ileocolic o.
    inferior o's of caroticotympanic
      canaliculi
    o. of inferior vena cava
    internal urethral o.
    interventricular o.
    o. to lesser sac of peritoneum
    o. for lesser superficial
      petrosal nerve
    nasal o. of facial skeleton
    o. of omental bursa
    orbital o., o. of orbital cavity,
      anterior
    ovarian o. of uterine tube
    o. of parotid duct
    o. of pelvis, inferior
    o. of pelvis, superior
    pharyngeal o. of auditory
      tube
    pharyngeal o. of eustachian
      tube
    piriform o.
    o. of pulmonary trunk
    pyloric o.
    o. of sacral canal, inferior
    saphenous o.
    semilunar o. of ethmoid bone
    o. for smaller superficial
      petrosal nerve
    o. of sphenoidal sinus
    o. of stomach, anterior
    tendinous o.
    thoracic o., inferior
    thoracic o., lower
    thoracic o., superior
    thoracic o., upper
    tympanic o. of auditory tube
    o. for tympanic branch of
      glossopharyngeal nerve
    o. of tympanic canal, superior
    uterine o. of uterine tube
    o. for vena cava
    o. of vermiform appendix
    vertical o.
    vesicourethral o.
    o. of Vieussens
open-mouth
open sky vitrectomy
operability
operable
operant
operate
operating microscope

operation
>> Abbe o.
>> Adams o.
>> Akin o.
>> Albee o.
>> Aldridge fascial sling o.
>> Alexander o.
>> Ammon o.
>> anastomotic o.
>> Andrews thoracoplasty o.
>> Aries-Pitanguy mastopexy o.
>> Arruga string o.
>> Auchincloss mastectomy o.
>> Babcock o.
>> Badgley spinal fusion o.
>> Baldwin vaginoplasty o.
>> Bankart o. for shoulder instability
>> Bankart-Bristow o. for shoulder instability
>> Barkan goniotomy o.
>> Barraquer o. for cataract
>> Barwell hernia repair o.
>> Basset o.
>> Bassini o.
>> Bateman bipolar endoprosthesis o.
>> Bateman hemiarthroplasty o.
>> Belsey Mark IV fundoplication o.
>> Bentall o.
>> Billroth I o., Billroth II o.
>> Bischof II myelotomy o.
>> Blalock-Hanlon o.
>> Blalock-Taussig o.
>> bloodless o.
>> Blount o.
>> Boari o.
>> Bondy radical mastoidectomy o.
>> Bosworth o. for acromioclavicular joint dislocation
>> Boyd o.
>> Braun anastomosis o.
>> Braun enteroenterostomy o.
>> Bricker ileal conduit o. for urinary diversion
>> Bristow o. for shoulder instability
>> Bristow-Latarjet o. for shoulder instability
>> Brock valvotomy o.
>> Brown o.
>> Browne urethroplasty o.

operation *(continued)*
>> Burch o. for stress urinary incontinence
>> Burow 8-to-S-plasty o.
>> buttonhole o.
>> Cabrol o.
>> Cairns trabeculectomy o.
>> Caldwell-Luc antrostomy o.
>> Carrel o.
>> Cecil-Culp hypospadias repair o.
>> Chaput osteotomy o.
>> Charles o. for lymphedema
>> Chopart amputation o.
>> Clagett open-window thoracostomy o.
>> Cloward spinal decompression o.
>> Colonna arthroplasty o.
>> Cooper ligament o.
>> Cooper lung volume reduction o.
>> cosmetic o.
>> Crawford o. for aneurysm repair, types I–III
>> Cronin o. for cleft palate
>> Cutler-Beard o. for eyelid reconstruction
>> Daniel rhinoplasty o.
>> Darrach o.
>> decompression o.
>> Delorme o. for rectal prolapse
>> Denis Browne o.
>> Denker o.
>> Derlacki o.
>> Döderlein (Doderlein) osteotomy o. for femoral derotation
>> Dohlman endoscopic Zenker diverticulotomy o.
>> Dohlman o. for keratopathy
>> Duhamel-Haddad o. for chagasic megacolon
>> Duplay o. for hypospadias repair
>> Duplay-Snodgrass o. for hypospadias repair
>> Dupuy-Dutemps dacryocystorhinostomy o.
>> Eden-Hybbinette o.
>> Elmslie-Trillat o. for patellar instability
>> Eloesser o. for bronchopleural fistula
>> Emmet o. for ingrown nails

O

operation *(continued)*
 equilibrating o.
 Evans o. for ankle instability
 exploratory o.
 face-lift o.
 Fasanella-Servat o. for eyelid ptosis repair
 fenestration o.
 Finney pyloroplasty o.
 flap o.
 Fontan o.
 Fredet-Ramstedt o.
 Friedrich thyroplasty o.
 Gallie spinal fusion o.
 Gant-Miwa o. for rectal prolapse
 Gill o. for spondylolisthesis
 Gilliam suspension o. for retroversion of uterus
 Gillies o.
 Girard o.
 Girdlestone o.
 Glenn o.
 Goldthwait o.
 Gritti-Stokes amputation o.
 Hartmann o.
 Haultain o.
 Haynes-Anderson o.
 Heermann tympanoplasty o.
 Heineke-Mikulicz pyloroplasty o.
 Heineke-Mikulicz strictureplasty o.
 Heller myotomy o. for esophageal achalasia
 Hey Groves o.
 Hibbs spinal fusion o.
 Hoke o. for Achilles tendon lengthening
 Horton-Devine o. for hypospadias
 Hotchkiss o.
 interposition o.
 interval o.
 iris inclusion o.
 Irving o. for tubal ligation
 Jaboulay pyloroplasty o.
 Jatene arterial switch o.
 Kasai portoenterostomy o.
 keel o.
 Keller bunionectomy o.
 Keller-Brandes o. for hallux valgus
 Kelly o. for stress urinary incontinence

operation *(continued)*
 Kelly-Kennedy o.
 Kestenbaum-Anderson o.
 Kocher o. for reducing shoulder dislocation
 Kock o. for continent urinary diversion
 Kraske o. for rectal carcinoma
 Langenbeck o.
 Lapidus arthrodesis o.
 Latzko o.
 Le Fort colpocleisis o. for repair of uterine prolapse
 Le Fort osteotomy o.
 lip adhesion o.
 Lisfranc foot amputation o.
 Ludloff o.
 Lynch o.
 Madlener o.
 magnet o.
 Magnuson-Stack o. for shoulder instability
 major o.
 Manchester o. for uterine prolapse
 Marshall-Marchetti o.
 Marshall-Marchetti-Birch o.
 Marshall-Marchetti-Krantz (MMK) o.
 mastoid o.
 mastoid obliteration o.
 McBride o.
 McVay o. for repair of hernia
 Miles o.
 Millard o. for repair of cleft lip
 minor o.
 Mitchell o.
 Monaldi o.
 morcellement o.
 Moschcowitz o. for hernia repair
 Mules o.
 Mustard o. for correction of transposition of great vessels
 Nissen fundoplication o.
 open o.
 osteoplastic frontal sinus o.
 palatal pushback o.
 Patey o.
 Pereyra o. for urinary incontinence
 Phemister epiphysiodesis o.
 Pirogoff o. for amputation of foot
 plastic o.
 Polya o.

operation *(continued)*

    Pomeroy tubal ligation o.

    Potts o.

    Putti-Platt o. for shoulder instability

    radical o.

    radical antrum o.

    Ramstedt o.

    Rashkind o.

    Rastelli o.

    reconstructive o.

    Reverdin o.

    Roux-Elmslie-Trillat o. for patellar instability

    Roux-en-Y o.

    Roux-Goldthwait o. for patellar instability

    Santulli enterostomy o.

    Schauta radical vaginal hysterectomy o.

    Schauta-Amreich o.

    Scheie o.

    Schuknecht o.

    Senning o. for transposition of great vessels

    shelf o.

    shelving o.

    Shirodkar o.

    Sistrunk o.

    Skoog o.

    sling o.

    Smith-Petersen o.

    Smith-Robinson o. for spinal decompression

    Soave o.

    stapes mobilization o.

    Steindler o.

    string o.

    subcutaneous o.

    Syme amputation o.

    tack o.

    Tanzer o.

    Tennison o. for cleft lip repair

    Tennison-Randall o. for cleft lip repair

    Terson o. for removal of pterygium

    Tessier o. for craniofacial abnormalities

    Thiersch graft o.

    Thiersch-Duplay o.

    Torkildsen o.

    Toupet fundoplication o.

    uterine suspension o.

    vacuum extraction o.

operation *(continued)*

    Vineberg o.

    V-Y o.

    Wardill-Kilner palatoplasty o.

    Waterston o. for pulmonary stenosis

    Watson-Jones hip replacement o.

    Weaver-Dunn o. for acromioclavicular joint dislocation

    Webster-type face and neck lift o.

    Whipple pancreaticoduodenectomy o.

    Williams-Richardson vaginopexy o.

    Witzel gastrostomy o.

    Wolfe rhinoplasty o.

    W-Y o.

    Young o. for correction of penile epispadias

    Young-Dees o. for bladder neck reconstruction

    Young-Dees-Leadbeetter o. for bladder neck reconstruction

    Z-plasty o.

operative

    o. arteriography

    o. cholangiography

    delayed o. cholangiography

operator

opercular

operculate

operculectomy

operculitis

operculum (opercula)

    cartilaginous o.

    dental o.

    frontal o., o. frontale

    frontoparietal o., o. frontoparietale

    o. insulae

    occipital o.

    opercula of insula

    o. orbitale

    parietal o.

    temporal o., o. temporale

    trophoblastic o.

operon

    lack o.

OPG—oxypolygelatin

OPG/CPA—oculoplethysmography/ carotid phonoangiography

ophiasis

O

ophidic
ophidism
Ophiophagu hannah
ophiotoxemia
ophryon
ophryosis
ophthalmagra
ophthalmalgia
ophthalmatrophia
ophthalmectomy
ophthalmencephalon
ophthalmia
    actinic ray o.
    Brazilian o.
    catarrhal o.
    caterpillar o.
    o. eczematosa
    Egyptian o.
    electric o.
    o. electrica
    flash o.
    gonococcal o. of newborn
    gonorrheal o.
    granular o.
    hepatic o.
    jequirity o.
    metastatic o.
    migratory o.
    mucous o.
    o. neonatorum
    neuroparalytic o.
    o. nivialis
    o. nodosa
    periodic o.
    phlyctenular o.
    purulent o.
    scrofulous o.
    solar o.
    spring o.
    strumous o.
    sympathetic o.
    transferred o.
    ultraviolet ray o.
    varicose o.
ophthalmiac
ophthalmiatrics
ophthalmic
ophthalmic acid
ophthalmic Graves disease
ophthalmitic
ophthalmitis
    sympathetic o.
ophthalmoblennorrhea
ophthalmocele
ophthalmocopia

ophthalmodesmitis
ophthalmodiaphanoscope
ophthalmodiastimeter
ophthalmodonesis
ophthalmodynamometer
ophthalmodynamometry
ophthalmodynia
ophthalmoeikonometer
ophthalmograph
ophthalmography
ophthalmogyric
ophthalmoleukoscope
ophthalmolith
ophthalmologic, ophthalmological
ophthalmologist
ophthalmology
ophthalmomalacia
ophthalmometer
    Javal o.
ophthalmometroscope
ophthalmometry
ophthalmomycosis
ophthalmomyiasis
ophthalmomyitis
ophthalmomyositis
ophthalmomyotomy
ophthalmoneuritis
ophthalmoneuromyelitis
ophthalmoparalysis
ophthalmopathy
    dysthyroid o.
    endocrine o.
    external o.
    hyperthyroid o.
    infiltrative o.
    internal o.
    thyrotoxic o.
ophthalmophacometer
ophthalmophantom
ophthalmophlebotomy
ophthalmophthisis
ophthalmoplasty
ophthalmoplegia
    basal o.
    congenital o.
    diabetic o.
    exophthalmic o.
    o. externa
    external o.
    fascicular o.
    hyperthyroid o.
    o. interna
    internal o.
    internuclear o.
    nuclear o.

ophthalmoplegia *(continued)*
    orbital o.
    painful o.
    Parinaud o.
    partial o.
    o. partialis
    o. progressiva
    progressive external o.
    relapsing o.
    Sauvineau o.
    sensorimotor o.
    thyrotoxic o.
    total o.
    o. totalis
ophthalmoplegic
ophthalmoptosis
ophthalmoreaction
    Calmette o.
ophthalmorrhagia
ophthalmorrhea
ophthalmorrhexis
ophthalmoscope
    binocular o.
    direct o.
    Friedenwald o.
    ghost o.
    indirect o.
ophthalmoscopic
ophthalmoscopy
    binocular indirect o.
    direct o.
    indirect o.
    medical o.
    metric o.
ophthalmospectroscope
ophthalmospectroscopy
ophthalmostasis
ophthalmostat
ophthalmostatometer
ophthalmosteresis
ophthalmosynchysis
ophthalmothermometer
ophthalmotomy
ophthalmotonometer
ophthalmotonometry
ophthalmotoxin
ophthalmotrope
ophthalmotropometer
ophthalmotropometry
ophthalmovascular
ophthalmoxerosis
ophthalmoxyster
opian
opianine
opiate

Opie paradox
opioid
Opisocrosti bruneri
opisthe
opisthenar
opisthencephalon
opisthiobasial
opisthion
opisthionasial
opisthocranion
opisthogenia
opisthoglyphic
opisthognathism
opisthomastigote
opisthoporeia
opisthorchiasis
opisthorchid
Opisthorchis
    O. felineus
    O. noverca
    O. sinensis
    O. tenuicollis
    O. viverrini
opisthorchosis
opisthotic
opisthotonoid
opisthotonos fetalis
Opitz
    disease
    syndrome
opium
    crude o.
    denarcotized o.
    o. deodoratum
    deodorized o.
    granulated o.
    o. granulatum
    gum o.
    powdered o.
    o. pulveratum
OPK—optokinetic
opocephalus
opodidymus
opossum
Oppenheim
    amyotonia
    disease
    gait
    reflex
    sign
    syndrome
opponens
opportunist
opportunistic infection
opposition

O

OPRT—orotate
  phosphoribosyltransferase
OPS—outpatient service
opsialgia
opsin
opsinogenous
opsiometer
opsiuria
opsoclonia
opsoclonus
opsomyoclonus
opsonic
opsonification
opsonin
    immune o.
    normal o.
opsonization
opsonize
opsonocytophagic
opsonophilia
opsonophilic
optesthesia
optic
    o. atrophy
    o. axis
    o. chiasm
    o. cup
    o. disk
    o. foramen
    o. iridectomy
    o. keratoplasty
    o. nerve
    o. neuritis
    o. tract
    o. vesicle
optical
    o. esophagoscope
    o. microscope
optician
opticianry
opticoagnosia
    Wernicke subcortical o.
opticochiasmatic
opticociliary
    o. neurectomy
    o. neurotomy
opticofacial winking
  reflex
opticokinetic
opticonasion
opticopupillary
optics
    fiber o.
opticus
optimal

optimism
    therapeutic o.
optimization
optimize
optimum
optoacoustic
optochiasmic
Optochin
optogram
optokinetic nystagmus
  (OKN)
optomeninx
optometer
optometrist
optometry
optomyometer
optophone
optotype
OPV—oral poliovirus vaccine
OR—operating room
ora (orae)
    o. serrata retinae
ora (plural of os)
orad
Oragrafin
oral
    o. cholecystography
    o. mucosa
    o. panendoscope
    o. tori
    o. urography
orale
orality
oralogy
orange
    o. II
    o. III
    acid o. 10
    acridine o.
    ethyl o.
    o. G
    gold o.
    methyl o.
    Poirier o.
    victoria o.
    wool o.
orangeophil
orangutan
orb
orbicular
orbiculare
orbicularis (orbiculi)
    o. ciliaris muscle
    o. oculi muscle
    o. oculi reflex

orbicularis (orbiculi) *(continued)*
    o. oris
    o. oris muscle
    o. pupillary reflex
    o. reflex
orbit
orbita (orbitae)
orbital
    o. angiography
    o. apex
    o. cellulitis
    o. decompression
    o. fascia
    o. fat pads
    o. fissure
    o. floor
    o. floor fracture
    o. periosteum
    o. pseudotumor
    o. septum
orbitale
orbitalis
orbitography
orbitonasal
orbitonometer
orbitonometry
orbitopagus
orbitopathy
    dysthyroid o.
    Graves o.
orbitostat
orbitotemporal
orbitotomy
Orbivirus
orcein
orchella
orchialgia
orchichorea
orchidalgia
orchidectomy
orchidic
orchiditis
orchidoepididymectomy
orchidometer
    Prader o.
orchidoncus
orchidopathy
orchidopexy
orchidoplasty
orchidoptosis
orchidorrhaphy
orchidotomy
orchiectomy
orchiencephaloma
orchiepididymitis

orchil
orchilytic
orchiocatabasis
orchiocele
orchiodynia
orchiomyeloma
orchioncus
orchioneuralgia
orchiopathy
orchiopexy
orchioplasty
orchiorrhaphy
orchioscheocele
orchioscirrhus
orchiotomy
orchis
orchitic
orchitis
    acute pyogenic o.
    acute syphilitic o.
    metastatic o.
    mumps o.
    o. parotidea
    spermatogenic
      granulomatous o.
    traumatic o.
    o. variolosa
orchitolytic
orchotomy
orcinol
ORD—optical rotatory dispersion
order
    birth o.
    form-o.
orderly
ordinate
oreoselinum
orexia
orexigenic
orexis
ORF—open reading frame
organ
    absorbent o.
    accessory o's of eye
    acoustic o.
    adipose o.
    Bidder o.
    cell o.
    cement o.
    Chievitz o.
    o. of Corti
    critical o.
    cutaneous sense o's
    digestive o's
    effector o.

O

organ *(continued)*
 enamel o.
 end o.
 essential o. of thalamus
 extraperitoneal o.
 genital o's
 Golgi tendon o.
 gustatory o.
 intromittent o.
 Jacobson o.
 lateral line o's
 Marchand o.
 o's of mastication
 Meyer o.
 neurotendinous o.
 olfactory o.
 parapineal o.
 parenchymal o.
 parenchymatous o.
 pineal o.
 primitive fat o.
 reproductive o's
 retroperitoneal o.
 Rosenmüller o.
 rudimentary o.
 o. of Ruffini
 segmental o.
 sense o's
 sensory o's
 sex o.
 shock o.
 o. of smell
 o's of special sense
 spiral o.
 subcommissural o.
 subfornical o.
 target o.
 taste o.
 tendon o.
 terminal o.
 touch o's
 urinary o's
 vestibular o.
 vestibulocochlear o.
 vestigial o.
 o. of vision
 visual o.
 vomeronasal o.
 Weber o.
 o's of Zuckerkandl
organelle
 paired o.
organic brain syndrome (OBS)
organicism

organicist
organism
 Arizona o.
 consumer o's
 nitrifying o's
 nitrosifying o's
 pleuropneumonia-like o's
 transgenic o.
 Vincent o.
organization
 health maintenance o. (HMO)
 preferred provider o. (PPO)
 Professional Standards
  Review O. (PSRO)
 World Health O. (WHO)
organizer
 mesodermic o.
 nucleolar o.
 nucleolus o.
 primary o.
 procentriole o.
 secondary o.
 tertiary o.
organochlorine
organofaction
organoferric
organogel
organogenesis
organogenetic
organogenic
organography
organoid
organoleptic
organology
organoma
organomegaly
organomercurial
organometallic
organopathy
organopexy
organophilic
organophilism
organophosphate
organophosphorus
organotaxis
organotherapy
 heterologous o.
 homologous o.
organotrope
organotrophic
organotropic
organotropism
organotropy
organ-specific

organule
organum (organa)
    o. extraperitoneale
    organa genitalia
    organa genitalia feminina
      externa
    organa genitalia feminina
      interna
    organa genitalia masculina
      externa
    organa genitalia masculina
      interna
    o. genitalia muliebria
    o. gustatorium
    o. gustus
    organa oculi accessoria
    o. olfactorium
    o. olfactus
    o. retroperitoneale
    organa sensoria
    organa sensuum
    o. spirale
    o. subcommissurale
    o. subfornicale
    organa urinaria
    organa uropoëtica
    o. vestibulocochleare
    o. visuale
    o. visus
    o. vomeronasale
orgasm
    inhibited male o.
orgotein
orientation
    coronal o.
    double o.
    reality o.
    sagittal o.
    transverse o.
oriented
    alert and o. (AO)
    o. to time, place, and person
      (OTPP)
    o. to time, place, person, and
      situation
    o. times three, o. x3
orienting reflex
ORIF—open reduction and internal
    fixation
orifice
    abdominal o. of uterine tube
    aortic o.
    o. of aqueduct of vestibule,
      external

orifice *(continued)*
    atrioventricular o.
    auriculoventricular o.
    buccal o.
    cardiac o.
    o. of coronary sinus
    duodenal o. of stomach
    epiploic o.
    esophagogastric o.
    o. of external acoustic
      meatus
    external urethral o.
    o. of female urethra, external
    gastroduodenal o.
    golf-hole ureteral o.
    hymenal o.
    o. of male urethra
    o. of maxillary sinus
    mitral o.
    pharyngeal o. of auditory
      tube
    pilosebaceous o's
    pulmonary o.
    o. of pulp canal
    pyloric o.
    tricuspid o.
    tympanic o.
    o. of ureter
    ureteral o.
    o. of urethra
    uterine o. of uterine tube
    o. of uterus
    o. of uterus, external
    vaginal o.
    vesicourethral o.
    o. of Vieussens
orificia (plural of orificium)
orificial angle
orificium (orificia)
    o. externum uteri
    o. hymenis
    o. internum uteri
    o. ureteris
    o. urethrae externum
      muliebris
    o. urethrae externum virilis
    o. urethrae internum
    o. vaginae
oriform
origin
orinotherapy
oris
orlistat
Ormond disease

O

Orn—ornithine
ornithine
    o. aminotransferase
    o. carbamoyl phosphate (OCP)
      deficiency
    o. carbamoyltransferase
    o. decarboxylase
    o.-keto-acid aminotransferase
    o. transcarbamoylase
    o.-transcarbamylase (OTC)
ornithinemia
Ornithodoros
    O. hermsii
    O. parkeri
    O. rudis
    O. talaje
Ornithonyssus
    O. bacoti
    O. bursa
    O. sylviarum
ornithosis
oroantral
orolingual
oromandibular
oromaxillary
oromeningitis
oronasal
oropharyngeal catheter
oropharynx
Oropsylla
    O. idahoensis
    O. montana
    O. silantiewi
orosomucoid
orotate phosphoribosyltransferase
  (OPRT)
orotic acid
orotidine 5′-phosphate
    o. decarboxylase (ODC)
    o. pyrophosphorylase
orotidine 5′-phosphate
  decarboxylase
orotidine 5′-phosphate
  pyrophosphorylase
orotidylate decarboxylase
orotidylic acid
orotracheal tube
Oroya fever
Orr
    incision
    method
    technique
    treatment
orrhomeningitis
orris

Orr-Loygue technique
ORS—orthopedic surgery
Orsi-Grocco method
orth; ortho—orthopedics
Orth
    solution
    stain
orthergasia
Orthicon camera
ortho-acid
ortho-aminoazotoluene
orthoarteriotony
orthobiosis
orthocardiac
orthocephalic
orthocephalous
orthochorea
orthochromatic
orthochromia
orthochromic
orthochromophil
orthocresol
orthocytosis
orthodactylous
orthodentin
orthodeoxia
orthodiagram
orthodiagraph
orthodiagraphy
orthodichlorobenzene
orthodigita
orthodontia
orthodontic
orthodontics
    corrective o.
    interceptive o.
    preventive o.
    prophylactic o.
    surgical o.
orthodontist
orthodromic
orthogenesis
orthogenics
orthoglycemic
orthognathia
orthognathic
orthognathous
orthogonal
orthograde
orthoiodohippurate
orthokeratosis
orthokinetics
orthomelic
orthometer
orthomolecular

orthomorphia
orthomyxovirus
orthoneutrophil
orthopantograph
orthopantomograph
orthopantomography
orthopedic
orthopedics
    dental o.
    dentofacial o.
    functional jaw o.
orthopedist
orthopercussion
orthophenanthroline
orthophony
orthophoria
    asthenic o.
orthophoric
orthophosphate
orthophosphoric acid
orthophrenia
orthopia
orthoplast jacket
orthoplessimeter
orthopnea
    three-pillow o.
    two-pillow o.
orthopneic
orthopraxy
orthopsychiatry
Orthoptera
orthoptic
orthoptics
orthoptist
orthoptoscope
orthoradioscopy
orthorhombic
orthoroentgenography
orthorrhachic
orthoscope
orthoscopic
orthoscopy
orthosis (orthoses)
    ankle-foot o. (AFO)
    balanced forearm o.
    dynamic o.
    Engen extension o.
    flexor hinge o.
    functional o.
    halo o.
    hip-knee-ankle-foot o. (HKAFO)
    hyperextension o.
    ischial weightbearing
      (weight-bearing) o.
    knee-ankle-foot o. (KAFO)

orthosis (orthoses) *(continued)*
    lumbosacral o. (LSO)
    opponens o.
    patellar tendon-bearing o.
    pneumatic o.
    poster o.
    resting o.
    serial stretch o's
    SOMI (sternal-occipital-
      mandibular immobilizer) o.
    spinal o.
    standing o.
    static o.
    therapeutic o.
    thoracolumbosacral o. (TLSO)
    Toronto Legg-Perthes o.
orthostatic hypotension
orthostatism
orthostereoscope
orthosympathetic
orthotherapy
orthotic
orthotics
orthotist
orthotonos
orthotopic
orthovoltage
orthuria
Ortolani
    click
    sign
    test
Oryza sativa
oryzenin
os (ora)
    o. externum uteri
    incompetent cervical o.
    Scanzoni second o.
    ora serrata retinae
    o. of uterus, external
os (ossa)
    o. acetabuli
    o. acromiale
    o. acromiale secondarium
    o. basilare
    o. breve
    o. calcis
    o. capitatum
    ossa carpalia
    ossa carpi
    o. centrale
    o. coccygis
    o. coronae
    o. costae
    o. costale

O

os (ossa) *(continued)*
　o. coxae
　ossa cranialia
　ossa cranii
　o. cuboideum
　o. cuneiforme
　ossa digitorum manus
　ossa digitorum pedis
　o. epitympanicum
　o. ethmoidale
　o. femorale
　ossa fonticulorum
　o. frontale
　o. hamatum
　o. hyoideum
　o. ilii
　o. incae
　o. incisivum
　o. innominatum
　o. intercuneiforme
　o. intermedium
　o. intermetatarseum
　o. interparietale
　o. irregulare
　o. ischii
　o. japonicum
　o. lacrimale
　o. longum
　o. lunatum
　o. magnum
　o. mastoideum
　ossa metacarpalia
　o. multangulum majus
　o. multangulum minus
　o. nasale
　o. naviculare
　o. novum
　o. occipitale
　o. odontoideum
　o. orbiculare
　o. palatinum
　o. parietale
　o. pedis
　o. pelvicum
　o. penis
　o. peroneum
　o. pisiforme
　o. planum
　o. pneumaticum
　o. priapi
　o. pubis
　o. radiale
　o. sacrale
　o. sacrum
　o. scaphoideum

os (ossa) *(continued)*
　o. sedentarium
　ossa sesamoidea manus
　ossa sesamoidea pedis
　o. sphenoidale
　o. styloideum
　o. subtibiale
　ossa suprasternalia
　o. suturale
　ossa tarsalia
　ossa tarsi
　o. tarsi fibulare
　o. tarsi tibiale
　o. temporale
　ossa thoracis
　o. tibiale externum
　o. tibiale posterius
　o. trapezium
　o. trapezoideum
　o. triangulare
　o. trigonum
　o. triquetrum
　o. unguis
　o. vesalianum pedis
　ossa Wormi
　o. zygomaticum
Os—osmium
OS—
　　left eye (L. oculus sinister)
　　opening snap
　　oral surgery
OSA—obstructive sleep apnea
OSAS—obstructive sleep apnea
　syndrome
osazone
Osbil
Osborne
　　operation
　　wave
Osborne and Folin method
oschea
oscheal
oscheitis
oschelephantiasis
oscheocele
oscheohydrocele
oscheolith
oscheoma
oscheoncus
oscheoplasty
oscillating Bucky
oscillation
　　bradykinetic o.
　　damped o.
oscillator

oscillogram
oscillograph
oscillometer
oscillometric
oscillometry
oscillopsia
oscilloscope
oscitate
oscitation
osculum
Osgood operation
Osgood-Haskins test
Osgood-Schlatter
    disease
    syndrome
OSHA—Occupational Safety and
  Health Administration
O'Shaughnessy forceps
Osiander sign
Osler
    disease
    nodes
    sign
    syndrome II
    triad
Osler-Vaquez disease
Osler-Weber-Rendu
    disease
    syndrome
Oslo
    breakfast
    meal
    study
OSM—oxygen saturation
  meter
osmate
osmatic
osmesis
osmesthesia
osmic
osmic acid
osmicate
osmics
osmidrosis
osmification
osmiophilic
osmiophobic
osmium (Os)
    o. tetroxide
osmoconformer
osmolal
osmolality
    calculated serum o.
    urine o.
osmolar

osmolarity
osmole (Osm)
osmology
osmolute
osmometer
    freezing-point o.
    Hepp o.
    membrane o.
osmometry
osmonosology
osmophilic
osmophobia
osmophore
osmoreceptor
osmoregulation
osmoregulator
osmoregulatory
osmoscope
osmose
osmosis
    reverse o.
osmosology
osmostat
osmotaxis
osmotherapy
osmotic
osone
osphresiology
osphresiometer
osphresis
osphretic
osphyarthrosis
osphyomyelitis
osphyotomy
ossa (plural of os)
ossature
ossein
osselet
osseoalbumoid
osseoaponeurotic
osseocartilaginous
osseofibrous
osseointegrated implant
osseointegration
osseoligamentous
osseomucin
osseomucoid
osseosonometer
osseosonometry
osseous
    o. syphilis
    o. yaws
ossicle
    Andernach o's
    auditory o.

O

ossicle *(continued)*
    o's of Bertin
    epactal o.
    episternal o's
    intercalcar o.
    Kerckring o.
    pterion o.
    Riolan o's
    sphenoturbinal o.
    wormian o's
ossicula (plural of ossiculum)
ossicular
    o. chain
    o. disarticulation
    o. system
ossiculectomy
ossiculoplasty
ossiculotomy
ossiculum (ossicula)
    ossicula auditoria
    ossicula auditus
ossiferous
ossific
ossificans
ossification
    cartilaginous o.
    ectopic o.
    endochondral o.
    heterotopic o.
    intramembranous o.
    membranous o.
    metaplastic o.
    perichondral o.
    periosteal o.
ossifluence
ossiform
ossify
ossifying
ossiphone
ossis
OST—object sorting test
osteal
ostealgia
osteanabrosis
osteanaphysis
ostearthrotomy
ostectomy
osteectopia
osteite
osteitic
osteitis
    acute o.
    o. albuminosa
    alveolar o.
    apical o.

osteitis *(continued)*
    benign necrotizing o. of
      external auditory meatus
    carious o.
    o. carnosa
    caseous o.
    central o.
    chronic o.
    chronic nonsuppurative o.
    o. condensans
    o. condensans generalisata
    o. condensans ilii
    condensing o.
    cortical o.
    o. deformans
    fibrocystic o.
    o. fibrosa
    o. fibrosa circumscripta
    o. fibrosa cystica
    o. fibrosa cystica
      generalisata
    o. fibrosa disseminata
    o. fibrosa localisata
    o. fibrosa osteoplastica
    formative o.
    o. fragilitans
    o. fungosa
    Garré o.
    o. granulosa
    gummatous o.
    hematogenous o.
    multifocal o. fibrosa
    necrotic o.
    o. ossificans
    pagetoid o.
    parathyroid o.
    pedal o.
    polycystic o.
    productive o.
    o. pubis
    rarefying o.
    sclerosing o.
    secondary hyperplastic o.
    o. tuberculosa cystica
    o. tuberculosa multiplex
      cystoides
    typhoid o.
    vascular o.
ostembryon
ostempyesis
osteoacusis
osteoanagenesis
osteoanesthesia
osteoaneurysm
osteoarthritic

osteoarthritis
    o. deformans
    o. deformans endemica
    endemic o.
    erosive o.
    hyperplastic o.
    hypertrophic o.
    interphalangeal o.
    ochronotic o.
    primary generalized
      hypertrophic o.
osteoarthropathy
    familial o. of fingers
    hypertrophic o., idiopathic
    hypertrophic pneumic o.
    hypertrophic o., primary
    hypertrophic pulmonary o.
    idiopathic hypertrophic o.
    pneumogenic o.
    primary hypertrophic o.
    pulmonary o.
    secondary hypertrophic o.
    tabetic o.
osteoarthrosis juvenilis
osteoarticular
osteoblast
osteoblastic
osteoblastoma
osteocachectic
osteocachexia
osteocampsia
osteocartilaginous
osteocele
osteocementum
osteochondral
osteochondritis
    adolescent o.
    calcaneal o.
    o. deformans juvenilis
    o. deformans juvenilis dorsi
    o. dissecans
    o. ischiopubica
    juvenile deforming
      metatarsophalangeal o.
    o. necroticans
    o. ossis metacarpi et metatarsi
    syphilitic o.
    o. of the tarsal navicular
osteochondroarthropathy
osteochondrodysplasia
osteochondrodystrophia deformans
osteochondrodystrophy
    o. deformans
    familial o.
osteochondrofibroma

osteochondrolysis
osteochondroma
    fibrosing o.
osteochondromatosis
    Ollier o.
    synovial o.
osteochondromyxoma
osteochondropathia
    cretinoidea
osteochondropathy
    polyglucose (dextran) sulfate–
      induced o.
osteochondrophyte
osteochondrosarcoma
osteochondrosis
    o. deformans tibiae
    o. dissecans
osteochondrous
osteoclasia
osteoclasis
osteoclast
    Collin o.
osteoclastic
osteoclastoma
osteocomma
osteocope
osteocopic
osteocranium
osteocystoma
osteocyte
osteodentin
osteodentinoma
osteodermia
osteodesmosis
osteodiastasis
osteodynia
osteodysplasia
osteodysplasty of Melnick and
  Needles
osteodystrophia
    o. cystica
    o. fibrosa
    o. juvenilis
osteodystrophy
    Albright hereditary o.
    azotemic o.
    parathyroid o.
    renal o.
osteoectasia
    familial o.
osteoepiphysis
osteofibrochondrosarcoma
osteofibroma
osteofibromatosis
    cystic o.

O

osteofibrosis
osteofluorosis
osteogen
osteogenesis
    endochondral o.
    o. imperfecta
      congenita (OIC)
    o. imperfecta cystica
    o. imperfecta tarda
      (OIT)
    o. imperfecta (OI),
      types I–IV
    periosteal o.
osteogenetic
osteogenic
osteogram
osteography
osteohalisteresis
osteohydatidosis
osteohypertrophic nevus
  flammeus
osteoid
osteoinduction
osteolipochondroma
osteolipoma
osteolith
osteologia
osteologist
osteology
osteolysis
osteolytic
osteoma
    cavalryman's o.
    compact o.
    o. cutis
    o. dentale
    o. durum
    o. eburneum
    ethmoid sinus o.
    frontal sinus o.
    giant osteoid o.
    ivory o.
    maxillary o.
    o. medullare
    osteoid o.
    o. sarcomatosum
    sphenoidal sinus o.
    o. spongiosum
    spongy o.
    trabecular o.
osteomalacia
    antacid-induced o.
    anticonvulsant o.
    familial
      hypophosphatemic o.

osteomalacia (continued)
    hepatic o.
    infantile o.
    juvenile o.
    osteogenic o.
    puerperal o.
    renal tubular o.
    senile o.
osteomalacic
osteomatoid
osteomatosis
osteomere
osteometry
osteomiosis
osteomyelitic
osteomyelitis
    chronic hemorrhagic o.
    chronic sclerosing o.
    conchiolin o.
    diffuse sclerosing o.
    focal sclerosing o.
    Garré o.
    salmonella o.
    sclerosing
      nonsuppurative o.
    tuberculous spinal o.
    typhoid o.
    o. variolosa
osteomyelodysplasia
osteomyelography
osteomyelosclerosis
osteon
osteonecrosis
osteonectin
osteoneuralgia
osteonosus
osteo-odontoma
osteopath
osteopathia
    o. condensans
    o. condensans disseminata
    o. condensans generalisata
    o. hemorrhagica infantum
    o. hyperostotica congenita
    o. hyperostotica multiplex
      infantilis
    o. striata
osteopathic manipulative therapy
  (OMT)
osteopathology
osteopathy
    alimentary o.
    disseminated condensing o.
    hunger o.
    myelogenic o.

osteopathy *(continued)*
    scorbutic o.
    starvation o.
osteopecilia
osteopedion
osteopenia
    hyperthyroid o.
osteopenic
osteoperiosteal
osteoperiostitis
    alveolodental o.
osteopetrosis
    o. gallinarum
    o. tarda
osteophage
osteophagia
osteophlebitis
osteophony
osteophyma
osteophyte
    bridging o's
osteophytosis
    spinal o.
    subperiosteal o.
osteoplaque
osteoplasia
osteoplast
osteoplastic frontal sinus
    operation
osteoplastica
    tracheopathia o.
osteoplasty
osteopoikilosis
osteopoikilotic
osteoporosis
    o. circumscripta cranii
    o. of disuse
    juxta-articular o.
    postmenopausal o.
    post-traumatic o.
    senile o.
osteoporotic
osteopsathyrosis
osteoradionecrosis
osteorrhagia
osteorrhaphy
osteosarcoma
    juxtacortical o.
    parosteal o.
    telangiectatic o.
osteosarcomatous
osteosclerosis
    o. congenita
    o. fragilis
    o. fragilis generalisata

osteosclerosis *(continued)*
    o. myelofibrosis
osteosclerotic
osteoscope
osteoseptum
osteosis
    o. cutis
    o. eburnisans
      monomelica
    ivory o.
    parathyroid o.
    renal o.
osteosuture
osteosynovitis
osteosynthesis
osteotabes
osteotelangiectasia
osteothrombophlebitis
osteothrombosis
osteotome
    Albee o.
    Alexander o.
    Blount o.
    Bowen o.
    Campbell o.
    Carroll o.
    Carroll-Legg o.
    Carroll-Smith-Petersen o.
    Cherry o.
    Clayton o.
    Cloward o.
    Cobb o.
    Converse o.
    Cottle o.
    Crane o.
    Dingman o.
    Epstein o.
    Frazier o.
    Hibbs o.
    Hoke o.
    Kezerian o.
    Lambotte o.
    Lambotte-Henderson o.
    Legg o.
    Leinbach o.
    Mayfield o.
    Meyerding o.
    Miner o.
    Moore o.
    New-Lambotte o.
    Rowland o.
    Sheehan o.
    Silver o.
    Smith-Petersen o.
    Stille o.

O

osteotomy
    angulation o.
    block o.
    chevron o.
    Coventry o.
    cuneiform o.
    cup-and-ball o.
    Dega pelvic o.
    displacement o.
    dome o.
    hinge o.
    innominate o.
    intertrochanteric o.
    Lapidus o.
    Le Fort o. (I–III)
    linear o.
    Lorenz o.
    Macewen o.
    Mitchell o.
    pelvic o.
    sagittal ramus o.
    sagittal split o.
    Salter o.
    sandwich o.
    segmental alveolar o.
    Southwick o.
    step o.
    subtrochanteric o.
    total maxillary o.
    transtrochanteric o.
    vertical ramus o.
    visor o.
    visor/sandwich o.
osteotribe, osteotrite
osteotrite
osteotrophy
osteotylus
osteotympanic
Ostertag-type amyloidosis
osthexia, osthexy
ostia (plural of ostium)
ostial
ostium (ostia)
    o. abdominale tubae
      uterinae
    o. aortae
    o. aorticum
    o. appendicis vermiformis
    o. arteriosum cordis
    o. atrioventriculare dextrum
    o. atrioventriculare
      sinistrum
    o. cardiacum
    o. commune
    coronary o.

ostium (ostia) *(continued)*
    o. ileocaecale
    o. ileocecale
    o. internum uteri
    o. maxillare
    persistent o. primum
    o. pharyngeum tubae
      auditivae
    o. pharyngeum tubae
      auditoriae
    o. primum
    o. primum defect
    o. pyloricum
    o. secundum
    o. secundum defect
    o. sinus coronarii
    sinusoidal o.
    sphenoid o.
    sphenoidal o.
    o. trunci pulmonalis
    o. tympanicum tubae
      auditivae
    o. ureteris
    o. urethrae externum
      femininae
    o. urethrae externum
      masculinae
    o. urethrae internum
    o. uteri
    o. uterinum tubae uterinae
    o. vaginae
    o. valvae ilealis
    o. venae cavae inferioris
    o. venae cavae superioris
    o. venarum pulmonalium
    o. venosum cordis
ostomate
-ostomy
    colostomy
    gastrostomy
    ileostomy
    jejunostomy
    neostomy
    proctostomy
    sigmoidostomy
    ureterostomy
    vesicostomy
ostosis
ostraceous
ostracosis
ostreotoxism
Ostrum-Furst syndrome
O'Sullivan
    operation
    retractor

O'Sullivan-O'Connor
    retractor
    speculum
OT—
    occlusion time
    occupational therapy
    old tuberculin
    original tuberculin
    orotracheal
    otolaryngology
otacoustic
otagra
otalgia
    o. dentalis
    geniculate o.
    o. intermittens
    referred o.
    reflex o.
    secondary o.
    tabetic o.
otalgic
OTC—
    ornithine transcarbamoylase
    over-the-counter
    oxytetracycline
OTD—organ tolerance dose
otic capsule
Otis
    anoscope
    bougie
    sound
    urethrotome
otitic barotrauma
otitis
    adhesive o. media
    aviation o.
    barotraumatic o.
    catarrhal o.
    o. crouposa
    o. desquamativa
    o. diphtheritica
    secretory o. media
    o. externa
    o. externa, circumscribed
    o. externa circumscripta
    o. externa diffusa
    o. externa, diffuse
    o. externa, furuncular
    o. externa furunculosa
    o. externa hemorrhagica
    o. externa, malignant
    o. externa mycotica
    exudative o. media
    furuncular o.
    o. haemorrhagica

otitis *(continued)*
    influenzal o.
    o. interna
    o. labyrinthica
    malignant o. externa
    malignant external o.
    o. mastoidea
    o. media
    o. media, adhesive
    o. media catarrhalis acuta
    o. media catarrhalis
      chronica
    o. media, purulent
    o. media purulenta acuta
    o. media purulenta
      chronica
    o. media sclerotica
    o. media, secretory
    o. media serosa
    o. media, serous
    o. media suppurativa
    o. media, suppurative
    o. media vasomotorica
    mucosis o.
    mucosus o.
    o. mycotica
    mycotic o. externa
    necrotizing o. externa
    necrotizing external o.
    necrotizing o. media
    parasitic o.
    pneumococcal o. media
    purulent o.
    o. sclerotica
    serous o. media
    traumatic o.
    tuberculous o. media
    suppurative o. media
otoacariasis
otoantritis
otobiosis
otoblennorrhea
otocephalus
otocephaly
otocerebritis
otocleisis
otoconia
otoconite
otoconium
otocranial
otocranium
otocyst
otodynia
otoencephalitis
otoganglion

O

otogenic
otogenous
otography
otolaryngologist
otolaryngology
otolith
otolith apparatus
otolithiasis
otologic
otologist
otology
otomastoiditis
otomicroscope
otomicroscopy
otomucormycosis
otomyasthenia
otomycosis aspergillina
otomyiasis
otoneuralgia
otoneurologic
otoneurology
otopharyngeal tube
otoplasty
    Crikelair o.
    Mustardé o.
    Mustarde flap o.
otopolypus
otopyorrhea
otopyosis
otorhinolaryngologist
otorhinolaryngology
otorhinology
otorrhagia
otorrhea
    cerebrospinal fluid o.
otosalpinx
otosclerosis
    clinical o.
    cochlear o.
    obliterative o.
otosclerotic
otoscope
    Bruening o.
    Brunton o.
    pneumatic o.
    Siegle o.
    Toynbee o.
    Welch-Allyn o.
otoscopy
    pneumatic o.
otosis
otospongiosis
otosteal
otosteon
ototomy

ototoxic
ototoxicity
OTR—Ovarian Tumor Registry
Ottenheimer dilator
Otto
    disease
    pelvis
OU—each eye
    (L. oculus uterque)
Ouchterlony method
Oudin
    current
    resonator
oulectomy
oulitis
ounce
    apothecary's o. (oz. ap.)
    o. avoirdupois (oz.)
    fluid o. (fl. oz.)
    liquid o. (liq. oz.)
    troy o. (oz. t.)
OURQ—outer upper right
    quadrant
outbreak
outbreeding
outcross
Outerbridge
    ridge
    scale
outflow
    o. channels
    craniosacral o.
    thoracolumbar o.
    o. tract murmur
outfracture
outgrowth
    spore o.
outlay
outlet
    marital o.
    pelvic o.
    thoracic o.
outlier
outlimb
outpatient
outpocket
outpocketing
outpouching
    cardiac o. (CO)
    energy o.
    urinary o.
output
    average acoustic power o.
    basal acid o. (BAO)
    cardiac o. (CO)

output *(continued)*
    energy o.
    insensible fluid o.
    maximal acid o. (MAO)
    peak acid o. (PAO)
    stroke o.
    urinary o.
    work o. of the heart
out-toeing
OV—office visit
oval
    o. esophagoscope
    o. window
ovalbumin
ovalocytary
ovalocyte
ovalocytosis
ovaria (plural of ovarium)
ovarian
    o. ablation
    o. agenesis
    o. amenorrhea
    o. artery
    atretic o. follicle
    o. cancer, o. carcinoma
    controlled o.
      hyperstimulation
    controlled o. stimulation
    o. cycle
    o. cyclicity
    o. cyst
    o. duct
    o. dysmenorrhea
    o. endometriosis
    o. fimbria
    o. follicle
    o. hernia
    o. hormones
    o. hyperstimulation
      syndrome
    o. ligament
    o. pregnancy
    premature o. failure
    o. remnant syndrome
    o. reserve
    o. seminoma
    o. steroid
    o. stroma
    o. stromal hyperplasia
    o. tubes
    o. tumor
    o. varicocele
    o. vein syndrome
ovaricus
ovaries (plural of ovary)

ovariocele
ovariocentesis
ovariocyesis
ovariodysneuria
ovarioepilepsy
ovariogenic
ovariolytic
ovariopexy
ovariorrhexis
ovariosteresis
ovariotestis (ovotestis)
ovariotomy
    abdominal o.
    Beatson o.
    vaginal o.
ovarium (ovaria)
    o. bipartitum
    o. gyratum
    o. lobatum
    o. masculinum
ovary (ovaries)
    adenocystic o.
    embryonic o.
    oyster o's
    polycystic o.
OVD—occlusal vertical
  dimension
over-and-over suture
overbite
    deep o.
    horizontal o.
    vertical o.
overbreathing
overclosure
    reduced interarch
      distance o.
overcompensation
overcorrection
overdenture
overdetermination
overdominance
overdosage
overdose (OD)
overdrive
overeruption
overexposure
overextension
overflexion
overflow
overgraft
overgrafting
overgrowth
    bony o.
    candidal o.
    fungal o.

O

overgrowth *(continued)*
    yeast o.
overhang
Overholt
    elevator
    operation
Overholt-Jackson
  bronchoscope
overhydration
overinflation
    nonobstructive
      pulmonary o.
    obstructive pulmonary o.
overjet
overjut
overlap
    horizontal o.
    vertical o.
overlapping
    o. sutures
    o. shadow
overlay
    emotional o.
    psychogenic o.
overload
    aortic o.
    circulatory o.
    iron o.
overnutrition
overprotection
    maternal o.
overreaching
overresponse
overriding
overshooting
overstain
overstimulation
overstrain
Overstreet forceps
overstress
overt
over-the-counter medications
overtoe
overtone
    psychic o.
overtransfusion
overtube
    Christopher-Williams o.
overventilation
overvoltage
overweight
ovi (genitive of ovum)
ovicide
oviducal
oviduct

oviductal
oviferous
oviform
ovigenesis
ovigenetic
ovigenic
ovigenous
ovigerm
ovigerous
ovine
ovinia
oviparity
oviparous
oviposit
oviposition
ovipositor
ovisac
ovist
ovum
ovocyte
ovoflavin
ovogenesis
ovoglobulin
ovogonium
ovoid
    fetal o.
    Manchester o.
ovolytic
ovomucin
ovomucoid
ovoplasm
ovotestis
ovotransferrin
ovovitellin
ovoviviparity
ovoviviparous
ovula
ovular
ovulate
ovulation
    amenstrual o.
    anestrous o.
    paracyclic o.
    supplementary o.
ovulatory
ovule
    graafian o's
    Naboth o.
    primitive o.
    primordial o.
ovulogenous
ovulum (ovula)
ovum (ova)
    blighted o.
    Bryce-Teacher o.

ovum (ova) *(continued)*
    fertilized o.
    o. forceps
    Hertig-Rock ova
    holoblastic o.
    Mateer-Streeter o.
    meroblastic o.
    Miller o.
    permanent o.
    primitive o.
    primordial o.
    Rock ova
    unfertilized o.
O/W—oil in water
Owen
    catheter
    contour lines
    operation
    view
Owren
    deficiency
    disease
oxalaldehyde
oxalate
    ammonium o.
    balanced o.
    calcium o.
    potassium o.
oxalated
oxalation
oxalemia
oxalic acid
oxalism
oxaloacetate
oxaloacetic acid
oxalosis
oxalosuccinate
oxalosuccinic acid
oxaluria
oxaluric acid
oxalyl
oxalylurea
oxamide
ox cell hemolysin test
Oxford operation
oxgall
oxidant
    direct o.
    indirect o.
    primary o.
oxidase
    direct o. (oxygenase)
    indirect o. (peroxidase)
    mixed function o.
    primary o.

oxidase *(continued)*
    xanthine o.
oxidation
    aerobic o.
    anaerobic o.
    beta o.
    biological o.
    coupled o.
    omega o.
oxidation-reduction
oxidative
oxide
    arsenous o.
    diethyl o.
    stannic o.
oxidizable
oxidize
oxidoreductase
oxidoreduction
oxidosis
oxime
oximeter
    ear o.
    finger o.
    intracardiac o.
    pulse o.
    whole blood o.
oximetry
    finger o.
    pulse o.
oxim, oxime
oxoacid
oxo-acid-lyase
3-oxoacyl-ACP reductase
3-oxoacyl-ACP synthase
oxogestone phenpropionate
oxoglutarate dehydrogenase
    (succinyl-transferring)
2-oxoglutaric acid
2-oxoisovalerate dehydrogenase
    (lipoamide)
oxolinic acid
oxonium
5-oxoprolinase
    (ATP hydrolyzing)
5-oxoproline
5-oxoprolinuria
oxyachrestia
oxybenzene
oxybenzoic acid
oxyblepsia
oxybutyria
oxybutyricacidemia
oxycalorimeter
oxycephalic

O

oxycephaly
oxychloride
oxychlorosene sodium
oxycholine
oxychromatic
oxychromatin
oxycinesia
oxycyanide
oxydendron
oxyecoia
oxyesthesia
oxyetherotherapy
oxygen (O)
    blow-by o.
    o. carrier
    o. cisternography
    excess o.
    heavy o.
    high-pressure o.
    hyperbaric o. (HBO)
    molecular o.
    o. myelography
    nasal o.
    singlet o.
    o. therapy
    T-piece o.
oxygenase
oxygenate
oxygenated
oxygenation
    apneic o.
    extracorporeal membrane o.
      (ECMO)
    hyperbaric o.
oxygenator
    bubble o.
    disk o.
    film o.
    membrane o.
    pump-o.
    rotating-disk o.
    screen o.
oxygenic
oxygeusia
oxyhematin
oxyhematoporphyrin
oxyheme
oxyhemochromogen
oxyhemocyanine
oxyhemoglobin
    (HbO$_2$ [HBO2])
oxyhydrocephalus
oxyhyperglycemia
oxyiodide

oxylalia
oxymetholone
oxymyoglobin
oxymyohematin
oxynervon
oxyneurine
oxyntic
oxyopia
oxyopter
oxyosis
oxyosmia
oxyosphresia
oxyparaplastin
oxypathia
oxypathy
oxyphenylethylamine
oxyphil
oxyphilic
oxyphonia
oxyplasm
oxypurine
oxyrhine
oxysalt
oxyspore
oxytalan
oxytalanolysis calcium
oxytocia
oxytocic
oxytocin
    arginine o.
    o. challenge test (OCT)
    o. citrate
oxytocinase
oxytropism
oxyuriasis
oxyuricide
oxyurid
oxyurifuge
Oxyuris
    O. equi
    O. incognita
    O. vermicularis
oz.—ounce (avoirdupois)
Oz
    O. antigen
    O. isotypic determinant
oz. ap.—apothecary's ounce
ozena laryngis
ozenous
ozone
ozonometer
ozonophore
ozostomia
oz. t.—troy ounce

π—pi (Greek letter)
φ—phi (Greek letter; alphabetized as ph)
ρ—rho (Greek letter; alphabetized as r)
p—
    pico- [prefix]
    probability
    proton
    short arm of a chromosome
P—
    para
    partial
    phosphate
    phosphorus
    plasma
    position
    posterior
    postpartum
    premolar
    presbyopia
    pressure
    primipara
    protein
    pulse
    pupil
P.—
    Pasteurella
    Plasmodium
    Proteus
P—power
P_1—pulmonic first sound
P_2—pulmonic second sound
p24 antigen test
pA—picoampere
Pa—
    pascal(s)
    protactinium
PA—
    paralysis agitans
    pernicious anemia
    phakic-aphakic
    posteroanterior
    primary amenorrhea
    pulmonary artery
    pulpoaxial
PA; P.A.—physician's assistant
P&A—percussion and auscultation
Paas disease
PABA—*p*-aminobenzoic acid [p-, para-]
PAC—
    papular acrodermatitis of childhood

PAC— *(continued)*
    pericarditis, arthropathy, camptodactyly (syndrome)
    phenacetin, aspirin, caffeine
    premature atrial contraction
Pacchioni
    foramen
    fossae
    granulations
pacchionian
    p. corpuscles
    p. depressions
    p. foramen
    p. glands
    p. granula
    p. granulations
Pace knife
pacemaker
    AAI p.
    AAIR p.
    AAT p.
    Amtech-Killeen p.
    antitachycardia p.
    AOO p.
    Arco p.
    artificial p.
    artificial cardiac p.
    asynchronous p.
    asynchronous atrial p.
    asynchronous ventricular p.
    atrial asynchronous p.
    atrial demand inhibited p.
    atrial demand triggered p.
    atrial synchronous ventricular p.
    atrial synchronous ventricular inhibited p.
    Atricor p.
    atrioventricular junctional p.
    atrioventricular sequential p.
    automatic p.
    AV sequential p.
    bifocal demand p.
    Biotronik p.
    bipolar p.
    cardiac p.
    p. catheter
    Chardack-Greatbatch p.
    Coratomic p.
    Cordis p.
    Cordis Atricor p.
    Cordis-Ectocor p.
    Cordis fixed-rate p.

pacemaker *(continued)*
 Cordis Ventricor p.
 CPI Maxilith p.
 CPI Minilith p.
 Cyberlith p.
 DDD p.
 DDDR p.
 DDI p.
 demand p.
 diaphragmatic p.
 dual chamber p.
 DVI p.
 Ectocor p.
 ectopic p.
 Electrodyne p.
 electronic p.
 electrophrenic p.
 endocardial bipolar p.
 epicardial p.
 escape p.
 external p.
 fixed-rate p.
 fully automatic p.
 gastric p.
 General Electric p.
 p. of heart
 implantable p.
 implanted p.
 internal p.
 junctional p.
 latent p.
 lithium p.
 Nathan p.
 nuclear p.
 Omni-Atricor p.
 Omni-Ectocor p.
 Omni-Stanicor p.
 phrenic p.
 radio frequency p.,
  radiofrequency p.
 rate responsive p.
 runaway p.
 secondary p.
 shifting p.
 single chamber p.
 Spectrax programmable
  Medtronic p.
 Stanicor p.
 Starr-Edwards p.
 synchronous p.
 transthoracic p.
 transvenous p.
 unipolar p.
 universal p.
 uterine p.

pacemaker *(continued)*
 VAT p.
 VDD p.
 Ventricor p.
 ventricular p.
 ventricular asynchronous p.
 ventricular demand inhibited p.
 ventricular demand triggered p.
 VOO p.
 VVI p.
 VVIR p.
 VVT p.
 wandering p.
 wandering atrial p.
 Zoll p.
 Zyrel p.
 Zytron p.
pachyblepharon
pachyblepharosis
pachycephalia
pachycephalic
pachycephaly
pachycheilia
pachychromatic
pachydactyly
pachyderma
 p. lymphangiectatica
 p. vesicae
pachydermatocele
pachydermatous eosinophilic
 dermatitis
pachydermia
 laryngeal contact p.
 p. laryngis
 lymphangiectatic p.
 posterior hypertrophic p.
  of larynx
 p. verrucosa laryngis
pachydermic
 p. bullous skin
 p. skin
pachydermoperiostosis plicata
pachyglossia
pachygnathous
pachygyria
pachyleptomeningitis
pachymeninges
pachymeningitis
 cerebral p.
 p. cervicalis hypertrophica
 circumscribed p.
 external p.
 fibrinohemorrhagic p.
 hemorrhagic internal p.
 hypertrophic spinal p.

pachymeningitis *(continued)*
    internal p.
    p. intralamellaris
    purulent p.
    pyogenic p.
    serous internal p.
    spinal p.
    suppurative p.
    syphilitic p.
    syphilitic hyperplastic p.
    syphilitic hypertrophic p.
pachymeningopathy
pachymeninx (pachymeninges)
pachynsis
pachyntic
pachyonychia congenita
pachypelviperitonitis
pachyperiosteoderma
pachyperiostitis
pachyperitonitis
pachypleuritis
pachysalpingitis
pachysalpingo-ovaritis
pachytene
pachyvaginalitis
pachyvaginitis
    cystic p.
pacifier
pacing
    atrial p.
    cardiac p.
    diaphragm p.
    endocardial p.
    epicardial p.
    overdrive p.
    paired p.
    programmed p.
    sequential p.
    ventricular p.
pacinian
Pacini corpuscle
pack
    Bellow p.
    cold p.
    dry p.
    full p.
    half p.
    hot p.
    ice p.
    internuclear p.
    lap p.
    Mikulicz p.
    one sheet p.
    oropharyngeal p.
    partial p.

pack *(continued)*
    periodontal p.
    salt p.
    surgical p.
    three-quarters p.
    throat p.
    wet p.
    wet-sheet p.
packer
packing
    denture p.
    p. fraction
    Gelfoam p.
    iodoform gauze p.
    vaginal p.
pack-year
$PaCO_2$ [PaCO2]— partial pressure of carbon dioxide
pad
    abdominal p.
    Bichat fat p.
    buccal fat p.
    butterfly p.
    fat p.
    gum p's
    infrapatellar fat p.
    knuckle p's
    occlusal p.
    Passavant p.
    periarterial p.
    retrodiscal p.
    retromolar p.
    retropatellar fat p.
    synovial fat p.
Padgett
    dermatome
    graft
Paecilomyces
paecilomycosis
PAF—
    platelet-activating factor
    pulmonary arteriovenous fistula
PAFD—percutaneous abscess and fluid drainage
PAFib—paroxysmal atrial fibrillation
PAGE—polyacrylamide gel electrophoresis
Pagenstecher operation
Paget
    abscess
    abscess syndrome
    cell
    disease

Paget *(continued)*
  disease of bone
  disease of the nipple
  disease of penis
  juvenile syndrome
  mammary disease
  quiet necrosis
  syndrome (I)
  test
pagetic
  p. bones
  p. changes
  p. lesions
  p. lymphocytes
  p. monocytes
  p. osteoblasts
  p. osteosarcoma
  p. spinal stenosis
pagetic-like bone lesions
pagetoid
  p. Bowen disease
  p. cells
  p. cutaneous neoplasm
  p. dyskeratosis
  p. infiltration
  p. intraepidermal spread
  p. melanocytes
  p. melanomas
  p. neoplasm
  p. reticulosis
  p. reticulosis of
    Woringer-Kolopp
  p. spread
  p. squamous cell carcinoma
Paget-von Schroetter syndrome
pagophagia
PAH—
  p-aminohippurate [p-, para-]
  pulmonary artery hypertension
PAHA—*p*-aminohippuric acid
  [p-, para-]
Pahvant Valley
  fever
  plague
PAI—plasminogen activator
  inhibitor
PAIDS—pediatric AIDS
pain
  atypical facial p.
  bearing-down p.
  boring p.
  Brodie p.
  central p.
  Charcot p's
  cross-referred p.

pain *(continued)*
  dilating p's
  eccentric p.
  evoked contralateral p.
  expulsive p's
  false p's
  fulgurant p's
  gas p's
  girdle p.
  growing p's
  heterotopic p.
  homotopic p.
  hunger p.
  intermenstrual p.
  jumping p.
  labor p's
  lancinating p.
  lightning p's
  middle p.
  nerve p.
  phantom limb p.
  piercing p.
  postprandial p.
  precordial p.
  premonitory p's
  psychic p.
  psychogenic p.
  referred p.
  rest p.
  root p.
  shooting p's
  spot p's
  stabbing p.
  starting p's
  terebrant p.
  terebrating p.
  thalamic p.
  vasculosympathetic facial p.
  wandering p.
paint
  antiseptic p.
  Castellani p.
pairing
  base p.
  distributive p.
  exchange p.
  somatic p.
pajaroello tick
Pajot
  hook
  law
  maneuver
  method
PAL—posterior axillary line
palata (plural of palatum)

palatal
    p. elevator
    p. height index
    p. index
palate
    artificial p.
    p. bone
    bony p.
    bony hard p.
    cleft p.
    hard p.
    p. hook
    osseous p.
    pendulous p.
    pillars of soft p.
    premaxillary p.
    primary p.
    secondary p.
    smokers' p.
    soft p.
    submucous cleft p.
palati (genitive of palatum)
palatine
    anterior p. suture
    p. bone
    p. index
    median p. suture
    middle p. suture
    posterior p. suture
    transverse p. suture
palatitis
palatoethmoidal suture
palatoglossal
palatognathous
palatography
palatomaxillary
    p. index
    p. suture
palatomyography
palatonasal
palatopagus
palatopharyngeal incompetence
palatopharyngoplasty
palatoplasty
    coblation p.
    Furlow double-opposing Z-p.
    Kriens three-layer p.
    laser p.
    straight-line p.
    two-flap p.
    V-Y push-back p.
    Wardill-Kilner push-back p.
    Z-p.
palatoplegia
palatoproximal

palatorrhaphy
palatoschisis
palatum (palata)
    p. durum
    p. durum osseum
    p. fissum
    p. molle
    p. ogivale
    p. osseum
paleocerebellum
paleocortex
paleogenetic
paleopathology
paleosensation
paleostriatal syndrome
paleostriatum
paleothalamus
Palfyn suture
palikinesia
palilalia
palindrome
palindromic rheumatism
palingraphia
palinmnesis
palinopsia
palinphrasia
palisade
palladium (Pd)
pallanesthesia
pallesthesia
palliate
palliative
pallidal
    p. atrophy
    p. degeneration
    p. raphe nucleus
pallidectomy
pallidofugal fibers
pallidotomy
pallidum (pallida)
pallor
    buccal p.
    conjunctival p.
    cutaneous p.
    elevational p.
    optic disk p.
    optic nerve p.
    palmar p.
    temporal p.
palm
    p. of hand
    handball p.
    liver p.
    p. print
    tripe p.

P

palma (palmae)
    p. manus
    palmae plicatae
palmar
palmaris
palmate
palmature
Palmer
    dilator
    forceps
Palmer-Widen operation
palmital
palmitin
palmitoleic acid
palmitoyl-CoA hydrolase
palmomental reflex
palpable
palpate
palpation
    bimanual p.
    light touch p.
palpebra (palpebrae)
    p. inferior
    p. superior
    p. tertia
    tertius p.
palpebral
palpebralis
palpebrate
palpebration
palpebritis
palpitate
palpitation
palsy
    acute thyrotoxic bulbar p.
    atonic cerebral p.
    Bell p.
    bilateral cord p.
    birth p.
    brachial plexus p.
    bulbar p.
    cerebral p.
    craft p.
    cranial nerve p.
    creeping p.
    crossed leg p.
    diver's p.
    epidemic infantile p.
    Erb p.
    Erb-Duchenne p.
    facial p.
    hammer p.
    horizontal gaze p.
    hypotonic cerebral p.
    infantile cerebral p.
    infantile progressive bulbar p.

palsy *(continued)*
    inherited bulbar p.
    ischemic p.
    Klumpke p.
    Landry p.
    lateral popliteal p.
    lead p.
    minimal cerebral p.
    night p.
    occupational p.
    ocular p.
    painter's p.
    palate p.
    pharyngeal p.
    pressure p.
    printer's p.
    progressive supranuclear p.
    pseudobulbar p.
    radial p.
    Saturday night p.
    scrivener's p.
    shaking p.
    spastic bulbar p.
    supranuclear p.
    tardy median p.
    tardy ulnar p.
    Todd p.
    transverse p.
    ulnar p.
    unilateral cord p.
    wasting p.
Paltauf
    dwarf
    stain
PAM—
    phenylalanine mustard
    pulmonary alveolar
      macrophage(s)
    pyridine aldoxime methiodide
pampiniform
    p. body
    p. plexus
PAN—
    periodic alternating
      nystagmus
    polyarteritis nodosa
panacea
panacinar
panagglutinable
panagglutination
panagglutinin
panangiitis
    diffuse necrotizing p.
pananxiety
    analgesic p.
panarteritis nodosa

panarthritis
Panas operation
panatrophy
    Gowers p.
panautonomic
    p. dysfunction
    p. failure
    p. neuropathy
panbronchiolitis
pancake
    p. appearance
    p. compression
    p. flap
    p. kidney
    ^{13}C octanoic acid–labeled p.
       [carbon C 13]
pancarditis
    rheumatic p.
Pancoast
    operation
    suture
    syndrome
    tumor
pancolectomy
pancreas (pancreata)
    aberrant p.
    p. accessorium
    accessory p.
    annular p.
    divided p.
    p. divisum
    lesser p.
    unciform p.
    Willis p.
    Winslow p.
pancreatalgia
pancreatectomy
pancreatic
    acute p. necrosis
    p. artery
    p. autodigestion
    p. buds
    p. calculus
    p. cholera
    p. colic
    p. cyst
    p. diarrhea
    p. digestion
    p. diverticula
    p. duct
    p. enzyme therapy
    p. function test
    infectious p. necrosis
    p. juice
    p. lipase
    p. lithiasis

pancreatic *(continued)*
    p. lymph nodes
    p. notch
    p. oncofetal antigen
    p. panniculitis
    p. phlegmon
    p. pseudocyst
    p. rest
    p. sinus
    p. sphincter
    p. veins
pancreaticobiliary
    anomalous p. ductal union
    p. cancer
    p. cystic neoplasm
    p. junction
    p. malformation
    p. maljunction
    peroral retrograde p.
       ductography
    p. reflux
    p. stricture
    p. tract
    p. tree
pancreaticoduodenal
    p. arteries
    p. lymph nodes
    p. veins
pancreaticoduodenectomy
pancreaticoduodenostomy
pancreaticoenterostomy
pancreaticogastrostomy
pancreaticohepatic syndrome
pancreaticojejunostomy
pancreaticosplenic
    p. abscess
    p. ligament
    p. lymph nodes
pancreatin
pancreatis (genitive of pancreas)
pancreatitis
    acute p.
    acute hemorrhagic p.
    acute necrotic p.
    acute necrotizing p.
    calcareous p.
    centrilobar p.
    chronic p.
    chronic obstructive p.
    chronic relapsing p.
    edematous p.
    gallstone p.
    interstitial p.
    mumps p.
    perilobar p.
    purulent p.

P

pancreatoblastoma
pancreatoduodenectomy
pancreatoduodenostomy
pancreatoenterostomy
pancreatogenic
pancreatogenous fatty diarrhea
pancreatography
    endoscopic retrograde p.
pancreatolith
pancreatolithectomy
pancreatolithiasis
pancreatolithotomy
pancreatolysis
pancreatomegaly
pancreatopathy
pancreatoscopy
pancreatotomy
pancrelipase
pancreozymin
pancultured
pancytopenia
    aplastic p.
    congenital p.
    Fanconi p.
pandemic
Pander
    islands
    layer
    nucleus
pandiculation
Pándy
    reaction
    test
pandysautonomia
panel
    chemistry p.
    closed p.
    metabolic p.
    open p.
    patch p.
    urine drug p. (UDP)
panencephalitis
    Pette-Döring (Doering) p.
    subacute sclerosing p. (SSPE)
panendoscope
    cap-fitted p.
    French-McCarthy p.
    McCarthy Foroblique p.
    oral p.
panendoscopy
panesthesia
panesthetic
Paneth cells
pang
    breast p.
    brow p.

Pang forceps
panglossia
panhypogammaglobulinemia
panhypogonadism
panhypopituitarism
    prepubertal p.
panhysterectomy
panhystero-oophorectomy
panhysterosalpingectomy
panhysterosalpingo-oophorectomy
panic
    p. attack
    p. disorder
panimmunity
Panje
    voice button
    voice prosthesis
panmyeloid
panmyelopathy
    constitutional infantile p.
panmyelophthisis
panmyelosis
Panner disease
panneuritis epidemica
panneurosis
panniculectomy
panniculitis
    alpha$_1$-antitrypsin deficiency
        p. [alpha-1]
    calcifying p.
    cytophagic histiocytic p.
    eosinophilic p.
    factitial p.
    idiopathic nodular p.
    lipomembranous p.
    lobular p.
    lupus p.
    lupus erythematosus
      (LE) p.
    mesenteric p.
    nodular nonsuppurative p.
    pancreatic p.
    poststeroid p.
    relapsing febrile nodular
      nonsuppurative p.
    sclerosing p.
    septal p.
    subacute nodular migratory p.
    traumatic p.
    Weber-Christian p.
panniculus (panniculi)
    p. adiposus
    p. carnosus
    hanging p.
    p. morbidus
    overhanging p.

pannus
    degenerative p.
    glaucomatous p.
    periodontoid rheumatoid p.
      formation
    phlyctenular p.
    retro-odontoid p. formation
    p. siccus
    p. trachomatosus
panophthalmia
panophthalmitis
panoptic
pan-oral radiography
panoramic
    p. radiography
    p. tomography
Panorex
panosteitis
panotitis
panphobia
panproctocolectomy
panretinal photocoagulation
Pansch fissure
pansclerosis
pansensitive
panseptum
pansinuitis
pansinusectomy
pansinusitis
panspermia
panspermic
panspermy
pansystolic
    apical p. murmur
    diffuse, p. apical thrust
    harsh p. murmur
    loud p. murmur
    mild p. ejection murmur
    p. mitral regurgitation
    p. prolapse
    p. tricuspid valve
      regurgitation
pantalgia
pantaloon
    p. embolism
    p. hernia
pantanencephaly
pantankyloblepharon
pantatrophia
pantatrophy
pantetheine
panthodic
panting
pantograph
pantoic acid
pantomographic

pantomography
    concentric p.
    eccentric p.
pantothenate synthase
pantothenic acid
pantoyltaurine
pantropic virus
pants-over-vest repair
panturbinate
panuveitis
Panzer scissors
PaO_2 [PaO2]—partial pressure of
    oxygen (arterial pO_2)
PAO—peak acid output
PAOD—peripheral arteriosclerotic
    occlusive disease
Pap—Papanicolaou
PAP—
    peroxidase-antiperoxidase
    positive airway pressure
    primary atypical
      pneumonia
    prostatic acid phosphatase
    pulmonary alveolar
      proteinosis
    pulmonary artery
      pressure
Papanicolaou (Pap)
    smear
    stain
    test
Paparella tube
papaw, pawpaw
papaya
paper
    blue litmus p.
    Congo red p.
    filter p.
    indicator p.
    litmus p.
    potassium nitrate p.
    red litmus p.
    test p.
papilla (papillae)
    acoustic p.
    anal p.
    arcuate papillae of
      tongue
    Bergmeister p.
    bile p.
    calciform papillae
    capitate papillae
    circumvallate papillae
    clavate papillae
    papillae conicae
    conical papillae of tongue

P

papilla (papillae) *(continued)*
    p. corii
    p. of corium
    corolliform papillae of tongue
    dental p.
    dentinal p.
    p. dentis
    dermal p.
    p. dermatis
    p. dermis
    duodenal p.
    p. duodeni major
    p. duodeni minor
    p. duodeni Santorini
    filiform papillae
    papillae filiformes
    papillae foliatae
    foliate papillae
    fungiform papillae
    papillae fungiformes
    gingival p.
    p. gingivalis
    gustatory papillae
    hair p.
    ileal p.
    p. ilealis
    ileocecal p.
    p. incisiva
    incisive p.
    interdental p.
    p. interdentalis
    interproximal p.
    lacrimal p.
    p. lacrimalis
    lagenar p.
    lenticular papillae
    papillae lenticulares
    p. lentiformes
    lingual papillae
    papillae linguales
    major duodenal p.
    p. mammae
    mammary p.
    medial papillae of tongue
    minor duodenal p.
    p. of Morgagni
    nerve p.
    p. nervi optici
    obtuse papillae of tongue
    optic p.
    palatine p.
    parotid p.
    p. parotidea
    p. pili
    renal papillae

papilla (papillae) *(continued)*
    papillae renales
    retromolar p.
    p. of Santorini
    skin p.
    p. spiralis
    sublingual p.
    tactile papillae
    urethral p.
    papillae vallatae
    vallate papillae
    vascular p.
    p. of Vater
    villous papillae of tongue
papillary
papillate
papillation
papillectomy
papilledema
papilliferous
papilliform
papillitis
    necrotizing p.
    necrotizing renal p.
papilloadenocystoma
papillocarcinoma
papilloma
    bladder p.
    choroid plexus p.
    cutaneous p.
    ductal p.
    fibroepithelial p.
    hirsutoid p's of penis
    intracanalicular p.
    intracystic p.
    intraductal p.
    inverted p.
    inverted ductal p.
    inverted nasal p.
    inverted schneiderian p.
    p. of renal pelvis
    squamous p.
    squamous cell p.
    transitional cell p.
    villous p.
    p. virus
    vulvar p.
    warty p.
papillomacular bundle
papillomatosis
    confluent and reticulate p.
    juvenile laryngeal p.
    malignant p. of Degos
    recurrent respiratory p.
papillomatous

papillomavirus
    human p. (HPV)
Papillon-Lefèvre syndrome
papillopathy
    ischemic p.
papilloretinitis
papillosphincterotomy
papillotome
papillotomy
papillula
papovavirus
    lymphotropic p. (LPV)
Pappenheim
    hemoblast
    reagent
    stain
papular
    p. acne
    p. acrodermatitis
    p. amyloidosis
    p. angiodysplasia
    p. elastorrhexis
    p. mucinosis
    p. myxedema
    p. and nodular mucinosis
    p. rosacea
    p. urticaria
papulation
papule
    Gottron p's
    moist p.
    mucous p.
    painful piezogenic pedal p's
    pearly penile p.
    piezogenic p.
    prurigo p.
    pruritic urticarial p's and
      plaques of pregnancy
      (PUPPP)
    rheumatoid p's
    split p.
papuloerythematous
papuloerythroderma
    Ofuji p.
papuloid
papulonecrotic tuberculid
papulonodule
papulopustular
    p. acne
    p. rosacea
papulopustule
papulosis
    bowenoid p.
    lymphomatoid p.
    malignant atrophic p.

papulosquamous dermatoses
papulovesicle
papulovesicular
PAPVC—partial anomalous
    pulmonary venous connection
PAPVR—partial anomalous
    pulmonary venous return
papyraceous
    fetus p.
    villous p.
PAR—
    postanesthesia room
    pulmonary arteriolar
      resistance
para-aminobenzoate (PAB)
para-aminobenzoic acid (PABA)
    [p-, p-]
para-aminohippuric acid
    (PAH, PAHA)
para-aminohippuric acid
    synthetase
para-analgesia
para-anesthesia
para-aortic
    p. bodies
    p. fields
para-appendicitis
parabanic acid
parabulia
paracardiac
paracenesthesia
paracentesis
    abdominal p.
paracentetic
paracentral
paracerebellar
paracervical
paracervix
parachordal
    p. cartilages
    p. plate
paraclinical
paraclonus
Paracoccidioides brasiliensis
paracoccidioidomycosis
paracolic
    p. abscess formation
    p. adhesiolysis
    p. adhesions
    p. arcade
    p. fat plane
    p. gutter
    p. hernia
    p. lymph nodes
    p. mass

P

paracolic *(continued)*
  p. space
  p. sulcus
paracolpitis
paracolpium
paracortex
paracostal incision
paracoxalgia
paracrine
paracusia
  p. loci
  p. willisiana
paracusis of Willis
paracystic
paracystitis
paracystium
paradental
  p. cyst
  inflammatory p. cyst
paradentitis
paradentium
paradentosis
paradidymal
paradidymis
paradimethylaminobenzaldehyde
paradipsia
paradontosis
paradox
  neurotic p.
  Opie p.
  Weber p.
paradoxic, paradoxical
paradoxus
  pulsus p.
paraeccrisis
paraepilepsy
paraesophageal
parafalx
paraffin
  p. dressing
  p. section
paraffinoma
parafoveal
parafunction
parafunctional
paraganglioma
  medullary p.
  nonchromaffin p.
paraganglion (paraganglia)
  adrenergic p.
  aortic p.
  cardiac p.
  cholinergic p.
paragenitalis
parageusia

parageusic
paragglutination
paraglossia
paraglottic
  p. space
  p. space invasion
  p. tissues
paragnathus
paragnosis
paragonimiasis
parahemophilia
parahepatic
  p. arteriovenous malformation
  p. space
parahormone
para-hydroxyphenylpyruvic acid
  (PHPPA)
parahypnosis
parahypophysis
parainfectious
parainfluenza
parainfluenzal
parainguinal incision
parakeratinized
parakeratosis
  granular p.
  p. pustulosa
  p. variegata
parakinesia
parakinetic
paralalia literalis
paraldehyde
paralexia
paralexic
  neglect p. error
  p. response
  visual p. error
paralgesia
paralgesic
parallactic
parallagma
parallax
  binocular p.
  crossed p.
  direct p.
  heteronymous p.
  homonymous p.
  p. method
  stereoscopic p.
  uncrossed p.
  vertical p.
parallel
  p. attachment
  p. fibers
  p. grid

parallel *(continued)*
    p. rays
    Retzius p. striae
parallergic reaction
parallergy
paralogia
    thematic p.
paralogism
paralogy
paralysis (paralyses)
    abducens p.
    abducens-facial p., congenital
    p. of accommodation
    acute ascending spinal p.
    acute spinal p.
    p. agitans
    alcoholic p.
    alternate p.
    alternating p.
    anesthesia p.
    ascending p.
    association p.
    atrophic p.
    atrophic spinal p.
    Avellis p.
    axillary nerve p.
    Bell p.
    bilateral p.
    birth p.
    brachial p.
    brachial plexus p.
    brachiofacial p.
    Brown-Séquard p.
    bulbar p.
    central p.
    central facial p.
    centrocapsular p.
    cerebral p.
    cerebral spastic infantile p.
    common peroneal nerve p.
    complete p.
    compression p.
    congenital abducens-facial p.
    congenital p. of horizontal gaze
    conjugate p.
    crossed p.
    cruciate p.
    crural p.
    crutch p.
    cubital p.
    decubitus p.
    diaphragmatic p.
    diver's p.
    Duchenne p.
    Duchenne-Erb p.

paralysis (paralyses) *(continued)*
    Erb p.
    Erb-Duchenne p.
    facial p.
    false p.
    familial hyperkalemic
      periodic p.
    familial hypokalemic
      periodic p.
    familial periodic p.
    familial spastic p.
    femoral nerve p.
    flaccid p.
    functional p.
    p. of gaze
    general p.
    glossolabial p.
    glossopharyngolabial p.
    hereditary cerebrospinal p.
    hyperkalemic periodic p.
    hypoglossal p.
    hypokalemic periodic p.
    hysterical p.
    idiopathic p.
    idiopathic facial p.
    immune p.
    immunologic p.
    incomplete p.
    infantile p.
    infantile cerebral ataxic p.
    infantile cerebrocerebellar
      diplegic p.
    infantile spinal p.
    ischemic p.
    juvenile p.
    Klumpke p.
    labial p.
    labioglossolaryngeal p.
    labioglossopharyngeal p.
    laryngeal p.
    laryngeal abductor p.
    lead p.
    lingual p.
    local p.
    masticatory p.
    median p.
    medullary tegmental
      paralyses
    mimetic p.
    mixed p.
    motor p.
    muscular p.
    musculospiral p.
    myopathic p.
    neurogenic p.

P

paralysis (paralyses) *(continued)*
  normokalemic periodic p.
  nuclear p.
  obstetric p.
  obturator nerve p.
  ocular p.
  oculomotor p.
  organic p.
  palatal p.
  parturient p.
  periodic p.
  peripheral p.
  peroneal p.
  pharyngeal p.
  phonetic p.
  phrenic p.
  posticus p.
  progressive p.
  progressive bulbar p.
  pseudobulbar p.
  pseudohypertrophic muscular p.
  radial p.
  recurrent laryngeal nerve p.
  reflex p.
  sensory p.
  serratus anterior p.
  sleep p.
  spastic p.
  spastic spinal p.
  spinal p.
  spinomuscular p.
  superior laryngeal nerve p.
  supranuclear p.
  thyrotoxic periodic p.
  tick p.
  Todd p.
  tourniquet p.
  trigeminal p.
  ulnar nerve p.
  unilateral p.
  unilateral vocal cord p.
  vagal p.
  vasomotor p.
  vocal cord p.
  vocal fold p.
  wasting p.
  writer's p.
paralytic
  p. drug
  p. ectropion
  p. hip subluxation
  p. ileus
  p. lagophthalmos
  p. mydriasis
  partially p.

paralytic *(continued)*
  p. rabies
  p. shellfish poisoning
paralytogenic
paralyzant
paralyze
paralyzer
paramagnetic
  electron p. resonance
paramastitis
paramastoid
paramastoiditis
parameatal
paramedial
paramedian
  p. approach
  p. disk protrusion
  p. forehead flap
  p. herniation
  p. incision
  p. interfascial approach
  p. midbrain-thalamic infarction
  p. palate
  p. pontine infarction
  p. pontine tegmentum
    infarction
  p. sectoriectomy
  shallow-angle p. oblique
    catheter insertion
  p. thalamic stroke
paramedic
paramedical
paramenia
parameningeal
parameniscitis
parameniscus
parameter
  pharmacokinetic p's
parametria
parametrial
  p. cervical intraepithelial
    neoplasia
  p. disease
  p. excision
  p. extension
  p. invasion
  p. involvement
  p. lymph nodes
  p. mass
  p. metastases
  p. resection
  p. tissues
  p. tumor spread
parametrismus
parametritic

parametritis
    anterior p.
    posterior p.
parametrium
parametropathy
paramimia
paramnesia
paramolar
paramuscular incision
paramusia
paramyloidosis
paramyoclonus multiplex
paramyotonia
    ataxia p.
    p. congenita
    symptomatic p.
paramyotonus
paranalgesia
paranasal
paraneoplasia
paraneoplastic
    p. cerebellar degeneration
    p. Cushing syndrome
    p. dermatoses
    p. inflammatory neuropathy
    p. myelopathy
    p. opsoclonus-myoclonus
      syndrome
    p. optic neuropathy (PON)
    p. pemphigus
    p. retinopathy
    p. rheumatic disorder
    p. Sweet syndrome
    p. syndrome
paranephric
    p. abscess
    p. extension of renal abscess
    p. fasciae
    p. fat
    p. fluid collection
    p. lymph nodes
    progressive p. pseudotumor
    p. space
    p. water instillation
paranephritis
    lipomatous p.
paranephroma
paraneural
paranoia
    alcoholic p.
    amorous p.
    heboid p.
    litigious p.
    p. querulans
    querulous p.

paranoia *(continued)*
    p. simplex
    social p.
paranoiac
paranoic
    p. behavior
    p. hallucinatory psychosis
    p. hallucinatory state
    p. reaction
    p. state
paranoid
    p. delusions
    p. ideation
    p. personality disorder
    p. phantasies
    p. schizophrenia
    p. thinking
paranomia
    visual p.
paranormal
paranuclear
paranucleolus
paranucleus (paranuclei)
paraomphalic
paraoperative
paraoral
paraovarian
parapancreatic
paraparesis
    spastic p.
paraparetic
parapatellar
    p. arthrotomy
    p. incision
    medial p. approach
    p. portal
parapedesis
paraperitoneal nephrectomy
parapertussis
parapharyngeal
paraphasia
    central p.
    literal p.
    verbal p.
paraphasic
paraphemia
paraphenylenediamine
paraphernalia
paraphia
paraphilia
paraphiliac
paraphimosis
paraphobia
paraphonia puberum
paraphora

P

paraphrasia
paraphrenia
    p. confabulans
    p. expansiva
    involutional p.
    late p.
    p. phantastica
    p. systematica
paraphrenic
paraphyseal
paraphysis
parapineal
paraplasm
paraplasmic
paraplastic
paraplastin
paraplegia
    alcoholic p.
    ataxic p.
    cerebral p.
    cervical p.
    congenital spastic p.
    Erb spastic p.
    Erb syphilitic spastic p.
    familial spastic p.
    flaccid p.
    functional p.
    hereditary spastic p.
    hysterical p.
    infantile spastic p.
    peripheral p.
    Pott p.
    reflex p.
    senile p.
    South Indian p.
    spastic p.
    spastic p., congenital
    spastic p., infantile
    spastic p., primary
    p. superior
    syphilitic p.
    toxic p.
paraplegia-in-extension
paraplegia-in-flexion
paraplegic
paraplegiform
parapleuritis
parapneumonia
parapophysis
parapraxia
parapraxis (parapraxes)
paraproctitis
paraproctium
paraprofessional
paraprostatitis

paraprotein
paraproteinemia
parapsoriasis (parapsoriases)
    p. acuta
    acute p.
    atrophic p.
    p. atrophicans
    chronic p.
    p. en plaques
    p. guttata
    guttate p.
    large-plaque p.
    p. lichenoides
    p. lichenoides chronica
    p. maculata
    poikilodermatous p.
    poikilodermic p.
    retiform p.
    small-plaque p.
    p. variegata
    p. varioliformis
    p. varioliformis acuta
    p. varioliformis chronica
parapsychology
parapsychosis
parapyknomorphous
parapyle
parapyramidal
paraquat
parareaction
pararectal
    p. approach
    p. cavitary lesion
    p. fascial
    p. fossa
    p. hematoma
    p. incision
    p. lymph nodes
    p. mass
    p. paraganglioma
    p. space
    p. tumor
pararectus incision
parareflexia
pararenal
    p. aneurysm
    anterior p. space
    p. aortic aneurysm
    p. hyaline-vascular–type
      Castleman disease
    posterior p. space
    p. retroperitoneal space
    p. urinoma
pararosaniline pamoate
pararrhythmia

pararthria
parasacral
    p. abscess
    p. approach
    p. block
    p. electrical stimulation
    p. hernia
    p. injection
    p. sciatic nerve block
    p. sphincteroplasty
    p. transsphincteric approach
parasagittal
    p. cortex
    p. craniotomy
    p. distribution
    p. incision
    p. interlaminar epidural
      approach
    p. lesion
    p. meningioma
    p. plane
    p. region
    p. watershed territory
parasalpingeal
parasalpingitis
parascapular
    p. fasciocutaneous free flap
    p. flap graft
    free p. flap
    p. free tissue transfer
    free vascular p. graft
    p. incision
    p. musculature
parasecretion
parasellar
parasexual
parasexuality
parasinoidal
parasinusoidal
parasite
    accidental p.
    allantoic p.
    animal p.
    autochthonous p.
    cytozoic p.
    diheteroxenic p.
    ectophytic p.
    ectozoic p.
    endophytic p.
    entozoic p.
    eurytrophic p.
    facultative p.
    false p.
    hematozoic p.
    incidental p.

parasite *(continued)*
    intermittent p.
    karyozoic p.
    malarial p.
    obligate p.
    obligatory p.
    occasional p.
    periodic p.
    permanent p.
    specific p.
    spurious p.
    stenotrophic p.
    temporary p.
    teratoid p.
parasitemia
parasitic
parasiticidal
parasiticide
parasitifer
parasitism
    extracellular p.
    intracellular p.
    multiple p.
parasitization
parasitize
parasitoid
parasitologist
parasitology
parasitosis
parasitotropic
parasomnia
paraspadias
paraspasm
paraspasmus faciale
paraspecific
paraspinal
paraspinous
parasplenic
    p. abscess
    p. lymph nodes
    p. lymphoma
parasternal
    p. acquisition
    p. approach
    p. displacement
    p. echocardiogram
    p. incision
    p. intercostal ropivacaine block
    p. leads
    p. long-axis view
    p. lymph nodes
    p. muscles
    p. sentinel nodes
    p. short-axis view
    p. window

P

parastriate
parasuicide
parasympathetic
parasympathicotonia
parasympatholytic
parasympathomimetic
parasympathoparalytic
parasynovitis
parasystole
parataxic distortion
paratenic host
paratenon
paraterminal body
paratesticular
parathion-methyl
parathormone (PTH)
parathymia
parathyroid
parathyroidal
parathyroidectomize
parathyroidectomy (PTX)
parathyroidoma
parathyromatosis
parathyropathy
parathyrotropic
paratonia
paratonic
paratonsillar
    p. glands
    p. secretory glands
    p. space
paratope
paratose
paratrachoma
paratrophic
paratrophy
paratubal
    p. cyst
    p. neoplasm
paratuberculosis
paratuberculous
paratype
paratyphi
    Salmonella p. A, B, C
paratyphlitis
paratyphoid
paratypical
paraumbilical incision
paraungual
paraureteric
paraurethra
paraurethral
    p. cyst
    p. false track
    p. fluid collection

paraurethral *(continued)*
    p. leiomyoma
    p. ligaments
    p. mass
    p. metastatic
      adenocarcinoma
    p. myoma
    p. neuromodulation
    p. saccule
    p. Skene glands
    recurrent sterile p. abscess
    p. suspension
    p. tissue
    p. tumor
paraurethritis
parauterine
paravaginal
    p. hysterectomy
    p. incision
paravaginitis
paravalvular
    p. abscess
    p. leak
    p. leakage
    p. mitral regurgitation
paravenous
    p. approach
    p. injection
    p. pigmentation
    pigmented p. chorioretinal
      atrophy
    pigmented p. retinochoroidal
      atrophy
    p. retinochoroidal atrophy
paraventricular
    p. nucleus (PVN)
    p. regions
paravertebral
    p. abscess
    p. analgesia
    p. block
    p. injection
    p. muscles
    p. space
paravesical
    p. abscess
    p. space
paravitaminosis
para-Wernicke
    encephalopathy
paraxial
Paré suture
parectasis
parectropia
parencephalia

parencephalous
parenchyma
    p. glandulare prostatae
    hepatic p.
    p. of kidney
    p. of lens
    renal p.
    p. testis
parenchymal
    junctional p. defect
parenchymatitis
parenchymatous
    acute p. hepatitis
    p. cartilage
    p. disease
    p. goiter
    p. hematoma
    p. hemorrhage
    p. inflammation
    p. injection
    p. keratitis
    p. mastitis
    p. myocarditis
    p. myositis
    p. nephritis
    p. neurosyphilis
    p. salpingitis
    p. syphilis
    p. tissue
parent
parental
parenteral
    p. absorption
    p. alimentation
    p. diarrhea
    p. digestion
    p. hyperalimentation
    p. nutrition
    total p. alimentation
    total p. nutrition (TPN)
Parenti-Fraccaro syndrome
parenting
paresis
    botulinum toxin p.
    canal p.
    facial nerve p.
    general p.
    inherited spastic p.
    juvenile p.
    parturient p.
    vestibular canal p.
paresthesia
    Bernhardt p.
    postoperative p.
paresthetic

paresthetica
    meralgia p.
paretic
Parhad-Poppen needle
Parham band
parica
paries (parietes)
    p. anterior gastris
    p. anterior vaginae
    p. caroticus cavitatis tympani
    p. externus ductus cochlearis
    p. inferior orbitae
    p. jugularis cavitatis tympani
    p. labyrinthicus cavitatis
      tympani
    p. lateralis orbitae
    p. mastoideus cavitatis tympani
    p. medialis orbitae
    p. membranaceus cavitatis
      tympani
    p. membranaceus tracheae
    p. posterior gastris
    p. posterior vaginae
    p. superior orbitae
    p. tegmentalis cavitatis
      tympani
    p. tympanicus ductus cochlearis
    p. vestibularis ductus
      cochlearis
parietal
    p. cell vagotomy
    p. suture
parietitis
parietofrontal
parietomastoid suture
parieto-occipital suture
parietosphenoid
parietosplanchnic
parietosquamosal
parietotemporal suture
parietovisceral
Parinaud
    conjunctivitis
    oculoglandular syndrome
    ophthalmoplegia
    syndrome
pari passu
parity
Park
    speculum
    aneurysm
Parker
    clamp
    fluid
    incision

P

Parker *(continued)*
    knife
    retractor
    tube
Parker-Kerr
    basting stitch
    enteroenterostomy
    forceps
    suture
Parkinson
    complex
    crisis
    disease
    facies
    mask
    rigidity
    sign
    syndrome
parkinsonian
parkinsonism
    atherosclerotic p.
    drug-induced p.
    hemiplegic p.
    intoxication p.
    juvenile p.
    postencephalitic p.
    postencephalitis p.
    primary p.
    secondary p.
    symptomatic p.
    traumatic p.
    vascular p.
paroccipital
parolfactory
    anterior p. sulcus
    Broca p. area
    posterior p. sulcus
parolivary bodies
Parona space
paronychia
    acute p.
    Candida p.
    chronic p.
    herpetic p.
paronychial
    p. cracking
    p. cutaneous leishmaniasis
    p. erythema
    p. folds
    p. infection
    p. inflammation
    p. involvement
    p. lesion
    p. notches
    p. tissues

paronychomycosis
parophthalmia
parorchis
parorexia
parosmia
parosteal
    p. lesion
    p. lipoma
    p. osteochondromatous
      proliferation
    p. osteosarcoma
parosteitis
parosteosis
parotid
parotidean
parotidectomy
parotitis
    bacterial p.
    chronic recurrent p.
    epidemic p.
    postoperative p.
    staphylococcal p.
    suppurative p.
    viral p.
parous
parovarian cyst
parovariotomy
parovaritis
parovarium
paroxysm
paroxysmal
    p. atrial tachycardia
    benign p. peritonitis
    benign p. positional vertigo
    benign p. vertigo of childhood
    p. choreoathetosis
    chronic p. hemicrania
    p. cold hemoglobinuria
    familial p. choreoathetosis
    p. kinesigenic choreoathetosis
    p. nocturnal dyspnea (PND)
    p. nocturnal hemoglobinuria
      (PNH)
    p. proteinuria
    p. pulmonary edema
    p. sleep
    p. tachycardia
    p. trepidant abasia
    p. vertigo
parried
parrot
    p. beak deformity
    p.-beaked clawing of the nails
    p.-beaked nose
    p. beak nail

parrot *(continued)*
- p. disease
- p. fever
- p. tongue

Parry disease

parry fracture

Parry-Romberg syndrome

pars (partes)
- p. abdominalis aortae
- p. abdominalis ductus thoracici
- p. abdominalis musculi pectoralis majoris
- p. abdominalis oesophagi
- p. abdominalis ureteris
- p. alaris musculi nasalis
- p. alveolaris mandibulae
- p. anterior commissurae anterioris
- p. anterior dorsi linguae
- p. anterior faciei diaphragmaticae hepatis
- p. anterior fornicis vaginae
- p. anterior lobuli quadrangularis anterioris
- p. anularis vaginae fibrosae digitorum manus
- p. anularis vaginae fibrosae digitorum pedis
- p. aryepiglottica musculi arytenoidei obliqui
- p. ascendens aortae
- p. ascendens duodeni
- p. atlantica arteriae vertebralis
- p. atlantis arteriae vertebralis
- p. autonomica systematis nervosi peripherici
- p. basilaris ossis occipitalis
- p. basilaris pontis
- p. basalis arteriae pulmonalis dextrae
- p. basalis arteriae pulmonalis sinistrae
- p. buccopharyngea musculi constrictoris pharyngis superioris
- p. canalis nervi optici
- p. cardiaca gastris
- p. cartilaginea septi nasi
- p. cartilaginea systematis skeletalis
- p. cartilaginea tubae auditivae
- p. cartilaginea tubae auditoriae
- p. cavernosa arteriae carotidis internae

pars (partes) *(continued)*
- p. centralis systematis nervosi
- p. centralis ventriculi lateralis
- p. ceratopharyngea musculi constrictoris pharyngis medii
- p. cerebralis arteriae carotidis internae
- p. cervicalis arteriae carotidis internae
- p. cervicalis arteriae vertebralis
- p. cervicalis ductus thoracici
- p. cervicalis esophagi
- p. cervicalis medullae spinalis
- p. cervicalis oesophagi
- p. cervicalis tracheae
- p. chondropharyngea musculi constrictoris pharyngis medii
- p. ciliaris retinae
- p. clavicularis musculi pectoralis majoris
- p. coccygea medullae spinalis
- p. coeliacoduodenalis musculi suspensorii duodeni
- p. colli esophagi
- p. colli oesophagi
- p. compacta substantiae nigrae
- p. convoluta lobuli corticalis renis
- p. corneoscleralis reticuli trabecularis

partes corporis humani
- p. costalis diaphragmatis
- p. cranialis partis parasympathici divisionis autonomicae systematis nervosi
- p. cricopharyngea musculi constrictoris pharyngis inferioris
- p. cruciformis vaginae fibrosae digitorum manus
- p. cruciformis vaginae fibrosae digitorum pedis
- p. cuneiformis vomeris
- p. cupularis recessus epitympanici
- p. descendens aortae
- p. descendens duodeni
- p. dextra faciei diaphragmaticae hepatis
- p. distalis adenohypophyseos
- p. distalis lobi anterioris hypophyseos
- p. distalis partis prostaticae urethrae masculinae

P

pars (partes) *(continued)*
- p. dorsalis lobuli quadrangularis anterioris
- p. duralis fili terminalis
- p. extraocularis arteriae centralis retinae
- p. fibrosa
- p. flaccida membranae tympanicae
- p. funicularis ductus deferentis
- p. glossopharyngea musculi constrictoris pharyngis superioris
- p. granulosa
- p. hepatis dextra
- p. hepatis sinistra
- p. horizontalis arteriae cerebri mediae
- p. horizontalis duodeni
- p. iliaca fasciae iliopsoas
- p. inferior duodeni
- p. inferior nervi vestibularis
- p. inferior venae lingularis
- p. infraclavicularis plexus brachialis
- p. infralobaris rami posterioris
- p. infralobaris venae posterioris
- p. inguinalis ductus deferentis
- p. insularis arteriae cerebri mediae
- p. intercartilaginea rimae glottidis
- p. intermedia adenohypophyseos
- p. intermedia lobi anterioris hypophyseos
- p. intermedia urethrae masculinae
- p. intermembranacea rimae glottidis
- p. intersegmentalis
- p. intracranialis arteriae vertebralis
- p. intracranialis nervi optici
- p. intralaminaris nervi optici intraocularis
- p. intralobaris rami posterioris
- p. intralobaris venae posterioris
- p. intramuralis ureteris
- p. intramuralis urethrae masculinae
- p. intraocularis arteriae centralis retinae

pars (partes) *(continued)*
- p. intraocularis nervi optici
- p. intrasegmentalis
- p. iridica retinae
- p. labialis musculi orbicularis oris
- p. laryngea pharyngis
- p. lateralis arcus longitudinalis pedis
- p. lateralis fornicis vaginae
- p. lateralis ossis occipitalis
- p. lateralis ossis sacri
- p. lateralis venae lobi medii
- p. libera membri inferioris
- p. libera membri superioris
- p. lumbalis diaphragmatis
- p. lumbalis medullae spinalis
- p. lumbaris medullae spinalis
- p. magnocellularis nuclei rubri
- p. marginalis musculi orbicularis oris
- p. medialis arcus pedis longitudinalis
- p. medialis venae lobi medii
- p. membranacea septi interventricularis
- p. membranacea septi nasi
- p. membranacea urethrae masculinae
- p. mobilis septi nasi
- p. muscularis septi interventricularis
- p. mylopharyngea musculi constrictoris pharyngis superioris
- p. nasalis ossis frontalis
- p. nasalis pharyngis
- p. nervosa hypophyseos
- p. obliqua musculi cricothyroidei
- p. occlusa arteriae umbilicalis
- p. olfactoria cavitatis nasi
- p. opercularis gyri frontalis inferioris
- p. optica retinae
- p. oralis pharyngis
- p. orbitalis glandulae lacrimalis
- p. orbitalis gyri frontalis inferioris
- p. orbitalis musculi orbicularis oculi
- p. orbitalis nervi optici
- p. orbitalis ossis frontalis
- p. ossea septi nasi
- p. ossea systematis skeletalis

pars (partes) *(continued)*
- p. ossea tubae auditivae
- p. ossea tubae auditoriae
- p. palpebralis glandulae lacrimalis
- p. palpebralis musculi orbicularis oculi
- p. parasympathetica divisionis autonomici systematis nervosi
- p. parvocellularis nuclei rubri
- p. patens arteriae umbilicalis
- p. pelvica ductus deferentis
- p. pelvica partis parasympathici divisionis autonomicae systematis nervosi
- p. pelvica ureteris
- p. peripherica systematis nervosi
- p. petrosa arteriae carotidis internae
- p. petrosa ossis temporalis
- p. phrenicocoeliaca musculi suspensorii duodeni
- p. pialis fili terminalis
- p. plana corporis ciliaris
- p. plicata corporis ciliaris
- p. postcommunicalis arteriae cerebri anterioris
- p. postcommunicalis arteriae cerebri posterioris
- p. posterior commissurae anterioris
- p. posterior commissurae rostralis
- p. posterior dorsi linguae
- p. posterior faciei diaphragmaticae hepatis
- p. posterior fornicis vaginae
- p. posterior hepatis
- p. posterior lobuli quadrangularis anterioris
- p. postlaminaris nervi optici intraocularis
- p. postsulcalis dorsi linguae
- p. precommunicalis arteriae cerebri anterioris
- p. precommunicalis arteriae cerebri posterioris
- p. prelaminaris nervi optici intraocularis
- p. preprostatica urethrae masculinae
- p. presulcalis dorsi linguae
- p. prevertebralis arteriae vertebralis

pars (partes) *(continued)*
- p. profunda glandulae parotideae
- p. profunda musculi masseteris
- p. profunda musculi sphincteris ani externus
- p. profunda partis palpebralis musculi orbicularis oculi
- p. prostatica urethrae masculinae
- p. proximalis partis prostaticae urethrae masculinae
- p. psoatica fasciae iliopsoas
- p. pterygopharyngea musculi constrictoris pharyngis superioris
- p. pylorica gastris
- p. pylorica ventriculi
- p. recta musculi cricothyroidei
- p. recta tubuli renalis
- p. respiratoria cavitatis nasi
- p. reticularis substantiae nigrae
- p. retrolentiformis capsulae internae
- p. sacralis medullae spinalis
- p. scrotalis ductus deferentis
- p. sphenoidalis arteriae cerebri mediae
- p. spinalis nervi accessorii
- p. spongiosa urethrae masculinae
- p. squamosa ossis temporalis
- p. sternalis diaphragmatis
- p. sternocostalis musculi pectoralis majoris
- p. subcutanea musculi sphincteris ani externi
- p. sublentiformis capsulae internae
- p. superficialis glandulae parotideae
- p. superficialis musculi masseteris
- p. superficialis musculi sphincteris ani externus
- p. superior duodeni
- p. superior faciei diaphragmaticae hepatis
- p. superior nervi vestibularis
- p. superior venae lingularis
- p. supraclavicularis plexus brachialis
- p. sympathetica divisionis autonomici systematis nervosi
- p. tecta duodeni

P

pars (partes) *(continued)*
    p. tecta membranae
      tympanicae
    p. terminalis ilei
    p. thoracica aortae
    p. thoracica ductus thoracici
    p. thoracica esophagi
    p. thoracica medullae spinalis
    p. thoracica oesophagi
    p. thoracica systematis
      autonomici
    p. thoracica tracheae
    p. thyroepiglottica musculi
      thyroarytenoidei
    p. thyropharyngea musculi
      constrictoris pharyngis
      inferioris
    p. tibiocalcanea ligamenti
      collateralis medialis
    p. tibionavicularis ligamenti
      collateralis medialis
    p. tibiotalaris anterior ligamenti
      collateralis medialis
    p. tibiotalaris posterior
      ligamenti collateralis medialis
    p. transversa musculi nasalis
    p. transversa rami sinistri
      venae portae hepatis
    p. transversaria arteriae
      vertebralis
    p. triangularis gyri frontalis
      inferioris
    p. tuberalis adenohypophyseos
    p. tuberalis lobi anterioris
      hypophyseos
    p. tympanica ossis temporalis
    p. umbilicalis rami sinistri
      venae portae hepatis
    p. uterina tubae uterinae
    p. uvealis reticuli trabecularis
    p. vagalis nervi accessorii
    p. ventralis lobuli
      quadrangularis anterioris
    p. vertebralis faciei costalis
      pulmonis
Parsons disease
partal
partes (plural of pars)
parthenogenesis
    artificial p.
parthenophobia
partial
    frontolateral p. laryngectomy
    p. hysterectomy
    lateral p. laryngectomy

partial *(continued)*
    p. mastectomy
    p. pulpectomy
    p. stapedectomy
partialism
participant-observer
particle
particulate
Partipilo method
partition
    p. chromatography
    p. coefficient
    oropharyngeal p.
partitioning
    gastric p.
Partsch operation
parturient
    p. canal
    p. fever
    p. paralysis
    p. paresis
parturifacient
parturition
    double p.
parulis
parumbilical
parvilocular
parvocellular
    p. part of medial geniculate
      body
    p. part of red nucleus
    p. reticular nucleus
parvovirus
    human p. B19
    human p. RA-1
parvule
PAS—
    periodic acid–Schiff
    pulmonary artery stenosis
PASA—*p*-aminosalicylic acid
    [p-, para-]
PAS-C—*p*-aminosalicylic acid,
    crystallized [p-, para-]
pascal (Pa)
Pascheff conjunctivitis
Paschen
    bodies
    corpuscles
    granules
PASG—pneumatic antishock
    garment
Pasini-Pierini syndrome
PASM—periodic acid–silver
    methenamine
PAS (periodic acid–Schiff) reaction

passage
  adiabatic fast p.
  blind p.
  bouton de p.
  false p.
  serial p.
Passavant
  bar
  cushion
  pad
  ridge
passband
passenger
  child p. restraint
  p. mutation
  restrained p.
  unrestrained p.
passer
  BirdBeak suture p.
  cable p.
  Carter-Thompson suture p.
  foil p.
  Gore suture p.
  left rear p.
  pointed tendon p.
  right front p.
  right rear p.
  Scorpion suture p.
  wire p.
passerby
passive
  continuous p. motion (CPM)
  p. agglutination
  p. algolagnia
  p. anaphylaxis
  p. atelectasis
  p. clot
  p. congestion
  p. cutaneous anaphylaxis
    reaction
  p. edema
  p. eruption
  p. euthanasia
  p. exercise
  p. hemolysis
  p. hyperemia
  p. immunity
  p. immunization
  p. incontinence
  p. movement
  p. transfer
  p. tremor
passive-aggressive
passivism
passivity

paste
  antibiotic p.
  arsenical p.
  Ihle p.
  impression p.
  Lassar plain zinc p.
  Teflon p.
  Unna p.
  zinc oxide p.
  zinc oxide and salicylic acid p.
paster
PAS (periodic acid–Schiff) test
Pasteur
  effect
  method
  reaction
  theory
  vaccine
Pasteur-Chamberland filter
Pasteurella
  P. multocida
  P. pneumotropica
pasteurellosis
pasteurization
Pastia
  lines
  sign
pastille
  antibiotic p.
  nystatin p.
past-pointing
  p-p. arthroscopic knots
  p-p. gaze
  horizontal p-p.
  p-p. test
PAT—
  paroxysmal atrial tachycardia
  prism adaptation test
Patau syndrome
patch
  p. angioplasty
  ash-leaf p.
  birth control p.
  blood p.
  butterfly p.
  Carrel p.
  p. clamp
  contraceptive p.
  cotton-wool p's
  p. dressing
  p. electrode
  p. graft
  gray p. ringworm
  herald p.
  mucous p.

P

patch *(continued)*
    Peyer p's
    salmon p.
    sentinel p.
    shagreen p.
    Silastic p.
    Teflon p.
    p. test
    transdermal p.
    white p.
patchy
    p. alopecia areata
    p. areas of caseation
    p. areas of fibrosis
    p. atelectasis
    p. axonal neuropathies
    p. consolidation
    p. contrast enhancement
    p. distribution
    p. erythema
    p. erythematous rash
    p. ground-glass opacity
    p. hyperpigmentation
    p. infiltrates
    p. staining
patefaction
patella
    p. alta
    p. baja
    p. bipartita
    bipartite p.
    p. cubiti
    floating p.
    high-riding p.
    p. infera
    low-riding p.
    p. partita
    slipping p.
patellapexy
patellaplasty
patellar
    p. dislocation
    p. extension
    p. instability
    p. ligament
    p. luxation
    p. realignment surgery
    p. subluxation
    p. taping
    p. tendinopathy
    p. tendon
    p. tendon autograft
    p. tendon disruption
    p. tendon rupture
patellectomy

patelliform
patellofemoral
patency
    fallopian tube p.
    graft p.
    vein p.
    vessel p.
patent
    p. bronchus sign
    p. ductus arteriosus (PDA)
    p. foramen ovale
    p. urachus
Paterson
    brain clip forceps
    laryngeal cannula
    laryngeal forceps
    long-shank brain clip
    syndrome
Paterson-Brown-Kelly
  syndrome
Paterson-Kelly syndrome
Patey operation
path.—pathology
path
    alvear p.
    condyle p.
    generated occlusal p.
    incisor p.
    p. of insertion
    ionization p.
    lateral condyle p.
    milled-in p's
    occlusal p.
    p. of removal
pathergic
pathergy
pathetic
pathfinder probe
Pathfinder
    knife
    punch
    scissors
    spinal instrumentation
    surgical robot
pathoclisis
pathoformic
pathogen
pathogenesis
    drug p.
pathogenic
pathogenicity
pathognomonic symptom
pathologic
    p. anatomy
    p. cause

pathologic *(continued)*
p. changes
p. classification
p. continuum
p. criteria
p. diagnosis
p. factors
p. findings
p. fracture
p. gambler
p. liar
p. neovascularization
p. process
p. response
p. risk factors
p. specimen
p. substances
p. vascularization
pathologist
pathology
anatomic p.
cellular p.
chemical p.
clinical p.
comparative p.
dental p.
experimental p.
forensic p.
functional p.
general p.
geographical p.
internal p.
medical p.
molecular p.
oral p.
special p.
speech p.
surgical p.
pathomimesis
pathomorphism
pathoneurosis
pathophobia
pathophysiology
pathopsychosis
pathway
accessory p.
accessory conduction p.
afferent p.
alternative complement p.
amphibolic p.
anabolic p.
atrioventricular p.
auditory p's
biosynthetic p.
central auditory p.

pathway *(continued)*
circus p.
classical complement p.
coagulation p's
concealed accessory p.
corticopontocerebellar p's
dentato-rubro-olivary p.
dopaminergic nigrostriatal p.
efferent p.
Embden-Meyerhof p. of
glucose metabolism
Embden-Meyerhof-Parnas p.
extrinsic p. of coagulation
final common p.
gustatory p's
internuncial p.
intrinsic p. of coagulation
leukotriene p.
lipoxygenase p.
metabolic p.
motor p.
olfactory p's
optical p's
pentose phosphate p.
perforant p.
perforating p.
phosphogluconate p.
reaction p.
reentrant p.
sensory p.
visual p.
patient
p.-controlled analgesia
p.-controlled epidural analgesia
Paton needle holder
patricide
Patrick
cross-leg maneuver
sign
test
trigger areas
patrilineal
patroclinous
pattern
alveolar p.
arch p.
beam p.
biphasic p.
broken bough p.
butterfly p.
Christmas tree p.
cloverleaf p.
convolutional p.
corkscrew p.
cystic p.

P

pattern *(continued)*
    dicing p.
    dietary p's
    diffraction p.
    fingerprint p.
    full interference p.
    hair brush p.
    hanging-fruit p.
    haustral p.
    herring-bone p.
    honeycomb p.
    interference p.
    juvenile p.
    loop p.
    mimosa p.
    muscle p.
    occlusal p.
    optokinetic p.
    recruitment p.
    reduced interference p.
    rugal p.
    sedimentation p.
    signet ring p.
    sine wave p.
    skeletal p.
    sleep p.
    solid p.
    starry sky p.
    startle p.
    stimulus p.
    wax p.
    wear p.
    whorl p.
patterning
Patterson
    bronchoscopic forceps
    empyema forceps
    specimen forceps
    trocar
Patton dilator
patty
    cement p.
    cottonoid p.
patulous
pauciarticular
paucisynaptic
paucity
    p. of findings
    p. of speech
Paufique
    operation
    trephine
Paul
    test
    treatment

Paul-Bunnell test
Paul-Bunnell-Davidsohn test
Pauling-Corey helix
Paul-Mixter tube
paunch
pause
    cardiac p.
    compensatory p.
    post-extrasystolic p.
    sinus p.
Pautrier abscess
Pauwels operation
pavé
pavement
    p. cells
    p. epithelium
pavementing
pavex
pavilion
    p. of the ear
    p. of the oviduct
    p. of the pelvis
paving
    crazy p.
    p. stone degeneration
Pavlov
    pouch
    stomach
pavor
    p. diurnus
    p. nocturnus
Pavy disease
Pawlik
    fold
    grip
    triangle
Pawlow position
PAWP—pulmonary artery wedge
    pressure
pawpaw
Payr
    clamp
    disease
    method
    sign
    syndrome
Pb—lead
PB—pressure breathing
PBA—pulpobuccoaxial
PBC—primary biliary cirrhosis
PBC, PcB—point of basal
    convergence
PBF—pulmonary blood flow
PBG—porphobilinogen
PBI—protein-bound iodine

PBL—peripheral blood lymphocytes

PBN—paralytic brachial neuritis

PBPI—penile-brachial pressure index

PBS—phosphate-buffered saline

PBT$_4$—protein-bound thyroxine

PBV—
predicted blood volume
pulmonary blood volume

p.c.—after meals (L. post cibum)

PC—
platelet count
portacaval
pubococcygeus
pulmonic closure

PCA—
patient-controlled analgesia

PCB—paracervical block

PCc—periscopic concave

PCD—
phosphate-citrate-dextrose
posterior corneal deposits

PCE—pseudocholinesterase

PCEC—purified chick embryo cell (vaccine)

PCG—phonocardiogram

PCH—paroxysmal cold hemoglobinuria

pCi—picocurie(s)

PCI—
percutaneous coronary intervention
pneumatosis cystoides intestinalis

PCM—protein-calorie malnutrition

PCNL—percutaneous nephrostolithotomy

PCO—polycystic ovary

pCO$_2$; PCO$_2$; pCO2—partial pressure of carbon dioxide

PCP—
phencyclidine hydrochloride
Pneumocystis pneumonia

PCR—polymerase chain reaction

PCS—portacaval shunt

PCT—portacaval transposition

PCV—
packed cell volume
polycythemia vera

PCV-M—polycythemia vera with myeloid metaplasia

PCW—pulmonary capillary wedge

PCWP—pulmonary capillary wedge pressure

PCx—periscopic convex

PD—
Parkinson disease
patent ductus
phosphate dehydrogenase
plasma defect
poorly differentiated
postural drainage
potential difference
pressor dose
prism diopter
psychotic depression
pulmonary disease
pulpodistal
pupillary distance

PDA—
patent ductus arteriosus
posterior descending artery

PDD—pyridoxine-deficient diet

PDGF—platelet-derived growth factor

PDH—
packaged disaster hospital
phosphate dehydrogenase

PDI—periodontal disease index

PDLL—poorly differentiated lymphocytic lymphoma

PDR—
Physicians' Desk Reference
proliferative diabetic retinopathy

PE—
pharyngoesophageal
phenylephrine
physical examination
pleural effusion
polyethylene
probable error
pulmonary edema
pulmonary embolism

PEA—pulseless electrical activity

peak
biclonal p.
Bragg p.
p. expiratory flow rate (PEFR)
p. flow gauge
p. flow meter
kilovolts p. (kVp)
monoclonal p.

peak-to-peak
p-p. amplitude
p-p. amplitude of action potentials
p-p. interval

P

peak-to-peak *(continued)*
- p-p. movement
- p-p. variability

Péan
- clamp
- forceps
- incision
- operation
- position

pearl
- Bohn p's
- p. cyst
- Elschnig p's
- enamel p.
- epithelial p's
- Epstein p's
- horn p's
- keratin p. formation
- parakeratotic p.

Pearson
- correlation coefficient
- position

peau
- p. de chagrin (Fr. shagreen skin)
- p. d'orange (Fr. orange peel skin)

pebble beach sign

pebble-like
- p-l. papule
- p-l. stools

peccant

peccatiphobia

Pecquet
- cistern
- duct
- reservoir

pecten (pectines)
- p. of anal canal
- p. analis
- p. ossis pubis

pectenine

pectenitis

pectenosis

pectenotomy

pectic acid

pectin

pectinate
- p. ligament
- p. line
- p. muscles of atrium
- p. zone

pectineal
- p. crest of femur
- p. hernia
- p. ligament
- p. line
- p. muscle

pectiniform

pectization

pectora (plural of pectus)

pectoral
- p. axillary lymph nodes
- p. cavity
- p. ectopia cordis
- p. fascia
- p. fremitus
- p. girdle
- p. glands
- greater p. muscle
- lateral p. nerve
- p. limb
- p. lymph nodes
- medial p. nerve
- p. muscle
- p. myopathy
- p. reflex
- p. region
- p. ridge
- smaller p. muscle
- p. veins

pectoralgia

pectoralis
- p. lateralis nerve
- p. major muscle
- p. medialis nerve
- p. minor muscle

pectorals

pectoriloquy
- aphonic p.
- whispered p.
- whispering p.

pectorophony

pectous

pectunculus

pectus (pectora)
- p. carinatum
- p. excavatum
- p. gallinatum
- p. recurvatum

ped; peds—pediatrics

pedal
- absent p. pulses
- p. arteries
- p. bone
- p. edema
- p. lymphangiography
- p. osteitis
- palpable p. pulses
- p. pulses
- p. vasculature
- p. vessels

pederast

Pederson speculum

pedes (plural of pes)
pediatric
    p. dentistry
    p. neurology
    p. speculum
    p. ward
pediatrician
pediatrics
pedicel
pedicellate, pedicellated
pedicellation
pedicle
    p. clamp
    cone p.
    double p. flap
    epigastric p.
    p. flap
    p. graft
    p. of lung
    neurovascular p.
    p. screw
    vascular p.
    p. of vertebral arch
pedicled
pedicular
pediculate
pediculated
pediculation
pediculicide
Pediculoides ventricosus
pediculosis
    p. capitis
    p. corporis
    p. inguinalis
    p. palpebrarum
    p. pubis
pediculous
pediculus (pediculi)
    p. arcus vertebrae
    p. pulmonis
Pediculus
    P. humanus
    P. humanus capitis
    P. humanus corporis
    P. humanus humanus
    P. inguinalis
    P. pubis
pedicure
pedigree
pedionalgia
pedis
    dorsalis p. artery
    dorsalis p. pulse
peditis
pedodontics
pedodontist

pedometer
pedopathy
pedophilia
pedophobia
peduncle
    anterior p. of thalamus
    caudal p. of thalamus
    central p. of thalamus
    cerebellar p.
    cerebellar p., caudal
    cerebellar p., cranial
    cerebellar p., inferior
    cerebellar p., middle
    cerebellar p., pontine
    cerebellar p., rostral
    cerebellar p., superior
    p's of cerebellum
    cerebral p.
    p. of cerebrum
    p. of flocculus
    mammillary p.
    p. of mammillary body
    olfactory p.
    pineal p.
    p. of pineal body
    posterior p. of thalamus
    superior p. of thalamus
    thalamic p.
    p's of thalamus
peduncular
pedunculated
pedunculotomy
pedunculus (pedunculi)
    p. cerebellaris inferior
    p. cerebellaris medius
    p. cerebellaris superior
    p. cerebri
    p. flocculi
    p. thalamicus inferior
peel
    apple p. intestinal
      atresia
    banana p. exposure
    beta-hydroxy acid p.
    bitter orange p.
    chemical p.
    double p.
    facial p.
    glycolic acid p.
    intimal p.
    lemon p.
    lidocaine-tetracaine p.
    lip p.
    onion p. configuration
    phenol p.
    salicylic acid p.

P

peel-away sheath
peeling
PEEP—positive end-expiratory
　　pressure
Peet operation
PEF—peak expiratory flow
PEFR—peak expiratory flow rate
peg
　　bone p.
　　p. cells
　　cortical bone p.
　　nine-hole p. test
　　odontoid p.
　　rete p's
　　p. tooth
PEG—
　　percutaneous endoscopic
　　　gastrostomy
　　pneumoencephalogram
　　polyethylene glycol
　　pseudoexfoliation glaucoma
peg-and-socket suture
PEG tube
pelade
pelargonic acid
Pel crises
Pel-Ebstein
　　crisis
　　disease
　　fever
　　pyrexia
　　symptom
Pelger nuclear anomaly
Pelger-Huët nuclear anomaly
pelgeroid
peliosis
　　bacillary p.
　　p. hepatis
　　p. of liver
Pelizaeus-Merzbacher disease
pellagra
　　p. sine p.
　　typhoid p.
pellagral
pellagroid
pellagrose
pellagrous
pellant
pellate
Pellegrini disease
Pellegrini-Stieda disease
pellet
　　foil p.
pellicle
　　brown p.

pellicle (continued)
　　dental p.
pellicular
pelliculous
Pellizzi syndrome
pellucid zone
pelves (plural of pelvis)
pelvic
　　p. congestion syndrome
　　p. exenteration
　　p. inflammatory disease (PID)
　　p. inlet
　　p. osteotomy
　　p. outlet
　　p. plane diameter
　　p. thrombophlebitis
pelvicaliceal, pelvicalyceal
pelvicellulitis
pelvicephalography
pelvicephalometry
Pelvicol collagen implant
pelvifemoral
pelvifixation
pelvimetry
　　clinical p.
　　combined p.
　　CT p.
　　digital p.
　　external p.
　　instrumental p.
　　internal p.
　　manual p.
　　MRI p.
　　x-ray p.
pelvioperitonitis
pelvioplasty
pelviotomy
pelviperitonitis
pelvirectal
　　p. abscess
　　p. achalasia
pelvis (pelves)
　　android p.
　　angle of p.
　　anthropoid p.
　　assimilation p.
　　beaked p.
　　bifid p.
　　bony p.
　　brachypellic p.
　　contracted p.
　　cordate p.
　　cordiform p.
　　coxalgic p.
　　dwarf p.

pelvis (pelves) *(continued)*
    extrarenal p.
    false p.
    flat p.
    frozen p.
    funnel-shaped p.
    giant p.
    greater p.
    gynecoid p.
    high-assimilation p.
    infantile p.
    p. justo major
    p. justo minor
    juvenile p.
    kyphoscoliotic p.
    kyphotic p.
    large p.
    lesser p.
    lordotic p.
    low-assimilation p.
    p. major
    mesatipellic p.
    p. minor
    p. nana
    oblique p.
    obliquely contracted p.
    p. obtecta
    p. ossea
    osteomalacic p.
    Otto p.
    p. ovalis
    pithecoid p.
    p. plana
    platypellic p.
    platypelloid p.
    Prague p.
    pseudo-osteomalacic p.
    rachitic p.
    renal p.
    p. renalis
    Rokitansky p.
    round p.
    scoliotic p.
    simple flat p.
    small p.
    spider p.
    p. spinosa
    split p.
    spondylolisthetic p.
    p. spuria
    stove-in p.
    true p.
    p. of ureter
pelvisacral
pelvisacrum

pelviscope
pelviscopy
pelvisection
pelvisternum
pelvitrochanterian
pelviureteral
pelvospondylitis ossificans
Pemberton clamp
pemphigoid
    benign mucosal p.
    Brunsting-Perry p.
    bullous p.
    cicatricial p.
    dermolytic p.
    gestational p.
    p. lichen planus
    localized bullous p.
    ocular p.
pemphigus
    benign p. vegetans
    Brazilian p.
    familial benign p.
    p. erythematosus
    p. foliaceus
    herpetiform p.
    p. neonatorum
    ocular p.
    paraneoplastic p.
    South American p.
    p. vegetans
    p. vulgaris
    wildfire p.
pen
    Humalog p.
    Humulin p.
penalization
pendelluft
    p. flow
    p. respiration
Pendred
    disease
    syndrome
pendular
pendulous
pendulum
    Pulfrich p.
penectomy
penetrability
penetrance
    complete p.
    genetic p.
penetrant
penetrating
    p. graft
    p. keratoplasty (PKP)

P

penetrating *(continued)*
    p. ulcer
    p. ulcer of foot
    p. wound
penetration
    p. enhancer
    radiographic p.
    sperm p. assay
Penfield
    epilepsy
    syndrome
penial
penicillamine
penicillanic acid
penicilli (plural of penicillus)
penicilliary
penicillic acid
penicillin-fast
penicillinic acid
penicilliosis
Penicillium
    P. citreoviride
    P. citrinum
    P. claviforme
    P. cyclopium
    P. expansum
    P. leucopus
    P. melinii
    P. uticale
    P. viridicatum
penicillus (penicilli)
    penicilli arteriae splenicae
penile
    p. body
    p. brachial index (PBPI)
    p. clamp
    p. curvature
    deep p. fascia
    dorsal p. nerve block
      (DPNB)
    p. epispadias
    p. fascia
    p. hypospadias
    p. implant
    p. induration
    p. intraepithelial neoplasia
    nocturnal p. tumescence
      (NPT) test
    pearly p. papule
    p. prosthesis
    p. reflex
    p. root
    p. schwannoma
    p. squamous cell carcinoma
    superficial p. fascia

penile *(continued)*
    p. tumescence
    p. urethra
penis
    bifid p.
    body of p.
    bulb of p.
    buried p.
    p. captivus
    cavernous body of p.
    clubbed p.
    concealed p.
    congenital curvature of p.
    corkscrew p.
    dorsal deviated p.
    double p.
    glans p.
    head of p.
    inconspicuous p.
    induratio p. plastica
    p. palmatus
    prepuce of p.
    shaft of p.
    spiral deviation of p.
    webbed p.
penischisis
penitis
penniform
Pennington
    clamp
    elevator
    forceps
    speculum
Penn seroflocculation reaction
pennyroyal
penoscrotal
Penrose drain
pentachlorophenol
pentad
pentadactyl
pentalogy of Fallot
pentasomy
pentetreotide
    indium In 111 p.
pentose
    p. cycle
    p. phosphate pathway
    p. shunt
pentosemia
pentosuria
    alimentary p.
    benign p.
    essential p.
pentosuric
penumbra

Penzoldt-Fisher test
PEO—progressive external
  ophthalmoplegia
PEP—preejection period
PEPP—positive expiratory
  pressure plateau
pepper
    cayenne p.
    p. spray
Pepper
    neuroblastoma
    syndrome
    type
peppermint
pepsin A
pepsinogen
pepsinuria
peptic
    chronic p. esophagitis
    p. digestion
    p. esophagitis
    giant p. ulcer
    p. glands
    p. ulcer
peptidase
    leucine amino p.
peptide
    atrial natriuretic p. (ANP)
    p. bond
    brain natriuretic p. (BNP)
    C p.
    chemotactic p.
    corticotropin-like intermediate
      lobe p. (CLIP)
    N-formylmethionyl p's
    gastrin-releasing p.
    glucagon-like p.
    p. hydrolase
    leader p.
    opioid p.
    parathyroid hormone–like p.
    signal p.
    p. test
    vasoactive intestinal p. (VIP)
peptidergic fibers
peptiduria
    opioid p.
peptogenic
Peptostreptococcus anaerobius
PER—protein efficiency ratio
peracephalus
peracidity
peracute
per anum
percentile

perception
    color p. test
    depth p.
    distorted p.
    extrasensory p. (ESP)
    facial p.
    light and color p.
    limit of p.
    speech p.
    stereognostic p.
    subliminal p.
perceptive
perceptivity
perceptual
perchlorate
    p. discharge test
    potassium p.
perchloric acid
percipient
percolate
percolation
percolator
per contiguum
per continuum
percuss
percussible
percussion
    auscultation and p. (A&P)
    auscultatory p.
    bimanual p.
    chest wall p.
    comparative p.
    deep p.
    direct p.
    distal tingling on p.
    drop p.
    dullness to p.
    finger p.
    fist p.
    Goldscheider p.
    p. hammer
    immediate p.
    instrumental p.
    Korányi p.
    Lerch p.
    mediate p.
    Murphy p.
    p. myotonia
    pain to p.
    palpatory p.
    paradoxical p.
    pencil p.
    piano p.
    Plesch p.
    pleximetric p.

P

percussion *(continued)*
    respiratory p.
    slapping p.
    p. sound
    strip p.
    tangential p.
    threshold p.
    topographic p.
percussor
percutaneous
    p. abscess and fluid drainage (PAFD)
    p. antegrade pyelography
    p. antegrade urography
    p. biopsy
    p. catheter
    p. cholecystostomy
    p. cordotomy
    p. coronary intervention
    direct p. transhepatic cholangiography
    p. drainage
    p. endoscopic gastrostomy (PEG)
    p. epididymal sperm aspiration
    p. hepatobiliary cholangiography
    p. mitral commissurotomy (PMC)
    p. nephrostolithotomy (PCNL)
    p. pericardial catheter drainage
    p. radiofrequency rhizotomy
    p. rhizotomy
    p. testicular sperm aspiration
    p. transhepatic biliary drainage (PTBD)
    p. transhepatic cholangiodrainage
    p. transhepatic cholangiography (PTC)
    p. transhepatic portography
    p. transluminal angioplasty (PTA)
    p. transluminal atrial valvuloplasty (PTAV)
    p. transluminal coronary angioplasty (PTCA)
    p. transluminal mitral valvuloplasty (PTMV)
    p. transluminal renal angioplasty (PTRA)
    p. transtracheal bronchography

percutaneous *(continued)*
    p. ultrasonic lithotripsy
    p. umbilical blood sampling
    p. vertebroplasty
per cutem
Percy
    cautery
    forceps
perennial
Pereyra
    colposuspension
    needle
    operation
    procedure
Perez sign
perfectionism
perfilcon A
perflation
perflubron
perforans (perforantes)
    elastosis p. serpiginosa
    scleromalacia p.
    p. varicosis
perforate
perforated
perforating
    acquired p. dermatosis
    p. appendicitis
    p. arteries
    chronic p. pulp hyperplasia
    p. cutaneous nerve
    p. fasciculus
    p. fibers
    p. folliculitis
    p. fracture
    p. ulcer
    p. veins
    p. verruciform collagenoma
    p. wound
perforation
    apical p.
    bowel p.
    corneal p.
    mechanical p.
    p. of nasal septum
    pathologic p.
    root p.
    tympanic membrane p.
perforator
    Blot p.
    Lempert p.
    Royce p.
    Smellie p.
    Thornwald p.

perfrication
perfusate
perfuse
perfusion
    acid p. test
    p. cannula
    cerebral p. pressure
    esophageal acid p. test
    isolation-p. technique
    luxury p.
    myocardial p. imaging
    myocardial p. scintigraphy
    p. pressure
    regional p.
    p. scintigraphy
    p. study
    thallium-201 myocardial p.
      scintigraphy
    ventilation-p. ratio
    ventilation-p. scan
perfusionist
periacinal
periacinous
periadenitis mucosa necrotica
  recurrens
periadnexal dermis
periadventitial
periampullary
perianal
    p. abscess
    chronic p. Crohn disease
    p. fibroadenoma
    p. fistula
    p. hematoma
    p. incision
    p. mass
    p. papules
    p. reflex
    p. skin tags
    p. ulcer
periangiitis
periangiocholitis
periangioma
periaortic
periaortitis
periapex
periapical
periappendicitis decidualis
periappendicular
periaqueductal gray electrode
periareolar
    double-opposing p. flap
    p. fine-needle aspiration
    p. flap
    p. incision

periareolar *(continued)*
    p. pityriasis versicolor
    p. reduction mammaplasty
periarterial sympathectomy
periarteriolar
periarteritis
    disseminated necrotizing p.
    p. gummosa
    p. nodosa
    syphilitic p.
periarthric
periarthritis
    p. calcarea
    p. of shoulder
periarticular
periatrial
periauricular
periaxial
periaxillary
periaxonal
peribronchial cuffing
peribronchiolar
peribronchiolitis
peribronchitis
peribulbar
peribursal
pericaliceal
pericallosal
pericanalicular
pericapillary
pericapsular
pericardial
    p. angiosarcoma
    p. baffle
    p. cavity
    p. calcification
    p. cyst
    p. effusion
    p. fluid
    p. fremitus
    p. friction sound
    Ionescu-Shiley p. xenograft
    p. knock
    p. lymph nodes
    p. murmur
    p. peel
    p. reflection
    p. rub
    p. rupture
    p. sac
    p. serum
    p. sinus
    p. space
    p. tamponade
    p. window

P

pericardiectomy
pericardiocentesis
pericardiolysis
pericardiomediastinitis
    adhesive p.
pericardiophrenic
pericardiopleural
pericardiorrhaphy
pericardiostomy
pericardiotomy
pericarditic
pericarditis
    acute benign p.
    acute exudative p.
    acute fibrinous p.
    adhesive p.
    amebic p.
    bacterial p.
    bread-and-butter p.
    carcinomatous p.
    constrictive p.
    dry p.
    p. with effusion
    external p.
    fibrinous p.
    fibrous p.
    hemorrhagic p.
    idiopathic p.
    leukemic p.
    localized p.
    malignant p.
    mediastinal p.
    neoplastic p.
    p. obliterans
    obliterating p.
    purulent p.
    rheumatic p.
    septic p.
    serofibrinous p.
    suppurative p.
    tuberculous p.
    uremic p.
    viral p.
pericardium
    adherent p.
    bread-and-butter p.
    calcified p.
    decompression of p.
    empyema of p.
    p. fibrosum
    fibrous p.
    parietal p.
    p. serosum
    serous p.
    shaggy p.

pericardium *(continued)*
    visceral p.
pericardotomy
pericaval
pericecal
pericecitis
pericellular
pericemental
pericementitis
    apical p.
    chronic suppurative p.
pericementum
pericephalic
pericholangitis
pericholecystitis
    gaseous p.
perichondrial
perichondritis
perichondrium
perichondroma
perichord
perichordal
perichoroidal
pericolic
pericolitis
    p. dextra
    membranous p.
    p. sinistra
pericolpitis
periconchal
periconchitis
pericorneal
pericoronal
pericoronitis
pericostal suture
pericoxitis
pericranial
pericranitis
pericranium
pericystic
pericystitis
pericyte
pericytial
pericytoma
perideferentitis
peridendritic
peridens
peridermal
peridesmic
peridesmitis
peridesmium
perididymis
perididymitis
peridiverticular
peridiverticulitis

periductal
periduodenitis
peridural
periencephalitis
periencephalomeningitis
perienteric
perienteritis
periependymal
periepithelioma
periesophageal
periesophagitis
perifascicular
perifistular
perifocal
perifollicular
perifolliculitis
    p. capitis abscedens et
      suffodiens
    superficial pustular p.
perigangliitis
periganglionic
perigastric
perigastritis
periglandular
periglandulitis
periglial
periglossitis
periglottic
periglottis
perigraft
perihepatic
perihepatitis
    p. chronica hyperplastica
    gonococcal p.
perihernial
perihilar
perihypophysial,
  perihypophyseal
perijejunitis
perikeratic
perilabyrinth
perilabyrinthitis
perilaryngeal
perilaryngitis
perilenticular
perilesional
periligamentous
perilimbal incision
perilobar
perilobulitis
perilymphadenitis
perilymphangitis
perilymphatic
perimacular
perimastitis

perimedullary
perimeningitis
perimeter
    arc p.
    dental p.
    projection p.
perimetric
perimetritic
perimetritis
perimetrium
perimetrosalpingitis
    encapsulating p.
perimetry
    flicker p.
    quantitative p.
perimolysis
perimyelitis
perimyocarditis
perimyoendocarditis
perimyometrium
perimyositis
perimysial
perimysiitis
perimysium (perimysia)
    external p.
    p. externum
    internal p.
    p. internum
perinatal
perinatologist
perinatology
perineal
    p. body
    p. fascia
    p. fistula
    p. flexure
    p. fossa
    p. hernia
    p. hypospadias
    p. ligament
    p. lithotomy
    p. membrane
    p. muscles
    p. pad
    p. pearls
    p. pouch
    p. prostatectomy
    p. raphe
    p. region
    p. sensation
    p. space
    p. urethrotomy
perineocele
perineoplasty
perineorectal

P

perineorrhaphy
    Emmet-Studdiford p.
perineoscrotal
perineotomy
perineovaginal
perineovaginorectal
perineovulvar
perinephric
perinephritic
perinephritis
perinephrium
perineum
    anterior p.
    posterior p.
    watering-can p.
perineural
    p. anesthesia
    p. block
    p. channel
    p. fibroblastoma
perineurial cyst
perineuritic
perineuritis
perineurium
perinuclear
periocular
period
    prefunctional p.
    absolute refractory p.
    acceleration p.
    antepartum p.
    child-bearing p.
    critical p.
    D p.
    deceleration p.
    early neonatal p.
    eclipse p.
    ejection p.
    p. of emptying
    fertile p.
    p. of filling
    G_1 p., G_2 p. [G1, G2]
    p. of gestation
    gestational period
    half-life p.
    incubation p.
    induction p.
    intrapartum p.
    isoelectric p.
    isometric p.
    isometric p. of cardiac cycle
    p. of isometric contraction
    p. of isometric relaxation
    isovolumic p.
    lag p.
    latency p.

period *(continued)*
    latent p.
    M p.
    menstrual p.
    monthly p.
    neonatal p.
    oral p.
    perinatal p.
    postneonatal p.
    postpartum p.
    prenatal p.
    prodromal p.
    puerperal p.
    quarantine p.
    reaction p.
    refractory p.
    relative refractory p.
    reproductive p.
    S p.
    safe p.
    silent p.
    steady p.
    waiting p.
    Wenckebach p.
periodate
periodic
    p. acid
    p. lateralized epileptiform
        discharge (PLED)
periodicity
    diurnal p.
    lunar p.
    nocturnal p.
    subperiodic p.
periodontal
    p. disease
    p. probe
periodontics
periodontist
periodontitis
    acute local p.
    adult p.
    apical p.
    chronic apical p.
    chronic suppurative p.
    juvenile p.
    marginal p.
    prepubertal p.
    rapidly progressive p.
    simple p.
    p. simplex
    suppurative p.
periodontium (periodontia)
    p. insertionis
    p. protectionis
    p. protectoris

periodontology
periodontosis
periomphalic
perionychia
perionychium
perionyx
perioophoritis
perioophorosalpingitis
perioperative
periophthalmic
periophthalmitis
perioral
periorbital
periorbititis
periorchitis
    p. adhaesiva
    p. purulenta
periorchium
periorificial lentiginosis
periosteal elevator
periosteoedema
periosteoma
periosteomedullitis
periosteomyelitis
periosteophyte
periosteorrhaphy
periosteotome
    Alexander p.
    Alexander-Farabeuf p.
    Dean p.
    Fomon p.
    Joseph p.
periosteotomy
periosteous
periosteum
    alveolar p.
    p. alveolare
    p. cranii
periostitis
    p. albuminosa
    albuminous p.
    diffuse p.
    hemorrhagic p.
    p. hyperplastica
    p. interna cranii
    orbital p.
    precocious p.
periostosis
    hyperplastic p.
periostosteitis
periotic
periovular
peripachymeningitis
peripancreatic
peripancreatitis
peripapillary

peripartum
peripatellar
peripatetic
peripenial
peripharyngeal
peripherad
peripheral
    p. airway resistance
    p. ameloblastoma
    p. anesthesia
    p. angiography
    p. anterior synechia
    p. arteriography
    p. arteriosclerosis
    p. blood
    p. cholangiocarcinoma
    p. chondrosarcoma
    p. curve
    p. cyanosis
    p. edema
    p. fusion
    p. giant cell granuloma
    p. glioma
    p. iridectomy (PI)
    p. lesion
    p. necrosis
    p. nervous system (PNS)
    p. neuralgia
    p. neuritis
    p. neurofibromatosis
    p. neuroglia
    p. neuropathy
    p. neutropenia
    p. ossifying fibroma
    p. paralysis
    p. paraplegia
    p. polyarthritis
    p. pulses
    p. retina
    p. scotoma
    p. ulcerative keratitis
    p. uveitis
    p. vascular resistance
    p. venography
    p. vertigo
    p. vision
peripherally
periphery
periphlebitic
periphlebitis
    sclerosing p.
periphoria
periphrenitis
peripleural
peripleuritis
peripneumonia period

P

peripolar
periporitis
periportal
periproctitis
periprostatic
periprostatitis
peripyelitis
peripylephlebitis
peripyloric
periradicular
perirectal
perirectitis
perirenal
perirhinal
perisalpingitis
perisalpingo-ovaritis
perisalpinx
periscapular incision
perisclerium
perisigmoiditis
perisinuous
perisinusitis
perispermatitis serosa
perisplanchnic
perisplanchnitis
perisplenic
perisplenitis cartilaginea
perispondylic
perispondylitis
    Gibney p.
peristalsis
    mass p.
    retrograde p.
    reversed p.
    uterine p.
peristaltic
    p. reflex
    p. rush
peristaphyline
peristrumitis
peristrumous
perisynovial
perisynovitis
peritectomy
peritendineum
peritendinitis
    adhesive p.
    p. calcarea
    p. crepitans
    p. serosa
peritendinous
peritenon
peritenoneum
perithelial
perithelioma

perithelium
    Eberth p.
perithoracic
perithyroiditis
peritomize
peritomy
peritoneal
    p. abscess
    p. button
    p. cavity, greater
    p. cavity, lesser
    continuous ambulatory p.
        dialysis
    continuous cyclic p.
        dialysis
    p. dialysis
    p. equilibration test
    p. gliomatosis
    p. incision
    p. lavage
    p. mesothelioma
    p. mouse
    p. sac
    p. sclerosis
peritonealgia
peritonealize
peritoneocentesis
peritoneomuscular
peritoneopathy
peritoneopericardial
peritoneopexy
peritoneoplasty
peritoneoscope
    Wolf p.
peritoneoscopy
peritoneotome
peritoneotomy
peritoneovenous
peritoneum
    abdominal p.
    intestinal p.
    parietal p.
    urogenital p.
    visceral p.
peritonism
peritonitis
    acute sterile p.
    adhesive p.
    bacterial p.
    benign paroxysmal p.
    bile p.
    biliary p.
    Candida p.
    chemical p.
    chylous p.

peritonitis *(continued)*
    circumscribed p.
    coccidioidal p.
    diaphragmatic p.
    diffuse p.
    fungal p.
    gas p.
    general p.
    granulomatous p.
    localized p.
    meconium p.
    pelvic p.
    perforative p.
    periodic p.
    puerperal p.
    purulent p.
    sclerosing p.
    sclerosing encapsulating p.
    septic p.
    silent p.
    spontaneous bacterial p.
    traumatic p.
    tuberculous p.
peritonization
peritonize
peritonsillar
peritonsillitis
peritracheal
peritrochanteric
perityphlitis actinomycotica
periumbilical
periungual
periureteral
periureteric
periureteritis plastica
periurethral
periurethritis
periuterine
perivaginal
perivaginitis
perivascular
perivascularity
perivasculitis
perivenous
periventricular
perivertebral
perivesical
perivesicular
perivesiculitis
perivisceral
perivisceritis
perivitelline
perivulvar
Perkins tonometer
PERL—pupils equal, react to light

PERLA—pupils equal, react to
    light and accommodation
perlèche
Per-Lee tube
Perlia nucleus
Perls
    stain
    test
permanganate
permanganic acid
permeability
    p. constant
    differential p.
    magnetic p.
permeable
permeate
permeation
permissive
pernasal
pernicious
pernio
perniosis
perobrachius
perocephalus
perochirus
perodactylus
peromelia
peromelus
peronarthrosis
peroneal
    p. artery
    p. atrophy
    p. border of foot
    p. bursa
    p. lymph node
    p. muscle
    p. nerve
    p. paralysis
    p. retinaculum
    p. sinus of tibia
    p. spine of calcaneus
    p. veins
peroneotibial
peroneus
    p. accessorius digiti minimi
    p. accessorius quartus
peronia
peropus
peroral
    p. endoscopy
    p. retrograde
        pancreaticobiliary
        ductography
per os (p.o.) (L. by mouth)
perosseous

P

peroxidase
peroxide
perpendicular
perplexed
per primam intentionem
(L. by first intention)
per rectum
Perrin-Ferraton disease
Perritt forceps
PERRLA—pupils equal, round,
react to light and accommodation
Perroncito
    apparatus
    spirals
per se
per secundam intentionem (L. by
second intention)
persecuted
persecutory
perseverance
perseverate
perseveration
persistence
    hereditary p. of fetal
      hemoglobin (HPFH)
persona
personality
    affective p. disorder
    aggressive p.
    alternating p.
    amoral p.
    anancastic p.
    antisocial p. disorder
    as-if p.
    asthenic p.
    avoidant p. disorder
    borderline p. disorder
    compulsive p.
    cycloid p. disorder
    cyclothymic p. disorder
    dependent p. disorder
    disordered p.
    dissociative p.
    double p.
    dual p.
    dyssocial p.
    epileptoid p. disorder
    explosive p.
    histrionic p. disorder
    hysterical p.
    inadequate p.
    multiple p.
    narcissistic p. disorder
    obsessive p.
    obsessive-compulsive p.
      disorder

personality *(continued)*
    paranoid p. disorder
    passive p.
    passive-aggressive p.
    passive-dependent p.
    psychopathic p.
    sadistic p. disorder
    schizoid p. disorder
    schizothymic p.
    schizotypal p. disorder
    seclusive p.
    self-defeating p. disorder
    shut-in p.
    sociopathic p.
    split p.
    split-off p.
perspiratio insensibilis
perspiration
    insensible p.
    sensible p.
perspire
persuasion
persulfuric acid
pertechnetate sodium
Perthes
    disease
    incision
    test
Pertik diverticulum
per tubam
pertubation
perturbation
pertussis
pertussoid
perusal
per vaginam
perversion
    polymorphous p.
    sexual p.
pervert
pervious
pes (pedes)
    p. abductus
    p. adductus
    p. anserinus
    p. calcaneocavus
    p. cavovarus
    p. cavus
    p. equinovalgus
    equinovarus p.
    p. gigas
    p. hippocampi
    p. pedunculi
    p. planovalgus
    p. valgus
    p. varus

pessary
    air-ball p.
    cheek p.
    contraceptive p.
    cup p.
    diaphragm p.
    doughnut p.
    Emmet-Gellhorn p.
    Gariel p.
    Gehrung p.
    Gellhorn p.
    Hodge p.
    lever p.
    Mayer p.
    Menge p.
    porcelain p.
    prolapsed p.
    retroversion p.
    ring p.
    Smith p.
    Smith-Hodge p.
    stem p.
    Thomas p.
    Wylie p.
    Zwanck p.
pessimism
    therapeutic p.
pesticide
pestiferous
pestilence
pestilential
pestle
PET—
    positron emission tomography
        (scan)
    pre-eclamptic
        toxemia
petechia (petechiae)
    calcaneal petechiae
    perifollicular p.
petechial
Peters
    anomaly
    syndrome
Petersen operation
petiolate, petiolated
petiole
    epiglottic p.
petiolus epiglottidis
Petit
    canal
    hernia
    law
    ligament
    sinus
    suture

Petit *(continued)*
    triangle
petit mal
    atonic p.m.
    myoclonic p.m.
petit pas
Petrén
    diet
    treatment
Petri
    dish
    plate
    reaction
    test
petrifaction
pétrissage
petrobasilar suture
petroclinoid
petrolatum
    p. gauze dressing
    white p.
petroleum
    p. benzin
    p. ether
    p. jelly
petromastoid
petro-occipital fissure
petropharyngeus
petrosal
petrosectomy
petrositis
petrosphenobasilar
    suture
petrosphenoid
petrosphenooccipital suture of
    Gruber
petrosquamosal suture
petrous
    p. pyramid
    p. tips
Petruschky
    litmus whey
    spinalgia
PETT—
    pendular eye-tracking test
    positron emission transaxial
        tomography
Pettenkofer
    test
    theory
Petzetaki
    reaction
    test
Peutz-Jeghers syndrome
pexic
pexis

P

Peyer
    glands
    insulae
    patches
    plaques
peyote
Peyronie disease
Peyröt thorax
Pezzer
    catheter
    drain
PF—platelet factor
Pfannenstiel incision
PFC—plaque-forming cell
Pfeifer operation
Pfeiffer
    disease
    phenomenon
    reaction
    syndrome
Pfeiffer-Comberg method
PFGE—pulsed field gradient gel
    electrophoresis
PFK—phosphofructokinase
Pflüger (Pflueger)
    cords
    law
    tubes
PFQ—personality factor
    questionnaire
PFR—peak flow rate
PFT—pulmonary function test
PFU—plaque-forming unit(s)
Pfuhl sign
Pfuhl-Jaffe sign
pg—picogram(s)
PG—
    plasma triglyceride
    prostaglandin
    pyoderma gangrenosum
PGD_2, PGE_2, $PGF_2\alpha$, PGI_2, etc.
    [PGD2, etc.]—symbols for
    various prostaglandins
PGDH—phosphogluconate
    dehydrogenase
PGDR—plasma glucose
    disappearance rate
PGH—pituitary growth
    hormone
PGI—potassium, glucose, and
    insulin
PGK—phosphoglycerate kinase
PGL—persistent generalized
    lymphadenopathy
PGR—psychogalvanic response

PGTR—plasma glucose tolerance
    rate
φ—phi (Greek letter)
pH—hydrogen ion concentration
PH—
    past history
    personal history
    prostatic hypertrophy
    pulmonary hypertension
PHA—phytohemagglutinin
phacoanaphylactic endophthalmitis
phacoanaphylaxis
phacoantigenic uveitis
phacocele
phacocyst
phacocystectomy
phacocystitis
phacoemulsification
phacoerysis
phacoglaucoma
phacoid
phacoiditis
phacolysis
phacolytic
phacomalacia
phacomatosis
phacometachoresis
phacoplanesis
phacosclerosis
phacoscopy
phacotoxic uveitis
Phaenicia
    P. cuprina
    P. sericata
phagedena
phagedenic
    p. chancre
    p. ulcer
phagocyte
    alveolar p.
    endothelial p.
    fixed p.
    free p.
    habitual p's
    mononuclear p.
phagocytic
phagocytize
phagocytolysis
phagocytolytic
phagocytose
phagocytosis
    induced p.
    spontaneous p.
    surface p.
phagocytotic vesicle

phagomania
phagophobia
phakitis
phakoma
    retinal p.
phakomatosis (phakomatoses)
    Bourneville p.
phalangeal
    p. articulation
    p. bones
    p. fracture
    p. joints
    p. osteotomy
    p. shaft
phalangectomy
phalanges (plural of phalanx)
phalangette
    drop p.
phalangitis
phalangization
phalangophalangeal
phalangosis
phalanx (phalanges)
    Deiters phalanges
    phalanges digitorum manus
    phalanges digitorum pedis
    distal p.
    p. distalis digitorum manus
    p. distalis digitorum pedis
    phalanges of fingers
    p. media digitorum manus
    p. media digitorum pedis
    p. prima digitorum manus
    p. prima digitorum pedis
    proximal p.
    p. proximalis digitorum manus
    p. proximalis digitorum pedis
    p. secunda digitorum manus
    p. secunda digitorum pedis
    p. tertia digitorum manus
    p. tertia digitorum pedis
    phalanges of toes
    tufted p.
    ungual p. of fingers
    ungual p. of toes
Phalen
    maneuver
    sign
    test
phallalgia
phallectomy
phallic
phalliform
phallitis
phallodynia

phalloid
phalloidin, phalloidine
phalloncus
phalloplasty
    augmentation p.
    reconstructive p.
    Shaeer augmentation p.
    staged p.
    total p.
    ventral p.
phallotomy
phallus
Phaneuf
    forceps
    maneuver
phantasm
phantasy
phantogeusia
phantom
    p. hand
    p. limb
    p. pain
    p. pregnancy
phantosmia
pharmaceutic, pharmaceutical
pharmacist
pharmacokinetics
pharmacologic
pharmacology
pharmacomania
pharmacopeia
pharmacopeial
pharmacophobia
pharmacopsychosis
pharmacotherapeutics
pharmacotherapy
pharmacy
Pharm. D., Phar. D.—Doctor of
  Pharmacy
pharyngalgia
pharyngeal
    p. aponeurosis
    p. apparatus
    p. arches
    ascending p. artery
    p. bursa
    p. bursitis
    p. canal
    p. cartilage
    p. cavity
    p. diphtheria
    p. fistula
    p. glands
    p. hypophysis
    lateral p. space

P

pharyngeal *(continued)*
    p. membrane
    middle p. recess
    p. mucosal space
    p. muscles
    p. nerve
    p. phlegmon
    p. pituitary
    p. plexus
    p. pouch
    p. raphe
    p. reflex
    p. ridge
    p. septum
    p. space
    p. spine
    p. tonsil
    p. tubercle
    p. tunic
    p. veins
pharyngectasia
pharyngectomy
pharyngeus
pharyngism
pharyngismus
pharyngitic
pharyngitis
    acute p.
    aphthous p.
    atrophic p.
    chronic p.
    follicular p.
    gangrenous p.
    gonococcal p.
    p. herpetica
    hypertrophic p.
    membranous p.
    purulent p.
    recurrent p.
    p. sicca
    streptococcal p.
    ulcerative p.
    viral p.
pharyngocele
pharyngodynia
pharyngoepiglottic
    p. arch
    p. fold
pharyngoesophageal
    p. constriction
    p. diverticulum
    p. junction
    p. sphincter
pharyngoesophagoplasty
pharyngoesophagus
pharyngoglossal

pharyngolaryngeal
    p. carcinoma
    p. cavity
    p. dysesthesia
    p. elevation
    p. pain
    p. reconstruction
pharyngolaryngectomy
pharyngolaryngitis
pharyngolith
pharyngolysis
pharyngomaxillary
    p. abscess
    p. space
pharyngomycosis
pharyngonasal
    p. bleed
    p. cavity
    p. reflux
    p. regurgitation
    p. tract
pharyngo-oral regurgitation
pharyngopalatine
    p. arch
    p. muscle
pharyngoparalysis
pharyngopathy
pharyngoplasty
    Hynes p.
    lateral p.
    patch p.
    sphincter p.
pharyngoplegia
pharyngorhinoscopy
pharyngoscope
pharyngoscopy
pharyngospasm
pharyngostenosis
pharyngostoma
pharyngostomy
pharyngotome
pharyngotomy
    lateral p.
    open p.
    suprahyoid p.
    suture-guided
      transhyoid p.
    transhyoid p.
pharyngotonsillitis
pharyngotympanic
    p. cephalalgia
    p. tube
pharynx
    laryngeal p.
    oral p.
    white line of p.

phase
    p. of decline
    diastolic p. of concentration
    diastolic isometric p.
    ejection p.
    follicular p.
    G_1 p.
    G_2 p.
    lag p.
    late luteal p.
    latency p.
    latent p.
    luteal p.
    menstrual p.
    postmenstrual p.
    premenstrual p.
    progestational p.
    proliferative p. endometrium
    resting p.
    secretory p.
    systolic p. of concentration
    ventricular filling p.
phase-contrast
    p.-c. microscope
    p.-c. microscopy
phasic
PHC—posthospital care
Pheifer-Young retractor
Phelps operation
Phemister
    elevator
    graft
    incision
    operation
phenanthrene
phencyclidine hydrochloride (PCP)
phengophobia
Phenistix urine test strip
phenol
    camphorated p.
    p. liquefactum
    liquefied p.
    p. red
    p. sulfatase
phenolate, phenolated
phenolemia
phenolization
phenolsulfonphthalein (PSP)
phenoluria
phenomenology
phenomenon (phenomena)
    anaphylactoid p.
    Anderson p.
    aqueous-influx p.
    Arias-Stella p.
    arm p.

phenomenon (phenomena)
    (continued)
    Arthus p., p. of Arthus
    Aschner p.
    Ashman p.
    Aubert p.
    Austin Flint p.
    autokinetic visible light p.
    Babinski p.
    Becker p.
    Bell p.
    blood-influx p.
    booster p.
    Bordet-Gengou p.
    borrowing-lending
        hemodynamic p.
    Bowditch staircase p.
    brake p.
    break-off p.
    Chase-Sulzberger p.
    cheek p.
    clasp-knife p.
    cogwheel p.
    cold agglutination p.
    Cushing p.
    Dale p.
    Danysz p.
    dawn p.
    Debré p.
    Dejerine-Lichtheim p.
    Denys-Leclef p.
    d'Herelle p.
    doll's head p.
    Doppler p.
    Duckworth p.
    Erben p.
    erythrocyte adherence p.
    escape p.
    extinction p.
    face p.
    facialis p.
    fall-and-rise p.
    Felton p.
    fern p.
    Fick p.
    finger p.
    first-set p.
    flicker p.
    Frégoli p.
    Friedreich p.
    Galassi pupillary p.
    Gärtner p.
    Gengou p.
    glass-rod p., negative
    glass-rod p., positive
    Goldblatt p.

P

phenomenon (phenomena)
  (continued)
    Gowers p.
    Grasset p.
    Grasset-Gaussel p.
    Gunn pupillary p.
    halisteresis p.
    Hamburger p.
    Hammerschlag p.
    Hata p.
    Hecht p.
    Hektoen p.
    Herendeen p.
    Hering p.
    Hertwig-Magendie p.
    hip-flexion p.
    Hochsinger p.
    Hoffmann p.
    Holmes p.
    Holmes-Stewart p.
    Houssay p.
    Huebener-Thomsen-
      Friedenreich p.
    Hunt paradoxical p.
    iceberg p.
    immune-adherence p.
    intercritical epileptic p.
    interference p.
    interictal epileptic p.
    inverse Marcus Gunn p.
    inverted Marcus Gunn p.
    irradiation p.
    jaw-winking p.
    Kanagawa p.
    Katz-Wachtel p.
    Kienböck p.
    Kleist opposition motor p.
    Köbner (Koebner) p.
    Koch p.
    Koebner p.
    Kohnstamm p.
    Kühne muscular p.
    LE (lupus erythematosus)
      cell p.
    Leede-Rumpel p.
    Le Grand-Geblewics p.
    Leichtenstern p.
    Lewis p.
    Liacopoulos p.
    Liesegang p.
    lip p.
    Litten diaphragm p.
    Lucio p.
    Lust p.
    Marcus Gunn pupillary p.

phenomenon (phenomena)
  (continued)
    Meirowsky p.
    Mills-Reincke p.
    mucus extravasation p.
    negative glass rod p.
    Negro p.
    Neisser-Wechsberg p.
    no-reflow p.
    Orbeli p.
    orbicularis p.
    paradoxical diaphragm p.
    paradoxical p. of dystonia
    paradoxical pupillary p.
    peroneal-nerve p.
    Pfeiffer p.
    phi p.
    Piltz-Westphal p.
    pivot-shift p.
    Pool p.
    Porret p.
    positive glass rod p.
    pronation p.
    psi p.
    Purkinje p.
    Queckenstedt p.
    radial p.
    Raynaud p.
    rebound p.
    reclotting p.
    red cell adherence p.
    release p.
    Riddoch p.
    Rieger p.
    R on T p.
    Rumpel-Leede p.
    Rust p.
    Sanarelli p.
    satellite p.
    Schellong-Strisower p.
    Schlesinger p.
    Schramm p.
    Schultz-Charlton p.
    second-set p.
    Sherrington p.
    shot-silk p.
    Shwartzman p.
    Shwartzman-Sanarelli p.
    Somogyi p.
    Soret p.
    Souques p.
    springlike p.
    staircase p.
    Staub-Traugott p.
    Straus p.

phenomenon (phenomena) *(continued)*
  Strümpell p.
  p. of successive contrast
  Sulzberger-Chase p.
  Theobald Smith p.
  tibial p.
  tip-of-the-tongue p.
  toe p.
  treadmill p.
  Trousseau p.
  Tullio p.
  Twort-d'Herelle p.
  vacuum p.
  Wedensky p.
  Wenckebach p.
  Westphal p.
  Westphal-Piltz p.
  Wever-Bray p.
  Williams p.
phenotype
  Bombay p.
  Cellano p.
  dominant p.
  McLeod p.
  murine T-cell p.
phenotypic
phenozygous
phenylacetic acid
phenylacetylurea
  phenylalanine p. hydroxylase
  p. hydroxylase deficiency
  p. 4-monooxygenase
phenylalaninemia
phenylketonuria (PKU)
  atypical p.
  classic p.
  Følling (Folling) p.
  maternal p.
  transient p.
  variant p.
phenyllactic acid
phenylpyruvic acid
phenylthiourea
pheochrome
  p. body
  p. cells
pheochromoblast
pheochromoblastoma
pheochromocyte
pheochromocytoma
  malignant p.
pheresis
pheromone
phi—Greek letter
  (φ; alphabetized as ph)

Philip glands
Phillips
  bougie
  catheter
  clamp
philtrum
phimosis
  acquired p.
  clitoral p.
  labial p.
  pathologic p.
  physiologic p.
  p. vaginalis
phimotic
phlebalgia
phlebangioma
phlebarteriectasia
phlebectasia laryngis
phlebectasis
phlebectomy
phlebemphraxis
phlebitic septicemia
phlebitis
  adhesive p.
  blue p.
  obliterating p.
  obstructive p.
  plastic p.
  productive p.
  proliferative p.
  puerperal p.
  septic p.
  sinus p.
  suppurative p.
phleboclysis
  drip p.
  slow p.
phlebodynamometry
phlebogenous
phlebogram
phlebography
  ascending p.
  descending p.
phleboid
phlebolith
phlebolithiasis
phlebometritis
phlebophlebostomy
phleboplasty
phleborheography
phleborrhaphy
phleborrhexis
phlebosclerosis
  portal p.
phlebosis

P

phlebostasis
phlebostenosis
phlebothrombosis
phlebotome
phlebotomist
phlebotomize
phlebotomy
    bloodless p.
phlegm
phlegmasia
    p. alba dolens
    cellulitic p.
    p. cerulea dolens
    thrombotic p.
phlegmatic
phlegmon
    Holz p.
    pancreatic p.
    periurethral p.
    pharyngeal p.
phlegmonous
    p. abscess
    p. adenitis
    p. cellulitis
    p. enteritis
    p. gastritis
    p. mastitis
    p. vulvitis
phlogistic
phlogogenic
phlorhizin, phlorizin, phlorrhizin
phloroglucin
phloroglucinol
phloxine B
phlyctena (phlyctenae)
phlyctenar
phlyctenula (phlyctenulae)
phlyctenular
    p. conjunctivitis
    p. keratitis
    p. keratoconjunctivitis
    p. ophthalmia
    p. pannus
phlyctenule
phlyctenulosis
    allergic p.
    tuberculous p.
PHM—posterior hyaloid membrane
phobia
phobic
Phocas disease
phocomelia
phocomelus
phonal
phonasthenia

phonation
    subenergetic p.
    superenergetic p.
phonatory
phoneme
phonemic
phonendoscope
phonetic
phonic
phonism
phonoangiography
phonoauscultation
phonocardiogram (PCG)
phonocardiograph
    fetal p.
phonocardiographic
phonocardiography
    digital p.
    intracardiac p.
phonocatheter
phonocatheterization
    intracardiac p.
phonogram
phonophobia
phonopsia
phonorenogram
phonoscopy
phoria
phose
phosgene
phosgenic
phosis
phosphatase
    acid p.
    alkaline p.
    leukocyte alkaline p. (LAP)
    serum p.
phosphate
    p. acetyltransferase
    acid p.
    adenosine p.
    alkaline p.
    aluminum p.
    ammoniomagnesium p.
    ammonium p.
    antazoline p.
    calcium p.
    carbamoyl p. synthetase
    creatine p.
    glycerol p.
    guanidine p.
    high-energy p. bond
    inorganic p.
    low-energy p. bond
    magnesium p.

phosphate *(continued)*
    normal p.
    organic p.
    polyestradiol p.
    triple p.
phosphatemia
phosphatidic acid
phosphatidosis
phosphatidylcholine–sterol
    o-acyltransferase
phosphatidylethanolamine (PE)
phosphatidylinositol (PI)
    p. 4,5-bisphosphate (PIP$_2$)
    p. 4-phosphate (PIP)
phosphatidylserine (PS)
phosphaturia
phosphene
    accommodation p.
phosphide
    zinc p.
phosphine
phosphocreatine
phosphodiester bond
phosphodiesterase I
phosphoglobulin
phosphoglucokinase
phosphoglucomutase
phosphogluconate dehydrogenase
    (decarboxylating)
phosphoglucose isomerase
3-phosphoglyceraldehyde
phosphoglycerate
    p. kinase
    p. mutase
phosphoglyceric acid
phosphoglyceride
phosphoglyceromutase
phosphoglycoprotein
phosphoguanidine
phosphoinositide
phospholipase (A$_1$, A$_2$, B, C, D)
phospholipid
phospholipidemia
phosphomannose isomerase
phosphomolybdic acid
phosphomutase
phosphonate
phosphonolipid
phosphopenia
phosphoprotein
phosphoprotein phosphatase
phosphoptomaine
phosphopyruvate
    p. carboxykinase
    p. hydratase

phosphorated
phosphorescence
phosphorescent
phosphoriboisomerase
phosphoribosylamine
phosphoribosylpyrophosphate
    (PRPP)
    p. synthetase
phosphoribosyltransferase
phosphoric acid
    p.a., diluted
    p.a., glacial
phosphorism
phosphorolysis
phosphorus (P)
    amorphous p.
    black p.
    labeled p.
    ordinary p.
    p. necrosis
    p. P 32
    p. poisoning
    radioactive p.
    red p.
    white p.
    yellow p.
phosphorylase
    p. b kinase deficiency
    glycogen p.
    glycogen p. kinase
    hepatic p. deficiency
    hepatic p. kinase
    p. kinase
    liver p. deficiency
    liver p. kinase
        deficiency
    muscle p. deficiency
    nucleoside p.
    polynucleotide p.
    purine-nucleoside p.
phosphorylation
    oxidative p.
    substrate-level p.
phosphoserine
phosphosugar
phosphotransferase
phosphotriose
phosphotungstate
phosphotungstic acid
phosphuresis
phosphuretic
photalgia
photic
photism
photoablation

P

photoactinic
photoactive
photoallergen
photoallergic
photoallergy
photocauterization
photochemical
photochemotherapy
photocoagulation
photocoagulator
    Mira p.
    Zeiss p.
photoconductivity
photoconvulsive
photocutaneous
photodermatitis
    polymorphous p.
photodermatosis
photodisruption
photodynamic
photodynamics
photodynia
photodysphoria
photoelectric
photoerythema
photoesthetic
photofluorogram
photofluorographic
photofluorography
photofluoroscope
photofluoroscopy
photography
    fluorescein fundus p.
    fluorescence retinal p.
photoinactivation
photolabile
photoluminescence
photolysis
photolytic
photoma
photomagnetism
photometer
    flame p.
    flicker p.
    Förster p.
photometry
    flicker p.
    internal standard flame p.
photomicrography
photomicroscopy
photomyogenic
photon
    degraded p.
    p. densitometry
    gamma p.
photonuclear reaction

photo-onycholysis
photoparoxysmal
photoperceptive
photoperiodic
photoperiodism
photophilic
photophobia
photophobic
photophosphorylation
    cyclic p.
photophthalmia
    flash p.
photopia
photopic
photopigment
photoplethysmography
photoprotection
photopsia
photopsin
photoptarmosis
photoptometry
photoradiation
photoreaction
photoreactivation
photoreception
photoreceptive
photoreceptor
photorespiration
photoretinitis
photoretinopathy
photoscan
photoscopy
photosensitive
photosensitivity
photosensitization
    contact p.
photosensitize
photostable
phototaxis
phototherapy
    ultraviolet p.
photothermal
photothermy
phototoxic
phototoxicity
photuria
PHP—
    primary hyperparathyroidism
    pseudohypoparathyroidism
phrenalgia
phrenectomy
phrenemphraxis
phrenetic
phrenic
phrenicectomy
phreniclasia

phreniclasis
phrenic nerve
phrenicocostal
phrenicoexeresis
phreniconeurectomy
phrenicotomy
phrenicotripsy
phrenitis
phrenocolic
    p. ligament
    p. space
phrenocostal space
phrenodynia
phrenogastric
phrenoglottic
phrenohepatic
phrenology
phrenopericardial angle
phrenopericarditis
phrenoplegia
phrenoptosis
phrenospasm
phrenosplenic
phrygian cap
phrynin
phrynoderma
phrynolysin
phthalate
    cellulose acetate p.
    dimethyl p.
    hypromellose p.
phthalein
    alpha-naphthol p.
    orthocresol p.
    thymol
phthalic
    p. acid
    p. anhydride
phthalin
phthiriasis
    p. inguinalis
    p. palpebrarum
    pubic p.
    p. pubis
Phthirus pubis
phthisis
    aneurysmal p.
    p. bulbi
    p. corneae
phycoerythrin
phycomycete
phycomycosis
    p. entomophthorae
    subcutaneous p.
phylactic
phylaxis

phyllodes tumor
phylloid
phyma (phymata)
phymatous rosacea
physaliform
physaliphorous cells
physalis (physalides)
physallization
physeal
physiatrics
physiatrist
physical
physician
    admitting p.
    p. assistant
    attending p.
    emergency p.
    family p.
    resident p.
Physick
    operation
    pouches
physiognomic
    p. anatomy
    p. upper face index
physiologic
    p. amenorrhea
    p. anemia
    p. antidote
    p. atrophy
    p. congestion
    p. cup
    p. curettement
    p. dead space
    p. drift
    p. dwarf
    p. elasticity of muscle
    p. epilepsy
    p. hypertrophy
    p. hypogammaglobulinemia
    p. incompatibility
    p. jaundice
    p. leukocytosis
    p. murmur
    p. pacing
    p. proteinuria
    p. rest position
    p. retraction ring
    p. saline solution
    p. scotoma
    p. tooth migration
    p. tremor
physiological
    p. anatomy
    p. astigmatism
    p. crown

P

physiological *(continued)*
    p. diplopia
    p. memory
    p. polyspermy
    p. root
    p. sounds
    p. tetanus
physiologically balanced
  occlusion
physiologicoanatomical
physiologist
physiology
    antenatal p.
    applied p.
    aviation p.
    cellular p.
    comparative p.
    dental p.
    developmental p.
    general p.
    human p.
    morbid p.
    pathologic p.
physiolysis
physiometry
physiopathologic
physiopathology
physiotherapeutic
physiotherapeutist
physiotherapist
physiotherapy
physique
physis
physohematometra
physohydrometra
physometra
physopyosalpinx
physostigmine
    p. salicylate
    p. sulfate
physostigminism
phytagglutinin
phytalbumin
phytanic acid
    p.a. α-hydroxylase [alpha-]
    p.a. storage disease
4-phytase
phytobezoar
phytochinin
phytohemagglutinin (PHA)
phytohormone
phytoid
phytophotodermatitis
phytotrichobezoar
phytoxylin

pi—Greek letter
  (π; alphabetized as p)
PI—
    pacing impulse
    performance intensity
    periodontal index
    peripheral iridectomy
    phosphatidylinositol
    pre-induction (examination)
    present illness
    protamine insulin
    pulmonary incompetence
    pulmonary infarction
pia
    p. mater
    p. mater cranialis
    p. mater encephalis
    p. mater spinalis
PIA—plasma insulin activity
pia-arachnoid
    p-a. complex
    p-a. hemorrhage
    p-a. membrane
pia-glia
pial
pian
    p. bois
    hemorrhagic p.
piblokto
pica
PICA—
    posterior inferior cerebellar
      artery
    posterior inferior
      communicating artery
PICA aneurysm
PICC—peripherally inserted
  central catheter
Picchini syndrome
Piccolomini striae
pick
    apical p.
    Burch p.
    crane p.
    Rhein p's
    root p.
Pick
    adenoma
    atrophy
    bodies
    bundle
    cell
    convolutional atrophy
    disease
    retinitis

Pick *(continued)*
    syndrome
    vision
pickwickian syndrome
picoampere (pA)
picocurie(s) (pCi)
picogram(s) (pg)
picoliter (pl)
picomole (pmol)
picopicogram (ppg)
picornavirus
Picot speculum
picounit (pU)
picric acid jaundice
picrocarmine
picrogeusia
picronigrosin
picrosclerotine
picrotoxin
picrotoxinism
picture-frame–like
PICU—
    pediatric intensive care unit
    pulmonary intensive care unit
PID—pelvic inflammatory disease
PIDT—plasma-iron disappearance
    time
PIE—pulmonary interstitial
    emphysema
piebaldism
piebald skin
piece
pièce de résistance
piecemeal
pie crusting
piedra
    black p.
    white p.
Piedraia hortae
pie-in-the-sky defect
pier abutment
PIER—percutaneous intentional
    extraluminal recanalization
Pierce
    dissector
    elevator
    retractor
Pierce-O'Connor operation
Pierre Robin syndrome
Piersol point
piesesthesia
piezoelectric effect
piezogenic papules
PIF—
    peak inspiratory flow

PIF— *(continued)*
    prolactin-inhibiting factor
    proliferation-inhibitory factor
Piffard curet
PIFR—peak inspiratory flow rate
pigeon
    p. breast
    p. breeder's lung
    p. chest
    p. toe
piggyback
piggybacking
pigment
    age p.
    acute multifocal placoid p.
        epitheliopathy (AMPPE)
    bile p.
    blood p.
    p. cell
    p. cirrhosis
    cone p.
    endogenous p.
    exogenous p.
    fatty p.
    p. gallstone
    p. granules
    hematogenous p.
    hepatogenous p.
    p. incontinence
    lipid p.
    lipochrome p.
    malarial p.
    melanotic p.
    respiratory p's
    retinal p. epithelium
    p. seam
    visual p.
    wear and tear p.
pigmentary
    p. atrophy
    p. dilution
    p. epithelium
    p. glaucoma
    p. retinopathy
    p. system
pigmentation
    addisonian dermal p.
    arsenic p.
    exogenous p.
    gingival p.
    hematogenous p.
pigmented
    p. ameloblastoma
    p. basal cell carcinoma
    chronic p. purpura

P

pigmented *(continued)*
    p. epithelial layer
    p. epithelium of iris
    p. epithelium of retina
    p. hairy epidermal nevus
    idiopathic multiple p.
      hemorrhagic sarcoma
    p. line of the cornea
    p. liver
    p. mole
    p. nevus
    p. purpuric dermatitis
    p. purpuric dermatosis
    p. purpuric lichenoid dermatitis
    p. purpuric lichenoid dermatosis
    p. villonodular synovitis
pigmentosa
    pseudoretinitis p.
pigmentosum
    xeroderma p.
Pignet
    formula
    index
    standard
pigtail
    p. angiographic catheter
    aortic flush p. catheter
    Judkins p. catheter
PIH—prolactin-inhibiting hormone
PII—plasma inorganic iodine
piitis
pila (pilae)
pilar
pilary canal
pilaster of Broca
pilation
Pilcher hemostatic bag
pile
    sentinel p.
    thrombosed p.
pileus
pili
pilial
piliate
piliation
piliform
pilimiction
pill
    birth control p. (BCP)
    p. electrode
    p. esophagitis
    p. mass
    morning-after p.
    oral contraceptive p's (OCP)
    pep p.

pill *(continued)*
    radio p.
    p.-rolling tremor
pillar
    anterior p. of fauces
    anterior p. of fornix
    p. cells
    p's of diaphragm
    p's of organ of Corti
    posterior p. of fauces
    posterior p. of fornix
    p. projection
    p's of soft palate
pillet
Pilling
    bronchoscope
    tube
pillion
pillow
    Frejka p. splint
pill-rolling
pilobezoar
pilocystic
pilocytic
    p. astrocytoma
    juvenile p. astrocytoma
piloerection
pilomatricoma
pilomotor
pilonidal
    p. cyst
    p. dimple
    p. sinus
pilose
pilosebaceous
Piltz
    reflex
    sign
Piltz-Westphal phenomenon
pilula (pilulae)
pilular
pilule
pilus (pili)
    pili annulati
    pili canaliculi
    pili incarnati
    pili incarnati recurvi
    pili multigemini
    pili torti
    pili trianguli et canaliculi
pimelitis
pimeloma
pimelopterygium
pimelorthopnea
pimple

pin
    Bohlman p.
    Compere p.
    Ender p.
    friction-retained p.
    Hagie p.
    Hansen-Street p.
    Hatcher p.
    incisal guide p.
    Knowles p.
    Kuntscher p.
    Moore p.
    Pischel p.
    retention p.
    Rush p.
    self-threading p.
    Steinmann p.
    Street p.
    p. suture
    Turner p.
    von Saal p.
    Walker p.
    Zimmer p.
pinacyanol
Pinard
    maneuver
    sign
pince-ciseaux
pincers
pinch
    devil's p's
    p. graft
    p. grip strength
    key p.
    pulp p.
    p. strength
    p. test
    tip p.
    tip-to-tip p.
pinchcock mechanism
Pindborg tumor
pineal
    p. body
    p. cell
    p. eye
    p. germinoma
    p. gland
    p. peduncle
    p. recess
    p. stalk
    p. syndrome
    p. ventricle
pinealectomy
pinealism
pinealoblastoma

pinealocyte
pinealocytoma
pinealoma
    ectopic p.
pinealopathy
Pinel system
ping-pong fracture
pinguecula
pinhole
    p. aperture
    p. collimator
    p. fistula
    p. fracture
    p. pupil
    p. scintigraphy
    p. Snellen visual acuity test
    p. SPECT
    p. subtraction imaging
piniform
pink disease
pinkeye, pink eye, pink-eye
pink puffer
pinledge crown
pinna
pinnal
pinocyte
pinocytic
pinocytosis
pinosome
pins-and-needles sensation
Pins sign
pinta fever
pintid
pinworm
pioepithelium
pion beam
Piophila casei
Piotrowski sign
PIP—proximal interphalangeal
Piper forceps
pipestem sheathing
pipette
PIPJ—proximal interphalangeal
    joint
γ-pipradol [gamma-]
piqûre
Pirie
    bone
    transoral projection
piriform
    p. muscle
    p. recess
    p. sinus
Pirogoff
    amputation

P

Pirogoff *(continued)*
 angle
 operation
 triangle
piroplasmosis
Pirquet (von Pirquet)
 cutireaction
 reaction
 test
Pischel
 electrode
 pin
pisiform
 p. bone
 p. motion
pisiformis
pisimetacarpal ligament
pisotriquetral
 p. angle
 p. arthritis
 p. arthrodesis
 p. arthrography
 p. arthrosis
 p. complex
 p. dysfunction
 p. instability
 p. joint
 p. ligaments
 p. loose bodies
 p. osteoarthritis
 p. recess
 p. space
piston
 McGee p.
 Nitinol stapes p. prosthesis
 Shea p.
 Smart stapes p. prosthesis
 stapedectomy p.
 Teflon stapes p.
 titanium CLiP stapes p.
pit
 anal p.
 arm p.
 auditory p.
 basilar p.
 chrome p.
 coated p's
 costal p. of transverse process
 ear p.
 gastric p's of Frey
 Gaul p's
 Herbert p's
 inferior articular p. of atlas
 inferior costal p.
 lens p.

pit *(continued)*
 nasal p.
 oblong p. of arytenoid cartilage
 olfactory p.
 optic p.
 otic p.
 postanal p.
 pterygoid p.
 p. of the stomach
 superior articular p. of atlas
 suprameatal p.
 triangular p. of arytenoid
  cartilage
PIT—plasma iron transport
pitch
pith
Pitha forceps
pithecoid
pithing
Pitocin drip
PITR—plasma iron transport rate
Pitres
 sections
 sign
pitting edema
pituicyte
pituita
pituitarism
pituitary
 anterior p.
 p. disease
 p. fossa
 p. gland
 p.-hypothalamus
 pharyngeal p.
 posterior p.
 whole p.
pituitectomy
pityriasis
 acute lichenoid p.
 p. alba
 p. amiantacea
 p. circinata
 lichenoid p.
 p. lichenoides
 p. lichenoides acuta
 p. lichenoides chronica
 p. lichenoides et varioliformis
  acuta
 p. linguae
 p. maculata
 p. nigra
 p. rosea
 p. rotunda
 p. rubra

pityriasis *(continued)*
  p. rubra pilaris
  p. sicca
  p. simplex
  p. steatoides
  p. versicolor
pityroid
pivot
  p. joint
  occlusal p.
pivot-shift
  p-s. phenomenon
  p-s. sign
  p-s. test
pizzeria
PJRT—permanent junctional
  reciprocating tachycardia
PK—pyruvate kinase
PK; P-K—Prausnitz-Küstner
PKP—penetrating keratoplasty
PKU—phenylketonuria
PKV—killed poliomyelitis vaccine
pl—picoliter
PL—
  light perception
  phospholipid
  placental lactogen
  pulpolingual
PLA—pulpolinguoaxial
placebo
placenta (placentas, placentae)
  ablatio placentae
  abruptio placentae
  accessory p.
  p. accreta
  adherent p.
  annular p.
  battledore p.
  bidiscoid p., bidiscoidal p.
  bilobate p.
  bilobed p.
  p. bipartita
  bipartite p.
  central p. previa
  chorioallantoic p.
  choriovitelline p.
  circummarginate p.
  p. circumvallata
  circumvallate p.
  cirsoid p.
  p. cirsoides
  complete p. previa
  deciduate p.
  deciduous p.
  p. diffusa

placenta (placentas, placentae)
  (continued)
  p. dimidiata
  dimidiate p.
  discoid p.
  p. discoidea
  Duncan p.
  duplex p.
  endotheliochorial p.
  epitheliochorial p.
  p. fenestrata
  fetal p.
  fundal p.
  furcate p.
  hemochorial p.
  hemoendothelial p.
  horseshoe p.
  incarcerated p.
  incomplete p. previa
  p. increta
  labyrinthine p.
  lobed p.
  marginal p. previa
  maternal p.
  p. membranacea
  monochorionic p.
  multilobate p.
  multilobed p.
  p. multipartita
  p. nappiformis
  nondeciduate p.
  nondeciduous p.
  partial p. previa
  p. percreta
  p. previa
  p. previa centralis
  p. previa marginalis
  p. previa partialis
  p. reflexa
  p. reniformis
  retained p.
  Schultze p.
  p. spuria
  stone p.
  p. succenturiata
  succenturiate p.
  syndesmochorial p.
  total p. previa
  p. triloba
  trilobate p.
  p. tripartita
  tripartite p.
  p. triplex
  uterine pl
  velamentous p.

P

placenta (placentas, placentae)
  (continued)
    villous p.
    yolk-sac p.
    zonary p.
    zonular p.
placental
    p. abruption
    p. barrier
    p. circulation
    confined p. mosaicism
    p. cyst
    p. dysfunction syndrome
    p. dystocia
    p. edema
    p. forceps
    p. growth hormone
    p. hormones
    human p. lactogen
    p. insufficiency
    p. lobes
    p. membrane
    p. presentation
    p. septa
    p. sign
    p. souffle
    p. stage
    p. thrombosis
    p. tissue
    p. transfusion
    p. vascular anastomosis
    p. zone
placentitis
placentoid
Placido disk
    corneal topography
    videokeratography
placode
    auditory p.
    dorsolateral p's
    epibranchial p's
    lens p.
    nasal p.
    olfactory p.
    otic p.
placoid
plafond
plagiocephalic
plagiocephaly
plague
    ambulatory p.
    bubonic p.
    pulmonic p.
    septicemic p.
plain
    p. catgut suture

plain *(continued)*
    p. suture
planar
    echo p. imaging
    p. mammography
    p. MIBG imaging
    p. phase analysis
    p. positron imaging
    p. scintigraphy
    p. spin imaging
    p. xanthoma
planchet
plane
    Addison p's
    Aeby p.
    auricular p. of sacral bone
    auriculoinfraorbital p.
    axial p.
    axial p. of tooth
    axial wall p.
    axiolabiolingual p.
    axiomesiodistal p.
    Baer p.
    base p.
    bite p., biteplane, bite-plane
    Blumenbach p.
    Bolton-nasion p.
    Broadbent-Bolton p.
    Broca p.
    buccolingual p.
    Camper p.
    coronal p.
    cove p.
    cross-sectional p.
    cusp p.
    datum p.
    Daubenton p.
    eye-ear p.
    facial p.
    first parallel pelvic p.
    Frankfort horizontal p.
    frontal p.
    frontoparallel p.
    p. of the greatest pelvic
      dimension
    guide p.
    guiding p.
    Hensen p.
    Hodge p's
    horizontal p.
    p. of inlet of pelvis
    intercristal p.
    interiliac p.
    interparietal p. of occipital bone
    interspinal p.
    intertubercular p.

plane *(continued)*
  labiolingual p.
  Listing p.
  Ludwig p.
  mandibular p.
  mean foundation p.
  Meckel p.
  median p.
  median-raphe p.
  median-sagittal p.
  mesiodistal p.
  midclavicular p.
  midpelvic p.
  midsagittal p.
  Morton p.
  narrow pelvic p.
  nasion-postcondylar p.
  nuchal p.
  occipital p.
  occlusal p.
  p. of occlusion
  orbital p.
  orbital p. of frontal bone
  parasagittal p.
  pelvic p., narrow
  pelvic p. of greatest dimension
  pelvic p. of inlet
  pelvic p. of least dimension
  pelvic p. of outlet
  pelvic p., wide
  popliteal p. of femur
  principal p.
  p. of regard
  sagittal p.
  sella-nasion (SN) p.
  semicircular p. of frontal bone
  semicircular p. of parietal bone
  semicircular p. of squama
    temporalis
  SN (sella-nasion) p.
  p's of reference
  spinous p.
  sternal p.
  sternoxiphoid p.
  subcostal p.
  supracrestal p.
  suprasternal p.
  p. suture
  temporal p.
  thoracic p.
  tooth p.
  transpyloric p.
  transtubercular p.
  transverse p.
  umbilical p.
  vertical p.

plane *(continued)*
  visual p.
  wide pelvic p.
planigraphy
planimetric
planing
  root p.
planning
  family p.
planoconcave
planoconvex
planovalgus
planta
plantalgia
plantar
  p. dermatosis, juvenile
  p. fibromatosis
  p. hyperkeratosis
  p. inoculum
  p. nevi
  p. reflex
  p. wart
plantaris
plantation
plantiflexion
plantigrade
planum (plana)
  p. interspinale
  p. intertuberculare
  p. nuchale
  p. occipitale
  p. orbitale
  p. popliteum femoris
  p. semilunatum
  p. sphenoidale
  p. sternale
  p. subcostale
  p. supracristale
  p. temporale
  p. transpyloricum
planuria
plaque
  atheromatous p.
  attachment p's
  bacterial p.
  bacteriophage p.
  dental p.
  ear p.
  en plaque
  eosinophilic p.
  fibrofatty p.
  fibrous p.
  p.-forming cell assay
  p.-forming unit
  herald p.
  Hollenhorst p's

P

plaque *(continued)*
    p's jaunes
    Jerne p. assay
    Jerne p. technique
    large p. parapsoriasis
    p. morphea
    mucous p.
    neuritic p's
    pleural p's
    pruritic urticarial papules and
      p's of pregnancy
    p. psoriasis
    senile p's
    small p. parapsoriasis
    talc p's
    tuberculoma en p.
plasma
    antihemophilic human p.
    artificial p. extender
    blood p.
    p. cell balanitis
    p. cell dyscrasia
    p. cell granuloma
    p. cell hepatitis
    p. cell leukemia
    p. cell mastitis
    p. cell pneumonia
    p. cell tumor
    p. cell vulvitis
    citrated p.
    p. exchange
    fasting p. glucose
    flaming p. cell
    p. fraction
    fresh frozen p.
    p. iron clearance
    p. iron clearance half-time
    p. kallikrein
    p. membrane
    normal human p.
    oxalate p.
    pooled p.
    p. protein fraction
    rapid p. reagin test
    renal p. flow
    p. renin activity
    salt p.
    seminal p.
    p. therapy
    p. thromboplastin antecedent
    true p.
    p. volume expander
plasmablastic lymphoma
plasmacyte
plasmacytic lymphoma

plasmacytoid
    p. lymphocyte
    p. lymphocyte lymphoma
plasmacytoma
    cutaneous p.
    extramedullary p.
    multiple p. of bone
    solitary p.
plasmacytosis
plasmalemmal vesicle
plasmapheresis
plasmatic
    p. canal
    p. stain
plasminogen
Plasmodium
    P. falciparum
    P. malariae
    P. ovale
    P. vivax
plasmodium (plasmodia)
plasmoid humor
plastein
plaster
    adhesive p.
    dental p.
    impression p.
    model p.
    mustard p.
    p. of Paris
    salicylic acid p.
    sterile adhesive p.
plastic
    p. bronchitis
    p. clot
    p. cyclitis
    p. dressing
    p. induration
    p. inflammation
    p. iritis
    modeling p.
    p. phlebitis
    p. splint
    p. surgery
    p. suture
plasticity
plasticizer
plastogel
plastron
plate
    alar p.
    anal p.
    auditory p.
    axial p.
    basal p.

plate   951

plate *(continued)*
    base p.
    bite p., biteplate, bite-plate
    blood p. thrombus
    Blount p.
    bone p.
    butt p.
    cardiogenic p.
    chorionic p.
    clinoid p.
    compression p.
    cortical p.
    cough p.
    counting p.
    p. of cranial bone, inner
    p. of cranial bone, outer
    cribriform p.
    cribriform p. of ethmoid bone
    cuticular p.
    cutis p.
    dental p.
    die p.
    dorsal p.
    dorsolateral p.
    Eggers p.
    end p.
    end p. activity
    end p. noise
    end p. potential
    end p. spikes
    epiphyseal p.
    equatorial p.
    ethmovomerine p.
    expansion p. appliance
    facial p.
    floor p.
    foot p.
    force p.
    frontal p.
    frontonasal p.
    growth p.
    hand p.
    horizontal p. of palatine bone
    Ishihara p's
    Jewett p.
    jumping-the-bite p.
    Kessel p.
    Kingsley p.
    Kühne terminal p's
    Lane p's
    lateral mesoblastic p.
    lateral p. of pterygoid bone
    lawn p.
    lingual p.
    Mancini p's

plate *(continued)*
    McLaughlin p.
    meatal p.
    medullary p.
    metaphase p.
    middle p.
    Moe p.
    motor end p.
    muscle p.
    nail p.
    neural p.
    notochordal p.
    oral p.
    orbital p. of ethmoid bone
    orbital p. of frontal bone
    outer p. of cranial bone
    palatal p.
    paper p.
    parachordal p.
    parietal p.
    perpendicular p. of ethmoid
      bone
    perpendicular p. of palatine
      bone
    Petri p.
    polar p's
    pole p's
    pour p.
    prechordal p.
    prochordal p.
    pseudoisochromatic p.
    pterygoid p., lateral
    pterygoid p., medial
    quadrigeminal p.
    reticular p.
    roof p.
    safety p.
    segmental p.
    Sherman p.
    spiral p.
    spring p.
    streak p.
    subgerminal p.
    tantalum p.
    tarsal p's
    tectal p.
    terminal p.
    Thornton p.
    tympanic p.
    urethral p.
    vascular foot p.
    ventral p.
    ventrolateral p.
    vertical p. of palatine bone
    wing p.

P

plateau
    p. iris
    p. pulse
    p. speech
    tibial p.
    ventricular p.
    p. wave
platelet
    p.-activating factor
    p. adhesiveness
    p. agglutination
    p. agglutinin
    p. aggregation
    p. antigen
    blood p.
    p. cofactor (I, II)
    p. count
    p.-derived growth factor
    p. factors
    giant p.
    giant p. syndrome
    gray p.
    gray p. syndrome
    p. inhibitor
plateletpheresis
platelike
    p. atelectasis
    p. crystals
    p. inspissated seminal
        secretions
    p. mineralization
    p. osteoma cutis
    p. trabeculae
    waxy p. scales
plating
    replica p.
platinosis
platinum (Pt)
    p. chloride
    p. foil
platybasia
platycelous
platycephalic
platycephaly
platycnemia
platycnemic
platycoria
platycrania
platyglossal
platyhieric
platymeria
platymeric
platymorphia
platymorphic
platymyarian

platymyoid
platypellic pelvis
platypelloid
platypnea
platypodia
platyrrhine
platysmal reflex
platysma muscle
platyspondylia
platyspondylisis
platystaphyline
platystencephalic
platystencephaly
Plaut angina
Plaut-Vincent angina
PLD—platelet defect
pleasure
    function p.
    organ p.
PLED—periodic lateralized
    epileptiform discharge
pledget
    anesthetic-soaked p.
    antibiotic-soaked p.
    cottonoid p.   ·
    cotton wool p.
    felt p.
    gelatin sponge p.
    Gelfoam p.
    lintene p.
    saline-soaked p.
    Salivette cotton p.
    p. sandwich
    p. sponge
    Teflon p.
    wet p.
plegaphonia
pleiades
pleiotropic
    p. drug resistance
    p. gene
pleocytosis
pleokaryocyte
pleomorphic
    p. adenoma
    carcinoma ex p. adenoma
    p. fibroma
    p. lipoma
    p. liposarcoma
    p. lymphoma
    malignant p. adenoma
    p. rhabdomyosarcoma
    p. tumor
pleomorphism
pleomorphous

pleonexia
pleonosteosis
    Léri p.
pleonotia
pleoptics
plerosis
Plesch
    percussion
    test
Plesiomonas shigelloides
plesiomorphous
plessesthesia
plethora
    p. of complaints
    p. of medications
    p. of problems
plethoric
plethysmogram
plethysmograph
    body p.
    digital p.
    finger p.
plethysmography
    air-cuff p.
    dynamic venous p.
    electrical impedance p.
    impedance p. (IPG)
    inductive p.
    strain-gauge p.
    thermistor p.
    tympanic p.
    venous occlusion p.
pleura (pleurae)
    cervical p.
    costal p.
    p. costalis
    diaphragmatic p.
    p. diaphragmatica
    mediastinal p.
    p. mediastinalis
    parietal p.
    p. parietalis
    pericardiac p.
    p. pericardiaca
    pericardial p.
    p. pulmonalis
    pulmonary p.
    visceral p.
    p. visceralis
pleuracentesis
pleuracotomy
pleural
    p. canals
    p. cavity
    p. effusion

pleural *(continued)*
    p. fibrin balls
    p. fibrosis
    p. fremitus
    p. lavage
    p. mesothelioma
    p. mouse
    p. plaques
    p. pressure
    p. recesses
    p. rings
    p. rub
    p. sac
    p. shock
    p. space
pleuralgia
pleuralgic
pleurapophysis
pleurectomy
pleurisy
    acute p.
    adhesive p.
    basal p.
    benign dry p.
    blocked p.
    cholesterol p.
    chronic p.
    chyliform p.
    chyloid p.
    chylous p.
    circumscribed p.
    costal p.
    diaphragmatic p.
    diffuse p.
    double p.
    dry p.
    p. with effusion
    encysted p.
    epidemic p.
    epidemic benign dry p.
    epidemic diaphragmatic p.
    exudative p.
    fibrinous p.
    hemorrhagic p.
    ichorous p.
    indurative p.
    interlobular p.
    latent p.
    mediastinal p.
    metapneumonic p.
    plastic p.
    primary p.
    proliferating p.
    pulmonary p.
    pulsating p.

P

pleurisy *(continued)*
    purulent p.
    sacculated p.
    secondary p.
    serofibrinous p.
    serous p.
    single p.
    suppurative p.
    typhoid p.
    visceral p.
    wet p.
pleuritic
pleuritis
pleuritogenous
pleurobronchitis
pleurocele
pleurocentesis
pleurocentrum
pleurocholecystitis
pleurocutaneous
pleurodesis
pleurodont
pleurodynia
    epidemic p.
pleurogenic
pleurogenous
pleurography
pleurohepatitis
pleurolith
pleurolysis
pleuromelus
pleuroparietopexy
pleuropericardial
    p. folds
    p. membranes
    p. murmur
pleuropericarditis
pleuroperitoneal
    p. cavity
    p. folds
    p. foramen
    p. hernia
    p. hiatus
    p. membranes
    p. sinus
pleuropneumonia
pleuropneumonolysis
pleuropulmonary regions
pleurosomus
pleurothotonos
pleurotome
pleurotomy
pleurotyphoid
pleurovisceral
plexal

plexectomy
plexiform
Plexiglas implant
pleximetric
pleximetry
plexitis
    acute p.
plexogenic
plexopathy
    lumbar p.
plexor
plexus (plexus, plexuses)
    abdominal aortic p.
    p. anesthesia
    annular p.
    anococcygeal p.
    anserine p.
    p. anserinus
    anterior bronchial p.
    anterior esophageal p.
    anterior pulmonary p.
    anterolateral p. of Santorini
    aortic p., abdominal
    aortic p., thoracic
    p. aorticus
    p. aorticus abdominalis
    p. aorticus thoracalis
    p. aorticus thoracicus
    p. arteriae cerebri anterioris
    p. arteriae cerebri mediae
    p. arteriae chorioideae
    p. arteriae ovaricae
    Auerbach p.
    auricular p.
    p. auricularis posterior
    autonomic p's
    p. autonomici
    axillary lymphatic p.
    basilar p.
    p. basilaris
    Batson p.
    brachial p.
    p. brachialis
    bulbar p.
    cardiac p.
    cardiac p., anterior
    cardiac p., deep
    cardiac p., great
    cardiac p., superficial
    p. cardiacus
    p. cardiacus profundus
    p. cardiacus superficialis
    p. caroticus communis
    p. caroticus externus
    p. caroticus internus

plexus (plexus, plexuses) *(continued)*
  carotid p.
  carotid p., common
  carotid p., external
  carotid p., internal
  p. cavernosi concharum
  p. cavernosus
  p. cavernosus conchae
  cavernous p.
  cavernous p's of conchae
  celiac p.
  p. celiacus
  cephalic ganglionated p.
  cervical p.
  p. cervicalis
  p. cervicobrachialis
  choroid p.
  p. of choroid arteries
  p. choroideus
  p. choroideus ventriculi
    lateralis
  p. choroideus ventriculi quarti
  p. choroideus ventriculi tertii
  choroid p. of fourth ventricle
  choroid p., inferior
  choroid p. of lateral ventricle
  choroid p. of third ventricle
  coccygeal p.
  coccygeal vascular p.
  p. coccygeus
  p. coeliacus
  colic p., left
  colic p., middle
  colic p., right
  corneal p.
  p. coronarius cordis
  p. coronarius cordis anterior
  p. coronarius cordis posterior
  coronary p's, gastric
  coronary p. of heart, anterior
  coronary p. of heart, posterior
  coronary p's of stomach,
    superior
  crural p.
  Cruveilhier p.
  cystic p.
  deep cervical p.
  deep stroma p.
  deferential p.
  p. deferentialis
  dental p., inferior
  p. dentalis inferior
  p. dentalis superior
  dental p., superior
  diaphragmatic p.

plexus (plexus, plexuses) *(continued)*
  dorsal venous p. of foot
  dorsal venous p. of hand
  enteric p.
  p. entericus
  epigastric p.
  esophageal p.
  p. esophageus
  p. esophageus anterior
  p. esophageus posterior
  Exner p.
  external iliac p.
  external maxillary p.
  facial p.
  p. of facial artery
  p. facialis
  femoral p.
  p. femoralis
  fundamental p.
  p. gangliosus ciliaris
  gastric p's
  p. gastrici
  p. gastricus anterior
  p. gastricus inferior
  p. gastricus posterior
  p. gastricus superior
  gastroepiploic p., left
  p. haemorrhoidalis
  p. haemorrhoidalis medius
  p. haemorrhoidalis superior
  Heller p.
  hemorrhoidal p.
  hepatic p., p. hepaticus
  hypogastric p.
  hypogastric p., inferior
  hypogastric p., superior
  p. hypogastricus
  p. hypogastricus inferior
  p. hypogastricus superior
  ileocolic p.
  iliac p's, p. iliaci
  p. iliacus externus
  inferior thyroid p.
  inferior vesical p.
  infraorbital p.
  inguinal p.
  p. inguinalis
  p. intercavernosus
  intercavernous p.
  intermediate p.
  intermesenteric p.
  intermesenteric p.,
    lumboaortic
  p. intermesentericus
  internal carotid venous p.

P

plexus (plexus, plexuses) *(continued)*
  internal maxillary p.
  interradial p.
  intestinal p., submucous
  intraepithelial p.
  intramural p.
  p. intraparotideus
  intrascleral p.
  ischiadic p.
  Jacobson p.
  Jacques p.
  jugular p.
  p. jugularis
  Kiesselbach p.
  laryngeal p.
  lateral p.
  Leber p.
  left coronary p. of heart
  left gastroepiploic p.
  lienal p.
  p. lienalis
  lingual p.
  p. lingualis
  p. lumbalis
  lumbar p.
  p. lumbaris
  lumboaortic intermesenteric p.
  lumbosacral p.
  p. lumbosacralis
  lymphatic p.
  p. lymphaticus
  p. lymphaticus axillaris
  p. mammarius
  p. mammarius internus
  mammary venous p.
  p. maxillaris externus
  p. maxillaris internus
  maxillary p.
  mediastinal p.
  Meissner p.
  meningeal p.
  p. meningeus
  mesenteric p., inferior
  mesenteric p., superior
  p. mesentericus inferior
  p. mesentericus superior
  molecular p.
  myenteric p.
  p. myentericus
  nasopalatine p.
  nerve p.
  p. nervorum spinalium
  nervous p.
  obturator p.
  occipital p.

plexus (plexus, plexuses) *(continued)*
  p. occipitalis
  p. oesophagealis
  p. oesophageus
  ophthalmic p.
  p. ophthalmicus
  ovarian p.
  p. ovaricus
  pampiniform p.
  p. pampiniformis
  pancreatic p.
  p. pancreaticus
  pancreaticoduodenal p.
  Panizza p's
  parotid p. of facial nerve
  p. parotideus nervi facialis
  p. patellae
  patellar p.
  pelvic p.
  p. pelvicus
  p. pelvina
  periarterial p.
  p. periarterialis
  pericorneal p.
  periesophageal p. of veins
  perimuscular p.
  perimysial p.
  p. perivascularis
  pharyngeal p.
  p. pharyngealis
  pharyngeal p. of vagus nerve
  p. pharyngeus
  p. pharyngeus ascendens
  p. pharyngeus nervi vagi
  phrenic p.
  p. phrenicus
  popliteal p.
  p. popliteus
  posterior pulmonary p.
  p. pulmonalis
  preaortic p's
  presacral p.
  prevertebral p's
  primary p.
  prostatic p.
  prostaticovesical p.
  p. prostaticus
  pterygoid p.
  p. pterygoideus
  p. pudendalis
  p. pulmonalis anterior
  p. pulmonalis posterior
  pulmonary p.
  pyloric p.
  Quénu hemorrhoidal p.

plexus (plexus, plexuses) *(continued)*

Ranvier p.
p. of Raschkow
p. rectales inferiores
p. rectales medii
rectal p's, inferior
p. rectalis inferior
p. rectalis medius
p. rectalis superior
rectal p's, middle
rectal p., superior
Remak p.
renal p.
p. renalis
right coronary p. of heart
sacral p.
sacral p., anterior
p. sacralis
p. sacralis anterior
p. sacralis medius
sacral lymphatic p.
Santorini p.
Sappey subareolar p.
sciatic p.
sinocarotid p.
solar p.
spermatic p.
p. spermaticus
p. of spinal nerves
splenic p.
p. splenicus
Stensen p.
stroma p.
sub-basal p.
subclavian p.
p. subclavius
subendocardiac p.
subendocardial terminal p.
subepithelial p.
submolecular p.
submucosal p.
p. submucosus p.
submucous p.
subpapillary p.
subpapillary venous p.
subpericardial p.
subpleural mediastinal p.
subsartorial p.
p. subsartorialis
subserosal p.
p. subserosus
subtrapezius p.
superior thyroid p.
supraradial p.
suprarenal p.

plexus (plexus, plexuses) *(continued)*

p. suprarenalis
p. sympathici
p. temporalis superficialis
testicular p.
p. testicularis
thoracic aortic p.
thyroid p., inferior
thyroid p., superior
thyroid venous p.
tonsillar p.
Trolard p.
tympanic p.
p. tympanicus
unpaired thyroid p.
ureteric p.
p. uretericus
urorectal p.
uterine p.
uterine venous p.
p. uterinus
uterovaginal p.
p. uterovaginalis
uterovaginal venous p.
vaginal p.
p. vaginalis
vaginal venous p.
vascular p.
p. vasculosus
p. of vas deferens
p. venosus
p. venosus areolaris
p. venosus canalis hypoglossi
p. venosus caroticus internus
p. venosus foraminis ovalis
p. venosus mamillae
p. venosus prostaticus
p. venosus pterygoideus
p. venosus rectalis
p. venosus sacralis
p. venosus suboccipitalis
p. venosus uterinus
p. venosus vaginalis
p. venosus vertebralis
  externus anterior
p. venosus vertebralis
  externus posterior
p. venosus vertebralis internus
  anterior
p. venosus vertebralis internus
  posterior
p. venosus vesicalis
venous p.
venous p., areolar
venous p. of foot, dorsal

P

plexus (plexus, plexuses) *(continued)*
    venous p. in foramen magnum
    venous p. of foramen ovale
    venous p. of hand, dorsal
    venous p., hemorrhoidal
    venous p. of hypoglossal canal
    venous p., prostatic
    venous p., rectal
    venous p., sacral
    venous p., suboccipital
    venous p., uterine
    venous p., vaginal
    venous p., vesical
    vertebral p.
    p. vertebralis
    vertebral venous p.
    vesical p.
    p. vesicalis
    vesical venous p.
    vesicoprostatic p.
    vidian p.
    visceral p's
    p. visceralis
Pley forceps
plica (plicae)
    plicae alares
    p. aryepiglottica
    p. axillaris anterior
    p. axillaris posterior
    p. caecalis vascularis
    p. cecalis vascularis
    p. chordae tympani
    p. choroidea
    plicae ciliares
    plicae circulares
    p. cordae utero-inguinalis
    p. duodenalis
    p. duodenalis inferior
    p. duodenalis superior
    p. duodenojejunalis
    p. duodenomesocolica
    p. epigastrica
    epiglottic p.
    p. fimbriata
    plicae gastricae
    p. gastropancreatica
    p. glossoepiglottica lateralis
    p. glossoepiglottica mediana
    p. hepatopancreatica
    p. hypogastrica
    p. ileocaecalis
    p. incudialis
    p. interarytenoidea
    p. interureterica
    p. lacrimalis

plica (plicae) *(continued)*
    p. longitudinalis duodeni
    p. lunata
    p. mallearis anterior
    p. mallearis anterior
      membranae tympani
    p. mallearis anterior
      tunicae mucosae cavitatis
      tympanicae
    p. mallearis posterior
    p. mallearis posterior
      membranae tympani
    p. mallearis posterior
      tunicae mucosae cavitatis
      tympanicae
    p. malleolaris anterior
      membranae tympani
    p. malleolaris posterior
      membranae tympani
    p. membranae tympani
      externa anterior
    p. membranae tympani
      externa posterior
    p. nasi
    p. nervi laryngei
    p. nervi laryngei superior
    plicae palatinae transversae
    plicae palmatae
    p. palpebronasalis
    p. paraduodenalis
    p. pubovesicalis
    p. recti
    p. rectouterina
    p. rectouterina Douglasi
    p. salpingopalatina
    p. salpingopharyngea
    plicae semilunares coli
    p. semilunaris
    p. semilunaris conjunctivae
    p. semilunaris faucium
    p. sigmoidea coli
    p. spiralis
    p. stapedialis
    p. sublingualis
    suprapatellar p.
    p. supratonsillaris
    p. synovialis
    p. synovialis infrapatellaris
    p. synovialis patellaris
    plicae transversales recti
    p. triangularis
    p. umbilicalis
    p. umbilicalis lateralis
    p. umbilicalis medialis
    p. umbilicalis mediana

plica (plicae) *(continued)*
    p. ureterica
    plicae vaginae
    p. venae cavae sinistrae
    p. ventricularis
    p. vesicalis transversa
    p. vestibularis
    p. villosae gastricae
    plicae villosae gastris
    plicae villosae ventriculi
    p. vocalis
plicate
plicated tongue
plicating suture
plication
    caval p.
    full-thickness p.
    fundal p.
    Kelly p.
    suture p., p. suture
    total gastric vertical p.
Plicator
plicotomy
pliers
    Allen root p.
    crown-crimping p.
plinth
plop
    cardiac tumor p.
    late diastolic tumor p.
    left atrial tumor p.
    tumor p.
    vegetation p.
plot
    bull's-eye p.
    polar p.
plototoxin
PLP—proteolipid protein
PLS—prostaglandin-like substance
PLT—psittacosis-lymphogranuloma
  venereum-trachoma
plug
    Amplatzer vascular p. II
    anal p.
    anal fistula p.
    apical p.
    bone p.
    cervical p.
    corner p.
    epithelial p.
    fat p.
    felt p.
    fibrin p.
    hemostatic p.
    meconium p.

plug *(continued)*
    meconium p. syndrome
    mesh p.
    p. migration
    mucus p.
    osteochondral p. graft
    parakeratotic follicular p.
    polypropylene p.
    punctal p.
    silicon punctal p.
    SmartPLUG punctum p.
    Surgisis AFP anal
      fistula p.
    vaginal p.
    yolk p.
plugger
    amalgam p.
    gold p.
    root canal p.
plumbism
Plummer
    bougie
    dilator
    disease
    sign
    treatment
Plummer-Vinson
    dilator
    radium applicator
    syndrome
plumose
plumper
    lip p.
plumula
pluridirectional spiral
  tomography
plurifocal
pluriglandular adenomatosis
plurigravida
plurihormonal adenoma
plurilocular
plurinuclear
pluriorificial
pluripara
pluriparity
pluripolar
pluripotential
pluripotentiality
pluriresistant
pluritissular
plurivisceral
plutonium (Pu)
PLV—
    live poliomyelitis vaccine
    panleukopenia virus

P

PLV— *(continued)*
  phenylalanine-lysine-
    vasopressin
p.m.; PM—after noon (L. post
  meridian)
PM—
  after death (L. post mortem)
  pacemaker
  physical medicine
  presystolic murmur
  preventive medicine
  pulpomesial
PMA—
  papillary, marginal, attached
  progressive muscular atrophy
PMB—postmenopausal bleeding
PMC—
  percutaneous mitral
    commissurotomy
  pseudomembranous colitis
PMD—progressive muscular
  dystrophy
PMH—past medical history
PMI—
  point of maximal impulse
  point of maximal intensity
P mitrale
PML—
  polymorphous light eruption
  progressive multifocal
    leukoencephalopathy
PMMA—polymethyl methacrylate
PMN—polymorphonuclear
  neutrophil (leukocyte)
pmol—picomole
PMP—past menstrual period
PMR—
  physical medicine and
    rehabilitation
  polymyalgia rheumatica
  proton magnetic resonance
PMS—premenstrual syndrome
PN—
  percussion note
  periarteritis nodosa
  peripheral nerve
  peripheral neuropathy
  polyneuritis
  pyelonephritis
PNa—plasma sodium
PND—
  paroxysmal nocturnal
    dyspnea
  postnasal drainage
  postnasal drip

PNET—peripheral
  neuroectodermal tumor
pneumarthrography
pneumarthrosis
pneumatic
  p. antishock garment
  p. balloon dilator
  p. bone
  p. cell
  p. dilatation
  p. dilator
  p. hammer disease
  intermittent p. compression
    (IPC)
  p. lithotripsy
  p. massage
  p. orthosis
  p. otoscope
  p. otoscopy
  p. paracorporeal ventricular
    assist device
  p. prosthesis
  p. retinopexy
  p. skin flattening
  p. space
  p. tourniquet
pneumatization
  mastoid p.
pneumatized
pneumatocardia
pneumatocele
  p. cranii
  extracranial p.
  intracranial p.
  parotid p.
  scrotal p.
pneumatogram
pneumatometry
pneumatorrhachis
pneumatosis
  p. coli
  p. cystoides intestinalis
  p. cystoides
    intestinorum
  gastric p.
  intestinal p.
  p. intestinalis
  p. pulmonum
pneumaturia
pneumatype
pneumoalveolography
pneumoamnios
pneumoangiogram
pneumoangiography
pneumoarthrogram

pneumoarthrography
pneumobilia
pneumoblastoma
pneumobulbar
pneumobulbous
pneumocardial
pneumocardiogram
pneumocardiograph
pneumocardiography
pneumocele
pneumocentesis
pneumocephalus
pneumocholecystitis
pneumococcal
    p. empyema
    heptavalent p. conjugate
      vaccine
    p. meningitis
    p. nephritis
    p. pneumonia
    p. polysaccharide
    p. vaccine polyvalent
pneumococcemia
pneumococci
pneumococcic
pneumococcidal
pneumococcolysis
pneumococcosis
pneumococcosuria
pneumococcus (pneumococci)
pneumocolon
pneumoconiosis (pneumoconioses)
    antimony p.
    asbestos p.
    bauxite p.
    coal worker's p.
    p. of coal workers
    collagenous p.
    complicated p.
    diatomaceous earth p.
    fractional p.
    fuller's earth p.
    graphite p.
    hard metal p.
    hematite p.
    kaolin p.
    mica p.
    mixed dust p.
    noncollagenous p.
    polyvinyl chloride p.
    rheumatoid p.
    p. siderotica
    talc p.
    titanium dioxide p.
pneumocrania

pneumocranium
pneumocystiasis
pneumocystic
    p. infection
    p. lymphadenitis
Pneumocystis
    P. jiroveci
      [formerly *P. carinii*]
    P. pneumonia
    P. pneumonitis
pneumocystography
pneumocystosis
pneumocystotomography
pneumocyte
pneumoderma
pneumodynamics
pneumoempyema
pneumoencephalocele
pneumoencephalogram
pneumoencephalography (PEG)
    cerebral p.
    fractional p.
pneumoencephalomyelogram
pneumoencephalomyelography
pneumoencephalos
pneumoenteritis
pneumofasciogram
pneumofornix
pneumogastric nerve
pneumogastrography
pneumogram
pneumograph
pneumography
    cerebral p.
    retroperitoneal p.
pneumogynogram
pneumohemia
pneumohemopericardium
pneumohemothorax
pneumohydrometra
pneumohydropericardium
pneumohydrothorax
pneumokidney
pneumolith
pneumolithiasis
pneumology
pneumolysin
pneumolysis
pneumomalacia
pneumomassage
pneumomediastinogram
pneumomediastinography
pneumomediastinum
pneumomelanosis
pneumomycosis

P

pneumomyelography
pneumonectasis
pneumonectomy
pneumonedema
pneumonia
    abortive p.
    Acinetobacter p.
    acute p.
    acute eosinophilic p.
    acute interstitial p.
    adenovirus p.
    p. alba
    alcoholic p.
    amebic p.
    anaerobic p.
    anthrax p.
    apex p.
    apical p.
    Aspergillus p.
    aspiration p.
    atypical p.
    atypical bronchial p.
    atypical interstitial p.
    bacterial p.
    bilious p.
    bronchial p.
    brooder's p.
    Buhl desquamative p.
    Candida p.
    caseous p.
    catarrhal p.
    central p.
    cheesy p.
    chemical p.
    chickenpox p.
    chlamydial p.
    Chlamydia trachomatis p.
    Chlamydophila pneumoniae p.
    Chlamydophila psittaci p.
    chronic p.
    chronic eosinophilic p.
    chronic fibrous p.
    coccidioidal p.
    cold agglutinin p.
    congenital p.
    congenital aspiration p.
    contusion p.
    core p.
    Corrigan p.
    creeping p.
    croupous p.
    cryptogenic organizing p.
    cytomegalovirus p.
    deglutition p.
    Desnos p.
    desquamative p.

pneumonia *(continued)*
    desquamative interstitial p.
    diffuse lymphoid interstitial p.
    p. dissecans
    double p.
    Eaton agent p.
    embolic p.
    Enterobacter p.
    eosinophilic p.
    ephemeral p.
    Escherichia coli p.
    ether p.
    fibrinous p.
    fibrous p.
    Friedländer p.
    Friedländer bacillus p.
    fungal p.
    gangrenous p.
    giant cell p.
    giant cell interstitial p.
    glanders p.
    gram-negative p.
    Haemophilus influenzae p.
    Hecht p.
    herpes simplex virus p.
    hypostatic p.
    indurative p.
    influenzal p.
    influenza virus p.
    inhalation p.
    p. interlobularis purulenta
    interstitial p.
    interstitial plasma cell p.
    intrauterine p.
    Klebsiella p.
    Legionella p.
    legionnaires' p.
    lingular p.
    lipid p.
    lipoid p.
    lobar p.
    lobular p.
    Löffler p.
    Louisiana p.
    lymphocytic interstitial p.
    lymphoid interstitial p.
    p. malleosa
    massive p.
    measles virus p.
    meningococcal p.
    metastatic p.
    migratory p.
    Moraxella p.
    Moraxella catarrhalis p.
    Mycoplasma p.
    mycoplasmal p.

pneumonia *(continued)*
   necrotizing p.
   Neisseria meningitidis p.
   neonatal p.
   Nocardia p.
   obstructive p.
   oil aspiration p.
   organizing p.
   parainfluenza virus p.
   parenchymatous p.
   Pasteurella multocida p.
   Pittsburgh p.
   plague p.
   plasma cell p.
   pleuritic p.
   pleurogenetic p.
   pleurogenic p.
   pneumococcal p.
   Pneumocystis p. (PCP)
   primary atypical p.
   Proteus p.
   Pseudomonas aeruginosa p.
   purulent p.
   Q fever p.
   radiation p.
   respiratory syncytial
     virus p.
   rheumatic p.
   Rhodococcus equi p.
   Riesman p.
   secondary p.
   septic p.
   Serratia p.
   staphylococcal p.
   Stoll p.
   streptococcal p.
   superficial p.
   suppurative p.
   terminal p.
   thrush p.
   toxemic p.
   transplantation p.
   traumatic p.
   tuberculous p.
   tularemic p.
   typhoid p.
   unresolved p.
   usual interstitial p.
   varicella p.
   varicella zoster p.
   ventilator-associated p.
   viral p.
   wandering p.
   white p.
   woolsorter's p.
pneumonic

pneumonitis
   acute interstitial p.
   acute lupus p.
   Ascaris p.
   aspiration p.
   chemical p.
   cholesterol p.
   desquamative interstitial p.
   eosinophilic p.
   granulomatous p.
   hypersensitivity p.
   interstitial p.
   kerosene p.
   lymphocytic interstitial p.
   malarial p.
   manganese p.
   mercury p.
   Pneumocystis p.
   radiation p.
   trimellitic anhydride p.
   uremic p.
pneumonocele
pneumonocentesis
pneumonocyte
   granular p's
   membranous p's
pneumonolipoidosis
pneumonolysis
pneumonomoniliasis
pneumonopathy
   eosinophilic p.
pneumonopexy
pneumonoresection
pneumonorrhaphy
pneumonosis
pneumonotherapy
pneumonotomy
pneumoparotitis
pneumopathy
pneumopericarditis
pneumopericardium
pneumoperitoneal
pneumoperitoneum
   diagnostic p.
   transabdominal p.
pneumoperitonitis
pneumopexy
pneumophagia
pneumophonia
pneumophrasia
   dysrhythmias p.
pneumoplasty
   reduction p.
pneumoplethysmography
pneumopleuritis
pneumopleuroparietopexy

P

pneumoprecordium
pneumopreperitoneum
pneumopyelogram
pneumopyelography
pneumopyopericardium
pneumopyothorax
pneumorachicentesis
pneumorachis
pneumoradiography
    retroperitoneal p.
pneumoresection
pneumoretroperitoneum
pneumorrhagia
pneumoscrotum
pneumoserosa
pneumoserothorax
pneumosilicosis
pneumosinus dilatans
pneumotachometer
pneumotachygraph
pneumotaxic center
pneumotherapy
pneumothermomassage
pneumothorax
    artificial p.
    catamenial p.
    clicking p.
    closed p.
    diagnostic p.
    extrapleural p.
    induced p.
    open p.
    pressure p.
    primary spontaneous p.
    secondary spontaneous p.
    spontaneous p.
    tension p.
    therapeutic p.
    traumatic p.
    valvular p.
pneumotomography
pneumotomy
pneumotropic
pneumotropism
pneumovirus
pneusis
PNH—paroxysmal nocturnal
  hemoglobinuria
PNI—psychoneuroimmunology
PNPB—positive-negative–pressure
  breathing
PNS—
    partial nonprogressing stroke
    peripheral nervous system
p.o.; PO—by mouth, orally (L. per os)

pO_2; pO2; PO_2—partial pressure of
  oxygen
PO—
    parieto-occipital
    period of onset
    phone order
POA—
    pancreatic oncofetal antigen
    point of application
POB—place of birth
POC—
    point of care
    postoperative care
    postoperative course
pock
    p. lesion
    p.-like scar
    p. mark, pockmark
    p. mark–like, pockmark-like
pocket
    absolute p.
    p. chamber
    complex p.
    compound p.
    endocardial p's
    gingival p.
    infrabony p.
    intra-alveolar p.
    intrabony p.
    nuclear p.
    pacemaker p.
    periodontal p.
    p. probe
    pyorrhea p.
    Rathke p.
    regurgitant p's
    relative p.
    retraction p.
    Seessel p.
    simple p.
    subcrestal p.
    suprabony p.
    supracrestal p.
    supragingival p.
    true p.
    p's of Zahn
pockmark
poculum Diogenis
POD—
    place of death
    postoperative day
podagra
podagral
podagric
podagrous

podalgia
podalic version
podarthritis
podedema
podencephalus
podiatric medicine
podiatrist
podiatry
podium (podia)
podoconiosis
podocyte slit diaphragm
pododerm
pododermatitis
pododynamometer
pododynia
podogram
podograph
podopompholyx
podotrochlitis
podotrochlosis
PODx—preoperative diagnosis
pogoniasis
pogonion
pOH—hydroxide ion concentration
Pohl test
poikiloblast
poikilocyte
poikilocythemia
poikilocytosis
poikiloderma
    p. atrophicans vasculare
    bullous acrokeratotic p.
    Civatte p.
    congenital p.
    p. congenitale
    hereditary acrokeratotic p.
    p. vasculare atrophicans
poikilodermatomyositis
poikilodermatous parapsoriasis
poikilosmosis
poikilosmotic
poikilostasis
poikilotherm
poikilothermal
poikilothermic
poikilothermism
poikilothermy
poikilothrombocyte
poikilothymia
poinsettia
point
    p. A
    absolute near p.
    absorbent p.
    acupuncture p.

point *(continued)*
    Addison p.
    alveolar p.
    apophysiary p.
    p. Ar
    p. of Arrhigi
    auricular p.
    p. B
    p. Ba
    Barker p.
    p. of basal convergence
      (PcB, PBC)
    p. of Béclard
    p. Bo
    Boas p.
    boiling p.
    Bolton p.
    Bolton registration p.
    Brewer p.
    Broadbent registration p.
    Broca p.
    Cannon p.
    cardinal p's
    p. of centricity
    Chauffard p.
    cold rigor p.
    condenser p.
    conjugate p.
    contact p.
    convenience p.
    p. of convergence
    convergence near p.
    corresponding p's
    Cova p.
    craniometric p.
    critical p.
    crossover p.
    p. D
    deaf p.
    de Mus p.
    Desjardins p.
    p. of direction
    disparate p's
    p. of dispersion
    p. of divergence
    dorsal p.
    p's douloureux
    E p.
    p. of election
    end p.
    Erb p.
    eye p.
    far p.
    p. of fixation
    flash p.

P

point *(continued)*
    focal p.
    freezing p.
    fusion p.
    Galliot p.
    glenoid p.
    growing p.
    Guéneau de Mussy's p.
    gutta-percha p.
    Hallé p.
    Hartmann p.
    Hartmann critical p.
    heat-rigor p.
    hinge-axis p.
    Hirschfeld silver p.
    homologous p.
    hysteroepileptogenous p.
    hysterogenic p.
    ice p.
    identical p's
    image p.
    p. of incidence
    incisal p.
    isobestic p.
    isoelectric p.
    isoionic p.
    J p.
    jugal p.
    jugomaxillary p.
    Keen p.
    Kienböck-Adamson p's
    Kocher p.
    Krafft p.
    lacrimal p.
    Lanz p.
    leak p.
    Mackenzie p.
    malar p.
    p. of maximal impulse (PMI)
    maximum occipital p.
    McBurney p.
    McEwen p.
    median mandibular p.
    Méglin p.
    melting p.
    mental p.
    metopic p.
    midinguinal p.
    motor p.
    Munro p.
    Mussy p.
    nasal p.
    near p.
    near p., absolute
    near p., relative

point *(continued)*
    neutral p.
    nodal p's
    normal boiling p.
    O p.
    object p.
    occipital p.
    ossification p.
    ossification p., primary
    ossification p., secondary
    P p.
    painful p's
    paper p.
    Pauly p.
    phrenic-pressure p.
    Piersol p.
    pour p.
    preauricular p.
    pressure p.
    pressure-arresting p.
    pressure-exciting p.
    principal p's
    p. of proximal contact
    p. R
    Ramond p.
    reflection p.
    refraction p.
    p. of regard
    registration p.
    retromandibular
      tender p.
    p. of reversal
    Robson p.
    root canal p.
    p. SE
    set p.
    silver p.
    p. SO
    spinal p.
    start p.
    stereoidentical p's
    subnasal p.
    subtemporal p.
    p. of Sudeck
    supra-auricular p.
    supraclavicular p.
    supranasal p.
    supraorbital p.
    sylvian p.
    tender p.
    thermal death p.
    trigger p.
    triple p.
    Trousseau apophysiary p's
    Valleix p's

point *(continued)*
    vital p.
    Vogt p.
    Vogt-Hueter p.
    Voillemier p.
    Weber p.
    p. Z
    Ziemssen motor p.
pointer
    back p.
    hip p.
pointillage
Poirier
    glands
    line
Poiseuille
    law
    space
poise unit
poison
    acrid p.
    acronarcotic p.
    acrosedative p.
    arrow p.
    catalyst p.
    contact p.
    corrosive p.
    fatigue p.
    fish p.
    fugu p.
    gonyaulax p.
    hemotropic p.
    irritant p.
    p. ivy
    mitotic p.
    muscle p.
    narcotic p's
    p. oak
    paralytic shellfish p.
    puffer p.
    sedative p's
    shellfish p.
    p. sumac
    toot p.
    vascular p.
    whelk p.
poison control center (PCC)
poisoning
    acetaminophen p.
    acetanilid p.
    acetylsalicylic acid p.
    akee p.
    alcohol p.
    aluminum p.
    aminopyrine p.

poisoning *(continued)*
    amphetamine p.
    aniline p.
    anticholinergic p.
    antimony p.
    arsenic p.
    aspirin p.
    barbiturate p.
    barium p.
    benzene p.
    beryllium p.
    bismuth p.
    blood p.
    bongkrek p.
    boron p.
    botulism food p.
    bromide p.
    broom p.
    buckthorn p.
    cadmium p.
    callistin shellfish p.
    carbamate p.
    carbon disulfide p.
    carbon monoxide p.
    carbon tetrachloride p.
    cheese p.
    chemical fume p.
    chloral hydrate p.
    chronic fluoride p.
    chronic fluorine p.
    cobalt p.
    copper p.
    corncockle p.
    coyotillo p.
    cyanide p.
    cyanobacteria p.
    darnel p.
    djenkol bean p.
    dural p.
    elasmobranch p.
    ergot p.
    esowasure-gai p.
    fish p.
    fluoroacetate p.
    food p.
    fugu p.
    Gymnothorax p.
    heavy metal p.
    hydrogen sulfide p.
    iodine p.
    iron p.
    larkspur p.
    lead p.
    loco p.
    manganese p.

P

poisoning *(continued)*
 meat p.
 mercury p.
 milk p.
 mushroom p.
 mussel p.
 naphthol p.
 neurotoxic shellfish p.
 nicotine p.
 nitroaniline p.
 nutmeg p.
 organophosphorus compound p.
 oxalate p.
 oxygen p.
 paraldehyde p.
 paralytic shellfish p.
 paraquat p.
 parathyroid p.
 petroleum distillate p.
 phenol p.
 phenothiazine p.
 phenytoin p.
 phosphorus p.
 potato p.
 puffer p.
 puffer fish p.
 ricin p.
 salicylate p.
 salmon p.
 salmonella food p.
 saturnine p.
 sausage p.
 scombroid p.
 scopolamine p.
 shellfish p.
 silver p.
 spider p.
 staphylococcal food p.
 strychnine p.
 tempeh p.
 tetrachloroethane p.
 tetraodon p.
 thallium p.
 thorn apple p.
 tobacco p.
 trinitrotoluene (TNT) p.
 whelk p.
 zinc p.
poisonous
Poisson distribution
Poisson-Pearson formula
poker spine
pokeweed
Poland
 anomaly
 syndrome

polarimeter
polarimetry
polariscope
polariscopic
polariscopy
polaristrobometer
polarity
 circular p.
 dynamic p.
 elliptical p.
 operon p.
 plane p.
 rotatory p.
 p. therapy
polarization
 angle of p.
 circular p.
 elliptical p.
 linear p.
 plane p.
 rotatory p.
polarize
polarizer
polarizing
 p. microscope
 rectified p. microscope
polarogram
polarographic
polarography
Polaroid
pole
 anterior p. of eyeball
 anterior p. of lens
 apical p.
 caudal p.
 caudal p. of testis
 cephalic p.
 cranial p.
 cranial p. of testis
 frontal p. of cerebral
  hemisphere
 frontal p. of hemisphere of
  cerebrum
 inferior p. of kidney
 inferior p. of testis
 lower p. of kidney
 lower p. of testis
 negative p.
 occipital p. of cerebral
  hemisphere
 occipital p. of hemisphere of
  cerebrum
 pelvic p.
 placental p.
 positive p.
 posterior p. of eyeball

pole *(continued)*
> posterior p. of lens
> superior p. of kidney
> superior p. of testis
> temporal p. of cerebral hemisphere
> temporal p. of hemisphere of cerebrum
> tubular p. of renal corpuscle
> twin p's
> upper p. of kidney
> upper p. of testis
> urinary p. of renal corpuscle
> vascular p. of renal corpuscle
> vascular p. of renal glomerulus

poli (genitive and plural of polus)

policeman
> p. stirring rod
> p. transfer tool

policeman's tip

policlinic

polio—poliomyelitis

poliocidal

polioclastic

poliodystrophia
> p. cerebri
> p. cerebri progressiva infantalis

poliodystrophy
> Christensen-Krabbe progressive infantile cerebral p.
> progressive cerebral p.

polioencephalitis
> p. acuta hemorrhagica
> p. acuta infantum
> acute bulbar p.
> bulbar p.
> p. infectiva
> inferior p.
> p. of Marie-Strümpell
> posterior p.
> superior hemorrhagic p.
> Wernicke acute p.

polioencephalomalacia

polioencephalomeningomyelitis

polioencephalomyelitis

polioencephalopathy
> Alpers p.

polioencephalotropic

poliomyelitic

poliomyeliticidal

poliomyelitis
> abortive p.
> acute anterior p.

poliomyelitis *(continued)*
> acute lateral p.
> anterior p.
> ascending p.
> bulbar p.
> bulbospinal p.
> cerebral p.
> chronic anterior p.
> encephalitic p.
> endemic p.
> epidemic p.
> nonparalytic p.
> paralytic p.
> postinoculation p.
> post-tonsillectomy p.
> postvaccinal p.
> spinal p.
> spinal paralytic p.
> spinobulbar p.
> p. virus

poliomyelopathy

polioneuromere

poliosis
> p. circumscripta
> p. eccentrica

poliovirus
> p. muris
> p. vaccine inactivated
> p. vaccine live oral

Polisar-Lyons tube

polishing
> p. disk
> glycine powder air-p.
> interproximal p.
> p. paste
> scaling and p.
> sodium bicarbonate air-p.

polisography

Politzer
> bag
> cone
> speculum
> test
> treatment

politzerization
> negative p.

polkissen

pollakidipsia

pollakiuria

pollen

pollenogenic

pollex (pollices)
> p. extensus
> p. flexus
> p. pedis

P

pollex (pollices) *(continued)*
    p. valgus
    p. varus
pollical
pollicis
    abductor p. brevis muscle
    abductor p. longus muscle
    adductor p. muscle
    extensor p. brevis muscle
    extensor p. longus muscle
    flexor p. brevis muscle
    flexor p. longus muscle
    opponens p. muscle
pollicization
pollicomental reflex
pollinic
pollinium
pollinosis
pollodic
pollutant
    outdoor air p.
pollution
    air p. index
    environmental p.
    noise p.
    particulate air p.
polonium (Po)
poltophagy
polus (poli)
    p. anterior bulbi oculi
    p. anterior lentis
    p. frontalis hemispherii cerebri
    p. inferior renis
    p. inferior testis
    p. occipitalis hemispherii
      cerebri
    p. posterior bulbi oculi
    p. posterior lentis
    p. superior renis
    p. superior testis
    p. temporalis hemispherii
      cerebri
poly—polymorphonuclear leukocyte
poly A—
    polyadenylate
    polyadenylic acid
Polya
    gastroenterostomy
    operation
polyacid
polyacrylamide gel electrophoresis
polyacrylonitrile
polyadenitis
    malignant p.
polyadenoma

polyadenomatosis
polyadenopathy
polyadenosis
polyadenous
polyadenylate
polyadenylated
polyadenylation
polyadenylic acid
polyagglutinability
polyalcoholism
polyalveolar lobe
polyamide
polyamine
polyandry
polyangiitis
    microscopic p.
    p. overlap syndrome
polyarcuate diaphragm
polyarteritis nodosa (PAN)
polyarthric
polyarthritis
    acute rheumatic p.
    chlamydial p.
    chronic secondary p.
    chronic villous p.
    p. destruens
    epidemic p.
    migratory p.
    peripheral p.
    p. rheumatica
    rheumatoid p.
    septic p.
    tuberculous p.
polyarthropathy
polyarthrosis
polyarticular gout
polyavitaminosis
polyaxon
polyaxonic
polybasic acid
polyblennia
polybrominated biphenyl
polycellular
polycentric
polycentricity
polycheiria
polychemotherapy
polychlorinated biphenyl (PCB)
polycholia
polychondritis
    p. chronica atrophicans
    chronic atrophic p.
    relapsing p.
polychondropathia
polychondropathy

polychrest
polychromasia
polychromatia
polychromatic
    p. cells
    p. erythroblast
    p. erythrocyte
    p. normoblast
polychromatocyte
polychromatocytosis
polychromatophil
polychromatophilia
polychromatophilic
polychromatosis
polychrome methylene blue
polychromemia
polychromic
polychromophil
polychromophilia
polyclinic
polyclinical
polyclonal
    p. activator
    p. antibody
    p. hypergammaglobulinemia
    p. hyperglobulinemia
polycoria
    p. spuria
    p. vera
polycrotic pulse
polycrotism
polycyclic
polycyesis
polycystic
    p. hydatid disease
    p. kidney disease
    p. kidneys
    p. liver disease
    p. ovaries
    p. ovary disease
    p. ovary syndrome
    p. renal disease
polycyte
polycythemia
    absolute p.
    appropriate p.
    benign p.
    chronic relative p.
    compensatory p.
    familial p.
    hypertonic p.
    p. hypertonica
    inappropriate p.
    myelopathic p.
    primary p.

polycythemia *(continued)*
    relative p.
    p. rubra
    p. rubra vera
    secondary p.
    splenomegalic p.
    spurious p.
    stress p.
    p. vera
polydactylia
polydactylism
polydactyly
Polydek suture
polydeoxyribonucleotide synthase
  (ATP)
polydextrose
polydimethylsiloxane
polydioxanone
polydipsia
    p., polyuria, and polyphagia
    psychogenic p.
polydispersoid
polydrug
polydysplasia
    hereditary ectodermal p.
polydysplastic epidermolysis
  bullosa dystrophica
polydysspondylism
polydystrophic
polydystrophy
    pseudo-Hurler p.
polyelectrolyte
polyembryoma
polyembryony
polyemia
    p. aquosa
    p. hyperalbuminosa
    p. polycythaemica
    p. serosa
polyendocrine
polyendocrinoma
polyendocrinopathy
polyene acids
polyergic
polyester suture
polyesthesia
polyesthetic
polyethylene
    p. catheter
    p. drain
    p. suture
    p. terephthalate
polyfilament suture
polygalactia
polygalin

P

polygamous
polygamy
polyganglionic
polygene
polygenic
polyglandular
polyglobulism
polygnathus
polygram
polygraph
    Keeler p.
polygyny
polygyria
polyhedral
polyheteroxenous
polyhexose
polyhidrosis
polyhybrid
polyhydramnios
polyhydric
polyhydruria
polyhypermenorrhea
polyhypomenorrhea
polyidrosis
polyinfection
polyionic
polykaryocyte
polyketide
polykinety
polyleptic
polylobular
polylysine
polymacon
polymastia
polymelia
polymelus
polymenorrhea
polymer
    addition p.
    condensation p.
polymerase
polymeria
polymeric
polymerization
polymerize
polymetacarpia
polymetatarsia
polymethyl methacrylate
    (PMMA)
polymicrobial
polymicrogyria
polymicrolipomatosis
polymicrotome
polymodal
polymorph

polymorpha
polymorphic
polymorphism
    balanced p.
    chromosome p.
    genetic p.
    restriction fragment length p.
      (RFLP)
    transient p.
polymorphocellular
polymorphocyte
polymorphonuclear
    p. basophil
    p. eosinophil
    filament p.
    p. leukocyte
    p. neutrophil
    nonfilament p.
polymyalgia
    p. arteritica
    p. rheumatica
polymyarian
polymyoclonus
polymyopathy
polymyositis
    acute p. with
      myoglobinuria
    hemorrhagic p.
    trichinous p.
polynesic
polyneuralgia
polyneural innervation
polyneuritic
polyneuritis
    acute febrile p.
    acute idiopathic p.
    acute infective p.
    acute postinfectious p.
    alcoholic p.
    anemic p.
    ascending p.
    p. cerebralis menieriformis
    cranial p.
    diabetic p.
    endemic p.
    p. endemica
    p. gallinarum
    Guillain-Barré p.
    infectious p.
    Jamaica ginger p.
    postinfectious p.
    p. potatorum
    progressive hypertrophic p.
    triorthocresyl phosphate p.
polyneuromyositis

polyneuronitis
    acute postinfectious p.
    erythredema p.
polyneuropathy
    acromegalic p.
    acute febrile p.
    acute postinfectious p.
    alcoholic p.
    amyloid p.
    anemic p.
    arsenic p., arsenical p.
    buckthorn p.
    carcinomatous p.
    chronic inflammatory
      demyelinating p. (CIDP)
    cranial p.
    critical illness p.
    demyelinating p.
    diabetic p.
    diphtheritic p.
    erythredema p.
    familial amyloid p.
    familial recurrent p.
    inflammatory demyelinating p.
    isoniazid p.
    lead p.
    nutritional p.
    paraneoplastic p.
    porphyric p.
    recurrent p.
    relapsing p.
    symmetrical p.
    symmetrical sensory p.
    uremic p.
polyneuroradiculitis
polynuclear
    p. aromatic hydrocarbons
      (PAHs)
    p. cells
    p. eosinophils
    p. giant cells
    p. infiltrates
    p. leukocyte-predominant
      pleocytosis
    p. leukocytes
    p. lymphocytes
    p. megakaryocytes
    p. neutrophils
    p. platinum complexes
    single p. polymorphisms (SNPs)
polynucleate, polynucleated
    p. cells
polynucleolar
polynucleolus
polynucleotidase

polynucleotide
    p. adenylyltransferase
    p. ligase
    p. phosphatase
    p. phosphorylase
polyodontia
polyol dehydrogenase
polyoma
polyomavirus
polyonychia
polyopia, polyopsia
    binocular p.
    p. monophthalmica
polyopsia
polyorchidism
polyorchis
polyorexia
polyostotic
polyotia
polyovular
polyovulatory
polyp
    adenomatous p.
    antrochoanal p.
    aural p.
    cardiac p.
    cervical p.
    choanal p's
    colonic p.
    cutaneous fibrous p.
    endocervical p.
    endometrial p's
    fibrinous p.
    fibrous p.
    fleshy p.
    p. forceps
    gelatinous p.
    gum p.
    Hopmann p.
    hydatid p.
    hyperplastic p.
    inflammatory p.
    intestinal p.
    juvenile p's
    laryngeal p.
    p's of larynx
    leiomyomatous p.
    lipomatous p.
    lymphoid p's
    mucosal p.
    myomatous p.
    nasal p's
    neoplastic p.
    non-neoplastic p.
    osseous p.

P

polyp *(continued)*
    pedunculated p.
    pedunculated juvenile p.
    retention p's
    sessile p.
    tooth p.
polypapilloma tropicum
polyparasitism
polyparesis
polypathia
polypectomy
polypeptidase
polypeptide
    gastric inhibitory p. (GIP)
    pancreatic p.
    vasoactive intestinal p. (VIP)
polypeptidemia
polypeptidorrhachia
polyperiostitis hyperesthetica
polyphagia
    polydipsia, polyuria, and p.
polyphalangia
polypharmaceutic
polypharmacy
polyphase
polyphasic
polyphenic
polypheny
polyphobia
polyphosphate
polyphyletic
polyphyletism
polyphyletist
polyphyodont
polypi (plural of polypus)
polypiferous
polypiform
polypionia
polyplastic
polyplegia
polypleurodiaphragmotomy
polyploid
polyploidy
polypnea
polypneic
polypodia
polypoid
polypoidosis
polyporin
polyporous
polyposia
polyposis
    acquired multiple p.
    adenomatous p. coli
    attenuated p. coli

polyposis *(continued)*
    cap p.
    p. coli
    colonic p.
    familial p.
    familial adenomatous p.
      (FAP)
    familial p. coli
    familial intestinal p.
    gastric p.
    p. gastrica
    gastric juvenile p. (GJP)
    gastrointestinal p.
    hereditary mixed p. syndrome
      (HMPS)
    intestinal p.
    intestinal hamartomatous p.
    p. intestinalis
    juvenile p. syndrome
    multiple familial p.
    multiple lymphomatous p.
    MUTYH adenomatous p.
    nasal p.
    nonfamilial juvenile p.
    p. ventriculi
polypotome
polypotrite
polypous
polypragmasy
polypropylene
    p. mesh
    monofilament p. suture
    p. plug
    p. suture
    p. tape
polyptychial
polypus (polypi)
    p. angiomatodes
    p. cysticus
    p. hydatidosus
    p. telangiectodes
polyradiculitis
polyradiculoneuritis
    acute p.
    acute idiopathic p.
polyradiculoneuropathy
    acute inflammatory
      demyelinating p.
    acute postinfective p.
    chronic inflammatory p.
    chronic relapsing p.
    inflammatory acute p.
    inflammatory demyelinating p.
polyribonucleotide
    nucleotidyltransferase

polyribosome
polyrrhea
polysaccharidase
polysaccharide
    p. A
    p. B
    bacterial p's
    core p.
    gastric p.
    immune p's
    O-specific p.
    pneumococcus p.
    specific p's
polysarcia
polysarcous
polyscelia
polyscelus
polysclerosis
polyscope
polysensitivity
polysensory
polyserositis
    familial recurrent p.
    idiopathic p.
    periodic p.
    recurrent p.
    tuberculous p.
polysialia
polysinusectomy
polysinusitis
polysomatic
polysomaty
polysome
polysomia
polysomic
polysomnography
    nocturnal p.
polysomus
polysomy
polysorbate
polyspermia
polyspermism
polyspermy
polyspike-wave
polysplenia
polystichia
polystyrene
polysuspensoid
polysynaptic
polysynbrachydactyly
polysyndactyly
polysynovitis
polysyphilide
polytef
polytendinitis

polytendinobursitis
polytene
polytenization
polytenosynovitis
polyteny
polytetrafluoroethylene (PTFE, Teflon)
polythelia
polythetic
polytocous
polytomogram
polytomographic
polytomography
polytrauma
polytrichia
polytrichosis
polytrophia
polytrophic
polytropic
polytypic
polyunguia
polyunsaturated fatty acids (PFAs)
polyuria
    nocturnal p.
    polydipsia, p., and polyphagia
polyuridylic acid
polyvalent
polyvinyl
    p. acetate
    p. alcohol
    p. bougie
    p. chloride (PVC)
    p. drain
polyvinylacetate
polyvinylbenzene
pneumoconiosis
pomade
pomatum
POMC—pro-opiomelanocortin
Pomeroy
    method
    operation
POMP—prednisone, Oncovin, methotrexate, 6-mercaptopurine
Pompe disease
pomphoid
pompholyhemia
pompholyx
pomphus
POMR—problem-oriented medical record
pomum adami
ponceau 3 B
Poncet
    disease

P

Poncet *(continued)*
    operation
    rheumatism
ponderable
ponderal index
pondostatural
ponesiatrics
Ponfick shadow
Ponka technique
ponograph
ponos
pons (pontes)
    p. cerebelli
    p. et cerebellum
    p. hepatis
    p. oblongata
    p. tarini
    p. varolii
pons-oblongata
Pontiac fever
pontibrachium
pontic
ponticular
ponticulus (ponticuli)
    p. auriculae
    p. hepatis
    p. promontorii
pontile
pontine
    p. gaze
    p. lesion
pontis
    basis p.
pontobulbar
pontobulbia
pontocerebellar angle tumor
pontomedullary
pontomesencephalic
pontoon spica cast
pontopeduncular
pool
    abdominal p.
    gene p.
    metabolic p.
    metabolite p.
    recirculating lymphocyte p.
Pool [eponym]
    phenomenon
    tube
Pooling Project Study
Pool-Schlesinger sign
POP—
    plasma oncotic pressure
    plaster of Paris
popcorn-like

poples
popliteal
    p. artery
    p. fascia
    p. incision
    p. ligament
    p. muscle
    p. nerve
    p. region
    p. space
popliteus
    p. minor muscle
    p. tendon
pop-off needle
Poppen clamp
Poppen-Blalock clamp
poppy
population
    closed p.
    Segi p.
    standard p.
POR—problem-oriented record
poradenitis
    p. nostras
    subacute inguinal p.
    p. venerea
poradenolymphitis
poral
porcelain
    dental p.
    p. gallbladder
porcelaneous
porcine
    Carpentier-Edwards p.
      xenograft
    p. collagen mesh
    p.-derived skin substitute
    Hancock p. xenograft
    p. heterograft
    p. valve
    p. xenograft
pore
    acoustic p., external
    acoustic p., internal
    acoustic p., osseous, external
    acoustic p., osseous, internal
    alveolar p's
    biliary p.
    birth p.
    Galen p.
    genital p.
    gustatory p.
    interalveolar p's
    Kohn p.
    mammary p.

pore *(continued)*
    nuclear p's
    slit p's
    sweat p.
    taste p.
    urinary p.
    p's of Vieussens
porencephalia
porencephalic
porencephalitis
porencephaly
    schizocephalic p.
    traumatic p.
Porges-Hermann-Perutz reaction
Porges-Meier
    reaction
    test
pori (genitive and plural of porus)
porin
poriomania
porion
pork insulin
pornographomania
pornolagnia
porocele
porocephaliasis
porofocon
porokeratosis
    disseminated superficial
      actinic p.
    p. excentrica
    p. of Mantoux
    p. of Mibelli
    p. palmaris et plantaris
      disseminata
porokeratotic
poroma
    eccrine p.
poroplastic
porosis
    cerebral p.
porosity
porotic
porotomy
porous
porphin
porphobilin
porphobilinogen
    p. deaminase
    p. synthase
porphobilinogenuria
porphyria
    acquired p.
    acute p.
    acute intermittent p. (AIP)

porphyria *(continued)*
    congenital erythropoietic p.
      (CEP)
    congenital photosensitive p.
    p. cutanea tarda (PCT)
    p. cutanea tarda hereditaria
    p. cutanea tarda symptomatica
    cutaneous p.
    cutaneous hepatic p.
    erythrohepatic p.
    erythropoietic p.
    p. erythropoietica
    hepatic p.
    p. hepatica
    hepatoerythropoietic p. (HEP)
    intermittent acute p.
    mixed p.
    ovulocyclic p.
    photosensitive p.
    South African genetic p.
    Swedish genetic p.
    symptomatic p.
    p. variegata
    variegate p. (VP)
porphyrinemia
porphyrinogen
porphyrinopathy
porphyrinuria
porphyrismus
porphyrization
porphyroxine
porphyruria
Porro
    cesarean section
    hysterectomy
    operation
Porro-Veit operation
porta (portae)
    p. hepatis
    p. labyrinthi
    p. lienis
    p. of lung
    p. omenti
    p. of omentum
    p. pulmonis
    p. renis
    p. of spleen
portacaval
portal
    p. of entry
    hepatic p.
    intestinal p.
    intestinal p., anterior
    intestinal p., posterior
    p. portography

P

portal *(continued)*
>   velopharyngeal p.
>   p. venography

porte-aiguille
portepolisher, porte-polisher
Porter
>   forceps
>   sign

Porter-Silber chromogens test
Porteus maze test
portio (portiones)
>   p. dura paris septimi
>   p. intermedia nervi acustici
>   p. major nervi trigemini
>   p. minor nervi trigemini
>   p. mollis paris septimi
>   p. supravaginalis cervicis
>   p. vaginalis cervicis

portiplexus
portligature
portoenterostomy
portogram
portography
>   percutaneous transhepatic p.
>   portal p.
>   splenic p.
>   umbilical p.

portosystemic shunt
portovenogram
portovenography
Portuguese man-o'-war
port wine birthmark
porus (pori)
>   p. acusticus externus
>   p. acusticus externus osseus
>   p. acusticus internus
>   p. acusticus internus osseus
>   p. galeni
>   p. gustatorius
>   p. opticus
>   p. sudoriferus

pos.—positive
Posada mycosis
Posada-Wernicke disease
position
>   abduction p.
>   acromion anterior p.
>   acromion posterior p.
>   Adams p.
>   adduction p.
>   Albert p.
>   anatomical p.
>   AP (anteroposterior) p.
>   arm-extension p.
>   batrachian p.

position *(continued)*
>   Bertel p.
>   Blackett-Healy p.
>   Bonner p.
>   Boyce p.
>   Bozeman p.
>   Brickner p.
>   Broden p.
>   bronchoscopic p.
>   brow anterior p.
>   brow-down p.
>   brow posterior p.
>   brow transverse p.
>   brow-up p.
>   Buie p.
>   cadaveric p.
>   Caldwell p.
>   Camp-Coventry p.
>   Casselberry p.
>   centric p.
>   cis p.
>   Cleaves p.
>   coiled p.
>   cross-table lateral p.
>   decerebrate p.
>   decorticate p.
>   decubitus p.
>   Depage p.
>   depressive p.
>   dorsal p.
>   dorsal elevated p.
>   dorsal inertia p.
>   dorsal lithotomy p.
>   dorsal recumbent p.
>   dorsal rigid p.
>   dorsosacral p.
>   Duncan p.
>   eccentric p.
>   Edebohls p.
>   electrical heart p.
>   Elliot p.
>   emprosthotonos p.
>   English p.
>   erect p.
>   eversion p.
>   extension p.
>   Feist-Mankin p.
>   fetal p.
>   Fick p.
>   Fleischner p.
>   flexion p.
>   flipper p.
>   Fowler p.
>   Friedman p.
>   frogleg p.

position *(continued)*
    froglegged p.
    froglike p.
    frontal anterior p.
    frontal posterior p.
    frontal transverse p.
    frontoanterior p.
    frontoposterior p.
    frontotransverse p.
    Fuchs p.
    p. of function
    Gaynor-Hart p.
    genucubital p.
    genufacial p.
    genupectoral p.
    Grashey p.
    Haas p.
    head dependent p.
    heart p.
    Hickey p.
    high pelvic p.
    hinge p.
    hinge p., condylar
    hinge p., mandibular
    hinge p., terminal
    horizontal p.
    hornpipe p.
    inlet p.
    intercuspal p.
    inversion p.
    Isherwood p.
    jackknife p.
    Johnson p.
    Jones p.
    kidney p.
    knee-chest p.
    knee-elbow p.
    kneeling-squatting p.
    Kraske p.
    Kurzbauer p.
    Laquerriére-Pierquin p.
    lateral p.
    lateral decubitus p.
    lateral prone p.
    lateral recumbent p.
    lateroabdominal p.
    Law p.
    Lawrence p.
    leapfrog p.
    Leonard-George p.
    Lewis p.
    ligamentous p.
    Lilienfeld p.
    Lindblom p.
    lithotomy p.

position *(continued)*
    Lorenz p.
    Mayer p.
    Mayo-Robson p.
    mentoanterior p.
    mentoposterior p.
    mentotransverse p.
    mentum anterior p.
    mentum posterior p.
    mentum transverse p.
    Miller p.
    Moynihan p.
    neck extension p.
    Noble p.
    Nölke p.
    nuchal hitch p.
    oblique p.
    occipitoanterior p.
    occipitoposterior p.
    occipitosacral p.
    occipitotransverse p.
    occiput anterior p.
    occiput posterior p.
    occiput sacral p.
    occiput transverse p.
    occlusal p.
    opisthotonos p.
    orthopnea p.
    orthopneic p.
    orthotonos p.
    Owen p.
    PA (posteroanterior) p.
    Pawlow p.
    Péan p.
    Pearson p.
    persistent occiput posterior p.
    physiologic rest p.
    posterior border p.
    primary p. of gaze
    Proetz p.
    prone p.
    protrusive p.
    recumbent p.
    rest p.
    reverse Waters p.
    Robson p.
    Rose p.
    sacroanterior p.
    sacroposterior p.
    sacrotransverse p.
    sacrum anterior p.
    sacrum posterior p.
    sacrum transverse p.
    Samuel p.
    scapula anterior p.

P

position *(continued)*
    scapula posterior p.
    scapuloanterior p.
    scapuloposterior p.
    Schüller p.
    scorbutic p.
    Scultetus p.
    semiaxial p.
    semierect p.
    semi-Fowler p.
    semiprone p.
    semireclining p.
    semirecumbent p.
    Settegast p.
    shoe-and-stocking p.
    Simon p.
    Sims p.
    Staunig p.
    Stecher p.
    Stenvers p.
    Stern p.
    submentovertex p.
    supine p.
    Tarrant p.
    Taylor p.
    terminal hinge p.
    Titterington p.
    Towne p.
    trans p.
    Trendelenburg p.
    tripod p.
    Twining p.
    upright p.
    Valentine p.
    verticosubmental p.
    Walcher p.
    Waters p.
    Waters p., reverse
    Wigby-Taylor p.
    Wolfenden p.
positioner
    tooth p.
positive
    p. Bing (test)
    biologic false p.
    false p.
positrocephalogram
positron
    p.-coincidence
    p. decay
    p. emission tomography (PET)
    p. emission transaxial
      tomography (PETT)
    p. emission transverse
      tomography (PETT)

Posner
    reaction
    test
Posner-Schlossman syndrome
posologic
posology
Possum (Patient-Operated Selector
    Mechanism)
post.—posterior
post
    abutment p.
    implant p.
    p. mortem
    status p.
postabortal
postacidotic
postalbumin
postanesthetic
postanoxic
postapoplectic
postauditory
postaurale
postauricular
    p. abscess
    p. area
    p. artery
    p. artery island flap
    p. ecchymosis
    p. fistula
    p. flap
    p. flip-flop flap
    p. full-thickness skin graft
    p. incision
    p. inferiorly based pedicled
      flap
    p. infratemporal fossa approach
    p. keloid
    p. nodular fasciitis
    p. nodule
    pull-through p. flap
    p. reflex
    p. region
    p. sinus
    p. skin biopsy
    p. sulcus
    p. turn-over flap
    p. tympanoplasty
    p. wound dehiscence
postaxial
    p. acrofacial dysostosis
    p. duplication
    p. muscle
    p. polydactyly
postbrachial
postbrachium

postbulbar
- p. area
- p. biopsy
- p. duodenal obstruction
- p. duodenal ulceration
- p. duodenum
- p. region
- p. stenosis
- p. ulcer

postcapillary
- p. segment
- p. venous filling pressure
- p. venules

postcardinal
postcardiotomy syndrome
postcava
postcaval
- p. lymph nodes
- p. recess
- p. segment
- p. shunt
- p. ureter
- p. vein

postcecal
postcentral
postcentralis
postcibal
post cibum
postcisterna
postcoital
- p. bleeding
- p. cervicovaginal sample
- p. contraception
- p. contraceptive
- p. headache
- p. hypersensitivity reaction
- p. interval
- p. test
- p. vaginal bleeding

post coitum
postconceptual
- p. age
- p. week

postcondylare
postconvulsive
- p. coma
- p. EEG
- p. hypoxic damage
- p. prefrontal slow-wave activity
- p. stupor

postcornu
postcranial
postcubital
postdiastolic
postdicrotic

postdiptheric
postdormital
postdormitum
postductal
- p. acidosis
- p. aortic coarctation
- p. oxygen saturation
- p. peripheral perfusion index
- p. pulse oximetry

postecdysis
postembryonic
postencephalic
postepileptic
- p. paralysis
- p. psychosis

posteriad
posterior
- acute p. ganglionitis
- p. chamber
- p. communicating artery
- p. incision
- p. nephrectomy
- p. palatine suture
- p. rhinoscopy
- p. rhizotomy
- p. sclerotomy
- p. tympanotomy

posteriorly
posteroanterior (PA) view
posteroclusion
posteroexternal
posteroinferior
posterointernal
posterolateral
- p. accessory pathway
- p. approach
- p. aspect
- p. branch
- p. bundle of anterior cruciate ligament
- p. corner deficiency
- p. corner of the knee
- p. corner reconstruction
- p. diaphragmatic hernia of Bochdalek
- p. fusion
- p. graft fixation device
- p. incision
- p. instability
- p. lumbar disk herniation
- p. lumbar fusion
- p. pin placement
- p. recess of the knee
- p. region
- p. rotatory instability

P

posterolateral *(continued)*
    p. stability
    p. surface
    p. thoracotomy
    p. tunnel
    p. vein
posteromedial
    p. approach
    p. aspect
    p. bundles of the posterior
      cruciate ligament
    p. capsule
    p. commissure
    p. compression-bending
    p. corners of the knee
    p. direction
    p. myocutaneous flap
    p. neurovascular bundle
    p. osteophyte
    p. papillary muscle
    p. parietal cortex
    p. parietal lobe
    p. portal
    p. stress fractures
posteromedian
posteroparietal
posterosuperior
posterotemporal
postesophageal
postexposure
post–fatty meal cholecystography
postfebrile
postganglionic
postglenoid
postglomerular
posthemiplegic
posthepatic
posthepatitic
postherpetic
posthetomy
posthioplasty
posthippocampal
posthitis
postholith
posthumous
posthyoid
posthypnotic
posthypoglycemic
posthypophysis
posthypoxic
postictal
    p. catecholamine surge
    p. epileptic dysfunction
    p. headache
    p. period

postictal *(continued)*
    p. psychosis
    p. psychotic episodes (PIPEs)
    p. recovery
    p. state
    p. transient hyperammonemia
posticus
postinfective
postirradiation
postischial
postmalarial
postmastectomy
postmastoid
postmature
postmaturity
postmaxillary
postmediastinal
postmediastinum
postmeiotic
postmenopausal
postmenstrual
postmesenteric
postminimus (postminimi)
postmitotic
postmortal
postmortem
postmyocardial infarction
postnares
postnarial
postnaris
postnasal
postnatal
    p. development
    p. developmental delay
    p. emmetropization
    p. growth delay
    p. growth retardation
    p. HIV transmission
    p. period
    p. weight gain
postnatal-onset
    p-o. failure to thrive
    p-o. short stature
postneuritic
postop.—postoperative
postoperative
    p. analgesia
    p. bleeding
    p. cholangiography
    p. complication
    p. day
    p. hemorrhage
    p. hypotony
    p. infection
    p. nausea and vomiting

postoperative *(continued)*
    p. pain
    p. period
    p. recovery
    p. stay
postovulatory
postpalatal
postpalatine
postparalytic
postpartum
    p. blues
    p. complications
    p. depression
    p. depressive symptoms
    p. eclampsia
    p. followup
    p. hemorrhage
    p. infection
    p. pain
    p. psychosis
    p. psychotic episode
    p. urinary incontinence
    p. uterine atony
postphlebitic
postpituitary
postpleuritic
postpneumonic
postpolio
postpontile
postprandial
postpubertal
postpuberty
postpump syndrome
postpyramidal
postrelease radiography
postrenal
postrolandic
postscarlatinal
postsinusoidal
postsphenoid
postsphygmic
postsplenic
poststenotic
postsylvian
postsynaptic
postsystolic
postthrombotic
posttraumatic
posttussive
postulate
    Ehrlich p.
    Koch p's
postural
    p. contraction
    p. drainage system

postural *(continued)*
    p. proteinuria
    p. reflex
    p. syncope
    p. tremor
    p. vertigo
posture
    chin-down p.
    upright p.
posturing
    catatonic p.
    decerebrate p.
    decorticate p.
    dystonic limb p.
    extensor p.
    face-down p.
    flexor p.
    postoperative p.
    prone p.
    symmetric tonic p.
    tonic limb p.
posturography
postvaccinal
postvaccinial
postvital
postvoid radiography
postzone
postzoster
postzygotic
potable
Potain trocar
potash
    caustic p.
    sulfurated p.
potassemia
potassic
potassium (K)
    p. acetate
    p. acid tartrate
    p. alum
    p. *p*-aminobenzoate [p-, para-]
    p. aspartate and magnesium
        aspartate
    p. bicarbonate
    p. bichromate
    p. bitartrate
    p. bromide
    p. carbonate
    p. chlorate
    p. chloride (KCl)
    p. citrate
    p. cyanide
    p. dichromate
    p. dihydrogen phosphate
    p. ferricyanide

P

potassium (K) *(continued)*
    p. glucaldrate
    p. gluconate
    p. glycerophosphate
    p. guaiacolsulfonate
    p. hydroxide
    p. iodate
    p. iodide
    p. mercuric iodide
    p. metaphosphate
    p. nitrate
    p. oxalate
    p. penicillin G
    p. perchlorate
    p. permanganate
    p. phenoxymethyl penicillin
    p. phosphate
    p. phosphate, dibasic
    p. phosphate, monobasic
    propicillin p.
    prospective p. Triplex
    radioactive p.
    reactive p. Triplex
    p. sodium tartrate
    p. sorbate
    p. sulfate
    p. tartrate
    p. thiocyanate
    p. Triplex
potbelly
potency
potent
potential
    action p. (AP)
    after-p.
    after-p., negative
    after-p., positive
    average evoked p.
    bioelectric p.
    biotic p.
    brain stem auditory evoked p.
      (BAEP)
    chemical p.
    cochlear p.
    cochlear microphonic p.
    compound action p.
    demarcation p.
    p. difference
    early vertex p.
    electrocortical p.
    electrode p.
    electrotonic p.
    endocochlear p.
    evoked p. (EP)
    evoked cortical p's

potential *(continued)*
    excitatory postsynaptic p.
      (EPSP)
    fasciculation p.
    fibrillation p's
    generator p.
    giant p.
    p. gradient
    ground p.
    hyperpolarizing p.
    inhibitory postequilibrium p.
    inhibitory postsynaptic p.
    injury p.
    late vertex p.
    life p.
    membrane p.
    miniature end-plate p's
    morphogenetic p.
    motor unit p. (MUP)
    motor unit action p. (MUAP)
    myopathic p.
    negative summating p.
    Nernst p.
    nerve p.
    oxidation-reduction p.
    pacemaker p.
    polyphasic p.
    polyspike p.
    postsynaptic p's
    receptor p.
    redox p.
    reinnervation p.
    reproductive p.
    resting p.
    ripple p.
    sensory p.
    sensory nerve action p. (SNAP)
    serrated action p.
    somatosensory evoked p. (SEP)
    spike p.
    spinal evoked p.
    standard electrode p.
    standard reduction p.
    streaming p.
    summating p.
    transmembrane p.
    utricular DC p.
    vertex p.
    visual evoked p. (VEP)
    visual evoked cortical p.
potentialization
potentiation
    paradoxical p.
    post-tetanic p.
potentiator

potentiometer
potentize
potification
potion
potomania
Pott
- abscess
- aneurysm
- curvature
- disease
- dwarfism
- fracture
- gangrene
- paralysis
- paraplegia
- puffy tumor
- syndrome (I, II)
- tumor
Pottenger sign
Potter
- disease
- facies
- treatment
- version
Potter-Bucky
- diaphragm
- grid
Potts
- anastomosis
- clamp
- operation
- rib shears
- scissors
- shunt
Potts-Niedner clamp
Potts-Smith
- clamp
- forceps
- scissors
Potts-Smith-Gibson operation
pouch
- abdominovesical p.
- allantochorionic p's
- anal p.
- anterior p. of Tröltsch (Troeltsch)
- branchial p.
- Broca p.
- craniobuccal p.
- craniopharyngeal p.
- Denis Browne p.
- p. of Douglas
- enterocoelic p.
- gill p.
- guttural p's

pouch *(continued)*
- Hartmann p.
- Heidenhain p.
- hepatorenal p.
- hyomandibular p.
- ileocecal p.
- Koch p.
- laryngeal p.
- Morison p.
- neurobuccal p.
- obturator p.
- paracystic p.
- pararectal p.
- paravesical p.
- Pavlov p.
- perineal p., deep
- perineal p., superficial
- pharyngeal p.
- Physick p's
- posterior p. of Tröltsch (Troeltsch)
- Prussak p.
- Rathke p.
- rectouterine p.
- rectovaginal p.
- rectovesical p.
- Seessel p.
- superficial perineal p.
- uteroabdominal p.
- uterovesical p.
- vesicouterine p.
- visceral p.
- Willis p.
- Zenker p.
poudrage
- pleural p.
- talc p.
poultice
pound (lb.)
pound-force (lbf.)
Poupart
- ligament
- line
- shelving edge
Poutasse forceps
poverty of movement
Powassan virus
powder
- absorbable dusting p.
- aluminum hydroxide p.
- bleaching p.
- blood-plasma p.
- p. of chalk, aromatic
- p. of chalk, aromatic, with opium

P

powder *(continued)*
    chalk p., compound
    Dalmatian insect p.
    Dover p.
    dusting p.
    dusting p., absorbable
    effervescent p's, compound
    furazolidone and nifuroxime p.
    glycyrrhiza p., compound
    Goa p.
    impalpable p.
    iodochlorhydroxyquin p.,
      compound
    licorice p., compound
    p. of liquorice, compound
    methylbenzethonium
      chloride p.
    methylbenzethonium chloride
      topical p.
    nystatin topical p.
    Persian insect p.
    Seidlitz p's
    senna p., compound
    Sippy p. (No. 1 or 2)
    sodium bicarbonate and
      calcium carbonate p.
    sodium bicarbonate and
      magnesium oxide p.
    talcum p.
    tissue p.
    tolnaftate p.
    tolnaftate topical p.
    triacetin p.
    zinc sulfate p., compound
power
    acoustic p.
    buffering p.
    candle p.
    carbon dioxide–combining p.
    CO_2–combining p. [CO2-]
    defining p.
    dioptric p.
    resolving p.
    stopping p.
Power operation
Power and Wilder method
pox
    Kaffir p.
    wart p.
Pozzi operation
PP—
    near point (L. punctum
      proximum) of accommodation
    partial pressure
    permanent partial

PP— *(continued)*
    pink puffer
    postpartum
    private practice
    prothrombin-proconvertin
    proximal phalanx
    pulse pressure
PPA—phenylpyruvic acid
ppb—parts per billion
PPB—
    platelet-poor blood
    positive-pressure breathing
PPBS—postprandial blood sugar
PPC—progressive patient care
PPCA—proserum prothrombin
    conversion accelerator
PPCF—plasmin prothrombin-
    converting factor
PPD—purified protein derivative
    (of tuberculin)
PPD-S—purified protein
    derivative–standard
ppg—picopicogram(s)
PPH—
    postpartum hemorrhage
    primary pulmonary
      hypertension
PP_i—pyrophosphate
PPLO—pleuropneumonia-like
    organisms
ppm—parts per million
PPNG—penicillinase-producing
    Neisseria gonorrhoeae
PPO—preferred provider
    organization
PPP—pentose phosphate pathway
PPR—Price precipitation reaction
PPT—pressure pain threshold
PPTT—
    prepubertal testicular tumor
    pressure pain tolerance
      threshold
P pulmonale syndrome
PPV—positive-pressure ventilation
PQ—permeability quotient
Pr—
    presbyopia
    prism
PR—
    far point (L. punctum
      remotum) of accommodation
    partial remission
    peer review
    peripheral resistance
    pregnancy rate

PR— *(continued)*
    public relations
    pulmonic regurgitation
    pulse rate
PRA—plasma renin activity
practice
    best p's
    contract p.
    family p.
    general p.
    group p.
    individual p.
    panel p.
    prepaid group p.
    private p.
    solo p.
practitioner
    general p.
    indigenous p.
    nurse p. (NP)
Prader-Labhart-Willi syndrome
Prader-Willi syndrome
praecox
    dementia p.
pragmatagnosia
pragmatamnesia
Prague maneuver
prandial
praseodymium (Pr)
pratique
Pratt
    anoscope
    curet
    dilator
    director
    hook
    probe
    scissors
    sound
    speculum
Pratt-Smith forceps
Prausnitz-Küstner
    reaction
    test
praxis
PRBV—placental residual blood
  volume
PRCs—packed red cells
PRD—postradiation dysplasia
preadaptation
preagonal
pre-AIDS
prealbumin
    thyroxine-binding p. (TBPA)
preanesthesia

preanesthetic
preaortic
preataxic
preaurale
preauricular
preaxial
prebacillary
prebase
prebeta-lipoprotein
    sinking p.
prebetalipoproteinemia
prebiotic
prebladder
prebrachial
prebrachium
precancerous
precapillary
precarcinogen
precarcinomatous
precardinal
precarious
precartilage
precava
precede
precementum
precentral
precession
prechiasmal
prechordal
precipitable
precipitant
precipitate
    alum p.
    immune p.
    keratic p's
    p. labor
    mutton-fat keratic p's
    pigmented keratic p's
    white p.
precipitately
precipitation
    electrostatic p. of dust
    group p.
    isoelectric p.
    salt p.
    tuberculin p. (TP)
precipitin
    p. curve
    p. reaction
precipitinogen
precipitous
    p. drop
    p. rise
precipitously
precision

P

preclinical
preclival
preclotting
precocious puberty
precocity
    heterosexual p.
    isosexual p.
    sexual p.
    skeletal p.
    true sexual p.
precognition
precollagenous
precoma
precommissural
precommissure
preconscious
preconvulsant
preconvulsive
precordial
    p. electrocardiography
    p. honk
precordialgia
precorneal
precornu
precostal
precritical
precuneal
precuneate
precuneus
precursor
    mast cell p.
predation
predator
predentin
predetector
prediabetes
prediastole
prediastolic
predicrotic
predigestion
predilection
predispose
predisposing
predisposition
    convulsive p.
    epileptic p.
prediverticular
predormital
predormitum
preductal
preeclampsia
    superimposed p.
preeclamptic
preejection
preepiglottic

preexcitation
    ventricular p.
pre-exposure
prefibrotic
preformation
preformationist
prefrontal lobotomy
prefunctional
preganglionic
pregenital
preglomerular
pregnancy
    abdominal p.
    afetal p.
    ampullar p.
    angular p.
    bigeminal p.
    broad ligament p.
    cervical p.
    combined p.
    compound p.
    cornual p.
    ectopic p.
    entopic p.
    exochorial p.
    extra-amniotic p.
    extrauterine p.
    fallopian p.
    false p.
    gemellary p.
    heterotopic p.
    hydatid p.
    hysterical p.
    incomplete p.
    interstitial p.
    intraligamentary p.
    intraligamentous p.
    intramural p.
    intraperitoneal p.
    intrauterine p.
    isthmic p.
    membranous p.
    mesenteric p.
    molar p.
    multiple p.
    mural p.
    nervous p.
    ovarian p.
    ovarioabdominal p.
    oviductal p.
    parietal p.
    phantom p.
    plural p.
    post-term p.
    primary ovarian p.

pregnancy *(continued)*
    prolonged p.
    pseudointraligamentary p.
    sarcofetal p.
    sarcohysteric p.
    spurious p.
    stump p.
    term p.
    tubal p.
    tuboabdominal p.
    tuboligamentary p.
    tubo-ovarian p.
    tubouterine p.
    twin p.
    uteroabdominal p.
    utero-ovarian p.
    uterotubal p.
pregnane
pregnanetriol
pregnant
pregnene
pregnenolone
pregonium
prehallux
prehensile
prehension
prehepatic
prehepaticus
Prehn sign
prehormone
prehyoid
prehypophysis
preictal
preinduction
preinsula
preinvasive
preiotation
Preiser disease
Preisz-Nocard bacillus
prejudice
prekallikrein
prelacteal
preleptotene
preleukemia
preleukemic
prelimbic
prelocalization
prelocomotion
premalignant
premature
prematurity
premaxilla
premaxillary suture
premedical
premedicant

premedication
premeiotic
premelanosome
premenarchal
premenarche
premenopausal
premenstrua
premenstrual
premenstruum
premitotic
premolar
premonitory
premorbid
premortal
premunition
premunitive
premyeloblast
premyelocyte
prenarcosis
prenarcotic
prenares
prenasale
prenatal
preneoplastic
preoccipital
preoedipal
preop.—preoperative
preoperculum
preoptic
preovulatory
preoxygenation
prep—prepare
preparalytic
preparation
    allergenic protein p's
    biomechanical p.
    cavity p.
    corrosion p.
    cover-glass p.
    cytologic filter p.
    hanging-drop p.
    heart-lung p.
    impression p.
    Langendorff p.
    proteolytic p's
    surgical p.
    touch p.
preparatory iridectomy
preparetic
prepartal
prepatellar
prepatency
prepatent
preperception
preperitoneal

P

preplacental
prepollex
preponderance
    p. of data
    p. of evidence
    ventricular p.
prepotential
prepped and draped
preprandial
preprocessing
preprohormone
preproinsulin
preprophage
preproprotein
preprosthetic
preprotein
prepubertal
prepuberty
prepuce
    p. of clitoris
    p. of penis
    redundant p.
preputial
preputiotomy
preputium
    p. clitoridis
    p. penis
prepyloric
prerectal lithotomy
prerenal azotemia
prerennin
prereproductive
preretinal
presacral neurectomy
presbyatrics
presbycardia
presbycusis
presbyesophagus
presbyope
presbyophrenia
presbyopia
presbyopic
prescapula
prescapular
presclerotic
prescribe
prescription
    p. drug coverage
    p. drug program
    shotgun p.
presecretory
presection suture
presegmenter
presenile melanosis
presenility

presenium
present
presentation
    acromion p.
    antigen p.
    arm p.
    breech p.
    breech p., complete
    breech p., double
    breech p., frank
    breech p., incomplete
    breech p., single
    brow p.
    cephalic p.
    compound p.
    p. of the cord
    double-footling p.
    face p.
    footling p.
    footling breech p.
    frank breech p.
    full breech p.
    funic p.
    funis p.
    hand and head p.
    knee breech p.
    longitudinal p.
    mentoanterior face p.
    oblique p.
    parietal p.
    pelvic p.
    placental p.
    polar p.
    shoulder p.
    single footling p.
    torso p.
    transverse p.
    trunk p.
    vertex p.
    vertex-vertex p.
preservative
presinusoidal
presomite
prespermatid
presphenoid
presphygmic
prespondylolisthesis
press
    French p.
pressometer
    Jarcho p.
pressor
pressoreceptive
pressoreceptor
pressosensitive

pressosensitivity
 reflexogenic p.
pressure
 absolute p.
 after p.
 airway p.
 alveolar p.
 ambulatory venous p.
 amniotic p.
 arterial p.
 atmosphere p.
 atmospheric p.
 back p.
 barometric p.
 biting p.
 blood p.
 brain p.
 capillary p.
 central venous p. (CVP)
 cerebrospinal p.
 colloid osmotic p.
 continuous positive airway p.
  (CPAP)
 critical p.
 critical closing p.
 diastolic p.
 p. dressing
 dry p. dressing
 endocardial p.
 expiratory p.
 filtration p.
 hydrostatic p.
 hyperbaric p.
 p. of ideas
 imbibition p.
 inspiratory p.
 inspiratory triggering p.
 interstitial p.
 intra-abdominal p.
 intracranial p. (ICP)
 intramyometrial p.
 intraocular p.
 intrapulmonary p.
 intraspinal p.
 intrathecal p.
 intrathoracic p.
 intratympanic p.
 intraventricular p.
 maximum safety p.
 mean circulatory filling p.
 minimum safety p.
 mutation p.
 nasal continuous positive
  airway p. (CPAP)
 negative p.

pressure *(continued)*
 negative end-expiratory p.
 occlusal p.
 oncotic p.
 osmotic p.
 osmotic p., effective
 partial p.
 perfusion p.
 portal venous p.
 positive p.
 positive end-expiratory p.
  (PEEP)
 posterior p.
 pulmonary p.
 pulmonary artery wedge p.
  (PAWP)
 pulmonary capillary wedge p.
  (PCWP)
 pulse p.
 radiation p.
 selection p.
 solution p.
 p. of speech
 splenic pulp p.
 standard p.
 subambient p.
 subatmospheric p.
 surface p.
 systolic p.
 thought p.
 tissue p.
 transairway p.
 transmural p.
 transpulmonary p.
 transthoracic p.
 vapor p.
 venous p.
 ventilator p.
 water vapor p.
 wedge p.
 wedged hepatic vein p.
 zero end-expiratory p.
pressure ring
 Walsh p.r.
presternum
prestriate
presubiculum
presumptive
presuppurative
presylvian
presymptom
presymptomatic
presynaptic
presystole
presystolic

P

pretarsal
pretectal
pretectum
preterm
preterminal
prethyroideal
prethyroidean
pretibial
pretracheal
pretuberculosis
preurethritis
prevalence
    period p.
    point p.
prevention
preventive
    p. healthcare
    p. intervention
    p. measures
    p. medicine
    p. therapy
    p. treatment
preventorium
preventriculosis
preventriculus
prevertebral
prevertiginous
prevesical
    retropubic p. prostatectomy
previable
previtamin H
Prévost
    law
    sign
Preyer
    reflex
    test
prezonular
prezygapophysis
prezygotic
PRF—prolactin-releasing factor
PRFM—prolonged rupture of fetal
   membranes
PRH—prolactin-releasing hormone
PRI—phosphoribose isomerase
priapism
    secondary p.
priapitis
priapus
Price-Jones
    curve
    method
Price-Thomas
    clamp
    forceps

prickles
prickly heat
Priessnitz
    bandage
    compress
primacy
    genital p.
    phallic p.
primal
primary suture
primed
primer
    cavity p.
primigravid
primigravida
    elderly p.
primip.—primipara
primipara
primiparity
primiparous
primitiae
primitivation
primitive
primordial
    p. follicle
    p. germ cells
primordium (primordia)
    genital p.
    lens p.
    uterovaginal p.
primverose
Prince
    forceps
    scissors
princeps
principal
    p. aspect
    p. reason
    p. symptom
principle
    active p.
    Bragg-Gray p.
    conservation of energy p.
    Doppler p.
    Fick p.
    follicle-stimulating p.
    Huygens p.
    immediate p.
    Le Chatelier p.
    luteinizing p.
    mass action p.
    melanophore dilating p.
    organic p.
    pleasure p.
    pleasure-pain p.

principle *(continued)*
    proximate p.
    reality p.
    repetition-compulsion p.
    Venturi p.
    watermelon seed p.
Prinos verticellatus
Prinzmetal angina
prion
prism
    adamantine p's
    p. diopter
    enamel p's
    Maddox p.
    Nicol p.
    Risley p.
prisma (prismata)
    prismata adamantina
prismatic
prismoid
prismoptometer
prismosphere
PRIST—paper
  radioimmunosorbent test
Pritchard cannula
Pritikin punch
privilege
    admitting p's
    bathroom p's
    conversion p.
    staff p's
PRL; Prl—prolactin
p.r.n.; prn; PRN—as necessary
proaccelerin
proactivator
    C3 p. (C3PA)
proamnion
proangiotensin
proatlas
probability
    birth order p.
    conditional p.
    posterior p.
    prior p.
    reproduction p.
    significance p.
probacteriophage
proband
probe
    Anel p.
    Arbuckle p.
    Bakes p.
    Barr fistula p.
    Barr rectal p.
    blood flow p.

probe *(continued)*
    blunt p.
    Bowman lacrimal p.
    Brackett p.
    Buie p.
    bullet p.
    Bunnell p.
    calibrated p.
    Desjardins p.
    drum p.
    Earle p.
    electric p.
    eyed p.
    Fenger p.
    fiberoptic p.
    Girdner electric p.
    heat p.
    hot-tip p.
    Kron bile duct p.
    lacrimal p.
    Larry rectal p.
    Lilienthal p.
    Mayo p.
    memory p.
    molecular
      hybridization p.
    Moynihan p.
    nuclear p.
    Ochsner p.
    oligonucleotide p.
    periodontal p.
    pocket p.
    Pratt p.
    priapus p.
    root canal p.
    Rosen p.
    scintillation p.
    scissors p.
    Spencer p.
    telephonic p.
    Theobald p.
    ultrasound p.
    uterine p.
    vertebrated p.
    Welch-Allyn p.
    WHO (World Health
      Organization) periodontal p.
    Williams p.
    Yankauer p.
    Ziegler p.
procallus
procarboxypeptidase
procarcinogen
procatarctic
procatarxis

P

procedure
    Anderson p.
    Aries-Pitanguy p.
    Bosworth p.
    Bristow p.
    Brock p.
    Buie p.
    Campbell p.
    Cleveland p.
    Cockett p.
    Dale p.
    Darrach p.
    DePalma staple p.
    Ewart p.
    exteriorization p.
    Feulgen p.
    Fontan p.
    four-flap p.
    Girard p.
    Glenn p.
    Gomori-Takamatsu p.
    Hartmann p.
    Hassab p.
    Heitz-Boyer p.
    Hummelsheim p.
    Husni p.
    Ilizarov leg-lengthening p.
    Jannetta p.
    Jensen p.
    Kazanjian p.
    Kestenbach-Anderson p.
    Kestenbaum p.
    Knapp p.
    Kuhnt-Szymanowski p.
    Ladd p.
    Lester Martin p.
    Linton p.
    May p.
    Merindino p.
    Mikulicz p.
    Mohs p.
    Mustard p.
    Nichol p.
    Ober-Barr p.
    obliteration p.
    Palma p.
    Pereyra p.
    Potts p.
    Puestow p.
    Puestow-Gillesby p.
    push-back p.
    Rashkind o.
    Sauvé-Kapandji p.
    second-look p.
    Senning p.

procedure *(continued)*
    shelf p.
    Shirodkar p.
    Soave p.
    Stamey p.
    stereotaxic p.
    Sugiura p.
    Swenson pull-through p.
    Tanner p.
    Temple p.
    Valsalva p.
    V-Y p.
    Womack p.
    Zancolli p.
proceed
procelous
procentriole
procephalic
procercoid
procerus
process
    A.B.C. p.
    accessory p. of lumbar vertebrae
    accessory p. of sacrum, spurious
    acromial p., acromion p.
    acute p. of helix
    alar p.
    alar p. of sacrum
    aliform p.
    aliform p. of sphenoid bone
    alveolar p.
    alveolar p. of mandible
    alveolar p. of maxilla
    ameloblastic p.
    anconeal p.
    anconeal p. of ulna
    angular p. of frontal bone,
        external
    anterior p. of malleus
    articular p.
    articular p. of axis, anterior
    articular p. of coccyx, false
    articular p. of sacrum, spurious
    ascending p's of vertebrae
    auditory p.
    axillary p.
    axillary p. of mammary gland
    axis-cylinder p.
    basilar p.
    Beccari p.
    p. of Blumenbach
    bremsstrahlung p.
    calcaneal p.
    calcanean p.
    capitular p.

process *(continued)*

    p. of cartilage of nasal septum, posterior

    caudate p.

    caudate p. of caudate lobe

    ciliary p's

    Civinini p.

    Civinini's p. of external pterygoid plate

    clinoid p.

    cochleariform p.

    condylar p.

    condylar p. of mandible

    condyloid p.

    condyloid p. of vertebrae, inferior

    condyloid p. of vertebrae, superior

    conoid p.

    coracoid p.

    coracoid p. of scapula

    coronoid p.

    coronoid p. of mandible

    coronoid p. of ulna

    costal p.

    cubital p.

    cubital p. of humerus

    deep p. of submandibular gland

    Deiters p.

    dendritic p.

    dental p.

    dentoid p.

    dentoid p. of axis

    descending p's of vertebrae

    ensiform p.

    ensiform p. of sphenoid bone

    ensiform p. of sternum

    epiphyseal p.

    ethmoidal p.

    ethmoidal p. of inferior nasal concha

    ethmoidal p. of Macalister

    facial p.

    facial p. of parotid

    falciform p.

    falciform p. of cerebellum

    falciform p. of cerebrum

    falciform p. of fascia lata

    falciform p. of fascia pelvis

    falciform p. of rectus abdominis muscle

    falciform p. of sacrotuberal ligament

    floccular p.

    folian p.

process *(continued)*

    p. of Folius

    foot p.

    frontal p.

    frontal p., external

    frontal p. of maxilla

    frontal p. of zygomatic bone

    frontonasal p.

    frontosphenoidal p.

    funicular p.

    globular p.

    Gottstein basal p.

    greater p. of ethmoid bone

    hamate p.

    hamular p.

    hamular p. of lacrimal bone

    hamular p. of sphenoid bone

    hamular p. of unciform bone

    head p.

    incisive p.

    inferior articular p.

    inframalleolar p.

    inframalleolar p. of calcaneus

    infraorbital p.

    infundibular p.

    Ingrassia p.

    intercondylar p.

    intercondylar p. of tibia

    internal p. of humerus

    intrajugular p.

    intrajugular p. of occipital bone

    intrajugular p. of temporal bone

    jugular p.

    jugular p. of occipital bone, lateral

    jugular p. of occipital bone, middle

    jugular p. of occipital bone, posterior, of Krause

    lacrimal p.

    lateral p.

    lateral p. of calcaneus

    lateral p. of malleus

    lateral p. of talus

    lateral p. of tuberosity of calcaneus

    lenticular p.

    lenticular p. of incus

    lentiform p.

    long p. of malleus

    lumbocostal p.

    lumbocostal p. of lumbar vertebra

    malar p.

    mammillary p.

P

process *(continued)*

mammillary p's of sacrum, oblique
mammillary p. of temporal bone
mammillary p. of vertebrae
mandibular p.
marginal p.
marginal p. of malar bone
mastoid p.
maxillary p.
maxillary p. of inferior nasal concha
maxillary p. of palatine bone
medial p.
medial angular p.
medial angular p. of frontal bone
medial p. of tuberosity of calcaneus
mental p.
middle clinoid p.
muscular p.
muscular p. of arytenoid cartilage
nasal p.
nasal p. of frontal bone
nasal p. of inferior turbinate bone
nasal p., lateral
nasal p., median
neutron absorption p.
notochordal p.
oblique p.
oblique p. of vertebrae, inferior
oblique p. of vertebrae, superior
occipital p.
occipital p. of occipital bone
p. of odontoblast
odontoblastic p.
odontoid p.
odontoid p. of axis
olecranon p.
olecranon p. of ulna
orbital p.
orbital p. of palatine bone
palatal p.
palatine p.
palatine p., lateral
palatine p., median
palatine p. of maxilla
papillary p.
papillary p. of liver
paracondyloid p.
paracondyloid p. of occipital bone

process *(continued)*

paramastoid p.
paramastoid p. of occipital bone
paroccipital p.
paroccipital p. of occipital bone
petrosal p.
petrosal p., anterior
petrosal p., middle
petrosal p., posterior superior
postauditory p.
posterior clinoid p.
posterior p. of talus
postglenoid p.
postmeatal p.
postmeatal p. of temporal bone
primary p.
pterygoid p.
pterygopalatine p.
pterygoquadrate p.
pterygospinous p.
pyramidal p.
pyramidal p. of palatine bone
random p.
Rau p.
ravian p.
restiform p. of Henle
retromandibular p.
schizophrenic p.
secondary p.
small p. of Soemmering
sphenoidal p.
sphenoidal p. of palatine bone
spinous p.
spinous p. of sacrum, spurious
spinous p. of tibia
spinous p. of vertebra
Stieda p.
stochastic p.
styloid p.
styloid p. of fibula
styloid p. of radius
styloid p. of temporal bone
styloid p. of third metacarpal bone
styloid p. of ulna
sucker p.
superior articular p.
superior articular p. of sacrum
superior articulating p.
supracondylar p.
supracondylar p. of humerus
synovial p.
temporal p.
temporal p. of mandible
temporal p. of zygomatic bone

process *(continued)*

- Todd p.
- Tomes p.
- transverse p.
- transverse p. of sacrum
- transverse p. of vertebrae, accessory
- trochlear p.
- trochlear p. of calcaneus
- unciform p.
- unciform p. of scapula
- uncinate p.
- uncinate p. of ethmoid bone
- uncinate p. of lacrimal bone
- uncinate p. of pancreas
- uncinate p. of unciform bone
- uncinate p's of vertebra
- ungual p.
- ungual p. of third phalanx of foot
- vaginal p.
- vaginal p. of sphenoid bone
- vaginal p. of styloid
- vaginal p. of temporal bone
- vermiform p.
- vermiform p. of cerebellum
- vertebral p.
- vocal p.
- xiphoid p.
- xiphoid p. of sphenoid bone
- zygomatic p.
- zygomatic p. of frontal bone
- zygomatic p. of maxilla
- zygomatico-orbital p.
- zygomatic p. of temporal bone

processing

- signal p.

processor

- array p.

processus (processus)

- p. accessorii spurii
- p. accessorius
- p. accessorius vertebrarum lumbalium
- p. alaris ossis ethmoidalis
- p. alveolaris maxillae
- p. anterior mallei
- p. anterior mallei Folii
- p. articularis
- p. articularis inferior vertebrarum
- p. articularis superior ossis sacri
- p. articularis superior vertebrarum
- p. axillaris

processus (processus) *(continued)*

- p. axillaris glandulae mammariae
- p. brevis incudis
- p. brevis mallei
- p. calcaneus
- p. calcaneus ossis cuboidei
- p. caudatus
- p. caudatus hepatis
- p. ciliares
- p. clinoideus anterior
- p. clinoideus medius
- p. clinoideus posterior
- p. cochleariformis
- p. condylaris
- p. condylaris mandibulae
- p. condyloideus
- p. condyloideus mandibulae
- p. coracoideus
- p. coracoideus scapulae
- p. coronoideus
- p. coronoideus mandibulae
- p. coronoideus ulnae
- p. costalis
- p. costalis vertebrae
- p. costarius
- p. costarius vertebrae
- p. e cerebello ad medullam
- p. e cerebello ad pontem
- p. e cerebello ad testes
- p. ethmoidalis
- p. ethmoidalis conchae nasalis inferioris
- p. falciformis
- p. falciformis ligamenti sacrotuberalis
- p. Ferreini lobuli corticalis renis
- p. frontalis
- p. frontalis maxillae
- p. frontalis ossis zygomatici
- p. frontosphenoidalis
- p. frontosphenoidalis ossis zygomatici
- p. gracilis
- p. of Ingrassia
- p. intrajugularis
- p. intrajugularis ossis occipitalis
- p. intrajugularis ossis temporalis
- p. jugularis
- p. jugularis ossis occipitalis
- p. lacrimalis
- p. lacrimalis conchae nasalis inferioris
- p. lateralis

P

processus (processus) *(continued)*
- p. lateralis glandulae mammariae
- p. lateralis mallei
- p. lateralis tali
- p. lateralis tuberis calcanei
- p. lenticularis incudis
- p. mammillaris
- p. marginalis
- p. marginalis ossis zygomatici
- p. mastoideus
- p. mastoideus ossis temporalis
- p. maxillaris
- p. maxillaris conchae nasalis inferioris
- p. medialis
- p. medialis tuberis calcanei
- p. muscularis
- p. muscularis cartilaginis arytenoideae
- p. orbitalis
- p. orbitalis ossis palatini
- p. palatinus maxillae
- p. papillaris
- p. papillaris hepatis
- p. paramastoideus
- p. paramastoideus ossis occipitalis
- p. phalangeus
- p. posterior cartilaginis septi nasi
- p. posterior sphenoidalis
- p. posterior tali
- p. pterygoideus
- p. pterygoideus ossis sphenoidalis
- p. pterygospinosus
- p. pterygospinosus Civinini
- p. pyramidalis
- p. pyramidalis ossis palatini
- p. retromandibularis
- p. retromandibularis glandulae parotidis
- p. sphenoidalis
- p. sphenoidalis ossis palatini
- p. sphenoidalis septi cartilaginei
- p. spinosus
- p. spinosus vertebrarum
- p. styloideus
- p. styloideus fibulae
- p. styloideus ossis metacarpalis III (tertii)
- p. styloideus ossis temporalis
- p. styloideus radii
- p. styloideus ulnae

processus (processus) *(continued)*
- p. supracondylaris humeri
- p. supracondyloideus humeri
- p. supraepicondylaris humeri
- p. temporalis
- p. temporalis ossis zygomatici
- p. transversus
- p. transversus vertebrarum
- p. trochlearis calcanei
- p. uncinatus
- p. uncinatus ossis ethmoidalis
- p. uncinatus pancreatis
- p. vaginalis
- p. vaginalis ossis sphenoidalis
- p. vaginalis peritonei
- p. vaginalis testis
- p. vermiformis
- p. vocalis
- p. xiphoideus
- p. zygomaticus
- p. zygomaticus maxillae
- p. zygomaticus ossis frontalis
- p. zygomaticus ossis temporalis

procheilon
prochondral
prochordal
prochorion
prochromosome
procidentia uteri
proclination
procoagulant
procollagen
- p.-lysine, 2-oxoglutarate 5-dioxygenase
- p.-lysine 5-dioxygenase
- p. peptidase
- p.-proline, 2-oxoglutarate 4-dioxygenase
- p. *N*-proteinase

procollagenase
proconceptive
procondylism
proconvertin
procreation
procreative
proctalgia fugax
proctatresia
proctectasia
proctectomy
proctencleisis
procteurynter
procteurysis
proctitis
- epidemic gangrenous p.
- factitial p.
- p. obliterans

proctitis *(continued)*
  pseudoinfectious p.
  radiation p.
  traumatic p.
  ulcerative p.
proctocele
proctococcypexy
proctocolectomy
proctocolitis
proctocolonoscopy
proctocolpoplasty
proctocystocele
proctocystoplasty
proctocystotome
proctocystotomy
proctodeum
proctodynia
proctogenic
proctologic
proctologist
proctology
proctoparalysis
proctoperineoplasty
proctoperineorrhaphy
proctopexy
proctoplasty
proctoplegia
proctopolypus
proctoptosis
Proctor
  elevator
  retractor
proctorrhagia
proctorrhaphy
proctorrhea
proctoscope
  ACMI p.
  Boehm p.
  Fansler p.
  Gabriel p.
  Goldbacher p.
  Hirschman p.
  Hirschman-Martin p.
  Kelly p.
  Lieberman p.
  Montague p.
  Newman p.
  Pruitt p.
  Strauss p.
  Tuttle p.
  Vernon-David p.
  Welch-Allyn p.
  Yeoman p.
proctoscopic speculum
proctoscopy
proctosigmoid

proctosigmoidectomy
proctosigmoiditis
proctosigmoidopexy
proctosigmoidoscope
proctosigmoidoscopy
proctospasm
proctostasis
proctostat
proctostenosis
proctostomy
proctotome
proctotomy
  external p.
  internal p.
  linear p.
proctovalvotomy
procumbent
procursive
procurvation
procuticle
prodroma (plural of prodromon)
prodromal
prodrome
  epileptic p.
prodromic
prodromon (prodroma)
pro-drug
product
  addition p.
  cleavage p.
  contact activation p.
  decay p.
  end p.
  fibrinolytic split p's
  fission p.
  gene p., primary
  spallation p's
  substitution p.
production
  ectopic hormone p.
  pair p.
productive
proecdysis
proelastase
proemial
proencephalus
proencephaly
proenzyme
proerythroblast
proerythrocyte
proestrogen
Proetz position
professional
  allied health p.
  P. Standards Review
    Organization (PSRO)

professor
profibrinolysin
Profichet
    disease
    syndrome
profilactin
profile
    antigenic p.
    biochemical p.
    biophysical p.
    blood p.
    facial p.
    health p.
    histochemical p.
    liver p.
    personality p.
    prognathic p.
    retrognathic p.
    urethral pressure p. (UPP)
profiler
    beam p.
profilin
profilometry
    urethral pressure p.
profluvium seminis
profound
    p. anemia
    p. debility
    p. hematuria
profundaplasty
profundus
progamous
progastrin
progenia
progenital
progeny
progeria
Progestasert IUD
progestational
progesteroid
progesterone
progestogen
progestomimetic
proglossis
proglottid
proglumide
prognathism
    mandibular p.
prognathometer
prognathous
prognose
prognosis
prognostic
prognosticate

prognostician
progonoma
    melanotic p.
progranulocyte
    early p.
progravid
progression
    backward p.
    cross-legged p.
    metadromic p.
progressive
prohistiocyte
prohormone
proinflammatory
proinsulin
projection
    anteroposterior (AP) p.
    anteroposterior lordotic p.
    apical lordotic p.
    axial p.
    axillary p.
    ball-catcher p.
    basilar p.
    biplane p.
    blow-out view p.
    Caldwell p.
    Chassard-Lapiné p.
    Chausse III p.
    cone-down p.
    craniocaudad p.
    cross-sectional transverse p.
    dorsoplantar p.
    eccentric p.
    erect fluoro spot p.
    erroneous p.
    essential p.
    flexion, extension p.
    p. formula
    frontal p.
    geniculostriate p.
    half-axial p.
    Heinig p.
    Hermodsson p.
    Hughston p.
    impersonal p.
    inferior-superior p.
    inferior-superior tangential p.
    inferosuperior axial p.
    intraoral p.
    L5–S1 p.
    lateral oblique axial p.
    lateral transcranial p.
    lateral transfacial p.
    lateromedial oblique p.

projection *(continued)*
    Lauenstein and Hickey p.
    Laurin p.
    left anterior oblique
      (LAO) p.
    left posterior oblique
      (LPO) p.
    Low-Beers p.
    lumbosacral p.
    medial oblique axial p.
    mediolateral p.
    Merchant p.
    mortise p.
    navicular p.
    neuronal p.
    notch p.
    oblique p.
    oblique lateral p.
    open-mouth p.
    parieto-orbital p.
    pillar p.
    Pirie transoral p.
    pontocerebellar p.
    posteroanterior (PA) p.
    posteroanterior lordotic p.
    recumbent lateral p.
    right anterior oblique
      (RAO) p.
    right posterior oblique
      (RPO) p.
    scaphoid p.
    Schüller p.
    semiaxial p.
    semiaxial anteroposterior p.
    semiaxial transcranial p.
    Settegast p.
    skyline p.
    Stenvers p.
    stereo right lateral p.
    stress p.
    Stryker notch p.
    submentovertex p.
    submentovertical axial p.
    sunrise p.
    superoinferior p.
    swimmer's p.
    tangential p.
    Templeton and Zim carpal
      tunnel p.
    thalamocortical p's
    third p. of Chausse
    Towne p.
    transtabular AP p.
    transtabular PA p.

projection *(continued)*
    transthoracic p.
    tunnel p.
    verticosubmental p.
    Waters p.
    West Point p.
    p. x-ray microscope
prokaryoblast
prokaryon
prokaryosis
prokaryote
prokaryotic
prolabium
prolactin
prolamin
prolapse
    acute cervical disk p.
    anal p.
    p. of anterior lip of cervix
    p. of anus
    p. of the cord
    p. of female urethra
    frank p.
    p. of intervertebral
      disk
    p. of the iris
    lumbar disk p.
    mitral valve p.
    Morgagni p.
    occult p. of cord
    rectal p.
    p. of rectum
    uterine p.
    p. of uterus
    vaginal p.
prolapsus
    p. ani
    p. recti
    p. uteri
Prolene suture
prolepsis
proleptic
proleukocyte
prolidase
prolidase deficiency
proliferate
proliferation
    bile duct p.
    fibroplastic p.
    mesangial p.
proliferative
prolific
proligerous
prolinase

P

proline
> p. dehydrogenase
> p. dipeptidase
> p. hydroxylase
> p. hydroxyproline glycinuria-5-oxidase

prolinemia
prolotherapy
prolyl
> p. dipeptidase
> p. hydroxylase

prolymphoblast
prolymphocyte
PROM—
> premature rupture of membranes
> prolonged rupture of membranes

promanide
promastigote
promegakaryocyte
promegaloblast
prometaphase
promethium (Pm)
promine
prominence
> Ammon scleral p.
> cephalic p.
> p. of facial canal
> laryngeal p.
> p. of lateral semicircular canal
> mallear p. of tympanic membrane
> spiral p.
> styloid p.
> tubal p.

prominentia (prominentiae)
> p. canalis facialis
> p. canalis semicircularis lateralis
> p. foraminalis
> p. frontonasalis
> p. laryngea
> p. mallearis membranae tympani
> p. malleolaris membranae tympani
> p. mandibularis
> p. spiralis
> p. styloidea

promitosis
promonocyte
promontorium (promontoria)
> p. cavitatis tympanicae
> p. faciei
> p. ossis sacri
> p. tympani

promontory
> p. of the middle ear
> pelvic p.
> p. of sacrum
> tympanic p.
> p. of tympanic cavity

promoter
> eosinophil stimulator p.

promotion
promyeloblast
promyelocyte
pronase
pronate
pronation
pronatoflexor
pronator
pronator-supinator
prone
pronephros
prong
pronograde
pronometer
pronormoblast
> Sabin p.

pronucleus
> female p.
> male p.

pro-opiomelanocortin (POMC)
pro-otic
proovarium
prop
> dental p.

propagate
propagation
propagative
propalinal
propane
propanidid
propanolide
propargyl
propenyl
propepsin
propeptone
propeptonuria
proper
> p. lamina
> p. ligament
> p. membrane

properitoneal
property
> colligative p.

prophage
prophase
prophenpyridamine
prophylactic
prophylactodontics

prophylaxis
    causal p.
    chemical p.
    clinical p.
    collective p.
    Credé p.
    dental p.
    drug p.
    gametocidal p.
    individual p.
    mechanical p.
    oral p.
    serum p.
    suppressive p.
prophyrism
propionate carboxylase
propionibacter
Propionibacterium
    P. acnes
    P. granulosum
    P. jensenii
    P. propionicum
propionicacidemia
propionitrile
propionylcholine
propionyl-CoA carboxylase
proplasmacyte
proplasmin
Proplast
proplastid
propons
proporphyrinogen oxidase
proportion
    femininity p.
    masculinity p.
    mutant p.
    optimal p.
proportional counter
proposita (propositae)
propositus (propositi)
propoxur
proprietary
proprioception
proprioceptive
proprioceptor
propriospinal
proprotein
proptometer
proptosis
propulsion
propylene
    p. dressing
    p. glycol
    p. oxide
pro re nata (p.r.n.)
prorennin

prorubricyte
prosecretin
prosect
prosection
prosector
prosencephalon
prosocoele
prosodemic
prosody
prosopagnosia
prosopalgia
prosopalgic
prosopantritis
prosopectasia
prosophenosia
prosoplasia
prosopoanoschisis
prosopodiplegia
prosopodysmorphia
prosoponeuralgia
prosopopagus
prosopoplegia
prosopoplegic
prosoposchisis
prosopospasm
prosoposternodymia
prosoposternodymus
prosoposternopagus
prosopothoracopagus
prostaglandin (PG)
    p. D_2 (PGD_2) [D2]
    p. E_1 (PGE_1) [E1]
    p. E_2 (PGE_2) [E2]
    p. endoperoxide synthase
    p. $F_2\alpha$ ($PGF_2\alpha$) [F2-alpha]
    p. $F_2\alpha$ tromethamine
      [F2-alpha]
    p. G_2 (PGG_2) [G2]
    p. H_2 (PGH_2) [H2]
    p. I_2 (PGI_2) [I2]
      (prostacyclin)
    p. synthase
    p. synthetase
prostalene
prostanoic acid
prostanoid
prostata
prostatalgia
prostatauxe
prostate
prostatectomy
    perineal p.
    radical p.
    radical retropubic p.
    retropubic p.
    retropubic prevesical p.

P

prostatectomy *(continued)*
    suprapubic p. (SPP)
    suprapubic transvesical p.
    transurethral p.
prostatelcosis
prostatic
    benign p. hyperplasia (BPH)
    benign p. hypertrophy (BPH)
prostaticovesical
prostaticovesiculectomy
prostatism
    vesical p.
prostatisme sans prostate
prostatitic
prostatitis
    allergic p.
    bacterial p.
    eosinophilic p.
    fungal p.
    granulomatous p.
    nonspecific granulomatous p.
    tuberculous p.
prostatocystitis
prostatocystotomy
prostatodynia
prostatography
prostatolith
prostatolithotomy
prostatomegaly
prostatometer
prostatomy
prostatomyomectomy
prostatorrhea
prostatotomy
prostatotoxin
prostatovesiculectomy
prostatovesiculitis
prostaxia
prosternation
prosthesis (prostheses)
    Alvarez p.
    Angelchik p.
    antireflux p.
    aortic p.
    Ashley breast p.
    Aufranc-Turner p.
    Austin Moore p.
    Bateman p.
    Beall mitral valve p.
    Bechtol hip p.
    biliary p.
    Björk-Shiley aortic valve p.
    Björk-Shiley convexoconcave
      60-degree valve p.
    Björk-Shiley floating-disk p.

prosthesis (prostheses) *(continued)*
    Blom-Singer voice p.
    Braunwald p.
    CAD (computer-assisted
      design) p.
    caged-ball p.
    Capetown aortic valve p.
    Cartwright p.
    Charnley p.
    Charnley-Mueller hip p.
    Charnley total hip p.
    cleft palate p.
    conventional single-axis knee p.
    Cooley p.
    Cronin p.
    Cutter-SCDK p.
    Cutter-Smeloff cardiac valve p.
    Dacron p.
    DeBakey p.
    dental p.
    DePalma p.
    DePuy p.
    discoid aortic p.
    disk-valve p.
    Duromedics p.
    Edwards p.
    Eicher p.
    endoskeletal p.
    exoskeletal p.
    feeding p.
    Geomedic p.
    geometric p.
    Giliberty p.
    Gott p.
    Guepar p.
    Harken p.
    heart valve p.
    Heyer-Schulte p.
    House p.
    Hufnagel p.
    Hydroflex penile p.
    Ionescu-Shiley p.
    Judet p.
    Kay-Shiley p.
    knitted vascular p.
    Lillehei-Kaster p.
    Lippman p.
    MacIntosh p.
    Magovern p.
    Matchett-Brown p.
    maxillofacial p.
    McKee-Farrar p.
    McKeever p.
    mitral p.
    modular p.

prosthesis (prostheses) *(continued)*
  Moore p.
  Mueller p.
  Munster p.
  myoelectric p.
  Neer p.
  Neville p.
  Niebauer p.
  ocular p.
  Panje voice p.
  penile p.
  pneumatic p.
  SACH (solid-ankle, cushioned-heel) foot p.
  SE (Starr-Edwards) p.
  semirigid p.
  Sheehy-House p.
  Shier p.
  Silastic testicular p.
  Smeloff-Cutter p.
  Smith-Petersen p.
  speech-aid p.
  Starr-Edwards p.
  Swanson p.
  Syme p.
  Teflon p.
  Thompson p.
  tilting-disk p.
  total ossicular replacement p. (TORP)
  Townley p.
  tracheoesophageal fistula voice button p.
  trileaflet aortic p.
  Vanghetti p.
  Vitallium p.
  Wada p.
  Walldius p.
  Weavenit p.
  Wesolowski p.
  woven vascular p.
  Zimaloy p.
  Zimmer p.
prosthetic
prosthetics
  dental p.
  denture p.
  facial p.
  maxillofacial p.
prosthetist
prosthion (PR)
prosthodontics
prosthodontist
prosthokeratoplasty
prostrate

prostration
  heat p.
  nervous p.
protactinium (Pa)
protagon
protalbumose
protaminase
protan
protandrous
protandry
protanomal
protanomalous
protanomaly
protanope
protanopia
protanopic
protanopsia
protean
protease
protection
  Caldwell p.
  passive p.
protective
protector
  Arruga p.
  hearing p.
  LATS (long-acting thyroid stimulator) p.
  nipple p.
protein
  p. A
  α-chain p. [alpha-]
  A, G, S p.
  alcohol-soluble p.
  allosteric p.
  amyloid A (AA) p.
  amyloid light chain (AL) p.
  autologous p.
  bacterial p.
  bacterial cellular p.
  Bence Jones p.
  binding p.
  bone morphogenetic p.
  p. C
  C4 binding p.
  calcium-binding p.
  carrier p.
  cationic p's
  coagulated p.
  coat p.
  complete p.
  compound p.
  conjugated p.
  constitutive p's
  control p's

P

protein *(continued)*
    cord p's
    corticosteroid-binding p.
    C-reactive p.
    denatured p.
    derived p.
    encephalitogenic p.
    eosinophil major basic p.
    fibrillar p.
    fibrous p.
    floating p.
    G p.
    Gc p.
    globular p.
    guanyl-nucleotide–binding p.
    Hektoen, Kretschmer, and
        Welker p.
    heme-thiolate p.
    heterologous p.
    p. hydrolysate
    immune p's
    incomplete p.
    insoluble p.
    iodized p.
    iron-sulfur p.
    p. kinase
    liquid p.
    p. lysine 6-oxidase
    M p.
    maintenance p.
    matrix p.
    mild silver p.
    myelin basic p. (MBP)
    myeloma p.
    native p.
    nonhistone chromosomal p.
    nonstructural p.
    partial p.
    periplasmic binding p's
    plasma p's
    plasma p. fraction
    R p.
    racemized p.
    retinol-binding p. (RBP)
    ribonuclear p.
    p. S
    serum p's
    serum amyloid A (SAA) p.
    silver p.
    simple p.
    staphylococcal p. A
    strong silver p.
    synthetic p.
    Tamm-Horsfall p.
    thyroid-binding p.

protein *(continued)*
    thyroxine-binding p.
    transport p.
    whole p.
    p. Z
proteinaceous
proteinase
proteinemia
    Bence Jones p.
    broad-beta p.
    floating-beta p.
protein-glutamine
    γ-glutamyltransferase [gamma-]
proteinic
proteinochrome
proteinogenous
proteinology
proteinosis
    lipid p.
    lipoid p.
    pulmonary alveolar p.
    tissue p.
proteinphobia
proteinuria
    accidental p.
    adventitious p.
    anoxemic p.
    asymptomatic p.
    athletic p.
    Bence Jones p.
    benign p.
    cardiac p.
    colliquative p.
    cyclic p.
    dietetic p.
    digestive p.
    effort p.
    emulsion p.
    enterogenic p.
    essential p.
    exercise p.
    false p.
    febrile p.
    functional p.
    gestational p.
    globular p.
    gouty p.
    hematogenous p.
    hemic p.
    intermittent p.
    intrinsic p.
    isolated p.
    light-chain p.
    lordotic p.
    march p.

proteinuria *(continued)*
    mixed p.
    nephrogenous p.
    nonselective p.
    orthostatic p.
    overflow p.
    palpatory p.
    paroxysmal p.
    persistent p.
    physiologic p.
    postrenal p.
    postural p.
    p. praetuberculosa
    prerenal p.
    pretuberculous p.
    pseudo-p.
    pyogenic p.
    regulatory p.
    renal p.
    residual p.
    selective p.
    serous p.
    transient p.
    true p.
proteinuric
proteoclastic
proteolipid
proteolysis
proteolytic
proteometabolic
proteometabolism
proteopepsis
proteopeptic
proteopexic
proteopexy
proteose
proteosemia
proteosuria
proter
Proteroglypha
proteroglyphic
protest
    masculine p.
Proteus
    P. mirabilis
    P. penneri
    P. vulgaris (serovars: Ox-2,
      Ox-19, Ox-K)
prothallus
prothrombin
prothrombinase
    extrinsic p.
    intrinsic p.
prothrombinogen
prothrombinogenic

prothrombinopenia
prothrombokinase
prothymocyte
protiodide
protirelin
protist
    eukaryotic p.
    higher p.
    lower p.
    prokaryotic p.
protium
protoalbumose
protoanemonin
protobiology
protoblast
protoblastic
protobrochal
protocatechuic acid
protochloride
protochlorophyll
protochondral
protochondrium
protochordate
protocol
    Balke p.
    Bruce p.
    Bruce treadmill p.
    citrovorum rescue p.
    clinical p.
    Ellestad p.
    fast-track p.
    leucovorin rescue p.
    maintenance p.
    Memorial Sloan-Kettering p.
    modified Bruce p.
    Naughton treadmill p.
    neon particle p.
    standardized p.
    Sugarbaker p.
    surveillance p.
    test p.
protocooperation
protodiastole
protodiastolic
protoduodenum
protoelastin
protoelastose
protofibril
protofilament
protogaster
protoglobulose
protogonocyte
protogynous
protogyny
protoheme

P

protohemin
protometer
proton
  p. beam (Bragg peak)
  p. spectroscopy
protonate
protoneuron
protonitrate
proto-oncogene
protopathic
protopecten
protophyllin
protopianoma
protopine
protoplasia
protoplasm
  functional p.
  granular p.
  superior p.
protoplasmic
protoplasmolysis
protoplast
protoporphyria
  erythrohepatic p.
  erythropoietic p.
protoporphyrinemia
protoporphyrinogen
  oxidase
protoporphyrinuria
protoproteose
protopsis
protosalt
protospasm
protospore
protostoma
protostome
protosulfate
protosyphilis
Prototheca
  P. wickerhamii
  P. zopfii
protothecosis
prototroph
prototrophic
prototrophy
prototropy
prototype
protoveratrine
protoverine
protovertebra
protoxide
protozoacide
protozoagglutinin
protozoal
protozoan
protozoiasis

protozoology
  clinical p.
protozoon
protozoophage
protozootherapy
protract
protraction
  mandibular p.
  maxillary p.
protractor
  Robinson p.
protransglutaminase
protrusio acetabuli
protrusion
  acetabular p.
  bimaxillary p.
  bimaxillary dentoalveolar p.
  intervertebral disk p.
  intrapelvic p.
  lateral p.
protrypsin
protuberance
  Bichat p.
  p. of chin
  external occipital p.
  frontal p.
  laryngeal p.
  mental p.
  natiform p.
  occipital p.
  occipital p., transverse
  palatine p.
  parietal p.
  tubal p.
protuberant
  p. abdomen
  p. nodule
protuberantia
  p. laryngea
  p. mentalis
  p. occipitalis externa
  p. occipitalis interna
proud
  cross-pin p.
  cross-pin left too p.
  p. flesh
  p. nebula
Proud syndrome
pro-UK—prourokinase
Proust-Lichtheim maneuver
proventriculus
Providence forceps
Providencia
  P. alcalifaciens
  P. rettgeri
  P. stuartii

provider
 preferred p. organization (PPO)
proviral
provirus
provisional
provitamin D
provocative
Prowazek bodies
Prowazek-Greeff bodies
proxemics
proximad
proximal
proximalis
proximally
proximate
proximoataxia
proximobuccal
proximoceptor
proximolabial
proximolingual
proxy
prozonal
prozone
PRP—
 panretinal photocoagulation
 pityriasis rubra pilaris
 platelet-rich plasma
 progesterone receptor proteins
 Psychotic Reaction Profile
PRPP—phosphoribosyl-
 pyrophosphate
PRRE—pupils round, regular, and
 equal
PRT—phosphoribosyltransferase
PRU—peripheral resistance unit
prual
pruinate
Pruitt
 anoscope
 proctoscope
prune-belly syndrome
pruned hilum
pruned-tree
 p.-t. appearance
 p.-t. arteriogram
prune juice sputum
pruriginous
prurigo
 p. agria
 Besnier p., p. of Besnier
 Besnier p. of pregnancy
 p. chronica multiformis
 dermographic p.
 p. estivalis
 p. ferox
 flexural p.

prurigo *(continued)*
 p. gestationis
 p. gestationis of Besnier
 p. of Hebra
 Hutchinson summer p.
 p. infantilis
 leukodermic p.
 melanotic p.
 p. mitis
 nodular p.
 p. nodularis
 polymorphic p.
 p. simplex
 summer p.
 summer p. of Hutchinson
 p. universalis
 p. vulgaris
 winter p.
pruritic
pruritogenic
pruritus
 p. ani
 aquagenic p.
 autotoxic p.
 Duhring p.
 p. gravidarum
 p. hiemalis
 p. scroti
 senile p.
 p. senilis
 symptomatic p.
 uremic p.
 p. vulvae
Prussak
 fibers
 pouch
 space
prussiate
prussic acid
Pryor-Péan retractor
ψ—psi (Greek letter)
ps—per second
PS—
 performing scale (IQ)
 periodic syndrome
 phosphatidylserine
 physical status
 plastic surgery
 Porter-Silber (chromogen)
 pulmonary stenosis
 pyloric stenosis
P/S—polyunsaturated-saturated
 fatty acid ratio
PSA—prostate-specific antigen
psalterial
psalterium

P

psammocarcinoma
psammoma bodies
psammomatous
psammosarcoma
psammotherapy
psammous
psauoscopy
PSC—
    Porter-Silber chromogen
    primary sclerosing
      cholangitis
PSD—peptone-starch-dextrose
pselaphesia
psellism
pseudacousma
pseudalbuminuria
pseudamnesia
pseudaphia
pseudarthritis
pseudarthrosis
pseudencephalus
pseudesthesia
pseudinoma
pseudoabscess
pseudoacanthosis nigricans
pseudoacephalus
pseudoachondroplasia
pseudoacromegaly
pseudoactinomycosis
pseudoagglutination
pseudoaggression
pseudoagrammatism
pseudoagraphia
pseudoalbuminuria
pseudoalleles
pseudoallelic
pseudoallelism
pseudoalveolar
pseudoamenorrhea
pseudoanaphylactic
pseudoanaphylaxis
pseudoanemia angiospastica
pseudoaneurysm
pseudoangina
pseudoankylosis
pseudoanodontia
pseudoantagonist
pseudoaphasia
pseudoapoplexy
pseudoappendicitis
pseudo–Argyll Robertson pupil
pseudo–Argyll Robertson syndrome
pseudoarthrosis
pseudoarticulation
pseudoastereognosis

pseudoasthma
pseudoathetosis
pseudoatrophoderma colli
pseudo-Babinski sign
pseudobacillus
pseudobacterium
pseudobasedow
pseudobronchiectasis
pseudobulbar
pseudocartilage
pseudocartilaginous
pseudocast
pseudocele
pseudocephalocele
pseudochancre redux
pseudocholecystitis
pseudocholesteatoma
pseudocholinesterase (PCE)
pseudochorea
pseudochromesthesia
pseudochromhidrosis
pseudochromosome
pseudochylous
pseudocirrhosis
pseudoclaudication
pseudoclonus
pseudocoarctation of the aorta
pseudocolloid
pseudocoloboma
pseudocoma
pseudocopulation
pseudo–corpus luteum
pseudocowpox
pseudocoxalgia
pseudocrisis
pseudocroup
pseudocryptorchidism
pseudocyesis
pseudocylindroid
pseudocyst
    p's of lung
    pancreatic p.
    pararenal p.
    pulmonary p's
pseudodecidua
pseudodelirium
pseudodementia
    hysterical p.
pseudodextrocardia
pseudodiabetes
    stress p.
pseudodiastolic
pseudodiphtheria
pseudodominance
pseudodominant

pseudodysentery
pseudoedema
pseudoelastin
pseudoembryonic
pseudoemphysema
pseudoencephalomalacia
pseudoendometritis
pseudoeosinophil
pseudoephedrine
pseudoepilepsy
pseudoepiphysis
pseudoerosion
pseudoerysipelas
pseudoexfoliation
pseudoexophoria
pseudoexophthalmos
pseudoexstrophy
pseudofarcy
pseudofluctuation
pseudofolliculitis barbae
pseudofracture
pseudofructose
pseudoganglion
    Bochdalek p.
    Cloquet p.
    Valentin p.
pseudogene
   dispersed p.
   processed p.
pseudogestation
pseudogeusesthesia
pseudogeusia
pseudoglanders
pseudoglioma
pseudoglobulin
pseudoglottic
pseudoglottis
pseudoglucosazone
pseudogonorrhea
pseudogout
pseudographia
pseudogynecomastia
pseudohallucination
pseudohaustration
pseudohelminth
pseudohemagglutination
pseudohematuria
pseudohemiacardius
pseudohemophilia hepatica
pseudohemoptysis
pseudohereditary
pseudohermaphrodism
pseudohermaphrodite
   female p.
   male p.

pseudohermaphroditism
   female p.
   male p.
pseudohernia
pseudoheterotopia
pseudo-Hurler
   disease
   polydystrophy
pseudohydrocephalus
   traumatic internal p.
pseudohydrocephaly
pseudohydronephrosis
pseudohyoscyamine
pseudohyperkalemia
pseudohypertrichosis
pseudohypertrophic
pseudohypertrophy
   muscular p.
pseudohypoaldosteronism
pseudohyponatremia
pseudohypoparathyroidism
pseudohypophosphatasia
pseudohypothyroidism
pseudoicterus
pseudoincontinence
pseudoinfarction
pseudoinfluenza
pseudointima
pseudoisochromatic
pseudoisocyanin
pseudojaundice
pseudokeratin
pseudolamellar
pseudoleukemia
    p. gastrointestinalis
    p. lymphatica
pseudolipoma
pseudolithiasis
pseudologia fantastica
pseudoluxation
pseudolymphoma of Spiegler-Fendt
pseudomalignancy
pseudomamma
pseudomania
pseudomasturbation
pseudomegacolon
pseudomelanoma
pseudomelanosis
pseudomelia paraesthetica
pseudomembrane
pseudomembranelle
pseudomembranous
pseudomeningitis
pseudomenopause
pseudomenstruation

P

pseudomethemoglobin
pseudomicrocephalus
pseudomicrocephaly
pseudomilium
pseudomonad
Pseudomonas
    P. aeruginosa
    P. alcaligenes
    P. fluorescens
    P. pseudoalcaligenes
    P. putida
    P. stutzeri
pseudomorphine
pseudomotivation
pseudomotor
pseudomucin
pseudomucinous
pseudomyasthenia
pseudomycelium
pseudomyiasis
pseudomyopia
pseudomyotonia
pseudomyxoma
  peritonei
pseudomyxovirus
pseudonarcotic
pseudonarcotism
pseudoneoplasm
pseudoneuritis
pseudoneuroma
pseudoneuronophagia
pseudonucleolus
pseudonystagmus
pseudo-obstruction
    idiopathic intestinal p.
    intestinal p.
pseudo-ochronosis
pseudo-optogram
pseudo-osteomalacia
pseudo-ovum
pseudopapilledema
pseudoparalysis
    p. agitans
    arthritic general p.
    congenital atonic p.
    generalized alcoholic p.
    Parrot p.
    syphilitic p.
pseudoparaplegia
pseudoparasite
pseudoparesis
pseudoparkinsonism
pseudopelade of Brocq
pseudopellagra
pseudopeptone

pseudopericardial
pseudoperitonitis
pseudophakia
    p. adiposa
    p. fibrosa
pseudophakodonesis
pseudophlegmon
    Hamilton p.
pseudophotesthesia
pseudophyllid
pseudophyllidean
pseudoplasm
pseudoplasmodium
pseudoplegia
pseudopneumonia
pseudopocket
pseudopod
pseudopodiospore
pseudopodium
  (pseudopodia)
pseudopoliomyelitis
pseudopolycythemia
pseudopolymelia
    p. paraesthetica
    paresthetic p.
pseudopolyp
pseudopolyposis
pseudoporencephaly
pseudo-Pott disease
pseudopregnancy
pseudoprognathism
pseudoproteinuria
pseudopsia
pseudopsychosis
pseudopterygium
pseudoptosis
pseudoptyalism
pseudopuberty
    heterosexual p.
    isosexual p.
    precocious p.
pseudoreaction
pseudoreduction
pseudoreminiscence
pseudoretinitis pigmentosa
pseudorheumatism
pseudorickets
pseudorosette
pseudosarcoid
pseudosarcoma
pseudoscarlatina
pseudosclerema
pseudoscleroderma
pseudosclerosis
    Jakob spastic p.

pseudosclerosis *(continued)*
    Neumayer amyotrophic
      lateral p.
    spastic p.
    p. spastica
    Strümpell-Westphal p.
    Westphal-Strümpell p.
pseudoscrotum
pseudosenility
pseudosign
pseudosmallpox
pseudosmia
pseudosolution
pseudostoma
pseudostrabismus
pseudostratified
pseudostrophanthin
pseudostructure
pseudosyncope
pseudotabes
    diabetic p.
    pupillotonic p.
pseudotetanus
pseudothorax
pseudothrill
pseudotoxin
pseudotrachoma
pseudotrismus
pseudotropine
pseudotruncus arteriosus
pseudotubercle
pseudotuberculoma
    silicotic p.
    p. silicoticum
pseudotuberculosis hominis
  streptothrica
pseudotubule
pseudotumor
    p. cerebri
    orbital p.
pseudo-Turner
  syndrome
pseudotympanites
pseudotyphus
pseudouremia
pseudouridine
pseudouridylate
pseudouridylic acid
pseudovacuole
pseudovalve
pseudoventricle
pseudovermicule
pseudovermiculus
pseudovertigo
pseudovillus

pseudovirion
pseudovitamin B_{12}
pseudovoice
pseudovomiting
pseudoxanthoma elasticum
PSG—
    peak systolic gradient
    presystolic gallop
PSGN—poststreptococcal
  glomerulonephritis
PSH—past surgical history
psi—
    Greek letter (ψ; alphabetized
    as ps)
    pounds per square inch
psicofuranine
psilosis pigmentosa
psittacine
psittacosis
psoas
    p. abscess
    p. fascia
    p. muscle
    p. shadow
    p. sign
psodymus
psoitis
psophogenic
psoralen
psorenteritis
psoriasiform
psoriasis
    annular p.
    p. annularis
    p. annulata
    p. arthopica
    arthritic p.
    p. arthropathica
    Barber p.
    p. buccalis
    p. circinata
    circinate p.
    p. diffusa
    discoid p.
    p. discoidea
    p. discoides
    erythrodermic p.
    exfoliative p.
    p. figurata
    figurate p.
    flexural p.
    follicular p.
    p. follicularis
    generalized pustular p.
    p. geographica

P

psoriasis *(continued)*
    p. guttata
    guttate p.
    p. gyrata
    gyrate p.
    inverse p.
    p. inveterata
    p. linguae
    localized pustular p.
    napkin p.
    nummular p.
    p. nummularis
    p. orbicularis
    p. ostracea
    ostraceous p.
    palmar p.
    p. palmaris et
      plantaris
    palmoplantar p.
    p. of palms and soles
    plantar p.
    plaque p.
    provoked p.
    p. punctata
    pustular p.
    rupioid p.
    p. rupioides
    seborrheic p.
    ungual p.
    p. universalis
    unstable p.
    volar p.
    von Zumbusch p.
    p. vulgaris
    Zumbusch p.
psoriatic
psorophthalmia
PSP—
    periodic short pulse
    phenolsulfonphthalein
    positive spike pattern
    progressive supranuclear
      palsy
PSRO—Professional Standards
  Review Organization
PSS—progressive systemic
  sclerosis
PST—penicillin, streptomycin,
  tetracycline
PSVT—paroxysmal
  supraventricular
  tachycardia
psy; psych—
    psychiatric
    psychiatry

psychalgia
psychalgic
psychanalysis
psychanopsia
psychataxia
psyche
psychedelic
psychergograph
psychiatric
psychiatrist
psychiatry
    biological p.
    community p.
    comparative p.
    consultation liaison p.
    cross-cultural p.
    cultural p.
    descriptive p.
    dynamic p.
    existential p.
    experimental p.
    forensic p.
    geriatric p.
    industrial p.
    liaison p.
    occupational p.
    organic p.
    orthomolecular p.
    phenomenological p.
    political p.
    preventive p.
    social p.
    transcultural p.
psychic
psychoacoustics
psychoactivator
psychoactive
psychoanaleptic
psychoanalysis
    adlerian p.
    classic p.
    jungian p.
psychoanalyst
psychoanalytic
psychoanalyze
psychoauditory
psychobiological
psychobiologist
psychobiology
psychocatharsis
psychocortical
psychocutaneous
psychodiagnosis
psychodiagnostics
psychodometer

psychodometry
psychodrama
psychodynamics
    adaptational p.
psychodysleptic
psychoepilepsy
psychogalvanic
psychogalvanometer
psychogender
psychogenic
psychogeriatric
psychogeriatrician
psychogeriatrics
psychognosis
psychognostic
psychogogic
psychogram
psychograph
psychohistory
psychoinfantilism
psychokinesia
psychokinesis
psychokyme
psycholagny
psycholepsy
psycholeptic
psycholinguistics
psychologic, psychological
psychologist
psychology
    abnormal p.
    adlerian p.
    analytic p., analytical p.
    animal p.
    applied p.
    behavioristic p.
    child p.
    clinical p.
    cognitive p.
    community p.
    comparative p.
    counseling p.
    criminal p.
    depth p.
    developmental p.
    dynamic p.
    environmental p.
    experimental p.
    gestalt p., Gestalt p.
    humanistic p.
    individual p.
    industrial p.
    infant p.
    Janet p.
    jungian p.

psychology *(continued)*
    physiologic p.
    social p.
psychometric
psychometrician
psychometry
psychomotor
psychoneural
psychoneurosis
  (psychoneuroses)
    defense p.
    p. maidica
    obsessive-compulsive p.
    paranoid p.
psychonomics
psychonomy
psychopath
    sexual p.
psychopathia sexualis
psychopathic
psychopathology
psychopathosis
psychopathy
psychopharmacology
psychophonasthenia
psychophysical
psychophysics
psychophysiologic
psychophysiology
psychoplegia
psychoplegic
psychopneumatology
psychopolitics
psychoprophylactic
psychoprophylaxis
psychoreaction
psychorhythmia
psychorrhea
psychorrhexis
psychosedation
psychosedative
psychosensorial
psychosensory
psychosexual
psychosexuality
psychosis (psychoses)
    affective p.
    alcoholic psychoses
    alcoholic polyneuritic p.
    alternating p.
    p. of association
    atypical p.
    bipolar p.
    bipolar affective p.
    brief reactive p.

P

psychosis (psychoses) *(continued)*
    bromide p.
    buffoonery p.
    Cheyne-Stokes p.
    chronic epileptic p.
    circular p.
    climacteric p.
    depressive p.
    drug p.
    functional p.
    gestational p.
    housewife's p.
    hysterical p.
    ICU p.
    idiophrenic p.
    induced p.
    involutional p.
    Korsakoff p.
    manic p.
    manic-depressive p.
    organic p.
    paranoiac p.
    paranoid p.
    periodic p.
    polyneuritic p.
    p. polyneuritica
    postpartum p.
    prison p.
    puerperal p.
    reactive p.
    reactive-depressive p.
    schizoaffective p.
    schizophrenic p.
    schizophreniform p.
    senile p.
    situational p.
    symbiogenic p.
    symbiotic p.
    symbiotic infantile p.
    tardive p.
    toxic p.
    unipolar p.
    Wernicke-Korsakoff p.
    windigo p.
psychosocial
psychosomatic
psychosomimetic
psychostimulant
psychosurgery
psychosyndrome
    focal brain p.
psychosynthesis
psychotechnics
psychotherapeutics
psychotherapist

psychotherapy
    brief p.
    contractual p.
    directive p.
    dynamic p.
    existential p.
    family p.
    group p.
    hypnotic p.
    personologic p.
    psychoanalytic p.
    suggestive p.
    supportive p.
    transactional p.
psychotic
psychotogen
psychotogenic
psychotomimetic
psychotropic
psychroalgia
psychroesthesia
psychrometer
    sling p.
psychrophile
psychrophilic
psychrophobia
psychrophore
psychrotherapy
pt—
    patient
    pint
PT—
    parathyroid
    paroxysmal tachycardia
    permanent and total
    physical therapist
    physical therapy
    physical training
    pneumothorax
    prothrombin time
PTA—
    persistent truncus
      arteriosus
    plasma thromboplastin
      antecedent
    post-traumatic amnesia
    prior to admission
    prior to arrival
PTAH—phosphotungstic acid–
    hematoxylin (stain)
ptarmic
ptarmus
PTAV—percutaneous transluminal
    atrial valvuloplasty
PTB—prior to birth

PTBD—percutaneous transhepatic biliary drainage
PTBD catheter
PTC—
    percutaneous transhepatic cholangiography
    plasma thromboplastin component (factor IX)
PTCA—percutaneous transluminal coronary angioplasty
PTD—permanent and total disability
PTE—
    parathyroid extract
    pulmonary thromboembolism
PTEN—pentaerythritol tetranitrate
pteridine
pterin deaminase
pterion
pternalgia
pteroic acid
pteropterin
pteroyl
pteroylglutamate
pterygium (pterygia)
    p. colli
    congenital p.
    p. unguis
pterygoid
pterygomandibular
pterygomaxillary
pterygopalatine
PTF—plasma thromboplastin factor
PTFE—polytetrafluoroethylene
PTH—
    parathyroid hormone
    post-transfusion hepatitis
pthiriasis pubis
PTHS—parathyroid hormone secretion (rate)
PTI—persistent tolerant infection
PTM—post-transfusion mononucleosis
PTMA—
    phenyltrimethylammonium
PTMV—percutaneous transluminal mitral valvuloplasty
ptomaine
ptomainemia
ptomainotoxism
ptomatopsia
ptomatopsy
ptomatropine

ptomatropism
ptosed
ptosis
    p. adiposa
    false p.
    Horner p.
    p. of kidney
    p. lipomatosis
    morning p.
    renal p.
    p. sympathetica
    p. sympathica
    traumatic p.
    waking p.
ptotic
PTP—
    post-tetanic potentiation
    prior to program
PTR—peripheral total resistance
PTRA—percutaneous transluminal renal angioplasty
PTT—
    particle transport time
    partial thromboplastin time
PTU—propylthiouracil
PTX—parathyroidectomy
ptyalagogue
ptyalectasis
ptyalin
ptyalism
    mercurial p.
ptyalize
ptyalocele
    sublingual p.
ptyalogenic
ptyalography
ptyalolithiasis
ptyalolithotomy
ptyaloreaction
ptyalorrhea
ptyalose
ptyocrinous
pubarche
puberphonia
pubertal
pubertas praecox
puberty
    delayed p.
    precocious p.
    pseudoprecocious p.
puberulic acid
pubes (pubes)
pubescence
pubescent

P

pubic
  p. bone
  inferior p. ligament
  inferior p. ramus
  p. lice
  p. ligament of Cowper
  p. phthiriasis
  p. rami
  p. region
  superior p. ligament
  superior p. ramus
  p. symphysis
  p. trichomycosis
  p. tubercle
pubioplasty
pubiotomy
pubis (genitive of pubes)
  symphysis p.
publicly
pubocavernosus
pubocervical
pubococcygeal
pubococcygeus
pubofemoral
puboperitonealis
puboprostatic
puborectal
pubotibial
pubotransversalis
pubovesical
pubovesicalis
PUD—peptic ulcer disease
pudendagra
pudendal
pudendum (pudenda)
  female p.
  p. femininum
  p. muliebre
Pudenz
  reservoir
  shunt
  tube
  valve
Pudenz-Heyer valve
pudic
PUE—pyrexia of unknown etiology
Puente disease
puericulture
puerile
puerilism
puerpera
puerperal
puerperalism
puerperant
puerperium
Puestow-Gillesby procedure

Puestow procedure
PUFA—polyunsaturated fatty
  acid(s)
puff
  chromosome p.
  veiled p.
puffer
  chubby p. syndrome
  pink p.
puffing
Pugh nail
pugil, pugillus
puits de Devergie
pulex (pulices)
Pulfrich
  pendulum
  phenomenon
pulicicide
pulicosis
pulley suture
pull-out wire suture
pull-through
  ileoanal p-t. anastomosis
  p-t. operation
pulmo (pulmones)
  p. dexter
  p. sinister
pulmoaortic
pulmogram
pulmolith
pulmometer
pulmometry
pulmonale
  cor p.
pulmonary
  p. abscess
  p. agenesis
  p. alveolus
  p. amyloidosis
  p. angiography
  p. anthrax
  p. arborization
  p. arteriography
  p. artery wedge pressure
    (PAWP)
  p. ascariasis
  p. aspergillosis
  p. atresia
  p. blastomycosis
  p. candidiasis
  p. congestion
  p. cryptococcosis
  p. diffusion
  p. edema
  p. ejection clicks
  p. embolic disease

pulmonary *(continued)*
- p. embolism
- p. eosinophilia
- p. fibrosis
- p. function
- p. function test (PFT)
- p. gangrene
- p. hemosiderosis
- p. histoplasmosis
- p. hypertension
- p. infarction
- p. lymphangiectasia
- p. maturity
- p. mucormycosis
- p. neoplasm
- p. nodulosis
- p. pedicle
- p. perfusion
- p. resection
- p. sarcoidosis
- p. sequestration
- p. sulcus
- p. suppuration
- p. surfactant
- p. telangiectasia
- p. thromboembolism
- p. thromboses
- p. toilet
- transventricular p. valvotomy
- p. valve
- p. valvotomy
- p. vascular markings
- p. vascular redistribution
- p. vasculature
- p. veno-occlusive disease
- p. venules

pulmonate
pulmonectomy
pulmones (plural of pulmo)
pulmonic
- p. atresia
- p. murmur
- p. plaque
- p. stenosis

pulmonis
pulmonitis
pulmonohepatic
pulmonologist
pulmonology
pulmonoperitoneal
pulmotor
pulp
- coronal p.
- dead p.
- dental p.
- devitalized p.

pulp *(continued)*
- digital p.
- enamel p.
- exposed p.
- hair p.
- mummified p.
- necrotic p.
- nonvital p.
- putrescent p.
- radicular p.
- red p.
- p. of spleen
- splenic p.
- tooth p.
- vertebral p.
- vital p.
- white p.

pulpa (pulpae)
- p. coronale
- p. coronalis
- p. dentis
- p. lienalis
- p. lienis
- p. radicularis
- p. splenica

pulpal
pulpalgia
pulpectomy
- partial p.

pulpiform
pulpitis (pulpitides)
- anachoretic p.
- closed p.
- hyperplastic p.
- open p.

pulpless
pulpoaxial
pulpobuccoaxial
pulpodistal
pulpolabial
pulpolingual
pulpolinguoaxial
pulpomesial
pulpotomy
pulpy
pulsate
pulsatile
pulsation
- expansile p.
- suprasternal p.

pulsator
- Bragg-Paul p.

pulse
- abdominal p.
- abrupt p.
- allorhythmic p.

P

pulse *(continued)*

- alternating p.
- anacrotic p.
- anadicrotic p.
- anatricrotic p.
- apical p.
- arachnoid p.
- atrial liver p.
- atrial venous p.
- atriovenous p.
- auriculovenous p.
- Bamberger bulbar p.
- biferious p.
- bigeminal p.
- bisferious p.
- cannon-ball p.
- capillary p.
- carotid p.
- catacrotic p.
- catadicrotic p.
- catatricrotic p.
- centripetal venous p.
- collapsing p.
- cordy p.
- Corrigan p.
- coupled p.
- decurtate p.
- p. deficit
- dicrotic p.
- digitalate p.
- dropped-beat p.
- elastic p.
- entoptic p.
- epigastric p.
- equal p.
- febrile p.
- filiform p.
- formicant p.
- frequent p.
- full p.
- funic p.
- gaseous p.
- gate p.
- guttural p.
- hard p.
- hepatic p.
- high-tension p.
- hyperdicrotic p.
- infrequent p.
- intermittent p.
- irregular p.
- jerky p.
- jugular p.
- jugular p. sphygmography
- Kussmaul p.

pulse *(continued)*

- Kussmaul Monneret p.
- labile p.
- low-tension p.
- Monneret p.
- monocrotic p.
- mouse tail p.
- nail p.
- paradoxical p.
- parvus et tardus p.
- pedal p.
- pistol-shot p.
- plateau p.
- polycrotic p.
- pulmonary p.
- quadrigeminal p.
- quick p.
- Quincke p.
- radial p.
- respiratory p.
- retrosternal p.
- Riegel p.
- running p.
- sharp p.
- short p.
- slow p.
- soft p.
- strong p.
- tense p.
- thready p.
- tremulous p.
- tricrotic p.
- trigeminal p.
- trip-hammer p.
- undulating p.
- unequal p.
- vagus p.
- venous p.
- ventricular venous p.
- vermicular p.
- vibrating p.
- water-hammer p.
- wiry p.

pulse-height analyzer
pulseless disease
pulsellum (pulsella)
pulsion
pulsus (pulsus)

- p. abdominalis
- p. aequalis
- p. alternans
- p. biferiens
- p. bigeminus
- p. bisferiens
- p. celer

pulsus (pulsus) *(continued)*
- p. contractus
- p. cordis
- p. debilis
- p. deficiens
- p. deletus
- p. differens
- p. duplex
- p. durus
- p. filiformis
- p. formicans
- p. fortis
- p. frequens
- p. heterochronicus
- p. intercurrens
- p. irregularis perpetuus
- p. magnus
- p. magnus et celer
- p. mollis
- p. monocrotus
- p. oppressus
- p. paradoxus
- p. parvus
- p. parvus et tardus
- p. plenus
- p. pseudo-intermittens
- p. rarus
- p. tardus
- p. trigeminus
- p. undulosus
- p. vacuus
- p. venosus
- p. vibrans

pultaceous
pulverization
pulverulent
pulvinar
- p. thalami
- p. tunicae internae segmenti
  arterialis anastomosis
  arteriovenae glomeriformis

pulvinate
pulvis
pumice
pump
- air p.
- Alvegniat p.
- blood p.
- breast p.
- calcium p.
- cardiac balloon p.
- Carrel-Lindbergh p.
- dental p.
- Emerson p.
- infusion p.

pump *(continued)*
- infusion-withdrawal p.
- intra-aortic balloon p.
- Lindbergh p.
- McGaw p.
- muscle p.
- Na+-K+ p.
- p.-oxygenator
- peristaltic p.
- rotary p.
- saliva p.
- sodium p.
- sodium-potassium p.
- stomach p.

puna
punch
- Acufex p.
- Adler p.
- Ainsworth p.
- Berens p.
- Brock p.
- Castroviejo p.
- cervical p. biopsy clamp
- Citelli-Meltzer atticus p.
- Deyerle p.
- Gass scleral p.
- Hajek-Skillern p.
- Hartmann p.
- Hoffmann p.
- Holth p.
- Kerrison p.
- Keyes biopsy p.
- Keyes dermal p.
- kidney p.
- Lermoyez p.
- Meltzer p.
- Mosher p.
- Murphy kidney p.
- Myles p.
- pin p.
- plate p.
- Pritikin p.
- rubber dam p.
- Rubin-Holth p.
- Spencer p.
- sphenoidal p.
- Spies p.
- Takahashi p.
- Turkel p.
- Wagner p.
- Walton p.
- Watson-Williams p.
- Wilde p.
- Yankauer p.

punchdrunk

P

punched-out
punctate
punctiform
punctograph
punctuation
    Schüffner p.
punctum (puncta)
    p. caecum
    puncta dolorosa
    lacrimal p.
    p. lacrimale
    puncta lacrimalia
    p. luteum
    p. nasale inferius
    p. ossificationis
    p. ossificationis primarium
    p. ossificationis secundarium
    p. proximum
    p. remotum
    puncta vasculosa
punctumeter
puncture
    bone marrow p.
    cisternal p.
    Corning p.
    cranial p.
    epigastric p.
    exploratory p.
    gland p.
    intracisternal p.
    Kronecker p.
    lumbar p. (LP)
    Marfan epigastric p.
    pericardial p.
    Quincke p.
    spinal p.
    splenic p.
    sternal p.
    subdural p.
    suboccipital p.
    suprapubic p.
    thecal p.
    tibial p.
    tracheoesophageal p.
    transethmoidal p.
    ventricular p.
pungent
Punnett square
PUO—pyrexia of unknown origin
pupil
    Adie p.
    Argyll Robertson p.
    artificial p.
    Behr p.
    bounding p.

pupil *(continued)*
    Bumke p.
    cat-eye p., cat's eye p.
    cornpicker's p.
    double p.
    fixed p.
    Horner p.
    Hutchinson p.
    keyhole p.
    Marcus Gunn p.
    multiple p.
    myotonic p.
    pinhole p.
    pseudo-Argyll Robertson p.
    Robertson p.
    skew p.
    stiff p.
    tonic p.
pupilla
pupillary
pupillatonia
pupilloconstriction
pupillograph
pupillography
pupillometer
pupillometry
pupillomotor
pupilloplegia
pupilloscope
pupilloscopy
pupillostatometer
pupillotonia
pupiparous
pupivorous
PUPPP—pruritic urticarial papules
    and plaques of pregnancy
pura (plural of pus)
Purcell retractor
purchase point
Purdy
    method
    test
purgation
purgative
    saline p.
purge
purging
    bingeing and p.
puriform
purine
    amino p.
    methyl p's
    p.-nucleoside phosphorylase
    p. 5'-nucleotidase
purinemia

purinemic
purinolytic
purinometer
puris (genitive of pus)
Purkinje
  cells
  fibers
  image
  layer
  network
  phenomenon
  shift
  vesicle
Purkinje-Sanson mirror images
purohepatitis
puromucous
purple
  bromcresol p.
  visual p.
purpura
  p. abdominalis
  actinic p.
  acute vascular p.
  allergic p.
  anaphylactoid p.
  p. angioneurotica
  p. annularis telangiectodes
  p. arthritica
  athrombocytopenic p.
  autoimmune
    thrombocytopenic p.
  benign hyperglobulinemic p.
  brain p.
  p. bullosa
  cachectic p.
  p. cachectica
  cocktail p.
  dependent
    nonthrombocytopenic p.
  drug p.
  dysproteinemic p.
  essential p.
  factitious p.
  fibrinolytic p.
  p. fibrinolytica
  p. fulminans
  hemogenic p.
  p. hemorrhagica
  Henoch p.
  Henoch-Schönlein (Henoch-
    Schoenlein) p.
  hypergammaglobulinemic p.
  hyperglobulinemic p.
  p. hyperglobulinemica
  idiopathic p.

purpura *(continued)*
  idiopathic thrombocytopenic
    p. (ITP)
  p. iodica
  itching p.
  Landouzy p.
  lung p. with nephritis
  p. maculosa
  Majocchi p.
  malignant p.
  mechanical p.
  p. nervosa
  p. of newborn
  nonpalpable p.
  nonthrombocytopenic p.
  orthostatic p.
  palpable p.
  p. pigmentosa chronica
  psychogenic p.
  p. pulicans
  p. pulicosa
  p. rheumatica
  Schönlein (Schoenlein) p.
  Schönlein-Henoch
    (Schoenlein-Henoch) p.
  p. scorbutica
  secondary thrombocytopenic p.
  senile p., p. senilis
  p. simplex
  steroid p.
  symptomatic p., p.
    symptomatica
  thrombocytopenic p. (TP)
  p. thrombolytica
  thrombopenic p.
  thrombotic p.
  thrombotic
    thrombocytopenic p.
  thrombotic thrombohemolytic p.
  p. urticans
  p. variolosa
  vascular p.
  Waldenström
    hyperglobulinemic p.
purpureaglycoside C
purpuric acid
purpuriferous
purpurin
purpurine
purpurinuria
purpurogenous
purr
purring
pursestring suture
purshianin

pursuit
  saccadic p.
Purtscher
  angiopathic retinopathy
  disease
  syndrome
purulence
purulent
puruloid
pus (pura)
  anchovy sauce p.
  blue p.
  burrowing p.
  cheesy p.
  curdy p.
  green p.
  ichorous p.
  laudable p.
  p. laudandum
  sanious p.
  p. tube
Pusey emulsion
pushback
  palatal p.
push plus
pustula (pustulae)
  p. maligna
pustular
pustulation
pustule
  amniotic p's
  compound p.
  malignant p.
  multilocular p.
  postmortem p.
  primary p.
  secondary p.
  simple p.
  spongiform p.
  spongiform p. of Kogoj
  unilocular p.
pustulosis
  acral p.
  p. palmaris
  p. palmaris et plantaris
  palmoplantar p.
  p. vacciniformis acuta
  p. varioliformis acuta
putamen
putative
Putnam type
Putnam-Dana syndrome
putrefaction
putrefactive
putrefy

putrescence
putrescent
putrescentia uteri
putrescine
putrid
Putti
  rasp
  syndrome
Putti-Platt
  arthroplasty
  operation
putty
  Horsley p.
Puusepp
  operation
  reflex
PUVA—psoralens and
  ultraviolet A
Puzo method
PV—
  peripheral vascular
  peripheral vein
  peripheral vessels
  plasma volume
  polycythemia vera
  portal vein
  postvoiding
P&V—pyloroplasty and vagotomy
PVA—polyvinyl alcohol
PVC—
  polyvinyl chloride
  postvoiding cystogram
  premature ventricular
    contraction
  pulmonary venous congestion
PVC (polyvinyl chloride)
  pneumoconiosis
PVD—peripheral vascular disease
PVE—partial vein embolization
PVF—portal venous flow
PVP—
  penicillin V potassium
  peripheral vein plasma
  portal venous pressure
PVP-I—povidone-iodine
PVR—
  peripheral vascular resistance
  pulmonary vascular resistance
PVS—premature ventricular
  systole
PVT—
  paroxysmal ventricular
    tachycardia
  portal vein thrombosis
PW—posterior wall

PWA—person with AIDS
PWB—partial weightbearing
   (weight-bearing)
PWC—physical work capacity
PWI—posterior wall infarction
PWM—pokeweed mitogen
Px—
   physical examination
   pneumothorax
   prognosis
PXE—pseudoxanthoma elasticum
pyarthrosis
pyelectasia
pyelectasis
pyelic
pyelitic
pyelitis
   acute p.
   calculous p.
   calculous pyelonephritis
   chronic p.
   cystic p.
   p. cystica
   defloration p.
   encrusted p.
   p. glandularis
   p. granulosa
   p. gravidarum
   hematogenous p.
   hemorrhagic p.
   suppurative p.
   urogenous p.
pyelocaliceal
pyelocaliectasis
pyelocystitis
pyelocystostomosis
pyelofluoroscopy
pyelogram
   dragon p.
   hydrated p.
   infusion p.
   intravenous p.
   retrograde p.
pyelography
   air p.
   antegrade p.
   ascending p.
   p. by elimination
   drip p.
   drip infusion p.
   p. by elimination
   excretion p.
   infusion p.
   intravenous p. (IVP)
   lateral p.

pyelography *(continued)*
   percutaneous antegrade p.
   respiration p.
   retrograde p.
   washout p.
pyeloileocutaneous
pyelointerstitial
pyelolithotomy
pyelometry
pyelonephritis
   acute p.
   acute nonobstructive p.
   ascending p.
   asymptomatic p.
   calculous p.
   chronic p.
   chronic bacterial p.
   emphysematous p.
   hematogenous p.
   p. of pregnancy
   xanthogranulomatous p.
pyelonephrosis
pyelopathy
pyelophlebitis
pyeloplasty
pyeloscopy
pyelostomy
pyelotomy
pyelotubular
pyeloureteral
pyeloureterectasis
pyeloureteritis cystica
pyeloureterogram
pyeloureterography
pyeloureterolysis
pyeloureteroplasty
pyelovenous
pyemesis
pyemia
   arterial p.
   cryptogenic p.
   otogenous p.
   portal p.
pyemic
Pyemotes ventricosus
pyencephalus
pyesis
pygal
pygalgia
pygmalionism
pygmy
pygoamorphus
pygodidymus
pygomelus
pygopagus parasiticus

P

pygopagy
pyic
pyknic
pyknocyte
pyknocytoma
pyknocytosis
pyknodysostosis
pyknoepilepsy
pyknometer
pyknometry
pyknomorphous
pyknophrasia
pyknoplasson
pyknosis
pyknosomatic
pyknotic
pyla
pylar
Pyle disease
pylephlebectasis
pylephlebitis
    adhesive p.
pylethrombophlebitis
pylethrombosis
pylic
pylon
pyloralgia
pylorectomy
pyloric
    p. antrum
    p. artery
    p. atresia
    p. canal
    p. constriction
    p. diaphragm
    p. glands
    hypertrophic p. stenosis
    p. lymph nodes
    p. membrane
    p. obstruction
    p. olive
    p. opening
    p. orifice
    p. outlet
    p. outlet obstruction
    p. sphincter
    p. sphincter muscle
    p. stenosis
    p. string sign
    p. valve
    p. vein
    p. web
pyloristenosis
pyloritis
pylorodilator

pylorodiosis
pyloroduodenitis
pylorogastrectomy
pyloromyotomy
    Fredet-Ramstedt p.
pyloroplasty
    double p.
    Finney p.
    Heineke-Mikulicz p.
    Horsley p.
    Jaboulay p.
    Judd p.
    Ramstedt p.
    vagotomy and p. (V&P)
pyloroscopy
pylorospasm
    congenital p.
    reflex p.
pylorostomy
pylorotomy
pylorus
Pynchon
    applicator
    speculum
    tube
pyoarthrosis
pyoblennorrhea
pyocalix
pyocele
    frontal sinus p.
pyocelia
pyocephalus
    external p.
    internal p.
pyochezia
pyocin
pyococcic
pyococcus
pyocolpocele
pyocolpos
pyocyanase
pyocyanic
pyocyanin
pyocyanogenic
pyocyanosis
pyocyst
pyocystis
pyocyte
pyoderma
    chancriform p.
    p. chancriforme faciei
    p. faciale
    p. gangrenosum
    malignant p.
    oral p.

pyoderma *(continued)*
    primary p.
    secondary p.
    streptococcal p.
    p. vegetans
    p. verrucosum
    verrucous p.
pyodermatitis vegetans
pyodermatosis
pyogenesis
pyogenic
pyogenous
pyohemothorax
pyohydronephrosis
pyoid
pyolabyrinthitis
pyometra
pyometritis
pyometrium
pyomyoma
pyomyositis
    tropical p.
pyonephritis
pyonephrolithiasis
pyonephrosis
    calculous p.
pyonephrotic
pyo-ovarium
pyopericarditis
pyopericardium
pyoperitoneum
pyoperitonitis
pyophagia
pyophthalmia
pyophylactic
pyophysometra
pyoplania
pyopneumocholecystitis
pyopneumocyst
pyopneumohepatitis
pyopneumopericarditis
pyopneumopericardium
pyopneumoperitoneum
pyopneumoperitonitis
pyopneumothorax
pyopoiesis
pyopoietic
pyoptysis
pyopyelectasis
pyorrhea
    p. alveolaris
    paradental p.
    Schmutz p.
pyorrheal
pyorubin

pyosalpingitis
pyosalpingo-oophoritis
pyosalpingo-oothecitis
pyosalpinx
pyosapremia
pyosclerosis
pyosepticemia
pyosis
    Corlett p., p. of Corlett
    p. of Manson
pyospermia
pyostatic
pyostomatitis vegetans
pyothorax
    subphrenic p.
pyotoxinemia
pyoumbilicus
pyourachus
pyoureter
pyovesiculosis
pyoxanthine
pyoxanthose
pyrabrom
pyracin
pyrahexyl
pyramid
    age-sex p.
    anterior p. of medulla
      oblongata
    p. of Arnold
    p. of cerebellum
    p. of Ferrein
    p. of kidney
    Lalouette p.
    p. of light
    Malacarne p.
    p's of Malpighi
    p. of medulla oblongata
    medullary p.
    olfactory p.
    petrous p.
    population p.
    posterior p. of medulla
      oblongata
    renal p.
    star p.
    p. of temporal bone
    p. of thyroid
    p. of tympanum
    p. of vermis
    p. of vestibule
    Wistar p's
pyramidale
pyramidalis
pyramidal tractotomy

P

pyramides
pyramidotomy
   spinal p.
pyramis (pyramides)
   p. cerebelli
   pyramides Malpighii
   p. medullae oblongatae
   p. ossis temporalis
   pyramides renales
   pyramides renales
    Malpighii
   p. vermis
   p. vestibuli
pyran
pyranose
pyranoside
pyranyl
pyrazine
pyrectic
pyrene
pyrenoid
pyrenolysis
pyrethrin
pyrethroid
pyrethron
pyrethrum
pyretic
pyretogen
pyretogenesis
pyretogenetic
pyretogenic
pyretogenous
pyretography
pyretology
pyretolysis
pyretotherapy
pyretotyphosis
pyrexia (pyrexiae)
   heat p.
   Pel-Ebstein p.
pyrexial
pyrexin
pyridoxic acid
pyridoxilated
pyridoxine
   p. dehydrogenase
   p. phosphate
pyridoxol phosphate
pyrimidine
pyrinoline
pyrithiamine
pyroborate
pyroboric acid
pyrocatechol
pyrodextrin

pyrogen
   bacterial p.
   endogenous p.
   exogenous p.
   leukocytic p.
pyrogenic
pyroglobulin
pyroglobulinemia
pyroglutamase
pyroglutamate
pyroglutamate hydrolase
pyroglutamic acid
pyrolagnia
pyroligneous
pyrolysis
pyromania
   erotic p.
pyrometer
pyrone
pyronin
   p. B
   p. G
   p. Y
pyronine
pyroninophilia
pyroninophilic
pyrophobia
pyrophos
pyrophosphatase
   inorganic p.
pyrophosphate
   ferric p.
   stannous p.
pyrophosphate ribose-P-synthetase
pyrophosphokinase
pyrophosphomevalonate
pyrophosphoric acid
pyrophosphorolysis
pyrophosphorylase
pyrophosphotransferase
pyrosis
pyrotic
pyroxylin
pyrrole
pyrrolidine
pyrroline
pyrroline-5-carboxylate
   reductase
pyrrolnitrin
pyrroloporphyria
pyruvate
   p. carboxylase (PC)
   p. carboxylase deficiency
   p. decarboxylase
   p. dehydrogenase (lipoamide)

pyruvate *(continued)*
    p. dehydrogenase complex (PDHC) deficiency
    p. kinase (PK)
    p. kinase deficiency, erythrocyte
pyruvemia
pyruvic acid
pythiosis
pythogenesis
pythogenic
pythogenous
pyuria
    abacterial p.
    miliary p.
PZ—pancreozymin
PZA—pyrazinamide
PZ-CCK—pancreozymin-cholecystokinin
PZI—protamine zinc insulin

Q

q—long arm of a chromosome
q—probability of an alternative event
q.—each; every (L. quaque)
Q—
    query
    ubiquinone
Q—
    electric charge
    heat
    reaction quotient
Q_{10}—temperature coefficient
q.a.m.—every morning (L. quaque ante meridiem)
QC—quinine-colchicine
q.d.—every day, daily (L. quaque die)
Q fever
q.h.—every hour (L. quaque hora)
q.2 h.—every two hours
q.3 h.—every three hours
q.4 h.—every four hours
q.h.s.—at bedtime (L. quaque hora somni)
q.i.d.—four times a day (L. quater in die)
q.o.d.—every other day
QP—Quanti-Pirquet reaction
QRS
    alternans
    axis
    changes
    complex
    duration
    interval
    loop

QRS *(continued)*
    morphology
    onset
    score
    vector
    wave
QRZ—wheal reaction time
qt.—quart
Q-tip test
Quaaludes
quack
quackery
quacksalver
quadrangle
quadrangular
    q. body
    q. cartilage
    q. cartilage flap
    q. cartilage paddle
    q. fontanelle
    q. ligament
    q. lobule of cerebellum
    q. membrane
    q. resection of posterior leaflet
    q. shape
    q. space
    q. space syndrome
quadrant
    contralateral q.
    dental q.
    q. hemianopia
    left lower q. (LLQ)
    left upper q. (LUQ)
    lower nasal q.
    q. pain

quadrant *(continued)*
 posteroinferior q. perforation
  of tympanic membrane
 q. resection
 right lower q. (RLQ)
 right upper q. (RUQ)
 q. scaling
 q. swelling
 temporal q.
 q's of the tympanic membrane
 q. ultrasonic debridement
 upper temporal retinal q.
 visual field q.
quadrantal
quadrantanopia
quadrantanopsia
quadrantectomy
quadrantic
quadrate
quadratipronator
quadrature detector
quadratus
quadribasic
quadriceps
 q. artery of femur
 q. boot
 q. femoris muscle
 q. gait
 q. jerk
 q. reflex
quadricepsplasty
quadricuspid
quadridentate
quadridigitate
quadrigemina
quadrigeminal
quadrigeminum (quadrigemina)
quadrilateral
 q. cartilage
 q. flap
 q. frame
 q. ligament
 q. plate
 q. Q-shaped skin flap
 q. skin flap
 q. space
 q. space syndrome
 vowel q.
quadrilocular
quadripara
quadriparesis
quadripartite
quadriplegia
quadriplegic
quadripolar

quadrisect
quadrisection
quadritubercular
quadrivalent
quadruplets
Quain
 degeneration
 fatty heart
quale
qualimeter
qualitative
qualitive
quality
quandary
quanta
quantal
quantification
quantile
quantimeter
quantitate
quantitative computed tomography
quantity
 vectorial q.
quantization
quantize, quantized
quantum (quanta)
 q. of light
 q. theory
quarantine
 measles q.
 q. period
 voluntary q.
quart (qt.)
quartan
 double q.
 triple q.
quartana
 q. duplex
 q. triplex
quarter
 false q.
 three-q. crown
quartet
quartile
quartisect
quartisternal
quartz
 cold q. lamp
 q. fiber post
 q. glass
 hot q. lamp
 q.-tungsten-halogen lamp
quasidiploid
quasidominance
quasidominant

quassation
quassia
quassin
quaternary
Quatrefages angle
queasy
Queckenstedt
    maneuver
    phenomenon
    sign
    test
Queckenstedt-Stookey test
quellung
quenching
    color q.
    fluorescence q.
    thermal q.
Quénu-Muret sign
Quénu plexus
quercetin-3-rutinoside
querulous
queue
Quevedo forceps
Queyrat erythroplasia
quick
    q. of the fingernail
    q. pulse
    q. recovery
Quick test
quick-change nosepiece
quick-cure resin
quickening
quicklime
quick-setting epoxy cement
quiescent
    q. cancer cells
    q. Crohn disease
    q. hematopoietic stem cells
    q. primary bone lymphoma
    q. state
    q. transplant glomerulopathy
quillaia
quillain
quilt
    q. suture
    q. venoplasty technique
quilted suture
quinaldic acid
quinaldinic acid
quinaquina
Quincke
    angioedema
    capillary pulsation
    disease
    edema

Quincke (continued)
    meningitis
    pulse
    puncture
    sign
    syndrome
quinestrol
quinhydrone
quinic acid
quinidine
    q. gluconate
    q. polygalacturonate
    q. sulfate
quinine
    β-q.
    q. ethylcarbonate
    q. sulfate
quininism
quininize
quinoid
quinol
quinoline
quinolone antibiotic
quinone
quinonoid
quinovin
Quinquaud
    decalvans folliculitis
    disease
    sign
quinquecuspid
quinquetubercular
quinquevalent
quinquina
quinsy
    lingual q.
quintan
quintessence
quintile
quintipara
quintisternal
quintuplet
Quisling hammer
quoad vitam [L. so far as life is concerned]
quotidian
quotient
    achievement q.
    albumin q.
    Ayala q.
    blood q.
    caloric q.
    D q.
    developmental q.
    D/N (dextrose/nitrogen) q.

Q

quotient *(continued)*
>   growth q.
>   intelligence q. (IQ)
>   phonation q.
>   protein q.
>   rachidian q.

quotient *(continued)*
>   reaction q.
>   respiratory q.
>   spinal q.
>   spinal reaction
> q.v.— which see (L. quod vide)

R

ρ—
>   rho (Greek letter)
>   electric charge density
>   mass density

℞ [R_x, Rx]—
>   prescription
>   take (L. recipe)

r—
>   drug resistance
>   ring chromosome

r—
>   correlation coefficient
>   distance radius

R.—Rickettsia

R—
>   radical
>   Rankine scale
>   rate
>   Réaumur scale
>   rectal
>   regression coefficient
>   remote
>   resistance
>   respiration
>   respiratory exchange
>   rhythm
>   right
>   Rinne test
>   rub

RA—
>   renal artery
>   rheumatoid arthritis
>   right arm
>   right atrial
>   right atrium

R_A; R_{AW}—airway resistance
RabAvert rabies vaccine
rabbeting
rabbit stools
rabicidal

rabid
rabies
>   dumb r.
>   furious r.
>   paralytic r.
>   r. vaccine

rabiform
raccoon eyes
racemase
racemate
racemic
>   r. calcium pantothenate
>   r. epinephrine
>   r. form
>   r. modification

racemization
racemose
rachialbuminimetry
rachialgia
rachianesthesia
rachicentesis
rachidial
rachidian
rachigraph
rachilysis
rachiocampsis
rachiocentesis
rachiochysis
rachiocyphosis
rachiodynia
rachiokyphosis
rachiomyelitis
rachiopagus
rachiopathy
rachioscoliosis
rachiotome
rachiotomy
rachiresistance
rachiresistant
rachis

rachisagra
rachischisis
    r. partialis
    r. posterior
    r. totalis
rachisensibility
rachisensible
rachitic
    r. metaphysis
    r. rosary
rachitis
    r. fetalis annularis
    r. fetalis anularis
    r. fetalis micromelica
    r. tarda
rachitism
rachitogenic
racial
Racine syndrome
raclage
raclopride C 11
racquet
    r. conjunctival flap
    r. ear
    r. flap
    r. incision
racquet-handle shape
racquet-shaped
    r-s. cytosome
    r-s. malignant cells
    r-s. Nucleotome
rad—radiation adsorbed dose
rad per second (rad/s)
RAD—right axis deviation
radectomy
radiability
radiable
radiad
radial
    r. artery
    r. bone
    r. cells of Müller
    r. cleavage
    r. clubhand
    r. collateral artery
    r. collateral ligament
    r. condyle
    r. crest
    deep r. nerve
    r. depression
    r. deviation
    r. drift
    r. eminence of wrist
    r. fibers
    r. glia

radial *(continued)*
    r. groove
    r. growth phase
    r. head of humerus
    r. hemimelia
    r. immunodiffusion
    r. incision
    inverted r. reflex
    r. keratotomy (RK)
    r. ligament
    r. malleolus
    r. nerve
    r. notch
    r. paralysis
    superficial r. nerve
radialis
radiant energy
radiate
radiathermy
radiatio (radiationes)
    r. acustica
    r. corporis callosi
    r. optica
    r. thalami anterior
    r. thalami centralis
    r. thalami inferior
    r. thalami posterior
radiation
    α r. [alpha]
    r. absorbed dose (rad)
    r. absorption
    acoustic r.
    actinic r.
    adaptive r.
    r. alopecia
    annihilation r.
    auditory r.
    β r. [beta]
    background r.
    backscattered r.
    r. barrier
    beta r.
    braking r.
    bremsstrahlung r.
    r. burn
    r. cataract
    Cerenkov r. production
    characteristic r.
    r. chimera
    r. colitis
    r. of corpus callosum
    corpuscular r.
    cosmic r.
    r. counter
    cyclotron r.

R

radiation *(continued)*
  r. cystitis
  r. dermatitis
  r. detector
  direct r.
  dose equivalent r.
  electromagnetic r.
  r. energy
  r. enteritis
  r. enteropathy
  r. equivalent man
  r. erythema
  r. esophagitis
  r. esophagus
  r. exposure
  r. fibrosis
  fractionated r.
  γ r. [gamma]
  r. gastritis
  geniculocalcarine r.
  geniculotemporal r.
  r. of Gratiolet
  hard r.
  r. hepatitis
  heterogeneous r.
  homogeneous r.
  Huldshinsky r.
  r. illness
  infrared r.
  r. injury
  r. intensity
  interstitial r.
  ionization r.
  ionizing r.
  irritative r.
  K-r.
  r. keratosis
  L-r.
  r. leakage
  Maxwell theory of r.
  mitogenetic r.,
    mitogenic r.
  r. monitor
  monochromatic r.
  monoenergetic r.
  r. myelitis
  r. myelopathy
  natural r.
  r. necrosis
  r. nephritis
  r. neuritis
  nonionizing r.
  nuclear r.
  occipitothalamic r.
  occupational r.

radiation *(continued)*
  r. oncology
  optic r.
  r. osteitis
  r. pericarditis
  photochemical r.
  photon theory of r.
  r. physics
  r. pneumonia
  r. pneumonitis
  primary r.
  r. proctitis
  r. protection
  protracted r. exposure
  pyramidal r.
  recoil r.
  remnant r.
  Rollier r.
  scattered r.
  secondary r.
  r. sickness
  specific r.
  r. spectrum
  spontaneous r.
  striatothalamic r.
  supervoltage r.
  r. syndrome
  r. synovectomy
  tegmental r.
  thalamic r's
  thalamic r., anterior
  thalamic r., caudal
  thalamic r., central
  thalamic r., inferior
  thalamic r., posterior
  thalamic r., superior
  thalamostriate r.
  thalamotemporal r.
  r's of thalamus
  r. therapy
  thermal r.
  r. thyroiditis
  r. toxicity
  ultraviolet r.
  useful-beam r.
  visual r.
  r. warning symbol
  Wernicke r.
  white r.
  r. window
radical
  r. antrum operation
  Auchincloss modified r.
    mastectomy
  extended r. mastectomy

radical *(continued)*
>   Halsted r. mastectomy
>   r. hysterectomy
>   Latzko r. hysterectomy
>   r. mastectomy (RM)
>   r. mastoidectomy
>   r. maxillary antrostomy
>   modified r. mastectomy
>   modified r. mastoidectomy
>   r. nephrectomy
>   r. operation
>   r. prostatectomy
>   r. retropubic prostatectomy
>   Schauta r. vaginal
>   hysterectomy
>   Wertheim r. hysterectomy

radical
>   acid r.
>   alcohol r.
>   color r.
>   free r.
>   oxygen r.

radical-ion
radices (plural of radix)
radiciform
radicis (genitive of radix)
radicle
>   bile duct r.
>   biliary r.
>   intercostal nerve r.
>   portal vein r.

radicotomy
radicula
radiculalgia
radicular
radiculectomy
radiculitis
>   acute r.
>   *Borrelia*-associated r.
>   *Borrelia burgdorferi* r.
>   cervical r.
>   chemical r.
>   herpes zoster r.
>   lower extremity r.
>   lumbar r.
>   lumbosacral r.
>   sacral r.
>   S1 r.
>   spinal r.
>   transient r.

radiculoganglionitis
radiculomedullary
radiculomeningomyelitis
radiculomyelopathy
radiculoneuritis

radiculoneuropathy
>   hypertrophic interstitial r.

radiculopathy
>   brachial r.
>   cervical r.
>   spinal r.
>   spondylotic caudal r.

radiectomy
radii (genitive and plural of radius)
radioablation
radioactinium
radioactive
>   r. balloon method
>   r. constant
>   r. decay
>   r. disintegration
>   r. effluents
>   r. element
>   r. equilibrium
>   r. fallout
>   r. gallium
>   r. gases
>   r. half-life
>   r. indicator
>   r. iodine
>   r. iodine uptake test
>   r. isotope
>   r. label
>   r. nuclide
>   r. series
>   r. source
>   r. tag
>   r. thorium
>   r. tracer

radioactivity
>   artificial r.
>   induced r.
>   natural r.

radioallergosorbent test (RAST)
radioautogram
radioautography
radiobicipital
radiobiological
radiobiologist
radiobiology
radiocalcium
radiocarbon
radiocarcinogenesis
radiocardiogram
radiocardiography
radiocarpal
radiocarpus
radiochemical purity
radiochemistry
radiochemotherapy

R

radiochroism
radiochromatography
radiocinematograph
radiocobalt
radiocolloid
radiocurability
radiocurable
radiocystitis
radiode
radiodense
radiodensity
radiodermatitis
radiodiagnosis
radiodiagnostics
radiodigital
radiodontics
radiodontist
radiodosimetry
radioecology
radioelectrocardiogram
radioelectrocardiograph
radioelectrocardiography
radioelement
radioencephalogram
radioencephalography
radioenzymatic
radioepidermitis
radioepithelioma
radioepithelitis
radiofrequency, radio
  frequency
    r. ablation (RFA)
    r. bistoury
    r. catheter ablation
    r. coagulation
    r. coil
    r. denervation
    r. energy
    intravascular ultrasound-
      derived r. analysis
    r. neurotomy
    r. pacemaker
    percutaneous r. rhizotomy
    percutaneous r.
      thermocoagulation
    plasma-mediated r.
    r. pulse
    pulsed r.
    r. therapy
    r. thermocoagulation
    r. treatment
radiogenesis
radiogenic
radiogold seed
radiogram

radiograph
  bite-wing r.
  cephalometric r.
  extraoral r.
  intraoral r.
  lateral oblique jaw r.
  lateral ramus r.
  lateral skull r.
  maxillary sinus r.
  occlusal r.
  panoramic r.
  periapical r.
  submental vertex r.
  submentovertex r.
  survey r.
  Towne projection r.
  Waters projection r.
  Waters view r.
radiographic
  r. analysis
  r. assessment
  r. density
  r. effect
  r. evaluation
  r. evidence
  r. examination
  r. findings
  r. followup
  r. measurements
  r. projection
  r. results
  r. review
  r. study
radiography
  biomedical r.
  body section r.
  computed digital r. (CDR)
  contrast r.
  digital r.
  digital subtraction r.
  double-contrast r.
  electron r.
  gamma r.
  mass r.
  mass miniature r.
    (MMR)
  mucosal relief r.
  neutron r.
  pan-oral r.
  panoramic r.
  postrelease r.
  postvoid r.
  sectional r.
  selective r.
  serial r.

radiography *(continued)*
 spot film r.
 stereoscopic r.
radiohumeral
 r. bursitis
 r. index
radioimmunity
radioimmunoassay (RIA)
radioimmunodetection
radioimmunodiffusion
radioimmunoelectrophoresis
radioimmunoimaging
radioimmunoprecipitation
radioimmunoscintigraphy
radioimmunosorbent assay (RIA)
radioindicator
radioiodinated
radioiodine
radioiron
radioisotope
 carrier-free r.
 r. image
 r. renal excretion test
 r. scanning
 r. synovectomy
radiokymography
radiolabeled
 r. anti-CD45 antibodies
 r. anti-VEGF antibody
 r. anti-VEGF-A-mAb
 r. DNA probe
 r. drug tracer
 r. fatty acids
 r. ferritin
 r. leukocytes
 r. marker
 r. metaiodobenzylguanidine
  scintigraphy (MIBG)
 r. monoclonal antibodies
 r. oligonucleotide ligation
  assay
 r. platelets
 r. probe
 r. RNA probe
radiolead
radiolesion
radioligand
radiologic, radiological
 class r. characteristics
 r. criteria
 r. diagnosis
 r. evaluation
 r. evidence
 r. features
 r. findings

radiologic, radiological *(continued)*
 r. followup
 r. imaging
 r. procedure
 r. study
radiologist
radiology
 dental r.
 interventional r.
 nuclear r.
 oral r.
radiolucency
 central r.
 circumferential r.
 intracoronal r.
 multilocular r.
 oval r.
 periapical r.
 pericoronal r.
 peri-implant r.
 periprosthetic r.
 round-shaped r.
 triangular-shaped r.
 unilocular r.
radiolucent
 r. areas
 r. lesion
 r. linear structure
 r. lines
 r. metaphyseal bands
 r. osteolytic lesion
 r. stone
 r. zone
radiolus
radiolysis
radiometer
radiometric analysis
radiomicrometer
radiomimetic
radiomuscular
radiomutation
radionecrosis
radionephrography
radioneuritis
radionitrogen
radionuclide
 r. angiocardiography
 r. angiography
 r. cardiography
 r. cholescintigraphy
 r. cisternography
 r. cystography
 r. emission tomography
 metastable r.
 parent r.

R

radionuclide *(continued)*
    r. scanning
    r. venography
    r. ventriculography
    r. voiding cystourethrography
radiopacity
radiopalmar
radiopaque
    r. branched stone
    r. capsule
    r. catheter
    r. clips
    r. eccentric halo
    r. gelified ethanol
    injectable r. polypropylene
      fumarate cement
    r. marker
    r. marker balls
    r. marker BBs
    r. mass
    r. material
    r. mesh
    r. nanoparticles
    r. platinum stent markers
    r. renal stone
    r. staghorn stone
    r. steel balls
    transverse r. lines
    r. urinary tract stones
radiopathology
radiopelvimetry
radiopharmaceutic,
    radiopharmaceutical
radiopharmacology
radiopharmacy
radiophobia
radiophosphorus
radiophotography
radiophylaxis
radiophysics
radioplastic
radiopotassium
radiopotentiation
radiopraxis
radiopulmonography
radioreaction
radioreceptor assay
radiorenography
radioresistance
radioresistant
radioresponsive
radioscope
radioscopy
radiosensitive
radiosensitivity

radiosensitizer
radiosodium
radiospirometry
radiostereoassay
radiostereoscopy
radiostrontium
radiosulfur
radiosurgery
radiotelemetry
radiotellurium
radiothanatology
radiotherapeutics
radiotherapist
radiotherapy
    adjuvant r.
    arc r.
    computerized r.
    conformal r.
    contact r.
    extended field r.
    external beam r.
    fast neutron r.
    hemibody r.
    high-voltage r.
    hyperfractionated r.
    interstitial r.
    intracavitary r.
    intraoperative r.
    inverted Y field r.
    involved field r.
    mantle field r.
    megavoltage r.
    neoadjuvant r.
    orthovoltage r.
    preoperative r.
    supervoltage r.
    whole-body r.
radiothermy
radiothorium
radiothyroxine
radiotomy
radiotoxemia
radiotracer
radiotransparency
radiotransparent
radiotropic
radiotropism
radioulnar
    r. deviation
    r. interosseous ligament
    r. interosseous membrane
    r. joint
    r. synostosis
    r. union
radisectomy

radium F (RaF)
radius (radii)
    Bohr r.
    r. curvus
    r. fixus
    radii of lens, radii lentis
    radii medullares
    van der Waals r.
radix (radices)
    r. anterior ansae cervicalis
    r. anterior nervi spinalis
    r. arcus vertebrae
    r. basalis anterior venae
        basalis communis
    r. clinica
    r. cochlearis nervi
        vestibulocochlearis
    radices craniales nervi
        accessorii
    r. dentis
    r. dorsalis nervi spinalis
    r. facialis
    r. inferior ansae cervicalis
    r. inferior nervi
        vestibulocochlearis
    r. intermedia ganglii
        pterygopalatini
    r. lateralis nervi mediani
    r. lateralis tractus optici
    r. linguae
    r. medialis nervi mediani
    r. medialis tractus optici
    r. mesenterii
    r. motoria nervi spinalis
    r. motoria nervi trigemini
    r. nasalis
    r. nasi
    r. nasociliaris ganglii ciliaris
    r. oculomotoria ganglii ciliaris
    r. parasympathetica ganglii
        ciliaris
    r. parasympathetica ganglii otici
    r. parasympathetica ganglii
        pterygopalatini
    r. parasympathetica ganglii
        sublingualis
    r. parasympathetica ganglii
        submandibularis
    r. parasympathetica
        gangliorum pelvicorum
    r. penis
    r. pili
    radices plexus brachialis
    r. posterior ansae cervicalis
    r. posterior nervi spinalis

radix (radices) *(continued)*
    r. pulmonis
    r. sensoria ganglii ciliaris
    r. sensoria ganglii otici
    r. sensoria ganglii
        pterygopalatini
    r. sensoria ganglii
        submandibularis
    r. sensoria nervi spinalis
    r. sensoria nervi trigemini
    r. spinales nervi accessorii
    r. superior ansae cervicalis
    r. superior nervi
        vestibulocochlearis
    r. sympathetica ganglii
        ciliaris
    r. sympathetica ganglii
        pterygopalatini
    r. unguis
    r. ventralis nervi spinalis
    r. vestibularis nervi
        vestibulocochlearis
radon Rn 219
Radovici
    reflex
    sign
RAE—right atrial enlargement
Raeder syndrome
RAF—rheumatoid arthritis factor
raffinose
rage
    sham r.
ragocyte
RAH—right atrial hypertrophy
RAI—radioactive iodine
raigan
raillietiniasis
Raimist sign
Rainey
    tube
    tubule
RAIU—radioactive iodine uptake
rale
    amphoric r's
    atelectatic r's
    bibasilar r's
    border r's
    bronchial r's
    bubbling r's
    cavernous r's
    cellophane r's
    clicking r's
    collapse r's
    consonating r's
    crackling r's

R

rale *(continued)*
    crepitant r's
    r. de retour
    dry r's
    extrathoracic r's
    gurgling r's
    guttural r's
    r. indux
    inspiratory r's
    laryngeal r's
    marginal r's
    metallic r's
    moist r's
    mucous r's
    r. muqueux
    pleural r's
    r. redux
    sibilant r's
    Skoda r's
    sonorous r's
    subcrepitant r's
    tracheal r's
    Velcro r's
    vesicular r's
    whistling r's
Ralks
    adapter
    clamp
    drill
    elevator
Rally pack
Ramadier operation
ramal
Raman effect
ramex
rami (genitive and plural of ramus)
ramicotomy
ramification
ramiform
ramify
Ramirez shunt
ramisection
ramitis
ramollissement
Ramon flocculation test
Ramond
    point
    sign
ramose
rampart
    maxillary r.
Ramsay Hunt
    disease
    syndrome
Ramsden eyepiece

Ramstedt
    dilator
    operation
    pyloroplasty
ramulus (ramuli)
ramus (rami)
    r. accessorius arteriae
      meningeae mediae
    r. acetabularis arteriae
      circumflexae femoris medialis
    r. acetabularis arteriae
      obturatoriae
    r. acromialis arteriae
      suprascapularis
    r. acromialis arteriae
      thoracoacromialis
    rami alveolares superiores
      posteriores nervi maxillaris
    rami anastomotici
    r. anastomoticus arteriae
      lacrimalis cum arteria
      meningea media
    r. anastomoticus arteriae
      meningeae mediae cum
      arteria lacrimali
    r. anterior arteriae
      obturatoriae
    r. anterior arteriae
      pancreaticoduodenalis
      inferioris
    r. anterior arteriae recurrentis
      ulnaris
    r. anterior arteriae renalis
    r. anterior ductus hepatici dextri
    rami anteriores nervorum
      cervicalium
    rami anteriores nervorum
      lumbalium
    rami anteriores nervorum
      sacralium
    rami anteriores nervorum
      thoracicorum
    r. anterior nervi auricularis
      magni
    r. anterior nervi coccygei
    r. anterior nervi cutanei
      antebrachii medialis
    r. anterior nervi obturatorii
    r. anterior nervi spinalis
    r. anterior sulci lateralis cerebri
    anterior rami of thoracic nerves
    r. anterior venae pulmonalis
      dextrae superioris
    r. anterior venae pulmonalis
      sinistrae superioris

ramus (rami) *(continued)*

r. apicalis venae pulmonalis dextrae superioris

r. apicoposterior venae pulmonalis sinistrae superioris

r. articularis

rami articulares arteriae descendentis genicularis

r. ascendens arteriae circumflexae femoris lateralis

r. ascendens arteriae circumflexae femoris medialis

r. ascendens arteriae circumflexae ilium profundae

r. ascendens arteriae segmentalis anterioris pulmonis dextri

r. ascendens arteriae segmentalis anterioris pulmonis sinistri

r. ascendens arteriae segmentalis posterioris pulmonis dextri

r. ascendens arteriae segmentalis posterioris pulmonis sinistri

r. ascendens rami superficialis arteriae transversae colli

r. ascendens sulci lateralis cerebri

rami atriales arteriae coronariae dextrae

r. atrialis anastomoticus rami circumflexi arteriae coronariae sinistrae

r. atrialis intermedius arteriae coronariae dextrae

rami auriculares anteriores arteriae temporalis superficialis

r. auricularis arteriae auricularis posterioris

r. auricularis arteriae occipitalis

r. auricularis nervi vagi

r. basalis tentorii arteriae carotidis internae

rami bronchiales arteriae thoracicae internae

rami bronchiales nervi vagi

ramus (rami) *(continued)*

rami buccales nervi facialis

rami calcanei laterales nervi suralis

rami calcanei mediales nervi tibialis

rami calcanei ramorum malleolarium lateralium arteriae fibularis

r. calcarinus arteriae occipitalis medialis

rami capsulares arteriae renis

rami cardiaci cervicales inferiores nervi vagi

rami cardiaci cervicales superiores nervi vagi

rami cardiaci thoracici nervi vagi

r. carpalis dorsalis arteriae radialis

r. carpalis dorsalis arteriae ulnaris

r. carpalis palmaris arteriae radialis

r. carpalis palmaris arteriae ulnaris

rami celiaci nervi vagi

r. chiasmaticus arteriae communicantis posterioris

rami choroidei posteriores laterales arteriae cerebri posterioris

rami choroidei ventriculi tertii arteriae choroideae anterioris

r. cingularis arteriae callosomarginalis

r. circumflexus arteriae coronariae sinistrae

r. circumflexus fibularis arteriae tibialis posterioris

r. clavicularis arteriae thoracoacromialis

rami clivales partes cerebralis arteriae carotidis internae

rami coeliaci nervi vagi

r. colicus arteriae ileocolicae

r. colli nervi facialis

r. communicans arteriae fibularis

r. communicans arteriae peroneae

r. communicans cochlearis nervi vestibularis

R

ramus (rami) *(continued)*

r. communicans fibularis nervi
fibularis communis

r. communicans nervi facialis
cum nervo glossopharyngeo

r. communicans nervi
glossopharyngei cum ramo
auriculari nervi vagi

r. communicans nervi
intermedii cum nervo vago

r. communicans nervi
intermedii cum plexu
tympanico

r. communicans nervi lacrimalis
cum nervo zygomatico

r. communicans nervi mediani
cum nervo ulnari

r. communicans nervi
nasociliaris cum ganglio
ciliari

r. communicans nervi vagi
cum nervo glossopharyngeo

r. communicans peroneus
nervi peronei communis

r. communicans ulnaris nervi
radialis

rami communicantes

rami communicantes nervi
auriculotemporalis cum
nervo faciali

rami communicantes nervi
lingualis cum nervo
hypoglosso

rami communicantes
nervorum spinalium

r. coni arteriosi arteriae
coronariae dextrae

rami corporis amygdaloidei
arteriae choroideae
anterioris

r. corporis callosi dorsalis
arteriae occipitalis medialis

rami corporis geniculati
lateralis arteriae choroideae
anterioris

r. costalis lateralis arteriae
thoracicae internae

r. cricothyroideus arteriae
thyroideae superioris

r. cutaneus

r. cutaneus anterior nervi
iliohypogastrici

r. cutaneus lateralis nervi
iliohypogastrici

r. cutaneus nervi obturatorii

ramus (rami) *(continued)*

r. deltoideus arteriae
profundae brachii

r. deltoideus arteriae
thoracoacromialis

rami dentales arteriae
alveolaris inferioris

rami dentales arteriarum
alveolarium superiorum
anteriorum

rami dentales inferiores
plexus dentalis inferioris

rami dentales superiores
plexus dentalis superioris

r. descendens arteriae
circumflexae femoris
lateralis

r. descendens arteriae
occipitalis

r. dexter arteriae hepaticae
propriae

r. dexter venae portae hepatis

r. digastricus nervi facialis

r. dorsalis arteriae subcostalis

r. dorsalis nervi coccygei

rami duodenales arteriae
pancreaticoduodenalis
superioris anterioris

rami epididymales arteriae
testicularis

r. externus nervi accessorii

r. externus nervi laryngei
superioris

r. femoralis nervi
genitofemoralis

r. frontalis anteromedialis
arteriae callosomarginalis

r. frontalis arteriae meningeae
mediae

r. frontalis arteriae temporalis
superficialis

r. frontalis posteromedialis
arteriae callosomarginalis

rami ganglionares
trigeminales arteriae
carotidis internae

rami gastrici arteriae
gastroomentalis dextrae

r. genitalis nervi
genitofemoralis

rami genus capsulae internae
arteriae choroideae
anterioris

rami gingivales inferiores
plexus dentalis inferioris

ramus (rami) *(continued)*

    rami gingivales superiores
      plexus dentalis superioris

    rami glandulares arteriae
      facialis

    rami glandulares arteriae
      maxillaris externae

    rami glandulares arteriae
      thyreoideae inferioris

    r. glandularis anterior arteriae
      thyreoideae superioris

    r. glandularis lateralis arteriae
      thyreoideae superioris

    r. glandularis posterior arteriae
      thyreoideae superioris

    rami globi pallidi arteriae
      choroideae anterioris

    rami helicini arteriae uterinae

    r. hypothalamicus arteriae
      communicantis posterioris

    r. ilealis arteriae ileocolicae

    r. iliacus arteriae iliolumbalis

    r. inferior nervi oculomotorii

    r. inferior ossis ischii

    r. infrahyoideus arteriae
      thyroideae superioris

    r. infrapatellaris nervi sapheni

    rami interganglionares trunci
      sympathici

    r. internus nervi accessorii

    r. internus nervi laryngei
      superioris

    ischiopubic r.

    r. of ischium

    rami isthmi faucium nervi
      lingualis

    r. of jaw

    rami labiales posteriores
      arteriae pudendae internae

    rami labiales superiores nervi
      infraorbitalis

    rami laryngopharyngei ganglii
      cervicalis superioris

    r. lateralis ductus hepatici
      sinistri

    r. lateralis interventricularis
      anterioris arteriae
      coronariae sinistrae

    r. lateralis nasi arteriae
      facialis

    r. lateralis nervi supraorbitalis

    rami lienales arteriae lienalis

    rami linguales nervi
      glossopharyngei

    rami linguales nervi hypoglossi

ramus (rami) *(continued)*

    rami linguales nervi lingualis

    r. lumbalis arteriae
      iliolumbalis

    rami malleolares laterales
      arteriae fibularis

    rami malleolares mediales
      arteriae tibiales posterioris

    rami mammarii laterales
      arteriae thoracicae lateralis

    r. mandibulae

    r. marginalis dexter arteriae
      coronariae dextrae

    r. marginalis mandibulae
      nervi facialis

    r. marginalis sinister rami
      circumflexi arteriae
      coronariae sinistrae

    r. marginalis tentorii arteriae
      carotidis internae

    rami mastoidei arteriae
      auricularis posterioris

    r. mastoideus arteriae
      occipitalis

    r. medialis ductus hepatici
      sinistri

    r. medialis nervi supraorbitalis

    rami mediastinales arteriae
      thoracicae internae

    r. membranae tympani nervi
      auriculotemporalis

    r. meningeus anterior arteriae
      ethmoidalis anterioris

    r. meningeus arteriae occipitalis

    r. meningeus nervi
      mandibularis

    r. meningeus nervi vagi

    rami mentales nervi mentalis

    rami musculares arteriae
      vertebralis

    rami musculares nervi
      axillaris

    rami musculares nervi
      femoralis

    rami musculares nervi
      fibularis profundi

    rami musculares nervi
      fibularis superficialis

    rami musculares nervi mediani

    rami musculares nervi
      musculocutanei

    rami musculares nervi peronei
      profundi

    rami musculares nervi peronei
      superficialis

R

ramus (rami) *(continued)*

rami musculares nervi radialis
rami musculares nervi tibialis
rami musculares nervi ulnaris
r. musculi stylopharyngei
    nervi glossopharyngei
r. mylohyoideus arteriae
    alveolaris inferioris
rami nasales externi nervi
    infraorbitalis
rami nasales interni nervi
    ethmoidalis anterioris
rami nasales interni nervi
    infraorbitalis
r. nervi oculomotorii arteriae
    communicantis posterioris
r. nodi atrioventricularis
    arteriae coronariae dextrae
r. nodi sinuatrialis arteriae
    coronariae dextrae
rami nuclei rubri arteriae
    choroideae anterioris
rami nucleorum hypothalami
    arteriae choroideae
    anterioris
rami occipitales arteriae
    occipitalis
r. occipitalis nervi auricularis
    posterioris
r. occipitotemporalis arteriae
    occipitalis medialis
rami oesophagei arteriae
    gastricae sinistrae
rami oesophagei arteriae
    thyroideae inferioris
rami omentales arteriae
    gastroomentalis dextrae
r. orbitalis arteriae meningeae
    mediae
r. ossis pubis
r. ovaricus arteriae uterinae
r. palmaris nervi mediani
r. palmaris nervi ulnaris
r. palmaris profundus arteriae
    ulnaris
r. palmaris superficialis
    arteriae radialis
rami palpebrales inferiores
    nervi infraorbitalis
rami palpebrales nervi
    infratrochlearis
rami pancreatici arteriae
    lienalis
rami pancreatici arteriae
    pancreaticoduodenalis
    superioris anterioris

ramus (rami) *(continued)*

rami pancreatici arteriae
    splenicae
r. parietalis arteriae
    meningeae mediae
r. parietalis arteriae occipitalis
    medialis
r. parietalis arteriae
    temporalis superficialis
r. parietooccipitalis arteriae
    occipitalis medialis
rami parotidei nervi
    auriculotemporalis
rami parotidei venae facialis
r. parotideus arteriae
    auricularis posterioris
r. parotideus arteriae
    temporalis superficialis
rami pectorales arteriae
    thoracoacromialis
rami pedunculares arteriae
    cerebri posterioris
r. perforans arteriae fibularis
rami perforantes arteriae
    thoracicae internae
rami perforantes arteriarum
    metatarsearum plantarium
r. pericardiacus nervi
    phrenici
rami peridentales arteriae
    alveolaris inferioris
rami perineales nervi cutanei
    femoris posterioris
r. petrosus arteriae meningeae
    mediae
r. petrosus superficialis
    arteriae meningeae mediae
rami pharyngei nervi
    glossopharyngei
rami pharyngei nervi vagi
r. pharyngeus arteriae canalis
    pterygoidei
rami phrenicoabdominales
    nervi phrenici
r. posterior arteriae
    obturatoriae
r. posterior arteriae
    pancreaticoduodenalis
    inferioris
r. posterior arteriae
    recurrentis ulnaris
r. posterior arteriae renalis
r. posterior ductus hepatici
    dextri
rami posteriores nervorum
    cervicalium

ramus (rami) *(continued)*

  rami posteriores nervorum lumbalium

  rami posteriores nervorum sacralium

  rami posteriores nervorum thoracalium

  r. posterior nervi coccygei

  r. posterior nervi cutanei antebrachii medialis

  r. posterior nervi obturatorii

  r. posterior sulci lateralis cerebri

  r. posterolateralis dexter arteriae coronariae dextrae

  r. profundus arteriae circumflexae femoris medialis

  r. profundus arteriae gluteae superioris

  r. profundus arteriae plantaris medialis

  r. profundus arteriae transversae colli

  r. profundus nervi plantaris lateralis

  r. profundus nervi radialis

  r. profundus nervi ulnaris

  rami prostatici arteriae vesicalis inferioris

  rami pterygoidei arteriae maxillaris

  r. pubicus arteriae epigastricae inferioris

  r. pubicus arteriae obturatoriae

  r. of pubis

  r. of pubis, ascending

  r. of pubis, descending

  rami radiculares arteriae vertebralis

  rami renales nervi vagi

  rami renales plexus coeliaci

  r. renalis nervi splanchnici minoris

  rami sacrales laterales arteriae sacralis medianae

  r. saphenus arteriae descendentis genus

  r. saphenus arteriae genus descendentis

  rami scrotales posteriores arteriae pudendae internae

  rami septales anteriores arteriae ethmoidalis anterioris

ramus (rami) *(continued)*

  rami septales posteriores arteriae sphenopalatinae

  r. septi nasi arteriae labialis superioris

  r. sinister arteriae hepaticae propriae

  r. sinister venae portae hepatis

  r. sinus carotici nervi glossopharyngei

  r. spinalis arteriae intercostalis posterioris primae

  r. spinalis arteriae intercostalis posterioris secundae

  r. spinalis arteriae iliolumbalis

  r. spinalis arteriae sacralis lateralis

  r. spinalis arteriae subcostalis

  rami spinalis arteriae vertebralis

  rami spinales rami dorsalis arteriae intercostalis posterioris

  r. spinalis venae intercostalis posterioris

  r. spinalis venarum intercostalium posteriorum (IV–XI)

  rami splenici

  rami splenici arteriae splenicae

  r. stapedius arteriae auricularis posterioris

  rami sternales arteriae thoracicae internae

  rami sternocleidomastoidei arteriae occipitalis

  r. sternocleidomastoideus arteriae thyroideae superioris

  r. stylohyoideus nervi facialis

  rami subendocardiales

  rami subscapulares arteriae axillaris

  rami substantiae nigrae arteriae choroideae anterioris

  rami substantiae perforatae anterioris arteriae choroideae anterioris

  r. superficialis arteriae circumflexae femoris medialis

  r. superficialis arteriae gluteae superioris

  r. superficialis arteriae plantaris medialis

R

ramus (rami) *(continued)*

    r. superficialis arteriae transversae colli

    r. superficialis nervi plantaris lateralis

    r. superficialis nervi radialis

    r. superficialis nervi ulnaris

    rami superiores nervi transversi colli

    r. superior nervi oculomotorii

    r. superior ossis pubis

    r. superior rami profundi arteriae gluteae superioris

    r. superior venae pulmonalis dextrae inferioris

    r. superior venae pulmonalis sinistrae inferioris

    r. suprahyoideus arteriae lingualis

    r. temporalis anterior arteriae cerebri mediae

    rami temporales anteriores arteriae occipitalis lateralis

    rami temporales intermedii arteriae occipitalis lateralis

    rami temporales medii arteriae occipitalis lateralis

    rami temporales nervi facialis

    r. temporales posteriores arteriae occipitalis lateralis

    rami temporales superficiales nervi auriculotemporalis

    r. temporalis medius arteriae cerebri mediae

    r. temporalis posterior arteriae cerebri mediae

    r. temporooccipitalis arteriae cerebri mediae

    r. tentorii nervi ophthalmici

    rami terminales inferiores arteriae cerebri mediae

    rami terminales superiores arteriae cerebri mediae

    rami thymici arteriae thoracicae internae

    r. thyrohyoideus ansae cervicalis

    r. tonsillae cerebelli arteriae inferioris posterioris cerebelli

    r. tonsillares arteriae facialis

    rami tonsillares nervi glossopharyngei

    rami tonsillares nervorum palatinorum minorum

ramus (rami) *(continued)*

    r. tonsillaris arteriae maxillaris externi

    rami tracheales arteriae thoracicae internae

    rami tracheales arteriae thyroideae inferioris

    rami tracheales nervi laryngei recurrentis

    rami tractus optici arteriae choroideae anterioris

    r. transversus arteriae circumflexae femoris lateralis

    r. transversus arteriae circumflexae femoris medialis

    r. tubalis plexus tympanici

    rami tubarii arteriae ovaricae

    r. tubarius arteriae uterinae

    r. tubarius plexus tympanici

    rami tuberis cinerei arteriae choroideae anterioris

    rami ureterici arteriae ductus deferentis

    rami ureterici arteriae ovaricae

    rami ureterici arteriae renalis

    rami ureterici arteriae testicularis

    rami vaginales arteriae rectalis mediae

    rami vaginales arteriae uterinae

    rami ventrales nervorum cervicalium

    rami ventrales nervorum lumbalium

    rami ventrales nervorum sacralium

    rami ventrales nervorum thoracicorum

    r. ventralis nervi coccygei

    r. ventralis nervi spinalis

    ventral rami of thoracic nerves

    r. vermis superior arteriae superioris cerebelli

    rami vestibulares

    rami vestibulares arteriae auditivae internae

    rami vestibulares arteriae labyrinthi

    r. vestibularis posterior arteriae vestibulocochlearis

    r. viscerales

ramus (rami) *(continued)*
    rami zygomatici nervi facialis
    r. zygomaticofacialis nervi
      zygomatici
    r. zygomaticotemporalis nervi
      zygomatici
Ranawat sign
rancid
rancidify
rancidity
Randall
    curet
    operation
    plaques
    sign
    stone forceps
Randolph cannula
random
randomization
randomize
Raney
    clip
    curet
    drill
    forceps
Raney-Crutchfield tongs
range
    r. of accommodation
    r. of audibility
    audiofrequency r.
    r. of convergence
    dynamic r.
    r. of hearing
    interquartile r.
    r. of motion
    normal r.
    partial r.
    reference r.
    r. of sensibility
    thermal comfort r.
rank
Ranke
    angle
    complex
    formula
    stages
Rankin
    clamp
    forceps
    retractor
Ransohoff
    operation
    sign
Ranson criteria for severity of
  acute pancreatitis

ranula
    pancreatic r.
ranular
Ranvier
    crosses
    nodes
    segment (internode)
    tactile disk
Ranzewski clamp
RAO—right anterior oblique
  (projection)
RAP—
    rheumatoid arthritis
      precipitin
    right atrial pressure
rape
    date r.
    statutory r.
raphania
raphe (raphae)
    abdominal r.
    amniotic r.
    r. anococcygea
    anococcygeal r.
    anogenital r.
    buccal r.
    r. corporis callosi
    lateral palpebral r.
    median r. of medulla oblongata
    r. mediana medullae
      oblongatae
    r. mediana pontina
    median r. of neck, posterior
    median r. of perineum
    median r. of pons
    r. medullae oblongatae
    r. of medulla oblongata
    r. mesencephali
    midpalatine r.
    r. palati
    palatine r.
    palpebral r.
    r. palpebralis lateralis
    r. penis
    perineal r.
    r. perinealis
    r. perinei
    r. of perineum
    pharyngeal r.
    r. pharyngis
    r. of pharynx
    r. of pons
    r. pontis
    pterygomandibular r.
    r. pterygomandibularis

R

raphe (raphae) *(continued)*
  scrotal r.
  r. scrotalis
  r. scroti
  r. of scrotum
raphes (genitive of raphe)
rapid biplane angiocardiography
Rappaport classification
rapport
rarefaction
  bone r.
RAS—
  renal artery stenosis
  renin-angiotensin system
  reticular activating system
Rasch sign
rash
  ammonia r.
  antitoxin r.
  astacoid r.
  brown-tail r.
  butterfly r.
  canker r.
  caterpillar r.
  diaper r.
  drug r.
  enema r.
  heat r.
  heliotrope r.
  hydatid r.
  lobster r.
  medicinal r.
  mulberry r.
  napkin r., nappy r.
  nettle r.
  rose r.
  scarlet r.
  serum r.
  summer r.
  sun r.
  vaccination r.
  wandering r.
Rashkind
  operation
  procedure
rasion
Rasmussen aneurysm
rasp
  Aufricht r.
  Aufricht-Lipsett r.
  Beck r.
  Berne r.
  Cottle r.
  Fomon r.
  Good r.

rasp *(continued)*
  Lewis r.
  Maltz r.
  Maltz-Lipsett r.
  Putti r.
  Wiener-Pierce r.
raspatory
RAST—radioallergosorbent test
Rastelli operation
rate
  abortion r.
  absorption r.
  adjusted r.
  adjusted death r.
  admission r.
  age-specific r.
  age-specific birth r.
  age-specific death r.
  age-specific fertility r.
  age-specific marital fertility r.
  age-specific mortality r.
  attack r.
  background counting r.
  basal metabolic r.
  base r.
  beam uniformity r.
  birth r.
  Boeckh r.
  Boeckh-Kuczynski r.
  carrier r.
  case r.
  case fatality r.
  cause-specific death r.
  circulation r.
  conduction r.
  corrected survival r.
  counting r.
  crude r.
  crude annual general death r.
  crude annual live birth r.
  crude survival r.
  cumulative incidence r.
  death r.
  DEF r.
  discharge r.
  DMF r.
  dose r.
  early neonatal death r.
  effective fertility r.
  equivalent average death r.
  erythrocyte sedimentation r.
    (ESR)
  evolutionary r.
  false-negative r.
  false-positive r.

rate *(continued)*
  fatality r.
  female reproduction r.
  fertility r.
  fetal death r.
  five-year survival r.
  flow r.
  frame r.
  general r.
  general fertility r.
  glomerular filtration r. (GFR)
  gross female reproduction r.
  growth r.
  heart r.
  incidence r.
  infant mortality r.
  instantaneous r.
  instantaneous growth r.
  intrinsic r. of natural increase
  Kuczynski r.
  lethality r.
  marital fertility r.
  marriage r.
  maternal mortality r.
  maximal midexpiratory flow r.
  maximum midexpiratory flow r.
  mendelian r.
  monthly fecundity r.
  morbidity r.
  mortality r.
  mutation r.
  natality r.
  r. of natural increase
  neonatal mortality r.
  net female reproductive r.
  nupitality r.
  oocyst r.
  output exposure r.
  parasite r.
  parity-specific birth r.
  peak expiratory flow r. (PEFR)
  peak inspiratory flow r.
  perinatal mortality r.
  plasma refilling r.
  population growth r.
  postneonatal death r.
  prevalence r.
  protein catabolic r.
  puerperal mortality r.
  pulse r.
  real-time r.
  relative survival r.
  replacement r.
  reproduction r.
  respiration r.

rate *(continued)*
  response r.
  secondary attack r.
  sedimentation r.
  sex-specific death r.
  sickness r.
  single nephron glomerular
      filtration r.
  slew r.
  specific r.
  specific birth r.
  specific death r.
  sporozoite r.
  standardized r.
  standardized death r.
  steroid metabolic clearance r.
  steroid production r.
  steroid secretory r.
  stillbirth r.
  survival r.
  total fertility r.
  true r. of natural increase
  Westergren sedimentation r.
rate meter
Rathke
  column
  cyst
  pocket
  pouch
  trabecula
  tumor
raticide
rating
  Apgar r.
  behavior r.
ratio
  absolute terminal innervation r.
  accommodative convergence-
      accommodation (AC/A) r.
  age dependency r.
  albumin/creatinine r.
  albumin-globulin (A/G) r.
  ALT/AST r.
  arm r.
  assimilation efficiency r.
  base r.
  base pair r.
  beam uniformity r.
  benefit-risk r.
  birth-death r.
  Blackburne-Peel r.
  body-weight r.
  cardiothoracic r.
  case fatality r.
  cell color r.

R

ratio *(continued)*

    channels r.
    child-woman r.
    clinical crown–clinical root r.
    concentration r.
    conduction r.
    conversion r.
    critical r.
    cross-products r.
    cup-to-disk r.
    curative r.
    death-to-case r.
    dependency r.
    dextrose-nitrogen (D/N) r.
    economic dependency r.
    expiratory exchange r.
    extraction r.
    F r.
    fatality r.
    fetal death r.
    fluorescein-protein (F/P) r.
    functional terminal
      innervation r.
    galvanic tetanus r.
    general fertility r.
    glucose-nitrogen (G/N) r.
    grid r.
    gyromagnetic r.
    hand r.
    helper-suppressor cell r.
    holdaway r.
    human blood r.
    [131]I conversion r. [131-I]
    innervation r.
    Insall-Salvati r.
    inspiratory-expiratory (I/E)
      phase time r.
    isophane r.
    karyoplasmic r.
    ketogenic-antiketogenic (K/A) r.
    lecithin-sphingomyelin (L/S) r.
    likelihood r.
    male/female r.
    masculinity r.
    mendelian r.
    middle-ear areal r.
    myeloid-erythroid (M/E) r.
    nuclear magnetogyric r.
    nucleocytoplasmic r.
    nucleoplasmic r.
    nutritive r.
    ocular micrometer r.
    odds r.
    ossicular lever r.
    parity progression r.

ratio *(continued)*

    peak-to-total r.
    polymorphonuclear-
      lymphocyte r.
    potency r.
    primary sex r.
    proportionate mortality r.
      (PMR)
    protein/creatinine r.
    protein efficiency r.
    protein-osmolar (P/O) r.
    radioactive iodide
      conversion r.
    relative risk r.
    respiratory exchange r.
    risk r.
    risk-benefit r.
    R/S r.
    saliva-to-plasma radioiodine r.
    sampling r.
    secondary sex r.
    sex r.
    signal-to-noise r.
    standardized morbidity r.
      (SMR)
    standardized mortality r.
      (SMR)
    stimulation r. (SR)
    target-to-nontarget r.
    therapeutic r.
    total cholesterol to HDL r.
    urea excretion r.
    urea reduction r.
    variance r.
    ventilation-perfusion (V/Q) r.
    zeta sedimentation r. (ZSR)

ration

    basal r.

rational

rationale

rationalization

Ratliff-Blake forceps

rat-tails

rattle

    death r.

rattlesnake

Rau (Ravius)

    apophysis

    process

Rauchfuss

    sling

    triangle

Rauscher leukemia virus

RAV—Rous-associated virus

Ravich cystoscope

ray

  α r's [alpha]
  actinic r.
  anode r's
  antirachitic r's
  astral r.
  β r's [beta]
  Bucky r's
  caloric r.
  canal r's
  cathode r's
  central r.
  characteristic r's
  characteristic fluorescent r's
  chemical r.
  convergent r.
  cortical r.
  cosmic r's
  δ-r's [delta]
  digital r.
  direct r.
  divergent r's
  Dorno r's
  dynamic r's
  erythema-producing r's
  Finsen r's
  fluorescent r's
  γ r's [gamma]
  glass r's
  Goldstein r's
  grenz r's
  hard r's
  heat r's
  incident r.
  indirect r's
  infrared r's
  infra roentgen r's
  intermediate r's
  Lenard r's
  luminous r's
  Lyman r's
  medullary r.
  parallel r's
  pigment-producing r's
  polar r.
  positive r's
  primary r's
  reflected r.
  refracted r.
  roentgen r's
  s r's
  Sagnac r's
  scattered r's
  Schumann r's
  secondary r.

ray *(continued)*

  soft r's
  ultraviolet r's
  ultra x-r.
  vertical r.
  vital r's
  W r's
  x-r's

Ray

  forceps
  mania
  speculum

Rayer disease
Rayleigh scattering law
Raymond apoplexy
Raymond-Cestan syndrome
Raynaud

  disease
  gangrene
  phenomenon
  syndrome

Ray-Parsons-Sunday elevator
Ray-Tec dressing
razor

  Occam r.

Rb—rubidium
RB—rating board
RBB—right bundle branch
RBBB—right bundle branch block
RBC—

  red blood cell(s)
  red blood cell count

RBC IT—red blood cell iron turnover
RBCV—red blood cell volume
RBF—renal blood flow
RBP—

  resting blood pressure
  retinol binding protein

RC—retrograde cystogram
RCA—

  radionuclide cerebral
    angiogram
  red cell aplasia
  regulator of complement
    activation
  right coronary artery

RCBV—regional cerebral blood
  volume
RCD—relative cardiac dullness
RCF—relative centrifugal force
RCM—right costal margin
RCR—respiratory control ratio
RCU—

  red cell utilization
  respiratory care unit

R

RCV—red cell volume
rd—rutherford
RD—
    retinal detachment
    right deltoid
RDA—
    recommended dietary
      allowance
    right dorsoanterior (position)
RDE—receptor-destroying enzyme
RDI—rupture-delivery interval
RDP—right dorsoposterior (position)
RDS—respiratory distress syndrome
RDW—red blood cell distribution
  width index
RE—
    regional enteritis
    reticuloendothelial
    retinol equivalent
    right eye
R&E—research and education
reablement
reabsorb
reabsorption
    facultative water r.
    intestinal r.
    obligatory water r.
    tubular r.
react
reactance
reactant
    acute phase r.
reaction
    accelerated r.
    acetic acid r.
    acid r.
    acrosome r.
    acute phase r.
    acute situational r.
    acute stress r.
    adjustment r.
    agglutination r.
    alarm r. (AR)
    alkaline r.
    allergic r.
    allograft r.
    alphanaphthol r.
    anamnestic r.
    anaphylactic r.
    anaphylactoid r.
    anaplerotic r.
    anergastic r.
    annihilation r.
    anniversary r.
    anthrone r.

reaction *(continued)*
    antibody-mediated cytotoxic
      hypersensitivity r.
    antibody-mediated
      hypersensitivity r.
    antigen-antibody r.
    antiglobulin r.
    anxiety r.
    argentaffin r.
    Arias-Stella r.
    arousal r.
    Arthus r.
    Arthus-type r.
    Ascoli r.
    associative r.
    autoimmune complement
      fixation r.
    axon r., axonal r.
    Bachman r.
    Bareggi r.
    Bekhterev (Bechterew) r.
    Bence Jones r.
    Berthelot r.
    bi-bi r.
    biomolecular r.
    biphasic r.
    Bittorf r.
    biuret r.
    Bloch r.
    blocking r.
    bombardment r.
    Bordet-Gengou r.
    Brieger cachexia r.
    browning r's
    Burchard-Liebermann r.
    cadaveric r.
    Calmette r.
    Cannizzaro r.
    capsular r.
    capsule swelling r.
    capture r.
    carbamino r.
    cascade r.
    Casoni r.
    cell-mediated
      hypersensitivity r.
    chain r.
    Chopra antimony r.
    chromaffin r.
    cockade r.
    colloidal gold r.
    complement fixation r.
    congenital leukemoid r.
    conglutination r.
    consensual r.

reaction *(continued)*
- consensual light r.
- conversion r.
- Coombs and Gell r.
- crisis r.
- cross r.
- Cushing r.
- cutaneous r.
- cytotoxic r.
- cytotoxic hypersensitivity r.
- Dale r.
- decidual r.
- defense r.
- r. of degeneration
- delayed hypersensitivity r.
- delayed-type hypersensitivity r.
- depot r.
- depressive r.
- dermatophytid r.
- dermotuberculin r.
- desmoplastic r.
- diazo r.
- Dick r.
- digitonin r.
- displacement r.
- dissociative r.
- dopa r.
- downgrading r.
- duplicative r.
- dysergastic r.
- Ebbecke r.
- eczematoid r.
- egg yellow r.
- Ehrlich aldehyde r.
- Ehrlich diazo r.
- electric r.
- eosinopenic r.
- equilibrium r.
- Erb r.
- erythrocyte sedimentation r.
- r. of exhaustion
- Fahraeus r.
- false-negative r.
- false-positive r.
- Felix-Weil r.
- Fernandez r.
- Feulgen r.
- fight-or-flight r.
- first-order r.
- flocculation r.
- focal r.
- foreign body r.
- r. formation
- Forssman antigen-antibody r.
- fuchsinophil r.

reaction *(continued)*
- Gangi r.
- gemistocytic r.
- Ghilarducci r.
- glycine-arginine r.
- Gmelin r.
- Goetsch skin r.
- gold r.
- graft-versus-host r. (GVHR)
- Grignard r.
- gross stress r.
- group r.
- Gruber r.
- Gruber-Widal r.
- Gubler r.
- Gunning r.
- hemagglutination-inhibition r.
- hemianopic pupillary r.
- hemoclastic r.
- Henle r.
- Herxheimer r.
- heteroclytic r.
- heterophil antibody r.
- Hill r.
- homograft r.
- hunting r.
- hyperkinetic r. of childhood
- hypersensitivity r.
- id r.
- r. of identity
- immediate hypersensitivity r.
- immune r.
- immune complex–mediated hypersensitivity r.
- immunity r.
- indirect light r.
- indirect pupillary r.
- indophenol r.
- infusion r.
- intracutaneous r.
- intradermal r.
- involutional psychotic r.
- isomorphous provocative r.
- Ito-Reenstierna r.
- Jaffé r.
- Jarisch-Herxheimer r.
- johnin r.
- Jolly r.
- Jones-Mote r.
- Keller-Killian r.
- Knaus r.
- Koch r.
- Kveim r.
- Lange r.
- late r.

R

reaction *(continued)*
 late phase r.
 lengthening r.
 lepra r.
 lepromin r.
 leukemic r., leukemoid r.
 Lewis r.
 Lieben r.
 Liebermann-Burchard r.
 ligase chain r.
 local r.
 local anesthetic r.
 Loeb decidual r.
 Loewi r.
 Lohmann r.
 lymphocyte transfer r.
 Machado-Guerreiro r.
 macrophage disappearance r.
 manic-depressive r.
 Mantoux r.
 Marañón r.
 Marchi r.
 Mátéfy r.
 Mazzotti r.
 Millon r.
 Mitsuda r.
 mixed agglutination r.
 mixed antiglobulin r.
 mixed leukocyte r.
 mixed lymphocyte r.
 Moeller r.
 Molisch r.
 Moloney r.
 Montenegro r.
 Morelli r.
 Moritz r.
 mouse tail r.
 myasthenic r.
 myotonic r.
 myotonic pupillary r.
 myotonoid r.
 Nadi r.
 Nagler r.
 near-point r.
 negative supporting r.
 negative therapeutic r.
 Neill-Mooser r.
 Neisser r.
 Neufeld r.
 neurotonic r.
 neutral r.
 Nile blue r.
 ninhydrin r.
 r. of nonidentity
 Nonne-Apelt r.
 normal lymphocytic transfer r.

reaction *(continued)*
 nuclear r.
 obsessive-compulsive r.
 Oestreicher r.
 ophthalmic r.
 orbicularis r.
 oxidase r.
 oxidation-reduction r.
 pain r.
 paradoxical pupillary r.
 parallergic r.
 Parish r.
 r. of partial identity
 PAS r.
 passive Arthus r.
 passive cutaneous
  anaphylaxis r.
 passive cutaneous Arthus r.
 Pasteur r.
 Paul-Bunnell r.
 periodic acid–Schiff (PAS) r.
 peroxidase r.
 Petri r.
 Petzetaki r.
 Pfeiffer r.
 phobic r.
 photochemical r.
 Pinkerton-Mooser r.
 Pirquet r.
 pneumococcus capsule
  swelling r.
 polymerase chain r.
 Porges-Pollatschek r.
 Porter-Silber r.
 positive supporting r.
 Posner r.
 Prausnitz-Küstner (P-K) r.
 precipitin r.
 primary r. of Nissl
 prozone r.
 pseudoallergic r.
 pseudomyotonic r.
 psychosomatic r.
 psychotic depressive r.
 puncture r.
 quantitative precipitin r.
 quellung r.
 rage r.
 redox r.
 retrobulbar pupil r.
 reversal r.
 reverse passive Arthus r.
 reversible r.
 righting r's
 Rivalta r.
 Roger r.

reaction *(continued)*
- Rubino r.
- Russo r.
- Sanarelli-Shwartzman r.
- sarcoid tissue r.
- Schardinger r.
- Schick r.
- Schultz-Charlton r.
- Schultz-Dale r.
- scrotal r.
- second-order r.
- second-set r.
- sedimentation r.
- Selivanoff (Seliwanow) r.
- serological r.
- serum r.
- serum sickness–like r.
- Sgambati r.
- shortening r.
- Shwartzman r., generalized
- Shwartzman r., localized
- sigma r.
- skin r.
- soluble immune complex r.
- spring r.
- startle r.
- statokinetic r.
- stemming r.
- Straus r.
- stress r.
- substitution r.
- supporting r's
- sympathetic stress r.
- Szent-Györgyi r.
- Tanret r.
- T cell–mediated hypersensitivity r.
- tendon r.
- thermonuclear r.
- thread r.
- thyroid function r.
- tilt r.
- toxin-antitoxin r.
- Trambusti r.
- transfusion r.
- trigger r.
- tuberculin r.
- tuberculin-type r.
- Turnbull blue r.
- upgrading r.
- vaccinoid r.
- vestibular pupillary r.
- vital r.
- Voges-Proskauer r.
- von Pirquet r.
- Waaler-Rose r.

reaction *(continued)*
- Wassermann r.
- Watson-Schwartz r.
- Weil-Felix r.
- Wernicke hemianopic r.
- wheal and erythema r.
- wheal and flare r.
- white-graft r.
- Widal r.
- Wolff-Calmette r.
- Wolff-Eisner r.
- xanthoproteic r.
- xanthydrol r.
- zed r.
- zero-order r.
- Zimmermann r.

reaction-formation

reactivate

reactivation of serum

reactivator
- cholinesterase r.

reactive

reactivity
- vascular r.

reactor
- nuclear r.
- universal r.

readiness
- explosion r.
- reading r.

reading
- lip r.
- speech r.
- wet r.

readthrough

reagent
- amino-acid r.
- arsenic–sulfuric acid r.
- Benedict r.
- benzidine r.
- Berthelot r.
- Bial r.
- biuret r.
- Black r.
- Bogg r.
- Bohme r.
- Bonchardat r.
- Brücke r.
- Cleland r.
- Cramer 2.5 r.
- Cross r.
- diazo r.
- dinitrosalicylic acid r.
- Ehrlich diazo r.
- formalin–sulfuric acid r.

R

reagent *(continued)*
    Fouchet r.
    Frohn r.
    general r.
    Gies biuret r.
    Grignard r.
    Hager r.
    Hahn oxine r.
    Haines' r.
    Ilosvay r.
    Izar r.
    Lloyd r.
    Mandelin r.
    Marme r.
    Marquis' r.
    Mayer r.
    Mecke r.
    Millon r.
    Mörner r.
    Moro r.
    Nadi r.
    Nakayama r.
    Nessler r.
    Ninhydrin r.
    Noguchi r.
    Obermayer r.
    Pappenheim r.
    Penzoldt r.
    Rosenthaler r.
    Schaer r.
    Scheibler r.
    Schiff r.
    Schweitzer r.
    Scott-Wilson r.
    selenious–sulfuric
      acid r.
    Sickledex r.
    Soldaini r.
    Spiegler r.
    splenic r.
    Sulkowitch r.
    Sumner r.
    Tanret r.
    Triboulet r.
    Tsuchiya r.
    Uffelmann r.
    vanadic–sulfuric acid r.
    Wolff r.
reagin
    atopic r.
reaginic
realgar
reality testing
real-time
    r.-t. echocardiography

real-time *(continued)*
    r-t. optical coherence
      tomography
    r-t. polymerase chain reaction
      (PCR)
reamer
    chamfer r.
    Küntscher r.
    Moore r.
    Rush r.
reamputation
reanimate
rearrangement
    Amadori r.
reattachment of pocket
Réaumur
    scale
    thermometer
rebase
rebound
    acid r.
    r. dystonia
    r. effect
    r. headache
    heparin r.
    HIV viral r.
    r. hyperglycemia
    r. insomnia
    r. overeating
    r. phenomenon
    r. relapse
    REM r.
    r. tenderness
    r. tenderness and guarding
    r. tonometry
    r. thrombocytopenia
    urea r.
    r. viremia
rebreather
    oxygen closed-circuit r.
    oxygen r. device
    partial r. face mask
rebreathing
    CO_2 r.
    mask r.
    r. protocol
    Read r. method
Rebuck skin window
  technique
recalcification
recalcitrant
    r. acute pancreatitis
    r. dermatitis
    r. disease
    r. dry eye syndrome

recalcitrant *(continued)*
  r. hemorrhage
  r. nonunion
  r. pain
  r. paronychia
  r. patient
  r. pemphigus vulgaris
  r. sinusitis
  r. to standard therapy
  r. vitiligo
recall
  free r.
Récamier
  curet
  operation
recanalization
recapitulation
recede
receive
receiver
receptaculum (receptacula)
  r. chyli
  r. ganglii petrosi
  r. Pecqueti
receptor
  α-adrenergic r's [alpha-]
  adrenergic r.
  alpha r's
  β-adrenergic r's [beta-]
  B-cell antigen r's
  beta r's
  beta-adrenergic r's
  cell-surface r.
  central r's
  cholinergic r's
  cold r.
  complement r's
  contact r.
  contiguous r.
  cutaneous r.
  cytokine r's
  distance r.
  dopaminergic r's
  equilibratory r's
  estrogen r. (ER)
  Fc r's
  γ-aminobutyric acid r's
    (GABA) [gamma-]
  genital r's
  G protein–coupled r's (GPCR)
  gravity r's
  gustatory r.
  hair follicle r's
  histamine r's
  histamine H_1 r. [H1]

receptor *(continued)*
  histamine H_2 r. [H2]
  homing r.
  IgE r's
  immune adherence r.
  insulin r's
  itch r.
  J-r's
  joint r.
  juxtacapillary r's
  length r.
  low-density lipoprotein
    (LDL) r's
  membrane r.
  muscarinic r's
  muscle r.
  N_1-r's [N1-]
  N_2-r's [N2-]
  nicotinic r's
  nonadapting r.
  nuclear r.
  olfactory r.
  opiate r.
  opioid r.
  orphan r.
  paciniform r's
  pain r.
  Pinkus-Iggo r.
  pressure r.
  progesterone r.
  P2X r's
  rapidly adapting r.
  ryanodine r.
  sensory r.
  slowly adapting r.
  static r's
  steroid r.
  steroid hormone r.
  stretch r.
  tactile r.
  taste r.
  T-cell antigen r's (TCR)
  tension r.
  thermal r.
  tissue r.
  touch r.
  transferrin r.
  vibration r.
  visual r.
  volume r's
  warmth r.
receptorology
recess
  accessory r. of elbow
  acetabular r.

R

recess *(continued)*
    anterior r. of interpeduncular
      fossa
    anterior r. of tympanic
      membrane
    aorticomediastinal r.
    Arlt r.
    attic r.
    azygoesophageal r.
    azygomediastinal r.
    cerebellopontile r.
    chiasmatic r.
    cochlear r. of vestibule
    conarial r.
    costodiaphragmatic r. of pleura
    costomediastinal r. of pleura
    duodenojejunal r.
    elliptical r. of vestibule
    epitympanic r.
    facial r.
    r. of fourth ventricle, lateral
    hepatoenteric r.
    hepatorenal r.
    Hyrtl r.
    incisive r.
    inferior duodenal r.
    inferior ileocecal r.
    inferior omental r.
    infundibular r.
    infundibuliform r.
    r. of infundibulum
    interpeduncular r.
    intersigmoidal r.
    labyrinthine r.
    laryngopharyngeal r.
    lateral r. of fourth ventricle
    lateral r. of nasopharynx
    lateral r. of rhomboid fossa
    r. of lesser omental cavity
    lienal r.
    mesenteric r.
    mesocolic r.
    middle pharyngeal r.
    nasopalatine r.
    r. of nasopharynx, lateral
    neuroporic r.
    optic r.
    optic r. of third ventricle
    paracolic r's
    paraduodenal r.
    r. of pelvic mesocolon
    peritoneal r's
    pharyngeal r., middle
    phrenicohepatic r's
    pineal r.

recess *(continued)*
    piriform r.
    pleural r's
    pneumatoenteric r.
    pontocerebellar r.
    posterior r. of interpeduncular
      fossa
    posterior r. of tympanic
      membrane
    Reichert r.
    retroannular r.
    retrocecal r.
    retroduodenal r.
    right subhepatic r.
    r. of Rosenmüller
    sacciform r. of articulation of
      elbow
    sacciform r. of distal
      radioulnar articulation
    saccular r.
    sphenoethmoidal r.
    spherical r. of vestibule
    splenic r.
    subhepatic r's
    suboptic r.
    subphrenic r's
    subpopliteal r.
    superior duodenal r.
    superior ileocecal r.
    superior omental r.
    superior r. of tympanic
      membrane
    suprapineal r.
    suprapyramidal r.
    supratonsillar r.
    Tarin r.
    Tarini r.
    triangular r.
    Tröltsch (Troeltsch) r's
    tubotympanic r.
    utricular r.
    r's of vestibule
recession
    angle r.
    bone r.
    clitoral r.
    gingival r.
    r. of ocular muscle
    tendon r.
recessive
recessiveness
recessus (recessus)
    r. anterior membranae
      tympanicae
    r. cerebellopontis

recessus (recessus) *(continued)*
    r. chiasmatis
    r. cochlearis vestibuli
    r. costodiaphragmaticus
        pleuralis
    r. costomediastinalis pleuralis
    r. duodenalis inferior
    r. duodenalis superior
    r. duodenojejunalis
    r. ellipticus vestibuli
    r. epitympanicus
    r. hepatorenalis
    r. ileocaecalis inferior
    r. ileocaecalis superior
    r. ileocecalis inferior
    r. ileocecalis superior
    r. inferior bursae omentalis
    r. inferior omentalis
    r. infundibularis
    r. infundibuli
    r. intersigmoideus
    r. lateralis fossae rhomboidei
    r. lateralis ventriculi quarti
    r. lienalis
    r. membranae tympani anterior
    r. membranae tympani
        posterior
    r. membranae tympani superior
    r. opticus
    r. paracolici
    r. paraduodenalis
    r. pharyngealis
    r. pharyngeus
    r. phrenicohepatici
    r. phrenicomediastinalis
    r. phrenicomediastinalis
        pleuralis
    r. pinealis
    r. piriformis
    r. pleurales
    r. pneumatoentericus
    r. posterior fossae
        interpeduncularis (Tarini)
    r. posterior membranae
        tympanicae
    r. pro utriculo
    r. retrocaecalis
    r. retrocecalis
    r. retroduodenalis
    r. sacciformis articulationis
        cubiti
    r. sacciformis articulationis
        radioulnaris distalis
    r. saccularis vestibuli
    r. sphenoethmoidalis

recessus (recessus) *(continued)*
    r. sphenoethmoidalis osseus
    r. sphericus vestibuli
    r. splenicus
    r. subhepatici
    r. subphrenici
    r. subpopliteus
    r. superior bursae omentalis
    r. superior membranae
        tympanicae
    r. superior omentalis
    r. supraopticus
    r. suprapinealis
    r. triangularis
    r. tubotympanicus
    r. utricularis vestibuli
    r. utriculi vestibularis
recidivation
recidivism
recidivist
recipe
recipient
    universal r.
recipiomotor
reciprocal
    r. anchorage
    r. arm
    r. beat
    r. force
    r. inhibition
    r. innervation
    r. interaction
    r. rhythm
reciprocation
    active r.
    passive r.
reciprocity
Recklinghausen (von
    Recklinghausen)
    canals
    disease of bone
    disease, central, type II
Recklinghausen-Appelbaum disease
reclination
Reclus disease
recognition
    cell r.
    immunologic r.
    multiple codon r.
    pattern r.
recoil
    passive r.
recombinant
    r. DNA
    hGH-r.

R

recombination
    bacterial r.
    intrachromosomal r.
    mitotic r.
    molecular r.
recommend
recommendation
recompression
reconditioning
reconstitution
reconstruction
    aortic r.
    arterial r.
    Bankart
    Brent eyebrow r.
    Bucknall r. of urethra
    image r. from projections
    Landolt eyelid r.
    Mladick ear r.
    Steffanoff ear r.
    Tagliacozzi nasal r.
    Tanzer auricle r.
    venous r.
    Wookey pharyngoesophageal r.
reconstructive
    r. operation
    r. phalloplasty
    r. rhinoplasty
reconstructor
    dynamic spatial r. (DSR)
recontour
record
    chew-in r., functional
    dental identification r.
    face-bow r.
    interocclusal r.
    interocclusal r., centric
    interocclusal r., eccentric
    interocclusal r., lateral
    interocclusal r., protrusive
    jaw relation r.
    maxillomandibular r.
    medical r.
    occluding centric relation r.
    patient r.
    problem-oriented r. (POR)
    profile r.
    protrusive r.
    terminal jaw relation r.
    unit r.
recorder
    pulse volume r.
    strip-chart r.
recording
    depth r.

recovery
    r. of cardiac function
    r. of impaired function
    postoperative r. time
    r. room
    r. score
    spontaneous r.
    r. stroke
    r. time
recrement
recrementitious
recrudescence
recrudescent
    r. coccidioidomycosis
    r. infection
    r. lesion
    r. nontyphoidal salmonella
    r. pain
    r. typhus
recruitment
    alveolar r.
    diminished r.
    r. factor
    follicle r.
    r. frequency
    r. interval
    loudness r.
    r. pattern
rectal
    r. lithotomy
    r. speculum
    r. trocar
    r. tube
    r. valvotomy
rectalgia
rectectomy
rectification
    full-wave r.
    half-wave r.
    spontaneous r.
rectified
rectifier
    thermionic r.
rectischiac
rectitis
rectoabdominal
rectoanal
rectocele
rectoclysis
rectococcygeal
rectococcypexy
rectocolitis
rectocutaneous
rectocystotomy
rectolabial

rectoperineorrhaphy
rectopexy
rectoplasty
rectoromanoscope
rectoromanoscopy
rectorrhaphy
rectoscope
rectoscopy
rectosigmoid
rectosigmoidectomy
rectosigmoiditis
rectosigmoidoscopy
rectostenosis
rectostomy
rectotome
rectotomy
rectourethral
rectouterine
rectovaginal
rectovesical lithotomy
rectovestibular
rectovulvar
rectum
rectus
    r. abdominis
    r. accessorius
    lateral r. incision
    r. muscle–splitting incision
recumbency
recumbent
recuperate
recuperation
recuperative
recur, recurred
recurrence
recurrent
recurvation
recurvatum
red
    alizarin r.
    alizarin r. S
    alizarin water-soluble r.
    aniline r.
    basic r. 2
    basic r. 9
    bordeaux r.
    bromphenol r.
    carmine r.
    cerasine r.
    chlorophenol r.
    Congo r.
    cotton r.
    cotton r. B
    cotton r. 4 B
    cotton r. C

red *(continued)*
    cresol r.
    dianil r. 4 C
    dianin r. 4 B
    direct r.
    direct r. 4 B
    indigo r.
    indoxyl r.
    magdala r.
    methyl r.
    naphthaline r.
    neutral r.
    oil r.
    oil r. IV
    oil r. O
    phenol r.
    provisional r.
    scarlet r.
    scarlet r. sulfonate
    senitol r.
    Sudan r.
    toluylene r.
    tony r.
    trypan r.
    vital r.
redecussate
red herring
redintegration
redislocation
Redivac
    drain
    drainage system
Redlich-Fisher miliary plaques
Redlich-Obersteiner area
redox
redressement
red Robinson catheter
red rubber catheter
reduce, reduced
reducible
reducing substance
reductant
reductase
    5α-r. [5-alpha-]
    lipoamide r.
reduction
    r. of chromosomes
    closed r.
    delayed r.
    r. en bloc
    r. en masse
    hydrostatic r.
    immediate r.
    lung volume r.
    r. mammaplasty

R

reduction *(continued)*
  meiotic r.
  meiotic r. of chromosomes
  mitotic r.
  open r.
  somatic r.
  somatic r. of chromosomes
  weight r.
redundancy
  gene r.
redundant
reduplicated
reduplication
reduviid
REE—resting energy
  expenditure
Reed cells, Dorothy Reed cells
Reed-Hodgkin disease
Reed and Muench method
Reed-Sternberg cells
reef
reefing
  stomach r.
reentrant
reentry
reepithelialization
Reese
  dermatome
  forceps
  operation
  syndrome
Rees-Ecker
  fluid
  solution
Reese-Ellsworth retinoblastoma
  classification (I–V)
Rees test
reexcitation
reexpand
REF—renal erythropoietic factor
refect
refection
refectious
referable
reference
referral
referred
refine
refixation
reflect
reflected
reflecting microscope
reflection
  pericardial r.
  specular r.

reflector
  dental r.
  specular r.
reflex
  abdominal r's
  abdominal cutaneous r.
  abdominocardiac r.
  Abrams r.
  Abrams heart r.
  acceleratory r.
  accommodation r.
  Achilles tendon r.
  acoustic r.
  acousticopalpebral r.
  acousticospinal r.
  acoustic stapedial r.
  acquired r.
  acromial r.
  adductor r.
  adductor r. of foot
  adductor r. of thigh
  allied r's
  anal r.
  anal wink r.
  ankle r.
  antagonistic r's
  antagonistic anterior tibial r.
    of Piotrowski
  anticus r.
  antigravity r.
  aortic r.
  aponeurotic r.
  Aschner r.
  atriopressor r.
  attention r. of pupil
  attitudinal r's
  audito-oculogyric r.
  auditory r.
  auditory-palpebral r.
  aural r.
  auricle r.
  auriculocervical nerve r.
  auriculopalpebral r.
  auriculopressor r.
  autonomic r.
  axon r.
  Babinski r.
  Babkin r.
  Bainbridge r.
  Balduzzi r.
  bar r.
  Barkman r.
  baroreceptor r's
  basal joint r.
  behavior r.

reflex *(continued)*

Bekhterev (Bechterew) deep r.
Bekhterev-Mendel r.
bending r.
Bezold r.
Bezold-Jarisch r.
biceps r.
Bing r.
bladder r.
blink r.
body-righting r.
bowing r.
brachioradialis r.
Brain quadrupedal r.
brainstem r's
bregmocardiac r.
Brissaud r.
Brudzinski r.
bulbocavernous r.
bulbomimic r.
bulbospongiosus r.
Capps r.
cardiac r.
cardiac depressor r.
carotid body r.
carotidosympathoatrial r.
carotidovagoatrial r.
carotidoventricular r.
carotid sinus r.
carpophalangeal r.
cat-eye r., cat's eye r.
celiac plexus r.
cephalopalpebral r.
cerebral cortex r.
cerebropupillary r.
Chaddock r.
chain r.
chin r.
chin-jerk r.
chocked r.
Chodzko r.
choked r.
ciliary r.
ciliospinal r.
clasping r.
clasp-knife r.
closed loop r.
cochleo-orbicular r.
cochleopalpebral r.
cochleopupillary r.
cochleostapedial r.
coital r.
coitus r.
cold pressor r.
concealed r.

reflex *(continued)*

conditioned r.
conjunctival r.
consensual r.
consensual light r.
contralateral r.
convergence r.
convergency r.
convulsive r.
coordinated r.
corneal r.
corneomandibular r.
corneomental r.
corneopterygoid r.
coronary r.
corticopupillary r.
costal arch r.
costal periosteal r.
costopectoral r.
cough r.
cranial r.
cremasteric r.
crossed r.
crossed adductor r.
crossed extensor r.
crossed flexor r.
crossed r. of pelvis
cuboidodigital r.
cutaneous r.
cutaneous pupillary r.
dartos r.
Darwin r.
darwinian r.
dazzle r.
deep r.
deep abdominal r's
deep reflex
deep tendon r's (DTRs)
defecation r.
defense r.
deglutition r.
delayed r.
deltoid r.
depressor r.
digital r.
direct r.
direct light r.
disynaptic r.
diving r.
doll's eye r.
dorsal r.
dorsocuboidal r.
dorsum pedis r.
ejaculation r.
elbow r.

R

reflex *(continued)*
- embrace r.
- emergency light r.
- enterogastric r.
- epigastric r.
- Erben r.
- erector spinae r.
- Escherich r.
- esophagosalivary r.
- extensor r.
- extensor thrust r.
- external auditory meatus r.
- external hamstring r.
- external oblique r.
- eyeball compression r.
- eyeball-heart r.
- eyelid closure r.
- facial r.
- faucial r.
- femoral r.
- femoroabdominal r.
- Ferguson r.
- finger flexor r.
- finger-thumb r.
- flexion r.
- flexion r. of leg
- flexor r., paradoxical
- flexor withdrawal r.
- flight r.
- fontanel r.
- fontanelle r.
- foveal r.
- foveolar r.
- front-tap r.
- fundus r.
- fusion r.
- gag r.
- gagging r.
- Galant r.
- galvanic skin r.
- Gamper bowing r.
- gastrocnemius r.
- gastrocolic r.
- gastroileac r.
- gastroileal r.
- gastropancreatic r.
- gastrosalivary r.
- Gault cochleopalpebral r.
- Geigel r.
- genital r.
- Gifford r.
- Gifford-Galassi r.
- glabellar tap r.
- glossary r.
- gluteal r.
- Gordon r.

reflex *(continued)*
- Gower-Henry r.
- grasp r., grasping r.
- great toe r.
- gripping r.
- Grünfelder (Gruenfelder) r.
- Guillain-Barré r.
- gustolacrimal r.
- H-r.
- Haab r.
- hamstring r.
- Head r.
- heart r.
- heel-tap r.
- heel r. of Weingrow
- Hering-Breuer r.
- Hirschberg r.
- Hoffmann r.
- Hughes r.
- hyperactive myotactic r.
- hypochondrial r.
- hypogastric r.
- hypothenar r.
- ileogastric r.
- inborn r.
- indirect r.
- infraspinatus r.
- inguinal r.
- inspiratory-inhibitory r.
- intercoronary r.
- internal hamstring r.
- interscapular r.
- intersegmental r.
- intestinal r.
- intestinointestinal r.
- inverted radial r.
- investigatory r.
- iris contraction r.
- ischemic r.
- jaw r.
- jaw jerk r.
- Joffroy r.
- Juster r.
- juvenile r.
- Kehrer r.
- Kisch r.
- knee flexion r.
- knee jerk r.
- Kocher r.
- labyrinthine r.
- labyrinthine righting r.
- lacrimal r.
- Laehr-Henneberg hard palate r.
- Landau r.
- laryngeal r.
- latent r.

reflex *(continued)*

laughter r.
let-down r.
lid r.
Liddell and Sherrington r.
light r.
lip r.
little toe r.
Livierato r.
local r.
lordosis r.
Lovén r.
lower abdominal r.
lower abdominal periosteal r.
lumbar r.
lung r.
Lust r.
macular r.
Magnus and de Kleijn neck r's
mandibular r.
Marey r.
Marinesco-Radovici r.
mark-time r.
mass r.
Mayer r.
McCarthy r.
McCormac r.
McDowall r.
medioplantar r.
mediopubic r.
menace r.
Mendel r.
Mendel-Bekhterev r.
Mendel dorsal r. of foot
metacarpohypothenar r.
metacarpothenar r.
metatarsal r.
micturition r.
middle ear r.
milk ejection r.
milk let-down r.
Mondonesi r.
monosynaptic r. (MSR)
Morley peritoneocutaneous r.
Moro r.
Moro embrace r.
motor r.
muscular r.
myenteric r.
myopic r.
myostatic r.
myotatic r.
nasal r.
nasofacial r.
nasolabial r.
nasomental r.

reflex *(continued)*

naso-ocular r.
nasopulmonary r.
near r.
neck r's
neck-righting r.
nociceptive r's
nociceptive r. of Riddoch and
    Buzzard
nose-bridge-lid r.
nose-eye r.
nostril r.
obliquus r.
ocular counter-rolling r.
ocular fixation r.
ocular righting r.
oculoauditory r.
oculoauricular r.
oculocardiac r.
oculocephalic r.
oculocephalogyric r.
oculogastric r.
oculopharyngeal r.
oculopupillary r.
oculosensory r.
oculovagal r.
oculovestibular r.
olecranon r.
open loop r.
Oppenheim r.
optical righting r.
opticofacial winking r.
opticopalpebral r.
orbicularis r.
orbicularis oculi r.
orbicularis oris r.
orbicularis pupillary r.
orbiculopupillary r.
orienting r.
pain r.
palatal r.
palatine r.
palmar r.
palm-chin r.
palmomental r.
palpebral r.
panting r.
paradoxical r.
paradoxical ankle r.
paradoxical extensor r.
paradoxical flexor r.
paradoxical patellar r.
paradoxical pupillary r.
paradoxical triceps r.
patellar r.
patelloadductor r.

R

reflex *(continued)*

pathologic r's
Pavlov r.
pectoral r.
Peiper r.
pendular r.
penile r.
penis r.
perception r.
perianal r.
pericardial r.
periosteal r.
periosteoradial r.
peristaltic r.
peritoneointestinal r.
pharyngeal r.
phasic r.
Philippson r.
pilomotor r.
Piltz r.
Piotrowski r.
placing r.
plantar r.
plantar flexor r.
platysmal r.
pollicomental r.
polysynaptic r.
positive supporting r.
postural r.
pressor r.
pressoreceptor r.
Preyer r.
primitive r.
pronator r.
proprioceptive r.
protective r.
protective laryngeal r.
psychic r.
psychocardiac r.
psychogalvanic r.
puboadductor r.
pulmonocoronary r.
pupillary r.
pupillary light r.
pupillary skin r.
Puusepp r.
pyelovesical r.
quadriceps r.
quadrupedal extensor r.
radial r.
radiobicipital r.
radioperiosteal r.
radiopronator r.
Radovici r.
rectal r.

reflex *(continued)*

rectoanal inhibitory r.
rectus abdominis r.
red r.
regional r.
Reimer r.
Remak r.
renal r.
renointestinal r.
renorenal r.
renoureteral r.
resistance r.
retrobulbar pupillary r.
retromalleolar r.
reversed pupillary r.
Riddoch mass r.
righting r.
Roger r.
Romberg r.
rooting r.
Rossolimo r.
Ruggeri r.
Saenger r.
scapular r.
scapulohumeral r.
Schäffer (Schaeffer) r.
Schunkel r.
scratch r.
scrotal r.
segmental r.
semimembranosus r.
semitendinosus r.
senile r.
sensory blinking r.
sexual r.
shot-silk r.
simple r.
sinus r.
skin r.
skin pupillary r.
sneezing r.
Snellen r.
snout r.
sole r.
sole-tap r.
somatointestinal r.
Somogyi r.
spinal r.
spino-adductor r.
stapedial r.
stapedius r.
startle r.
static r.
static adaptation r.
static attitudinal r.

reflex *(continued)*
    statokinetic r.
    statotonic r's
    stepping r.
    sternobrachial r.
    Stookey r.
    stretch r.
    Strümpell r.
    styloradial r.
    suborbital r.
    sucking r.
    suckling r.
    suck-swallow r.
    superficial r.
    superficial abdominal r.
    supination r.
    supinator r.
    supinator jerk r.
    supinator longus r.
    supporting r's
    supraorbital r.
    suprapatellar r.
    suprapubic r.
    supraumbilical r.
    swallowing r.
    tactile r.
    tapetal light r.
    tarsophalangeal r.
    tendon r.
    tensor fasciae latae r.
    testicular compression r.
    thigh crossed lengthening r.
    threat r.
    Throckmorton r.
    thumb r.
    tibialis posterior r.
    tibioadductor r.
    toe r.
    tonic r.
    tonic neck r.
    tonic plantar r.
    tonic vibration r.
    trained r.
    triceps r.
    triceps surae r.
    trigeminocervical r.
    trigeminofacial r.
    trigeminus r.
    trochanter r.
    Trömner (Troemner) r.
    tympanic r.
    ulnar r.
    unconditioned r.
    unloading r.
    upper abdominal periosteal r.

reflex *(continued)*
    upper deep abdominal r.
    urinary r's
    utricular r.
    vagal pupillary r.
    vagovagal r.
    vagus r.
    vascular r.
    vasomotor r.
    vasopressor r's
    vasovagal r.
    venorespiratory r.
    vertebra prominens r.
    vesical r.
    vesicointestinal r.
    vestibular r's
    vestibulo-ocular r.
    vestibulospinal r.
    virile r.
    visceral r.
    visceral traction r.
    viscerocardiac r.
    visceromotor r.
    viscerosensory r.
    viscerotrophic r.
    visual orbicularis r.
    visuocortical r.
    vomiting r.
    von Mering r.
    walking r.
    Wartenberg r.
    Weingrow r.
    Weiss r.
    Westphal-Piltz r.
    Westphal pupillary r.
    wink r.
    withdrawal r.
    wrist clonus r.
    wrist flexion r.
    zygomatic r.
reflexogenic
reflexograph
reflexology
reflexometer
reflexometry
reflexophil
reflux
    abdominojugular r.
    duodenogastric r.
    duodenogastroesophageal r.
    enterogastric r.
    esophageal r.
    r. esophagitis
    gastroesophageal r.
    (GER)

R

reflux *(continued)*
- gastroesophageal r. disease (GERD)
- hepatojugular (HJ) r.
- Hinman r.
- intrarenal r.
- laryngopharyngeal r.
- r. nephropathy
- pyelolymphatic r.
- pyelorenal r.
- pyelosinus r.
- pyelotubular r.
- pyelovenous r.
- valvular r.
- vesicoureteral r. (VUR)
- vesicoureteric r.

reformat

refract

refracta dosi

refractile

refraction
- cycloplegic r.
- double r.
- dynamic r.
- homatropine r.
- manifest r.
- ocular r.
- static r.

refractionist

refractive

refractivity

refractometer

refractometry

refractor

refractory
- absolute r. period
- r. anemia
- r. cast
- effective r. period
- r. epilepsy
- r. flask
- r. glaucoma
- r. illness
- r. normoblastic anemia
- pacemaker r. period
- r. pain
- r. period
- relative r. period
- r. rickets
- r. sprue
- r. state
- vitamin D–r. rickets

refracture

refrangibility

refrangible

refresh

refrigerants

refrigeration

refringent

Refsum
- disease
- syndrome

refusion

REG—radioencephalogram

regainer
- space r.

regainer-maintainer

regard

Regaud method

Regaud and Lacassagne technique

regeneration
- epimorphic r.
- morphallactic r.

regime
- Smith & Smith r.

regimen
- chemotherapeutic r.
- sanitary r.

regio (regiones)
- regiones abdominales
- r. analis
- r. antebrachialis
- r. antebrachialis anterior
- r. antebrachialis posterior
- r. antebrachii anterior
- r. antebrachii posterior
- r. auricularis
- r. axillaris
- r. brachialis
- r. brachialis anterior
- r. brachialis posterior
- r. brachii anterior
- r. brachii posterior
- r. buccalis
- r. calcanea
- regiones capitis
- r. carpalis
- r. carpalis anterior
- r. carpalis posterior
- regiones cervicales
- r. cervicalis anterior
- r. cervicalis lateralis
- r. cervicalis posterior
- regiones colli
- r. colli anterior
- r. colli lateralis
- r. colli posterior
- r. coxae
- r. cruralis anterior
- r. cruralis posterior

regio (regiones) *(continued)*
    r. cruris
    r. cruris anterior
    r. cruris posterior
    r. cubitalis
    r. cubitalis anterior
    r. cubitalis posterior
    r. deltoidea
    regiones dorsales
    r. dorsalis manus
    r. dorsalis pedis
    regiones dorsi
    r. epigastrica
    r. facialis
    r. femoralis
    r. femoralis anterior
    r. femoralis posterior
    r. femoris
    r. femoris anterior
    r. femoris posterior
    r. frontalis
    r. genualis anterior
    r. genualis posterior
    r. genus
    r. genus anterior
    r. genus posterior
    r. glutealis
    r. hypochondriaca
    r. hypogastrica
    r. hypothalamica anterior
    r. hypothalamica dorsalis
    r. hypothalamica intermedia
    r. hypothalamica posterior
    r. inframammaria
    r. infraorbitalis
    r. infrascapularis
    r. infratemporalis
    r. inguinalis
    r. lateralis
    r. lumbalis
    r. lumbaris
    r. mammaria
    r. manus
    r. mastoidea
    regiones membri inferioris
    regiones membri superioris
    r. mentalis
    r. metacarpalis
    r. metatarsalis
    r. nasalis
    r. nuchalis
    r. occipitalis
    r. olfactoria
    r. oralis
    r. orbitalis

regio (regiones) *(continued)*
    r. palmaris
    r. parietalis
    r. parotideomasseterica
    regiones pectorales
    r. pectoralis
    r. pectoralis lateralis
    r. pedis
    r. perinealis
    regiones plantares digitorum
      pedis
    r. plantaris
    regiones pleuropulmonales
    r. presternalis
    r. pubica
    r. respiratoria
    r. retromalleolaris lateralis
    r. retromalleolaris medialis
    r. sacralis
    r. scapularis
    r. sternocleidomastoidea
    r. surae
    r. suralis
    r. talocruralis anterior
    r. talocruralis posterior
    r. tarsalis
    r. temporalis
    regiones thoracicae anteriores
      et laterales
    r. umbilicalis
    r. urogenitalis
    r. vertebralis
    r. zygomatica
region
    abdominal r.
    r. of accommodation
    AN r.
    anal r.
    ankle r., anterior
    ankle r., posterior
    antebrachial r.
    antebrachial r., radial
    antebrachial r., ulnar
    antebrachial r., volar
    anterior antebrachial r.
    anterior r. of arm
    anterior brachial r.
    anterior crural r.
    anterior cubital r.
    anterior forearm r.
    anterior r. of forearm
    anterior hypothalamic r.
    anterior r. of knee
    anterior r. of leg
    anterior r. of neck

R

region *(continued)*
    anterior r. of wrist
    anterior thigh r.
    auricular r.
    axillary r.
    r's of back
    basilar r.
    brachial r.
    brachial r., anterior
    brachial r., posterior
    Broca r.
    buccal r.
    C r.
    calcaneal r.
    carpal r., anterior
    carpal r., posterior
    cervical r., anterior
    cervical r., lateral
    cervical r., posterior
    ciliary r.
    cingulate r.
    complementarity determining r.
    constant (C) r.
    core r.
    crural r., anterior
    crural r., posterior
    cubital r., anterior
    cubital r., posterior
    deltoid r.
    dorsal r's
    dorsal r. of foot
    dorsal lip r.
    elbow r.
    encephalic r.
    epigastric r.
    external r.
    extrapolar r.
    Fab r.
    facial r's
    Fc r.
    femoral r.
    focal r.
    foot r.
    framework r.
    frontal r.
    Geiger r.
    genitourinary r.
    gluteal r.
    gustatory r.
    hand r.
    heel r.
    hinge r.
    hip r.
    homogeneously staining r's
    homology r's

region *(continued)*
    hypencephalic r.
    hypervariable r's
    hypochondriac r.
    hypogastric r.
    hypothalamic r., anterior
    hypothalamic r., dorsal
    hypothalamic r., intermediate
    hypothalamic r., lateral
    hypothalamic r., posterior
    I r.
    iliac r.
    infraclavicular r.
    infrahyoid r.
    inframammary r.
    infraorbital r.
    infrascapular r.
    infraspinous r.
    infratemporal r.
    infundibulotubular r.
    inguinal r.
    intermediate hypothalamic r.
    ischiorectal r.
    K-r.
    knee r.
    lateral r.
    lateral abdominal r.
    lateral r. of neck
    leg r.
    r's of leg, anterior and posterior
    limbic r.
    locus control r.
    lumbar r.
    mammary r.
    mammillary r.
    mastoid r.
    mental r.
    metacarpal r.
    metatarsal r.
    motor r.
    mylohyoid r.
    myotube r. of intrafusal fiber
    N r.
    r. of nape
    nasal r.
    NH r.
    nuchal r.
    nucleated r. of intrafusal fiber
    nucleolar organizing r.
    nucleolus organizing r.
    occipital r.
    ocular r.
    olecranal r.
    olecranon r.
    olfactory r.

region *(continued)*
    opticostriate r.
    oral r.
    orbital r.
    palmar r.
    parietal r.
    parietotemporal r.
    parotideomasseteric r.
    patellar r.
    pectoral r's
    pectoral r., lateral
    pelvic r.
    perichromatin r.
    perineal r.
    plantar r's of toes
    pleuropulmonary r's
    popliteal r.
    posterior antebrachial r.
    posterior r. of arm
    posterior brachial r.
    posterior crural r.
    posterior cubital r.
    posterior forearm r.
    posterior r. of forearm
    posterior
      hypothalamic r.
    posterior r. of knee
    posterior r. of leg
    posterior r. of neck
    posterior thigh r.
    posterior r. of wrist
    precordial r.
    prefrontal r.
    preoptic r.
    presternal r.
    presumptive r.
    pretectal r.
    proportional r.
    pseudoautosomal r.
    pterygomaxillary r.
    pubic r.
    respiratory r.
    retromalleolar r., lateral
    retromalleolar r., medial
    retromaxillary r.
    rolandic r.
    sacral r.
    sacrococcygeal r.
    scapular r.
    sensory r.
    sternocleidomastoid r.
    subauricular r.
    submandibular r.
    submaxillary r.
    submental r.

region *(continued)*
    subphrenic r.
    subscapular r.
    subthalamic r.
    supraclavicular r.
    suprainguinal r.
    supraomental r.
    supraoptic r.
    suprapubic r.
    supraspinous r.
    sural r.
    talocrural r., anterior
    talocrural r., posterior
    tegmental r.
    temporal r.
    trabecular r.
    trochanteric r.
    umbilical r.
    urogenital r.
    variable (V) r.
    vertebral r.
    vestibular r.
    V_H [V-H] r.
    V_L [V-L] r.
    volar r's of fingers
    volar r. of hand
    zygomatic r.
regional
regiones (plural of regio)
region of interest
register
    immunization r.
registrant
registrar
registration
    r. of functional form
    maxillomandibular r.
    occlusal r.
registry
    cancer r.
Regnoli operation
regression
    atavistic r.
    curvilinear r.
    linear r.
    multiple r.
    nonlinear r.
regressive
regular
regulation
    down-r.
    fertility r.
    menstrual r.
    ontogenetic r.
regulator

R

regulon
regurgitant
  r. area ratio
  effective r. orifice area
  r. flow
  r. fraction
  r. jet
  r. lesion
  r. menstruation
  mitral r. jet
  r. murmur
  r. pockets
  r. pressure gradient
  r. pump flow
  tricuspid r. jet velocity
  valvular r. lesion
  r. velocity
  r. volume
regurgitate
regurgitation
  aortic r. (AR)
  duodenal r.
  esophageal r.
  functional r.
  mitral r. (MR)
  pulmonic r. (PR)
  tricuspid r. (TR)
  valvular r.
  vesicoureteral r.
rehab—rehabilitation
rehabilitate
rehabilitation
  alaryngeal voice r.
  functional r.
  mouth r.
  occlusal r.
  oral r.
  vocational r.
rehabilitee
rehalation
Rehfuss
  method
  test
  tube
rehydration
Reich clamp
Reichel
  chondromatosis
  cloacal duct
Reichenheim-King operation
Reichert
  canal
  cartilage
  membrane
  method

Reichert (continued)
  recess
  scar
Reichmann
  disease
  syndrome
Reich-Nechtow
  clamp
  curet
  dilator
Reid
  baseline
  index
Reifenstein syndrome
Reil
  insula
  island
  ribbon
  sulcus
  trigone
Reilly bodies
Reiner-Beck snare
Reiner-Knight forceps
reinfection
reinforcement
  delayed r.
  differential r.
  fixed interval r.
  fixed ratio r.
  negative r.
  positive r.
  primary r.
  r. of reflex
  secondary r.
  r. of tendon reflexes
  variable interval r.
  variable ratio r.
reinforcer
reinforcing suture
reinfusate
reinfusion
Reinke
  crystalloids
  crystals
reinnervation
reinoculation
Reinsch test
reintegration
reintubation
reinversion
reinvocation
Reis-Bücklers disease
Reissner
  fiber
  membrane

Reitan-Indiana aphasic screening test
Reiter
    disease
    syndrome
reiterate
reiterature
rejection
    acute r.
    acute cellular r.
    acute renal transplant r.
    allograft r.
    cellular r.
    chronic r.
    chronic renal transplant r.
    first-set r.
    graft r.
    hyperacute r.
    hyperacute renal transplant r.
    immunologic r.
    second-set r.
rejoinder
rejuvenescence
Rekoss disk
relapse
    intercurrent r.
    mucocutaneous r.
    rebound r.
    risk of r.
relapsing
    chronic r. pancreatitis
    chronic r.
        polyradiculoneuropathy
    Dutton r. fever
    endemic r. fever
    epidemic r. fever
    r. febrile nodular
        nonsuppurative panniculitis
    r. immune thrombocytopenic
        purpura
    louse-borne r. fever
    r. multiple sclerosis
    r. myelitis
    r. polychondritis
    r. remitting multiple sclerosis
    tick-borne r. fever
    r. viral load
relation
    acentric r.
    buccolingual r.
    centric r.
    centric jaw r.
    convenience r. of teeth
    cusp-fossa r.
    dynamic r's

relation (continued)
    eccentric r.
    eccentric jaw r.
    eccentric jaw r., acquired
    Frank-Starling r.
    intermaxillary r.
    jaw r.
    jaw-to-jaw r.
    lateral occlusal r.
    length-tension r.
    mass-energy r.
    maxillomandibular r.
    median jaw r.
    median retruded jaw r.
    object r.
    occlusal r.
    occlusal jaw r.
    posterior border jaw r.
    protrusive jaw r.
    range-energy r.
    rest jaw r.
    ridge r.
    static r's
    unstrained jaw r.
    vertical r.
relationship
    blood r.
    confidential r.
    dose-effect r.
    dose-response r.
    linear r.
relative
    first-degree r.
    second-degree r.
    third-degree r.
relativistic mass
relaxant
    muscle r.
    smooth muscle r.
relaxation
    isometric r.
    isovolumetric r.
    longitudinal r.
    mecystatic r.
    r. suture
relaxin
relaxing incision
relearning
release
    contracture r.
    laryngeal r.
reliability
relief
    gingival r.
    r. incision

R

relieve
reline
relucence
reluxation
rem—roentgen-equivalent-man
REM—rapid eye movement
Remak
    axon
    band
    fibers
    ganglion
    paralysis
    plexus
    reflex
    sign
    symptom
    type
remediable
    surgically r.
remedial
remedy
    Bach r's, Bach flower r's
    concordant r's
    inimic r's
    Rescue R.
    specific r.
    tissue r's
remineralization
reminiscent
remission
    Legroux r.
remit
remittence
remittent
remnant
    acroblastic r.
    allantoic r.
    dermal r.
remodeling
    bone r.
remotivation
removal
    pulp r.
REMP—roentgen equivalent–man
  period
remyelination
ren
    r. mobilis
    r. unguliformis
renal
    r. agenesis
    r. angiography
    r. arteriography
    r. artery
    r. blastema

renal *(continued)*
    r. calculi
    r. cell carcinoma
    r. cortex
    r. cortical necrosis
    r. cyst
    r. cystic disease
    r. dysgenesis
    r. dysplasia
    r. ectopia
    r. failure
    r. fascia
    r. function
    r. hyperplasia
    r. insufficiency
    intravenous r. angiography
    r. lithiasis
    r. medulla
    r. osteodystrophy
    r. papillae
    r. parenchyma
    r. pedicle
    r. pelvis
    percutaneous transluminal r.
      angioplasty (PTRA)
    r. plexus
    r. pouch
    r. rickets
    r. sinus
    r. toxicity
    r. transplant
    r. transplantation
    r. tubular acidosis
    r. tubular necrosis
    r. tubule
    r. vein
    r. vein thrombosis
    r. venogram
renaturation
Rendu tremor
Rendu-Osler-Weber
    disease
    syndrome
renicapsule
reniculus (reniculi)
reniform
renin
    r. angiotensin system
    big r.
    r. substrate
reninism
    primary r.
reninoma
renipelvic
reniportal

renis
rennet
rennin
renocortical
renocutaneous
renocystogram
renogastric
renogenic
Renografin-60, Renografin-76
renogram
    isotope r.
    radionuclide r.
renography
    emission r.
renointestinal
renopathy
renoprival
renotrophic
renotropic
renovascular
renown
Renshaw inhibition
reovirus
reoxidation
reoxygenation
repair
    Belsey r.
    Brown-McDowell r. of cleft lip
    Cecil r.
    Cecil-Culp r. of hypospadias
    central episiotomy and r. (CER)
    DuVries hammer toe r.
    excision r.
    Lich-Gregoire r.
    Lichtenstein hernia r.
    Matsner median episiotomy
      and r.
    pants-over-vest r.
    Rose-Thompson r.
reparative
repatency
repellent
repeller
repercolation
repercussion
repercussive
reperfusion
reperitonealize
repertoire
repetatur
repetition
repetition time (TR)
replacement
    isomorphous r.
    reciprocal r.

replacer
    Green r.
replant
replantation
    finger r.
    intentional r.
    microsurgical r.
    penile r.
    scalp r.
    r. surgery
    tooth r.
replenisher
repletion
replicase
replicate
replication
    conservative r.
    DNA r.
    nonconservative r.
    semiconservative r.
replicon
repolarization
reposition
repositioning
    jaw r.
    muscle r.
repositor
repository
representation
    sensorimotor r.
repression
    catabolite r.
    coordinate r.
    endproduct r.
    enzyme r.
repressor
    active r.
    inactive r.
reproduction
reproductive
repullulation
repulsion
    capillary r.
requirement
    minimum daily r. (MDR)
RER—rough endoplasmic
    reticulum
RES—reticuloendothelial system
rescinnamine
rescue
    citrovorum r.
    folinic acid r.
    leucovorin r.
resect
resectable

R

resection
- abdominoperineal r. (APR)
- antral r.
- bladder neck r.
- block r.
- colon r. (CR)
- endocardial r.
- gastric r. (GR)
- Girdlestone r.
- levator r.
- mandibular r.
- massive bowel r. syndrome
- maxillary r.
- Mikulicz r.
- pulmonary r.
- root r., root-end r.
- septal r.
- sleeve r.
- submucosal r.
- submucous r. (SMR)
- submucous r. of nasal septum
- submucous r. and rhinoplasty (SMRR)
- submucous r. of vocal cord
- transurethral r. (TUR)
- transurethral r. of bladder (TURB)
- transurethral r. of bladder tumor (TURBT)
- transurethral r. of prostate (TURP)
- transurethral prostatic r.
- wedge r.

resectoscope
- Baumrucker r.
- Bumpus r.
- cold punch r.
- Iglesias r.
- McCarthy r.
- Stern-McCarthy r.
- Thompson r.

resectoscopy

reserve
- alkali r.
- alkaline r.
- bone marrow r.
- breathing r.
- cardiac r.
- contractile r.
- lifetime r.
- ovarian r.
- renal r.
- respiratory r.

reservoir
- cardiotomy r.
- chromatin r.

reservoir *(continued)*
- continent ileal r.
- continent urinary r.
- ileoanal r.
- r. of infection
- Koch r.
- Kock r.
- Mainz pouch urinary r.
- Ommaya r.
- Pecquet r.
- Pudenz r.
- Rickham r.
- Rickham-Salmon r.

resettlement
- occupational r.

reshaping

residency

resident

residua (plural of residuum)

residual
- postvoiding r.

residue
- acceptable pesticide r.
- day r.
- pesticide r.

residuum (residua)
- gastric r.

resilience

resiliency

resilient

resin
- acrylic r's
- activated r.
- anion-exchange r.
- A-stage r.
- autopolymer r.
- azure A carbacrylic r.
- carbacrylamine r's
- cation exchange r.
- cholestyramine r.
- cold-curing r.
- composite r.
- copolymer r.
- C-stage r.
- cyanoacrylate r.
- direct filling r.
- epoxy r.
- guaiacum r.
- heat-curing r.
- ion exchange r.
- ionomer r.
- jalap r.
- light-activated r.
- light-cured r.
- phentermine r.
- podophyllum r.

resin *(continued)*
  polyamine-methylene r.
  polyester r.
  quick-cure r.
  quinine carbacrylic r.
  self-curing r.
  styrene r.
  sulfonated
    polystyrene r.
  synthetic r.
  thermoset r.,
    thermosetting r.
  vinyl r.
resinoid
resinous
res ipsa loquitur
resistance
  acquired radiation r.
  airway r.
  androgen r.
  basilar membrane r.
  capillary r.
  cogwheel r.
  complete androgen r.
  drug r.
  ego r.
  electrical r.
  environmental r.
  expiratory r.
  glucocorticoid r.
  hybrid r.
  id r.
  incomplete androgen r.
  input r.
  insulin r.
  internal r.
  mineralocorticoid r.
  multidrug r.
  multiple drug r.
  natural r.
  peripheral r.
  peripheral vascular r.
  phenotypic r.
  pleiotropic drug r.
  pulmonary r.
  pulmonary vascular r.
  superego r.
  total peripheral r.
  total pulmonary r.
  vascular r.
  venous r.
resistant
resistive magnet
resistivity
resistor
resite

resolution
  angular r.
  axial r.
  azimuthal r.
  depth r.
  energy r.
  lateral r.
  longitudinal r.
  range r.
  spatial r.
  transverse r.
resolve
resolvent
resonance
  amphoric r.
  bandbox r.
  bell-metal r.
  r. capture
  cavernous r.
  cough r.
  cracked-pot r.
  electron paramagnetic r. (EPR)
  electron spin r. (ESR)
  hydatid r.
  magnetic r. angiography (MRA)
  nasal r.
  nuclear magnetic r. (NMR)
  osteal r.
  proton magnetic r. (PMR)
  shoulder-strap r.
  skodaic r.
  tympanic r.
  tympanitic r.
  vesicular r.
  vesiculotympanic r.
  vesiculotympanitic r.
  vocal r. (VR)
  whispering r.
  wooden r.
resonant
resonator
  Oudin r.
resorb
resorbent
resorcin
resorcinism
resorcinolphthalein
resorption
  apical root r.
  bone r.
  external root r.
  gingival r.
  horizontal r.
  idiopathic r.
  internal r.
  physiologic r.

R

resorption *(continued)*
    rear r.
    root r.
    surface root r.
    tooth r., external
    tooth r., internal
    tubular r.
    undermining r.
    vertical r.
respirable
respiration
    abdominal r.
    absent r.
    accelerated r.
    aerobic r.
    amphoric r.
    anaerobic r.
    artificial r.
    asthmoid r.
    ataxic r.
    Austin Flint r.
    Biot r.
    Bouchut r.
    bronchial r.
    bronchocavernous r.
    bronchovesicular r.
    cavernous r.
    cell r.
    cellular r.
    cerebral r.
    Cheyne-Stokes r.
    cogwheel r.
    collateral r.
    controlled diaphragmatic r.
    Corrigan r.
    costal r.
    diaphragmatic r.
    diffusion r.
    direct r.
    divided r.
    electrophrenic r. (EPR)
    external r.
    fetal r.
    forced r.
    granular r.
    harsh r.
    indefinite r.
    intermittent positive-pressure
      r. (IPPR)
    internal r.
    interrupted r.
    jerky r.
    Kussmaul r.
    Kussmaul-Kien r.
    labored r.

respiration *(continued)*
    meningitic r.
    metamorphosing r.
    mouth-to-mouth r.
    nervous r.
    paradoxical r.
    pendelluft r.
    periodic r.
    placental r.
    puerile r.
    r. pyelography
    rude r.
    Seitz metamorphosing r.
    slow r.
    spontaneous r's
    stertorous r.
    supplementary r.
    suppressed r.
    thoracic r.
    tidal r.
    tissue r.
    transitional r.
    tubular r.
    vesicular r.
    vesiculocavernous r.
    vicarious r.
    wavy r.
respirator
    BABYbird r.
    Bird r.
    cabinet r.
    cuirass r.
    demand r.
    Drinker r.
    Engström r.
    negative-pressure r.
    protective r.
respiratory
    r. acidosis
    r. arrest
    r. bronchiolitis
    r. center drive
    r. distress
    r. distress syndrome (RDS)
    r. insufficiency
    r. paralysis
    r. rate
    r. scoring system
    r. syncytial virus (RSV)
    r. system
    r. tract
    r. tract mucosa
respirometer
    Wright r.
respirometry

respondeat superior
response
 acute phrase r.
 allergic r.
 anal r.
 anamnestic r.
 anticipatory r.
 Arthus r.
 auditory brainstem r. (ABR)
 autoimmune r.
 average evoked r.
 Babinski r.
 blink r.
 booster r.
 brain stem evoked r. (BSER)
 conditioned r. (CR)
 corneal r.
 Cornell r.
 decremental r.
 decrementing r.
 delayed r.
 delayed conditioned r.
 disinhibition r.
 dose r.
 dynamic r.
 electrodermal r.
 evoked r.
 extensor plantar r.
 F r.
 flare r.
 frequency r.
 fright r.
 galvanic skin r.
 ice water r.
 immediate r.
 immune r.
 immune r., primary
 immune r., secondary
 incremental r.
 inflammatory r.
 isomorphic r.
 lysogenic r.
 lytic r.
 M r.
 memory r.
 middle latency r.
 orienting r.
 paradoxical cold r.
 placing r.
 positive Babinski r.
 postauricular r.
 primary immune r.
 psychogalvanic r. (PGR)
 psychogalvanic skin r.
 quantal r.

response *(continued)*
 rage r.
 recall r.
 relaxation r.
 reticulocyte r.
 Rinne r.
 secondary immune r.
 second-set r.
 somatosensory evoked r. (SER)
 startle r.
 stretch r.
 thalamic r.
 triple r.
 triple r. (of Lewis)
 unconditioned r. (UR)
 vestibular placing r.
 wheal and flare r.
 wink r.
responsibility
 criminal r.
rest
 aberrant r.
 adrenal r.
 bed r.
 carbon r.
 caudal medullary r.
 cingulum r.
 embryonic r.
 epithelial r.
 fetal r.
 incisal r.
 lingual r.
 Malassez r.
 mesonephric r.
 nephrogenic r.
 occlusal r.
 pancreatic r.
 precision r.
 recessed r.
 semiprecision r.
 suprarenal r.
 surface r.
 Walthard cell r's
restaurateur
restbite
restenosis
 false r.
 true r.
restibrachium
restiform
restis
restitutio
 r. ad integrum
 r. integrum
restitution

R

restoration
  buccal r.
  cast r.
  crown r.
  cusp r.
  direct r.
  facial r.
  indirect r.
  pin-ledge r.
  prosthetic r.
restorative
restoratives
restraint
  chemical r.
  mechanical r.
  medicinal r.
  MHC r.
restriction
  intrauterine growth r.
    (IUGR)
  MHC r.
resultant
resupination
resuscitation
  active compression-
    decompression r.
  cardiac r.
  cardiopulmonary r.
    (CPR)
  colloid r.
  crystalloid r.
  expired air r. (EAR)
  fluid r.
  r. of the heart
  hypertonic r.
  mouth-to-mouth r.
  mouth-to-nose r.
  oral r.
resuscitator
  cardiopulmonary r.
resuture
retainer
  continuous bar r.
  direct r.
  Hawley r.
  indirect r.
  intracoronal r.
  matrix r.
  space r.
retard
  expiratory r.
retardation
  cultural-familial mental r.
  fetal growth r.
  intrauterine growth r.

retardation (continued)
  mental r.
  mental r., borderline
  mental r., mild
  mental r., moderate
  mental r., profound
  mental r., severe
  psychomotor r.
  psychosocial r.
retch
retching
rete (retia)
  acromial r.
  r. acromiale
  r. arteriosum
  r. arteriosum dermidis
  r. arteriosum subpapillare
  articular r.
  articular cubital r.
  r. articulare cubiti
  r. articulare genus
  articular r. of elbow
  articular r. of knee
  calcaneal r.
  r. calcaneum
  r. canalis hypoglossi
  carpal r., dorsal
  r. carpale dorsale
  r. carpi dorsale
  r. cutaneum
  dermal r.
  r. dorsale pedis
  dorsal venous r. of foot
  dorsal venous r. of hand
  r. foraminis ovalis
  r. of Haller, r. halleri
  r. lymphocapillare
  r. malleolare laterale
  r. malleolare mediale
  malleolar r., lateral
  malleolar r., medial
  malpighian r.
  r. mirabile
  r. mirabile of kidney
  r. mucosum
  r. nasi
  r. olecrani
  r. ovarii
  r. patellae
  patellar r.
  r. patellare
  r. patellaris
  plantar r.
  plantar venous r.
  r. subpapillare

rete (retia) *(continued)*
 subpapillary r.
 r. testis
 r. testis (halleri)
 r. of urine
 r. vasculosum
 r. vasculosum articulare
 retia venosa vertebrarum
 retia venosa vertebrarum
  retention
 r. venosum
 r. venosum dorsale manus
 r. venosum dorsale pedis
 r. venosum plantare
retention
 bladder r.
 r. catheter
 denture r.
 direct r.
 indirect r.
 surgical r.
 r. suture
 urinary r.
 r. of urine
retethelioma
retia (plural of rete)
retial
reticula (plural of reticulum)
reticular
 r. dermis
 r. erythematous mucinosis
reticulate
reticulation
 dust r.
reticulin M
reticulitis
reticulocyte count
reticulocytogenic
reticulocytopenia
reticulocytosis
reticuloendothelial
 r. blockade
 r. system
reticuloendothelioma
reticuloendotheliosis
 leukemic r.
reticuloendothelium
reticulohistiocytary
reticulohistiocytoma of Crosti
reticulohistiocytosis
 multicentric r.
reticuloid
 actinic r.
reticulolymphosarcoma
reticuloma

reticulonodular
reticuloperithelium
reticulopituicyte
reticuloplasmocytoma
reticulopodium (reticulopodia)
reticulosis
 benign r.
 benign inoculation r.
 benign lymphocytic r.
 bony r.
 epidermotropic r.
 familial hemophagocytic r.
 familial histiocytic r.
 histiocytic medullary r.
 inflammatory r.
 lipomelanic r.
 lipomelanotic r.
 malignant midline r.
 midline malignant r.
 medullary r.
 pagetoid r.
 polymorphic r.
 primary r. of brain
reticulospinal
reticulothelium
 agranular r.
reticulotomy
reticulum (reticula)
 agranular endoplasmic r.
 arachnoid r.
 r. cell carcinoma
 Chiari r.
 Ebner r.
 endoplasmic r.
 granular endoplasmic r.
 reticula lienis
 nuclear r.
 rough endoplasmic r.
 sarcoplasmic r.
 smooth endoplasmic r.
 splenic r.
 stellate r.
 r. trabeculare
 r. trabeculare anguli
  iridocornealis
 r. trabeculare sclerae
 transitional endoplasmic r.
retiform parapsoriasis
retina
 cilial r.
 cilioiridial r.
 coarctate r.
 r. commotio
 detached r.
 detachment of r.

R

retina *(continued)*
    iridial r.
    Kandori fleck r.
    leopard r.
    nasal r.
    physiologic r.
    shot silk r.
    temporal r.
    tessellated r.
    tigroid r.
    watered-silk r.
retinaculum (retinacula)
    r. of arcuate ligament
    r. capsulae articularis coxae
    caudal r.
    r. caudale
    r. costae ultimae
    retinacula cutis
    extensor r. of foot, inferior
    extensor r. of foot, superior
    extensor r. of hand
    r. extensorum manus
    fibular r., inferior
    fibular r., superior
    flexor r. of ankle
    flexor r. of foot
    flexor r. of hand
    r. flexorum manus
    r. of hip joint
    r. ligamenti arcuati
    r. musculorum extensorum
      inferius pedis
    r. musculorum extensorum
      manus
    r. musculorum extensorum
      superius pedis
    r. musculorum fibularium
      inferius
    r. musculorum fibularium
      superius
    r. musculorum flexorum manus
    r. musculorum flexorum pedis
    r. musculorum peronaeorum
      inferius
    r. musculorum peroneorum
      inferius
    r. musculorum peroneorum
      superius
    r. patellae laterale
    r. patellae mediale
    patellar r., lateral
    patellar r., medial
    peroneal r., inferior
    peroneal r., superior
    r. tendinum

retinaculum (retinacula) *(continued)*
    r. tendinum musculorum
      extensorum
    r. tendinum musculorum
      extensorum inferius
    r. tendinum musculorum
      extensorum superius
    r. tendinum musculorum
      flexorum
    retinacula unguis
    Weitbrecht r.
retinal
    11-*cis* r.
    all-*trans* r.
    r. detachment
    fluorescence r. photography
    r. isomerase
    r. pigment epithelium
    r. tear
retinaldehyde
retinene
retinitis
    actinic r.
    albuminuric r.
    r. albuminurica
    apoplectic r.
    azotemic r.
    central angiospastic r.
    r. centralis serosa
    r. circinata
    circinate r.
    Coats r.
    cytomegalovirus r.
    diabetic r.
    disciform r.
    exudative r.
    r. gravidarum
    gravidic r.
    r. haemorrhagica
    hypertensive r.
    Jacobson r.
    Jensen r.
    leukemic r.
    metastatic r.
    nephritic r.
    Pick r.
    r. pigmentosa
    r. pigmentosa sine pigmento
    r. proliferans
    proliferating r.
    r. punctata albescens
    punctate r.
    renal r.
    r. sclopetaria
    serous r.

retinitis *(continued)*
    simple r.
    solar r.
    splenic r.
    r. stellata
    striate r.
    suppurative r.
    syphilitic r.
    r. syphilitica
    uremic r.
    Wagener r.
retinoblastoma
retinocerebelloangiomatosis
retinochoroid
retinochoroiditis
    birdshot r.
    r. juxtapapillaris
    toxoplasmic r.
retinocytoma
retinodialysis
retinograph
retinography
retinoid
retinol
retinomalacia
retinopapillitis
retinopathy
    actinic r.
    AIDS-associated r.
    apoplectic r.
    arteriosclerotic r.
    background r.
    background diabetic r.
    bull's eye r.
    central angiospastic r.
    central disk-shaped r.
    central serous r.
    chloroquine r.
    circinate r.
    diabetic r.
    eclamptic r.
    exudative r.
    hemorrhagic r.
    HIV-associated r.
    hypertensive r.
    Keith-Wagener r.
    leukemic r.
    macular r.
    nonproliferative r.
    pigmentary r.
    r. of prematurity
    proliferative r.
    proliferative diabetic r.
    Purtscher angiopathic r.
    purulent r.

retinopathy *(continued)*
    renal r.
    rubella r.
    septic r.
    sickle cell r.
    splenic r.
    stellate r.
    suppurative r.
    thioridazine r.
    toxemic r. of pregnancy
retinopexy
    pneumatic r.
retinophotoscopy
retinopiesis
retinoschisis
retinoscope
    Copeland r.
retinoscopy
retinosis
retinotopic
retinotoxic
retisolution
retispersion
retoperithelium
retort
retract
retractile
retraction
    clot r.
    gingival r.
    head r.
    lid r.
    mandibular r.
    massive vitreous r.
    systolic r.
    uterine r.
retractor
    abdominal r.
    Adson r.
    Agrikola r.
    Allison r.
    Allport r.
    Alm r.
    Amoils r.
    Andrews r.
    Army-Navy r.
    Aufricht r.
    Austin r.
    Balfour r.
    Balfour r. with fenestrated
      blade
    Balfour self-retaining r.
    Ballantine hemilaminectomy r.
    Bankart r.
    Barrett-Adson r.

R

retractor *(continued)*

Barr self-retaining rectal r.
Beardsley esophageal r.
Beckman r.
Beckman-Adson laminectomy r.
Beckman-Eaton laminectomy r.
Beckman goiter r.
Beckman self-retaining r.
Belfield wire r.
Benedict r.
Bennett r.
Berens r.
Berna infant abdominal r.
Bernay tracheal r.
Bethune phrenic r.
Billroth ovarian r.
Blount r.
Brantley-Turner r.
Brawley r.
Brewster r.
Brown r.
Bucy r.
Buie-Smith r.
Byford r.
Campbell r.
Carroll self-retaining spring r.
Carter r.
Castallo r.
Castroviejo r.
Chandler r.
Cherry r.
Cloward r.
Cloward-Hoen r.
cobra r.
Cole r.
Cone r.
contour r.
Cooley r.
Coryllos r.
Cottle r.
Cottle-Neivert r.
Crawford r.
Crile r.
Cushing r.
Davidoff (Davidov) r.
Davidson r.
Davis r.
Deaver r.
DeBakey-Balfour r.
DeBakey-Cooley r.
DeLee r.
D'Errico r.
D'Errico-Adson r.
Desmarres r.
Dingman r.
Doyen r.

retractor *(continued)*

Eastman r.
Elschnig r.
Emmet r.
Farr r.
Ferguson-Moon r.
Ferris-Smith r.
Ferris-Smith-Sewall r.
Fink r.
flexible shaft r.
Foss r.
Franz r.
Frazier r.
Frazier hook r.
French S-shaped r.
Friedman r.
Gelpi r.
Gibson-Balfour r.
Gifford r.
Glenner r.
Goelet r.
Goldstein r.
Gosset r.
Gradle r.
Green r.
Grieshaber r.
Groenholm r.
Gross r.
Gross-Pomeranz-Watkins r.
Guttmann r.
Haight r.
Hajek r.
Hamby r.
Harrington r.
Harrington-Pemberton r.
Hartstein r.
Haslinger r.
Heaney r.
Heaney-Simon r.
Hedblom r.
Henner r.
Hibbs r.
Hill-Ferguson r.
Hillis r.
Hohmann r.
House-Urban r.
Israel r.
Jackson r.
Jacobson r.
Jansen r.
Judd r.
Judd-Masson r.
Kelly r.
Kerrison r.
Killian-King r.
King r.

retractor *(continued)*
    Kirby r.
    Klemme r.
    Knapp r.
    Kocher r.
    Kocher-Crotti r.
    Krasky r.
    Kronfeld r.
    Lahey r.
    Latrobe r.
    Legueu r.
    Lempert r.
    Linton r.
    Little r.
    Lothrop r.
    Love r.
    Luer r.
    Lukens r.
    Luongo r.
    Martin r.
    Masson-Judd r.
    Mayo r.
    Mayo-Collins r.
    Mayo-Lovelace r.
    McGannon r.
    Meller r.
    Meyer r.
    Meyerding r.
    Millin-Bacon r.
    Moorehead r.
    Mueller r.
    Murphy r.
    Neivert r.
    Oldberg r.
    O'Sullivan r.
    O'Sullivan-O'Connor r.
    palate r.
    Parker r.
    periosteal r.
    Pheifer-Young r.
    Pierce r.
    Proctor r.
    Pryor-Péan r.
    Purcell r.
    rake r.
    Rankin r.
    rib r.
    Richardson r.
    Richardson-Eastman r.
    Rigby r.
    Rizzo r.
    Rizzuti r.
    Robinson r.
    Rochester-Ferguson r.
    Rollet r.
    Ross r.

retractor *(continued)*
    Roux r.
    Sachs r.
    Schuknecht r.
    Scoville r.
    self-retaining r.
    Semb r.
    Senn r.
    Senn-Dingman r.
    Shambaugh r.
    Sheldon r.
    Shurly r.
    Sims r.
    Sims-Kelly r.
    Sistrunk r.
    Sloan r.
    Sluder r.
    Smith-Buie r.
    Snitman r.
    Stevenson r.
    Sweet r.
    Taylor r.
    Theis r.
    tonsil pillar r.
    Tower r.
    Tuffier r.
    Tuffier-Raney r.
    Ullrich r.
    Veenema r.
    vein r.
    Volkmann r.
    Walker r.
    Walter-Deaver r.
    Webster r.
    Weinberg r.
    Weitlaner r.
    Wesson r.
    White-Proud r.
    Wolfson r.
    Wullstein r.
    Yasargil r.
    Young r.
retrad
retreat
    vegetative r.
retrenchment
retrieval
    information r.
retroaction
retroauricular
    r. approach
    r. area
    r. calvarial bone island flap
    r. fistula
    r. flap
    r. incision

R

retroauricular *(continued)*
    r. myoperiosteal graft
    pedicled r. island flap
    r. region
    reverse-flow r. island flap
    r. skin-cartilage composite graft
    r. skin island
    r. sulcus
retrobuccal
retrobulbar
retrocalcaneobursitis
retrocatheterism
retrocecal
retrocedent
retrocervical
retrocessed
retrocession of uterus
retroclination
retrocochlear
retrocolic
retrocollic
retrocollis
retroconduction
retrocrural
retrocursive
retrodeviation
retrodisplacement
retroduodenal
retrodural
retrofilling
retroflexed
retroflexion of uterus
retrogasserian
    r. neurectomy
    r. neurotomy
    r. rhizotomy
retrognathia
retrognathic
retrograde
    r. amnesia
    r. angiocardiography
    r. aortography
    r. approach
    balloon-occluded r.
       transvenous obliteration
    r. cannulation
    r. cardioangiography
    r. catheter
    r. cystography
    r. cystourethrography
    r. ejaculation
    endoscopic r.
       cholangiopancreatography
       (ERCP)
    endoscopic r. pancreatography

retrograde *(continued)*
    r. fashion
    r. flow
    r. nail insertion
    peroral r. pancreaticobiliary
       ductography
    r. pulmonary embolectomy
    r. pulmonary vein perfusion
    r. pyelography
    r. reflux
    r. urethrogram
    r. urography
    r. venography
retrography
retrogression
retroillumination
retroinfection
retroinsular
retroiridian
retrojection
retrolabyrinthine
retrolental
retrolenticular
retrolisthesis
retromammary
retromandibular
retromastoid
retromolar
retromorphosis
retronasal
retro-ocular
retro-orbital
retropatellar
retroperitoneal
    r. pneumography
    r. pneumoradiography
retroperitoneum
retroperitonitis
retropharyngeal
retropharyngitis
retropharynx
retroplacental
retroplasia
retroposed
retroposition
retropubic
    r. prevesical prostatectomy
    radical r. prostatectomy
retropulsion
retrorsine
retrosinus
retrosplenial
retrospondylolisthesis
retrostalsis
retrosternal

retrosymphysial
retrotarsal
retrourethral catheterization
retrouterine
retroversioflexion
retroversion
    acetabular r.
    anteversion-r.
    glenoid r.
    humeral head r.
    r. index
    uterine r., r. of uterus
retroverted
    r. acetabulum
    r. coccyx
    r. ears
    r. epiglottis
    r. hemipelvis
    r. implant
    r. pelvis
    r. and retroflexed uterus
    r. uterus
retrovesical
retrovirus
    human lymphotrophic r.
    lymphotropic r.
retrusion
    mandibular r.
Rett syndrome
Retter needle
return
    r. flow hemostatic
      catheter
    venous r.
Retzius
    cavity
    fibers
    foramen
    lines
    parallel striae
    space
    striae
    stripes
    veins
Reuss
    color charts
    tables
Reuter tube
revaccination
revascularization
    myocardial r.
revehent veins
Reverdin
    graft
    needle

Reverdin *(continued)*
    operation
reversal
    epinephrine r.
    r.-formation
    r. of gradient
    sex r.
reverse-bevel laryngoscope
reverse transcriptase
reversible
reversion
    antigenic r.
    genotypic r.
    Mantoux r.
    phenotypic r.
    true r.
revertant
revision
    r. canal wall down
      mastoidectomy
    surgical r.
    r. total hip arthroplasty
    r. total joint arthroplasty
    ventricular outflow tract r.
    W-plasty r.
    Z-plasty r.
revival
revivescence
revivification
revolute
revolution
    demographic r.
revulsant
revulsion
revulsive
reward
    token r.
rewarming
Rexed laminae
Reye syndrome
Reynals permeability factor
Reynold test
RF—
    radiofrequency, radio
      frequency
    Reitland-Franklin unit
    relative fluorescence
    releasing factor
    rheumatoid factor
RFA—
    right femoral artery
    right frontoanterior (position)
RFB—retained foreign body
RFLA—rheumatoid factor–like
  activity

R

RFLP—restriction fragment length polymorphism
RFP—right frontoposterior (position)
RFS—renal function study
RFT—
    right frontotransverse (position)
    rod-and-frame test
RFW—rapid-filling wave
RG—right gluteal
RGP—rigid gas-permeable (contact lens)
rh—rheumatic
Rh—rhesus factor
Rh −, Rh neg—rhesus factor–negative
Rh +, Rh pos—rhesus factor–positive
Rh
    antibody
    blood group
    blood type
    factor
    immunization
    incompatibility
    isoantigen
RH—
    relative humidity
    releasing hormone
rhabditic dermatitis
rhabditiform
Rhabditis
    R. hominis
    R. intestinalis
    R. niellyi
    R. pellio
    R. strongyloides
rhabdoid suture
rhabdomyoblast
rhabdomyoblastoma
rhabdomyochondroma
rhabdomyolysis
    exertional r.
    familial paroxysmal r.
    idiopathic r.
rhabdomyoma
rhabdomyomyxoma
rhabdomyosarcoma
rhabdos
rhabdosarcoma
    renal r.
rhabdosphincter
rhabdovirus
rhacoma
rhaebocrania
rhaeboscelia

rhaebosis
rhagades
rhagadiform
rhagiocrine
rhagionid
rhamninose
rhamnose
rhamnoside
RHD—relative hepatic dullness
rhegma
rhegmatogenous
Rhein picks
Rheinberg microscope
rhenium (Re)
rheobase
rheoencephalography
rheology
rheometry
rheonome
rheoscope
rheostat
rheostosis
rheotachygraphy
rheotaxis
    negative r.
    positive r.
rheotome
rheotrope
rheotropism
rhesus (Rh)
    r. factor
    r. isoimmunization
rheuma
rheumatalgia
rheumatic
    r. disease
    r. factor
    r. fever
    r. heart disease
    r. pneumonia
rheumatid
rheumatism
    acute articular r.
    apoplectic r.
    articular r., acute
    articular r., chronic
    Besnier r.
    cerebral r.
    chronic articular r.
    desert r.
    gonorrheal r.
    r. of the heart
    Heberden r.
    inflammatory r.
    lumbar r.

rheumatism *(continued)*
    MacLeod capsular r.
    muscular r.
    nodose r.
    nonarticular r.
    osseous r.
    palindromic r.
    Poncet r.
    subacute r.
    synovial r.
    tuberculous r.
    visceral r.
rheumatismal
rheumatogenic
rheumatoid
    r. arthritis (RA)
    r. factor
    r. nodule
    r. vasculitis
rheumatologic
rheumatologist
rheumatology
rheumatosis
rheumic
rhexis
rhigosis
rhigotic
rhinal
rhinalgia
rhinallergosis
rhinectomy
    total r.
rhinedema
rhinencephalic
rhinencephalon
rhinenchysis
rhinesthesia
rhineurynter
rhinion
rhinism
rhinitis
    acute r.
    acute catarrhal r.
    allergic r.
    anaphylactic r.
    atopic r.
    atrophic r.
    r. caseosa
    catarrhal r.
    chronic r.
    chronic catarrhal r.
    croupous r.
    dyscrinic r.
    fibrinous r.
    gangrenous r.

rhinitis *(continued)*
    granulomatous r.
    hypertrophic r.
    inclusion body r.
    infectious r.
    infective r.
    influenzal r.
    intrinsic r.
    r. medicamentosa
    membranous r.
    necrotic r.
    non-airflow r.
    nonseasonal allergic r.
    perennial r.
    perennial allergic r.
    periodic r.
    polypoid r.
    porcine inclusion
      body r.
    pseudomembranous r.
    purulent r.
    seasonal allergic r.
    scrofulous r.
    r. sicca
    suppurative r.
    syphilitic r.
    tuberculous r.
    vasomotor r.
rhinoanemometer
rhinoantritis
rhinobyon
rhinocanthectomy
rhinocephalus
rhinocephaly
rhinocheiloplasty
rhinocleisis
rhinocoele
rhinodacryolith
rhinodymia
rhinodynia
rhinoentomophthoromycosis
rhinogenous
rhinohyperplasia
rhinokyphectomy
rhinokyphosis
rhinolalia
    r. aperta
    r. clausa
    open r.
rhinolaryngitis
rhinolaryngology
rhinolith
rhinolithiasis
rhinologist
rhinology

R

rhinomanometer
rhinomanometry
rhinommectomy
rhinomycosis
rhinonecrosis
rhinonemmeter
rhinoneurosis
rhinopathia vasomotoria
rhinopathy
　　vasomotor r.
rhinopharyngeal
rhinopharyngitis mutilans
rhinopharyngocele
rhinopharyngolith
rhinopharynx
rhinophonia
rhinophycomycosis
rhinophyma
rhinoplastic
rhinoplasty
　　augmentation r.
　　Carpue r.
　　English r.
　　Indian r.
　　Italian r.
　　Joseph r.
　　reconstructive r.
　　submucous resection and r.
　　　(SMRR)
　　tagliacotian r.
　　Tagliacozzi r.
rhinopolypus
rhinorrhagia
rhinorrhaphy
rhinorrhea
　　cerebrospinal fluid
　　　(CSF) r.
rhinosalpingitis
rhinoscleroma
rhinoscope
rhinoscopic
rhinoscopy
　　anterior r.
　　median r.
　　posterior r.
rhinosinusitis
rhinosporidiosis
Rhinosporidium seeberi
rhinostegnosis
rhinostenosis
rhinotomy
　　lateral r.
rhinoviral
rhinovirus
rhizanesthesia

rhizodontropy
rhizodontrypy
rhizoid
rhizolysis
rhizomelia
rhizomelic
rhizomeningomyelitis
rhizomere
rhizoneure
Rhizopus
　　R. oryzae
　　R. rhizopodoformis
rhizotomy
　　anterior r.
　　chemical r.
　　dorsal r.
　　glycerol r.
　　percutaneous r.
　　percutaneous radiofrequency r.
　　posterior r.
　　retrogasserian r.
　　trigeminal r.
RHL—right hepatic lobe
RHLN—right hilar lymph node
rhm—roentgen(s) (per) hour
　(at one) meter
Rh_{null} syndrome [Rh-null]
rho
　　Greek letter
　　　(ρ; alphabetized as r)
　　Spearman r.
rhodamine
　　r. B
　　r. isothiocyanate
rhodanate
rhodanese
rhodanic acid
rhodanine
Rhodin fixative
rhodium (Rh)
Rhodnius prolixus
rhodogenesis
rhodomycin
rhodophylactic
rhodophylaxis
rhodopsin
Rhodotorula
　　R. glutinis
　　R. rubra
rhodotorulosis
rhodotoxin
RhoGAM test
rhombencephalic
rhombencephalitis
rhombencephalon

rhombocoele
rhomboid
    Michaelis r.
rhombomere
rhonchal, rhonchial
rhonchial
rhonchus (rhonchi)
    audible rhonchi
    bibasilar rhonchi
    bilateral rhonchi
    coarse rhonchi
    diffuse rhonchi
    expiratory rhonchi
    faint rhonchi
    few rhonchi
    harsh rhonchi
    high-pitched rhonchi
    humming rhonchi
    inspiratory rhonchi
    low-pitched rhonchi
    marked rhonchi
    musical rhonchi
    occasional rhonchi
    post-tussive inspiratory
      rhonchi
    rare rhonchi
    scattered rhonchi
    sibilant rhonchi
    sonorous rhonchi
    upper respiratory rhonchi
    whistling rhonchi
rhoptry
rhotacism
Rh sensitization
rhubarb
Rhus
    R. diversiloba
    R. radicans
    R. toxicodendron
    R. vernix
rhus dermatitis
rhythm
    accelerated atrioventricular
      (AV) junctional r.
    accelerated idioventricular r.
    agonal r.
    alpha r.
    atrial r.
    atrial escape r.
    atrioventricular r.
    atrioventricular (AV)
      junctional r.
    atrioventricular (AV)
      junctional escape r.
    atrioventricular (AV) nodal r.

rhythm *(continued)*
    Berger r.
    beta r.
    bigeminal r.
    biologic r.
    biological r.
    cantering r.
    cardiac r.
    circadian r.
    circamensual r.
    circannual r.
    circaseptan r.
    circus r.
    coronary sinus r.
    coupled r.
    delta r.
    ectopic r.
    escape r.
    fetal r.
    gallop r.
    gallop r., systolic
    gamma r.
    idionodal r.
    idioventricular r.
    infradian r.
    junctional r.
    junctional escape r.
    mu r.
    nodal r.
    nyctohemeral r.
    parasystolic r.
    pendulum r.
    quadrigeminal r.
    quadruple r.
    reciprocal r.
    reciprocating r.
    reentrant r.
    reversed r.
    sinoatrial r.
    sinus r.
    sinusoidal r.
    supraventricular r.
    theta r.
    train-wheel r.
    triple r.
    ultradian r.
    ventricular r.
    ventricular escape r.
rhythmic
    aberrant r. activity
    r. artifact
    r. contractions
    r. cortical myoclonus
    r. delivery of chemotherapy
      drugs

R

rhythmic *(continued)*
    r. handgrip exercise
    high-frequency r. cortical
      myoclonus
    intermittent r. delta activity
    r. movement disorder
    multifocal r. myoclonic jerks
    r. notched theta waves
    r. pattern
    r. theta-delta activity
    r. twitching
rhythmical
    r. nystagmus
    r. vasomotion
rhythmically
rhythmicity
    circadian r.
    slow wave r.
rhytidectomy
rhytidoplasty
rhytidosis
RI—
    recession index
    regional ileitis
    respiratory illness
RIA—radioimmunoassay
rib
    abdominal r's
    asternal r's
    bicipital r.
    bifid r.
    branched r.
    cervical r.
    false r's
    floating r's
    fused r.
    slipping r.
    spurious r's
    sternal r's
    sternebral r.
    Stiller r.
    true r's
    vertebral r's
    vertebrochondral r's
    vertebrocostal r's
    vertebrosternal r's
    Zahn r's
ribbon
    r. gut suture
    r. of Reil
    r. stools
    synaptic r.
rib contractor
    Bailey r.c.
    Bailey-Gibbon r.c.
    Sellor r.c.

rib cutter
    Bethune r.c.
Ribes ganglion
ribodesose
riboflavin kinase
ribofuranose
ribofuranosyladenine
ribofuranosylcytosine
ribofuranosylguanine
ribonuclear protein
ribonuclease
    r. I
    r. II
    pancreatic r.
    r. S
ribonucleic acid (RNA)
    heterogenous nuclear RNA
      (hnRNA)
    messenger RNA (mRNA)
    ribosomal RNA (rRNA)
    transfer RNA (tRNA)
ribonucleoprotein
ribonucleoside diphosphate
    reductase
ribonucleotide reductase
riboprine
ribopyranose
ribose
    r. nucleic acid
    r.-5-phosphate isomerase
    r.-phosphate
      pyrophosphokinase
riboside
ribosomal
ribosome
ribosuria
ribosylthymine
5-ribosyluracil
ribothymidine
ribovirus
rib shears
    Bethune r.s.
    Giertz-Shoemaker r.s.
    Gluck r.s.
    Moure-Coryllos r.s.
    Potts r.s.
    Shoemaker r.s.
rib spreader
    Burford r.s.
    Finochietto r.s.
    Harken r.s.
    Lemmon r.s.
    Lilienthal-Sauerbruch r.s.
    Rienhoff-Finochietto r.s.
    Tuffier r.s.
    Wilson r.s.

rib stripper
  Dorian r.s.
ribulose-phosphate 3-epimerase
Ricard amputation
rice
  r. polishings
  white r.
Richards
  curet
  screw
Richardson
  retractor
  sign
  suture
  technique
Richardson-Eastman retractor
Richards-Rundle syndrome
Richet
  aneurysm
  fascia
  operation
Richner-Hanhart syndrome
Richter
  hernia
  suture
  syndrome
Richter-Monro line
ricinism
ricinoleic acid
rickets
  acute r.
  adult r.
  anticonvulsant r.
  autosomal dominant vitamin
    D–resistant r.
  beryllium r.
  celiac r.
  familial hypophosphatemic r.
  familial vitamin D–resistant r.
  fat r.
  fetal r.
  hemorrhagic r.
  hepatic r.
  hereditary hypophosphatemic
    r. with hypercalciuria
  hypophosphatemic r.
  late r.
  lean r.
  oncogenous r.
  pancreatic r.
  pseudodeficiency r.
  pseudovitamin D–deficiency r.
  refractory r.
  renal r.
  resistant r.
  scurvy r.

rickets (continued)
  tardy r.
  vitamin D–dependent r.,
    type I
  vitamin D-dependent r.,
    type II
  vitamin D–refractory r.
  vitamin D–resistant r.
rickettsemia
Rickettsia
  R. africae
  R. akari
  R. australis
  R. conorii
  R. honei
  R. japonica
  R. parkeri
  R. prowazekii
  R. rickettsii
  R. sennetsu
  R. sibirica
  R. typhi
  R. typhi (mooseri)
rickettsia (rickettsiae)
rickettsial
rickettsialpox
rickettsicidal
rickettsiology
rickettsiosis
  canine r.
  north Asian tick-borne r.
rickettsiostatic
Rickham reservoir
Rickham-Salmon reservoir
rictal
rictus
RID—radial immunodiffusion
Riddoch
  phenomenon
  syndrome
Ridell operation
rider's
  r. bone
  r. bursa
  r. leg
  r. muscles
  r. sprain
  r. tendon
ridge
  alveolar r.
  alveolar r., residual
  anal r.
  apical ectodermal r.
  basal r.
  bicipital r., anterior
  bicipital r., external

R

ridge *(continued)*
- bicipital r., internal
- bicipital r., outer
- bicipital r., posterior
- buccocervical r.
- buccogingival r.
- bulbar r's
- carotid r.
- cerebral r's of cranial bones
- deltoid r.
- dental r.
- dermal r's
- digital r's
- edentulous r.
- epicondylic r., lateral
- epicondylic r., medial
- epipericardial r.
- fingerprint r.
- ganglion r.
- gastrocnemial r.
- genital r.
- germ r.
- gluteal r. of femur
- gonadal r.
- healing r.
- r. of humerus
- incisal r.
- interarticular r. of head of rib
- interosseous r.
- interosseous r. of fibula
- interosseous r. of radius
- interosseous r. of tibia
- interosseous r. of ulna
- intertrochanteric r.
- interureteric r.
- linguocervical r., linguogingival r.
- longitudinal r. of hard palate
- Mall r.
- mammary r.
- r. of mandibular neck
- marginal r.
- medullary r.
- mesonephric r.
- middle r. of femur
- milk r.
- mylohyoid r.
- r. of neck of rib
- nephrogenic r.
- neural r.
- r. of nose
- oblique r.

ridge *(continued)*
- oblique r's of scapula
- palatine r's, transverse
- papillary r's
- Passavant r.
- pectoral r.
- pharyngeal r.
- pterygoid r.
- pulmonary r.
- radial r. of wrist
- residual r.
- residual alveolar r.
- rete r's
- rough r. of femur
- semicircular r.
- semicircular r. of parietal bone, inferior
- semicircular r. of parietal bone, superior
- skin r's
- sphenoid r.
- sublingual r.
- superciliary r.
- supinator r.
- supplemental r.
- supracondylar r., of humerus, lateral
- supracondylar r., of humerus, medial
- supraepicondylar r. of humerus, lateral
- supraepicondylar r. of humerus, medial
- supracondylar r., lateral
- supracondylar r., medial
- supraorbital r.
- suprarenal r.
- synaptic r.
- taste r's
- temporal r.
- tentorial r.
- transverse r.
- transverse r's of sacrum
- transverse r's of vaginal wall
- trapezoid r.
- triangular r.
- tubercular r. of sacrum
- ulnar r. of wrist
- urethral r.
- urogenital r.
- wolffian r.

ridge lap

ridging

Ridley sinus

Ridlon operation
Ridpath curet
Riecker bronchoscope
Riedel
    disease
    lobe
    struma
    thyroiditis
Rieder
    cell
    cell leukemia
    lymphocyte
    paralysis
    syndrome
Riegel pulse
Rieger
    anomaly
    dysgenesis
    syndrome
Riegler test
Riehl melanosis
Rienhoff
    clamp
    forceps
Riesman
    myocardosis
    pneumonia
    sign
Rietti-Greppi-Micheli anemia
Rieux hernia
RIF—right iliac fossa
Rift Valley fever
Riga-Fede disease
Rigby retractor
Riggs disease
right-angle
    r.-a. mattress suture
    r.-a. telescope
right-eyed
right-handed
right-sided angiocardiography
rigid gas-permeable (RGP)
    contact lens
rigidity
    α-r. [alpha-]
    anatomical r.
    cadaveric r.
    catatonic r.
    cerebellar r.
    clasp-knife r.
    cogwheel r.
    congenital articular r.
    decerebrate r.
    decorticate r.
    extrapyramidal r.

rigidity (continued)
    γ-r. [gamma-]
    hemiplegic r.
    hysterical r.
    lead-pipe r.
    muscular r.
    mydriatic r.
    nuchal r.
    pallidal r.
    paratonic r.
    parkinsonian r.
    pathologic r.
    postmortem r.
    spasmodic r.
    spastic r.
RigiScan
    device
    measurement
    penile tumescence monitor
rigor
    acid r.
    calcium r.
    heat r.
    instantaneous r. mortis
    r. mortis
    r. nervorum
    r. tremens
    water r.
rigors
RIH—right inguinal hernia
RIHSA—radioactive iodinated
    human serum albumin
Riley virus
Riley-Day
    dysautonomia
    syndrome
Riley-Shwachman syndrome
Riley-Smith syndrome
rim
    r. of abrasion
    bite r., bite-r.
    r. incision
    occlusion r.
    record r.
rima (rimae)
    r. ani, r. clunium
    r. glottidis
    r. glottidis cartilaginea
    r. glottidis membranacea
    intercartilaginous r.
    intermembranous r.
    r. oris
    r. palpebrarum
    r. pudendi
    r. respiratoria

R

rima (rimae) *(continued)*
    r. vestibuli
    r. vocalis
    r. vulvae
RIMA—
    right internal mammary
        anastomosis
    right internal mammary
        artery
rimae (plural of rima)
rimal
rimose
rimula
RIND—reversible ischemic
    neurologic disability
Rindfleisch
    cells
    folds
RINE—reversible ischemic
    neurologic event
ring
    Abbe r's
    abdominal r.
    abdominal inguinal r.
    abdominal r., deep
    abdominal r., external
    abdominal r., internal
    abdominal r., superficial
    Albl r.
    amnion r.
    anal r.
    annular r's
    annular r. of Gerlach
    anorectal r.
    apical r.
    atrial r.
    atrioventricular r's,
    atrioventricular valve r's
    Balbiani r.
    Bandl r.
    benzene r.
    Bickel r.
    Bonaccolto scleral r.
    r. of bone
    Braun r.
    Cabot r's
    Cannon r.
    carbocyclic r.
    cardiac lymphatic r.
    Carpentier r.
    casting r.
    ciliary r. of iris
    circumaortic venous r.
    closing r. of Winkler-
        Waldeyer

ring *(continued)*
    Coats r.
    common tendinous r.
    conjunctival r.
    constriction r.
    contact r.
    contractile r.
    contraction r.
    coronary r.
    crural r.
    cytoplasmic r.
    Döllinger tendinous r.
    Donder r.
    Duran r.
    Effler r.
    esophageal r.
    esophageal contraction r.
    esophagogastric r.
    Falope r.
    femoral r.
    fibrocartilaginous r. of
        tympanic membrane
    fibrous r's of heart
    fibrous r., interpubic
    fibrous r. of intervertebral disk
    Fleischer keratoconus r.
    Fleischer-Strümpell r.
    Flieringa r.
    r. forceps
    r. fracture
    furan r.
    germ r.
    glaucomatous r.
    Graefenberg r.
    halo r.
    hernial r.
    heterocyclic r.
    homocyclic r.
    hymenal r.
    infancy r.
    inguinal r.
    inguinal r., deep
    inguinal r., external
    inguinal r., internal
    inguinal r., superficial
    interpubic fibrous r.
    r. of iris, greater
    r. of iris, lesser
    isocyclic r.
    Kayser-Fleischer r.
    Landolt r.
    left fibrous r. of heart
    Liesegang r's
    Löwe r.
    Lower r's

ring *(continued)*
    lower esophageal contraction r.
    lymphoid r.
    Maxwell r.
    middle r.
    mitral r.
    mitral valve r.
    neonatal r.
    Newton r's
    nucleoplasmic r.
    Ochsner r.
    olive r.
    pathologic retraction r.
    pericorneal lymphatic r.
    periosteal bone r.
    pelvic r.
    physiologic retraction r.
    pleural r's
    polar r.
    posterior limiting r.
    pyran r.
    retraction r.
    right fibrous r. of heart
    Schatzki r.
    Schwalbe anterior border r.
    scleral r.
    r. scotoma
    sewing r.
    signet r.
    Soemmering r.
    subchorial closing r.
    tantalum r.
    tendinous r., common
    terminal r.
    tonsillar r.
    tracheal r's
    tricuspid r.
    tricuspid valve r.
    tympanic r.
    umbilical r.
    vascular r.
    venous r. of Haller
    r. of Vieussens
    Vossius lenticular r.
    Waldeyer tonsillar r.
    Wimberger r.
    Zinn r.
ring-bone
    low r.
Ringer
    injection, lactated
    irrigation
    lactate
    mixture
    solution, lactated

ring-knife
Ring-McLean catheter
ringworm
    anthropophilic r.
    r. of axillae
    r. of the beard
    black-dot r.
    r. of the body
    crusted r.
    ectothrix r.
    endothrix r.
    r. of the face
    r. of the feet
    geophilic r.
    gray-patch r.
    r. of the groin
    r. of the hand
    honeycomb r.
    hypertrophic r.
    r. of the nails
    Oriental r.
    r. of the scalp
    Tokelau r.
Rinne
    response
    test, modified
Riolan
    anastomosis
    arch
    bone
    muscle
    nosegay
    ossicle
RIP—radioimmunoprecipitation
RIPA—radioimmunoprecipitation
  assay
riparian
ripe cataract
ripple voltage
RISA—radioactive iodinated serum
  albumin
Risdon
    extraoral incision
    wire
risk
    absolute r.
    assumption of r.
    attributable r.
    r.-benefit ratio
    competing r.
    empiric r.
    genetic r.
    insurable r.
    population attributable r.
    relative r.

R

Risley prism
Risser
    cast
    jacket
RIST—radioimmunosorbent test
Ristella melaninogenica
risus sardonicus
RITC—rhodamine isothiocyanate
Ritchie tenaculum
Ritgen
    maneuver
    method
Ritter
    disease
    fiber
ritual
RIU—radioactive iodine uptake
rivalry
    binocular r.
    retinal r.
    sibling r.
Rivalta
    reaction
    test
Riva-Rocci sphygmomanometer
Rivers cocktail
Rives splenectomy
Riviere sign
rivinian
Rivinus
    canals
    ducts
    foramen
    gland
    incisure
    membrane
    notch
    segment
rivus lacrimalis
riziform
Rizzo retractor
Rizzuti retractor
RK—
    radial keratotomy
    right kidney
RKY—roentgen kymography
RL—
    right leg
    right lung
RLC—residual lung capacity
RLD—related living donor
RLE—right lower extremity
RLF—retrolental fibroplasia
RLL—right lower lobe (of lung)
RLN—recurrent laryngeal nerve

RLP—radiation-leukemia-
    protection
RLQ—right lower quadrant
RLS—Ringer lactated solution
RM—
    radical mastectomy
    respiratory movement
RMA—right mentoanterior
    (position)
R-meter
RMK—rhesus monkey kidney
RML—right middle lobe
RMP—
    rapidly miscible pool
    right mentoposterior (position)
RMS—root-mean-square
RMT—
    retromolar trigone
    right mentotransverse
    (position)
RMV—respiratory minute volume
RN, R.N.—registered nurse
RNA—ribonucleic acid
RNA
    ambisense RNA
    RNA amplification technique
    antisense RNA (asRNA)
    complementary RNA (cRNA)
    DNA-directed RNA
        polymerase
    RNA-directed DNA
        polymerase
    RNA-directed RNA
        polymerase
    heterogenous nuclear RNA
    RNA-induced silencing
        complex
    informational RNA
    RNA interference
    messenger RNA
    negative-sense RNA
    nuclear RNA (nRNA)
    polycistronic messenger RNA
    RNA polymerase
    positive-sense RNA
    precursor RNA
    pre-mRNA, pre-messenger
        RNA
    pre-rRNA, pre-ribosomal RNA
    pre-tRNA, pre-transfer RNA
    RNA processing
    RNA replicase
    ribosomal RNA (rRNA)
    small interfering RNA
        (siRNA)

RNA *(continued)*
    small nuclear RNA (snRNA)
    small nucleolar RNA
        (snRNA)
    soluble RNA
    RNA splicing
    template RNA
    transfer RNA (tRNA)
    RNA virus
RNAi—RNA interference
RNA nucleotidyltransferase
RNase
RND—radical neck dissection
RNP—ribonucleoprotein
RO—Ritter-Oleson (technique)
RO, R/O—rule out
ROA—right occipitoanterior
    (position)
roach
Robb forceps
Robert
    ligament
    pelvis
Roberts
    applicator
    esophagoscope
    forceps
    laryngoscope
    operation
    test
Robertshaw tube
Robertson
    forceps
    knife
    pupil
    sign
robertsonian translocation
Robin
    anomalad
    syndrome
Robinson
    catheter, red
    disease
    protractor
    retractor
    stone dislodger
Robinul
Robison ester dehydrogenase
Robles disease
roborant
Robson
    line
    point
    position
robust

robustness
ROC—receiver operating
    characteristics (curve)
Rochester
    awl
    connector
    elevator
    forceps
    knife
    needle
Rochester-Carmalt forceps
Rochester-Ewald forceps
Rochester-Ferguson
    retractor
    scissors
Rochester-Mixter forceps
Rochester-Ochsner forceps
Rochester-Péan forceps
Rochester-Rankin forceps
Rochon-Duvigneaud
    syndrome
rocker-bottom foot
Rockey
    cannula
    clamp
    endoscope
    forceps
Rockey-Davis incision
rocking microtome
Rock-Mulligan hood
rod
    analyzing r.
    Auer r.
    basal r.
    r. of Corti
    Cotrel-Dubousset r.
    enamel r's
    germinal r.
    Harrington r.
    r's of Heidenhain
    House r.
    Knodt r.
    König (Koenig) r's
    Luque r.
    Maddox r's
    Meckel r.
    muscle r.
    olfactory r.
    Reichmann r's
    retinal r.
    Rush r.
rodent
rodenticide
rodentine
rodocaine

R

Roeder
  forceps
  treatment
Roederer
  ecchymosis
  obliquity
roentgen (R)
  r.-equivalent-man (rem)
  r. kymography (RKY)
  r's per second (R/s)
  r. tube
roentgenocinematography
roentgenogram
roentgenograph
roentgenographic
roentgenography
  body section r.
  double-contrast r.
  magnification r.
  mass r.
  mucosal relief r.
  sectional r.
  selective r.
  spot film r.
roentgenologic,
  roentgenological
roentgenologist
roentgenology
roentgenolucent
roentgenometer
roentgenometry
roentgenopaque
roentgenoparent
roentgenoscope
roentgenoscopy
roentgenotherapy
  intraoral r.
roentgen rays
roentgentherapy
  intraoral r.
  intravaginal r.
roflurane
Roger
  bruit
  disease
  dissector
  murmur
  reaction
  reflex
  sphygmomanometer
  symptom
Roger-Josué test
Rogers sphygmomanometer
Röhl (Roehl) marginal
  corpuscles

Roida tube
Rokitansky
  disease
  diverticulum
  hernia
  kidney
  pelvis
Rokitansky-Aschoff sinus
Rokitansky-Cushing ulcer
Rokitansky-Küster-Hauser
  syndrome
Rolandi
  substantia r.
rolandic fissure
Rolando
  angle
  cells
  fasciculus
  line
  tubercle
role
  gender r.
role-playing
Rolf
  forceps
  lance
rolfing
roll
  cotton r.
  iliac r.
  jelly r.
  scleral r.
  r. tube
roller
Roller nucleus
Rollet
  chancre
  incision
  irrigator
  retractor
  syndrome
Rollier
  radiation
  treatment
ROM—
  range of motion
  rupture of membranes
Romaña sign
Romanowsky
  method
  stain
Romberg
  disease
  facial hemiatrophy
  sign

Romberg *(continued)*
> spasm
> station
> syndrome
> test
> trophoneurosis

Romberg-Howship syndrome
rombergism
ROMI—rule out myocardial
  infarction
rongeur
> Adson r.
> Beyer r.
> Cloward r.
> Converse r.
> DeVilbiss r.
> duckbill r.
> Dufourmentel r.
> gooseneck r.
> Hartmann r.
> Hartmann-Herzfeld r.
> Hoffmann r.
> Husks r.
> Ivy r.
> Kerrison r.
> Leksell r.
> Lombard-Boies r.
> Love-Gruenwald r.
> Rowland r.
> Ruskin r.
> Schlesinger r.
> Spurling r.
> Stille-Luer r.
> Tobey r.
> Whiting r.

ronnel
Rood method
roof
> r. of fourth ventricle
> r. of lateral ventricle
> r. of mouth
> r. of nasal cavity
> nasopharyngeal r.
> r. of nasopharynx
> r. of orbit
> r. of skull
> r. of third ventricle
> r. of tympanic cavity
> r. of tympanum

room
> anechoic r.
> birthing r.
> consulting r.
> delivery r.
> emergency r.

room *(continued)*
> intensive therapy r.
> labor r.
> operating r.
> postdelivery r.
> predelivery r.
> recovery r.

rooming-in
Roosevelt clamp
Roos test
root
> anatomical r.
> r's of ansa cervicalis
> anterior r. of ansa cervicalis
> anterior r. of spinal nerve
> anterior r. of zygomatic
>   process of temporal bone
> r. of aorta, aortic r.
> r. of arch of vertebra
> belladonna r.
> bitter r.
> r. of brachial plexus
> clinical r.
> r. of clitoris
> cochlear r. of acoustic nerve
> cochlear r. of vestibulocochlear
>   nerve
> cranial r's of accessory nerve
> r. curettement
> deadly nightshade r.
> descending r. of trigeminal
>   nerve
> dorsal r.
> dorsal r. of spinal nerve
> facial r., r. of facial hair
> r. of hair
> inferior r. of ansa cervicalis
> inferior r. of vestibulocochlear
>   nerve
> intermediate r. of olfactory
>   trigone
> internal olfactory r.
> lateral and medial r's of
>   olfactory trigone
> lateral r. of median nerve
> lateral r. of optic nerve
> licorice r.
> lingual r.
> long r. of ciliary ganglion
> r. of lung
> mandrake r.
> medial r. of median nerve
> medial r. of optic tract
> mesencephalic r. of trigeminal
>   nerve

R

root *(continued)*

r. of mesentery
middle r. of zygomatic process
motor r.
motor r. of ciliary ganglion
motor r. of mandibular nerve
motor r. of spinal nerve
motor r's of submandibular
    ganglion
motor r. of trigeminal nerve
r. of nail
nasociliary r. of ciliary
    ganglion
nerve r's
nerve r., motor
nerve r., sensory
r. of nose
oculomotor r. of ciliary
    ganglion
r. of optic tract, lateral
r. of optic tract, medial
orizaba jalap r.
orris r.
r. of otic ganglion
palatine r.
parasympathetic r. of ciliary
    ganglion
parasympathetic r. of otic
    ganglion
parasympathetic r. of
    pterygopalatine ganglion
parasympathetic r. of
    sublingual ganglion
parasympathetic r. of
    submandibular ganglion
penile r.
r. of penis
posterior r. of ansa cervicalis
posterior r. of zygomatic
    process of temporal bone
psychological r.
puccoon r.
red r.
r. resection
retained r.
sensory r. of ciliary ganglion
sensory r. of mandibular
    nerve
sensory r. of otic ganglion
sensory r. of pterygopalatine
    ganglion
sensory r. of spinal nerve
sensory r. of submandibular
    ganglion
sensory r. of trigeminal nerve

root *(continued)*

short r. of ciliary ganglion
spinal r's
spinal r's of accessory nerve
r's of spinal nerve
r. of spinal nerves, anterior
r. of spinal nerves, motor
r. of spinal nerves, posterior
r. of spinal nerves, sensory
spinal vestibular r.
superior r. of ansa cervicalis
superior r. of vestibulocochlear
    nerve
sweet r.
sympathetic r's of ciliary
    ganglion
sympathetic r. of
    pterygopalatine ganglion
third r. of zygomatic process
r. of tongue
r. of tooth
ventral r.
ventral r. of spinal nerve
vestibular r. of acoustic nerve
vestibular r. of auditory nerve
vestibular r. of
    vestibulocochlear nerve
r. of vestibulocochlear nerve,
    inferior
r. of vestibulocochlear nerve,
    superior
root canal probe
rootlet
    flagellar r.
root-splitting forceps
ROP—right occipitoposterior
    (position)
Roper cannula
Rorschach test
ROS—review of systems
rosacea
    acne r.
    erythematotelangiectatic r.
    r. fulminans
    granulomatous r.
    inflammatory r.
    lupoid r.
    ocular r.
    papular r.
    papulopustular r.
    phymatous r.
    steroid r.
    vascular r.
rosacic acid
rosamicin

rosaniline
rosary
    rachitic r.
rose bengal
Rose
    operation
    position
Rose-Bradford kidney
rosein
Rosen
    explorer
    incision
    knife
    needle
    operation
    probe
    separator
    tube
Rosenbach
    disease
    erysipeloid
    law
    sign
    syndrome
Rosenburg operation
Rosenmüller (Rosenmueller)
    body
    curet
    fossa
    gland
    node
    organ
Rosenthal
    canal
    speculum
    syndrome
    test
    vein
Rosenzweig test
roseola
    r. infantilis
    r. infantum
    syphilitic r.
    r. typhosa
    r. urticata
roseolous
Roser
    mouth gag
    sign
Roser-Braun sign
Rose-Thompson
    operation
    repair
rosette
    E r.

rosette *(continued)*
    EA r.
    EAC r.
    Homer Wright r.
    malarial r.
    Wintersteiner r.
Rose-Waaler test
rosin
rosolic acid
Ross
    black spores
    bodies
    retractor
Rossbach disease
Rosser hook
Rossolimo
    reflex
    sign
Rostan asthma
rostra (plural of rostrum)
rostrad
rostral
rostralis
rostrate
rostriform
rostrum (rostrums, rostra)
    r. corporis callosi
    r. of corpus callosum
    r. of sphenoid
    sphenoidal r.
    r. sphenoidale
ROT—right occipitotransverse
  (position)
rotameter
rotary
rotate
rotating
    r. anode tube
    r. anoscope
    r. frame of reference
    r.-hinge arthroplasty
    r. laryngoscope
rotation
    clockwise r. of heart
    counterclockwise r. of heart
    external r.
    internal r.
    lateral r.
    manual r.
    medial r.
    molecular r.
    optical r.
    renal r.
    specific r.
    torsional r.

R

rotation *(continued)*
    van Ness r.
    wheel r.
rotational tomography
rotationplasty
rotator
rotatory
Rotavirus (antigen groups A–F)
rotavirus gastroenteritis
Rotch sign
rotenone
rotexed
rotexion
Roth
    disease
    spots
    syndrome
    vas aberrans
Roth-Bernhardt
    disease
    syndrome
Roth-Bielschowsky syndrome
Rothera test
Rothia
    R. dentocariosa
    R. mucilaginosa
Rothmann-Makai syndrome
Rothmund syndrome
Rothmund-Thomson syndrome
rotoextraction
Rotor syndrome
rotoscoliosis
Rotter
    nodes
    test
Rotunda treatment
rouge
Rouge operation
Rouget
    bulb
    cells
    muscle
rough
roughage
Roughton-Scholander
  method
Rougnon-Heberden disease
Rouleau
round bur
roundworm
Rous
    sarcoma
    test
Roussy-Dejerine syndrome
Roussy-Lévy
    disease

Roussy-Lévy *(continued)*
    hereditary ataxic dystasia
    syndrome
routing
    contralateral r. of signals
    (CROS)
Roux
    gastroenterostomy
    retractor
    serum
Roux-en-Y
    anastomosis
    cystojejunostomy
    gastrectomy
    gastroenterostomy
    gastrojejunostomy
    jejunal loop incision
    operation
Roux-Goldthwait operation
Rovsing sign
Rowland
    forceps
    osteotome
    rongeur
Rowntree-Geraghty test
Royce perforator
Royle operation
Rp—pulmonary resistance
RP—
    reactive protein
    refractory period
    resting pressure
    rest pain
    retinitis pigmentosa
    retrograde pyelogram
RPA—right pulmonary artery
RPCF, RPCFT—Reiter protein
  complement fixation test
RPE—retinal pigment epithelium
RPF—renal plasma flow
RPG—retrograde pyelogram
RPGN—rapidly progressive
  glomerulonephritis
rpm—revolutions per minute
RPM—rapid processing mode
  [par speed screens]
RPO—right posterior oblique
  (projection)
RPR—rapid plasma reagin (test)
RPR-CT—rapid plasma reagin
  circle card test
RPS—renal pressor substance
RPV—right pulmonary vein
RQ—
    recovery quotient
    respiratory quotient

RR—
    radiation response
    recovery room
    renin release
    respiratory rate
    response rate
R&R—rest and recuperation
RRA—radioreceptor assay
RR&E—round, regular, and equal
RR-HPO—rapid recompression–
    high-pressure oxygen
rRNA—ribosomal RNA
RRP—relative refractory period
RRR—renin-release rate
r_s—Spearman rank correlation
    coefficient
RS—
    rating schedule
    respiratory syncytial
    right side
R/s—roentgen(s) per second
RSA—
    relative specific activity
    right sacroanterior (position)
RSB—right sternal border
RSC—rested-state contraction
RScA—right scapuloanterior
    (position)
RScP—right scapuloposterior
    (position)
RSNA—Radiological Society of
    North America
RSP—right sacroposterior
    (position)
RSR—regular sinus rhythm
rSr complex
RST—
    radiosensitivity test
    right sacrotransverse
    (position)
RSTL—relaxed skin tension line
RSV—
    respiratory syncytial virus
    right subclavian vein
    Rous sarcoma virus
RS virus
rt—right
RT—
    radiation therapy,
      radiotherapy
    reaction time
    reading test
    recreational therapy
    right thigh
    room temperature
rT_3—reverse triiodothyronine

RTA—renal tubular acidosis
RTD—routine test dilution
RTF—
    replication and transfer
    resistance transfer factor
RTx—radiation therapy
RU—
    rat unit
    resistance unit
    retrograde urogram
    right upper
    roentgen unit
rub
    friction r.
    pericardial r.
    pericardial friction r.
    pleural r.
    pleural friction r.
    pleuritic r.
    pleuropericardial r.
rubber
    r. band (also: rubber-band)
    r. suture
rubber dam drain
rubber-shod clamp
rubedo
rubefacient
rubella scarlatinosa
rubelliform
rubeola
    r. notha
    r. scarlatinosa
rubeosis
    r. iridis
    r. retinae
ruber
ruberous
rubescent
rubidium (Rb) and ammonium
    bromide
rubidomycin
rubiginose, rubiginous
Rubin
    cannula
    clamp
    operation
    test
    tube
Rubin-Holth punch
Rubinstein syndrome
Rubinstein-Taybi
    syndrome
Rubivirus
Rubner
    law
    test

R

rubor
    dependent r.
ruborous
rubra
rubreserine
rubriblast
rubric
rubricyte
rubrobulbar
rubrocerebellar
rubroglioclandin
rubro-olivary
rubroreticular
rubrospinal
rubrothalamic
rubrous
rubrum Congo
ructus
Rud syndrome
rudiment
    r. of corpus striatum
    hair r.
    hepatic r.
    hippocampal r.
    lens r.
    r. of vaginal process
rudimentary
rudimentum (rudimenta)
    r. processus vaginalis
rue
RUE—right upper
  extremity
Ruffini
    brushes
    corpuscles
    cylinder
    end-organ
rufous
ruga (rugae)
    gastric rugae
    rugae gastricae
    rugae palatinae
    palatine rugae
    r. of scrotum
    rugae of stomach
    r. of urinary bladder
    rugae of vagina
    rugae vaginales
    rugae vesicae biliaris
    rugae vesicae felleae
rugal pattern
rugate
Ruggeri
    reflex
    sign

rugine
    Lempert r.
rugitus
rugose, rugous
rugosity
rugous
RUL—right upper lobe
  (of lung)
rule
    r. of bigeminy
    delivery date r.
    dermatomal r.
    r. of fourths
    His r.
    r. of nines
    octet r.
    r. of outlet
    phase r.
rumble
    diastolic r.
Rumel
    clamp
    forceps
    tourniquet
rumination
    obsessive r.
ruminative
Rummo disease
Rumpel-Leede
    phenomenon
    sign
    test
Rumpf sign
Rundles-Falls
    anemia
    syndrome
Runeberg
    anemia
    disease
    formula
    type
running continuous
    suture
runoff
rupia escharotica
rupial
rupioid
rupture
    artificial r. of membranes
      (AROM)
    defense r.
    extracapsular r.
    r. of gravid uterus
    incidental r.
    intracapsular r.

rupture *(continued)*
    r. of membranes (ROM)
    premature r. of membranes
      (PROM)
    prolonged r. of membranes
      (PROM)
    spontaneous r.
    traumatic r.
    r. of tympanic membrane
RUQ—right upper quadrant
RUR—resin-uptake ratio
RURTI—recurrent
  upper respiratory tract
  infection
Rusch laryngoscope
Ruschelit bougie
Rusconi anus
Rush
    mallet
    pin
    reamer
    rod
Ruskin
    forceps
    rongeur
Russe bone graft
Russell
    bodies
    corpuscles
    double-sugar agar
    effect
    forceps
    syndrome
    traction
    viper
    viper venom
Russian
    forceps
    spring-summer
      encephalitis
Russo
    reaction
    test
Rust [eponym]
    disease
    phenomenon
    sign
    syndrome
rusty
    r. expectoration
    r. sputum
ruthenium (Ru)
rutherford (Rd)
rutherfordium (Rf)
rutidosis

rutin
rutinose
rutoside
Ruysch
    disease
    glomeruli
    glomerulus
    membrane
    muscle
    tube
    tunic
    veins
ruyschian membrane
RV—
    rat virus
    residual volume
    respiratory volume
    right ventricle
    rubella virus
RVA—rabies vaccine absorbed
RVAD—right ventricular assist
  device
RVB—red venous blood
RVD—relative vertebral
  density
RVE—right ventricular
  enlargement
RVEDP—right ventricular
  end-diastolic pressure
RVH—right ventricular
  hypertrophy
RVR—
    renal vascular resistance
    resistance to venous return
RVRA—
    renal vein renin activity
    renal vein renin assay
RVRC—renal vein renin
  concentration
RVS—
    Relative Value Schedule
    Relative Value Study
RVT—renal vein thrombosis
RW—ragweed
Rx (℞, R_x)—
    prescription
    take (L. recipe)
    therapy
    treatment
rye
    spurred r.
Rye classification of Hodgkin
  disease
Ryerson tenotome
Ryle tube

R

Σ—sigma (Greek letter)
s—sample standard deviation
S—
    sacral (vertebra)
    spherical lens
    subject
    Svedberg unit
S—entropy
S.—
    Salmonella
    Schistosoma
    Spirillum
    Staphylococcus
    Streptococcus
S_1–S_4 (S1–S4)—heart sounds
S1–S5—sacral vertebrae 1–5
s^{-1}—reciprocal second
SA—
    salicylic acid
    sarcoma
    secondary amenorrhea
    serum albumin
    sinoatrial
    Stokes-Adams
SAA—severe aplastic anemia
SA attack
saber-cut incision
saber-legged
Sabin
    megaloblast
    pronormoblast
    vaccine
Sabin-Feldman test
sabinism
sabinol
Sabolich Socket System
Sabouraud
    dextrose agar
    dextrose broth
    glucose agar
    plates
sabulous
saburra
saburral amaurosis
sac
    abdominal s.
    air s.
    allantoic s.
    alveolar s's
    amniotic s.
    anal s.
    aneurysmal s.
    aortic s.
    chorionic s.

sac *(continued)*
    conjunctival s.
    dental s.
    dural s.
    embryonic s.
    enamel s.
    endolymphatic s.
    epiploic s.
    gestation s.
    greater s. of peritoneum
    heart s.
    hernial s.
    Hilton s.
    lacrimal s.
    laryngeal s.
    lesser s. of peritoneal cavity
    lymphatic s's
    omental s.
    peritoneal s., greater
    peritoneal s., lesser
    pleural s.
    posterior lymph s's
    preputial s.
    pudendal s.
    retroperitoneal lymph s.
    serous s.
    splenic s.
    synovial s.
    tear s.
    tubotympanic s.
    vaginal s.
saccade
saccadic
    s. intrusion
    s. latency
    s. movement
    s. pursuit
    s. reaction time
    s. response
    s. slowing
    s. velocity
saccate
saccharate, saccharated
saccharephidrosis
saccharic acid
saccharide
    O-linked s.
saccharification
    Einhorn s.
    fermentation s.
    Lohnstein s.
saccharimeter
    fermentation s.
    s. test

saccharin
    s. calcium
    s. sodium
    s. test
saccharine disease
saccharinol
saccharocoria
saccharolytic
saccharometabolic
saccharometabolism
saccharomyces
Saccharomyces
    S. carlsbergensis
    S. cerevisiae
    S. fragilis
    S. pastorianus
saccharomycetes
saccharomycetic
saccharomycetolysis
saccharopine dehydrogenase
saccharopinemia
saccharopinuria
Saccharopolyspora rectivirgula
saccharose
sacci (genitive and plural
   of saccus)
sacciform recess
saccular
    s. aneurysm
    s. bronchiectasis
    s. gland
    s. nerve
    s. recess
    terminal s. period
    terminal s. phase
sacculated
    s. bladder
    s. pleurisy
sacculation
    cecal s's
    colic s's
    s's of colon
    uterine s.
saccule
    air s's
    alveolar s's
    laryngeal s.
    s. of larynx
    terminal s's
sacculi (genitive and plural of
   sacculus)
sacculitis
    anal s.
sacculocochlear canal
sacculotomy

sacculoutricular
    s. canal
    s. duct
sacculus (sacculi)
    sacculi of Beale
    s. dentis
    s. laryngis
saccus (sacci)
    s. anticus
    s. conjunctivalis
    s. endolymphaticus
    s. lacrimalis
    s. medius
    s. posticus
    s. profundus perinei
    s. subcutaneus perinei
    s. superior
    s. vaginalis
SACH—solid-ankle,
   cushioned-heel (foot prosthesis)
Sachs
    cannula
    disease
    guard
    needle
    retractor
    spatula
    suction tube
sacrad
sacral
sacralgia
sacralization
    lumbar s.
sacrarthrogenic
sacrectomy
sacrifice
sacrilegious
sacroanterior
sacrococcygeal
sacrococcyx
sacrocolpopexy
    abdominal s.
sacrocoxalgia
sacrocoxitis
sacrodynia
sacroiliac
sacroiliitis
    pyogenic s.
sacrolisthesis
sacrolumbar
sacroperineal
sacroposterior
sacropromontory
sacrosciatic
sacrospinal

S

sacrotomy
sacrotransverse
sacrouterine
sacrovertebral
sacrum
    assimilation s.
    tilted s.
sactosalpinx
SAD—
    seasonal affective disorder
    small airways disease
    source to axis distance
saddle
    s. angle
    s. area
    s. back
    s. block anesthesia
    bounded s.
    s. connector
    denture base s.
    s. depression
    s. emboli
    free-end s. prosthesis
    s. joint
    medial malleolar s.
    s. nose deformity
    s. pulmonary embolism
    s.-shaped uterus
    thumb s.
saddleback fever
sadism
    anal s.
    oral s.
    phallic s.
    sexual s.
sadist
sadistic
sadomasochism
sadomasochistic
Saemisch
    operation
    section
    ulcer
Saenger
    macula
    operation
    reflex
    sign
    suture
Saethre-Chotzen syndrome
Safar bronchoscope
safranin O, safranine O
Saf-T-Coil
sagacious
sagacity

sagittal
    s. axis
    s. border of parietal bone
    s. depth
    s. diameter
    s. fontanelle
    s. groove
    inferior s. sinus
    s. margin of parietal bone
    median s. plane
    s. planes
    posterior s. anorectoplasty
    s. ramus osteotomy
    s. section
    s. sinus
    s. slice fracture
    s. split osteotomy
    s. splitting of mandible
    s. sulcus
    superior s. sinus
    s. suture
    s. synostosis
sagittalis
sago
SAH—subarachnoid hemorrhage
Sahli
    method
    reaction
    test
St. Anthony's
    disease
    fire
St. Clair-Thompson curet
St. Jude (St. Jude Medical,
  SJM)
    Atlas (V-193) implantable
      cardioverter defibrillator
    bileaflet mechanical heart
      valve
    Biocor bovine pericardial
      bioprosthesis
    Epic heart valve bioprosthesis
    Regent heart valve
      prosthesis
St. Louis encephalitis (virus)
salaam
    s. activity
    s. convulsion
    s. seizures
    s. spasm
Sala cells
salad
    word s.
salamander
salamandrine

Saldino-Noonan syndrome
Salibi clamp
salicylamide
salicylanilide
salicylate
    choline s.
    magnesium s.
    s. meglumine
    methyl s.
    octyl s.
    phenyl s.
    physostigmine s.
    sodium s.
    trolamine s.
salicylated
salicylemia
salicylic acid
    s.a. collodion
    s.a. plaster
    zinc oxide and s.a. paste
salicylism
salicylsulfonic acid
salicyluric acid
salient
    s. characteristics
    s. clinical aspects
    s. factors
    s. features
    s. findings
salifiable
salify
salimeter
saline
    s. agglutinin
    s. antibody
    s. cathartic
    hypertonic s.
    hypotonic s.
    s. infusion
    s. laxatives
    normal s. (NS)
    physiologic s. solution
    s. solution
salinity
salinometer
saliva
    artificial s.
    chorda s.
    ganglionic s.
    lingual s.
    parotid s.
    ropy s.
    sublingual s.
    submaxillary s.
    s. substitute

saliva *(continued)*
    sympathetic s.
salivant
salivaria
salivarian
salivaris
    caruncula s.
salivary
    s. capsule
    s. corpuscle
    s. digestion
    s. ducts
    external s. gland
    s. fistula
    s. glands
    s. gland virus
    inferior s. nucleus
    internal s. gland
    major s. gland
    minor s. gland
    s. stone
    superior s. nucleus
salivate
salivation
salivator
salivatory
    caudal s. nucleus
    inferior s. nucleus
    rostral s. nucleus
salivolithiasis
Salkowski
    method
    test
salmon
    s. patch
    s. poisoning
Salmonella enterica subsp.
    enterica, serovar *Enteritidis*
salmonellal
salmonellosis
salol
salpingectomy
    abdominal s.
    bilateral s.
    ipsilateral s.
    laparoscopic s.
    left s.
    partial s.
    right s.
    total s.
    unilateral total s.
salpingemphraxis
salpinges (plural of salpinx)
salpingian dropsy
salpingion

S

salpingitic
salpingitis
    chronic interstitial s.
    eustachian s.
    follicular s.
    gonococcal s.
    hemorrhagic s.
    hypertrophic s.
    s. isthmica nodosa
    mural s.
    nodular s.
    parenchymatous s.
    s. profluens
    pseudofollicular s.
    purulent s.
    tuberculous s.
salpingocele
salpingogram
salpingography
salpingolysis
salpingo-oophorectomy
salpingo-oophoritis
salpingo-oophorocele
salpingo-oothecitis
salpingo-ovariectomy
salpingo-ovariotomy
salpingopalatine fold
salpingoperitonitis
salpingopexy
salpingopharyngeal
    s. fold
    s. muscle
salpingoplasty
salpingorrhaphy
salpingoscope
salpingoscopy
salpingostomatomy
salpingostomatoplasty
salpingostomy
salpingotomy
    laparoscopic s.
    linear s.
salpingoureteral
salpinx (salpinges)
    s. auditiva
salsalate
salt
    acid s.
    artificial s.
    artificial Carlsbad s.
    artificial Kissingen s.
    basic s.
    bile s's
    bone s's
    buffer s.

salt *(continued)*
    Carlsbad s.
    common s.
    complex s.
    diuretic s.
    double s.
    effervescent s's
    effervescent artificial Vichy s.
    Epsom s's
    halide s.
    haloid s.
    iodized s.
    neutral s.
    normal s.
    Plimmer s.
    Preston s.
    Rochelle s.
    Seignette s.
    Wurster s's
saltation
saltatorial
saltatory
    s. chorea
    s. conduction
    s. evolution
    s. progression
    s. spasm
    s. tic
Salter
    fracture (I–VI)
    incremental lines
    operation
    osteotomy
salting in
salting out
saltpeter
    Chile s.
    s. paper
salubrious
saluresis
saluretic
salutary
salute
    allergic s.
    iron s. sign
    s. splint
saluting chorea
salvage therapy
salve
    lip s.
    Norwegian spruce resin s.
    topical s.
salvo
    s. of action potentials
    s. of activity

salvo *(continued)*
    s. of antral pressure waves
    s. of data
    ventricular tachycardia s.
salvo-free period
Salzmann nodular corneal
    dystrophy
SAM—systolic anterior motion
samandarine
samarium (Sm)
sampling
    chorionic villus s. (CVS)
    systemic s.
Sam Roberts forceps
Samuel position
Sanarelli phenomenon
sanative
sanatory
sand
    s. bath
    s. bodies
    brain s.
    s. flea
    hydatid s.
    intestinal s.
    s. tumor
sandalwood oil
sanded nucleus
Sanders
    bed
    disease
    epidemic keratoconjunctivitis
    forceps
    incision
    laryngoscope
    oscillating bed
Sanders-Brown-Shaw needle
sandfly
    s. fever
    s. fever virus
Sandhoff disease
Sandifer syndrome
Sandison-Clark chamber
sandpaper
    s. disk
    s. gallbladder
Sandrock test
Sandström
    bodies
    glands
sandwich
    s. assay
    s. osteotomy
    s. technique
    visor-s. osteotomy

Sandwith bald tongue
sandworm disease
sane
Sanfilippo
    disease
    syndrome
Sanger Brown ataxia
sang-froid
sanguicolous
sanguifacient
sanguiferous
sanguification
sanguimotor
sanguinarine
sanguine
sanguineous
    s. conjunctival discharge
    s. drainage
    s. infiltration
    s. pleural fluid
    s. secretions
    s. urine
    s. vaginal discharge
sanguinification
sanguinolent
sanguinopurulent
sanguis
sanies (sanies)
sanious pus
sanitary
sanitation
sanitization
sanitize
sanity
San Joaquin fever
San Joaquin Valley disease
Sansom sign
Sanson images
Santavuori disease
Santorini
    accessory duct
    canal
    cartilages
    fissures
    incisura
    ligament
    major caruncle
    muscle
    papilla
    parietal vein
    plexus
    tubercle
sap
SAP—
    serum alkaline phosphatase

S

SAP—*(continued)*
    systemic arterial pressure
saphena
    vena s. accessoria
    vena s. magna
    vena s. parva
saphenectomy
saphenofemoral
saphenography
saphenous
    accessory s. vein
    great s. vein
    s. hiatus
    s. loop fistula
    s. nerve
    s. opening
    small s. vein
    s. vein
sapid
sapogenin
saponaceous
saponifiable
saponification
    s. number
    s. value
saponify
saponin
    cholan s's
    triterpenoid s's
saporosity
sapotoxin
Sappey
    fibers
    ligament
    nucleus
    veins
sapphism
saprodontia
sapronosis
saprophagous
saprophilous
saprophyte
saprophytic bacterium
saprozoic
Sarbó sign
sarcoblast
sarcocarcinoma
sarcocele
sarcocyst
sarcocystin
Sarcocystis
    S. bovihominis
    S. suihominis
sarcocystosis
sarcofetal pregnancy

sarcogenic cells
sarcoglycan
sarcohysteric pregnancy
sarcoid
    Boeck s., s. of Boeck
    Darier-Roussy s.
    s. granuloma
    multiple benign s.
    necrotizing s. granulomatosis
    s. neuropathy
    Salem s.
    Schaumann s.
    Spiegler-Fendt s.
sarcoidosis
    acute s.
    beryllium s.
    Boeck s.
    cardiac s.
    cerebral s.
    s. cordis
    Danielssen-Boeck s.
    hypercalcemic s.
    intrathoracic s.
    muscular s.
    myocardial s.
sarcolemma
sarcolemmic
L-sarcolysin
sarcoma (sarcomas, sarcomata)
    adipose s.
    alveolar soft part s.
    ameloblastic s.
    botryoid s.
    s. botryoides
    chloromatous s.
    chondroblastic s.
    clear cell s. of kidney
    embryonal s.
    endometrial stromal s.
    epithelioid s.
    Ewing s.
    fascial s.
    fibroblastic s.
    giant cell s.
    granulocytic s.
    hemangioendothelial s.
    Hodgkin s.
    idiopathic multiple pigmented
        hemorrhagic s.
    immunoblastic s. of B cells
    immunoblastic s. of T cells
    Jensen s.
    Kaposi s.
    Kupffer cell s.
    leukocytic s.

sarcoma (sarcomas, sarcomata)
  (continued)
    lymphatic s.
    melanotic s.
    meningeal s.
    mixed cell s.
    multiple idiopathic
      hemorrhagic s.
    multipotential primary s. of bone
    myeloid s.
    neurogenic s.
    osteoblastic s.
    osteogenic s.
    osteolytic s.
    parosteal s.
    polymorphous s.
    pseudo–Kaposi s.
    reticulum cell s.
    Rous s.
    Rous s. virus
    soft tissue s.
    spindle cell s.
    synovial s.
    telangiectatic s.
sarcomagenic
sarcomata (plural of sarcoma)
sarcomatoid
sarcomatosis
    abdominal s.
    GIST (GI stromal tumor) s.
    intraperitoneal s.
    leptomeningeal s.
    low-grade s.
    non-GIST s.
    peritoneal s.
    pleural s.
    visceral s.
sarcomatous leptomeningitis
sarcomere
sarconeme
sarcopenia
Sarcophaga haemorrhoidalis
sarcoplasm
sarcoplasmic
    s. cone
    s. matrix
    s. reticulum
sarcoplast
sarcopoietic
Sarcoptes scabiei
sarcoptic
sarcoptidosis
sarcosine dehydrogenase
sarcosinemia
sarcosinuria

sarcosis
sarcosome
sarcostosis
sarcostyle
sarcotic
sarcotubules
sarcous
    s. element
    s. substance
sardonic
sarin
Sarot
    clamp
    forceps
sarsaparilla
sarsasapogenin
SAS—supravalvular aortic stenosis
sassafras
sat.—saturated
SAT—Scholastic Aptitude Test
SATA—spatial average temporal
  average
satellite
    s. abscess
    bacterial s.
    s. cell infection
    s. cell necrosis
    s. cells
    centriolar s.
    s. colony
    s. DNA
    s. lesion
    s. nodule
    perineuronal s.
    s. phenomenon
    s. potential
    s. probe
    s. virus
satellitism
    platelet s.
satellitosis
satiate, satiated
satiation
satiety
Satinsky
    clamp
    forceps
    scissors
Satterlee saw
saturated
    s. compound
    s. fat
    s. fatty acids
    s. hydrocarbon
    s. solution

S

saturation
- arterial oxygen s. (SaO2)
- blood oxygen s.
- s. color
- s. current
- s. deficit
- s. hybridization
- s. limit
- oxygen s.
- s. recovery technique
- transferrin s.

Saturday night palsy
saturnine
- s. encephalopathy
- s. gout
- s. nephropathy
- s. poisoning

saturnism
satyriasis
satyromania
sauce
- anchovy s. pus

saucer
- auditory s.

saucerization
saucerize
Sauer
- debrider
- forceps
- speculum
- tonsillectome

Sauerbruch prosthesis
Sauer-Sluder tonsillectome
Sauer vaccine
sauna bath
Saunders
- disease
- sign

sausage poisoning
Sauvineau ophthalmoplegia
Savage perineal body
Savary-Gilliard dilator
save, save that
savin oil
Savin operation
saw
- Adams s.
- Albee s.
- amputating s.
- bayonet s.
- Butcher s.
- Charriére bone s.
- Clerf s.
- Cottle s.
- crown s.

saw *(continued)*
- Farabeuf s.
- Gigli wire s.
- Gottschalk s.
- Hey s.
- Hey skull s.
- hole s.
- Joseph s.
- Joseph-Maltz s.
- Lamont s.
- Langenbeck (von Langenbeck) s.
- Maltz s.
- Myerson s.
- Satterlee s.
- separating s.
- Shrady s.
- Slaughter s.
- Stille-Gigli s.
- Stryker s.
- subcutaneous s.

Sawtell forceps
saw-tooth
saxifragant
saxitoxin
Saxtorph maneuver
Sayoc operation
Sayre
- apparatus
- jacket
- operation
- splint

SB—
- serum bilirubin
- sinus bradycardia
- Stanford-Binet (test)
- sternal border
- stillbirth

SBE—subacute bacterial endocarditis
SBF—splanchnic blood flow
SBFT—small bowel follow-through (x-ray)
SBP—systolic blood pressure
SBT—
- serum bacterial titer
- single-breath test

SBTI—soybean trypsin inhibitor
SC—
- sacrococcygeal
- scleral cautery
- semicircular
- semiclosed
- sickle cell
- sternoclavicular

SC— *(continued)*
 subclavian
 subconjunctival
 subcutaneous
 succinylcholine
 sugar-coated
SCA—single-chain antigen-binding
scab
scabbard trachea
scabetic
scabicide
scabies
 crusted s.
 Norwegian s.
 sarcoptic s.
scabietic
scala (scalae)
 s. of Löwenberg
 s. tympani
 s. vestibuli
scalar
 s. coupling
 s. effect
 s. electrocardiogram
scalariform
scald
scalded
 nonstaphylococcal s. skin syndrome
scale
 absolute s.
 absolute temperature s.
 adhesive s.
 Apgar s.
 ASIA s.
 Baumé s.
 Bayley s. of infant development
 Borg s.
 Brazelton behavioral s.
 Brief Psychiatric Rating S.
 Cattell Infant Intelligence S.
 Celsius s.
 centigrade s.
 Charriére s.
 Clark s.
 Columbia Mental Maturity S.
 Defensive Functioning S.
 developmental s.
 Dubowitz infant maturity s.
 Dunfermline s.
 Esterman s.
 Fahrenheit s.
 Fitzpatrick s.

scale *(continued)*
 French s.
 GAF (Global Assessment of Functioning) s.
 Gaffky s.
 Gesell developmental s's
 Glasgow Coma S.
 Glasgow Outcome S.
 gray s.
 Hamilton Depression Rating S.
 Karnofsky performance s.
 Karnofsky rating s.
 Kelvin s.
 Lund-Browder burn s.
 Matthew s.
 NIH s. of stroke severity
 Outerbridge osteoarthritis s.
 performance s.
 pH s.
 Rankine s.
 rating s.
 Réaumur s.
 Social and Occupational Functioning Assessment S.
 Sörensen s.
 Stanford-Binet intelligence s.
 Tanner developmental s.
 temperature s.
 Toronto western spasmodic torticollis rating s.
 Vineland social maturity s.
 visual analog s.
 Wechsler Adult Intelligence S. (WAIS)
 Wechsler Intelligence S. for Children (WISC)
 Zung depression s.
scalene
 anterior s. muscle
 anterior s. syndrome
 s. fascia
 middle s. muscle
 posterior s. muscle
 smallest s. muscle
 s. tubercle
scalenectomy
scalenotomy
scalenus
 s. anterior muscle
 s. anticus syndrome
 s. medius muscle
 s. minimum muscle
 s. posterior muscle

S

scaler
    chisel s.
    deep s.
    double-ended s.
    hoe s.
    sickle s.
    superficial s.
    ultrasonic s.
    watch-spring s.
scaling
    deep s.
    s. nodule
    s. plaque
    root s.
    subgingival s.
    ultrasonic s.
scalloped
    s. appearance
    s. bone
    s. border
    s. fenestration
    s. implant
    s. intestinal mucosal folds
    s. lesion
    s. nucleus
    s. pattern
    s. placenta
    s. true aortic annulus
    s. tumor margin
scalloping
    s. appearance
    s. artifact
    bony s.
    calvarial s.
    cortical s.
    s. of duodenal folds
    s. effect
    endosteal s.
    s. of folds
    iatrogenic placental s.
    irregular s.
    sacral s.
    s. of sacrum
    tongue s.
    vertebral body s.
    vertebral s. sign
    visceral s.
scalp
    dissecting cellulitis of s.
    double s.
    s. electrode
    gyrate s.
    s. pH
    ringworm of s.
    s. tourniquet
    s. vein needle

scalpel
    Jackson s.
    plasma s.
scaly
    s. erythematous plaque
    erythematous s. skin
    s. lesion
    s. macule
    s. papule
    s. patch
    red s. plaques
    s. scalp
scan
    A s.
    adrenal s.
    B s.
    bilirubin s.
    blood pool s.
    bone s.
    bone marrow s.
    brain s.
    C s.
    capillary blockade perfusion s.
    cardiac s.
    CAT (computed axial
       tomography) s.
    C-mode s.
    compound s.
    CT (computed tomography) s.
    DEXA (dual-energy x-ray
       absorptiometry) s.
    DISIDA
       (diisopropyliminodiacetic
       acid) s.
    dynamic CT s.
    EMI s.
    fluorescence s.
    gallium s.
    gamma s.
    hepatobiliary s.
    HIDA (hepatoiminodiacetic
       acid) s.
    isotope bone s.
    kidney s.
    krypton s.
    liver s.
    liver-spleen s.
    lung s.
    mechanical compound s.
    Meckel s.
    medronate s.
    MDCT (multidetector
       computed tomography) s.
    MUGA (multiple gated
       acquisition) s.
    multiple gated blood pool s.

scan *(continued)*

 multislice full line s.
 nongated CT s.
 nucleotide s.
 OCT (optic coherence tomography) s.
 perfusion s.
 perfusion lung s.
 PET (positron emission tomography) s.
 PIPIDA hepatobiliary s.
 Positron s.
 PYP (pyrophosphate) s.
 radioactive s.
 radionuclide s.
 RAI (radioactive iodine) s.
 renal s.
 RISA (radioactive iodinated serum albumin) s.
 salivary gland s.
 sector s.
 selective excitation line s.
 single sweep s.
 SPECT (single photon emission computed tomography) s.
 spleen s.
 ^{99m}Tc-labeled macroaggregated albumin (MAA) s.
 ^{99m}Tc-PIPIDA s., technetium-99m PIPIDA
 technetium s.
 thallium 201 s.
 thallium myocardial s.
 thyroid s.
 ventilation s.
 ventilation-perfusion (V/Q) s.

scandium (Sc)

scanner

 CT body s.
 duplex s.
 EMI s.
 gated s. CT
 General Electric CT/T7 800 s.
 mechanical real-time s.
 Medx s.
 multicrystal whole-body s.
 neurodiagnostic s.
 nuclear s.
 PET (positron emission tomography) s.
 radioisotope s.
 rectilinear s.
 scintillation s.
 small-parts s.
 tomographic s.

scanner *(continued)*

 tomographic multiplane s.
 whole-body s.

scanning

 A-mode (amplitude modulation) s.
 B-mode (brightness modulation) s.
 bone marrow s.
 brain s.
 cine CT s.
 compound s.
 confocal laser s. microscopy
 contiguous s.
 CT (computed tomography) s.
 s. electron microscope
 FDG-PET (^{18}F-fluorodeoxyglucose positron emission tomography) s.
 full line s.
 gallium s.
 gamma s.
 infarct avid s.
 lacrimal s.
 s. laser ophthalmoscopy
 s. laser polarimetry
 line s.
 linear s.
 s. microscope
 M-mode (time-motion) s.
 multiplanar s.
 nuclear s.
 nucleotide s.
 perfusion s.
 point s.
 postablation radioiodine whole body s.
 radioisotope s.
 radionuclide s.
 real-time s.
 renal s.
 rotate-rotate s.
 rotate-stationary s.
 sector s.
 sensitive point s.
 s. sequence
 single-pass s.
 s. spot
 three-phase bone s.
 s. transmission electron microscopy
 transverse s.
 ventilation-perfusion (V/Q) s.
 water path s.
 whole-body s.

S

scansion
scanty
   s. amount
   s. details
   s. eosinophils
   s. evidence
   s. growth
   s. history
   s. information
   s. intraabdominal fat
   s. menses
Scanzoni
   maneuver
   operation
scapha
   eminence of s.
scaphion
scaphocephalia
scaphocephalic
scaphocephalism
scaphocephalous
scaphocephaly
scaphocuneiform ligaments
scaphohydrocephalus
scaphohydrocephaly
scaphoid
   s. abdomen
   s. bone of foot
   s. bone of hand
   s. fossa
   s. megalourethra
   s. scapula
scaphoiditis
   tarsal s.
scapholunate advanced collapse
SCA proteins
scapula (scapulae)
   alar s.
   s. alata
   s. anterior position
   elevated s.
   Graves s.
   s. posterior position
   scaphoid s.
   spine of s.
   winged s.
scapulalgia
scapular
   s. bone
   s. extremity of clavicle
   descending s. artery
   s. head of triceps muscles
   s. line
   s. nerve
   s. notch

scapular *(continued)*
   s. reflex
   s. region
   transverse s. artery
   s. tuberosity of Henle
scapulary
scapulectomy
scapuloanterior position
scapuloclavicular joint
scapulocostal syndrome
scapulodynia
scapulohumeral
   s. bursitis
   s. muscular dystrophy
   s. reflex
scapuloperoneal muscular dystrophy
scapulopexy
scapuloposterior position
scapulothoracic
scapus (scapi) pili
scar
   acne s's
   apical s.
   appendectomy s.
   s. band lysis
   s. border zone
   s. bridle
   burn s.
   conspicuous s.
   corneal s.
   cortical s.
   fibrotic s. tissue
   s. formation
   hypertrophic s.
   hysterectomy s.
   inconspicuous s.
   s.-induced contracture
   infarct s.
   lower-segment cesarean s.
   mature s.
   s.-related ventricular
     tachycardia
   s. revision
   s. rupture
   s. sarcoidosis
   smallpox vaccination s.
   surgical s.
   tattoo s.
   three-dimensional s. mapping
   s. tissue
   tissue paper s.
   ulceration s.
   Vancouver S. Scale
   vertical s.
   white s. of ovary

SCAR—subclinical acute rejection
Scardino
    ureteropelvioplasty
    uteropelvioplasty
Scardino-Prince
  ureteropelvioplasty
scarf
    crescentic inverted s. osteotomy
    Mayor s.
    s. osteotomy
    s. pin aspiration
    s. pin foreign body
    s. pin inhalation
    s. prepuce
    s.-ring sign
    s. sign
scarification
    branding s.
    chemical s.
    corneal s.
    epidermal s.
    religious s.
    ritual s.
scarifier
    Desmarres s.
scarify
scarlatina
scarlatinal nephritis
scarlatiniform
scarlatinoid
scarlet
    Biebrich s.
    s. fever
    s. G
    s. R
    s. red
Scarpa
    canals
    fascia
    fluid
    foramina
    ganglion
    hiatus
    ligament
    liquor
    membrane
    method
    nerve
    operation
    sheath
    staphyloma
    triangle
scarring
    acne s.
    adventitial s.

scarring *(continued)*
    s. alopecia
    chorioretinal s.
    s. and contracture
    extensive s.
    hypertrophic s.
    lung s.
    marked s.
    minimal s.
    permanent s.
    pleural s.
    prone to s.
    recurring s. aphthae
    renal s.
    scalp s.
    severe s.
    significant s.
    soft tissue s.
    web s.
SCAT—
    sheep cell agglutination test
    sickle cell anemia test
scatologic
scatology
    telephone s.
scatoma
scatophagy
scatophilia
scatoscopy
scatter
    s. analysis
    coherent s.
    s. correction
    forward s.
    s.-induced cupping artifact
    s.-induced noise
    s.-induced streak artifact
    light s.
    s. radiation
    repolarization s.
    ventilation-perfusion s.
    x-ray s.
scattered radiation
scattering
    acoustic s.
    coherent s.
    Rayleigh s.
    small-angle x-ray s.
    tip-enhanced Raman s.
    ultrasound s.
scavenger
    s. cell
    nitric oxide (NO) s.
    oxidant s.
    s. receptor

S

SCBA—self-contained breathing
  apparatus
SCD—service-connected disability
ScDA—right anterior scapular
  (L. scapulodextra anterior)
  (position)
ScDP—right posterior scapular
  (L. scapulodextra posterior)
  (position)
scenario
SCFA—short-chain fatty acids
SCG—serum chemistry graft
Schaefer (Schäfer)
    bladder outlet obstruction grade
    classification
Schaeffer
    ethmoid curet
    mastoid curet
Schafer method
Schäffer
    collaterals
    collateral synapses
    fixative
    reflex
Schaffer test
Schall tube
Schamberg
    dermatosis
    disease
    extractor
    progressive pigmented
      purpuric dermatosis
    purpura
Schanz
    disease
    operation
    syndrome
Schardinger
    enzyme
    reaction
Schatzki ring
Schatz maneuver
Schaudinn fluid
Schaumann
    benign lymphogranuloma
    bodies
    disease
    sarcoid, sarcoidosis
    syndrome
Schauta
    operation
    radical vaginal hysterectomy
Schauta-Amreich
    operation
    vaginal hysterectomy

Schauta-Wertheim operation
Schede operation
schedule
    S. for Affective Disorders and
      Schizophrenia (SADS)
    Diagnostic Interview S.
    fixed interval s.
    fixed ratio s.
    Gesell developmental s.
    s. of reinforcement
    sleep-wake s. disorder
    variable interval s.
    variable ratio s.
Scheibe deafness
Scheie
    cannula
    cautery
    knife
    operation
    syndrome
Scheinmann forceps
schema
schematic
scheme
Scheuermann
    disease
    kyphosis
    syndrome
Schick
    reaction
    sign
    test
Schiff
    biliary cycle
    reagent
    test
Schilder
    disease
    encephalitis
Schilder-Addison complex
Schiller
    test
    tumor
Schilling
    blood count
    leukemia
    test
Schimek operation
Schimmelbusch disease
Schindler
    esophagoscope
    gastroscope
Schiotz tonometer
Schirmer test
schistasis

schistocormia
schistocormus
schistocyte
schistocytosis
schistomelia
schistomelus
schistosis
Schistosoma
  S. haematobium
  S. intercalatum
  S. japonicum
  S. mansoni
  S. mekongi
schistosomal
  s. bladder carcinoma
  s. dermatitis
  s. dysentery
  s. granuloma
schistosome
schistosomia
schistosomiasis
  bladder s.
  cerebral s.
  cutaneous s.
  eastern s.
  genitourinary s.
  hepatic s.
  s. intercalatum
  intestinal s.
  s. japonica
  Manson s.
  s. mansoni
  Oriental s.
  pulmonary s.
  rectal s.
  urinary s.
  vesical s.
  visceral s.
schistosomicidal
schistosomicide
schistosomus
schizamnion
schizaxon
schizencephalic
schizencephaly
schizoaffective
schizocyte
schizocytosis
schizogenesis
schizogenous
schizogony
schizogyria
schizoid personality disorder
schizokinesis
schizonychia

schizophasia
schizophrenia
  acute s.
  ambulatory s.
  atypical s.
  borderline s.
  catatonic s.
  childhood s.
  disorganized s.
  hebephrenic s.
  latent s.
  nuclear s.
  paranoid s.
  prepsychotic s.
  process s.
  prodromal s.
  pseudopsychopathic s.
  reactive s.
  residual s.
  schizoaffective s.
  simple s.
  undifferentiated s.
schizophrenic
  acute s. episode
schizophreniform disorder
schizoprosopia
schizotaxia
schizothorax
schizotonia
schizotrichia
schizotropic
schizotypal personality
  disorder
Schlatter
  disease
  operation
  sprain
Schlatter-Osgood disease
Schlein-type elbow
  arthroplasty
Schlemm
  canal
  ligaments
Schlepper
Schlesinger
  forceps
  phenomenon
  rongeur
  sign
Schlichter test
Schlichting dystrophy
Schmalz operation
Schmidel
  anastomosis
  ganglion

S

Schmidt
  keratitis
  syndrome
Schmidt-Lanterman
  clefts
  incisures
  segment
Schmincke tumor
Schmitz bacillus
Schmorl
  body
  disease
  furrow
  node
  nodule
Schmutz pyorrhea
schneiderian membrane
Schneider nail
Schober test
Schoemaker
  clamp
  gastroenterostomy
  line
Schoenberg forceps
Scholz
  disease
  sclerosis
Scholz-Bielschowsky-Henneberg
  sclerosis
Scholz-Greenfield disease
Schönbein
  reaction
  test
Schönlein (Schoenlein)
  disease
  purpura
Schönlein-Henoch
  (Schoenlein-Henoch)
  disease
  purpura
  syndrome
Schott
  bath
  treatment
Schottmüller (Schottmueller)
  disease
  fever
Schramm phenomenon
Schreger
  band
  lines
  striae
  zones
Schroeder
  disease
  fibers

Schroeder *(continued)*
  forceps
  operation
  scissors
  syndrome
  tenaculum
  test
Schrön granule
Schrön-Much granules
Schrötter (Schroetter) chorea
Schubert forceps
Schuchardt
  incision
  operation
Schuchardt-Pfeifer operation
Schüffner
  dots
  granules
  punctuation
  stippling
Schuknecht
  excavator
  hook
  knife
  operation
  retractor
  speculum
  stapedectomy
Schüller
  disease
  phenomenon
  position
  stain
  syndrome
  view
Schüller-Christian
  disease
  syndrome
Schultz
  angina
  disease
  syndrome
Schultz-Charlton
  phenomenon
  reaction
  test
Schultz-Dale
  reaction
  technique
Schultze
  acroparesthesia
  bundle
  cells
  fold
  mechanism
  method

Schultze *(continued)*
    placenta
    sign
    tract
    type
Schultze-Chvostek sign
Schultze-type acroparesthesia
Schutz
    bundle
    clip
    forceps
    micrococcus
    tract
Schwabach test
Schwachman syndrome
Schwalbe
    corpuscles
    fissure
    foramen
    nucleus
    olivary peduncle of s.
    ring
    sheath
    space
    line
Schwann
    cell
    membrane
    nucleus
    sheath
    substance
    white substance
schwannoma
    granular cell s.
    malignant s.
schwannosis
Schwartz
    clip
    forceps
    hook
Schwartz-Bartter syndrome
Schwartze
    mastoidectomy
    operation
    sign
Schwartz-Jampel
    myotonia
    syndrome
Schwartzman
    phenomenon
    reaction
Schwartzman-Sanarelli
    phenomenon
Schwarz
    activator
    appliance

Schwediauer disease
Schweigger forceps
Schweigger-Seidel sheath
Schweizer forceps
Schweizer-Foley Y-plasty
Schweninger-Buzzi
    anetoderma
SCI—structured clinical
    interview
sciage
scialyscope
Scianna blood group
sciatic
    s. artery
    s. block
    s. bursa
    Fajersztajn crossed s. sign
    greater s. foramen
    greater s. notch
    s. hernia
    lesser s. foramen
    lesser s. notch
    s. nerve
    s. neuralgia
    s. neuritis
    s. scoliosis
    s. spine
    s. tuber
sciatica
SCID—severe combined
    immunodeficiency
SCIDS—severe combined
    immunodeficiency
    syndrome
science
    behavioral s.
    forensic s.
scientist
scieropia
scilla
scillabiose
scillaren
scilliroside
scimitar
    isolated s. vein anomaly
    s. sacrum
    s. shadow
    s. sign
    s. syndrome
    s. vein stenosis
scintiangiography
    dynamic radionuclide s.
    hepatic s.
    hepatobiliary s.
    quantitative s.
    renal s.

S

scintiangiography *(continued)*
   99mTC-DTPA s.
   technetium Tc 99m RBC
     gated s.
scintigram
scintigraphic
scintigraphy
   acute infarct s.
   bone s.
   exercise thallium s.
   gallium citrate s.
   gated blood pool s.
   infarct avid s.
   111In-labeled
     leukocyte s.
   metaiodobenzylguanidine
     (MIBG) s.
   myocardial perfusion s.
   nuclear s.
   perfusion s.
   planar s.
   renal s.
   99mTC-depreotide s.
   99mTC-DPD s.
   99mTC-MDP s.
   technetium TC 99m
     pyrophosphate s.
   technetium TC 99m
     tetrofosmin s.
   thallium-201 myocardial
     perfusion s.
   thallium perfusion s.
   thyroidal lymph node s.
   ventilation s.
scintillating scotoma
scintillation
   s. camera
   s. counter
   s. counting technique
   s. crystal
   liquid s. counting
   s. probe
   s. scanner
scintiphotograph
scintiphotography
scintiphotosplenoportography
scintirenography
scintiscan
scintiscanner
Scion image analysis
scirrhoid
scirrhous
   s. carcinoma
   s. cord
scirrhus

scissile bond
scission
scissoring
scissors
   Adson s.
   Aebli s.
   Barraquer s.
   Barraquer-DeWecker
     iris s.
   Bellucci s.
   Berens s.
   s. bite
   Boettcher s.
   Braun s.
   Brooks s.
   Buie s.
   Burnham s.
   canalicular s.
   cannula s.
   Castroviejo s.
   Cooley s.
   corneoscleral s.
   Cottle s.
   Craafoord s.
   Craig s.
   craniotomy s.
   Dandy s.
   Dean s.
   Deaver s.
   DeBakey s.
   DeBakey-Metzenbaum s.
   DeWecker iris s.
   Doyen s.
   Emmet s.
   Esmarch s.
   Ferguson s.
   Fomon s.
   Fox s.
   s. gait
   Harrison s.
   House s.
   iris s.
   Irvine s.
   Jackson s.
   Jacobson s.
   Jones s.
   Jorgenson s.
   Joseph s.
   Katzin s.
   Kelly s.
   Kirby s.
   Knapp s.
   Knight s.
   Knowles s.
   Lagrange s.

scissors *(continued)*
s. leg
Lejeune s.
Lillie s.
Lister s.
Liston s.
Littauer s.
Litwak s.
Lynch s.
Mayo s.
Mayo-Harrington s.
Mayo-Noble s.
Mayo-Sims s.
McClure s.
McGuire s.
McLean s.
McPherson s.
McPherson-Castroviejo s.
McPherson-Vannas s.
Metzenbaum s.
Metzenbaum-Lipsett s.
Miller s.
Morse s.
s. movement
Nelson s.
New s.
Northbent s.
Noyes-Shambaugh s.
Nugent-Gradle s.
Ochsner s.
Panzer s.
Potts s.
Potts-Smith s.
Pratt s.
Prince s.
s. probe
Rochester-Ferguson s.
Satinsky s.
Schroeder s.
Seiler s.
Shortbent s.
Sims s.
Sistrunk s.
Smart s.
Smellie s.
Spencer s.
Stevens s.
Stevenson s.
stitch s.
Strully s.
Sweet s.
Taylor s.
Thorek s.
Thorek-Feldman s.
Thorpe s.

scissors *(continued)*
Thorpe-Castroviejo s.
Thorpe-Westcott s.
Toennis s.
umbilical s.
Vannas s.
Verhoeff s.
Walker s.
Westcott s.
Wester s.
Wilmer s.
scissors-bite crossbite
scissura
longitudinal s.
middle s.
transverse s.
scissural
SCK—serum creatine
kinase
ScLA—left anterior scapular
(L. scapulolaeva anterior)
(position)
sclera (sclerae)
blue s.
scleradenitis
scleral
Ammon s. prominence
s. buckle
s. buckling
s. canal
s. contact lens
s. crescent
s. ectasis
s. framework
s. furrow
s. icterus
s. lens
s. limbus
s. plexus
s. rigidity
s. ring
s. roll
s. spur
s. staphyloma
s. trabecula
s. tunnel incision
s. veins
scleratitis
scleratogenous
sclerectasia
sclerectasis
sclerectoiridectomy
sclerectoiridodialysis
sclerectome
sclerectomy

S

scleredema
    s. adultorum
    Buschke s.
    s. neonatorum
sclerema adiposum
sclerencephaly
scleriasis
scleriritomy
scleritis
    anterior s.
    brawny s.
    diffuse s.
    necrotizing s.
    nodular s.
    posterior s.
scleroadipose
sclerochoroiditis
    s. anterior
    s. posterior
scleroconjunctival
scleroconjunctivitis
sclerocornea
sclerocorneal junction
sclerodactylia
sclerodactyly
scleroderma
    circumscribed s.
    diffuse s.
    generalized s.
    linear s.
    localized s.
    progressive s.
    s. renal crisis
    systemic s.
sclerodermatomyositis
sclerodermatous
sclerodermoid
sclerogenic
sclerogenous
sclerogummatous
scleroid
scleroiritis
sclerokeratitis
sclerokeratoiritis
sclerokeratosis
scleroma
scleromalacia perforans
scleromere
scleromyxedema
scleronychia
scleronyxis
sclero-oophoritis
sclero-oothecitis
sclerophthalmia
scleroplasty

scleroprotein
sclerosal
sclerosant
sclerose, sclerosed
sclérose en plaques
sclerosing
    s. agent
    s. basal cell carcinoma
    s. cholangitis
    chronic s. thyroiditis
    diffuse s. osteomyelitis
    s. encapsulating peritonitis
    s. epithelial hamartoma
    focal s. osteomyelitis
    s. hemangioma
    s. inflammation
    s. injection
    s. keratitis
    mammary s. adenosis
    s. mastoiditis
    s. myeloma
    s. nonsuppurative osteomyelitis
    s. osteitis
    s. panniculitis
    s. periphlebitis
    s. peritonitis
    primary s. cholangitis
    s. solution
    subacute s.
      leukoencephalopathy
    subacute s. panencephalitis
    s. sweat duct carcinoma
    van Bogaert s. leukoencephalitis
sclerosis
    amyotrophic lateral s. (ALS)
    anterolateral s.
    aortic s.
    arterial s.
    arteriolar s.
    Baló concentric s.
    bone s.
    central areolar choroidal s.
    cerebral s.
    choroidal s.
    combined s.
    concentric s.
    cortical s.
    dentinal s.
    diaphyseal s.
    diffuse s.
    diffuse cerebral s.
    diffuse mesangial s.
    diffuse systemic s.
    disseminated s.
    endocardial s.

sclerosis *(continued)*
    Erb s.
    familial centrolobar s.
    focal s.
    focal glomerular s.
    gastric s.
    glomerular s.
    hippocampal s.
    hyperplastic s.
    lateral s.
    lenticular nuclear s.
    lobar s.
    medial calcific s.
    mesial temporal s.
    miliary s.
    Mönckeberg s.
    multiple s. (MS)
    nodular s.
    nuclear s.
    Pelizaeus-Merzbacher s.
    peritoneal s.
    posterolateral s.
    primary lateral s.
    primary systemic s.
    progressive systemic s.
      (PSS)
    subendocardial s.
    systemic s.
    tuberous s.
    unicellular s.
    valvular s.
    vascular s.
    venous s.
    ventrolateral s.
scleroskeleton
sclerostenosis
sclerostomy
    full-thickness s.
    inner s. wound
sclerotherapy
    catheter-delivered s.
    catheter-directed s.
    compression s.
    doxycycline s.
    endoscopic s.
    foam s.
    injection s.
    percutaneous s.
    transcatheter foam s.
    ultrasound-guided s.
    vein s.
sclerotia
sclerotic
    s. acid
    s. bodies

sclerotic *(continued)*
    s. cells
    s. coat
    s. degeneration
    s. dentin
    senile nuclear s. cataract
    s. teeth
sclerotica
sclerotitis
sclerotium
sclerotization
sclerotized
sclerotogenous layer
sclerotome
    Curdy s.
sclerotomy
    anterior s.
    s. incision
    posterior s.
    right-hand s.
    s. suture
sclerous tissues
ScLP—left posterior scapular
    (L. scapulolaeva posterior)
    (position)
scolecoid
scoliokyphosis
scoliorachitic
scoliosiometry
scoliosis
    Brissaud s.
    cicatricial s.
    congenital s.
    coxitic s.
    empyematic s.
    fixed s.
    functional s.
    habit s.
    inflammatory s.
    ischiatic s.
    myopathic s.
    osteopathic s.
    paralytic s.
    rachitic s.
    rheumatic s.
    sciatic s.
    static s.
    structural s.
scoliosometer
scoliotic pelvis
scoliotone
scolopsia
scombroid poisoning
scombrotoxic
scombrotoxin

S

scoop
    Arlt s.
    Beck gastrostomy s.
    Berens s.
    Daviel s.
    Desjardins s.
    Ferguson s.
    Ferris s.
    Knapp s.
    Lewis s.
    Luer-Korte s.
    Mayo s.
    Mayo-Robson s.
    Moore s.
    Moynihan s.
    Mules s.
    Wilder s.
scoparin
scoparius
scopes
    amblyoscope
    amnioscope
    anomaloscope
    anorthoscope
    anoscope
    arthroscope
    auriscope
    binoscope
    bronchofiberscope
    bronchoscope
    colonoscope
    colposcope
    culdoscope
    cystoscope
    cystourethroscope
    endoscope
    esophagoscope
    fibercolonoscope
    fibergastroscope
    fiberscope
    fluoroscope
    gastroscope
    gonioscope
    haploscope
    hypopharyngoscope
    hysterocolposcope
    hysteroscope
    keratoscope
    laparoscope
    laryngoscope
    laryngostroboscope
    mediastinoscope
    microscope
    nasopharyngoscope
    nasoscope
    nephroscope

scopes *(continued)*
    ophthalmoscope
    otomicroscope
    otoscope
    peritoneoscope
    pharyngoscope
    photofluoroscope
    photomicroscope
    proctoscope
    proctosigmoidoscope
    resectoscope
    retinoscope
    rhinoscope
    salpingoscope
    sigmoidoscope
    spectroscope
    sphincteroscope
    stereoscope
    stethoscope
    thoracoscope
    tracheoscope
    ultramicroscope
    ureterocystoscope
    urethroscope
    uteroscope
    vaginoscope
    ventriculoscope
    Visuscope
scopolagnia
scopophilia
scopophobia
Scopulariopsis brevicaulis
scopulariopsosis
scorbutic
scorbutigenic
scorbutus
score
    Agatston calcium s.
    AIS (Abbreviated
        Injury Scale) s.
    APACHE s.
    Apgar s.
    Bishop s.
    Canadian s.
    disability status s.
    Dubowitz s.
    GRSEQ (Gambling Refusal
        Self-Efficacy Questionnaire) s.
    Glasgow coma s.
    Gleason grading s.
    Gleason-sum s.
    high upper lip bite test s.
    JHAAC (Johns Hopkins
        Allergy and Asthma
        Composite) severity s.
    injury severity s.

score *(continued)*
 Kurtzke disability status s.
 LAP (leukocyte alkaline
  phosphatase) s.
 muscle strength s.
 NIHSS (NIH Stroke Scale) s.
 pain s.
 patient satisfaction s.
 perfusion s.
 pneumonia severity index s.
 Ramsay sedation s.
 recovery s.
 sedation s.
 Silverman s.
 standardized s.
 TIMI (Thrombolysis in
  Myocardial Infarction) risk s.
 visual function s.
 z score
scoring
scorpion
scorpionism
scotochromogen
scotochromogenic
scotochromogenicity
scotodinia
scotoma (scotomata)
 absolute s.
 annular s.
 arcuate s.
 aural s.
 s. auris
 Bjerrum s.
 cecocentral s.
 central s.
 centrocecal s.
 color s.
 flittering s.
 hemianopic s.
 mental s.
 motile s's
 negative s.
 paracentral s.
 peripapillary s.
 peripheral s.
 physiologic s.
 positive s.
 relative s.
 ring s.
 scintillating s.
 Seidel s.
 suppression s.
scotomatous
scotometer
 Bjerrum s.
scotometry

scotophilia
scotophobia
scotopia
scotopic
 s. adaptation
 s. vision
scotopsin
Scott
 cannula
 speculum
Scoville
 clip
 forceps
 retractor
Scoville-Lewis clip
scratcher
 Kratz s.
scratch-type incision
screen
 Bjerrum s.
 s. craze artifact
 dream s.
 fluorescent s.
 Hess-Lees s.
 intensifying s.
 oral s.
 skin s.
 SOGS-R (Revised South Oaks
  Gambling) S.
 solar s.
 s. test
 tangent s.
 urine drug s. (UDS)
 vestibular s.
screening
 antibody s.
 baseline s.
 cancer s.
 chest s.
 s. colonoscopy
 Denver Developmental S.
  test
 diabetes s.
 genetic s.
 heavy metal s.
 HIV (human
  immunodeficiency virus) s.
 HPV (human papilloma
  virus) s.
 hypertension s.
 lung cancer s.
 s. mammography
 mass s.
 multiphasic s.
 multiple s.
 neonatal s.

S

screening *(continued)*
    prenatal s.
    prescriptive s.
    skin cancer s.
    s. study
    s. test
    toxicological s.
    s. x-ray
screw
    Basile s.
    Bosworth s.
    Collison s.
    Coventry s.
    dentin s.
    Eggers s.
    expansion s.
    Kristiansen s.
    Leinbach s.
    McAtee s.
    McLaughlin s.
    Richards hip s.
    Sherman s.
    Thornton s.
    Vitallium s.
    Zimmer s.
Scribner shunt
scribomania
scrobiculate
scrobiculus cordis
scrofula
scrofular conjunctivitis
scrofuloderma
    bilateral ocular s.
    multifocal s.
    ocular s.
    recalcitrant s.
    symmetrical s.
scrofulous
    s. keratitis
    s. ophthalmia
scroll ear
scrotal
    s. arteries
    s. fat necrosis
    s. hemangioma
    s. hematocele
    s. hernia
    s. hydrocele
    s. ligament
    s. lymphangioma
    s. nerves
    s. raphe
    s. reflex
    s. septum
    s. swellings

scrotal *(continued)*
    s. tongue
    s. veins
scrotectomy
scroti
    elephantiasis s.
    pruritus s.
    raphe s.
scrotitis
scrotocele
scrotoplasty
scrotum
    angiokeratoma of s.
    bifid s.
    lymph s.
    watering-can s.
scruple
scrupulosity
SCT—sex chromatin test
SCU—special care unit
Scudder
    clamp
    forceps
Scully tumor
sculpt
sculptured nose
scultetus (bandage)
Scultetus position
scu-PA—single chain urokinase-
    type plasminogen activator
scurrile
scurrilous
scurvy
    alpine s.
    biochemical s.
    hemorrhagic s.
    infantile s.
    land s.
    sea s.
    subclinical s.
scutate
scute
    tympanic s.
scutiform
scutular
scutulum
scutum pectoris
scybalous
scybalum (scybala)
SD—
    septal defect
    sero-defined (antigens)
    serologically defined (antigens)
    skin dose
    spontaneous delivery

SD— *(continued)*
    standard deviation
    sudden death
S/D—systolic-to-diastolic ratio
SDA—right anterior sacral
   (L. sacrodextra anterior)
   (position)
SDCL—symptom distress checklist
SDE—specific dynamic effect
SDP—right posterior sacral
   (L. sacrodextra posterior)
   (position)
SDS—
    Self-Rating Depression Scale
    sudden death syndrome
SDS-PAGE—SDS–polyacrylamide
  gel electrophoresis
SDT—right transverse sacral
   (L. sacrodextra transversa)
   (position)
SE—Starr-Edwards (prosthesis)
sea fan
    s.f. neovascular formation
    s.f. neovascularization
    s.f. pattern
seagull bruit
seal
    border s.
    crimp s.
    double s.
    peripheral s.
    posterior palatal s.
    velopharyngeal s.
sealant
    dental s.
    fissure s.
    pit and fissure s.
sealer
    endodontic s.
    root canal s.
sealing
    fissure s.
seam
    osteoid s.
    pigment s.
searcher
    Allport s.
    Allport-Babcock s.
Searcy tonsillectome
Seashore test
seasickness
seat
    basal s.
    rest s.
seaweed

sebaceous
    s. adenocarcinoma
    s. adenoma
    s. carcinoma
    s. cyst
    s. epithelioma
    s. follicle
    s. glands
    s. horn
    s. hyperplasia
    s. nevus
    s. nevus syndrome
Sebileau
    bands
    hollow
    muscle
sebocyte
sebogenesis
sebopoiesis
seborrhea
    s. adiposa
    s.-like dermatitis
    s.-like dermatosis
    eczematoid s.
    facial s.
    nasolabial s.
    s. sicca
seborrheal
seborrheic
    s. alopecia
    s. dermatitis
    s. eczema
    s. keratosis
    s. psoriasis
    s. wart
seborrhiasis
sebostasis
sebotropic
sebum
    cutaneous s.
    s. palpebrale
secede
Seckel
    dwarf
    syndrome
seclusio pupillae
second (s, sec.)
    gray per s.
    inverse s.
    milliampere s. (mAs)
    reciprocal s.
secondaries
secondary
    s. abutment
    s. adhesion

S

secondary *(continued)*
- s. aldosteronism
- s. amenorrhea
- s. amyloidosis
- s. apnea
- s. asphyxia
- s. atelectasis
- s. attack rate
- s. axis
- s. biliary cirrhosis
- s. bronchi
- s. bronchial buds
- s. bronchitis
- s. buffering
- s. cardiomyopathy
- s. care
- s. cataract
- s. cause
- s. chemoprophylaxis
- s. choana
- chronic s. polyarthritis
- s. constriction
- s. curvatures of spine
- s. cuticle
- s. cyst
- s. degeneration
- s. dental caries
- s. dentin
- s. dentition
- s. deviation
- s. dextrocardia
- s. diagnosis
- s. drowning
- s. dysmenorrhea
- s. epileptogenic focus
- s. fracture
- s. gain
- s. gangrene
- s. glaucoma
- s. gout
- s. granule
- s. hemochromatosis
- s. host
- s. hydrocephalus
- s. hyperparathyroidism
- s. hyperplastic osteitis
- s. hypertension
- s. hypogonadism
- s. hypothyroidism
- s. immune response
- s. impotence
- s. impression
- s. infection
- s. infertility
- s. keratitis

secondary *(continued)*
- s. livedo reticularis
- s. lymphedema
- s. myeloid metaplasia
- s. myxedema
- s. narcissism
- s. nodule
- s. nystagmus
- s. oocyte
- s. optic atrophy
- s. ossification center
- s. ossification point
- s. otalgia
- s. ovarian follicles
- s. pacemaker
- s. palate
- s. pneumonia
- s. polycythemia
- s. priapism
- s. reinforcer
- s. renal calculus
- s. sensation
- s. sequestrum
- s. shock
- s. spontaneous pneumothorax
- s. sterility
- s. suture
- s. syphilis
- s. thrombocytopenic purpura
- s. tuberculosis
- s. tympanic membrane
- s. villus
- s. vitreous

second intention
second-look laparotomy
secreta
secretagogue
secrete
secretin
- s. family
- gastric s.
- s. injection test
- intravenous s. test
- s. stimulation test
- s. test

secretin-cholecystokinin test
secretin-pancreozymin test
secretion
- antilytic s.
- external s.
- gastric s's
- internal s.
- neurohumoral s.
- paralytic s.

secretoinhibitory

secretomotor nerve
secretor
secretory
    s. canaliculus
    s. capillary
    s. coil
    s. component deficiency
    s. compound
    s. cyst
    s. diarrhea
    s. duct
    s. granules
    s. IgA
    s. nerve
    s. otitis media
    s. vesicles
sectile
sectio (sectiones)
    sectiones cerebellares
    sectiones cerebelli
    sectiones corporum
      quadrigeminorum
    sectiones hypothalami
    sectiones hypothalamicae
    sectiones isthmi
    s. mediana
    sectiones medullae oblongatae
    sectiones medullae spinalis
    sectiones mesencephali
    sectiones mesencephalicae
    sectiones pedunculi cerebri
    sectiones pontis
    sectiones telencephali
    sectiones telencephalicae
    sectiones thalamicae et
      metathalamicae
    sectiones thalami et
      metathalami
section
    abdominal s.
    celloidin s.
    cervical cesarean s.
    classic cesarean s.
    coronal s.
    corporeal cesarean s.
    cross s.
    extraperitoneal cesarean s.
    frontal s.
    frozen s.
    ground s.
    Latzko cesarean s.
    low cervical cesarean s.
    lower segment cesarean s.
    Munro Kerr cesarean s.
    paraffin s.

section *(continued)*
    perineal s.
    Pitres s's
    pituitary stalk s.
    Porro cesarean s.
    postmortem cesarean s.
    radical cesarean s.
    root s.
    Saemisch s.
    sagittal s.
    semithin s.
    serial s.
    step s.
    transperitoneal cesarean s.
    transverse cesarean s.
    trigeminal root s.
    ultrathin s.
sectional
    cross-s. study
    s. impression
    s. method
    s. radiography
    s. roentgenography
sectiones (plural of sectio)
sectioning
    complete s.
    longitudinal s.
    optical s.
    optical axial s.
    partial s.
    sequential s.
    serial s.
    serial perpendicular s.
    step s.
    surgical s.
    tooth s.
    transverse s.
sector
    s. iridectomy
    Sommer s.
sectorial
secundam
    per s. intentionem
secundigravida
secundina (secundinae)
secundines
secundipara
secundiparity
secundiparous
secundum
    s. artem
    ostium s. defect
SED—
    skin erythema dose
    spondyloepiphyseal dysplasia

S

sedate, sedated
sedation
- adequate s.
- ambulatory s.
- conscious s.
- continuous deep s.
- depth of s.
- dexmedetomidine s.
- excessive s.
- level of s.
- light s.
- moderate s.
- office-based dental s.
- opioid s.
- propofol s.
- Ramsay s. score
- s. score

sedative
- cardiac s.
- cerebral s.
- s. effect
- gastric s.
- general s.
- intestinal s.
- nerve trunk s.
- nervous s.
- s. poisons
- respiratory s.
- spinal s.
- vascular s.

Seddon nerve graft
sedentary
Sédillot
- elevator
- operation

sediment
- s. tube
- urinary s.

sedimentable
sedimentation
- s. coefficient
- s. constant
- erythrocyte s.
- erythrocyte s. rate
- erythrocyte s. reaction
- s. rate
- Ritchie formalin–ethyl acetate s.
- s. time
- s. tube
- Westergren s. rate
- Wintrobe s. rate
- zeta s. ratio

sedimentator
sedoheptulose 7-phosphate

sed rate—sedimentation rate
seed
- brachytherapy s.
- cardamom s.
- celery s.
- grape s. extract
- s. implant brachytherapy
- iodine I 125 seed implant
- s. markers
- melon s. body
- s. metastases
- plantago s.
- psyllium s.
- s. pulmonary metastases
- radiogold s.
- radon s.
- sunflower s.
- s. tick
- s. wart

Seessel
- pocket
- pouch

Séglas type
segment
- arterial s. of glomeriform arteriovenous anastomosis
- arterial s's of kidney
- basal s.
- body s.
- bronchopulmonary s.
- cardiac s.
- ceratobranchial s.
- connecting s.
- cranial s's
- differential s.
- epibranchial s.
- equatorial s.
- Fc s.
- frontal s.
- hepatic s's
- hypobranchial s.
- initial s.
- interannular s.
- intermaxillary s.
- internodal s.
- s's of kidney
- lingular s.
- s's of liver
- lower s. cesarean section
- lower uterine s.
- medullary s.
- mesoblastic s.
- muscle s.
- neural s.
- occipital s.

segment *(continued)*
> pairing s's
> parietal s.
> pharyngobranchial s.
> posterior s.
> PQ s.
> P-R s.
> pubic s. of the pelvis
> Ranvier s.
> renal s.
> rivinian s.
> s. of Rivinus
> rod s.
> RS-T s.
> sacral s.
> Schmidt-Lanterman s.
> spinal s's.
> s's of spinal cord
> ST s.
> Ta s.
> thick s.
> thin s.
> TP s.
> TP-Q s.
> upper uterine s.
> uterine s.
> venous s. of glomeriform
>   arteriovenous anastomosis
> venous s's of kidney
> venous s's of liver

segmenta (plural of
  segmentum)

segmental
> s. alveolar osteotomy
> s. anesthesia
> s. arterial mediolysis
> s. arteries
> s. atelectasis
> s. bronchi
> s. bronchus
> s. buds
> s. demyelination
> s. dilatation
> s. fracture
> s. glomerulonephritis
> s. hyalinizing vasculitis
> s. lentiginosis
> s. lines
> s. mastectomy
> s. medullary artery
> s. neuritis
> s. neuropathy
> s. plate
> s. reflex
> s. renal hyperplasia

segmental *(continued)*
> s. sensory dissociation
> s. tubules
> s. veins
> s. vitiligo
> s. zone

segmentation
> s. cavity
> complete s.
> s. contraction
> haustral s.
> metameric s.
> s. movement
> s. nucleus
> partial s.
> regular s.
> rhythmic s.
> signal s.
> s. sphere
> unequal s.

segmented neutrophils
  (segs, segmenteds)

segmenter

segmentum (segmenta)
> s. arteriale anastomosis
>   arteriovenae
>   glomeriformis
> segmenta bronchopulmonalia
> segmenta hepatis
> segmenta medullae spinalis
> segmenta renalia
> s. venosum anastomosis
>   arteriovenae
>   glomeriformis

Segond
> forceps
> spatula

segregation
> nuclear s.

segregator
> Cathelin s.
> Harris s.

segs—segmented neutrophils

Séguin
> sign
> signal symptom

Sehrt
> clamp
> compressor

Seidel
> scotoma
> sign

Seidelin bodies

Seidlitz powder test

Seiffert forceps

S

Seiler
- formula
- knife
- scissors

Seip-Lawrence syndrome

Seitelberger
- disease
- dystrophy
- syndrome

Seitz metamorphosing respiration

seizure
- absence s.
- adversive s.
- astatic s.
- atonic s.
- audiogenic s.
- automatic s.
- autonomic s.
- centrencephalic s.
- cerebral s.
- clonic s.
- complex partial s.
- febrile s.
- focal s.
- focal motor s.
- generalized s.
- generalized tonic-clonic s.
- hysterical s.
- jacksonian s.
- major motor s.
- minor motor s.
- myoclonic s.
- neonatal s.
- partial s.
- partial complex s.
- partial onset s.
- psychogenic s.
- psychomotor s.
- reflex s.
- reflex anoxic s.
- sensory s.
- serial s's
- simple partial s.
- sylvian s.
- tonic s.
- tonic-clonic s.
- traumatic s.
- uncinate s.
- uremic s.

Seldinger
- approach
- catheterization
- method
- needle
- technique

Seldinger *(continued)*
- technique, balloon-assisted
- technique, modified
- technique, percutaneous
- technique, transfemoral
- technique, ultrasound-guided
- wire, knotted

selection

selective
- s. antegrade cerebral perfusion
- s. arteriography
- highly s. vagotomy
- s. coronary angiography
- s. radiography
- s. roentgenography
- s. vagotomy
- s. venography

selectivity

seleniferous

selenious acid

selenite broth

selenium (Se)
- s. 75
- s. poisoning
- s. sulfide
- vitamin E–s. deficiency syndrome

selenomethionine

selenomethylnorcholesterol

selenosis

Seletz cannula

self
- idealized s.
- true s.

self-absorption

self-analysis

self-assertion

self-awareness

self-care

self-consciousness

self-defeating personality disorder

self-efficacy

self-esteem

self-healing
- s-h. juvenile cutaneous mucinosis
- multiple s-h. squamous epithelioma

self-hypnosis

self-image

self-infection

self-limited disease

self-limiting

self-observation

self-quenched counter tube

self-recognition
self-retaining
 s-r. atrial retractor
 s-r. catheter
 s-r. clip
 s-r. elastic abdominal
  retractor
 s-r. expanded PTFE-silicone
  tube
 s-r. gastric balloon port
 s-r. laryngoscope
 s-r. lighted retractor
 s-r. retractor
 s-r. ring retractor
 s-r. T incision
 s-r. titanium clip stapes
  prosthesis
 s-r. transconjunctival
  chandelier endoilluminator
 s-r. ureteral stent
self-tolerance
Selivanoff (Seliwanow)
 reaction
 test
sella (sellae)
 empty s.
 empty s. syndrome
 s. turcica
sellar
Sellick maneuver
Sellor
 knife
 rib contractor
Selsun Blue shampoo
Selter disease
Selverstone clamp
Selye
 adaptation syndrome
 syndrome
SEM—scanning electron
 microscopy
semantic
semantics
Semb
 forceps
 operation
 retractor
semeiology
semeiotic
semen
semenuria
semialdehyde
 α-aminoadipic s. synthase
  [alpha-]
 glutamic-γ-s. [-gamma-]

semialdehyde *(continued)*
 succinate s.
 succinate-s. dehydrogenase
  deficiency
semicanal
 s. of auditory tube
 s. of humerus
 s. of tensor tympani muscle
semicanalis (semicanales)
 s. musculi tensoris
  tympani
 s. tubae auditivae
 s. tubae auditoriae
semicartilaginous
semicircular
 bony s. canal
 s. ducts
 s. incision
 s. line of Douglas
 s. lines
 membranous s. canal
 s. planes
 s. ridge
semiclosed anesthesia
semicoma
semicomatose
semiconscious
semicrista incisiva
semiflexed incision
semiflexion
semifluctuating
semi-Fowler position
semilunar
 s. bodies
 s. bone
 s. cartilage
 s. cusps of aortic valve
 s. cusps of pulmonary valve
 s. fascia
 s. fasciculus
 s. fibrocartilages
 s. fold of conjunctiva
 s. fold of fauces
 s. folds of colon
 s. fossa of ulna
 s. ganglion
 s. incision
 s. line
 s. lobes
 s. lobule
 s. notch of mandible
 s. notch of scapula
 s. notch of ulna
 s. opening of ethmoid bone
 s. space

S

semilunar *(continued)*
    s. sulcus of radius
    s. valve
semilunare
semiluxation
semimembranous
seminal
    s. colliculus
    s. crest
    s. ducts
    excretory duct of s. gland
    s. fluid
    s. gland
    s. gland duct
    s. granules
    s. hillock
    s. plasma
    s. vesicle
    s. vesicle calculus
    s. vesicle cyst
    s. vesiculitis
    s. vesiculotomy
semination
seminiferous
    convoluted s. tubules
    s. cords
    s. epithelium
    straight s. tubules
    s. tubule dysgenesis
    s. tubules
seminoma
    anaplastic s.
    classical s.
    ovarian s.
    spermatocytic s.
seminomatous
    s. testicular neoplasm
    s. testicular tumor
seminormal solution
seminuria
semiopen anesthesia
semiotics
semioval center
semiovale
    centrum s.
semipennate muscle
semipenniform
semipermeable membrane
semiplegia
semiprecision
    s. attachment
    s. test
semiprivate room
semipronation
semiprone position

semirecumbent
semirigid prosthesis
semis
semispinalis
    s. capitis muscle
    s. cervicis muscle
    s. muscle
    s. thoracis muscle
semispinal muscle
semistarvation
semisulcus (semisulci)
semisupination
semisupine position
semisynthetic
semitendinosus muscle
semitendinous bursa
Semken forceps
Semliki Forest
    encephalitis
    virus
Semon law
Semon-Hering
    hypothesis
    theory
Semon-Rosenbach law
Senear-Usher
    disease
    syndrome
senecio disease
Senecio poisoning
senescence
    dental s.
senescent
    s. alopecia
    s. CD4+
    s. CD8+
    premature s. fibroblasts
    s. T cells
Sengstaken tube
Sengstaken-Blakemore tube
senile
    atrophic s. gingivitis
    s. amyloidosis
    s. angioma
    s. ankylosing hyperostosis
      of spine
    s. arteriosclerosis
    s. atrophoderma
    s. atrophy
    s. atrophy of skin
    s. cataract
    s. chorea
    s. coxitis
    s. degeneration
    s. delirium

senile *(continued)*
    s. dementia
    s. disciform macular
      degeneration
    s. ectropion
    s. elastosis
    s. emphysema
    s. exudative macular
      degeneration
    s. gangrene
    s. halo
    s. involution
    s. keratoma
    s. keratosis
    s. lentigines
    s. lentigo
    s. macular exudative choroiditis
    s. neuropathy
    s. nuclear sclerotic cataract
    s. osteomalacia
    s. osteoporosis
    s. paraplegia
    s. plaques
    s. pruritus
    s. psychosis
    s. purpura
    s. reflex
    s. tremor
    s. vaginitis
    s. vulvovaginitis
senilis
    arcus s.
senilism
senility
Senn
    forceps
    operation
    retractor
Senn-Dingman retractor
Senning
    operation
    procedure
sennoside (A and B)
senopia
sensation
    articular s.
    chromatic s.
    cincture s.
    color s.
    common s.
    concomitant s.
    cutaneous s.
    delayed s.
    dermal s.
    eccentric s.

sensation *(continued)*
    epigastric s.
    external s.
    form s.
    general s.
    generalized epileptic somatic s.
    girdle s.
    gnostic s's
    internal s.
    joint s.
    kinesthetic s.
    light s.
    objective s.
    palmesthetic s.
    pressure s.
    primary s.
    proprioceptive s.
    protopathic s.
    radiating s.
    referred s.
    reflex s.
    secondary s.
    seventh s.
    skin s.
    space s.
    stereognostic s.
    strain s.
    subjective s.
    tactile s.
    time s.
    tone s.
    transferred s.
    vascular s.
    visceral s.
    s. of warmth
sense
    body s.
    chemical s.
    color s.
    contact s.
    dermal s.
    distance s.
    s. of equilibrium
    external s.
    form s.
    internal s.
    interoceptive s's
    joint s.
    joint position s.
    kinesthetic s.
    labyrinthine s.
    light s.
    motion s.
    movement s.
    muscle s.

S

sense *(continued)*
    muscular s.
    obstacle s.
    pain s.
    s. of pitch
    position s.
    posture s.
    pressure s.
    proprioceptive s.
    seventh s.
    sixth s.
    somatic s's
    space s.
    special s.
    static s.
    stereognostic s.
    tactile s.
    temperature s.
    time s.
    tone s.
    vestibular s.
    vibration s.
    visceral s.
sensibility
    articular s.
    binaural s.
    bone s.
    common s.
    cortical s.
    cutaneous s.
    deep s.
    dissociation s.
    electromuscular s.
    epicritic s.
    gnostic s.
    interoceptive s.
    joint s.
    kinesthetic s.
    mesoblastic s.
    muscular s.
    myotatic s.
    nervous s.
    pallesthetic s.
    palmesthetic s.
    proprioceptive s.
    protopathic s.
    recurrent s.
    somesthetic s.
    splanchnesthetic s.
    touch s.
    two-point s.
    uterine s.
    vibratory s.
sensibilization
sensible

sensiferous
sensitive
sensitivity
    analytical s.
    antibiotic s.
    antimicrobial s.
    autoerythrocyte s.
    deep s.
    delayed s.
    diagnostic s.
    differential s.
    plane s.
    point s.
    proportional s.
    thermal s.
    trophic s.
    vibratory s.
sensitization
    active s.
    autoerythrocyte s.
    passive s.
    photodynamic s.
    Rh s.
sensitized
sensitizer
sensomotor
sensor
sensorial
sensoriglandular
sensorimotor
    s. arc
    s. area
    s. neuropathy
sensorimuscular
sensorineural
    s. hearing loss
    s. stimulus
    s. tinnitus
sensorium
    s. commune
    general s.
sensorivascular
sensorivasomotor
sensory
    s. amusia
    s. aphasia
    s. apraxia
    s. areas
    s. association area
    s. ataxia
    s. cell
    s. centers
    compound s. nerve action
      potential
    s. decussation

sensory *(continued)*
    s. deficit
    Denny-Brown s.
      neuropathy
    s. deprivation
    s. epilepsy
    s. fibers
    s. ganglion
    s. gating
    s. hairs
    s. hearing loss
    hereditary motor and s.
      neuropathy
    hereditary s. neuropathy
    s. image
    s. latency
    s. lemniscus
    s. loss
    s. neglect
    s. nerve
    s. nerve root
    s. neuron
    s. neuropathy
    s. nucleus
    s. overload
    s. paralysis
    s. paralytic bladder
    s. pathway
    peripheral s. neuron
    s. potential
    primary s. neuron
    s. radicular neuropathy
    s. receptor
    s. regions
    s. root
    s. seizure
    somatic s. area
    somatic s. component
    splanchnic s. component
    s. stimulation
    symmetrical s. polyneuropathy
    s. tract
    s. transduction
    s. tunic of eyeball
    visceral s. component
sentence
    Babcock s.
sentient
sentinel
    s. clot
    s. gland
    s. loop
    s. node
    s. node biopsy
    s. patch

sentinel *(continued)*
    s. pile
    s. tumor
Senturia speculum
SEP—
    sensory evoked potential
    somatosensory evoked potential
    systolic ejection period
separation
    A/C (acromioclavicular) joint s.
    s. anxiety
    s. anxiety disorder
    eschar s.
    s. of placenta
    shoulder s.
separator
    Horsley s.
    House s.
    Rosen s.
sepsin
sepsis
    burn wound s.
    catheter s.
    gas s.
    incarcerated s.
    oral s.
    postabortal s.
    postanginal s.
    puerperal s.
septa (plural of septum)
    Bertin s.
    placental s.
    s. of testis
septal
    aortic s. defect
    aorticopulmonary s. defect
    s. area
    s. arteries
    asymmetrical s. hypertrophy
    atrial s. aneurysm
    atrial s. defects
    s. cartilage of nose
    s. cells
    costophrenic s. lines
    s. cusp of right
      atrioventricular valve
    s. defect
    s. gingiva
    interventricular s. arteries
    lateral s. nucleus
    medial s. nucleus
    s. myocardial infarction
    s. nuclei
    s. panniculitis
    s. resection

S

septal *(continued)*
    s. space
    triangular s. nucleus
    ventricular s. defect
septanose
septate
    s. hymen
    s. uterus
septation
septatome
septectomy
    balloon atrial s.
septi (genitive of septum)
    depressor s. nasi muscle
septic
    s. abortion
    s. arthritis
    s. bursitis
    s. disease
    s. embolization
    s. endocarditis
    s. fever
    s. infarct
    s. knee
    s. necrosis
    s. peritonitis
    s. phlebitis
    s. polyarthritis
    s. shock
    Simon s. factor
    s. sore throat
    s. wound
septicemia
    acute fulminating
      meningococcal s.
    bronchopulmonary s.
    Bruce's s.
    coliform s.
    cryptogenic s.
    Escherichia coli s.
    hemorrhagic s.
    metastasizing s.
    perinatal s.
    phlebitic s.
    plague s.
    puerperal s.
    sputum s.
septicemic
    s. abscess
    s. colibacillosis
    s. pasteurellosis
    s. plague
    s. tularemia
septicopyemia

septicopyemic
septigravida
septimetritis
septineuritis
    Nicolau s.
septipara
septivalent
septomarginal
    s. fasciculus
    s. tract
septonasal
septo-optic dysplasia
septoplasty
septorhinoplasty
septostomy
    atrial s.
    balloon atrial s.
    Rashkind balloon atrial s.
septotome
septotomy
septulum (septula)
    septula testis
septum (septa)
    alveolar s.
    s. alveoli
    aorticopulmonary s.
    atrial s.
    atrioventricular s. of heart
    s. of auditory tube
    bony s. of eustachian canal
    bony s. of nose
    s. bulbi urethrae
    s. canalis musculotubarii
    cartilaginous s. of nose
    cervical s., intermediate
    cloacal s.
    Cloquet s.
    s. corporum cavernosorum
      clitoridis
    crural s.
    deviated nasal s.
    dorsal median s.
    Douglas s.
    enamel s.
    femoral s.
    s. of frontal sinuses
    gingival s.
    s. glandis penis
    s. of glans penis
    iliopectineal s.
    interalveolar s.
    interatrial s. of heart
    interdental s.
    interlobular s.

septum (septa) *(continued)*

    intermuscular s., crural, anterior

    intermuscular s., crural, posterior

    intermuscular s. of arm, external

    intermuscular s. of arm, internal

    intermuscular s. of arm, lateral

    intermuscular s. of arm, medial

    intermuscular s. of leg, anterior

    intermuscular s. of leg, posterior

    intermuscular s. of thigh, external

    intermuscular s. of thigh, lateral

    intermuscular s. of thigh, medial

    s. intermusculare anterius cruris

    s. intermusculare brachii laterale

    s. intermusculare brachii mediale

    s. intermusculare cruris anterius

    s. intermusculare cruris posterius

    s. intermusculare femoris laterale

    s. intermusculare femoris mediale

    s. intermusculare humeri laterale

    s. intermusculare humeri mediale

    s. intermusculare posterius cruris

    interradicular s.

    interventricular s. of heart

    Körner (Koerner) s.

    lingual s.

    s. linguae

    s. lucidum

    median s. of spinal cord, dorsal

    s. medianum dorsale medullae spinalis

    s. medianum posterius medullae spinalis

    mediastinal s.

    membranous s. of nose

    s. mobile nasi

septum (septa) *(continued)*

    s. of musculotubal canal

    nasal s.

    s. nasale

    s. nasi

    s. nasi osseum

    neural s.

    s. of nose

    osseous s. of nose

    s. pectiniforme

    pellucid s.

    s. pellucidum

    s. penis

    pharyngeal s.

    precommissural s.

    s. primum

    rectovaginal s.

    s. rectovaginale

    rectovesical s.

    s. rectovesicale

    scrotal s.

    s. of scrotum

    s. secundum

    s. sinuum frontalium

    s. sinuum sphenoidalium

    sphenoidal s.

    s. of sphenoidal sinuses

    spiral s.

    spurious s.

    subarachnoidal s.

    septa of testis

    s. of tongue

    tracheoesophageal s.

    transverse s. of ampulla

    s. transversum

    true s.

    urogenital s.

    urorectal s.

    s. of ventricles of heart

    ventricular s.

    s. verum

septuplet

seq.—

    sequela

    sequestrum

sequel

sequela (sequelae)

sequence

    adenoma-carcinoma s.

    amniotic band s.

    consensus s.

    flanking s.

    gene s.

    insertion s. (IS)

S

sequence *(continued)*
    intervening s.
    oligohydramnios s.
    pulse s.
    signal s.
    targeting s.
sequence-tagged site (STS) map
sequential
    s. analysis
    atrioventricular (AV) s.
      pacemaker
    s. chemotherapy
    s. determinant
    s. mechanism
sequestered
    s. antigens
    s. disk
sequestra (plural of sequestrum)
sequestral
sequestrant
sequestration
    biochemical s.
    bronchopulmonary s.
    corneal s.
    disk s.
    extralobar s.
    intralobar
    pulmonary s.
sequestrectomy
sequestrotomy
sequestrum (sequestra)
    corneal s.
    s. forceps
    primary s.
    secondary s.
    tertiary s.
sequoiosis
SER—
    somatosensory evoked response
    systolic ejection rate
sera (plural of serum)
serendipitous
serendipity
Sereny test
Sergent white adrenal line
serial
    s. dilution
    s. EKGs
    s. extraction
    s. passage
    s. radiography
    s. section
    s. seizures
    s. stretch orthoses
serially

serialograph
series
    basophil s., basophilic s.
    eosinophil s., eosinophilic s.
    erythrocyte s., erythrocytic s.
    gastrointestinal (GI) s.
    granulocyte s., granulocytic s.
    Hofmeister s.
    homologous s.
    leukocytic s.
    lymphocyte s., lymphocytic s.
    lyotropic s.
    monocyte s., monocytic s.
    myelocytic s.
    myeloid s.
    neutrophil s., neutrophilic s.
    plasmacyte s., plasmacytic s.
    radioactive s.
    small-bowel s.
    thrombocyte s., thrombocytic s.
serine
    s. endopeptidase
    s. hydroxymethyltransferase
    s. protease
    s. protease inhibitor
    s. proteinase
    s./threonine kinase
    s.-type carboxypeptidase
seroalbuminous
seroconversion
seroconvert
seroculture
serocystic
serodiagnosis
serodiagnostic
seroenteritis
seroepidemiology
sero-fast
serofibrinous
    s. pericarditis
    s. pleurisy
serofibrous
seroflocculation
serogroup
serolipase
serologic test for syphilis (STS)
serological reaction
serologist
serology
    diagnostic s.
    forensic s.
seroma
seromembranous
seromucosa
    glandula s.

seromucoid
seromucous gland
seromucus
seromuscular suture
seromyotomy
seronegative
seronegativity
serophilic
seroplastic inflammation
seropneumothorax
seropositive
seropositivity
seroprevalence
seroprognosis
seropurulent
seropus
seroreaction
serorelapse
seroresistance
seroresistant
seroreversal
seroreversion
serosa
serosal fold
serosamucin
serosanguineous
seroserous suture
serositis (serositides)
 adhesive s.
 multiple serositides
serosity
serosurvey
serosynovial
serosynovitis
serotherapy
serothorax
serotonin
 selective s. reuptake inhibitor
  (SSRI)
 s. syndrome
 s.-norepinephrine reuptake
  inhibitor (SNRI)
serotoninergic
serotype
 heterologous s.
 homologous s.
serous
 acute diffuse s. choroiditis
 acute s. labyrinthitis
 s. atrophy
 s. borderline tumor
 s. canal
 s. capsule of spleen
 s. cavity
 s. cell

serous *(continued)*
 central s. retinopathy
 s. coat
 s. coat of esophagus
 s. coat of gallbladder
 s. coat of large intestine
 s. coat of liver
 s. coat of small intestine
 s. coat of stomach
 s. coat of urinary bladder
 s. cyclitis
 s. cyst
 s. cystadenocarcinoma
 s. cystadenoma
 s. diarrhea
 s. fluid
 s. gland
 s. hepatosis
 s. infiltration
 s. inflammation
 s. iritis
 s. layer
 s. layer of esophagus
 s. layer of gallbladder
 s. layer of large intestine
 s. layer of liver
 s. layer of small intestine
 s. layer of stomach
 s. ligament
 s. membrane
 s. otitis media
 s. pericarditis
 s. pleurisy
 s. retinal detachment
 s. retinitis
 s. sac
 s. synovitis
serovaccination
serovar
serpent
serpentine
 s. aneurysm
 s. asbestos
 s. biatrial thrombus
 s. cords
 s. flow voids on MR image
 giant s. aneurysm
 s. incision
 s. thrombus
 s. vessel
serpiginous
 s. areas of flow void
 s. borders
 s. chorioretinitis
 s. choroiditis

S

serpiginous *(continued)*
    s. choroidopathy
    s. corneal ulcer
    s. hypodensities
    s. intrathrombus flow voids
    s. keratitis
    s. lesion
    s. low signal intensity line
    s. mass
    s. morphology
    s. thrombus
    s. tunneling
    s. vascular structure
serrated
    s. action potential
    s. border
    s. curet
    s. edge
    s. suture
Serratia
    S. liquefaciens
    S. marcescens
    S. odorifera
    S. rubidaea
serration
serratus anterior muscle
Serre operation
serrefine
    Blair s.
    s. clamp
Serres
    angle
    glands
Sertoli
    cell
    column
    tumor
Sertoli cell–only syndrome
Sertoli-Leydig cell tumor
serum (serums, sera)
    s. acid phosphatase
    active s.
    s. albumin
    alkaline blood s.
    s. alkaline phosphatase
    s. alpha-fetoprotein (AFP)
    s. amyloid A protein
    s. amyloid P component
    antianthrax s.
    antibotulinus s.
    anticholera s.
    anticomplementary s.
    anticrotalus s.
    antidiphtheria s.
    anti-gas-gangrene s.

serum (serums, sera) *(continued)*
    antiglobulin s.
    antilymphocyte s. (ALS)
    antimeningococcus s.
    antipneumococcus s.
    antirabies s.
    antisnakebite s.
    antitetanic s. (ATS)
    antithymocyte s.
    antitoxic s.
    s. bactericidal activity test
    bacteriolytic s.
    blister s.
    s. blocking factor
    blood s.
    blood grouping s's
    s. carnosinase deficiency
    s. cholinesterase
    convalescence s.
    convalescent s.
    despeciated s.
    s. diagnosis
    s. disease
    s. eruption
    foreign s.
    s. gastrin test
    s. globulins
    s. hepatitis
    s. hepatitis antigen
    heterologous s.
    homologous s.
    hyperimmune s.
    immune s.
    inactivated s.
    s. lactis
    Löffler (Loeffler) blood s.
    lymphatolytic s.
    monospecific s.
    monovalent s.
    multipartial s.
    s. neuritis
    s. neuropathy
    s. neutralization test
    normal s.
    normal human s.
    North American
       antisnakebite s.
    s. paralysis
    pericardial s.
    polyvalent s.
    pooled s.
    pregnancy s.
    s. proteins
    s. prothrombin conversion
       accelerator

serum (serums, sera) *(continued)*
    quality control s.
    Sclavo s.
    s. shock
    s. sickness
    s. sickness-like reaction
    s. sickness-like syndrome
    specific s.
    s. therapy
    s. thrombotic accelerator
    truth s.
    unheated s. reagin test
    s. urate level
    s. urea nitrogen (SUN)
    s. uric acid
    von Behring (Behring) s.
    Widal s. test
    Yersin s.
serum-fast
servomechanism
SES—socioeconomic status
sesame
    s. oil
    s. seed
sesamoid
    s. bones of foot
    s. bones of hand
    s. cartilage of larynx
    s. cartilage of vocal
      ligament
    s. cartilages of nose
sesamoiditis
sesquioxide
sesquisulfate
sesquisulfide
sessile
set
    Barraquer-Krumeich-Swinger
      refractive s.
    mental s.
    phalangeal s.
    preparatory s.
SET—systolic ejection time
seta (setae)
setaceous
setiferous
setigerous
seton operation
set-point
Settegast position
setup
    diagnostic s.
Seutin bandage
Sever disease
sewage

Sewall
    chisel
    forceps
sex
    s. cells
    s. chromatin test
    chromosomal s.
    s. chromosomes
    s. cords
    s. cord–stromal tumors
    s. cycle
    s. determination
    endocrinologic s.
    s. factor
    female s. hormone
    genetic s.
    genital s.
    s. gland
    gonadal s.
    s. hormone–binding globulin
    s. hormones
    s.-influenced inheritance
    s.-influenced trait
    s. linkage
    s.-linked gene
    s.-linked inheritance
    s.-linked trait
    male s. hormone
    morphological s.
    nuclear s.
    psychological s.
    primary s. characteristics
    s. ratio
    s. reversal
    secondary s. characteristics
    social s.
    s. steroid
sexdigitate
sexivalent
sexology
sextant
sextigravida
sextipara
Sexton knife
sextuplet
sexual
    s. abuse
    s. arousal
    s. arousal disorder
    s. aversion disorder
    s. deviant
    s. deviation
    s. differentiation
    s. dimorphism
    s. disorder

S

sexual *(continued)*
    s. drive
    s. dysfunction
    hypoactive s. desire disorder
    s. infantilism
    s. intercourse
    s. masochism
    s. pain disorder
    s. precocity
    s. reflex
    s. sadism
    substance-induced s.
      dysfunction
sexuality
sexualization
sexually
    s. transmitted disease (STD)
    s. transmitted infection
Sézary
    cell
    erythroderma
    reticulosis
    syndrome
Sf, S$_f$—Svedberg flotation unit(s)
SF—
    shell fragment
    shrapnel fragment
    spinal fluid
    synovial fluid
SFEMG—single-fiber
  electromyography
SFP—screen filtration pressure
SFS—split-function study
SFT—skinfold thickness
SFW—
    shell fragment wound
    shrapnel fragment wound
SG—
    serum globulin
    skin graft
    specific gravity
SGA—small for gestational age
Sgambati
    reaction
    test
SH—
    serum hepatitis
    sex hormone
    sinus histiocytosis
    social history
    surgical history
Shaaf forceps
shadow
    acoustic s.
    artifactual s.

shadow *(continued)*
    bat's wing s.
    s. cell
    s. curve
    eye s.
    heart s.
    iris s.
    miliary s.
    s. nucleus
    overlap s.
    Ponfick s.
    psoas s.
    Purkinje s's
    snowstorm s.
    soft tissue s.
    sound s.
    s. test
shadow-casting
Shaeffer rigid orthosis
Shafer sign
Shaffer modification of Barkan
  knife
shaft
    s. of femur
    s. of fibula
    hair s.
    s. of humerus
    s. of metacarpal bone
    s. of metatarsal bone
    s. of penis
    s. of phalanx of fingers
    s. of phalanx of toes
    s. of radius
    s. of rib
    s. of tibia
    s. of ulna
shaggy
    s. chorion
    s. pericardium
shagreen
    s. lesion
    s. patch
    s. plaque
    s. skin
shakes
    helium s.
    spelter s.
    Teflon s.
Shallcross forceps
Shambaugh
    adenotome
    elevator
    headrest
    hook
    incision

Shambaugh *(continued)*
    irrigator
    needle
    operation
    retractor
Shambaugh-Derlacki
    chisel
    elevator
Shambaugh-Lempert knife
sham-feeding
shank
shape
    baseball bat s.
    cricket bat s.
shaping
Shapleigh curet
sharp curettage
Sharpey fibers
sharp-toothed tenaculum
shave
    lip s.
Shaver disease
Shaw stripper
Shea
    curet
    drill
    hook
    irrigator
    knife
    stapedectomy
    tube
shear
Shearer forceps
Shearing lens
shears
    bandage s.
    Lebsche s.
    Liston s.
    malleus s.
sheath
    arachnoid s.
    axillary s.
    bulbar s.
    carotid s.
    caudal s.
    chordal s.
    common synovial flexor s.
    common s. of tendons of
      peroneal muscles
    common s. of testis and
      spermatic cord
    crural s.
    dentinal s.
    dural s.
    enamel prism s.

sheath *(continued)*
    enamel rod s.
    endoneurial s.
    epithelial s.
    s. of eyeball
    fascial s. of prostate
    femoral s.
    fibrous s's of fingers
    fibrous s. of kidney
    fibrous s. of liver
    fibrous s. of optic nerve
    fibrous s. of spermatozoon
    fibrous s. of tendon
    fibrous s's of toes
    Henle s.
    Hertwig s., s. of Hertwig
    intermeningeal s. of optic
      nerve
    s. of Key and Retzius
    lamellar s.
    Mauthner s.
    medullary s.
    meningeal s's of optic nerve
    mitochondrial s.
    mucous s's
    mucous s., intertubercular
    mucous s. of tendon
    mucous s's of tendons of
      fingers
    mucous s's of tendons of toes
    myelin s.
    Neumann s., s. of Neumann
    neurilemmal s.
    notochordal s.
    nucleated s.
    s. of optic nerve, internal
    s. of optic nerve, outer
      meningeal
    outer meningeal s. of optic
      nerve
    peel-away s.
    periarterial lymphatic s.
    periarterial lymphoid s. (PALS)
    periesophageal s.
    perinephric s.
    perivascular s.
    pial s.
    s. of plantar tendon of long
      peroneal muscle
    prism s.
    s. of prostate
    rectus s.
    s. of rectus abdominis muscle
    rod s.
    root s.

S

sheath *(continued)*
    Scarpa s.
    Schwalbe s.
    s. of Schwann
    Schweigger-Seidel s.
    s's of optic nerve
    spiral s.
    s. of styloid process
    s. syndrome
    synovial s.
    synovial s. of bicipital groove
    synovial s. of intertubercular
      groove
    synovial s. of tendon
    synovial s. of tendons of foot
    tendinous s.
    tendinous s's of flexor muscles
      of fingers
    tendinous s's of flexor muscles
      of toes
    tendinous s. of leg
    tendon s.
    tendon s. of anterior tibial
      muscle
    tendon s's of long extensor
      muscles of toes
    tendon s's of long flexor
      muscles of toes
    tendon s. of posterior tibial
      muscle
    s. of thymus
    thyroid s.
sheathed catheter
Sheehan
    chisel
    disease
    osteotome
    syndrome
Sheehan-Dodge technique
Sheehy
    knife
    syndrome
    tube
Sheehy-House prosthesis
sheepskin dressing
sheet
    β-s. [beta-]
    β-pleated s. [beta-]
    draw s.
    drip s.
    pleated s.
    secretory s.
Sheets lens
Sheldon retractor
Sheldon-Pudenz dissector
Sheldon-Spatz needle

shelf
    Blumer s.
    buccal s.
    dental s.
    mesocolic s.
    s. operation
    palatal s.
    palatine s.
    rectal s.
shell
    electron s.
shellac
shell shock
shelving
    s. incision
    s. operation
Shenstone tourniquet
Shenton
    arch
    line
Shepard tube
Shepherd fracture
Sherman
    plate
    screw
    unit
Sherman-Bourquin unit
    (of vitamin B_2)
Sherman-Munsell unit
    (of vitamin A)
Sherrington law
SHG—synthetic human gastrin
shiatsu
Shibley sign
shield
    amputation s.
    Buller s.
    circumcision s.
    Dalkon s.
    embryonic s.
    eye s.
    Faraday s.
    Fox s.
    Fuller s.
    heat s.
    lead s.
    lead gonad s.
    nipple s.
    oral s.
    phallic s.
    skull s.
shielding
Shier prosthesis
shift
    antigenic s.
    axis s.

shift *(continued)*
    chemical s.
    chloride s.
    Doppler s.
    s. down
    frame s.
    s. of Hamburger
    isohydric s.
    midline s.
    permanent threshold s.
    phase s.
    Purkinje s.
    regenerative blood s.
    temporary threshold s.
    s. to the left
    s. to the right
shifting dullness
Shiga
    bacillus
    dysentery
    toxin
Shigella
    S. boydii
    S. dysenteriae
    S. flexneri
    S. sonnei
shigellosis
Shiley tube
shin
    bucked s's
    cucumber s.
    saber s.
    sore s's
    s. splints
shinbone
Shiner tube
shingles
Shirodkar
    needle
    operation
    procedure
shiver
shivering
SHML—sinus histiocytosis with
    massive lymphadenopathy
SHO—secondary hypertrophic
    osteoarthropathy
shock
    acoustic s.
    anaphylactic s.
    anaphylactoid s.
    anesthesia s.
    apoplectic s.
    asthmatic s.
    bacteremic s.
    burn s.

shock *(continued)*
    cardiac s.
    cardiogenic s.
    cerebral s.
    culture s.
    declamping s.
    deferred s.
    delayed s.
    diastolic s.
    electric s.
    electrotherapeutic s.
    endotoxic s.
    endotoxin s.
    Forssman s.
    heart s.
    hematogenic s.
    hemoclastic s.
    hemorrhagic s.
    histamine s.
    hypoglycemic s.
    hypovolemic s.
    insulin s.
    irreversible s.
    neural s.
    neurogenic s.
    obstetric s.
    oligemic s.
    osmotic s.
    paralytic s.
    peptone s.
    pleural s.
    postoperative s.
    primary s.
    protein s.
    secondary s.
    septic s.
    serum s.
    shell s.
    spinal s.
    surgical s.
    testicular s.
    toxic s.
    traumatic s.
    vasogenic s.
Shoemaker
    clamp
    rib shears
Shohl and Pedley method
Shohl solution
Shone
    anomaly
    complex
    syndrome
Shope
    fibroma
    papilloma

S

Shortbent scissors
shortsighted
shortsightedness
short-windedness
shot
    booster s.
shot-compressor
shotted suture
shotty lymph nodes
shoulder
    s. blade
    bull's eye s.
    s. disarticulation
    drop s.
    s. dystocia
    s.-elbow-wrist-hand orthosis
    frozen s.
    s. girdle
    hand-s. syndrome
    s. joint
    knocked-down s.
    linguogingival s.
    loose s.
    periarthritis of s.
    s. presentation
    round s's
    s. separation
    s. slip, slipped s.
    s.-strap incision
    stubbed s.
Shouldice herniorrhaphy
show
    bloody s.
shower
    s. of echoes
    s. of emboli
    uric acid s.
shrapnel
Shrapnell membrane
shrinkage
shrinker
    stump s.
shudder
shuffle
shunt
    aortopulmonary s.
    arteriovenous (AV) s.
    Buselmeier s.
    cardiovascular s.
    cavomesenteric s.
    Denver s.
    dialysis s.
    Drapanas s.
    endolymphatic s.
    endolymphatic-mastoid s.

shunt *(continued)*
    end-to-side s.
    Glenn s.
    hexose monophosphate s.
    Holter s.
    internal s.
    intracardiac s.
    Javid s.
    left-to-right s.
    LeVeen peritoneovenous s.
    Linton s.
    lymphaticovenous s.
    mesoatrial s.
    mesocaval s.
    otic-periotic s.
    parietal s.
    pentose s.
    peritoneosubarachnoid s.
    peritoneothecal s.
    peritoneovenous s.
    PFTE
      (polyfluorotetraethylene) s.
    portacaval s.
    portorenal s.
    portosystemic s.
    postcaval s.
    Pudenz s.
    pulmonary s.
    Quinton-Scribner s.
    Ramirez s.
    renal-splenic venous s.
    reversed s.
    right-to-left s.
    salpingothecal s.
    Scribner s.
    side-to-side s.
    Silastic ventriculoperitoneal s.
    splenorenal s.
    splenorenal s., distal
    Stookey-Scarff s.
    subduroperitoneal s.
    subduropleural s.
    Thomas s.
    Thomas appliqué s.
    Torkildsen s.
    transjugular intrahepatic
      portosystemic s. (TIPS)
    ureterothecal s.
    ventriculoatrial s.
    ventriculojugular s.
    ventriculoperitoneal s.
    ventriculopleural s.
    ventriculovenous s.
    Warren s.
    Waterston s.

shunting
    left-to-right ductus s.
Shurly retractor
shuttle
    glycerol phosphate s.
    malate-aspartate s.
Shwachman syndrome
Shwachman-Diamond syndrome
Shwartzman-Sanarelli
  phenomenon
Shy-Drager syndrome
SI—
    International System of Units
      (Fr. Système International
      d'Unités)
    sacroiliac
    self-inflicted
    serum iron
    soluble insulin
    stimulation index
SIADH—syndrome of
  inappropriate antidiuretic
  hormone
sialaden
sialadenectomy
sialadenitis
    chronic nonspecific s.
sialadenography
sialadenoma papilliferum
sialadenopathy
    benign lymphoepithelial s.
sialadenosis
sialadenotomy
sialagogic
sialagogue(s)
sialectasia
sialectasis
sialic acid
sialism, sialismus
sialitis
sialoadenectomy
sialoadenitis
sialoadenotomy
sialoaerophagy
sialoangiectasis
sialoangiitis
sialoangiography
sialocele
sialodochitis
sialodochoplasty
sialoductitis
sialogenous
sialogram
sialography
sialolith

sialolithiasis
sialolithotomy
sialometry
sialomucin
sialophagia
sialorrhea pancreatica
sialoschesis
sialostenosis
sialosyrinx
Sia water test
sibilant
    s. articulation
    s. fricatives
    s. phonemes
    s. rales
    s. rhonchi
    s. sounds
    s. wheezing sound
Sibley-Lehninger test
sibling
sibship
Sibson
    aponeurosis
    fascia
    furrow
    groove
    notch
    vestibule
Sicard syndrome
siccus
SICD—serum isocitric
  dehydrogenase
sick bay
sickle cell
    s.c. anemia
    s.c. dactylitis
    s.c. disease
    s.c.–hemoglobin C disease
    s.c.–hemoglobin D disease
    s.c. nephropathy
    s.c.–thalassemia disease
    s.c. trait
sickled
sicklemia
sicklemic
sickler
sickness
    acute serum s.
    acute sleeping s.
    aerial s.
    air s.
    altitude s.
    aviation s.
    balloon s.
    car s.

S

sickness *(continued)*
>   compressed-air s.
>   decompression s.
>   drug-induced serum s.
>   high-altitude s.
>   laughing s.
>   morning s.
>   motion s.
>   mountain s.
>   radiation s.
>   salt s.
>   sea s.
>   secondary radiation s.
>   serum s.
>   sleeping s.
>   space s.
>   stiff s.
>   sweating s.
>   three-day s.
>   vomiting s.
>   x-ray s.

SICU—surgical intensive care unit
SID—sudden infant death
Sidbury syndrome
side
>   balancing s.
>   s. effect
>   functioning s.
>   nonfunctioning s.
>   working s.

side-bone
side-cutting
sideroblast
>   ringed s.

sideroblastic
siderocyte
siderocytosis
sideroderma
siderofibrosis
sideropenia
sideropenic
siderophilous
siderosilicosis
siderosis
>   Bantu s.
>   s. bulbi
>   s. conjunctivae
>   hepatic s.
>   nutritional s.
>   pulmonary s.
>   urinary s.

siderotic
side-shift
side wall
sidewinder catheter

SIDS—sudden infant death
>   syndrome

Siegbahn unit
Siegert sign
Siegle
>   otoscope
>   pneumatic ear speculum

siemens (S) unit
Siemerling nucleus
Sierra-Sheldon tracheotome
Sieur
>   sign
>   test

sieve
>   s. graft
>   molecular s.

sievert (Sv)
sig.—significant
SIg—surface immunoglobulin
sigh
>   s. rate
>   s. syndrome

sighing
>   irrepressible persistent s.
>   s. respirations

sight
>   day s.
>   far s.
>   line of s.
>   long s.
>   near s.
>   night s.
>   old s.
>   second s.
>   short s.

sigma
>   Greek letter
>   (Σ; alphabetized as s)
>   s. angle
>   s. method
>   s. virus

sigmatism
sigmoid
>   s. arteries
>   s. cartilages
>   s. cavity of radius
>   s. cavity of ulna
>   s. colectomy
>   s. colon
>   s. conduit
>   s. cystoplasty
>   s. flexure
>   s. folds of colon
>   s. fossa
>   s. fossa of temporal bone

sigmoid *(continued)*
    s. fossa of ulna
    s. groove of temporal bone
    s. kidney
    s. lymph nodes
    s. mesocolon
    s. notch
    s. notch of ulna
    s. sinus
    s. sulcus
    s. veins
    s. volvulus
sigmoidectomy
sigmoiditis
sigmoidocystoplasty
sigmoidopexy
sigmoidoproctostomy
sigmoidorectostomy
sigmoidoscope
    Boehm s.
    Buie s.
    disposable s.
    fiberoptic s.
    Frankfeldt s.
    Kelly s.
    KleenSpec s.
    Lieberman s.
    Montague s.
    Solow s.
    Tuttle s.
    Vernon-David s.
    Welch-Allyn s.
    Yeoman s.
sigmoidoscopic
sigmoidoscopy
sigmoidosigmoidostomy
sigmoidostomy
sigmoidotomy
sigmoidovesical
Sigmund glands
sign
    Aaron s.
    Abadie s.
    Abrahams s.
    accessory s.
    Achilles tendon s.
    Ahlfeld s.
    air bronchogram s.
    air crescent s.
    air-cushion s.
    air dome s.
    Allis s.
    Alri s.
    Amoss s.
    anatomical snuffbox s.

sign *(continued)*
    Andral s.
    André Thomas s.
    Anghelescu s.
    antecedent s.
    anterior drawer s.
    anterior tibial s.
    anticus s.
    Apley s.
    Argyll Robertson pupillary s.
    Arroyo s.
    assident s.
    associated abduction s.
    associated adduction s.
    Auenbrugger s.
    Aufrecht s.
    auscultatory s's
    Auspitz s.
    Babinski toe s.
    Baccelli s.
    Baillarger s.
    Balduzzi s.
    Ballance s.
    Ballet s.
    Bamberger s.
    banana s.
    bandage s.
    Bárány s.
    Bard s.
    Barré s.
    Barré pyramidal s.
    Bastian-Bruns s.
    Battle s.
    Beccaria s.
    Becker s.
    Béclard s.
    Beevor s.
    Béhier-Hardy s.
    Bekhterev s.
    Bell s.
    Bergara-Wartenberg s.
    Berger s.
    Bergman s.
    Bespaloff s.
    Bethea s.
    Bezold s.
    Biederman s.
    Biernacki s.
    Bikele s.
    Bing s.
    Biot s.
    Bird s.
    Bjerrum s.
    Blatin s.
    Blumberg s.

S

sign *(continued)*
- Boas s.
- Bolt s.
- Bonnet s.
- Bordier-Fränkel s.
- Borsieri s.
- Boston s.
- Bouillaud s.
- Bouveret s.
- bowler hat s.
- Boyce s.
- Bozzolo s.
- Bragard s.
- Branham s.
- Braun-von Fernwald s.
- Braunwald s.
- Braxton-Hicks s.
- Brenner s.
- Broadbent inverted s.
- Brockenbrough s.
- Brodie s.
- Brown s.
- Brown Kelly s.
- Brown-Séquard s.
- Brudzinski s.
- Brunati s.
- Bruns s.
- Bryant s.
- Burton s.
- Calkins s.
- camelot s.
- candlewax s.
- Cantelli s.
- Capps s.
- Carabelli s.
- cardinal s's
- cardiorespiratory s.
- Carman s.
- Carman-Kirklin meniscus s.
- Carnett s.
- Carvallo s.
- caviar s.
- Cegka s.
- Cestan s.
- Chaddock s.
- Chadwick s.
- chandelier s.
- Charcot s.
- Cheyne-Stokes s.
- Chilaiditi s.
- chin-retraction s.
- Chvostek s.
- Chvostek-Weiss s.
- Clark s.
- Claude hyperkinesis s.

sign *(continued)*
- clavicular s.
- claw hand s.
- Cleeman s.
- clenched fist s.
- closed fist s.
- cobra head s.
- Codman s.
- cogwheel s.
- coiled spring s.
- coin s.
- Cole s.
- Collier s.
- colon cutoff s.
- Comby s.
- commemorative s.
- Comolli s.
- complementary opposition s.
- compressed tissue s.
- Conillaud s.
- contralateral s.
- Coopernail s.
- Cope s.
- Corrigan s.
- coughing s.
- Courtois s.
- Courvoisier s.
- Cowen s.
- crescent s.
- Crichton-Browne s.
- Crowe s.
- Cullen s.
- Cumbo s.
- curtain s.
- Dalrymple s.
- D'Amato s.
- dance s.
- Danforth s.
- Darier s.
- Dawbarn s.
- Dejerine s.
- de la Camp s.
- Delbet s.
- Delmege s.
- Demarquay s.
- Demianoff s.
- de Musset s.
- Dennie s.
- Desault s.
- d'Espine s.
- Dew s.
- Diakiogiannis s.
- diaphragm s.
- Dieuaide s.

sign *(continued)*

distal tingling on pressure (DTP) s.
Dixon Mann s.
doll's eye s.
Dorendorf s.
dorsocuboidal s.
double-bubble s.
double-contour s.
doublet s.
doughnut s.
drawer s.
Drummond s.
DTP (distal tingling on pressure) s.
Dubois s.
Duchenne s.
Duckworth s.
Dugas s.
Duncan-Bird s.
Dupuy-Dutemps s.
Dupuy-Dutemps and Cestan s.
Dupuytren s.
Duroziez s.
Dutemps-Cestan s.
E s.
echo s.
Elliot s.
Ellis s.
Ely s.
Enroth s.
Erb s.
Erben s.
Erichsen s.
Escherich s.
Eustace Smith s.
Ewart s.
Ewing s.
external malleolar s.
extinction s.
eyelash s.
fabere (flexion, abduction, external rotation, extension) s.
facial s.
fadir s.
Faget s.
Fajersztajn crossed sciatic s.
fan s.
fat pad s.
Federici s.
femoral s.
figure three s.
finger spread s.
Finkelstein s.
fistula s.

sign *(continued)*

flag s.
floating-tooth s.
flush-tank s.
Foerster s.
fontanelle s.
forearm s.
formication s.
Fournier s.
Fränkel s.
Friedreich s.
Froment paper s.
frontal release s.
front tap s.
Fuchs s.
Gaenslen s.
Galeazzi s.
Gangolphe s.
Gauss s.
Gianelli s.
Gifford s.
Gilbert s.
glabellar tap s.
Glasgow s.
Gobiet s.
Goggia s.
Golden s.
Goldstein s.
Goldthwait s.
Gonda s.
Goodell s.
Gordon s.
Gorissenne s.
Gorlin s.
Gottron s.
Gowers s.
Graefe (von Graefe) s.
Grancher s.
Granger s.
Grasset s.
Grasset-Bychowski s.
Grasset-Gaussel-Hoover s.
Grey Turner s.
Griesinger s.
Griffith s.
grip s.
Grocco s.
Gubler s.
Guilland s.
Gunn crossing s.
Gunn pupillary s.
Günzberg s.
Guye s.
Guyon s.
Hahn s.

S

sign *(continued)*
  Halban s.
  Hall s.
  halo s.
  Hamilton s.
  Hamman s.
  harlequin s.
  Harris s.
  Hatchcock s.
  Haudek s.
  Hawkins s.
  Heberden s's
  Hefke-Turner s.
  Hegar s.
  Heilbronner s.
  Heim-Kreysig s.
  Helbing s.
  Hennebert s.
  Hennings s.
  Hertwig-Magendie s.
  Hicks s.
  Higouménaki s.
  Hill s.
  Hirschberg s.
  Hochsinger s.
  Hoehne s.
  Hoffmann s.
  Holmes s.
  Homans s.
  Hoover s.
  Hope s.
  Horn s.
  Horner s.
  Horsley s.
  Howship-Romberg s.
  Hoyne s.
  Hueter fracture s.
  Huntington s.
  Hutchinson s.
  hyperkinesis s.
  interossei s.
  Itard-Cholewa s.
  Jaccoud s.
  Jackson s.
  Jacquemier s.
  Jendrassik s.
  Joffroy s.
  Jolly s.
  jugular s.
  Kanavel s.
  Kantor string s.
  Karplus s.
  Keen s.
  Kehr s.
  Kellock s.

sign *(continued)*
  Kelly s.
  Kerandel s.
  Kergaradec s.
  Kernig s.
  Kerr s.
  Kestenbaum s.
  Kleist s.
  Klemm s.
  Klippel-Feil s.
  Klippel-Weil s.
  Kluge s.
  Knies s.
  Kocher s.
  Koplik s.
  Kreysig s.
  Krisovski (Krisowski) s.
  Kussmaul s.
  Küstner s.
  Ladin s.
  Laënnec s.
  Lafora s.
  Langoria s.
  Lasègue s.
  Laugier s.
  leg s.
  Le Gendre s.
  leg flexion s.
  Leichtenstern s.
  lemon s.
  Lennhoff s.
  Leri s.
  Leser-Trélat s.
  levator s.
  Levine clenched-fist s.
  Lhermitte s.
  Lichtheim s.
  ligature s.
  Liget s.
  Linder s.
  Litten s.
  Livierato s.
  Lloyd s.
  Lockwood s.
  Loenen s.
  Lombardi s.
  long tract s.
  Lorenz s.
  Lucas s.
  Ludloff s.
  Lust s.
  Macewen s.
  Magendie s.
  Magendie-Hertwig s.
  Magnan s.

sign *(continued)*
    Mahler s.
    Maisonneuve s.
    Mann s.
    Mannkopf s.
    Marañón s.
    Marcus Gunn pupillary s.
    Marfan s.
    Marie s.
    Marie-Foix s.
    Marinesco s.
    May s.
    Mayor s.
    McBurney s.
    McCarthy s.
    McClintock s.
    McCort s.
    McGinn-White s.
    McMurray s.
    Means s.
    Meltzer s.
    Mendel-Bekhterev s.
    meniscus s.
    Mennell s.
    Mercedes-Benz s.
    Meunier s.
    Mexican hat s.
    Milian s.
    Mingazzini s.
    Minor s.
    Mirchamp s.
    Möbius (Moebius) s.
    Moniz s.
    Morquio s.
    Moschcowitz s.
    Mosler s.
    moulage s.
    Moutard-Martin s.
    Müller s.
    Munson s.
    Murphy s.
    Musset s.
    Myerson s.
    neck s.
    Negro s.
    Neri s.
    newspaper s.
    niche s.
    Nicoladoni s.
    Nikolsky s.
    nostril s.
    Nothnagel s.
    nuchal s.
    Ober s.
    objective s's

sign *(continued)*
    obturator s.
    oil-drop s.
    Oliver s.
    Olshausen s.
    Oppenheim s.
    orange-peel s.
    orbicularis s.
    Ortolani s.
    Osiander s.
    Osler s.
    palmoplantar s.
    Parkinson s.
    Parrot s.
    Pastia s.
    patent bronchus s.
    Patrick s.
    Pemberton s.
    Pende s.
    Perez s.
    peroneal s.
    Petruschky s.
    Pfuhl s.
    Pfuhl-Jaffe s.
    Phalen s.
    physical s's
    Piltz s.
    Pinard s.
    Pins s.
    Piotrowski s.
    Piskacek s.
    Pitres s.
    pivot-shift s.
    placental s.
    platysma s.
    plumb-line s.
    Plummer s.
    pneumatic s.
    Pool-Schlesinger s.
    Porter s.
    posterior drawer s.
    Potain s.
    Pottenger s.
    Prehn s.
    Prévost s.
    pronation s.
    pseudo-Babinski s.
    pseudo-Graefe s.
    psoas s.
    puddle s.
    pyloric string s.
    pyramid s., pyramidal s.
    pyramidal tract s. of lower
        extremities
    Quant s.

S

sign *(continued)*

    Queckenstedt s.
    Quénu-Muret s.
    Quincke s.
    Quinquaud s.
    radialis s.
    Radovici s.
    railroad track s.
    Raimiste s.
    Ramond s.
    Randall s.
    Ransohoff s.
    Rasch s.
    Rasin s.
    Raynaud s.
    rebound s.
    Remak s.
    reservoir s.
    reversed three s.
    Revilliod s.
    Riesman s.
    rim s.
    rising sun s.
    Ritter-Rollet s.
    Riviere s.
    Robertson s.
    Roger counter s.
    Romaña s.
    Romberg s.
    Rommelaere s.
    root s.
    rope s.
    Rosenbach s.
    Roser s.
    Roser-Braun s.
    Rossolimo s.
    Rotch s.
    Rothschild s.
    Roux s.
    Rovighi s.
    Rovsing s.
    Rucker s.
    Ruggeri s.
    Rumpel-Leede s.
    Rumpf s.
    Rust s.
    Saenger s.
    sail s.
    Salmon s.
    Sansom s.
    Sarbó s.
    Saunders s.
    scarf s.
    Schepelmann s.
    Schick s.

sign *(continued)*

    Schlesinger s.
    Schultze s.
    Schultze-Chvostek s.
    Schwartze s.
    scimitar s.
    Seeligmüller (Seeligmueller) s.
    Séguin s.
    Seidel s.
    Seitz s.
    Semon s.
    setting-sun s.
    Shafer s.
    Shibley s.
    Siegert s.
    Signorelli s.
    Silex s.
    silhouette s.
    Simon s.
    Sisto s.
    Skoda s.
    Smith s.
    Snellen s.
    soft s's
    Somagyi s.
    Soto-Hall s.
    Souques s.
    Spalding s.
    spinal s., spine s.
    Spurling s.
    square root s.
    Squire s.
    stairs s.
    steeple s.
    Stellwag s.
    Sterles s.
    Sternberg s.
    Stewart-Holmes s.
    Stierlin s.
    Stimson s.
    Stokes s.
    Strauss s.
    string s.
    string-of-beads s.
    Strümpell s.
    Strunsky s.
    subjective s's
    Suker s.
    Sumner s.
    swinging flashlight s.
    tapir snout s.
    Tarnier s.
    Tay s.
    Theimich lip s.
    thermic s.

sign *(continued)*
 thigh s.
 Thomas s.
 Thomson s.
 Thornton s.
 three s.
 Throckmorton s.
 thumb s.
 thumbprint s.
 tibialis s.
 Tinel s.
 toe s.
 toe spread s.
 Tournay s.
 Traube s.
 Trendelenburg s.
 trepidation s.
 Tresilian s.
 Trimadeau s.
 Troisier s.
 trolley-track s.
 Trömner s.
 Trousseau s.
 Turner s.
 Turyn s.
 twin peak s.
 Uhthoff s.
 Unschuld s.
 Uriolla s.
 Valleix s.
 Vanzetti s.
 vein s.
 Vermel s.
 Vipond s.
 vital s's
 vitropressin s.
 Von Fernwald s.
 von Graefe s.
 von Monakow s.
 von Strümpell s.
 Wartenberg s.
 Warthin s.
 water lily s.
 Weber s.
 Wegner s.
 Weill s.
 Weiss s.
 Wenckebach s.
 Wernicke s.
 Westermark s.
 Westphal s.
 Widowitz s.
 Wilder s.
 Williams s.
 Williamson s.

sign *(continued)*
 Wilson pronator s.
 Wimberger s.
 Winterbottom s.
 Wintrich s.
 Wood s.
 Wreden s.
 Yergason s.
 Zaufal s.
signal
 Doppler velocity s.
 magnetic resonance s.
 nuclear s.
 sensory s.
 s.-to-noise ratio (S/N)
signature
 tumor s.
signe
 s. de journal
 s. de la bandera
 s. de peau d'orange
signet-ring pattern
significance
 statistical s.
significant
Signorelli sign
SIJ—sacroiliac joint
silafilcon A
Silastic
 coronary artery cannula
 cup
 implant
 injection
 mushroom catheter
 patch
 testicular prosthesis
 ventriculoperitoneal shunt
silence
 electrical s.
 electrocerebral s.
silent
 s. allele
 s. angina
 s. area
 s. gallstones
 s. gap
 s. gene
 s. ischemia
 s. mastoiditis
 s. mutation
 s. myocardial infarction
 s. period
 s. thyroiditis
Silex sign
Silfverskiold syndrome

S

silhouette
 cardiac s.
 cardiopericardial s.
 cardiovascular s.
 s. sign
silica
 s.-bonded investment
 s. gel
silicate
 aluminum s.
 s. cement
 magnesium s.
 magnesium aluminum s.
silicatosis
silicea
siliceous, silicious
 purified s. earth
silicic
 s. acid
 s. anhydride
silicoanthracosis
silicofluoride
silicon (Si)
 s. carbide
 colloidal s. dioxide
 s. dioxide
 s. fluoride
silicone
 s. liquid
 s. oil
 s. synovitis
silicophosphate cement
silicoproteinosis
silicosiderosis
silicosis
 infective s.
silicotic granuloma
silicotuberculosis
siliqua olivae
siliquose
silk
 artificial s. keratitis
 black s. suture
 braided s. suture
 floss s.
 s. gelatin
 shot-s. phenomenon
 shot-s. reflex
 shot-s. retina
 surgical s.
 s. suture
 watered-s. retina
 water-s. reflex
 white s. suture
silken crepitus

silkworm
 s. gut suture
 s. moth
silo filler's disease
Silva-Costa operation
Silvadene
silver (Ag)
 s. chloride
 colloidal s.
 colloidal s. iodide
 s. iodide
 methenamine s.
 mild s. protein
 s. nitrate
 strong s. protein
 s. sulfadiazine
 toughened s. nitrate
Silver
 bunionectomy
 operation
 osteotome
 syndrome
Silverman
 needle
 score
Silver-Russell syndrome
silver-spoon deformity
silver wire
 s.w. effect
 s.w. suture
Simcoe lens
Similac
similia similibus
 curantur
simillimum
Simmonds
 disease
 speculum
 syndrome
Simmons catheter
Simon
 disease
 foci
 incision
 operation
 position
 septic factor
 sign
 suture
Simonart
 band
 thread
simple
 s. mastectomy (SM)
 s. mastoidectomy

simple *(continued)*
    s. microscope
    s. nephrectomy
    s. suture
Simpson
    forceps
    lamp
    light
    sound
Simpson-Luikart forceps
Sims
    anoscope
    curet
    depressor
    position
    retractor
    scissors
    sound
    speculum
    suture
Sims-Kelly retractor
simulation
simulator
    electrocardiographic s.
    space s.
Simulium
    S. damnosum
    S. neavei
    S. ochraceum
    S. venustum
simultagnosia, simultanagnosia
simultaneous
    s. cancer
    s. decrease
    s. increase
    s. placement
    s. procedure
    s. surgery
SIMV—synchronized intermittent
  mandatory ventilation
sin [without]
sincalide
sincipital
sinciput
sine-wave pattern
singer's nodes (nodules)
single
    s. ascertainment
    s. breath test
    s. chamber pacemaker
    s. chamber pacing
    s. cone method
    s. diffusion
    s. expirate
    s. fiber electromyography

single *(continued)*
    s. fiber needle electrode
    s. nephron glomerular
      filtration rate
    s. radial diffuse
    s. support phase
    s. syndactyly
    s. system ureterocele
    s. ventricle
single-armed suture
single-blind clinical trial
single-breath nitrogen washout test
single-cell gel electrophoresis
single-chain
    s.-c. antigen-binding proteins
      (SCA proteins)
    s.-c. urokinase–type
      plasminogen activator
single-photon emission computed
  tomography (SPECT)
singlet
    s. oxygen
    s. state
Singleton incision
single-tooth, single-toothed
    s.-t. forceps
    s.-t. tenaculum
Singley forceps
singly
singular canal
singultation
singultous
singultus
sinister
sinistrad
sinistral
sinistrality
sinistrocardia
sinistrocerebral
sinistrocular
sinistrocularity
sinistrogyration
sinistromanual
sinistropedal
sinistrotorsion
sinoaortic
sinoatrial (SA)
    s. block
    s. bradycardia
    s. ganglion
    s. nodal artery
    s. node
    s. rhythm
    s. valve
sinobronchitis

S

Sinografin
sinography
sinomenine
sinopulmonary
sinoscopy
sinospiral fibers
sinovaginal bulb
sinoventricular
Sinskey lens
sinuate
sinuatrial
sinuous
sinus (sinus, sinuses)
    accessory s's of the nose
    air s.
    anal s's
    anterior s's
    anterior s. of atlas
    s. of anterior chamber
    s. aortae
    aortic s.
    Arlt s.
    s. arrest
    s. arrhythmia
    s. arrhythmia, nonrespiratory
    s. arrhythmia, respiratory
    articular s. of atlas
    s. barotrauma
    basilar s.
    s. beat
    s. block
    s. of Bochdalek
    s. bradycardia
    branchial s.
    Breschet s.
    s. caroticus
    carotid s.
    carotid s. massage
    carotid s. reflex
    carotid s. syncope
    carotid s. syndrome
    s. catarrh
    s. cavernosus
    cavernous s.
    cavernous s. syndrome
    cavernous s. thrombosis
    cerebral s.
    cervical s.
    circular s.
    s. circularis iridis
    coccygeal s.
    confluence of s's
    s. coronarius
    coronary s.
    coronary s. electrogram

sinus (sinus, sinuses) *(continued)*
    cortical s's
    costal s's of sternum
    costodiaphragmatic s.
    costomediastinal s. of pleura
    costophrenic s.
    cranial s's
    Cuvier s's
    dental s.
    dermal s.
    draining s.
    dural s.
    s's of dura mater
    endodermal s. tumor
    s. epididymidis
    Eternod s.
    ethmoid s's, ethmoidal s's
    s. ethmoidales
    Forssell s.
    frontal s.
    functional endoscopic s.
      surgery (FESS)
    s. ganglion
    Guérin s.
    s. histiocytosis
    s. histiocytosis with massive
      lymphadenopathy
    Huguier s.
    s. intercavernosus anterior
    s. intercavernosus posterior
    intercavernous s's
    intermediate s's
    s. of kidney
    lacteal s's
    lactiferous s's
    laryngeal s.
    s. of larynx
    lateral s.
    Lauth s.
    s. lienalis
    longitudinal s., inferior
    longitudinal s., superior
    lymph s's
    lymphatic s's
    s. of Maier
    marginal s's
    s. marginalis
    mastoid s's
    s. maxillaris
    maxillary s.
    maxillary s. radiograph
    s. medii
    medullary s's
    Meyer s.
    middle s's

sinus (sinus, sinuses) *(continued)*
  s. of Morgagni
  mucous s's of male urethra
  nail s.
  nasal s's
  s. nerve
  s. nodal reentry
  s. node
  s. node electrogram
  oblique s. of pericardium
  s. obliquus pericardii
  occipital s.
  s. occipitalis
  opening of coronary s.
  opening of frontal s.
  opening of sphenoid s.
  oral s.
  orifice of coronary s.
  orifice of maxillary s.
  paranasal s's
  s. paranasales
  parasinoidal s.
  s. pause
  pericardial s.
  s. pericardii
  peroneal s. of tibia
  Petit s.
  petrosal s., inferior
  petrosal s., superior
  s. petrosquamosus
  s. petrosus inferior
  s. petrosus superior
  s. phlebitis
  phrenicocostal s.
  s. phrenicocostalis
  pilonidal s.
  piriform s.
  s. pleurae
  pleural s.
  pleuroperitoneal s.
  s. pocularis
  posterior s's
  s. posterior cavitatis
    tympanicae
  preauricular s.
  prostatic s.
  s. of pulmonary trunk
  pyriform s.
  rectal s's
  s. rectus
  s. reentrant tachycardia
  renal s.
  renal s. cyst
  renal s. lipomatosis
  s. reunions

sinus (sinus, sinuses) *(continued)*
  rhomboid s.
  rhomboid s. of Henle
  s. rhythm
  Ridley s.
  Rokitansky-Aschoff s.
  sacrococcygeal s.
  sagittal s., inferior
  s. sagittalis inferior
  s. sagittalis superior
  sagittal s., superior
  sick s. syndrome
  sigmoid s.
  soleal s's
  sphenoid s., sphenoidal s.
  sphenoparietal s.
  s. of spleen
  splenic s.
  s. standstill
  straight s.
  subarachnoidal s's
  subcapsular s's
  s. tachycardia
  tarsal s.
  tentorial s.
  terminal s.
  s. thrombosis
  tonsillar s.
  s. tonsillaris
  s. tract
  transverse s. of dura mater
  transverse s. of pericardium
  s. transversus durae
    matris
  s. transversus pericardii
  traumatic s.
  s. trunci pulmonalis
  s. tympani
  tympanic s.
  s. of tympanic cavity,
    posterior
  s. unguis
  unroofed coronary s.
  urachal s.
  urogenital s.
  s. urogenitalis
  uterine s's
  uteroplacental s.
  s. of Valsalva
  s. of venae cavae
  s. venosus
  s. venosus defect
  s. venosus sclerae
  venous s.
  venous s's of dura mater

S

sinus (sinus, sinuses) *(continued)*
 venous s. of sclera
 s. ventriculi
sinusal
 aortic s. aneurysm
sinusitis
 barotraumatic s.
 chronic caseous s.
 ethmoid s.
 ethmoidal s.
 frontal s.
 fungal s.
 hyperplastic s.
 intracranial s.
 maxillary s.
 orbital s.
 papillary s.
 paranasal s.
 sphenoid s., sphenoidal s.
 viral s.
sinusoid
 discontinuous s.
 fenestrated s.
 hepatic s.
 myocardial s's
sinusoidal
 s. capillary
 s. circulation
 s. current
 s. ostium
 s. vessel
 s. wave
 s. waveform
sinusoscopy
sinusotomy
sinuspiral
sinuventricular
siphon
 s. caroticum
 carotid s.
 Duguet s.
siphonage
Sipple syndrome
Sippy
 diet
 dilator
 method
 treatment
Sips
 distribution
 plot
sireniform fetus
sirenomelia
sirenomelus
SIRS—soluble immune response
 suppressor

SISI—short increment sensitivity
 index (test)
sister
Sister Mary Joseph nodule
Sistrunk
 operation
 retractor
 scissors
site
 active s.
 allosteric s.
 antibody-combining s.
 antigen-binding s.
 antigen-combining s.
 binding s's
 catalytic s.
 combining s.
 donor s.
 fragile s.
 graft donor s.
 hypersensitive s.
 immunologically
  privileged s's
 marker s.
 mutable s.
 nucleotide replacement s.
 operator s.
 peptidyl s.
 privileged s's
 receptor s.
 recipient s.
 restriction s.
sitology
sitomania
sitophobia
sitosterol
β-sitosterolemia [beta-]
sitotaxis
sitotoxin
sitotoxism
sitotropism
situation
 untenable s.
situs (situs)
 s. inversus
 s. inversus abdominalis
 s. inversus thoracis
 s. inversus viscerum
 s. perversus
 s. solitus
 s. transversus
SIW—self-inflicted wound
size
 achieved family s.
 completed family s.
 field s.

size *(continued)*
 French s.
 sample s.
Sjögren
 disease
 syndrome
Sjögren-Larsson syndrome
Sjöqvist
 method
 operation
 tractotomy
skatole
skatoxyl
Skeele curet
skein
 Holmgren s's
 test s's
skeletal
 s. dysplasia
 s. emphysema
 s. fixation
 s. fluorosis
 s. growth factor
 s. muscle
 s. system
 s. tissue
 s. traction
 s. tuberculosis
skeletin
skeletization
skeletogenous
 s. cell
 s. layer
skeletogeny
skeleton
 appendicular s.
 articulated s.
 axial s.
 cardiac s.
 fibrous s. of heart
 s. hand
 s. of heart
 s. membri inferioris liberi
 s. membri superioris liberi
 thoracic s.
 s. thoracis
 s. of thorax
 visceral s.
skeletonization
skeletonize, skeletonized
skeletopia, skeletopy
Skene
 curet
 ducts
 forceps
 glands

skenitis
skew
 s. deviation
 s. distribution
 s. pupils
skewfoot
skewness
skiagram
skiametry
skiascope
skiascopy
Skillern
 forceps
 fracture
skimming
 plasma s.
skin
 alligator s.
 bronzed s.
 citrine s.
 s. clip
 collodion s.
 crocodile s.
 elastic s.
 farmers' s.
 fish s.
 freeze-dried s.
 glabrous s.
 glossy s.
 India rubber s.
 lax s.
 loose s.
 lyophilized s.
 marble s.
 nail s.
 parchment s.
 piebald s.
 pig s.
 porcupine s.
 sailors' s.
 scalded s.
 shagreen s.
skin lifter
 Amico s.l.
Skinner classification
skip
 s. areas
 s. lesion
 s. tomography
skipper
 cheese s.
Sklar-Schiotz tonometer
Skoda
 rale
 sign
 tympany

S

skodaic
- s. resonance
- s. tympany

Skoog operation

SKSD—streptokinase-streptodornase

skull
- Alpert s.
- cloverleaf s.
- hot-cross-bun s.
- lacuna s.
- maplike s.
- membranous s.
- natiform s.
- steeple s.
- stenobregmatic s.
- sutures of s.
- s. tongs
- tower s.
- West-Engstler s.
- West lacuna s.

skullcap

SL—
- sensation level
- sublingual

SLA—left anterior sacral (L. sacrolaeva anterior) (position)

slant of occlusal plane

Slaughter saw

SLD, SLDH—serum lactate dehydrogenase

SLE—systemic lupus erythematosus

sleep
- activated s.
- active s.
- crescendo s.
- D s.
- deep s.
- delta-wave s.
- desynchronized s. (DS)
- dreaming s.
- dreamless s.
- electric s.
- electrotherapeutic s.
- fast-wave s.
- hypnotic s.
- non–rapid eye movement (NREM) s.
- orthodox s.
- paradoxical s.
- paroxysmal s.
- pontine s.
- prolonged s.
- quiet s.
- rapid eye movement (REM) s.

sleep *(continued)*
- rhomboencephalic s.
- rolandic s.
- S s.
- slow-wave s.
- synchronized s.
- twilight s.

sleep apnea
- obstructive s.a. (OSA)
- s.a. syndrome

sleeplessness

sleeptalking

sleepwalking

sleeve
- s. lobectomy
- Watzke s.

slice
- CT s.
- s. geometry
- s. selection

slide
- histology s.
- microscope s.

sliding microtome

sling
- Glisson s.
- levator s.
- mandibular s.
- s. operation
- pterygomasseteric s.
- pubovaginal s.
- pulmonary artery s.
- pulmonary s. syndrome
- s. psychrometer
- Rauchfuss s.
- s. ring complex
- suburethral s.
- s. suture
- s. and swathe
- Teare s.
- vaginal wall s.

slit
- s. diaphragm
- filtration s's
- filtration s. membrane
- s. membrane
- pharyngeal s.
- podocyte s. diaphragm
- s. pores
- s. scanography
- stenopeic s.
- vulvar s.

slit lamp
- s.l. biomicroscopy
- s.l. examination

slit lamp *(continued)*
    Gullstrand s.l.
    s.l. microscope
slit-scanning elevation topography
SLKC—superior limbic
    keratoconjunctivitis
SLN—superior laryngeal nerve
SLO—streptolysin-O
Sloan
    incision
    retractor
Slocum operation
slope
    E to F s.
    lower ridge s.
    mandibular anteroposterior
        ridge s.
    s. culture
slotted laryngoscope
slough
    blackish s.
    cutaneous s.
    fibrinous s.
    fibrous s.
    graft s.
    necrotic s.
    s. off
    skin s.
    yellow s.
    wound s.
sloughing
slow
    s. activity
    s. axonal transport
    s. channel
    s. filling wave
    s. muscle
    s. pulse
    s. twitch
    s. twitch muscle fibers
    s. wave
    s. wave sleep
slowing
    AF (atrial fibrillation) s.
    saccadic s.
SLP—left posterior sacral
    (L. sacrolaeva posterior)
SLR—straight leg raising
SLRT—straight leg-raising test
SLT—left transverse sacral
    (L. sacrolaeva transversa)
    (position)
Sluder
    adenotome
    disease

Sluder *(continued)*
    guillotine tonsillectomy
        method
    neuralgia
    operation
    retractor
    syndrome
    tonsillar guillotine
    tonsillectome
Sluder-Demarest tonsillectome
Sluder-Jansen mouth gag
Sluder-Sauer
    tonsillar guillotine
    tonsillectome
sludge
    activated s.
    biliary s.
sludged blood
sludging of blood
slurry
    activated charcoal s.
    activated charcoal and
        sorbitol s.
    aqueous s.
    calcium citrate malate
        (CCM) s.
    charcoal s.
    deferoxamine-charcoal s.
    injectable cartilage s.
    oral s.
    talc s.
    s. of thrombin-soaked Gelfoam
slyke unit
SM—
    simple mastectomy
    submucous
    systolic murmur
SMA—
    sequential multiple analyzer
        [SMA 6/60, SMA 12/60, SMA
        20/60]
    superior mesenteric artery
SMAC—sequential multiple
    analyzer plus computer [SMAC
    7, SMAC 12, SMAC 20]
SMAF—Specific Macrophage
    Arming Factor
small
    s. airways disease
    s. B-cell lymphoma
    s. bowel enema
    s. bowel follow-through
    s. cell carcinoma
    s. cell osteosarcoma
    s. cleaved cell lymphoma

S

small *(continued)*
    s. intestine
    s. lymphocytic lymphoma
    s. lymphocytic T-cell
      lymphoma
    s. noncleaved cell lymphoma
    s. pelvis
    s. plaque parapsoriasis
    s. trochanter
    s. vessel vasculitis
small-for-gestational-age infant
smallpox
    confluent s.
    discrete s.
    fulminant s.
    hemorrhagic s.
    s.-lunged emphysema
    mild s.
    ordinary s.
    s. vaccine
    s.-vessel disease
    s. virus
Smart
    forceps
    scissors
Smead-Jones closure
smear
    bronchoscopic s.
    buccal s.
    buffy coat s.
    cervical s.
    cul-de-sac s.
    cytologic s.
    FGT (female genital tract)
      cytologic s.
    fungi s.
    Nickerson medium s.
    Papanicolaou (Pap) s.
    TB s.
    Tzanck s.
    VCE (vagina, ectocervix, and
      endocervix) s.
Smedberg drill
smegma
    s. bacillus
    s.-producing glands
smegmalith
smegmatic
smell
    s. hallucination
    s. prodrome
    sweet pleasant s.
Smellie
    method
    perforator

Smellie-Veit maneuver
Smeloff-Cutter prosthesis
smilacin
smile
    s. arc
    gummy s.
    s. incision
    s. length
    modified s. index
    natural s.
    posed s.
    sardonic s.
smiling
    s. depression
    s. hydatid
    s. incision
Smiley-Williams needle
Smillie
    knife
    meniscotome
    meniscotomy
    nail
Smith
    clip
    dislocation
    expressor
    forceps
    fracture
    hook
    operation
    pessary
    sign
    test
Smith-Buie retractor
Smith-Green knife
Smith-Hodge pessary
Smith-Kuhnt operation
Smith-Kuhnt-Szymanowski
    operation
Smith-Lemli-Opitz syndrome
Smith-Petersen
    nail
    operation
    osteotome
    prosthesis
Smith-Robinson operation
Smith & Smith regime
Smith-Strang disease
Smithwick
    forceps
    operation
SMo—stainless steel with
    molybdenum
SMo brace
smog

smoke
    mainstream s.
    second-hand s.
    sidestream s.
smoking
    passive s.
SMON—subacute
    myelo-opticoneuropathy
SMR—submucous resection
SMRR—submucous resection and
    rhinoplasty
SMR speculum
smudging
Sn—tin
SN—suprasternal notch
S/N—signal-to-noise ratio
snake
    poisonous s.
    venomous s.
snap
    mitral opening s.
    tricuspid opening s.
SNAP—sensory nerve action
    potential
snare
    basket s.
    Bosworth s.
    Brown s.
    Bruening s.
    Eves tonsillar s.
    Frankfeldt s.
    Krause s.
    Lewis s.
    Myles s.
    nasal s.
    Norwood s.
    Reiner-Beck s.
    Storz-Beck s.
    tonsil s.
    Tydings s.
    Wilde-Bruening s.
    Wright s.
SNB—scalene node biopsy
Sneddon-Wilkinson disease
sneeze
    allergen-induced s.
    cold air–induced s.
    nasally obstructed s.
    photic s. reflex
    photic s. response
    s. reflex
    s. syncope
Snellen
    chart
    implant

Snellen *(continued)*
    operation
    reform eye
    tests
    test type
SNF—skilled nursing facility
Snider match test
Snitman retractor
SNM—Society of Nuclear
    Medicine
snore
snoring
    S. Bed Partner Survey
    disruptive s.
    habitual s.
    s. index
    loud s. with breathing pauses
    quiet s.
    s. scale
    self-reported s.
    sonorous s.
snow
    s. blindness
    carbon dioxide s.
    falling s. sign on Doppler
        sonography
    s. flurry of emboli
    s. white sign on colonoscopy
snowball opacities
snowballs
snowbanks
snowblindness
snowboarder
snowboarding
snowflake
    s. cataract
    s. vitreoretinal
        degeneration
snowglobe sign
snowman
    s. protrusions in retinal
        pigment epithelium (RPE)
    s. sign of total anomalous
        pulmonary venous return
    s. sign in thrombotic
        thrombocytopenic purpura
        (TTP)
snowmobiling
snowstorm
    s. appearance of scattered
        microcalcifications
    s. shadow
snowy
SNS—sympathetic nervous
    system

snuffbox
    anatomical s.
snuffles
Snyder
    Surgivac drainage system
    Surgivac suction tube
Snyder test
SO—salpingo-oophorectomy
SOA-MCA—superficial
    occipital artery to middle
    cerebral artery
soap
    antibacterial s.
SOAP—Subjective, Objective,
    Assessment, Plan [format for
    medical reports]
soapstone
Soave
    operation
    procedure
SOB—shortness of breath
SOC—sequential-type oral
    contraceptive
socialization
socia parotidis
Socin operation
socioacusis
sociobiologic, sociobiological
sociogenic
sociologist
sociology
sociometry
sociopath
sociopathic
sociopathy
sociotherapy
socket
    adjustable s.
    dry s.
    Dundee s.
    eye s.
    infected s.
    partial-contact s.
    plug-fit s.
    septic s.
    suction s.
    tooth s's
    total-contact s.
soda
    baking s.
    bicarbonate of s.
    caustic s.
    chlorinated s.
    s. lime
sodii (genitive of sodium)

sodium (Na)
    s. acetate
    s. acetate C 11
    s. acid phosphate
    s. alginate
    s. alizarinsulfonate
    s. ascorbate
    s. aurothiomalate
    s. benzoate
    s. bicarbonate
    s. biphosphate
    s. bisulfite
    s. borate
    s. calcium edetate
    s. carbonate
    s. chloride (NaCl)
    s. chromate
    s. chromate Cr 51
    s. citrate
    dibasic s. phosphate
    s. dodecyl sulfate
    s. fluoride
    s. fluosilicate
    s. folate
    s. glutamate
    s. hydroxide
    s. hypochlorite
    s. hyposulfite
    s. iodide
    s. iodide I 123 (I 125, I 131)
    s. ipodate
    s. lactate
    s. lauryl sulfate
    s. metabisulfite
    s. monofluorophosphate
    s. nitrate
    s. nitrite
    s. nitroferricyanide
    s. nitroprusside
    s. para-aminosalicylate
    s. perborate
    s. pertechnetate Tc 99m
    s. phosphate
    s. phosphate P 32
    s. polyphosphate
    s. polystyrene sulfonate
    potassium s. tartrate
    s. propionate
    s. pyroborate
    s. salicylate
    s. silicofluoride
    s. stearate
    s. stibocaptate
    s. sulfate
    s. sulfite

sodium (Na) *(continued)*
    s. tetraborate
    s. tetradecyl sulfate
    s. thiamylal
    s. thiosulfate
    s. trimetaphosphate
sodium-potassium adenosine
  triphosphatase
sodomist
sodomy
Soemmering
    foramen
    gray substance
    ring
    spot
Sofield operation
softening
    anemic s.
    s. of the brain
    colliquative s.
    gray s.
    green s.
    s. of heart
    hemorrhagic s.
    inflammatory s.
    mucoid s.
    pyriform s.
    red s. of brain
    s. of the stomach
    white s.
    yellow s.
soja bean
sola (plural of solum)
solanaceous
solanine
solanoid
Solanum carolinense
solar
    s. cheilitis
    s. dermatitis
    s. elastosis
    s. erythema
    s. keratosis
    s. lentigo
    nasal s. dermatitis
    s. plexus
    s. pruritus
    s. purpura
    s. retinitis
    s. screen
    s. spectrum
    s. therapy
    s. urticaria
solarium
solder

sole
sole plate, sole-plate
solid
    s. ameloblastoma
    s. bone
    color s.
    s. cystic hidradenoma
    s. cystic tumor of pancreas
    s. edema
    s. extract
    gas-s. chromatography (GSC)
    s. pulmonary edema
    s. solution alloy
    s. teratoma
    s. vision
solipsism
solipsistic
solitary
    s. angiokeratoma
    s. bone cyst
    s. bundle
    s. cells of Meynert
    s. fasciculus
    s. fibrous tumor
    s. follicles
    s. glands of intestine
    s. keratoacanthoma
    s. myeloma
    s. neurofibroma
    s. nodule
Solow sigmoidoscope
solubility
solubilize
soluble
    alcohol-s. protein
    s. blue 3M
    fat-s. vitamins
    s. fiber
    s. fluorescein
    s. gum-resin
    s. indigo blue
    s. ligature
    specific s. substance
    s. starch
    s. toxin
    water-s. vitamins
solute
solution
    alcoholic s.
    aluminum acetate topical s.
    aluminum subacetate topical s.
    ammonia s.
    anisotonic s.
    anticoagulant citrate
      dextrose s.

S

solution *(continued)*
   anticoagulant citrate
     phosphate dextrose s.
   anticoagulant heparin s.
   antipyrine and benzocaine s.
   antiseptic s.
   aqueous s.
   auxiliary s.
   balanced electrolyte s.
   balanced salt s.
   Brompton s.
   Buckberg
   buffer s.
   Burnett s.
   carbolfuchsin topical s.
   cardioplegic s.
   carmine s.
   centinormal s.
   citrated Locke s.
   coal tar topical s.
   colloid s., colloidal s.
   compound iodine s.
   comprehensive s.
   contrast s.
   crystal violet s.
   cyanocobalamin Co 57 s.
   cyanocobalamin Co 60 s.
   Czapek-Dox s.
   Dakin s., modified
   Darrow s.
   decimolar s.
   decinormal s.
   dexamethasone sodium
     phosphate ophthalmic s.
   diluted ammonium hydroxide s.
   disclosing s.
   double-normal s.
   epinephrine s.
   ferric subsulfate s.
   fiftieth-normal s.
   fixative s.
   formaldehyde s.
   formol-Zenker s.
   gentian violet topical s.
   gold Au 198 s.
   Gowers s.
   gram molecular s.
   half-normal saline s.
   hundredth-normal s.
   hydrogen peroxide topical s.
   hydroxypropyl methylcellulose
     ophthalmic s.
   hyperbaric s.
   hypertonic s.
   hypobaric s.

solution *(continued)*
   hypotonic s.
   iodine topical s.
   isobaric s.
   lactated Ringer s.
   Locke s.
   magnesium citrate oral s.
   methoxsalen topical s.
   methylcellulose ophthalmic s.
   methylrosaniline chloride s.
   modified Dakin s.
   molal s., molar s.
   molecular disperse s.
   normal s.
   normal saline s.
   ophthalmic s.
   physiologic salt s.
   physiologic sodium chloride s.
   Ringer s., lactated
   saline s.
   salt s.
   saturated s.
   sclerosing s.
   seminormal s.
   sodium chloride s.
   sodium fluoride and acidulated
     phosphate topical s.
   sodium fluoride oral s.
   sodium hypochlorite s.
   sodium iodide I 125 s.
   sodium iodide I 131 s.
   sodium pertechnetate
     Tc 99m s.
   sodium phosphate P 32 s.
   sodium radioiodide s.
   standard s.
   strong ammonia s.
   stronger ammonium
     hydroxide s.
   strong iodine s.
   supersaturated s.
   tenth-normal s.
   test s's
   thousandth-normal s.
   triple antibiotic s.
   volumetric s.
   Ziehl-Neelsen carbolfuchsin s.
solvable
solvate
solvation
solvency
solvent
   lipid s.
   polar s.
solvolysis

SOM—serous otitis media
somal
somalin
somatalgia
somatasthenia
somatesthesia
somatesthetic
somatic
    s. afferent fibers
    s. agglutinin
    s. antigen
    s. cavity
    s. cells
    s. death
    s. delusion
    s. efferent fibers
    s. fibers
    s. hallucination
    s. hypermutation
    s. layer
    s. motor component
    s. muscle
    s. nerve fibers
    s. nerves
    s. nervous system
    s. pain
    s. senses
    s. sensory area
    s. sensory component
somaticovisceral
somatization disorder
somatochrome
somatoderm
somatodidymus
somatodymia
somatoform
somatogenic
somatognosis
somatogram
somatomammotropin
    chorionic s.
somatomegaly
somatometry
somatomotor
    primary s. area
somatopagus
somatopathic
somatopathy
somatophrenia
somatoplasm
somatopleural
somatopleure
somatopsychic
somatoschisis
somatoscopy

somatosensory
    s. area
    s. epilepsy
    s. evoked potential (SEP)
    s. evoked response (SER)
somatosexual
somatosplanchnic angle
somatosplanchnopleuric
somatostatin cells
somatostatinoma
somatotherapy
somatotonia
somatotopagnosia
somatotrope
    s. adenoma
    s. cell
somatotropin
    s. release-inhibiting factor
    s. release-inhibiting
        hormone
    s.-releasing hormone
somatotropinoma
somatotype
somatotyping
Somers forceps
SOMI—sternal occipital
   mandibular immobilizer
SOMI brace
somnambulance
somnambulation
somnambulism
somnambulist
somnifacient
somniferous
somnific
somniloquence
somniloquism
somniloquist
somniloquy
somnocinematograph
somnolence
somnolent
somnolentia
Somogyi
    effect
    phenomenon
    reflex
    unit
sonde coudé
Sondermann canals
Sones coronary catheter
sonic
sonicate
sonication
Sonne dysentery

S

Sonnenschein speculum
sonogram
sonographer
sonographic
sonography
>   Acuson computed s.
>   Acuson transvaginal s.

sonolucency
sonolucent
sonorous
>   s. breathing
>   s. quality
>   s. rales
>   s. rhonchi
>   s. snoring
>   s. voice

Soonawalla uterine elevator
SOP—standard operating
  procedure
sophisticate
sophistication
sophomore
sopor
soporiferous
soporific
soporous
sorbefacient
sorbic acid
sorbitol
sorbose
sordes (sordes)
sore
>   bed s.
>   canker s.
>   chrome s.
>   cold s., coldsore
>   denture s.
>   desert s.
>   hard s.
>   mixed s.
>   pressure s.
>   primary s.
>   soft s.
>   umballa s.
>   veldt s.
>   venereal s.

Soresi cannula
Soret
>   band
>   effect
>   phenomenon

sore throat
>   clergyman's s.t.
>   epidemic streptococcal s.t.
>   hospital s.t.

sore throat *(continued)*
>   putrid s.t.
>   septic s.t.
>   spotted s.t.
>   streptococcal s.t.
>   ulcerated s.t.

sorter
>   fluorescence-activated cell s.
>   (FACS)

Soto-Hall sign
Sotos syndrome
Sottas disease
souffle
>   cardiac s.
>   fetal s.
>   funic s.
>   funicular s.
>   placental s.
>   splenic s.
>   umbilical s.
>   uterine s.

sound
>   adventitious s's
>   aortic second s. (A_2 [A2])
>   atrial s.
>   auscultatory s's
>   bandbox s.
>   Beatty-Bright friction s.
>   bell s.
>   Bellocq s.
>   bellows s.
>   Benique s.
>   bottle s.
>   bronchial breath s's
>   Campbell s.
>   cardiac s's
>   cavernous voice s.
>   coin s.
>   cracked-pot s.
>   cranial cracked-pot s.
>   Davis s.
>   diastolic s.
>   Dittel s.
>   dive-bomber s.
>   eddy s's
>   ejection s's
>   entotic s's
>   esophageal s.
>   first heart s. (S_1)
>   flapping s.
>   fourth heart s. (S_4)
>   Fowler s.
>   friction s.
>   gallop s. (S_3, S_4)
>   Guyon s.

sound *(continued)*

    heart s's (first through
      fourth, S_1–S_4)
    Jewett s.
    Korotkoff s.
    lacrimal s.
    Le Fort s.
    metallic s.
    muscle s.
    Otis s.
    peacock s.
    percussion s.
    pericardial friction s.
    physiologic s's, physiological s's
    pistol-shot s.
    post-tussis suction s.
    Pratt s.
    pulmonic second s. (P_2)
    respiratory s.
    Santini booming s.
    second s., aortic (A_2)
    second heart s. (S_2)
    second s., pulmonic (P_2)
    S_3 gallop s.
    S_4 gallop s.
    shaking s.
    Simpson s.
    Sims s.
    subjective s.
    succussion s's
    third heart s.
    tick-tack s's
    to-and-fro s.
    urethral s.
    uterine s.
    Van Buren s.
    vesicular breath s's
    Walther s.
    water-wheel s.
    white s.
    Winternitz s.
    xiphisternal crunching s.

source

    point s.

Sourdille operation
Southey trocar
Southey-Leech tube
Southwick osteotomy
Souttar tube
souvenir

    s. infection
    s. knife

soya
soybean
soy sauce

SP—

    shunt procedure
    skin potential
    suprapubic
    symphysis pubis
    systolic pressure

S/P, SP—status post
SPA—suprapubic aspiration
space

    alveolar dead s.
    anatomical dead s.
    anatomic dead s.
    antecubital s.
    apical s.
    arachnoid s.
    axillary s.
    Blessig s's
    Bogros s.
    Bowman s.
    bregmatic s.
    Burns s.
    capsular s.
    cartilage s's
    cell s's
    chyle s's
    circumlental s.
    Colles s.
    complemental s.
    corneal s's
    cupola s.
    cupular s.
    Czermak s's
    dead s.
    dead s., anatomical
    s's in dentin
    s's of Disse
    Disse s's
    Douglas s.
    epicerebral s.
    epidural s.
    episcleral s.
    epispinal s.
    epitympanic s.
    escapement s's
    extradural s.
    extraperitoneal s.
    filtration s.
    follicular s.
    Fontana s.
    freeway s.
    globular s's of Czermak
    H s.
    haversian s.
    Henke s.
    His perivascular s.

S

space *(continued)*
    Holzknecht s.
    iliocostal s.
    interarytenoid s.
    intercostal s.
    intercristal s.
    intercrural s.
    interdental s.
    interfascial s.
    interglobular s's
    interglobular s's (of Owen)
    interlamellar s's
    intermesoblastic s.
    intermetacarpal s's
    intermetatarsal s's
    interocclusal s.
    interosseous s's
    interosseous s's of metacarpus
    interosseous s's of
      metatarsus
    interpeduncular s.
    interpleural s.
    interproximal s.
    interproximate s.
    interradicular s.
    interseptal s.
    interstitial s.
    intervaginal s.
    intervaginal s's of optic nerve
    intervillous s.
    intra-adventitial s.
    intracapsular s.
    intracristal s.
    intrapial s.
    intravesical s.
    Kiernan s's
    Kiesselbach s.
    Kretschmann s.
    Larrey s's
    leeway s.
    Lesshaft s.
    lymph s.
    lymphatic s.
    Magendie s's
    marrow s.
    mechanical dead s.
    Meckel s.
    mediastinal s.
    medullary s.
    meningeal s.
    midpalmar s.
    mitochondrial membrane s.
    Mohrenheim s.
    Nance leeway s.
    Nuel s's

space *(continued)*
    palmar s.
    paraglottic s.
    parapharyngeal s.
    pararectal s.
    pararenal s.
    parasinoidal s's
    paravesical s.
    paraxial s.
    Parona s.
    pelvocrural s.
    perforated s., anterior
    perforated s., posterior
    periaxial s.
    perichoroidal s.
    perilymphatic s.
    perineal s., deep
    perineal s., superficial
    perineural s.
    perineuronal s.
    perinodal s.
    perinuclear s.
    periotic s.
    peripharyngeal s.
    periplasmic s.
    perisinusoidal s's
    peritoneal s.
    perivascular s.
    perivitelline s.
    personal s.
    pharyngomaxillary s.
    phrenocostal s.
    physiologic dead s.
    pia-arachnoid s.
    placental blood s.
    plantar s.
    pleural s.
    pleuroperitoneal s.
    pneumatic s.
    Poiseuille s.
    popliteal s.
    postnasal s.
    postperforated s.
    postpharyngeal s.
    preepiglottic s.
    preperitoneal s.
    preputial s.
    presacral s.
    prestyloid s.
    prevertebral s.
    prevesical s.
    prezonular s.
    proximal s.
    proximate s.
    Prussak s.

space *(continued)*
- pterygomandibular s.
- pulp s.
- quadrangular s.
- quadrilateral s.
- relief s.
- respiratory dead s.
- retrobulbar s.
- retrocardiac s.
- retroinguinal s.
- retromylohyoid s.
- retro-ocular s.
- retroperitoneal s.
- retropharyngeal s.
- retropubic s.
- Retzius s., s. of Retzius
- Schwalbe s's
- semilunar s.
- septal s.
- subarachnoid s.
- subchorial s.
- subdural s.
- subepicranial s.
- subgingival s.
- submaxillary s.
- subphrenic s.
- subumbilical s.
- suprahepatic s's
- suprapubic s.
- suprasternal s.
- Tarin s.
- Tenon s.
- thenar s.
- thiocyanate s.
- third s.
- thyrohyal s.
- Traube s.
- Tröltsch (Troeltsch) s's
- urogenital s.
- Virchow-Robin s's
- vitelline s.
- web s.
- Westberg s.
- zonular s's

spacer

spacing
- third s.

spadelike

Spaeth operation

SPAI—steroid protein activity index

Spalding sign

Spalding-Richardson
- hysterectomy
- operation

spallation

span
- attention s.
- auditory s.
- liver s.

Spanish windlass

Spanlang-Tappeiner syndrome

spar
- Iceland s.

sparganosis

sparganum

Sparine

sparing
- aortic valve–s. reimplantation
- bladder s.
- blood s.
- bone s.
- limb-s. surgery
- macular s.
- muscle s.
- nephron-s. surgery
- organ-s. surgery
- parenchymal-s. resection
- protein s.
- rectum s.
- sacral s.
- skin s.

spark
- direct s.

sparteine

spartium

spasm
- s. of accommodation
- arterial s.
- athetoid s.
- bowing s.
- bronchial s.
- cadaveric s.
- carpopedal s.
- cerebral s.
- clonic s.
- clonic facial s.
- coronary artery s.
- cynic s.
- dancing s.
- diffuse esophageal s.
- epidemic transient diaphragmatic s.
- esophageal s.
- facial s.
- fatigue s.
- fixed s.
- flexion s.
- flexor s.
- functional s.

S

spasm (continued)
glottic s.
habit s.
histrionic s.
infantile massive s's
inspiratory s.
intention s.
lock s.
malleatory s.
massive s.
masticatory s.
mimic s.
mixed s.
mobile s.
muscle s.
myopathic s.
nictitating s.
nodding s.
occupation s.
oculogyric s.
pantomimic s.
pedal s.
perineal s.
phonatory s.
postparalytic facial s.
professional s.
progressive torsion s.
recruitment s.
respiratory s.
retrocollic s.
Romberg s.
rotatory s.
salaam s.
saltatory s.
sewing s.
spinal accessory s.
stutter s.
synclonic s.
tailor's s.
tetanic s.
tonic s.
tonoclonic s.
torsion s.
toxic s.
vascular s.
West s.
winking s.
spasmodic
s. asthma
s. bladder
s. croup
s. dysmenorrhea
s. dysphonia
s. mydriasis
s. stricture

spasmodic (continued)
s. synkinesis
s. torticollis
spasmogen
spasmogenic
spasmolysis
spasmolytic
spasmophilic
spasmus nutans
spastic
s. abasia
s. aphonia
s. bladder
s. bulbar palsy
s. colon
congenital s. paraplegia
s. constipation
s. diplegia
s. dysarthria
s. dysphagia
s. dysuria
s. ectropion
s. entropion
Erb s. paraplegia
s. flatfoot
s. gait
s. hemiplegia
hereditary s. paraplegia
s. ileus
infantile s. paraplegia
inherited s. paresis
s. miosis
s. paralysis
s. paraplegia
paraplegic s. gait
spasticity
cerebral s.
clasp-knife s.
inherited periodic s.
spatial
s. disorientation
s. vector
s. vectorcardiography
spatium (spatia)
spatia anguli iridis
(Fontanae)
spatia anguli iridocornealis
s. episclerale
s. extraperitoneale
s. intercostale
s. interfasciale (Tenoni)
spatia interglobularia
spatia interossea metacarpi
spatia interossea metatarsi
s. intervaginale

spatium (spatia) *(continued)*
    spatia intervaginalia nervi
      optici
    s. perichoroideale
    s. perilymphaticum
    s. peripharyngeum
    s. profundum perinei
    s. retroperitoneale
    s. retropharyngeum
    s. retropubicum
    s. subdurale
    s. superficiale perinei
    spatia zonularia
spatula
    Berens s.
    Castroviejo s.
    Cushing s.
    Davis s.
    Elschnig s.
    s. foot
    Jacobson s.
    Knapp s.
    Lindner s.
    s. mallei
    McPherson s.
    s. needle
    Sachs s.
    Segond s.
    Tauber s.
    tongue s.
    Wheeler s.
    Woodson s.
spatular
spatulate
spatulation
SPBI—serum protein-bound
  iodine
SPCA—serum prothrombin
  conversion accelerator
SPE—serum protein
  electrophoresis
speaking tube
Spearman
    rank correlation coefficient
    rho
spearmint
specialist
    clinical nurse s.
    nurse s.
specialization
specialize
specialty
specific
    s. activity
    s. gravity

specificity
    carrier s.
    diagnostic s.
    neuronal s.
specimen
    corrosion s.
    cytologic s.
speckle
    digital image s. correlation
      (DISC)
    s. filtering
    fluorescent s. microscopy
      (FSM)
    laser s.
    nuclear s's
    s. pattern
    s. reduction
    s. signal
speckled
    s. antinucleolar
      antibodies
    blue-s. secretions
    s. erythroplakia
    s. lentiginous nevus
    s. leukoplakia
    s. molecules
    s. pattern
    s. spleen
SPECT—single photon emission
  computed tomography
spectacles
    aspheric lenticular s.
    compound s.
    decentered s.
    divided s.
    half-glass s.
    industrial s.
    Masselon s.
    mica s.
    pantoscopic s.
    periscopic s.
    prismatic s.
    protective s.
    pulpit s.
    safety s.
    stenopeic s.
    tinted s.
    wire frame s.
spectra (plural of spectrum)
spectral
spectrocolorimeter
spectrofluorometer
spectrograph
    mass s.
    x-ray s.

S

spectrometer
  beta-ray s.
  gamma-ray s.
  infrared s.
  mass s.
  Mossbauer s.
  pulse-height s.
  scintillation s.
  x-ray s.
spectrometry
  pulse height s.
  tandem mass s.
  x-ray emission s.
spectrophotofluorometer
spectrophotometer
  absorption s.
spectrophotometry
  atomic absorption s.
  flame emission s.
spectropolarimeter
spectroscope
  direct vision s.
spectroscopic analysis
spectroscopy
  infrared s.
  magnetic resonance s.
  microabsorption s.
  nuclear magnetic resonance s.
  proton s.
spectrum (spectra)
  absorption s.
  action s.
  antibacterial s.
  antibiotic s.
  broad-s.
  chemical s.
  chromatic s.
  color s.
  continuous s.
  continuous x-ray s.
  electromagnetic s.
  excitation s.
  fluorescence s.
  fortification s.
  gaseous s.
  grafting s.
  invisible s.
  normal s.
  ocular s.
  prismatic s.
  pure s.
  solar s.
  thermal s.
  visible s.
  x-ray s.

SPECT scan
speculum (specula, speculums)
  Allingham rectal s.
  anal s.
  s. anoscope
  Aufricht s.
  aural s.
  Auvard-Remine s.
  Auvard weighted s.
  Barr anal s.
  Barraquer s.
  Barraquer-Colibri s.
  Barr rectal s.
  Beckman-Colver nasal s.
  Beckman nasal s.
  Berens s.
  Berlind-Auvard s.
  bivalve s., bivalved s.
  Boucheron s.
  Bozeman s.
  Brewer s.
  Brinkerhoff rectal s.
  Buie-Smith s.
  Castroviejo s.
  Chelsea-Eaton s.
  Chevalier Jackson s.
  Coakley s.
  Collin s.
  Converse s.
  Cook s.
  Cottle s.
  Cusco s.
  David s.
  DeVilbiss s.
  duckbill s., duck-billed s.
  Dudley-Smith s.
  Duplay s.
  Duplay-Lynch s.
  Eaton s.
  esophageal s.
  eye s.
  Fansler s.
  Farrior s.
  Fergusson s.
  Flannery s.
  Fränkel s.
  Garrigue s.
  Gerzog s.
  Goldbacher s.
  Graves s.
  Gruber s.
  Guild-Pratt s.
  Guttmann s.
  Guyton-Maumenee s.
  Guyton-Park s.

speculum (specula, speculums)
(continued)
  Halle s.
  Halle-Tieck s.
  Hartmann dewaxer s.
  Heffernan s.
  Helmont s.
  Henrotin s.
  Hinkle-James rectal s.
  Huffman-Graves s.
  Ingals s.
  Jonas-Graves s.
  Kahn-Graves s.
  Kelly s.
  Killian nasal s.
  Killian rectal s.
  Knapp s.
  Kramer s.
  Kyle s.
  Lancaster s.
  Lange s.
  Lempert-Colver endaural s.
  lid s.
  Lillie s.
  Lister-Burch s.
  Mahoney s.
  Martin s.
  Martin and Davy s.
  Mason-Auvard s.
  Mathews s.
  Maumenee-Park s.
  Mayer s.
  McHugh s.
  McPherson s.
  Mellinger s.
  Miller s.
  Mosher s.
  Mueller s.
  Murdock-Wiener s.
  Myles s.
  nasal s.
  nasopharyngeal s.
  Nott s.
  O'Sullivan-O'Connor s.
  Park s.
  Pederson s.
  pediatric s.
  Pennington s.
  Picot s.
  Politzer s.
  Pratt s.
  proctoscopic s.
  Pynchon s.
  Ray s.
  rectal s.

speculum (specula, speculums)
(continued)
  Rosenthal s.
  Sauer s.
  Scott s.
  Senturia s.
  Siegle pneumatic
    ear s.
  Simmonds s.
  Sims s.
  SMR s.
  Sonnenschein s.
  stop eye s.
  Thudichum nasal s.
  Toynbee s.
  Tröltsch s.
  urethral s.
  vaginal s.
  Vernon-David s.
  Vienna s.
  Weeks s.
  weighted s.
  Weisman-Graves s.
  Welch-Allyn s.
  Wiener s.
  Williams s.
  wire s.
  wire bivalve s.
  Yankauer s.
Spee curvature (curve)
speech
  alaryngeal s.
  ataxic s.
  clipped s.
  echo s.
  esophageal s.
  explosive s.
  incoherent s.
  interjectional s.
  jumbled s.
  mirror s.
  plateau s.
  pressured s.
  scamping s.
  scanning s.
  scattered s.
  slurred s.
  spastic s.
  staccato s.
  stuttering s.
  tangential s.
  telegraphic s.
speech-aid prosthesis
speechreading
Speed-Boyd operation

S

spell
    breath-holding s.
    syncopal s.
Spemann induction
Spence forceps
Spence-Adson forceps
Spencer
    probe
    punch
    scissors
Spencer-Parker vaccine
Spencer-Watson operation
Spencer Wells forceps
Spence tail
Spens syndrome
SPEP—serum protein
  electrophoresis
sperm
    s. agglutination test
    s. cell
    s.–cervical mucus contact test
    s. head
    s. immobilization test
    intracytoplasmic s. injection
    s. lysin
    microsurgical epididymal s.
      aspiration
    muzzled s.
    s. penetration assay
    percutaneous epididymal s.
      aspiration
    percutaneous testicular s.
      aspiration
    subzonal injection of s.
    subzonal insertion of s.
    s. swim-up method
    s. swim-up technique
    testicular s. extraction
    washed s.
    s. washing
spermatic
    s. artery
    s. canal
    s. cord
    s. duct
    s. fascia
    s. filament
    s. fistula
    s. nerve
    s. plexus
    s. vein
spermaticide
spermatid
spermatoblast
spermatocele
spermatocelectomy

spermatocidal
spermatocide
spermatocyst
spermatocyte
    primary s.
    secondary s.
spermatocytic seminoma
spermatocytogenesis
spermatocytoma
spermatogenesis
spermatogenic
    s. epididymitis
    s. granulomatous orchitis
spermatogenous
spermatogeny
spermatogone
spermatogonial cell
spermatogonium
spermatoid
spermatolysin
spermatolysis
spermatolytic
spermatopoietic
spermatozoa
spermatozoal
spermatozoid
spermatozoon
spermaturia
spermiation
spermicidal
    s. agent
    s. contraception
    s. gel
    s. sponge
spermicide
    5 nonoxynol-9 vaginal s.
    vaginal s.
spermidine
spermiduct
spermine
spermiogenesis
spermiogram
spermoblast
spermocytoma
spermolith
spermolysis
spermolytic
spermoneuralgia
spermoplasm
spermotoxic
spermotoxin
Spero forceps
SPF—
    specific pathogen-free
    split products of fibrin
sp gr—specific gravity

SPGR—spoiled GRASS
  [gradient recalled acquisition in
  a steady state]
sph—
    spherical
    spherical lens
SPH—secondary pulmonary
  hemosiderosis
sphenion (sphenia)
sphenocephalus
sphenocephaly
sphenoethmoid, sphenoethmoidal
    s. recess
    s. suture
sphenofrontal suture
sphenoid
    s. angle
    s. bone
    s. cell
    Koffler s.
    s. ostium
    s. ridge
    s. sinus
    s. sinusitis
    s. turbinate
sphenoidal
    s. angle of parietal bone
    s. crest
    s. emissary foramen
    s. fissure–optic anal
      syndrome
    s. fontanelle
    s. ligament
    s. margin
    s. process
    s. yoke
sphenoidale
    os s.
    planum s.
sphenoidectomy
    frontoethmoidal s.
sphenoiditis
sphenoidostomy
sphenoidotomy
sphenomalar suture
sphenomandibular ligament
sphenomaxillary
    s. ganglion
    s. suture
spheno-occipital,
  sphenooccipital
    s. fissure
    s. suture
spheno-orbital, sphenoorbital
    s. suture
sphenopagus

sphenopalatine
    s. artery
    s. canal
    s. foramen
    s. nerves
    s. notch of palatine
      bone
    s. rest
sphenoparietal
    s. sinus
    s. suture
sphenopetrosal
    s. fissure
    s. suture
sphenopharyngeal canal
sphenosis
sphenosquamosal
sphenosquamous suture
sphenotemporal
    s. margin of parietal
      bone
    s. suture
sphenotic
    s. center
    s. foramen
sphenoturbinal
    s. bone
    s. ossicle
sphenovomerine suture
sphenozygomatic suture
sphere
    attraction s.
    conflict-free ego s.
    embryotic s.
    s. granule
    neurosecretory s.
    segmentation s.
spherical
spherocyte
spherocytic
spherocytosis
    hereditary s.
spheroid
spheroidal
spherophakia-brachymorphia
  syndrome
spheroplast
spherule
    s's of Fulci
    rod s.
spherulin
sphincter
    anal s.
    anatomic s.
    s. ani
    artificial genitourinary s.

sphincter *(continued)*
    s. of bile duct
    s. of Boyden
    cardiac s.
    cardioesophageal s.
    choledochal s.
    s. of common bile duct
    cornual s.
    cricopharyngeal s.
    s. of duct of Wirsung
    duodenal s.
    esophageal s., lower
    esophageal s., upper
    esophagogastric s.
    external s. of anus
    s. of eye
    gastroesophageal s.
    Giordano s.
    Glisson s.
    Henle s.
    hepatic s.
    s. of hepatopancreatic ampulla
    Hyrtl s.
    ileal s.
    inguinal s.
    internal s. of anus
    s. iridis
    laryngeal s.
    Lütkens (Luetkens) s.
    s. muscle
    Nélaton s.
    O'Beirne s.
    s. oculi
    s. of Oddi
    s. oris
    ostial s.
    palatopharyngeal s.
    pancreatic s.
    pharyngoesophageal s.
    physiologic s.
    precapillary s.
    prepyloric s.
    s. pupillae
    pyloric s.
    rectal s.
    segmental s.
    smooth muscle s.
    s. spasm
    striated muscle s.
    tubal s.
    s. urethrae
    s. vaginae
    s. vesicae
sphincteral achalasia
sphincteralgia

sphincterectomy
sphincteric
sphincterismus
sphincteritis
sphincterolysis
sphincteroplasty
sphincteroscope
    Kelly s.
sphincteroscopy
sphincterotome
sphincterotomy
    choledochal s.
    internal s.
sphinganine
sphingogalactoside
sphingoin
sphingolipid activator protein
sphingolipidosis
    cerebral s.
    late-onset cerebral s.
sphingolipodystrophy
sphingomyelin
    lecithin-s. ratio
    s. lipidosis
    s. phosphodiesterase
sphingomyelinase
    deficiency
sphingomyelinosis
sphingophospholipid
sphingosine
sphygmic period
sphygmogram
sphygmographic
sphygmography
sphygmomanometer
spica
    s. bandage
    hip s.
spicular
spicularity
spiculated
    s. appearance
    s. lesion
    s. margins
    s. mass
    s. periosteal reaction
spiculation segmentation
spicule
    cemental s.
    s. segmentation
spiculum
spider
    arterial s.
    banana s.
    black widow s.

spider *(continued)*
>   brown recluse s.
>   s. burst
>   European wolf s.
>   funnel-web s.
>   jointed s.
>   lynx s.
>   vascular s.
>   wandering s.
>   wolf s.

Spieghel line

Spiegler
>   reagent
>   test
>   tumors

Spiegler-Fendt sarcoid

Spielmeyer-Vogt disease

Spies punch

spigelian hernia

Spigelius line

spike
>   cemental s.
>   centrotemporal s's
>   s. duration
>   end-plate s's
>   fever s.
>   focal s's
>   s. foci
>   glycemic s.
>   hypertensive intracranial
>   pressure (ICP) s.
>   interictal midline s's
>   intraocular pressure s.
>   M s.
>   midline s's
>   multiple s's
>   occipital s's
>   physiologic occipital s's
>   s. potential
>   slow s.
>   s. and slow wave complex
>   temperature s.
>   s. threshold
>   s. and wave activity
>   s.-wave discharges

spiked

spiking fever

spill
>   cellular s.
>   sugar s.
>   ureteral s. of indigo
>   carmine

spillage
>   urine glucose s.

Spiller syndrome

spilling
>   s. of protein
>   s. of sugar

spillway
>   occlusal s.

spin
>   s. echo
>   s.-lattice relaxation time
>   nuclear s.
>   s-s. relaxation time

spina (spinae)
>   s. bifida
>   s. bifida anterior
>   s. bifida aperta
>   s. bifida cystica
>   s. bifida manifesta
>   s. bifida occulta
>   s. bifida posterior
>   s. frontalis
>   s. helicis
>   s. iliaca anterior inferior
>   s. iliaca anterior superior
>   s. iliaca posterior inferior
>   s. iliaca posterior superior
>   s. intercondyloidea
>   s. ischiadica
>   s. ischialis
>   s. meatus
>   s. mentalis
>   s. mentalis inferior
>   s. nasalis anterior maxillae
>   s. nasalis ossis frontalis
>   s. nasalis ossis palatini
>   s. ossis sphenoidalis
>   spinae palatinae
>   s. scapulae
>   s. suprameatalis
>   s. suprameatica
>   s. tibiae
>   s. trochlearis
>   s. tympanica major
>   s. tympanica minor
>   s. ventosa

spinal
>   s. analgesia
>   s. anesthesia
>   s. aperture
>   s. apoplexy
>   s. arachnoid
>   s. arachnoiditis
>   s. arachnoid mater
>   s. arteriography
>   s. artery
>   s. ataxia
>   s. block

S

spinal *(continued)*
 s. canal
 s. caries
 s. column
 s. compression
 s. cord
 s. cord compression
 s. curvature
 s. dysraphism
 s. embolism
 s. filament
 s. fluid
 s. foramen
 s. fusion
 s. ganglion
 s. headache
 s. hemangioblastoma
 s. hemianesthesia
 s. hemiplegia
 s. induction
 s. laminae
 s. marrow
 s. meningitis
 s. meningocele
 s. miosis
 s. muscle
 s. mydriasis
 s. nerves
 s. orthosis
 s. pachymeningitis
 s. paralysis
 s. point
 s. poliomyelitis
 s. puncture
 s. pyramidotomy
 s. reflex
 s. reticular formation
 s. root of accessory nerve
 s. roots
 s. sedative
 s. segments
 s. shock
 s. sign
 s. stenosis
 s. stimulant
 s. subarachnoid block
 s. syphilis
 s. thrust
 s. tract of trigeminal nerve
 s. tuberculosis
 s. veins
spinalgia
 Petruschky s.
spinalis
 s. capitis muscle
 s. cervicis muscle

spinalis *(continued)*
 s. muscle
 s. thoracis muscle
spinate
spindle
 aortic s.
 Axenfeld-Krukenberg s.
 Bütschli nuclear s.
 central s.
 cleavage s.
 complex muscle s.
 enamel s's
 intermediate muscle s.
 Krukenberg s.
 mitotic s.
 muscle s.
 neuromuscular s.
 neurotendinal s.
 neurotendinous s.
 nuclear s.
 simple muscle s.
 sleep s's
 tandem s.
 tendon s.
 tigroid s's
 urine s's
spindling
spine
 alar s.
 angular s.
 anterior inferior iliac s.
 anterior superior iliac s.
 bamboo s.
 basilar s.
 cervical s.
 Civinini s.
 cleft s.
 dendritic s.
 dorsal s.
 ethmoidal s. of Macalister
 frontal s.
 s. of greater tubercle of
  humerus
 s. of helix
 hemal s.
 s. of Henle
 iliopectineal s.
 intercondyloid s.
 ischial s.
 s. of ischium
 kissing s's
 s. of lesser tubercle of humerus
 lumbar s.
 lumbosacral (LS) s.
 s. of maxilla
 meatal s.

spine *(continued)*
    nasal s., anterior
    nasal s. of frontal bone
    nasal s. of palatine bone
    nasal s., posterior
    neural s.
    obturator s.
    occipital s., external
    occipital s., internal
    palatine s's
    peroneal s. of calcaneus
    peroneal s. of os calcis
    pharyngeal s.
    poker s.
    posterior inferior iliac s.
    posterior palatine s.
    posterior superior iliac s.
    s. of pubic bone
    s. of pubis
    railway s.
    rigid s.
    sacral s.
    s. of scapula
    sciatic s.
    sphenoidal s.
    s. of sphenoid bone
    s. of Spix
    suprameatal s.
    thoracic s.
    s. of tibia
    tibial s.
    tibial s. of Macewen
    trochanteric s., greater
    trochanteric s., lesser
    trochlear s.
    tympanic s., anterior
    tympanic s., greater
    tympanic s., lesser
    tympanic s., posterior
    typhoid s.
    s. of vertebra
    vertebral s.
Spinelli operation
Spinhaler
spinifugal
spinipetal
spin-lattice relaxation time
spinnbarkeit
spinobulbar
spinocellular
spinocerebellar degenerative disease
spinocerebellum
spinocollicular
spinocortical
spinocostalis
spinoglenoid

spinomuscular
spinoneural
spinotectal tract
spinothalamic
    s. tract
    s. tractotomy
spinous
    s. layer
    s. plane
    s. process
    s. process of tibia
    s. process of vertebra
    spurious s. process of sacrum
spiradenoma
    eccrine s.
Spira disease
spiral
    s. arteries
    s. bandage
    bony s. lamina
    s. canal of cochlea
    s. canal of modiolus
    s. canal of Rosenthal
    s. cleavage
    s. computed tomography (CT)
    s. crest
    s. crest of cochlea
    Curschmann s's
    s. deviation of penis
    s. fold
    s. fracture
    s. ganglion
    Golgi-Rezzonico s.
    s. groove
    Herxheimer s's
    s. incision
    s. joint
    s. lamina
    lentula s.
    s. ligament of cochlea
    s. limbus
    s. line of femur
    s. membrane of cochlear duct
    s. modiolar artery
    s. organ
    Perroncito s's
    s. plate
    s. reverse bandage
    s. sulcus
    s. sulcus of humerus
    s. suture
    s.-tip catheter
    s. tubule
    s. valve of cystic duct
    s. visual field
    s. volumetric CT

S

spirillum fever
Spirillum minus
spirit
  aromatic s. of ammonia
  benzaldehyde s.
  camphor s.
  compound orange s.
  peppermint s.
  s's of turpentine
spirochetal jaundice
spirochete
spirochetemia
spirocheticidal
spirochetolytic
spirochetosis
spirocheturia
spirogram
spirography
spiroid
spiroma
spirometer
  Benedict-Roth s.
  Collins respirometer-s.
  Douglas bag s.
  Krogh apparatus s.
  Tissot s.
  Venturi meter s.
  Wright respirometer-s.
Spirometra
  S. erinaceieuropaei
  S. mansonoides
spirometric
spirometry
  bronchoscopic s.
  incentive s.
  Tri-Flow incentive s.
spittle
Spitzka
  nucleus
  tract
Spitzka-Lissauer
  column
  tract
Spitz nerve
Spix spine
SPL—sound pressure level
splanchnesthesia
splanchnesthetic sensibility
splanchnic
  s. block
  s. cavity
  s. ganglion
  s. layer
  s. mesoderm
  s. motor component

splanchnic *(continued)*
  s. nerves
  s. sensory component
  s. wall
splanchnicectomy
splanchnicotomy
splanchnocoele
splanchnocranium
splanchnoderm
splanchnomegaly
splanchnopleural
splanchnopleure
splanchnotomy
splash
  gastric s.
  succussion s.
S-plasty
splay legs
splayfoot
spleen
  accessory s.
  bacon s.
  cyanotic s.
  diffuse waxy s.
  enlarged s.
  flecked s. of Feitis
  floating s.
  Gandy-Gamna s.
  hyperreactive malarial s.
  s. index
  lardaceous s.
  movable s.
  porphyry s.
  sago s.
  speckled s.
  wandering s.
  waxy s.
splen accessorius
splenalgia
splenatrophy
splenectasis
splenectomize
splenectomy
  abdominal s.
  s. clamp
  Henry s.
  Rives s.
  subcapsular s.
splenectopia
splenelcosis
splenemia
splenemphraxis
splenial
  s. center
  s. gyrus

splenic
    s. abscess
    acute s. tumor
    s. anemia
    s. artery
    s. cords
    s. flexure of colon
    s. flexure syndrome
    s. fossa of omental sac
    s. lymph nodes
    s. mycosis
    s. portography
    primary s. neutropenia
    s. puncture
    s. reagent
    s. souffle
    s. tissue
    s. vein
    s. venography
splenicterus
spleniform
spleniserrate
splenitis
splenium corporis callosi
splenoblast
splenocele
splenocolic
splenocyte
splenodynia
splenogastric
    s. ligament
    s. omentum
splenogenous
splenogram
splenography
splenohepatomegaly
splenoid gland
splenolymphatic
splenolysis
splenoma
splenomalacia
splenomedullary
splenomegalic polycythemia
splenomegaly
    chronic s.
    congestive s.
    malarial s.
    tropical s.
splenometry
splenomyelogenous
splenomyelomalacia
splenonephric
splenonephroptosis
splenopancreatic
splenopathy

splenopexy
splenophrenic ligament
splenopneumonia
splenoportal hypertension
splenoportography
splenoptosis
splenorenal
    s. bypass
    s. ligament
    s. shunt
splenorrhagia
splenorrhaphy
splenosis
splenotomy
splenotoxin
splenulus
splenunculus
splice
splicing
    alternative s.
    DNA s.
    gene-s.
    RNA s.
splint
    abutment s.
    acrylic s.
    acrylic resin bite-guard s.
    Agnew s.
    air s.
    airplane s.
    anchor s.
    Anderson s.
    Angle s.
    Asch s.
    Ashhurst s.
    Balkan s.
    banjo traction s.
    Baylor s.
    Böhler s.
    Böhler-Braun s.
    Bond s.
    Bowlby s.
    Brant s.
    bridge s.
    Brown s.
    Buck s.
    buddy s.
    Bunnell s's
    Cabot s.
    caliper s.
    canine-to-canine lingual s.
    cap s.
    Carter s.
    cast bar s.
    cast cap s.

S

splint *(continued)*
- Chandler felt collar s.
- Chatfield-Girdleston s.
- coaptation s's
- cock-up s.
- Colles s.
- continuous clasp s.
- crib s.
- Curry s.
- Davis s.
- Denis Browne clubfoot s.
- DePuy s.
- diodontic s.
- dropfoot s.
- Dupuytren s.
- dynamic s.
- Eggers s.
- Engelmann s.
- Erich s.
- Essig-type s.
- fixed s.
- fixed partial denture s.
- Fox s.
- fracture s.
- Frejka pillow s.
- Friedman s.
- functional s.
- Futura s.
- Gilmer s.
- Gordon s.
- Hart s.
- hayrake s.
- Hodgen s.
- interdental s.
- Jones s.
- Kanavel cockup s.
- Kazanjian s.
- Keller-Blake s.
- Kingsley s.
- Kirschner wire s.
- labial s.
- ladder s.
- Lewin s.
- Lewin-Stern s.
- lingual s.
- Liston s.
- Love s.
- Mason-Allen s.
- Mayer s.
- Morris external fixation s.
- nasal s.
- open cap s.
- opponens s.
- pillow s.
- plaster s.

splint *(continued)*
- plastic s.
- poroplastic s.
- Porzett s.
- Roger Anderson s.
- Sayre s.
- shin s's
- Stader s.
- sugar-tong s.
- surgical s.
- talipes hobble s.
- Taylor s.
- therapeutic s.
- Thomas knee s.
- Tobruk s.
- Toronto s.
- traction s.
- Valentine s.
- volar s.
- Volkmann s.
- Wertheim s.
- Zimmer s.

splinter hemorrhage
splinting
split-sheath catheter
split-thickness
- s-t. flap
- s-t. skin graft

splitting
- fee s.
- s. of heart sounds
- sagittal s. of mandible

spoiled GRASS (gradient recalled acquisition in a steady state) (SPGR)
spoking
- cortical s.

spondee
spondylalgia
spondylarthritis ankylopoietica
spondylarthrocace
spondylarthropathy
spondylitic
spondylitis
- s. ankylopoietica
- ankylosing s.
- Bekhterev s.
- Bekhterev-Strümpell s.
- hypertrophic s.
- s. infectiosa
- Kümmell s.
- Marie-Strümpell s.
- muscular s.
- posttraumatic s.
- rheumatoid s.

spondylitis *(continued)*
    traumatic s.
    s. tuberculosa
    tuberculous s.
    s. typhosa
spondylizema
spondyloarthropathy
    seronegative s's
spondylocace
spondylodesis
spondylodynia
spondylolisthesis
    congenital s.
    degenerative s.
    dysplastic s.
    isthmic s.
    pathological s.
    traumatic s.
spondylolisthetic
spondylolysis
spondylomalacia traumatica
spondylopathy
    traumatic s.
spondyloptosis
spondylopyosis
spondyloschisis
spondylosis
    cervical s.
    s. chronica
      ankylopoietica
    degenerative s.
    lumbar s.
    rhizomelic s.
    s. uncovertebralis
spondylosyndesis
spondylotherapy
spondylothoracic dysplasia
spondylotic
    s. caudal radiculopathy
    s. cervical myelopathy
spondylotomy
spondylous
sponge
    Bernays s.
    s. biopsy
    Bunge s.
    fibrin s.
    s. forceps
    s.-holding forceps
    gauze s.
    gelatin s.
    s. implant
    medullary s. kidney
    peanut s.
    sodium s.

sponge *(continued)*
    spermicidal s.
    s. stick
    Weck s.
    Weck-cel s.
    white s. nevus
spongiform
spongioblast
spongioblastoma
    s. multiforme
    polar s.
    unipolar s.
spongiocyte
spongiocytoma
spongioid
spongioplasm
spongiosa
spongiosaplasty
spongiose urethra
spongiosis
    eosinophilic s.
spongiositis
spongiosum
    osteoma s.
    stratum s.
spongiotic
spongy
spontaneous
spool
spoon
    Bunge s.
    Cushing s.
    Daviel s.
    s. denture
    Elschnig s.
    s. excavator
    Gross s.
    Hess s.
    Kirby s.
    Knapp s.
    s. nail
    sharp s.
    Volkmann s.
sporadic
sporangial
sporangium (sporangia)
spore
sporiferous
Sporothrix schenckii
sporotrichosis
sporotrichotic
sports medicine
sport-specific exercise
sports-related injury
sporular

S

spot
  age s.
  ash leaf s.
  Bitot s.
  blind s.
  blue s.
  Brushfield s's
  café au lait s.
  Campbell de Morgan s.
  cherry-red s.
  cold s.
  cotton-wool s's
  deaf s.
  Elschnig s.
  eye s.
  s. film
  s.-film radiography
  flame s.
  focal s.
  Forchheimer s.
  Fordyce s.
  Forster-Fuchs s.
  Fuchs s.
  germinal s.
  s. grinding
  Harrison s. test
  hot s.
  hot s. imaging
  hot s. scan
  Janeway s.
  Koplik s's
  lance-ovate s.
  laser s. diameter
  lenticular s.
  light s.
  liver s.
  Mariotte s.
  Maxwell s.
  mental blind s.
  milk s.
  milky s.
  mongolian s.
  mononucleosis s. test
  mulberry s.
  orange s.
  pain s.
  pink s.
  rose s.
  Roth s's
  sacral s.
  Smith-McGuckin s.
  spongy s.
  Tardieu s.
  Tay s.
  trigger s.

spot (continued)
  typhoid s.
  warm s.
  wet w.
  white s. disease
  yellow s.
spot film
  s.f. device
  s.f. radiography
  s.f. roentgenography
  s.f. study
spotting
SPP—suprapubic
  prostatectomy
spraddle legs
sprain
  acromioclavicular s.
  deltoid s.
  rider's s.
  tibiofibular s.
  vertebral cervical s.
Spratt curet
spray
  ether s.
  lysine pitressin s.
  needle s.
  tyrothricin s.
spread
  electrotonic s.
  gene s.
  secondary s.
spreader
  gutta-percha s.
  Millin-Bacon s.
  root canal filling s.
  Wiltberger s.
Sprengel deformity
spring
  auxiliary s.
  bow s.
  closed s.
  coil s.
  finger s.
  Kesling s.
  loop s.
  open s.
  paddle s.
  separating s.
  uprighting s.
  Weiss s's
  Z s.
sprout
  nodal s.
  syncytial s's
sprouting

sprue
    celiac s.
    collagenous s.
    nontropical s.
    refractory s.
    tropical s.
    unclassified s.
sprue-former
SPTA—spatial peak temporal
  average
spud
    Corbett s.
    Davis s.
    Dix s.
    Fisher s.
    Francis s.
    Gross s.
    Hosford s.
    LaForce s.
    Walter s.
spur
    calcaneal s.
    cementum s.
    enamel s.
    heel s.
    occipital s.
    olecranon s.
    scleral s.
spurious
    s. findings
Spurling
    forceps
    rongeur
    sign
    test
spurring
Spurway syndrome
sputum
    albuminoid s.
    egg yolk s.
    globular s.
    green s.
    icteric s.
    moss-agate s.
    mucoid s.
    nummular s.
    prune juice s.
    rusty s.
    s. tube
    yellow-green s.
SPWB—Saunders Pharmaceutical
  Word Book
sq.—square
SQ—social quotient
SQ, subcu, subq—subcutaneous

squalene
squama (squamae)
    s. alveolaris
    external mental s.
    s. of frontal bone
    s. frontalis
    occipital s.
    s. occipitalis
    perpendicular s.
    superior occipital s.
    temporal s.
    s. of temporal bone
    s. temporalis
squamate
squamatization
squame
squamocellular
squamocolumnar junction
squamofrontal
squamomastoid suture
squamo-occipital bone
squamoparietal suture
squamopetrosal
squamosa
squamosal
squamosphenoid suture
squamotemporal
squamotympanic fissure
squamous
    adenoid s. cell carcinoma
    s. alveolar cells
    s. bone
    s. border of parietal bone
    s. carcinoma
    s. cell
    s. cell carcinoma
    s. epithelium
    s. hyperplasia
    intraepidermal s. cell
      carcinoma
    s. intraepithelial lesion
    s. margin of parietal bone
    s. metaplasia
    multiple self-healing s.
      epithelioma
    s. odontogenic tumor
    s. papilloma
    self-healing s. epithelioma
    simple s. epithelium
    stratified s. epithelium
    s. suture
    s. suture of cranium
squamozygomatic
square
    Punnett s.

S

square millimeter(s) (mm², sq mm)
squash-bite
squatting facet
squeeze
    s. dynamometer
    s. technique
    tussive s.
squid ink
squill
    red s.
    white s.
squillitic
squint
    accommodative s.
    comitant s.
    concomitant s.
    convergent s.
    divergent s.
    noncomitant s.
    upward and downward s.
SR—
    sarcoplasmic reticulum
    secretion rate
    sedimentation rate
    sensitization response
    sinus rhythm
    skin resistance
    superior rectus
    systemic resistance
    systems review
S-R—stimulus-response
SRF—somatotropin-releasing factor
SRFS—split renal function study
SRH—somatotropin-releasing
    hormone
sRNA—soluble RNA
SRP—short rib polydactyly
SRR—slow rotation room
SRS—slow-reacting substance
SRS-A—slow-reacting substance of
    anaphylaxis
SRT—
    sedimentation rate test
    speech reception threshold
SS—
    signs and symptoms
    soapsuds [enema]
    subaortic stenosis
SSA—sulfosalicylic acid (test)
Ssabanejew-Frank
    gastrostomy
    operation
SSc—systemic sclerosis
s-screen containing cassette
SSD—source to skin distance

SSE—soapsuds enema
SSKI—saturated solution of
    potassium iodide
SSP—Sanarelli-Shwartzman
    phenomenon
SSP, SSPE—subacute sclerosing
    panencephalitis
SSS—sick sinus syndrome
SSSS—staphylococcal scalded skin
    syndrome
SSU—sterile supply unit
ST—
    sinus tachycardia
    skin test
    standardized test
STA—serum thrombotic
    accelerator
stab (band, immature neutrophil)
stabilate
stabile
    heat s.
stability
    denture s.
    dimensional s.
stabilization
stabilizer
    endodontic s.
stable
stab wound
    s.w. drain
    s.w. incision
staccato
stachybotryotoxicosis
Stacke operation
Staderini nucleus
Stader splint
Stadie-Riggs microtome
staff
    attending s.
    consulting s.
    house s.
stage
    amphibolic s.
    anal s.
    bell s.
    cap s.
    cold s.
    eruptive s.
    exoerythrocytic s.
    expulsive s.
    first s. of labor
    fourth s. of labor
    genital s.
    hot s.
    imperfect s.

stage *(continued)*

    s's of labor (1–4)
    latency s.
    mechanical s.
    oral s.
    perfect s.
    phallic s.
    placental s.
    preeruptive s.
    preerythrocytic s.
    premenstrual s.
    prodromal s.
    prodromal s. of labor
    progestational s.
    proliferative s.
    pyretogenic s.
    rest s.
    resting s.
    ring s.
    rotation s. of labor
    second s. of labor
    stepladder s.
    sweating s.
    Tanner developmental s's
      (I–V)
    third s. of labor
    transitional pulp s.
    ugly duckling s. of mixed
      dentition

staging

    clinical s. of cancer
    clinical s. of lymphomas
    Greulich and Pyle bone age s.
    s. laparotomy
    Marshall and Tanner
      pubertal s.
    pathologic s. of lymphomas
    Rai s.
    TNM (tumor, node,
      metastasis) s.

Stahl ear No. 1 (or 2)

Stahr gland

stain

    acid s.
    acid-fast s. (AFS)
    acid fuchsin s.
    Albert diphtheria s.
    Alzheimer s.
    Anthony capsule s.
    auramine-rhodamine s.
    azan s.
    basic s.
    Benda s.
    Best carmine s.
    Bielschowsky s.

stain *(continued)*

    Bowie s.
    carbolfuchsin s.
    carbol–gentian violet s.
    Castaneda s.
    Ciaccio s.
    contrast s.
    counter s.
    Davenport s.
    Dieterle s.
    differential s.
    Ehrlich acid hematoxylin
    Ehrlich triacid s.
    electron s's
    Feulgen method
    Fontana s.
    Fontana-Masson s.
    Giemsa s.
    Gimenez s.
    Gomori s.
    Gomori methenamine–silver
      nitrate s.
    Gomori-Wheatley s.
    Goodpasture s.
    Gram s.
    Grocott-Gomori methenamine–
      silver nitrate s.
    Hale iron s.
    Harris hematoxylin
    heavy-metal s.
    Heidenhain iron hematoxylin s.
    hemalum s.
    hematoxylin-eosin s.
    hematoxylin-eosin-azure II s.
    Hiss capsule s.
    Hortega method
    India ink capsule s.
    iron hematoxylin method
    Kinyoun s.
    Leifson flagella s.
    Leishman s.
    lipoid s.
    lithium-carmine s.
    Loeffler alkaline methylene
      blue s.
    Luxol fast blue s.
    Macchiavello s.
    Mallory acid fuchsin, orange
      G, and aniline blue s.
    Mallory phloxine–methylene
      blue s.
    Mallory phosphotungstic
      acid–hematoxylin s.
    Mallory triple s.
    Masson s.

S

stain *(continued)*
- Masson trichrome s.
- Maximow s.
- May-Grünwald s. (Gruenwald)
- May-Grünwald-Giemsa s. (Gruenwald)
- metachromatic s.
- methenamine silver s.
- methyl green–pyronin (MGP) s.
- neutral s.
- nuclear s.
- Pal-Weigert method
- Papanicolaou s.
- Pappenheim s.
- PAS (periodic acid–Schiff) s.
- periodic acid–Schiff s. (PAS s.)
- phosphotungstic acid–hematoxylin s. (PTAH s.)
- plasmatic s.
- plasmic s.
- port-wine s.
- protoplasmic s.
- quinacrine fluorescent method
- Ranson pyridine silver s.
- resorcin-fuchsin s.
- reverse Giemsa method
- Romanovsky (Romanowsky) s.
- selective s.
- Seller s.
- Sternheimer-Malbin s.
- Sudan black B fat s.
- Truant auramine-rhodamine s.
- tumor s.
- Unna-Pappenheim s.
- van Gieson s.
- Verhoeff s.
- Verhoeff-van Gieson s.
- von Kossa s.
- Warthin-Starry silver s.
- Wayson s.
- Weigert fibrin s.
- Weigert iron hematoxylin s.
- Weigert neuroglia fiber s.
- Weigert resorcin-fuchsin s.
- Weil s.
- Wirtz-Conklin spore s.
- Wright s.
- Ziehl-Neelsen s.

staining
- bipolar s.
- corneal s.
- differential s.
- double s.
- fluorescent s.
- intravital s.

staining *(continued)*
- multiple s.
- negative s.
- polar s.
- postvital s.
- preagonal s.
- relief s.
- simple s.
- substantive s.
- supravital s.
- telomeric s.
- terminal s.
- triple s.
- vital s.

stainless steel suture

staircase phenomenon

stalk
- allantoic s.
- body s.
- cerebellar s.
- connecting s.
- s. of the epiglottis
- hypophysial (hypophyseal) s.
- infundibular s.
- neural s.
- optic s.
- pineal s.
- pituitary s.
- s. pouch
- s's of thalamus
- yolk s.

Stallard operation

staltic

STA-MCA—superficial temporal artery to middle cerebral artery

Stamey
- procedure
- test

stamina

Stamm
- gastrostomy
- method
- operation

stammer

stammering

stanch

standard
- Aub-Dubois s's
- Dubois s.
- Harris and Benedict s.
- international biological s.
- nylic s.
- Pignet's s.
- radioactive s.
- reference s.

standardization
    biologic s.
    direct s.
    indirect s.
    physiologic s.
standardize
standby
standing
standstill
    atrial s.
    auricular s.
    cardiac s.
    respiratory s.
    sinus s.
    ventricular s.
Stanford bioptome
Stanford-Binet test
Stanley bacillus
Stanmore shoulder arthroplasty
stannic
    s. chloride
    s. oxide
stanniferous
Stannius ligature
stannosis
stannous
    s. chloride
    s. fluoride
    s. pyrophosphate
    s. sulfur colloid
stannum (Sn)
Stanton disease
stapedectomy
    Guilford s.
    Hough s.
    House s.
    partial s.
    piston s.
    Schuknecht s.
    Shea s.
stapedial tenotomy
stapediolysis
stapedioplasty
stapediotenotomy
stapediovestibular
stapedotomy
stapes mobilization operation
staph—staphylococcus
staphisagria
staphisagrine
staphyline
staphylitis
staphylococcal
    s. endocarditis
    s. impetigo

staphylococcal *(continued)*
    s. mastitis
    s. parotitis
    s. pneumonia
    s. protein A
    s. scalded skin syndrome
      (SSSS)
    s. toxin
staphylococcemia
staphylococci (plural of
  staphylococcus)
staphylococcic
staphylococcin
staphylococcolysin
staphylococcosis
Staphylococcus
    S. aureus
    S. epidermidis
    S. haemolyticus
    S. hominis
    S. hyicus
    S. saprophyticus
    S. simulans
    S. viridans
staphyloderma
staphylokinase
staphylolysin
    α s., alpha s.
    β s., beta s.
    δ s., delta s.
    ϵ s., epsilon s.
    γ s., gamma s.
staphyloma
    annular s.
    anterior s.
    ciliary s.
    s. corneae
    s. corneae racemosum
    corneal s.
    equatorial s.
    intercalary s.
    posterior s.
    s. posticum
    projecting s.
    retinal s.
    Scarpa s.
    scleral s.
    uveal s.
staphylomatous
staphyloptosis
staphylorrhaphy
staphyloschisis
staphylotome
staphylotomy
staphylotoxin

S

Staple bronchoscope
stapler
 Blount s.
 TA-55 s.
staple suture
stapling
 gastric s.
star
 daughter s.
 dental s.
 lens s's
 mother s.
 polar s's
 s's of Verheyen
 Winslow s's
starch
 cassava s.
 corn s.
 pregelatinized s.
 soluble s.
stare
 postbasic s.
Stargardt
 disease
 syndrome
Stark line
Starling
 equation
 forces
 hypothesis
 law
 mechanism
Starr-Edwards
 pacemaker
 prosthesis
 valve
starry-sky pattern
starter
star test pattern
starvation
 salt s.
starve
stasis
 ileal s.
 intestinal s.
 papillary s.
 pressure s.
 s. syndrome
 urinary s.
 venous s.
stat., STAT—immediately
 (L. statim)
state
 absent s.
 acute confusional s.

state (continued)
 alcoholic paranoid s.
 alpha s.
 altered s's of
  consciousness
 anelectrotonic s.
 aneuploid s.
 anxiety s.
 anxiety tension s.
 borderline s.
 carrier s.
 central excitatory s.
 central inhibitory s.
 compulsive s.
 convulsive s.
 D s.
 delta s.
 dreamy s.
 epileptic s.
 epileptic clouded s.
 epileptic twilight s.
 excited s.
 Ganser s.
 ground s.
 haploid s.
 hypnagogic s.
 lacunar s.
 local excitatory s.
 metastable s.
 obsessive-ruminative s.
 persistent vegetative s.
 plastic s.
 pluripotent s.
 postepileptic s.
 refractory s.
 resting s.
 singlet s.
 split-brain s.
 steady s.
 subscurvy s.
 triplet s.
 twilight s.
 vegetative s.
State operation
statement
 antemortem s.
 uncertainty s.
static
statics
statim
station
 anterior s.
 s. of fetus
 olfactory s. of
  Broca

station *(continued)*
    posterior s.
    Romberg s.
stationary
statistic
    kappa s.
statistics
    bayesian s.
    Bose-Einstein s.
    distribution-free s.
    Fermi-Dirac s.
    health s.
    medical s.
    nonparametric s.
    vital s.
statoacoustic
statoconium (statoconia)
statokinetic
statokinetics
statural
stature
status
    absence s.
    s. asthmaticus
    s. calcifames
    s. choreicus
    s. convulsivus
    s. cribalis
    s. cribrosus
    s. criticus
    s. dysmyelinatus
    s. dysmyelinisatus
    s. dysraphicus
    s. epilepticus
    focal s.
    s. hemicranicus
    Karnofsky s.
    s. lacunaris
    s. lacunosus
    s. lymphaticus
    s. marmoratus
    mental s.
    myoclonic s.
    nutritional s.
    petit mal s.
    s. praesens
    psychomotor s.
    s. thymicolymphaticus
    s. thymicus
    s. verrucosus
    s. vertiginosus
Staub-Traugott
    effect
    test
Staude forceps

Staude-Moore forceps
Staunig position
staurion
stauroplegia
staurospore
staxis
stay
    s. suture
    s. of white line
STC—soft tissue calcification
STD—
    sexually transmitted
      disease
    skin test dose
    skin-to-tumor distance
    standard test dose
STE—subperiosteal tissue
  expander
steal
    extracranial s.
    intracerebral s.
    subclavian s.
    s. syndrome
    vascular s.
stearaldehyde
stearate
stearic acid
steariform
stearin
stearoptene
stearoyl-CoA desaturase
steatadenoma
steatite
steatitis
steatocele
steatocystoma multiplex
steatogenous
steatolysis
steatolytic
steatoma
steatomatosis
steatomatous
steatonecrosis
steatopygia
steatopygous
steatorrhea
    congenital pancreatic s.
    familial s.
    idiopathic s.
steatosis
    s. cardiaca
    s. cordis
    macrovesicular s.
    microvesicular s.
Stecher position

S

steel
   s. mesh suture
   stainless s. suture
Steele
   dilator
   murmur
Steele-Richardson-Olszewski
   disease
   syndrome
Steell murmur
Steenbock unit (of vitamin D)
steeple sign
Steffanoff ear reconstruction
stegnosis
stegnotic
Stein
   operation
   test
Stein-Abbe lip flap
Steinbrinck anomaly
Steindler operation
Steiner disease
Steinert
   disease
   myotonic dystrophy
   syndrome
Stein-Kazanjian lower lip flap
Stein-Leventhal syndrome
Steinmann
   extension
   forceps
   pin
steinstrasse
stella (stellae)
   s. lentis hyaloidea
   s. lentis iridica
stellate incision
stellectomy
stellula (stellulae)
   stellulae vasculosae winslowii
   stellulae of Verheyen
   stellulae verheyenii
Stellwag
   brawny edema
   sign
   symptom
stem
   brain s.
   infundibular s.
Stender dishes
Stenger test
stenion
stenobregmatic
stenocephalous
stenocephaly

stenochoria
stenocoriasis
stenocrotaphia
stenopeic iridectomy
stenose
stenosed
stenosing tenosynovitis
stenosis (stenoses)
   adult pyloric s.
   anorectal s.
   antral s.
   aortic s. (AS)
   aortic valve s.
   aqueduct s., aqueductal s.
   arterial s.
   bronchial s.
   buttonhole mitral s.
   calcified aortic s.
   caroticovertebral s.
   carotid s.
   choanal s.
   cicatricial s.
   congenital aortic s.
   congenital hypertrophic
     pyloric s.
   coronary s.
   coronary ostial s.
   critical s.
   cystic duct s.
   Dittrich s.
   esophageal s.
   fishmouth mitral s.
   granulation s.
   hypertrophic s.
   hypertrophic pyloric s.
   idiopathic hypertrophic
     subaortic s. (IHSS)
   infundibular s.
   infundibular pulmonary s.
   laryngeal s.
   lumbar canal s.
   meatal s.
   mitral s.
   muscular subaortic s.
   muscular subvalvular s.
   myocardial infundibular s.
   nasal s.
   papillary s.
   postdiphtheritic s.
   posterior s. of urethra
   postischemic s.
   post-tracheostomy s.
   preventricular s.
   pulmonary s. (PS)
   pulmonary artery s.

stenosis (stenoses) *(continued)*
    pulmonary valve s.
    pulmonic s.
    pyloric s.
    renal artery s.
    spinal s.
    subaortic s.
    subvalvular aortic s.
    supravalvular s.
    supravalvular
      aortic s.
    tracheal s.
    tricuspid s. (TS)
    valvular s.
    valvular pulmonic s.
    vertebral s.
stenostomia
stenothermic
stenothorax
stenotic
stenoxenous
Stensen
    canal
    duct
    experiment
    foramen
    plexus
Stenstrom foot flap
stent
    Carpentier s.
    double-J silicone s.
    foam rubber
      vaginal s.
    Gibbon ureteral s.
    pigtail s.
Stent [eponym]
    compound
    dressing
    mass
Stenvers
    position
    projection
    view
step
    Krönig (Kroenig) s's
    s. osteotomy
    rate-controlling s.
    rate-determining s.
    rate-limiting s.
stepping
    air s.
steradian (sr)
stercobilin
stercobilinogen
stercolith

stercoraceous
    s. abscess
    s. ulcer
    s. vomiting
stercoral
    s. appendicitis
    s. fistula
    s. tumor
stercoraria
stercorarian
stercoroma
stercorous
sterculia gum
stereoagnosis
stereoanesthesia
stereoarthrolysis
stereoauscultation
stereoblastula
stereocampimeter
stereochemical
stereochemistry
stereocilium (stereocilia)
stereocinefluorograph
stereocinefluorography
stereocolpogram
stereocolposcope
stereoencephalotome
stereoencephalotomy
stereofluoroscopy
stereognosis
stereognostic
stereogram
stereograph
stereography
stereoisomer
stereoisomeric
stereoisomerism
stereology
stereometer
stereometry
stereomonoscope
stereo-ophthalmoscope
stereo-orthopter
stereophantoscope
stereophorometer
stereophoroscope
stereophotomicrograph
stereoplasm
stereopsis
stereoradiogram
stereoradiograph
stereoradiography
stereoradiometry
stereoroentgenography
stereosalpingography

S

stereoscope
stereoscopic
    s. microscope
    s. radiography
    s. zonography
stereoscopy
stereoskiagraphy
stereospecific
stereospecificity
stereostroboscope
stereotactic
stereotaxic
stereotaxis
stereotaxy
stereotropic
stereotropism
stereotypy
Stereum
steric
sterilant
sterile, sterilely
sterilely
sterility
    absolute s.
    aspermatogenic s.
    dyspermatogenic s.
    female s.
    male s.
    normospermatogenic s.
    one-child s.
    partial s.
    primary s.
    relative s.
    secondary s.
    two-child s.
sterilization
    eugenic s.
    fractional s.
    intermittent s.
    tubal s.
sterilize
sterilizer
    steam s.
Sterisil
Steri-Strip
sternad
sternal-splitting incision
sternalgia
sternalis
Sternberg
    disease
    giant cells
    sign
Sternberg-Reed cells
sternebra

Stern needle
sternen
Stern-McCarthy
    electrotome
    resectoscope
sternoclavicular
sternoclavicularis
sternocleidal
sternocleidomastoid
sternocoracoid
sternocostal
sternocostalis
sternodymia
sternodymus
sternodynia
sternogoniometer
sternohyoid
sternohyoideus azygos
sternoid
sternomastoid
sterno-omphalopagus
sternopagia
sternopagus
sternopericardial
sternoscapular
sternoschisis
sternothyreoideus
sternothyroid
sternotomy
    median s.
sternotracheal
sternotrypesis
sternovertebral
sternoxiphoid
sternoxiphopagus
Stern position
sternum
    s. bifidum
    cleft s.
sternutation
sternutator
sternutatory
sternzellen
steroid
    s. 5α-reductase [5-alpha-]
    s. 11β-monooxygenase
    [11-beta-]
    s. 17α-monooxygenase
    [11-alpha-]
    s. 21-monooxygenase
    anabolic s.
    adrenal cortical s.,
    adrenocortical s.
    s. diabetes
    s. glaucoma

steroid *(continued)*
    gonadal s.
    s. hormones
    s. monooxygenase
    s. myopathy
    ovarian s.
    s. purpura
    s. receptor
    s. rosacea
    sex s.
    s. sulfatase
steroidogenesis
steroidogenic
sterol
stertor
    hen-cluck s.
stertorous
steryl sulfatase
stethalgia
stethogoniometer
stethograph
stethography
stethokyrtograph
stethomyositis
stethoparalysis
stethophone
stethopolyscope
stethoscope
    binaural s.
    Cammann s.
    DeLee-Hillis s.
    differential s.
    electronic s.
    esophageal s.
    Leff s.
stethoscopic
stethoscopy
stethospasm
Stevens
    forceps
    hook
    scissors
Stevens-Johnson
    disease
    syndrome
Stevenson
    clamp
    forceps
    retractor
    scissors
Stewart
    hook
    incision
Stewart-Holmes sign
Stewart-Morel syndrome

Stewart-Treves syndrome
STH—somatotropic hormone
sthenia
sthenic
sthenometer
sthenometry
stibamine glucoside
stibenyl
stibialism
stibiated
stibine
stibinic acids
stibium
stibocaptate
stibophen
stichochrome
stick
    sponge s.
    s. tie
    s.-tie suture
Sticker disease
Stieda
    disease
    fracture
    process
Stierlin
    sign
    symptom
Stifel figure
stiffness
    congenital spasmodic limb s.
    neck s.
stifle
stigma (stigmas, stigmata)
    s. of degeneracy
    follicular s.
    Giuffrida-Ruggieri s.
    Koplik s. of degeneration
    malpighian s's
    professional s's
    syphilitic s's
stigmasterol
stigmata (plural of stigma)
stigmatic
stigmatism
stigmatization
stigmatometer
stigmatophilia
stilalgin
stilbazium iodide
Stiles-Crawford effect
Still
    disease
    murmur
stillbirth

S

stillborn
Still-Chauffard syndrome
Stille
    clamp
    drill
    forceps
    osteotome
Stille-Gigli saw
Stille-Liston forceps
Stille-Luer
    forceps
    rongeur
Stiller rib
stillicidium
    s. narium
    s. urinae
Stilling
    canal
    column
    fibers
    fleece
    nucleus
    syndrome
stillingia
Stilling-Türk-Duane syndrome
Stilphostrol
Stim-U-Dents
stimulant
    alcoholic s.
    central s.
    cerebral s.
    diffusible s.
    general s.
    local s.
    nervous s.
    respiratory s.
    spinal s.
    topical s.
    uterine s.
    vascular s.
    vasomotor s.
stimulate
stimulation
    areal s.
    audio-visual-tactile s.
    biocular s.
    cerebellar s.
    direct s.
    faradic s.
    indirect s.
    intermittent photic s.
    magnetic s.
    nonspecific s.
    paradoxical s.
    paraspecific s.

stimulation *(continued)*
    photic s.
    punctual s.
    transcutaneous electrical
      nerve s. (TENS)
    vagus s.
stimulator
    Bimler s.
    cerebellar s.
    dorsal column s.
    electronic s.
    human thyroid adenylate
      cyclase s's (HTACS)
    interdental s.
    long-acting thyroid s.
      (LATS)
    nerve s.
stimulus (stimuli)
    adequate s.
    aversive s.
    chemical s.
    conditioned s. (CS)
    conditioning s.
    discriminative s.
    electric s.
    eliciting s.
    heterologous s.
    heterotopic s.
    homologous s.
    inadequate s.
    latent s.
    manifest s.
    maximal s.
    mechanical s.
    minimal s.
    morphogenetic s.
    nomotopic s.
    reinforcing s.
    square-wave s.
    subthreshold s.
    supraliminal s.
    supramaximal s.
    thermal s.
    threshold s.
    unconditioned s.
stimulus-response (S-R)
sting
    Irukandji s.
stinger
stippling
    basophilic s.
    basophilic s. of erythrocytes
    epiphyseal s.
    gingival s.
    malarial s.

stirrup
    Finochietto s.
    swivel s.
stitch
    glover s.
STK—streptokinase
STM—streptomycin
stochastic
Stock operation
Stocker needle
Stockholm box
stockinet, stockinette
    s. dressing
stocking
    compression s's
    Jobst s's
    T.E.D. s's
    thromboembolic disease
        (TED) s's
Stockman clamp
Stock-Spielmeyer-Vogt syndrome
Stoerk blennorrhea
stoichiology
stoichiometric
stoichiometry
stoke
Stokes
    amputation
    collar
    expectorant
    law
    lens
    operation
    sign
    syndrome
Stokes-Adams
    attack
    disease
    syndrome
Stokvis
    disease
    test
Stokvis-Talma syndrome
Stoll pneumonia
stoma
    Turnbull loop s.
stomach
    bilocular s.
    cardiac s.
    cascade s.
    cup-and-spill s.
    dumping s.
    hourglass s.
    leather bottle s.
    thoracic s.

stomach *(continued)*
    s. tube
    upside-down s.
    waterfall s.
    watermelon s.
stomachache
stomachal
stomachalgia
stomachic
stomachics
stomachodynia
stomal
stomata
stomatal
stomatalgia
stomatic
stomatitis (stomatitides)
    acute necrotizing s.
    allergic s.
    angular s.
    aphthobullous s.
    s. aphthosa
    aphthous s.
    s. arsenicalis
    bismuth s.
    catarrhal s.
    contact s.
    denture s.
    epidemic s.
    epizootic s.
    erythematopultaceous s.
    s. exanthematica
    fusospirochetal s.
    gangrenous s.
    gonococcal s.
    gonorrheal s.
    herpetic s.
    infectious s.
    s. intertropica
    lead s.
    s. medicamentosa
    membranous s.
    mercurial s.
    mycotic s.
    necrotizing ulcerative s.
    s. nicotina
    nonspecific s.
    recurrent aphthous s.
    s. scarlatina
    s. scorbutica
    syphilitic s.
    traumatic s.
    tropical s.
    ulcerative s.
    uremic s.

S

stomatitis (stomatitides) *(continued)*
    s. venenata
    vesicular s.
    Vincent s.
stomatocace
stomatocyte
stomatocytosis
stomatodynia
stomatodysodia
stomatogenesis
stomatoglossitis
stomatognathic
stomatography
stomatolalia
stomatological
stomatologist
stomatology
stomatomalacia
stomatomenia
stomatomy
stomatomycosis
stomatonecrosis
stomatonoma
stomatopathy
stomatoplastic
stomatoplasty
stomatorrhagia gingivarum
stomatoschisis
stomatoscope
stomatotyphus
stomion
stomocephalus
stomodeal
stomodeum
stomoschisis
stone
    artificial s.
    bladder s.
    blue s.
    chalk s.
    cystine s.
    dental s.
    diamond s.
    s. forceps
    kidney s.
    lathe s.
    lung s.
    metabolic s.
    pulp s.
    salivary s.
    s. searcher
    skin s's
    staghorn s.
    struvite s.

stone *(continued)*
    tear s.
    urate s.
    ureteral s.
    vein s.
    wheel s.
    womb s.
Stone [eponym]
    bunionectomy
    clamp
    forceps
stone dislodger
    Councill s.d.
    Davis s.d.
    Dormia s.d.
    Johnson s.d.
    Levant s.d.
    Robinson s.d.
    woven loop s.d.
Stone-Holcombe clamp
Stones implant
Stookey reflex
Stookey-Scarff
    operation
    shunt
stool
    acholic s.
    bilious s.
    caddy s.
    s. culture
    currant jelly s.
    fatty s.
    s. guaiac
    lienteric s.
    mucous s.
    pea soup s.
    pipe-stem s.
    rabbit s's
    ribbon s's
    rice-water s's
    sago-grain s.
    silver s.
    spinach s.
stop
    centric s.
    s. eye speculum
    glottal s.
    occlusal s.
    short s.
storax
storiform
storm
    thyroid s.
    thyrotoxic s.

Storm van Leeuwen chamber
Storz
    bronchoscope
    cystoscope
    hysteroscope
    magnet
Storz-Beck snare
STP—
    scientifically treated
        petroleum
    standard temperature and
        pressure
strabismic
strabismology
strabismometer
strabismometry
strabismus
    A s.
    absolute s.
    accommodative s.
    alternating s.
    bilateral s.
    binocular s.
    Braid s.
    comitant s.
    concomitant s.
    constant s.
    convergent s.
    cyclic s.
    s. deorsum vergens
    divergent s.
    dynamic s.
    external s.
    s. fixus
    incomitant s.
    intermittent s.
    internal s.
    kinetic s.
    latent s.
    manifest s.
    mechanical s.
    monocular s.
    monolateral s.
    muscular s.
    noncomitant s.
    nonconcomitant s.
    nonparalytic s.
    paralytic s.
    relative s.
    seesaw s.
    spasmodic s.
    suppressed s.
    s. sursum vergens
    unilateral s.

strabismus *(continued)*
    uniocular s.
    V s.
    vertical s.
strabometer
strabometry
strabotome
strabotomy
Strachan
    disease
    syndrome
Strachan-Scott syndrome
straggling
strahlen
straight tenaculum
strain
    cell s.
    heterologous s.
    homologous s.
    left ventricular s.
    s. pattern
    reference s.
    resistant s.
    right ventricular s.
    S s.
    T-s.
    vertebral cervical s.
    Vi s.
    wild-type s.
strainer
strain-gauge plethysmography
strait
    inferior pelvic s.
    pelvic s., inferior
    pelvic s., superior
    superior pelvic s.
Straith operation
straitjacket
stramonium
strand
    Billroth s's
    lateral enamel s.
    plus s.
strangalesthesia
strangle
strangles
strangulated
strangulation of bladder
stranguria
strangury
strap
    crib s.
    Montgomery s.
strapping

S

Strap procedure
Strasburger cell plate
Strassman
    forceps
    metroplasty
    phenomenon
    technique
    transverse fundal incision
    uterine forceps
Strassman-Jones operation
strata (plural of stratum)
stratification
stratified
stratiform
stratigram
stratigraphy
Stratte needle holder
stratum (strata)
    s. adamantinum
    s. basale endometrii
    s. basale epidermidis
    s. cinereum
    s. circulare gastris
    s. circulare membranae
      tympani
    s. circulare tunicae muscularis
      coli
    strata colliculi rostralis
    strata colliculi superioris
    s. compactum
    s. compactum endometrii
    s. corneum
    s. cutaneum membranae
      tympani
    s. eboris
    s. externum tunicae
      muscularis ductus deferentis
    s. externum tunicae
      muscularis ureteris
    s. externum tunicae
      muscularis vesicae
      urinariae
    s. fibrosum capsulae
      articularis
    s. fibrosum vaginae tendinis
    s. functionale
    s. functionale endometrii
    s. germinativum
    s. granulosum cerebelli
    s. granulosum epidermidis
    strata grisea et alba colliculi
      rostralis
    s. intermedium
    s. lacunosum

stratum (strata) *(continued)*
    s. lemnisci
    s. limitans externum
    s. limitans internum
    s. longitudinale gastris
    s. longitudinale tunicae
      muscularis coli
    s. longitudinale tunicae
      muscularis intestini tenuis
    s. lucidum epidermidis
    s. lucidum hippocampi
    s. malpighii
    s. medium tunicae muscularis
      ductus deferentis
    s. medium tunicae muscularis
      ureteris
    s. medium tunicae muscularis
      vesicae urinariae
    s. moleculare cerebelli
    s. moleculare hippocampi
    s. mucosum membranae
      tympani
    s. nervosum retinae
    s. neuronorum piriformium
    s. nucleare externum
    s. nucleare internum
    s. oriens hippocampi
    s. papillare dermidis
    s. pigmentosum retinae
    s. plexiforme cerebelli
    s. plexiforme externum
    s. pyramidale hippocampi
    s. reticulare corii
    s. reticulare dermidis
    s. spinosum
    s. spongiosum
    s. spongiosum endometrii
    s. submucosum
    s. subserosum
    s. subvasculare
    s. supravasculare
    s. synoviale capsulae
      articularis
    s. synoviale vaginae
      tendinis
    s. vasculare
    s. zonale thalami
Straus
    phenomenon
    reaction
    test
Strauss
    proctoscope
    sign

strawberry
    s. cervix
    s. mark
streak
    angioid s's
    fatty s.
    germinal s.
    Knapp s's
    medullary s.
    meningeal s.
    meningitic s.
    primitive s.
    s. retinoscope
streaking
stream
    axial s.
    blood s.
    s. of consciousness
    electron s.
    hair s's
streaming
    cytoplasmic s.
    protoplasmic s.
Street pin
strength
    biting s.
    dioptric s.
    ego s.
    ionic s.
strep—
    streptococcal
    streptococci
strepitus
strepogenin
streptamine
streptidine
streptoangina
streptobacilli
Streptobacillus
  moniliformis
streptobiosamine
streptocerciasis
streptococcal
streptococcemia
streptococci
streptococcicide
streptococcolysin
streptococcosis
streptococcus (streptococci)
    beta-hemolytic streptococci
    group A (B, C, etc.)
      streptococci
    hemolytic s.
    indifferent s.

streptococcus (streptococci)
  (continued)
    nonhemolytic s.
    viridans s.
Streptococcus
    S. acidominimus
    S. agalactiae
    S. anginosus
    S. bovis
    S. constellatus
    S. dysgalactiae subsp.
      equisimilis
    S. equinus
    S. intermedius
    S. lactis
    S. mitis
    S. mutans
    S. pneumoniae
    S. pyogenes
    S. salivarius
    S. sanguinis
    S. uberis
streptodermatitis
streptodornase
    streptokinase-s.
streptoduocin
streptogenin
streptohemolysin-streptodornase
  (SKSD)
streptokinase (SK)-streptodornase
  (SKSD)
streptoleukocidin
streptolydigin
streptolysin
    s. O
    s. S
    S. noursei
    S. orchidaceus
    S. orientalis
streptomicrodactyly
Streptomyces somaliensis
streptomycete
streptomycosis
streptonigrin
streptonivicin
streptose
streptosepticemia
streptozocin
streptozotocin
streptozyme test
stress
    s. film
    s. incontinence
    occlusal s.

stress *(continued)*
    post-traumatic s.
    s. test
    s. thallium-201
stress-breaker
stress-strain curve
stretcher
stretching
    pulse s.
stria (striae)
    acoustic striae
    striae albicantes
    striae of Amici
    striae atrophicae
    auditory striae
    striae ciliares
    s. diagonalis (Broca)
    striae distensae
    s. of Gennari
    Kaes s.
    Knapp striae
    s. of Lanci
    Langhans s.
    longitudinal s. of corpus
      callosum, lateral
    s. longitudinalis lateralis
      corporis callosi
    s. longitudinalis medialis
      corporis callosi
    s. mallearis membranae
      tympani
    s. malleolaris membranae
      tympani
    s. medullaris thalami
    medullary s. of corpus
      striatum, medial
    medullary striae of fourth
      ventricle
    medullary striae of rhomboid
      fossa
    medullary s. of thalamus
    meningitic s.
    Nitabuch s.
    striae olfactoriae
    olfactory striae
    olfactory s., intermediate
    Retzius parallel striae
    Rohr s.
    Schreger striae
    s. terminalis
    s. vascularis ductus cochlearis
    Wickham striae
striascope
striatal
striated

striation
    Baillarger s's
    basal s's
    s's of Frommann
    tabby cat s.
    tigroid s.
striatonigral
striatopallidal
striatum
stricture
    anal s.
    annular s.
    bridle s.
    cicatricial s.
    contractile s.
    esophageal s.
    false s.
    functional s.
    Hunner s.
    hysterical s.
    impassable s.
    impermeable s.
    irritable s.
    linear s.
    organic s.
    permanent s.
    rectal s.
    recurrent s.
    ring s.
    spasmodic s.
    spastic s.
    string s.
    temporary s.
stricturization
stricturotome
stricturotomy
strident
stridor
    congenital laryngeal s.
    expiratory s.
    inspiratory s.
    laryngeal s.
    s. serraticus
stridulous
string
    s. operation
    s. sign
string-halt sign
striocellular
striocerebellar
striomotor
striomuscular
strionigral
strip
    abrasive s.

strip *(continued)*
    amalgam s.
    lightning s.
    linen s.
    moving s.
    polishing s.
    separating s.
stripe
    s's of Baillarger
    endometrial s. (on sonogram of uterus)
    s. of Gennari
    s. of Kaes-Bekhterev
    Mees s's
    s's of Retzius
stripper
    Carroll forearm tendon s.
    Emerson s.
    external s.
    internal s.
    intraluminal s.
    Keeley s.
    Kurten s.
    Mayo s.
    Meyer s.
    Nabatoff s.
    Shaw s.
    thrombus s.
    vein s.
    Webb s.
    Wilson s.
    Wylie s.
stripping
    s. of membranes
    s. of pleura
strobila (strobilae)
strobilation
strobilocercus
strobiloid
strobilus
stroboscope
stroboscopic
    s. disk
    s. microscope
strobostereoscope
Stroganoff (Stroganov) treatment
stroke
    apoplectic s.
    atherothrombotic s.
    back s.
    cardioembolic s.
    cerebral s.
    completed s.
    developing s.
    embolic s.

stroke *(continued)*
    s. in evolution
    exertional heat s.
    heat s.
    heat s., exertional
    ischemic s.
    lacunar s.
    light s.
    lightning s.
    middle cerebral artery s.
    paralytic s.
    progressive s.
    sun s., sunstroke
    thrombotic s.
stroke-in-evolution
stroma (stromata)
    s. of cornea
    erythrocyte s.
    s. ganglii
    s. glandulae thyroideae
    s. iridis
    s. of iris
    lymphatic s.
    ovarian s.
    s. ovarii
    s. of ovary
    Rollet s.
    s. of thyroid gland
    vitreous s.
    s. vitreum
stromal
stromatin
stromatogenous
stromatolysis
stromatosis
    endometrial s.
Strömbeck
    incision
    mammaplasty
    operation
Stromeyer cephalhematocele
stromuhr
strongyle
strongyli
strongylid
strongyliform
Strongyloides
    S. intestinalis
    S. stercoralis
strongyloidiasis
strongylosis
strontium (Sr)
    s. chloride Sr 89
    radioactive s.
    s. Sr 85 nitrate

S

strontium (Sr) *(continued)*
  s. Sr 87m
  s. Sr 90
  s. with yttrium 90
strontiuresis
strontiuretic
strophanthidin
strophanthin
  G-s.
  s.-G
strophocephalus
strophocephaly
strophosomia
strophosomus
strophulus albidus
struck
structural
structure
  antigenic s.
  β s.
  covalent s.
  denture-supporting s's
  fine s.
  primary s.
  quaternary s.
  secondary s.
  tertiary s.
Strümpel (Struempel)
  ear alligator forceps
  ear punch forceps
  rongeur
struggle
  death s.
Strully scissors
struma
  s. aberrata
  cast iron s.
  s. colloides
  s. endothoracica
  s. fibrosa
  s. follicularis
  s. gelatinosa
  Hashimoto s.
  ligneous s.
  s. lingualis
  s. lymphomatosa
  s. nodosa
  s. ovarii
  s. parenchymatosa
  Riedel s.
  s. vasculosa
strumectomy
  median s.
strumiform
strumitis

strumous
Strümpell
  disease
  reflex
  sign
  type
Strümpell-Leichtenstern
  disease
  encephalitis
  hemorrhagic encephalitis
Strümpell-Marie disease
Strümpell-Westphal
  pseudosclerosis
Strunsky sign
Struthers ligament
struvite
Struyken forceps
strychnine
strychninism
strychninization
strychninomania
Stryker
  dermatome
  drill
  frame
  saw
STS—
  serologic test for syphilis
  Society of Thoracic Surgeons
ST-segment [adj.]
  ST-s. alternans
  ST-s. changes
  ST-s. elevation
STSG—split-thickness skin graft
STT—serial thrombin time
STU—skin test unit
Stuart-Bras
  disease
  syndrome
Stuart-Prower factor deficiency
  disease
Stubbs curet
study
  air s.
  air contrast s.
  barium meal s.
  blood flow s.
  case-control s.
  cine s.
  cohort s.
  cross-sectional s.
  cytogenetic s.
  cytological s.
  descriptive s.
  double-blind s.

study *(continued)*
    double-contrast s.
    dual-contrast s.
    enzyme s.
    experimental s.
    fat absorption s.
    gastrointestinal s.
    horizontal beam s.
    H reflex s.
    intervention s.
    iodized oil s.
    longitudinal s.
    lumbar, flexion, and extension s.
    motility s.
    opacification s.
    perfusion s.
    perirenal air s.
    phonation s.
    prospective s.
    quantitative regional lung
      function s.
    retrococcygeal air s.
    retroperitoneal air s.
    retrospective s.
    single-contrast s.
    spot film s.
    technetium albumin s.
      (TECA s.)
    tracer s.
    ventilation s.
    videotape s.
    washout s.
Stühmer (Stuehmer) disease
stump
    conical s.
    invaginated s.
    ischial-bearing s.
    tracheal s.
stun
stunt
stupefacient
stupefactive
stupor
    anergic s.
    benign s.
    Cairns s.
    catatonic s.
    delusion s.
    depressive s.
    epileptic s.
    Kahlbaum catatonic s.
    lethargic s.
    melancholic s.
    postconvulsive s.
    spike-wave s.

stuporous
sturdy
Sturge
    disease
    syndrome
Sturge-Kalischer-Weber syndrome
Sturge-Weber
    disease
    encephalotrigeminal
      angiomatosis
    syndrome
Sturge-Weber-Dimitri disease
Sturm
    conoid
    interval
Sturmdorf
    operation
    suture
stutter
stuttering
    labiochoreic s.
    urinary s.
stycosis
stye
    meibomian s.
    zeisian s.
stylet
    endotracheal s.
    lacrimal s.
styliform
styliscus
styloglossal
styloglossus
stylohyal
stylohyoid
styloid
styloiditis
stylomandibular
stylomastoid
stylomaxillary
stylomyloid
stylopodium
stylostaphyline
stylosteophyte
stylostixis
stylus
stymatosis
stypage
stype
stypsis
styptic
    Binelli s.
    chemical s.
    mechanical s.
    vascular s.

S

styptics
styramate
styrene
Styrofoam dressing
SU—sensation unit
SUA—serum uric acid
subabdominal
subabdominoperitoneal
subacetabular
subacetate
subacid
subacidity
subacromial
subacute
subalimentation
subanal
subanconeus
subaortic
subapical
subaponeurotic
subarachnoid
    s. anesthesia
    s. block
    s. cavity
    s. cisterns
    s. hemorrhage
    s. space
    spinal s. block
subarachnoiditis
    acute curable juvenile s.
subarcuate
subareolar
subastragalar
subastringent
subatloidean
subatomic
subaural
subaurale
subauricular
subaxial
subaxillary
subbasal
subbrachial
subbrachycephalic
subcalcareous
subcalcarine
subcallosal
subcapsular splenectomy
subcapsuloperiosteal
subcarbonate
subcartilaginous
subcentral
subception
subcerebellar
subcerebral

subchloride
subchondral
subchordal
subchorionic
subchoroidal
subchronic
subclass
subclavian
    s. artery
    s. catheter
subclavicular
subclinical
subclone
subcollateral
subconjunctival
subconscious
subconsciousness
subcoracoid
subcortex
subcortical
subcostal
    s. angle
    s. artery
    s. groove
    s. incision
    s. line
    s. muscles
    s. nerve
    s. plane
    s. vein
subcostalis (subcostales)
subcranial
subcrepitant
subcrepitation
subcu, subq, SQ—subcutaneous
subculture
subcurative
subcutaneous
    s. abscess
    s. acromial bursa
    s. bursa
    s. emphysema
    s. fat
    s. fatty tissue
    s. fracture
    s. infusion
    s. injection
    s. mastectomy
    s. operation
    s. phycomycosis
    s. pseudosarcomatous
      fibromatosis
    s. tissue
    s. wound
    s. zygomycosis

subcuticular
    s. suture
subcutis
subdelirium
subdeltoid
subdental
subdermal
subdiaphragmatic
subdorsal
subduct
subduction
subdural
    s. abscess
    s. cavity
    s. hematoma
    s. hemorrhage
    s. hygroma
    s. space
subendocardial
subendocardium
subendothelial
subendothelium
subendymal
subependymal
subependymoma
subepicardium
subepidermal
subepidermic
subepiglottic
subepithelial plexus
suberitin
suberosis
subextensibility
subfalcial
subfascial
subfecundity
subfertile
subfertility
subfissure
subflavous
subfoliar
subfolium
subfornical
subfrontal
subgaleal
subgallate
subgemmal
subgenus
subgerminal
subgingival curettage
subglenoid
subglossal
subglossitis
subglottic
subgranular

subgrondation
subgyrus
subhepatic
subhumeral
subhyaloid
subhyoid
    s. laryngotomy
    s. pharyngotomy
subhyoidean
subicteric
subicular
subiculum
    s. cornu ammonis
    s. hippocampi
    s. promontorii cavitatis
        tympanicae
    s. promontorii cavi tympani
    s. of promontory of tympanic
        cavity
subiliac
subilium
subinflammation
subinflammatory
subinguinal incision
subintern
subintimal
subintrance
subintrant
subinvolution
    chronic s. of uterus
subjacent
subject
subjective
subjectoscope
subjugal
sublabial antrotomy
sublation
sublatio retinae
sublesional
sublethal
sublimate
    corrosive s.
sublimation
sublime
subliminal
sublimis
subline
sublingual
sublinguitis
sublobe
sublobular
subluxate
subluxation
    atlantoaxial s.
    congenital s. of hip

S

subluxation *(continued)*
   s. of lens
     Volkmann s.
sublymphemia
submammary incision
submandibular
submania
submarginal
submaxilla
submaxillaritis
submaxillary
submedial
submedian
submembranous
submeningeal
submental lipectomy
submersion
submetacentric
submicroscopic, submicroscopical
submorphous
submucosa
submucosal
   s. leiomyoma
   s. resection
submucous
   s. cleft
   s. cleft palate
   s. cystitis
   s. fibroma
   s. layer
   s. layer of bladder
   s. layer of colon
   s. resection (SMR)
   s. resection of nasal septum
   s. resection and rhinoplasty
    (SMRR)
   s. resection of vocal cord
   s. ulcer
subnarcotic
subnasal
subnasale
subnasion
subnatant
subneural
subnitrate
subnormal
subnormality
   mental s.
subnotochordal
subnucleus
subnutrition
suboccipital
suboperculum
suboptic
suboptimal

suborbital
suborder
suboxidation
suboxide
subpapillary
subpapular
subparalytic
subparietal
subpatellar
subpectoral
subpeduncular
subpelviperitoneal
subpericardial
subperiosteal
subperiosteocapsular
subperitoneal
subperitoneoabdominal
subperitoneopelvic
subpetrosal
subpharyngeal
subphrenic
subphylum (subphyla)
subpial
subpituitarism
subplacenta
subplacental
subpleural
subpontine
subpopulation
subpreputial
subpubic
subpulmonary
subpulpal
subpyramidal
subrectal
subretinal
subrostral
subscaphocephaly
subscapular
subscleral
subsclerotic
subscription
subserosa
subserous
subset
subsibilant
subside
subsidence
subsigmoid
subsonic
subspecialty
subspecies
subspinale
subspinous
subsplenial

substage
substance
    α-s., alpha s.
    A s.
    acute phase s.
    adamantine s. of tooth
    agglutinating s.
    anterior perforated s.
    anterior pituitary–like s.
    antidiuretic s.
    anti-immune s.
    arborescent white s. of
      cerebellum
    β-s., beta s.
    B s.
    black s.
    blood group s's
    blood grouping specific s's
    bony s. of tooth
    C s.
    cement s.
    cementing s.
    central gray s.
    central gray s. of cerebrum
    central intermediate s. of
      spinal cord
    chromidial s.
    chromophil s.
    colloid s.
    compact s. of bones
    s. content
    controlled s.
    cortical s. of bone
    cortical s. of kidney
    cortical s. of lens
    cortical s. of lymph nodes
    cortical s. of suprarenal gland
    depressor s.
    exophthalmos-producing s.
    external s. of suprarenal gland
    filar s.
    gelatinous s. of posterior horn
      of spinal cord
    gelatinous s. of spinal cord
    glandular s. of prostate
    gray s.
    gray s. of cerebrum, central
    gray reticular s. of medulla
      oblongata
    gray s. of spinal cord
    ground s.
    H s.
    hyaline s.
    I s.
    interfibrillar s. of Flemming

substance *(continued)*
    interfilar s.
    intermediate gray s. of spinal
      cord, central
    intermediate gray s. of spinal
      cord, lateral
    intermediate s. of spinal cord
    internal s. of suprarenal gland
    interpeduncular perforated s.
    interprismatic s.
    interspongioplastic s.
    interstitial s.
    intertubular s. of tooth
    ivory s. of tooth
    ketogenic s.
    lateral intermediate s. of
      spinal cord
    s. of lens
    medullary s. of bone
    medullary s. of bone, red
    medullary s. of bone, yellow
    medullary s. of kidney
    medullary s. of suprarenal
      gland
    metachromatic s.
    molecular s.
    müllerian-inhibiting s.
    muscular s. of prostate
    neurosecretory s.
    s. of Nissl
    no-threshold s's
    onychogenic s.
    organ-forming s's
    s. P
    pellagra-preventing (P-P) s.
    perforated s., anterior
    perforated s., interpeduncular
    perforated s., posterior
    periaqueductal gray s.
    periventricular gray s.
    posterior perforated s.
    prelipid s.
    pressor s.
    proper s. of choroid
    proper s. of cornea
    proper s. of sclera
    proper s. of tooth
    red medullary s. of bone
    red s. of spleen
    reducing s's
    Reichert's s.
    released s.
    reticular s.
    reticular s. of medulla oblongata
    reticular s., white, of Arnold

S

substance *(continued)*
  Rolando gelatinous s.
  Rollett secondary s.
  rostral perforated s.
  sarcous s.
  Schwann white s.
  s. sensibilisatrice
  sensitizing s.
  slow-reacting s. of anaphylaxis (SRS-A)
  specific soluble s. (SSS)
  spongy s. of bone
  threshold s's
  thromboplastic s.
  tigroid s.
  trabecular s. of bone
  transmitter s.
  white s.
  white reticular s.
  white reticular s. of Arnold
  white s. of Schwann
  white s. of spinal cord
  yellow medullary s. of bone
  zymoplastic s.
substantia (substantiae)
  s. adamantina dentis
  s. alba
  s. alba medullae spinalis
  s. cinerea
  s. compacta ossium
  s. corticalis lentis
  s. corticalis ossium
  s. eburnea dentis
  s. ferruginea
  s. gelatinosa centralis
  s. gelatinosa (Rolandi)
  s. glandularis prostatae
  s. gliosa centralis
  s. grisea
  s. grisea centralis
  s. grisea medullae spinalis
  s. innominata
  s. innominata of Reichert
  s. intermedia centralis medullae spinalis
  s. intermedia lateralis medullae spinalis
  s. intertubularis dentis
  s. lentis
  s. muscularis prostatae
  s. nigra
  s. ossea dentis
  s. perforata anterior

substantia (substantiae) *(continued)*
  s. perforata interpeduncularis
  s. perforata posterior
  s. perforata rostralis
  s. propria corneae
  s. propria sclerae
  s. reticularis
  s. reticulofilamentosa
  s. spongiosa ossium
  s. trabecularis ossium
  s. visceralis secundaria medullae spinalis
substernal
substernomastoid
substituent
substitute
  Biobrane synthetic skin s.
  blood s.
  plasma s.
substitution
  creeping s. of bone
  gene s.
substitutive
substrain
substrate
  renin s.
substratum
substructure
  implant s.
subsulcus
subsulfate
subsultus tendinum
subsylvian
subsynaptic
subtalar
subtarsal
subtelocentric
subtemporal
subtenial
subtentorial
subterminal
subtertian
subtetanic
subthalamic
subthalamus
subthreshold
subthyroidism
subtile
subtilin
subtilisin
subtle
subtly
subtotal hysterectomy

subtraction
    s. angiography
    second order s.
    s. venography
subtrapezial
subtribe
subtrigonal
subtrochanteric
    s. incision
    s. osteotomy
subtrochlear
subtuberal
subtympanic
subtypical
subumbilical incision
subungual
subunit
    catalytic s.
    regulatory s.
suburethral
subvaginal
subvertebral
subvesical
subviral
subvitaminosis
subvitrinal
subvolution
subwaking
subzonal
subzygomatic
succagogue
succedaneous
succedaneum
succeed
succenturiate
succession
succi (plural of succus)
succinate
succinate-CoA ligase
succinate
  dehydrogenase
succinic acid
succinic semialdehyde
succinylcholine chloride
succinyl-CoA synthetase
succinylsulfathiazole
succorrhea
succulence
succus (succi)
    s. cerasi
    s. entericus
    s. gastricus
    s. pancreaticus
    s. prostaticus
    s. rubi idaei

succussion
    hippocratic s.
    s. splash
sucker
    Marshall surgical s.
sucking reflex
Sucquet-Hoyer
    anastomosis
    canal
sucralfate
sucrase
sucrate
sucroclastic octaacetate
sucrose
    s. α-D-glucohydrolase
    s. α-D-glucosidase
    s. octaacetate
    s. polyester
sucrosemia
sucrosuria
suction
    s. curettage
    DeLee s.
    s. dilatation and curettage
    (D&C)
    s. drain
    s. lipectomy
    post-tussive s.
    s. tube
    wall s.
    Wangensteen s.
suctioning
    endotracheal-bronchial s.
suction tube
    Adson s.t.
    Andrews-Pynchon s.t.
    Buie rectal s.t.
    Frazier s.t.
    Sachs s.t.
suctorial
SUD—
    sudden unexpected death
    sudden unexplained
    death
sudamen
sudamina
sudaminal
Sudan
    S. I–IV
    S. black B fat stain
    S. G
    S. red
    S. yellow G
sudanophil
sudanophilia

S

sudanophilic
sudanophilous
sudarium
sudation
sudatory
Sudeck
    atrophy
    critical point
    disease
    syndrome
Sudeck-Leriche syndrome
sudogram
sudomotor
sudor
sudoral
sudoresis
sudoriferous
sudorific
sudoriparous
sudorometer
SUDS—sudden unexplained death
   syndrome
suffocant
suffocate
suffocation
suffraginis
suffusion
sugar
    s. alcohol
    amino s.
    anhydrous s.
    barley s.
    beet s.
    blood s.
    burnt s.
    cane s.
    compressible s.
    confectioner's s.
    deoxy s.
    diabetic s.
    fruit s.
    invert s.
    reducing s.
    simple s.
    starch s.
    threshold s.
Sugar clip
sugar-tong splint
suggestibility
suggestible
suggestion
    hypnotic s.
    posthypnotic s.
suggillation
Sugiura procedure

suicidal
    s. ideation
    s. thoughts
suicide
    s. attempt, attempted s.
    immunologic s.
    psychic s.
suicidology
SUID—sudden unexplained infant
   death
suit
    antiblackout s.
    anti-G s.
    antishock s.
    body exhaust s.
    G s.
    pressure s.
    space s.
suite
    operating s.
Suker
    iris forceps
    sign
sulcal
sulcate
sulcation
sulci (plural of sulcus)
sulciform
sulculus (sulculi)
sulcus (sulci)
    alveolabial s.
    alveolingual s.
    alveolobuccal s.
    alveololabial s.
    alveololingual s.
    ampullary s.
    angular s.
    ansate s.
    anterolateral s.
    s. anterolateralis medullae
       oblongatae
    s. anterolateralis medullae
       spinalis
    anterolateral s. of medulla
       oblongata
    anterolateral s. of spinal cord
    s. anthelicis transversus
    aortic s.
    s. aorticus
    s. arteriae occipitalis
    s. arteriae subclaviae
    s. arteriae temporalis mediae
    s. arteriae vertebralis atlantis
    sulci arteriales
    sulci arteriosi

sulcus (sulci) *(continued)*
    atrioventricular s.
    s. of auditory tube
    s. of auricle, posterior
    s. auriculae posterior
    s. of auricular branch of vagus
      nerve
    basilar s. of occipital bone
    basilar s. of pons
    bicipital s.
    s. bicipitalis lateralis
    s. bicipitalis medialis
    s. bicipitalis radialis
    s. bicipitalis ulnaris
    bicipital s., lateral
    bicipital s., medial
    bicipital s., radial
    bicipital s., ulnar
    buccal s.
    bulbopontine s.
    s. bulbopontinus
    bulboventricular s.
    calcaneal s.
    s. calcanei
    calcarine s.
    s. calcarinus
    callosal s.
    callosomarginal s.
    s. canaliculi mastoidei
    s. caroticus ossis sphenoidalis,
      carotid s.
    carpal s.
    s. carpi
    central s. of cerebrum
    central s. of insula
    s. centralis cerebri
    s. centralis insulae
    cerebral s., lateral
    sulci cerebri
    sulci of cerebrum
    chiasmatic s.
    s. chiasmatis
    cingulate s.
    s. cingulatus
    s. cinguli
    s. of cingulum
    circular s. of insula
    collateral s.
    s. collateralis
    s. colli mandibulae
    s. coronarius cordis
    coronary s. of heart
    s. corporis callosi
    s. of corpus callosum
    s. costae

sulcus (sulci) *(continued)*
    costal s.
    costal s., inferior
    s. cruris helicis
    s. of crus of helix
    cuboid s.
    sulci cutis
    dorsolateral s.
    s. dorsolateralis medullae
      oblongatae
    s. dorsolateralis medullae
      spinalis
    dorsolateral s. of medulla
      oblongata
    dorsolateral s. of spinal cord
    s. ethmoidalis ossis nasalis
    ethmoidal s. of nasal bone
    s. of eustachian tube
    fimbriodentate s.
    frontal s., inferior
    s. frontalis inferior
    s. frontalis superior
    frontal s., superior
    s. of sigmoid sinus
    gingival s.
    s. gingivalis
    gingivobuccal s.
    gingivolingual s.
    gluteal s.
    greater palatine s.
    greater palatine s. of maxilla
    greater palatine s. of palatine
      bone
    s. of greater petrosal nerve
    habenular s.
    s. hamuli pterygoidei
    Harrison s.
    hemispheric s.
    s. hippocampalis
    s. hippocampi
    horizontal s. of cerebellum
    hypothalamic s.
    s. hypothalamicus
    s. for inferior petrosal sinus of
      occipital bone
    s. for inferior petrosal sinus of
      temporal bone
    infraorbital s. of maxilla
    infrapalpebral s.
    s. infrapalpebralis
    s. of innominate canal
    interarticular s. of
      calcaneus
    interarticular s. of talus
    interatrial s.

sulcus (sulci) *(continued)*

intermediate s. of spinal cord, dorsal

intermediate s. of spinal cord, posterior

s. intermedius dorsalis medullae spinalis

s. intermedius gastricus

s. intermedius posterior medullae spinalis

internal spiral s.

interparietal s.

intertubercular s. of humerus

interventricular s., anterior

interventricular s. of heart

interventricular s., inferior

s. interventricularis anterior

s. interventricularis inferior

s. interventricularis posterior

interventricular s., posterior

intraparietal s.

s. intraparietalis

Jacobson s.

labiodental s.

s. lacrimalis maxillae

s. lacrimalis ossis lacrimalis

lacrimal s. of lacrimal bone

lacrimal s. of maxilla

lateral s.

lateral bicipital s.

s. lateralis cerebri

s. lateralis mesencephali

s. lateralis pedunculi cerebri

lateral s. for lateral sinus of occipital bone

lateral s. for lateral sinus of parietal bone

lateral s. of medulla oblongata, anterior

lateral s. of medulla oblongata, posterior

lateral occipital s.

lateral s. for sigmoidal part of lateral sinus

lateral s. of spinal cord, anterior

lateral s. of spinal cord, posterior

s. of lesser petrosal nerve

s. limitans fossae rhomboideae

s. limitans insulae

s. limitans ventriculorum cerebri

lingual s.

longitudinal s. of heart

sulcus (sulci) *(continued)*

lunate s.

s. lunatus

mallear s. of temporal bone

malleolar s. of fibula

s. malleolaris fibulae

malleolar s. of temporal bone

malleolar s. of tibia

mandibular s.

marginal s.

s. of mastoid canaliculus

s. matricis unguis

s. of matrix of nail

medial bicipital s.

medial s. of crus cerebri

median s. of fourth ventricle

median s. of medulla oblongata, dorsal

median s. of medulla oblongata, posterior

median s. of spinal cord, dorsal

median s. of spinal cord, posterior

median s. of tongue

s. medianus dorsalis medullae oblongatae

s. medianus dorsalis medullae spinalis

s. medianus linguae

s. medianus posterior medullae oblongatae

s. medianus posterior medullae spinalis

s. medianus ventriculi quarti

meningeal sulci

mentolabial s.

s. mentolabialis

middle frontal s.

s. of middle temporal artery

s. of Monro

muscular s. of tympanic cavity

s. musculi flexoris hallucis longi calcanei

s. musculi flexoris hallucis longi tali

s. musculi peronaei ossis cuboidei

s. musculi subclavii

s. mylohyoideus mandibulae

mylohyoid s. of mandible

s. of nail matrix

nasal s., posterior

s. of nasal process of maxilla

nasofrontal s.

nasolabial s.

sulcus (sulci) *(continued)*

s. nasolabialis
s. nervi oculomotorii
s. nervi petrosi majoris
s. nervi petrosi minoris
s. nervi radialis
s. nervi spinalis
s. nervi ulnaris
nymphocaruncular s.
obturator s. of pubis
s. of occipital artery
occipital sulci, lateral
occipital sulci, superior
occipital s., transverse
occipitotemporal s.
s. occipitotemporalis
oculomotor s.
s. oculomotorius
s. olfactorius lobi frontalis
s. olfactorius nasi
olfactory s. of frontal lobe
olfactory s. of nose
optic s.
s. of optic chiasm
orbital sulci of frontal lobe
palatine sulci of maxilla
s. palatinus major maxillae
s. palatinus major ossis
    palatini
s. palatovaginalis
paracolic sulci
sulci paracolici
paraglenoid sulci of hip bone
paramedian s.
parietooccipital s.
s. parieto-occipitalis
parolfactory s., anterior
parolfactory s., posterior
petrobasilar s.
petrosal s. of occipital bone,
    inferior
petrosal s. of temporal bone,
    inferior
petrosal s. of temporal bone,
    posterior
petrosal s. of temporal bone,
    superior
s. petrosus inferior ossis
    occipitalis
s. petrosus inferior ossis
    temporalis
s. petrosus superior ossis
    temporalis
s. of pharyngeal tonsil
polar s.

sulcus (sulci) *(continued)*

pontobulbar s.
pontopeduncular s.
postcalcarine s.
postcentral s.
postclival s.
posterointermediate s. of
    spinal cord
s. posterolateralis medullae
    oblongatae
s. posterolateralis medullae
    spinalis
posterolateral s. of medulla
    oblongata
posterolateral s. of spinal cord
postnodular s.
postpyramidal s.
preauricular s.
precentral s.
precentral s. of cerebrum
prechiasmatic s.
s. prechiasmaticus
s. prechiasmatis
prepyramidal s.
prerolandic s.
s. promontorii cavitatis
    tympani
s. of pterygoid hamulus
pterygoid s. of pterygoid
    process
pterygopalatine s. of palatine
    bone
pterygopalatine s. of pterygoid
    process
s. pterygopalatinus processus
    pterygoidei
pulmonary s.
pulmonary s. of thorax
radial s. of humerus
s. for radial nerve
Reil s.
retroauricular s.
retrocentral s.
rhinal s.
s. rhinalis
rolandic s.
sagittal s.
s. sclerae
scleral s.
sclerocorneal s.
s. of semicanal of humerus
semilunar s. of radius
sigmoid s.
s. for sigmoid sinus of occipital
    bone

S

sulcus (sulci) *(continued)*

s. for sigmoid sinus of parietal bone

s. for sigmoid sinus of temporal bone

s. sinus petrosi inferioris ossis occipitalis

s. sinus petrosi inferioris ossis temporalis

s. sinus petrosi superioris

s. sinus sagittalis superioris

s. sinus sigmoidei

s. sinus sigmoidei ossis occipitalis

s. sinus sigmoidei ossis parietalis

s. sinus sigmoidei ossis temporalis

s. sinus transversi

sulci of skin

s. for spinal nerve

spiral s.

spiral s., external

spiral s. of humerus

spiral s., internal

s. spiralis

s. spiralis externus

s. spiralis internus

subclavian s.

s. for subclavian artery

s. for subclavian muscle

subclavian s. of lung

s. subclavius

s. for subclavian vein

s. subclavius pulmonis

subparietal s.

s. subparietalis

s. for superior petrosal sinus

supra-acetabular s.

s. supra-acetabularis

supraorbital s.

suprasplenial s.

suprasylvian s.

s. tali, s. of talus

temporal s.

sulci temporales transversi

temporal s., inferior

s. temporalis inferior

s. temporalis superior

s. temporalis transversus

temporal s., middle

temporal s., superior

temporal s. of temporal bone

temporal sulci, transverse

sulcus (sulci) *(continued)*

s. tendinis musculi flexoris hallucis longi calcanei

s. tendinis musculi peronei longi

s. for tendon of flexor hallucis longus muscle of calcaneus

s. for tendon of peroneus longus muscle

s. terminalis atrii dextri

s. terminalis linguae

terminal s. of right atrium

terminal s. of thalamus

terminal s. of tongue

s. of tongue

transverse s. of anthelix

transverse s. of heart

transverse s. of occipital bone

transverse s. of parietal bone

s. of transverse sinus

transverse s. of temporal bone

s. transversus ossis occipitalis

s. transversus ossis parietalis

s. tubae auditivae

s. tubae auditoriae

Turner s.

tympanic s.

tympanic s. of temporal bone

s. tympanicus ossis temporalis

s. for ulnar nerve

s. for umbilical vein

uvulonodular s.

s. valleculae

sulci for veins

s. for vena cava

s. venae cavae

s. venae subclaviae

s. venae umbilicalis

sulci venosi

venous sulci

ventral s. of spinal cord

s. ventrolateralis medullae oblongatae

s. ventrolateralis medullae spinalis

ventrolateral s. of spinal cord

vermicular s.

s. of vertebral artery of atlas

vertical s.

s. vomeris

vomerovaginal s.

s. vomerovaginalis

s. of wrist

sulfabenzamide

sulfacetic acid

sulfacid
sulfacytine
sulfadiazine
    s. silver
    s. sodium
sulfadoxine
sulfaethidole
sulfaguanidine
sulfalene
sulfamerazine
sulfameter
sulfamethazine
sulfamethizole
sulfamethoxazole
sulfamethoxypyridazine
sulfamethyldiazine
sulfamethylthiadiazole
sulfamido
sulfamidochrysoidine
sulfamine
sulfamonomethoxine
sulfamoxole
sulfan blue
sulfanilamide
sulfanilate
sulfanilic acid
sulfanilylsulfanilamide
sulfanitran
sulfanuria
sulfapyridine
sulfapyrimidine
sulfaquinoxaline
sulfasalazine
sulfatase
    multiple s. deficiency
sulfate
    acid s.
    basic s.
    chondroitin s.
    conjugated s's
    ethereal s's
    hydrogen s.
    mineral s's
    neutral s.
    normal s.
    preformed s's
sulfatemia
sulfatidase
sulfatide
sulfatidosis
sulfenic acid
sulfhemoglobin
sulfhemoglobinemia
sulfhydrate
sulfhydric acid

sulfhydryl
sulfide
    mercuric s.
sulfinic acid
sulfinide
sulfinpyrazone
sulfinyl
β-sulfinylpyruvic acid [beta-]
sulfisomidine
sulfisoxazole
    s. acetyl
    s. diolamine
sulfite oxidase
sulfmethemoglobin
sulfoacid
sulfoamino
sulfoconjugation
sulfocyanate
sulfocyanic acid
sulfogel
N-sulfoglucosamine sulfohydrolase
sulfohydrate
sulfoiduronate sulfatase
sulfolipid
sulfolithocholylglycine
sulfolithocholyltaurine
sulfolysis
sulfonamide
sulfonamidemia
sulfonamidocholia
sulfonamidotherapy
sulfonamiduria
sulfonate
sulfone
sulfonethylmethane
sulfonic
sulfonic acid
sulfonium
sulfonmethane
sulfonyl
sulfonylurea
sulfoprotein
sulfosalicylic acid
sulfosalt
sulfosol
sulfotransferase
sulfoxide
    methionine s.
sulfoxism
sulfur (S)
    colloidal s.
    s. dioxide
    flowers of s.
    s. hydride
    lac s.

S

sulfur (S) *(continued)*
    s. lotum
    s. monochloride
    precipitated s.
    radioactive s.
    roll s.
    s. S 35
    sublimed s.
    washed s.
    wetable s.
sulfurated
sulfurator
sulfuric acid
sulfuris
sulfurize
sulfurous acid
sulfurtransferase
sulfuryl
sulindac
sulisobenzone
sullage
suloctidil
sulpiride
sulprostone
sulthiame
Sulzberger-Garbe syndrome
sumac
    poison s.
    swamp s.
summation
    central s.
    s. gallop
    spatial s.
    temporal s.
summit
    s. of bladder
    s. of nose
Sumner
    reagent
    sign
sump
    Baylor s.
    s. drain
    s. drainage system
    s. tube
SUN—serum urea
  nitrogen
sunburn
Sunday [eponym] elevator
Sunday morning paralysis
sunspot
sunstroke
superabduction
superacid
superacidity

superacromial
superactivity
superacute
superalimentation
superalkalinity
superantigen
superaurale
Superblade
supercarbonate
supercentral
supercilia
superciliary
supercilium
superclass
supercoil
supercooled
superdistention
superduct
superego
superexcitation
superextended
superextension
superfamily
superfecundation
superfetation
superficial
    s. abscess
    s. basal cell carcinoma
    s. brachial artery
    s. bursa of knee
    s. bursa of olecranon
    s. calcaneal bursitis
    s. cardiac plexus
    s. cerebral veins
    s. cervical artery
    s. cervical fascia
    s. cervical lymph nodes
    s. chronic keratitis
    s. cleavage
    s. fascia
    s. fascia of perineum
    s. fascia of scrotum
    s. femoral arch
    s. femoral artery
    s. frostbite
    s. implantation
    s. inguinal lymph nodes
    s. inguinal ring
    s. investing fascia
    s. investing layer
    s. layer
    s. ligament of carpus
    s. line of cornea
    s. lymph nodes
    s. necrosis

superficial *(continued)*
>> s. nephron
>> s. peroneal nerve
>> s. popliteal lymph nodes
>> s. radial nerve
>> s. reflex
>> s. sacrococcygeal ligament
>> s. scaler
>> s. suture
>> s. vein

superficialis
superfissure
superflexion
superfunction
superhelix
superimposed
superimposition
superimpregnation
superinduce
superinfection
superinvolution
superior
>> s. laryngotomy
>> s. ramus
>> s. tracheotomy
>> s. vena cava (SVC)

superjacent
superlactation
superlethal
supermicroscope
supermotility
supernatant
supernate
supernormal
supernumerary
supernutrition
superolateral
superomedial
superovulation
superoxide
superparasite
superparasitic
superparasitism
superpetrosal
superphosphate
super-regeneration
supersalt
supersaturate
superscription
supersecretion
supersede
supersensitive
supersensitivity
>> disuse s.

supersensitization

supersoft
supersonic
supersonics
superspecies
supersphenoid
superstructure
>> implant s.

supersulcus
supervascularization
supervenosity
supervention
superversion
supervisor
supervitaminosis
supervoltage
supinate
supination of foot
supinator
supine
supplemental
supply
>> extrinsic nerve s.
>> intrinsic nerve s.

support
>> Abée s.
>> advanced cardiac life s.
>> advanced life s. (ALS)
>> advanced trauma life s.
>> basic life s. (BLS)
>> s. of the promontory
>> s. suture

supportive
suppository
>> glycerin s.

suppressant
suppression
>> otoacoustic s.
>> phenotypic s.

suppressor
>> amber s.
>> s. cell
>> codon-specific s.
>> crossover s.
>> soluble immune
>>   response s.

suppurant
suppurate
suppuration
>> alveodental s.

suppurative
supra-acromial
supra-anal
supra-aortic
supra-auricular
supra-axillary

S

suprabuccal
suprabulge
supracallosal
supracerebellar
supracerebral
supracervical
    s. hysterectomy
    s. incision
suprachoroid
suprachoroidea
supraciliary
supraclavicular
supraclavicularis
supraclinoid
supraclusion
supracondylar
supracostal
supracotyloid
supracranial
supradiaphragmatic
supraduction
supradural
supraepicondylar
supraepitrochlear
suprageniculate
supraglenoid
supraglottic laryngectomy
supraglottis
supragranular
suprahepatic
suprahilar
suprahyoid
suprailiac
suprainguinal
supraintestinal
supralethal
supraliminal
supralumbar
supramalleolar
supramammary
supramammillary
supramandibular
supramarginal
supramastoid
supramaxillary
supramaximal
suprameatal
supramental
supramentale
Supramid suture
supranasal
supranormal
supranuclear
supraoccipital
supraocular
supraomohyoid
supraoptic
supraoptimal
supraoptimum
supraorbital
suprapatellar
suprapelvic
suprapharmacologic
suprapineal
suprapontine
suprapromontorial
suprapubic
    s. catheterization
    s. cystotomy
    s. incision
    s. lithotomy
    s. prostatectomy (SPP)
    s. transvesical prostatectomy
suprarenal
suprarenalectomy
suprarenalism
suprarenalopathy
suprarenogenic
suprarenotropic
suprascapula
suprascapular
suprascleral
suprasegmental
suprasellar
supraseptal
supraspinal
supraspinous
suprastapedial
suprasternal
suprasternale
suprasterol
suprasylvian
supratemporal
supratentorial
suprathoracic
supratonsillar
supratrochlear
supraturbinal
supratympanic
supraumbilical incision
supravaginal hysterectomy
supravalvular
supraventricular
supravergence
supraversion
supravital
supraxiphoid
suprofen
sura
sural

suralimentation
surcingle
surdimute
surdimutism
surditas congenita
surdity
surexcitation
surface
  acromial articular s. of clavicle
  alveolar s.
  alveolar s. of maxilla
  anterior s.
  anterior s. of cornea
  anterior s. of eyelids
  anterior s. of iris
  anterior s. of kidney
  anterior s. of lens
  anterior s. of manubrium and gladiolus
  anterior s. of pancreas
  anterior s. of sacral bone
  anterior s. of scapula
  anterior s. of stomach
  anterior s. of suprarenal gland
  anterior talar articular s.
  anterior talar articular s. of calcaneus
  anteromedial s.
  anteromedial s. of humerus
  approximal s.
  articular s.
  articular s. of acetabulum
  articular s. of sacral bone, lateral
  axial s.
  basal s.
  basal s. of denture
  buccal s.
  carpal articular s.
  carpal articular s. of radius
  colic s.
  colic s. of spleen
  condyloid s.
  condyloid s. of tibia
  contact s.
  costal s.
  costal s. of lung
  costal s. of scapula
  cuboid articular s.
  cuboid articular s. of calcaneus
  denture foundation s.
  denture impression s.
  diaphragmatic s.
  diaphragmatic s. of heart
  diaphragmatic s. of liver

surface *(continued)*
  diaphragmatic s. of lung
  diaphragmatic s. of spleen
  distal s.
  dorsal s.
  dorsal s. of scapula
  extensor s.
  facial s.
  flexor s.
  foundation s.
  gastric s.
  gastric s. of spleen
  s. of heart, right
  impression s.
  incisal s.
  inferior s.
  inferior articular s. of tibia
  inferior s. of liver
  inferior s. of pancreas
  infratemporal s.
  infratemporal s. of maxilla
  interlobar s.
  interlobar s. of lung
  isodose s.
  labial s.
  lateral s.
  left s. of heart
  lingual s.
  masticatory s.
  medial s.
  medial s. of lung
  mediastinal s.
  mediastinal s. of lung
  mesial s.
  middle talar articular s. of calcaneus
  morsal s's
  occlusal s.
  occlusal s. of teeth
  occlusal s., working
  oral s.
  orbital s.
  orbital s. of sphenoid bone
  polished s.
  posterior s.
  posterior s. of cornea
  posterior s. of eyelids
  posterior s. of iris
  posterior s. of kidney
  posterior s. of lens
  posterior s. of pancreas
  posterior s. of sacral bone
  posterior s. of scapula
  posterior s. of stomach

S

surface *(continued)*
    posterior s. of suprarenal
      gland
    posterior talar articular s. of
      calcaneus
    proximal s.
    proximate s.
    pulmonary s. of heart
    renal s.
    renal s. of spleen
    renal s. of suprarenal gland
    right s. of heart
    sacropelvic s.
    sacropelvic s. of the ilium
    sternocostal s. of heart
    subocclusal s.
    superior s.
    superior articular s. of
      atlas
    superior articular s.
      of tibia
    superior s. of talus
    symphysial s.
    symphysial s. of pubis
    temporal s.
    temporal s. of frontal bone
    tentorial s.
    total body s.
    ventral s.
    ventral s. of scapula
    vestibular s.
    visceral s.
    visceral s. of liver
    visceral s. of spleen
surface-active
surfactant
    pulmonary s.
surfeit
surgeon
    acting assistant s.
    assistant s.
    attending s.
    barber s.
    contract s.
    dental s.
    district s.
    s. general
    house s.
    oral s.
    orthopedic s.
    post s.
surgery
    abdominal s.
    ambulatory s.
    anaplastic s.

surgery *(continued)*
    antiseptic s.
    arthroscopic s.
    aseptic s.
    aural s.
    bench s.
    bench work s.
    cardiac s.
    cardiovascular s.
    cineplastic s.
    clinical s.
    closed s.
    closed heart s.
    conservative s.
    cosmetic s.
    cryogenic s.
    day s.
    definitive s.
    dental s.
    dentofacial s.
    elective s.
    esthetic s.
    exploratory s.
    featural s.
    foot-plate s.
    general s.
    in-and-out s.
    laser s.
    major s.
    maxillofacial s.
    microvascular s.
    minor s.
    Mohs s.
    mucogingival s.
    open heart s.
    operative s.
    operative dental s.
    oral s.
    oral and maxillofacial s.
    orthopedic s.
    palliative s.
    peripheral vascular s.
    plastic s.
    psychiatric s.
    radical s.
    rapid in-and-out
      (RIO) s.
    reconstructive s.
    sonic s.
    stapes s.
    stereotactic s.
    stereotaxic s.
    structural s.
    thoracic s.
    transsexual s.

surgical
  s. microscope
  s. suture
  s. vagotomy
Surgicel gauze dressing
Surgilene suture
Surgilon suture
Surgilope suture
Surgivac
  drainage system, Snyder
  suction drainage system
surprise
surprisingly
surrogate
sursumduction
sursumvergence
sursumversion
suruçucu
surveillance
  epidemiologic s.
  immune s.
  immunological s.
survey
  Jenkins activity s.
surveying
surveyor
survival
  five-year s.
  red blood cell s.
survivorship
SUS—stained urinary sediment
susceptibility
  differential s.
  magnetic s.
susceptible
sushi
suspect
suspenopsia
suspensiometer
suspension
  alumina and magnesia oral s.
  ampicillin for oral s.
  betamethasone sodium
    phosphate and
    betamethasone acetate s.,
    sterile
  chloramphenicol palmitate
    oral s.
  chlorothiazide oral s.
  cholestyramine for oral s.
  Coffey s.
  colistin sulfate for oral s.
  colloid s.
  corticotropin zinc hydroxide
    injectable s.

suspension *(continued)*
  corticotropin zinc hydroxide
    s., sterile
  cortisone acetate ophthalmic s.
  cortisone acetate s., sterile
  cuff s.
  demeclocycline oral s.
  desoxycorticosterone pivalate
    s., sterile
  dicloxacillin sodium for oral s.
  diphenylhydantoin oral s.
  epinephrine oil s., sterile
  estradiol s., sterile
  extended insulin zinc s.
  hydrocortisone acetate
    ophthalmic s.
  hydrocortisone acetate s.,
    sterile
  hydrocortisone cypionate
    oral s.
  hydroxyzine pamoate oral s.
  ipodate calcium for oral s.
  s. laryngoscope
  s. laryngoscopy
  levopropoxyphene napsylate
    oral s.
  magaldrate oral s.
  magnesia and alumina oral s.
  medroxyprogesterone acetate
    s., sterile
  medrysone ophthalmic s.
  meprobamate oral s.
  methenamine mandelate
    oral s.
  methylprednisolone acetate
    injectable s.
  methylprednisolone acetate s.,
    sterile
  neomycin and polymyxin B
    sulfates and hydrocortisone
    otic s.
  nitrofurantoin oral s.
  novobiocin calcium oral s.
  oxytetracycline calcium oral s.
  penicillin G benzathine s.,
    sterile
  penicillin G procaine with
    aluminum stearate s., sterile
  penicillin G procaine s., sterile
  penicillin V benzathine oral s.
  penicillin V hydrabamine
    oral s.
  penicillin V for oral s.
  penicillin V potassium for
    oral s.

S

suspension *(continued)*
   phensuximide oral s.
   phenytoin oral s.
   prednisolone acetate s., sterile
   primidone oral s.
   progesterone s., sterile
   prompt insulin zinc s.
   propoxyphene napsylate oral s.
   propyliodone injectable oil s.
   propyliodone oil s., sterile
   propyliodone s., sterile
   protamine zinc insulin s.
   pyrantel pamoate oral s.
   pyrvinium pamoate oral s.
   salicylamide oral s.
   selenium sulfide detergent s.
   simethicone oral s.
   sitosterols s.
   sulfacetamide, sulfadiazine,
      and sulfamerazine oral s.
   sulfadimethoxine oral s.
   sulfamethizole oral s.
   sulfamethoxazole oral s.
   sulfisoxazole acetyl oral s.
   testolactone s., sterile
   testosterone s., sterile
   tetracycline oral s.
   thiabendazole oral s.
   triamcinolone acetonide s.,
      sterile
   triamcinolone diacetate s.,
      sterile
   triamcinolone hexacetonide s.,
      sterile
   trisulfapyrimidines oral s.
   troleandomycin oral s.
suspensoid
suspensorius
suspensory
sustentacular
sustentaculum (sustentacula)
   s. lienis
   s. tali, s. of talus
susurration
susurrus
   s. aurium
   s. murmur
Sutton
   disease
   nevus (nevi)
Sutton-Rendu-Osler-Weber
   syndrome
sutura (suturae)
   s. coronalis
   s. dentate

sutura (suturae) *(continued)*
   s. ethmoidolacrimalis
   s. ethmoidomaxillaris
   s. frontalis
   s. frontalis metopica
   s. fronto-ethmoidalis
   s. frontolacrimalis
   s. frontomaxillaris
   s. frontonasalis
   s. frontozygomatica
   s. harmonia
   s. incisiva
   s. infraorbitalis
   s. intermaxillaris
   s. internasalis
   s. lacrimoconchalis
   s. lacrimomaxillaris
   s. lambdoidea
   s. limbosa
   s. nasofrontalis
   s. nasomaxillaris
   s. occipitomastoidea
   s. palatina mediana
   s. palatina transversa
   s. palatoethmoidalis
   s. palatomaxillaris
   s. parietomastoidea
   s. plana
   s. sagittalis
   s. serrata
   s. spheno-ethmoidalis
   s. sphenofrontalis
   s. sphenomaxillaris
   s. sphenoorbitalis
   s. sphenoparietalis
   s. sphenosquamosa
   s. sphenovomeriana
   s. sphenozygomatica
   s. squamosa
   s. squamosa cranii
   s. squamosomastoidea
   s. temporozygomatica
   s. vera
   s. zygomaticomaxillaris
sutural
suturation
suture [anatomy]
   anterior palatine s.
   bony s.
   bregmatomastoid s.
   coronal s.
   cranial s's
   dentate s.
   denticulate s.
   endognathic s.

suture [anatomy] *(continued)*
   endomesognathic s.
   ethmoidolacrimal s.
   ethmoidomaxillary s.
   false s.
   flat s.
   frontal s.
   frontoethmoidal s.
   frontolacrimal s.
   frontomalar s.
   frontomaxillary s.
   frontonasal s.
   frontoparietal s.
   frontosphenoid s.
   frontozygomatic s.
   s. of Goethe
   incisive s.
   infraorbital s.
   interendognathic s.
   intermaxillary s.
   internasal s.
   interpalatine s.
   interparietal s.
   jugal s.
   lacrimoconchal s.
   lacrimoethmoidal s.
   lacrimomaxillary s.
   lacrimoturbinal s.
   lambdoid s., lambdoidal s.
   limbal s.
   limbous s.
   longitudinal s.
   longitudinal s. of palate
   malomaxillary s.
   mammillary s.
   mastoid s.
   median palatine s.
   metopic s.
   middle palatine s.
   nasal s.
   nasofrontal s.
   nasomaxillary s.
   occipital s.
   occipitomastoid s.
   occipitoparietal s.
   occipitosphenoidal s.
   palatine s., anterior
   palatine s., median
   palatine s., middle
   palatine s., posterior
   palatine s., transverse
   palatoethmoidal s.
   palatomaxillary s.
   parietal s.
   parietomastoid s.

suture [anatomy] *(continued)*
   parieto-occipital s.
   parietotemporal s.
   petrobasilar s.
   petrosphenobasilar s.
   petrosquamosal s.
   plane s.
   posterior palatine s.
   premaxillary s.
   rhabdoid s.
   sagittal s.
   serrated s.
   s's of skull
   sphenoethmoidal s.
   sphenofrontal s.
   sphenomalar s.
   sphenomaxillary s.
   spheno-occipital s.
   spheno-orbital s.
   sphenoparietal s.
   sphenopetrosal s.
   sphenosquamous s.
   sphenotemporal s.
   sphenovomerine s.
   sphenozygomatic s.
   squamomastoid s.
   squamoparietal s.
   squamosal s.
   squamosphenoid s.
   squamous s.
   squamous s. of cranium
   temporal s.
   temporomalar s.
   temporozygomatic s.
   transverse s. of Krause
   transverse palatine s.
   true s.
   tympanomastoid s.
   zygomaticofrontal s.
   zygomaticomaxillary s.
   zygomaticosphenoid s.
   zygomaticotemporal s.
suture-holding forceps
suture material
   0 s. [size zero]
   00 s., 2-0 s.
   000 s., 3-0 s.
   #1 s. [#2, #3, etc.]
   absorbable s.
   absorbable surgical s.
   Acutrol s.
   Alcon s.
   Atraloc s.
   black braided s.
   black silk s.

S

suture material *(continued)*
  braided s.
  cardiovascular s.
  catgut s.
  celluloid s.
  chromic catgut s.
  collagen s.
  Dacron s.
  Deknatel s.
  Dermalene s.
  Dermalon s.
  Dexon s.
  Dulox s.
  elastic s.
  Equisetene s.
  Ethibond s.
  Ethicon s.
  Ethiflex s.
  Ethilon s.
  Flaxedil s.
  Flexitone s.
  Flexon s.
  gut chromic s.
  horsehair s.
  Marlex s.
  Mayo linen s.
  Medrafil wire s.
  Mersilene s.
  monofilament s.
  multifilament s.
  multistrand s.
  nonabsorbable s.
  nonabsorbable surgical s.
  Nurolon s.
  nylon monofilament s.
  Pagenstecher linen thread s.
  plain s.
  plain catgut s.
  Polydek s.
  polyester s.
  polyethylene s.
  polyfilament s.
  polypropylene s.
  Prolene s.
  ribbon gut s.
  rubber s.
  silk s.
  silk-braided s.
  silkworm gut s.
  silver wire s.
  stainless steel s.
  staple s.
  steel mesh s.
  Supramid s.
  Surgilene s.

suture material *(continued)*
  Surgilon s.
  Surgilope s.
  tantalum wire s.
  Tevdek s.
  Thermo-flex s.
  Ti-Cron s.
  tiger gut s.
  unabsorbable s.
  Vicryl s.
  Viro-Tec s.
  white braided s.
  white silk s.
  wire s.
  Zytor s.
suture technique
  Albert s.
  Allison s.
  alternating s.
  anchoring s.
  angle s.
  Appolito s.
  apposition s.
  approximation s.
  arcuate s.
  Argyll Robertson s.
  Arlt s.
  atraumatic s.
  Axenfeld s.
  Babcock s.
  back-and-forth s.
  Barraquer s.
  baseball s.
  basilar s.
  bastard s.
  Béclard s.
  Bell s.
  biparietal s.
  blanket s.
  bolster s.
  Bozeman s.
  bregmatomastoid s.
  bridle s.
  bunching s.
  Bunnell s.
  buried s.
  button s.
  buttonhole s.
  cable wire s.
  capitonnage s.
  chain s.
  circular s.
  circumcision s.
  Coakley s.
  coaptation s.

suture technique *(continued)*
    cobbler's s.
    compound s.
    Connell s.
    continuous s.
    corneoscleral s.
    cruciform s.
    Cushing s.
    cushioning s.
    cutaneous s.
    cuticular s.
    Czerny s.
    Czerny-Lembert s.
    delayed s.
    delayed primary s.
    dermal s.
    double-armed s., doubly
        armed s.
    double-button s.
    Dupuytren s.
    edge-to-edge s.
    Emmet s.
    end-on mattress s.
    epineural s.
    everting s.
    everting interrupted s.
    far-and-near s.
    figure-of-eight s.
    fixation s.
    fore-and-aft s.
    Fothergill s.
    free ligature s.
    Frost s.
    furrier's s.
    Gaillard-Arlt s.
    Gambee s.
    Gély s.
    Gibson s.
    glover's s.
    Gould s.
    groove s.
    Gussenbauer s.
    guy s.
    Guyton-Friedenwald s.
    Halsted s.
    harelip s.
    Harris s.
    helical s.
    hemostatic s's
    horizontal mattress s.
    Horsley s.
    imbricated s.
    infolding s.
    implanted s.
    interlocking s.

suture technique *(continued)*
    interrupted s.
    intradermal s.
    intradermal mattress s.
    intradermic s.
    invaginating s.
    inverted s., inverting s.
    Ivalon s.
    Jobert s.
    Kalt s.
    kangaroo tendon s.
    Kelly s.
    Kirby s.
    Kirschner s.
    lace s.
    Le Dentu s.
    Le Fort s.
    Lembert s.
    lens s's
    ligation s.
    s. ligature
    Littré s.
    locking s.
    lock-stitch s.
    Löffler s.
    loop s.
    loop-on mucosa s.
    mattress s.
    mattress s., end-on
    mattress s., horizontal
    mattress s., intradermal
    mattress s., right-angle
    mattress s., vertical
    Maunsell s.
    Meigs s.
    near-and-far s.
    nerve s.
    noose s.
    over-and-over s.
    overlapping s's
    Palfyn s.
    Pancoast s.
    Paré s.
    Parker-Kerr s.
    peg-and-socket s.
    pericostal s.
    Petit s.
    pin s.
    plastic s.
    plicating s., plication s.
    presection s.
    primary s.
    pulley s.
    pull-out wire s.
    pursestring s.

S

suture technique *(continued)*
    quilt s., quilted s.
    reinforcing s.
    relaxation s.
    retention s.
    Richardson s.
    Richter s.
    right-angle mattress s.
    running continuous s.
    Saenger s.
    secondary s.
    seromuscular s.
    seroserous s.
    shotted s.
    Simon s.
    simple s.
    Sims s.
    single-armed s.
    sling s.
    spiral s.
    stay s.
    stick-tie s.
    Sturmdorf s.
    subcuticular s.
    superficial s.
    support s.
    surgical s.
    Taylor s.
    tendon s.
    tension s.
    Thiersch s.
    through-and-through s.
    Tom Jones s.
    tongue-and-groove s.
    traction s.
    transfixing s., transfixion s.
    twisted s.
    uninterrupted s.
    Verhoeff s.
    vertical mattress s.
    whipstitch s.
    Wölfler (Woelfler) s.
    Y-s.
    Z-s.
SUUD—sudden unexpected, unexplained death
Suzanne gland
Sv—sievert(s)
SV—
    sinus venosus
    stroke volume
    subclavian vein
SV40—simian virus 40
SVAS—supravalvular aortic stenosis

SVC—
    slow vital capacity
    superior vena cava
SVCG—spatial vectorcardiogram
SVD—
    spontaneous vaginal delivery
    spontaneous vertex delivery
svedberg unit (Sv, S)
SVM—syncytiovascular membrane
SVR—systemic vascular resistance
SVT—supraventricular tachycardia
SW—
    spiral wound
    stroke work
swab
    NIH s.
swaddler
    silver s.
swage
swager
swallow
    barium s.
    Hypaque s.
swallowing
    air s.
    infantile s.
    tongue s.
Swan syndrome (I, II)
Swan-Ganz catheter
Swanson
    operation
    prosthesis
swarming
swathe
swayback
swearing
    compulsive s.
sweat
    bloody s.
    blue s.
    fetid s.
    green s.
    night s.
    phosphorescent s.
sweating
    insensible s.
    sensible s.
Swediaur disease
Sweet
    forceps
    method
    retractor
    scissors
sweetener
    artificial s.

sweetgum
Sweet syndrome
swelling
    albuminous s.
    arytenoid s.
    blennorrhagic s.
    brain s.
    bulbar s's
    Calabar s's
    capsular s.
    cloudy s.
    familial fibrous s. of jaws
    fugitive s.
    genital s.
    glassy s.
    hunger s.
    Kamerun s's
    labial s.
    labioscrotal s.
    lateral lingual s's
    levator s.
    premenstrual s.
    scrotal s.
    Soemmering crystalline s.
    tropical s's
    tubular cloudy s.
    tympanic s.
    white s.
Swenson
    operation
    procedure
Swift disease
swimmer's
    s. dermatitis
    s. ear
    s. itch
    s. projection
    s. view
swing
    mood s's
    torsion s.
swing-bed
Swiss Alps appearance
Swiss-cheese endometrium
switch
    class s.
    selector s.
swoon
SWS—slow-wave sleep
Swyer syndrome
Swyer-James syndrome
Swyer-James-Macleod
  syndrome
sychnuria
sycosiform tinea barbae

sycosis
    s. barbae
    fulminant herpetic s.
    herpetic s.
    kerion-like s. barbae
    lupoid s.
    s. nuchae
    tinea s.
    s. vulgaris
Sydenham
    chorea
    cough
sylvatic
Sylvest disease
sylvian
    s. aqueduct syndrome
    s. fissure
sylviduct
Sylvius
    angle
    aqueduct (aqueduct of S.)
    cistern (cistern of S.)
    cistern of fossa of S.
    fissure (fissure of S.)
    fossa
    valve
    ventricle of S.
symbiology
symbionic
symbiont
symbiosis (symbioses)
symbiotic
symblepharon
    anterior s.
    posterior s.
    total s.
symblepharopterygium
symbol
    phallic s.
symbolia
symbolism
symbolization
symbolophobia
symbrachydactyly
symclosene
Syme
    amputation
    operation
    prosthesis
Symington body
symmelia
symmelus
Symmers
    disease
    fibrosis

S

symmetric, symmetrical
symmetry
    bilateral s.
    inverse s.
    radial s.
sympathectomize
sympathectomy
    cervical s.
    chemical s.
    lumbar s.
    lumbodorsal s.
    periarterial s.
sympathetic
    s. ganglia
    s. nervous system
    s. ophthalmia
    s. uveitis
sympatheticoparalytic
sympatheticotonic
sympathetoblast
sympathicoblast
sympathicoblastoma
sympathicogenic
sympathicogonioma
sympathicopathy
sympathicotherapy
sympathicotripsy
sympathicotropic
sympathicus
sympathin
sympathism
sympathizer
sympathoadrenal
sympathochromaffin
sympathogonioma
sympathogonium
  (sympathogonia)
sympatholytic
sympathomimetic
sympathoparalytic
sympathy
sympectothiene
sympectothion
symperitoneal
sympexion (sympexia)
symphalangia
symphalangy
symphalocephalus
symphoricarpus
symphyocephalus
symphyseal
symphyses (plural of symphysis)
symphysic
symphysiectomy
symphysiolysis

symphysiorrhaphy
symphysiotome
symphysiotomy
symphysis (symphyses)
    intervertebral s.
    s. intervertebralis
    s. mandibulae
    mandibular s.
    manubriosternal s.
    s. manubriosternalis
    s. mentalis
    s. menti
    pubic s.
    s. pubica
    s. xiphosternalis
symphysitis
symphysodactyly
symplasm
symplasmatic
symplex
sympodia
symport
symptom
    abstinence s's
    accessory s.
    acute on chronic s's
    Anton s.
    assident s.
    Bárány s.
    Béhier-Hardy s.
    Bekhterev (Bechterew) s.
    Berger s.
    Bonhoeffer s.
    Brauch-Romberg s.
    Buerger s.
    Burghart s.
    Capgras s.
    cardinal s.
    Castellani-Low s.
    characteristic s.
    Chvostek s.
    Colliver s.
    concomitant s.
    consecutive s.
    constitutional s.
    conversion s.
    crossbar s. of Fränkel
    deficiency s.
    delayed s.
    direct s.
    dissociation s.
    endothelial s.
    Epstein s.
    equivocal s.
    esophagosalivary s's

symptom *(continued)*
  factitious s.
  Frenkel s.
  Froin s.
  fundamental s.
  Ganser s.
  general s.
  Gordon s.
  gramophone s.
  guiding s.
  Haenel s.
  halo s.
  Huchard s.
  incarceration s.
  indirect s.
  induced s.
  Jonas s.
  Kussmaul s.
  labyrinthine s's
  Lade s.
  Liebreich s.
  local s.
  localizing s's
  Loewi s.
  Magendie s.
  Magnan s.
  negative s.
  neighborhood s.
  nostril s.
  objective s.
  Oehler s.
  passive s.
  pathognomonic s.
  Pel-Ebstein s.
  precursor s.
  precursory s.
  premonitory s.
  presenting s.
  prodromal s.
  prodromal epileptic s.
  rainbow s.
  rational s.
  reflex s.
  Remak s.
  Roger s.
  Romberg-Howship s.
  Seguin signal s.
  signal s.
  Skeer s.
  Sklowsky s.
  static s.
  subjective s.
  sympathetic s.
  systemic s.
  Trendelenburg s.

symptom *(continued)*
  Uhthoff s.
  Wernicke s.
  withdrawal s's
symptomatic
symptomatology
symptomatolytic
symptome
symptosis
symptothermal
sympus
  s. apus
  s. dipus
  s. monopus
synadelphus
synaetion
synalbumin
synalgia
synalgic
synanastomosis
synanthrin
synanthrose
synaphymenitis
synapse
  axoaxonic s.
  axodendritic s.
  axodendrosomatic s.
  axosomatic s.
  dendrodendritic s.
  electrotonic s.
  en passant s.
  false s.
  loop s.
  neuromuscular s.
  pericorpuscular s.
synapsis
synaptene
synaptic
synaptology
synaptosome
synarthrodial
synarthrophysis
synarthroses
synarthrosis
syncaine
syncanthus
syncaryon
syncelom
syncephalus
  asymmetros
synchesis
synchilia
synchiria
syncholia
synchondrectomy

S

synchondroseotomy
synchondrosis (synchondroses)
    anterior intraoccipital s.
    s. costae primae
    costoclavicular s.
    cranial synchondroses
    synchondroses of
      cranium
    synchondroses cranii
    s. of first rib
    intersphenoidal s.
    intraoccipital s., anterior
    s. intraoccipitalis anterior
    s. intraoccipitalis posterior
    intraoccipital s., posterior
    manubriosternal s.
    s. manubriosternalis
    neurocentral s.
    petrooccipital s.
    s. petrooccipitalis
    posterior intraoccipital s.
    synchondroses of skull
    sphenobasilar s.
    sphenoethmoidal s.
    s. sphenoethmoidalis
    spheno-occipital s.
    s. sphenooccipitalis
    s. sphenopetrosa
    sternal synchondroses
    synchondroses sternales
synchondrotomy
synchorial
synchronia
synchronism
synchronization of potentials
synchronous
synchrony
    bilateral s.
synchrotron
synchysis scintillans
synclinal
synclitic
syncliticism
synclitism
synclonus beriberica
syncopal
syncope
    Adams-Stokes s.
    cardiac s.
    carotid sinus s.
    cough s.
    defecation s.
    deglutition s.
    digital s.
    heat s.

syncope *(continued)*
    laryngeal s.
    micturition s.
    orthostatic s.
    postural s.
    stretching s.
    swallow s.
    tussive s.
    vasodepressor s.
    vasovagal s.
syncretio
syncytial
    s. alteration
    respiratory s. virus (RSV)
    s. trophoblast
syncytiolysin
syncytioma malignum
syncytiotoxin
syncytiotrophoblast
syncytium
syncytoid
syndactylous
syndactylus
syndactyly
    complete s.
    complicated s.
    double s.
    partial s.
    simple s.
    single s.
    triple s.
syndectomy
syndesine
syndesis
syndesmectomy
syndesmectopia
syndesmitis metatarsea
syndesmochorial
syndesmodiastasis
syndesmography
syndesmologia
syndesmology
syndesmoma
syndesmo-odontoid
syndesmopexy
syndesmophyte
syndesmoplasty
syndesmorrhaphy
syndesmosis (syndesmoses)
    syndesmoses columnae
      vertebralis
    dentoalveolar s.
    s. dentoalveolaris
    radioulnar s.
    s. radioulnaris

syndesmosis (syndesmoses)
  (continued)
    syndesmoses thoracis
    tibiofibular s.
    s. tibiofibularis
    s. tympanostapedia
    tympanostapedial s.
    s. tympanostapedialis
    syndesmoses of vertebral
      column
syndesmotomy
syndrome
    Aarskog s.
    Aarskog-Scott s.
    Aase s.
    abdominal muscle deficiency s.
    abruptio placentae s.
    abstinence s.
    abused child s.
    accelerated conduction s.
    Achard s.
    Achard-Thiers s.
    acid aspiration s.
    acquired cerebellar s.
    acquired immunodeficiency s.
      (AIDS)
    acute brain s.
    acute cervical
      centromedullary s.
    acute nephritic s.
    acute organic brain s.
    acute radiation s.
    acute respiratory distress s.
      (ARDS)
    acute retinal necrosis s.
    Adair Dighton s.
    Adams-Stokes s.
    addisonian s.
    adherence s.
    Adie s.
    adiposogenital s.
    adrenal virilism s.
    adrenogenital s.
    Adson s.
    adult respiratory distress s.
      (ARDS)
    afferent loop s.
    aglossia-adactylia s.
    Ahumada-del Castillo s.
    Aicardi s.
    akinetic-abulic s.
    Alajouanine s.
    Albright s.
    Albright-McCune-Sternberg s.
    alcoholic pseudo-Cushing s.

syndrome *(continued)*
    alcohol withdrawal s.
    Aldrich s.
    Alezzandrini s.
    Alice in Wonderland s.
    Allemann s.
    allergic vasculitis s.
    Alport s.
    Alström (Alstrom) s.
    alveolar-capillary block s.
    alveolar hypoventilation s.
    amnesic s., amnestic s.
    amnestic-confabulatory s.
    amniotic band s.
    amniotic fluid s.
    amniotic infection s. of Blane
    amyostatic s.
    Andersen s.
    androgen insensitivity s.
    androgenital s.
    Angelucci s.
    angiectid s.
    anginal s.
    angular gyrus s.
    ankyloglossia superior s.
    anorectal s.
    anorexia-cachexia s.
    anterior abdominal wall s.
    anterior cerebral s.
    anterior chamber cleavage s.
    anterior choroidal artery s.
    anterior compartment s.
    anterior cord s.
    anterior cornual s.
    anterior spinal artery s.
    anterior tibial compartment s.
    anterior tibial nerve s.
    anterolateral s.
    antibody deficiency s.
    anticholinergic s.
    Anton s.
    Anton-Babinski s.
    anxiety s.
    aortic arch s.
    aortoiliac steal s.
    Apert s.
    s. of approximate answers
    argentaffinoma s.
    Arnold-Chiari s.
    Arnold nerve reflex cough s.
    arthrogryposis s.
    Ascher s.
    Asherman s.
    Asherson s.
    asplenia s.

S

syndrome *(continued)*

- ataxia-telangiectasia s.
- auriculotemporal s.
- autoerythrocyte sensitization s.
- autoimmune polyendocrine-candidiasis s.
- Avellis s.
- Axenfeld s.
- Ayerza s.
- Baastrup s.
- Babinski s.
- Babinski-Fröhlich s.
- Babinski-Nageotte s., s. of Babinski-Nageotte
- Babinski-Vaquez s.
- bacterial overgrowth s.
- Balint s.
- Baller-Gerold s.
- ballooning mitral valve s.
- ball valve s.
- Bannwarth s.
- Bardet-Biedl s.
- bare lymphocyte s.
- Barlow s.
- Barraquer-Simons s.
- Barré-Guillain s.
- Barrett s.
- Bart s.
- Bartter s.
- basal cell nevus s.
- Bassen-Kornzweig s.
- battered child s.
- Bazex s.
- Bearn-Kunkel s.
- Bearn-Kunkel-Slater s.
- Beckwith s.
- Beckwith-Wiedemann s.
- Benedikt s.
- Berardinelli-Seip s.
- Bernard s.
- Bernard-Horner s.
- Bernard-Sergent s.
- Bernard-Soulier s. (BSS)
- Bernheim s.
- Bertolotti s.
- Biemond s., II
- Bing-Neel s.
- Björnstad s.
- Blackfan-Diamond s.
- blind loop s.
- BLM (buccal-lingual-masticatory) s.
- Bloch-Sulzberger s.
- Bloom s.
- blue diaper s.

syndrome *(continued)*

- blue toe s.
- body of Luys s.
- Boerhaave s.
- Bonnet-Dechaume-Blanc s.
- Börjeson s.
- Börjeson-Forssman-Lehmann s.
- Bouillaud s.
- Bourneville-Pringle s.
- Bouveret s.
- bowel bypass s.
- boxer's s.
- brachial s.
- Brachmann-de Lange s.
- bradycardia-tachycardia s.
- brain s.
- brain death s.
- branchial s.
- Brennemann s.
- Briquet s.
- Brissaud-Sicard s.
- Bristowe s.
- brittle bones s.
- brittle cornea s.
- broad thumb-hallux s.
- Brock s.
- Brown-Séquard s.
- Brown vertical retraction s.
- Bruns s.
- Brunsting s.
- Brushfield-Wyatt s.
- buccal-lingual-masticatory (BLM) s.
- Buckley s.
- Budd-Chiari s.
- bulbar s.
- Bürger-Grütz (Buerger-Gruetz) s.
- Burnett s.
- burning feet s.
- Buschke-Ollendorff s.
- Bywaters s.
- Caffey s.
- Caffey-Silverman s.
- calcarine artery s.
- callosal s.
- camptomelic s.
- Canada-Cronkhite s.
- Capgras s.
- Caplan s.
- capsular thrombosis s.
- capsulothalamic s.
- carcinoid s.
- carotid sinus s.
- carpal tunnel s. (CTS)

syndrome *(continued)*
    Carpenter s.
    cartilage-hair hypoplasia s.
    cat-eye s., cat's eye s.
    cat's cry s.
    cauda equina s.
    causalgia s.
    cavernous sinus s.
    celiac s.
    celiac band s.
    central cord s.
    centroposterior s.
    cerebellar s.
    cerebellomedullary
      malformation s.
    cerebellopontine angle s.
    cerebellopyramidal s.
    cerebellosympathetic s.
    cerebellothalamic s.
    cerebrocardiac s.
    cerebrohepatorenal s.
    cervical s.
    cervical disk s.
    cervical fusion s.
    cervical radicular s.
    cervical rib s.
    cervical tension s.
    cervicobrachial s.
    cervicothoracic outlet s.
    Cestan s.
    Cestan-Chenais s.
    Cestan-Raymond s.
    chancriform s.
    Charcot s.
    Charcot-Marie s.
    Charcot-Weiss-Baker s.
    Chédiak-Higashi s.
    Chiari s.
    Chiari-Arnold s.
    Chiari-Frommel s.
    chiasma s.
    chiasmatic s.
    Chilaiditi s.
    Chinese restaurant s. (CRS)
    cholesterol emboli s.
    chorea s.
    chorioretinopathy and pituitary
      dysfunction (CPD) s.
    Chotzen s.
    Christian s.
    Christ-Siemens-Touraine s.
    chromosome breakage s.
    chronic brain s.
    chronic organic brain s.
    chubby puffer s.

syndrome *(continued)*
    Churg-Strauss s.
    Citelli s.
    Clarke-Hadfield s.
    Claude s.
    Claude Bernard–Horner s.
    click s.
    click-murmur s.
    closed head s.
    Clouston s.
    cloverleaf skull s.
    cloverleaf skull deformity s.
    clumsy child s.
    Cockayne s.
    Cogan s.
    cold agglutinin s.
    Collet s.
    Collet-Sicard s.
    compartment s.,
      compartmental s.
    compression s.
    concussion s.
    congenital rubella s.
    Conn s.
    Conradi s.
    Conradi-Hünermann s.
    contiguous gene s.
    contracture s.
    conus s.
    Cornelia de Lange s.
    coronary failure s.
    coronary intermediate s.
    corpora quadrigemina s.
    corpora quadrigeminal s.
    corpus callosum s.
    s. of the corpus Luysii
    s. of corpus striatum
    Costen s.
    costochondral s.
    costoclavicular s.
    costoclavicular compression s.
    Cotard s.
    cough s.
    Courvoisier-Terrier s.
    couvade s.
    CPD (chorioretinopathy and
      pituitary dysfunction) s.
    craniocarpotarsal s.
    craniosynostosis–radial
      aplasia s.
    CREST s.
    Creutzfeldt-Jakob s.
    cricopharyngeal achalasia s.
    cri du chat
    Crigler-Najjar s.

S

syndrome *(continued)*
    s. of crocodile tears
    Cronkhite-Canada s.
    Cross s.
    Cross-McKusick-Breen s.
    CRST s.
    crus s.
    crush s.
    Cruveilhier-Baumgarten s.
    cryptophthalmia-syndactyly s.
    cryptophthalmos s.
    cubital s.
    cubital tunnel s.
    culture-specific s.
    Curtius s.
    Cushing s.
    cushingoid s.
    Cushing s. medicamentosus
    cutaneomucouveal s.
    Cyriax s.
    cystic duct stump s.
    DaCosta s.
    Danbolt-Closs s.
    Debré-Semelaigne s.
    defibrination s.
    Dejean s.
    Dejerine s.
    Dejerine-Klumpke s.
    Dejerine-Roussy s.
    de Lange s.
    del Castillo s.
    de Morsier s.
    dengue shock s.
    Dennie-Marfan s.
    Denny-Brown s.
    depersonalization s.
    deposed child s.
    depressive s.
    de Quervain s.
    DES (diethylstilbestrol) s.
    De Sanctis-Cacchione s.
    de Toni-Fanconi s.
    dialysis disequilibrium s.
    Diamond-Blackfan s.
    DIDMOAD s.
    diencephalic s.
    diethylstilbestrol
      (DES) s.
    DiGeorge s.
    Di Guglielmo s.
    disk s.
    Donohue s.
    Down s.
    Dresbach s.
    Dressler s.

syndrome *(continued)*
    dry eye s.
    Duane s.
    Dubin-Johnson s.
    Dubin-Sprinz s.
    Dubreuil-Chambardel s.
    Duchenne s.
    Duchenne-Erb s.
    dumping s.
    Duncan s.
    Dyke-Davidoff-Masson s.
    dysarthria–clumsy hand s.
    dyscontrol s.
    dysequilibrium s.
    dysmnesic s.
    dysplasia oculodentodigitalis s.
    dysplastic nevus s.
    dystocia-dystrophia s.
    Eagle-Barrett s.
    Eaton-Lambert s.
    ectopic ACTH s.
    ectopic corticotropin-releasing
      hormone s.
    ectrodactyly-ectodermal
      dysplasia-clefting (EEC) s.
    Eddowes s.
    Edwards s.
    EEC s.
    effort s.
    egg-white s.
    Ehlers-Danlos s.
    Eisenmenger s.
    Ekbom s.
    elbow pain s.
    elfin facies s.
    Ellis-van Creveld s.
    embryonic testicular
      regression s.
    EMG s.
    emotional deprivation s.
    empty nest s.
    empty sella s.
    encephalotrigeminal vascular s.
    endocrine polyglandular s.
    eosinophilia-myalgia s.
    eosinophilic s.
    epiphyseal s.
    erythrocyte autosensitization s.
    erythroderma-atopy–bamboo
      hair s.
    euthyroid sick s.
    Evans s.
    exomphalos-macroglossia-
      gigantism (EMG) s.
    external carotid steal s.

syndrome *(continued)*

    extrapyramidal s.
    Faber s.
    facet s.
    faciodigitogenital s.
    Fanconi s.
    Farber s.
    Farber-Uzman s.
    Favre-Racouchot s.
    Felty s.
    feminizing testes s.
    fertile eunuch s.
    fetal alcohol s.
    fetal aspiration s.
    fetal distress s.
    fetal face s.
    fetal hydantoin s.
    fetal postmaturity s.
    fetal warfarin s.
    Fèvre-Languepin s.
    fibrosing s.
    Fiessinger-Leroy-Reiter s.
    first arch s.
    Fisher s.
    Fitz-Hugh–Curtis s.
    fleck s's
    floppy infant s.
    floppy valve s.
    focal dermal hypoplasia s.
    Foix s.
    Foix-Alajouanine s.
    Forbes-Albright s.
    Forsius-Eriksson s.
    Förster s.
    Förster atonic-astatic s.
    Foster Kennedy s.
    four-day s.
    Foville s.
    fragile X s.
    Franceschetti s.
    Franceschetti-Jadassohn s.
    François s.
    Fraser s.
    Freeman-Sheldon s.
    Frey s.
    Friderichsen-Waterhouse s.
    Friedmann vasomotor s.
    Fröhlich s.
    Froin s.
    Frommel-Chiari s.
    frontal lobe s.
    Fuchs s.
    functional bowel s.
    functional prepubertal
      castrate s.

syndrome *(continued)*

    G s.
    Gailliard s.
    galactorrhea-amenorrhea s.
    Ganser s.
    Garcin s.
    Gardner s.
    Gardner-Diamond s.
    Gasser s.
    gasserian ganglion s.
    gastrocardiac s.
    gastrojejunal loop obstruction s.
    gay bowel s.
    Gélineau s.
    gender dysphoria s.
    general adaptation s.
    genital ulcer s.
    Gerstmann s.
    Gianotti-Crosti s.
    giant platelet s.
    Gilbert s.
    Gilles de la Tourette s.
    Gjessing s.
    glioma-polyposis s.
    s. of globus pallidus
    glucagonoma s.
    Goldenhar s.
    Goltz s.
    Goltz-Gorlin s.
    gonadal agenesis s.
    Good s.
    Goodman s.
    Goodpasture s.
    Gopalan s.
    Gordon s.
    Gorlin s.
    Gorlin-Goltz s.
    Gorlin-Psaume s.
    Gougerot-Blum s.
    Gougerot-Carteaud s.
    Gougerot-Nulock-Houwer s.
    Gowers s.
    gracilis s.
    Gradenigo s.
    Graham Little s.
    gray s.
    gray baby s.
    gray platelet s.
    gray spinal s.
    Greig s.
    Griscelli s.
    Grisel s.
    Grönblad (Groenblad)-
      Strandberg s.
    Gruber s.

S

syndrome *(continued)*

    Guillain-Barré s.
    Gunn s.
    gustatory sweating s.
    gynandrism s.
    gynecomastia-
      aspermatogenesis s.
    Hadfield-Clarke s.
    Hakim s.
    Hallermann-Streiff s.
    Hallermann-Streiff-
      François s.
    Hallopeau-Siemens s.
    Hamman s.
    Hamman-Rich s.
    hand-foot s.
    hand-foot-uterus s.
    Hand-Schüller-Christian s.
    hand-shoulder s.
    Hanhart s.
    Hanot-Chauffard s.
    happy-puppet s.
    Harada s.
    Hare s.
    harlequin color change s.
    Harris s.
    Hartnup s.
    heart-hand s.
    Heerfordt s.
    Heidenhain s.
    HELLP s. (hemolysis,
      elevated liver enzymes,
      and low platelet count
      occurring in association with
      preeclampsia)
    hemangioma-
      thrombocytopenia s.
    hemiparaplegic s.
    hemiplegia, hemiconvulsions,
      and epilepsy (HHE) s.
    hemisphere s.
    hemohistioblastic s.
    hemolytic uremic s.
    hemopleuropneumonic s.
    Hench-Rosenberg s.
    Henoch-Schönlein (Henoch-
      Schoenlein) s.
    hepatocerebral s.
    hepatorenal s.
    hereditary benign
      intraepithelial
      dyskeratosis s.
    Hermansky-Pudlak s.
    herniated disk s.
    herpes gestationis s.

syndrome *(continued)*

    high-pressure neurologic s.
      (HPNS)
    Hoffmann-Werdnig s.
    holiday heart s.
    Holmes-Adie
    Holt-Oram s.
    Homén s.
    Horner s.
    Horner-Bernard s.
    Horton s.
    Howel-Evans s.
    Hunt s.
    Hunter s.
    Hurler s.
    Hurler-Scheie s.
    Hutchinson s.
    Hutchinson-Gilford s.
    Hutchison s.
    hyaline membrane s.
    hydralazine lupus s.
    17-hydroxylase deficiency s.
    hyperabduction s.
    hyperactive child s.
      (HACS)
    hypercalcemia s.
    hypereosinophilic s.
    hypergonadotropic s.
    hyperimmunoglobulinemia E
      (hyper IgE) s.
    hyperkinetic s.
    hyperkinetic heart s.
    hyperlucent lung s.
    hyperophthalmopathic s.
    hypersensitive xiphoid s.
    hypersomnia-bulimia s.
    hypertelorism-hypospadias s.
    hyperventilation s.
    hyperviscosity s.
    hypoglossia-hypodactyly s.
    hypo-osmolar s.
    hypophysial (hypophyseal) s.
    hypophysiodiencephalic s.
    hypophysis s.
    hypoplastic left heart s.
      (HLHS)
    hypospadias-dysphagia s.
    hypothalamic s.
    hypothalamic chiasmal s.
    hypothalamic commissural s.
    hypothalamohypophysial
      (hypothalamohypophyseal) s.
    hypotonic infant s.
    iatrogenic Cushing s.
    ICE (iridocorneal-endothelial) s.

syndrome *(continued)*

idiopathic Fanconi s. of adults
idiopathic postprandial s.
idiopathic respiratory distress s.
iliac compression s.
Imerslund s.
Imerslund-Graesbeck s.
immotile cilia s.
immunodeficiency s.
impingement s.
s. of inappropriate antidiuretic
  hormone (SIADH)
infantile cortical hyperostosis s.
inferior pontine s.
inferior s. of red nucleus
infraclinoid s.
infundibular s.
infundibulohypophysial
  (infundibulohypophyseal) s.
inhibitory s.
inspissated bile s.
inspissated milk s.
internal capsule s.
internal carotid artery s.
intestinal polyposis–cutaneous
  pigmentation s.
intrauterine parabiotic s.
irritable bowel s. (IBS)
Isaacs s.
Ivemark s.
Jaccoud s.
Jackson s.
Jacod s.
Jacod-Negri s.
Jadassohn-Lewandowsky s.
Jahnke s.
jaw-winking s.
Jefferson s.
jejunal s.
Jervell and Lange-Nielsen s.
Jeune s.
Job s.
Johanson-Blizzard s.
jugular foramen s.
Kallmann s.
Kanner s.
Kartagener s.
Kasabach-Merritt s.
Kast s.
Kearns-Sayre s.
Kennedy s.
Kenny-Caffey s.
keratitis-ichthyosis-deafness
  (KID) s.
KID s.

syndrome *(continued)*

kidney rejection s.
Kiloh-Nevin s.
Kimmelstiel-Wilson s.
kinky hair s.
Kinsbourne s.
kleeblattschädel s.
Kleine-Levin s.
Klein-Waardenburg s.
Klinefelter s.
Klippel-Feil s.
Klippel-Trénaunay s.
Klippel-Trénaunay-Weber s.
Klumpke-Dejerine s.
knee pain s.
Kocher-Debré-Sémélaigne s.
Koerber-Salus-Elschnig s.
König (Koenig) s.
Korsakoff s.
Kostmann s.
Krause s.
Kugelberg-Welander s.
Kunkel s.
Ladd s.
Lambert-Eaton s.
Lambert-Eaton myasthenic s.
Landry s.
Langer-Giedion s.
Laron s.
Larsen s.
laryngeal-vertigo s.
lateral bulbar s.
lateral cord and associated
  anterior cornual s.
lateral medullary s.
lateral pontine s.
Launois s.
Laurence-Moon s.
Lawrence-Seip s.
lazy leukocyte s. (LLS)
left heart hypoplasia s.
Legg-Calvé-Perthes s.
Lennox s.
Lennox-Gastaut s.
Lenz s.
LEOPARD s.
Leredde s.
Leriche s.
Lermoyez s.
Lesch-Nyhan s.
levator s.
Lévy-Roussy s.
Leyden-Möbius s.
Lichtheim s.
Liddle s.

S

syndrome *(continued)*
>   Lightwood s.
>   Lignac s.
>   Lignac-Fanconi s.
>   limp infant s.
>   liver-kidney s.
>   locked-in s.
>   locker-room s.
>   loculation s.
>   locus niger s.
>   Löffler s.
>   long QT s.
>   Looser-Milkman s.
>   Lorain-Lévi s.
>   Louis-Bar s.
>   Löwe s.
>   lower radicular s.
>   Löwe-Terrey-MacLachlan s.
>   Lown-Ganong-Levine s.
>   low-salt s.
>   low-sodium s.
>   Lucey-Driscoll s.
>   lupus-like s.
>   Lutembacher s.
>   Lyell s.
>   lymphadenopathy s.
>   lymphoproliferative s.
>   lymphoreticular s's
>   Mackenzie s.
>   Macleod s.
>   Maffucci s.
>   malabsorption s.
>   malarial hyperreactive spleen s.
>   male Turner s.
>   malignant hyperthermia s.
>   Mallory-Weiss s.
>   mandibulo-oculofacial s.
>   manic s.
>   Marchesani s.
>   Marchiafava-Micheli s.
>   Marcus Gunn s.
>   Marcus Gunn jaw-winking s.
>   Marfan s.
>   Marie-Bamberger s.
>   Marinesco-Sjögren s.
>   Martorell s.
>   massive bowel resection s.
>   mastocytosis s.
>   maternal s.
>   maternal deprivation s. (MDS)
>   maternal obesity s.
>   Mauriac s.
>   Mayer-Rokitansky-Küster-
>   Hauser s.
>   McCune-Albright s.

syndrome *(continued)*
>   Meckel s.
>   Meckel-Gruber s.
>   meconium aspiration s.
>   meconium blockage s.
>   meconium plug s.
>   medial longitudinal fasciculus s.
>   median medullary s.
>   megacystic s.
>   megacystis-megaureter s.
>   megacystis-microcolon–
>   intestinal hypoperistalsis s.
>   (MMIHS)
>   Meige s.
>   Meigs s.
>   Melkersson s.
>   Melkersson-Rosenthal s.
>   MEN (multiple endocrine
>   neoplasia) s.
>   Mendelson s.
>   meningeal s.
>   meningococcic adrenal s.
>   Menkes s.
>   metameric s.
>   metastatic carcinoid s.
>   methionine malabsorption s.
>   Meyer-Schwickerath and
>   Weyers s.
>   micrognathia-glossoptosis s.
>   middle cerebral artery s.
>   middle lobe s.
>   midline s.
>   Mikulicz s.
>   milk-alkali s.
>   Milkman s.
>   Millard-Gubler s.
>   Miller s.
>   Miller Fisher s.
>   minimal brain dysfunction
>   (MBD) s.
>   minimal chronic brain s.
>   Minkowski-Chauffard s.
>   minor contusion s.
>   Minot-von Willebrand s.
>   mitral valve prolapse s.
>   Möbius s.
>   Mohr s. s.
>   Moore s.
>   morbid hunger s.
>   Morel s.
>   Morgagni-Adams-Stokes s.
>   morning glory s.
>   Morquio s.
>   Morris s.
>   Morton s.

syndrome *(continued)*
- Morvan s.
- Mosse s.
- motor radicular s.
- Mounier-Kuhn s.
- Mount s.
- Mount-Reback s.
- Moynahan s.
- Muckle-Wells s.
- mucocutaneous lymph node s. (MLNS)
- mucosal neuroma s.
- multiple endocrine neoplasia (MEN) s.
- multiple glandular deficiency s.
- multiple hamartoma s.
- multiple lentigines s.
- Münchausen s.
- Munchausen s. by proxy
- myasthenia gravis s.
- myasthenic s.
- myasthenic-myopathic s.
- myelofibrosis-osteosclerosis s.
- myeloproliferative s.
- myocardial postinfarction s.
- myokymia-hyperhidrosis s.
- myonephropathic metabolic s.
- myotonia congenita s.
- Naegeli s.
- Naffziger s.
- Nager s.
- nail-patella s.
- Nelson s.
- neocerebellar s.
- neonatal thymectomy s.
- nephrotic s.
- nerve compression s.
- Netherton s.
- Nettleship-Falls s.
- neurocutaneous s.
- neuroleptic malignant s.
- nevoid basal cell carcinoma s.
- nevoid basaloma s.
- Nezelof s.
- night-eating s.
- nitritoid s.
- Noack s.
- Nonne-Milroy-Meige s.
- nonpsychotic organic brain s.
- nonsense s.
- nonstaphylococcal scalded skin s.
- Noonan s.
- Nothnagel s.
- OAV (oculoauriculovertebral) s.

syndrome *(continued)*
- occipital horn s.
- ocular–mucous membrane s.
- oculoauriculovertebral (OAV) s.
- oculobuccogenital s.
- oculocerebral-hypopigmentation s.
- oculocerebrorenal s.
- oculocutaneous s.
- oculodentodigital (ODD) s.
- oculodento-osseous s.
- oculoglandular s.
- oculomandibulofacial s.
- oculopharyngeal s.
- oculovertebral s.
- oculovestibuloauditory s.
- ODD (oculodentodigital) s.
- odor-of-sweaty-feet s.
- OFD (oral-facial-digital) s. (types I–III)
- Ogilvie s.
- Oldfield s.
- olfactory groove s.
- OMM (ophthalmomandibulomelic) s.
- ophthalmomandibulomelic (OMM) s.
- ophthalmoplegia-ataxia-areflexia s.
- opticopyramidal s.
- oral-facial-digital, orofaciodigital (OFD) s. (types I–III)
- orbital apex s.
- organic anxiety s.
- organic brain s.
- organic delusional s.
- organic mental s.
- organic mood s.
- organic personality s.
- orogenital s.
- osteomyelofibrotic s.
- Ostrum-Furst s.
- otopalatodigital s.
- outlet s.
- ovarian-remnant s.
- ovarian vein s.
- overlap s.
- oversuppression s.
- overwear s.
- Paget-von Schroetter s.
- pain dysfunction s.
- painful arc s.
- painful bruising s.
- paleocerebellar s.

S

syndrome *(continued)*

- paleostriatal s.
- pallidal s.
- pallidomesencephalic s.
- Pancoast s.
- pancreatic cholera s.
- pancreatic insufficiency s.
- pancreaticohepatic s.
- pancytopenia-dysmelia s.
- papillary muscle s.
- Papillon-Lefevre s.
- paralysis agitans s.
- paramedian s.
- paramedian pontine s.
- paraneoplastic s.
- paratrigeminal s.
- parietal s.
- Parinaud s.
- Parinaud oculoglandular s.
- parkinsonian s.
- Parry-Romberg s.
- Patau s.
- Paterson s.
- Paterson–Brown Kelly s.
- Paterson-Kelly s.
- peduncular s.
- Pellegrini-Stieda s.
- Pellizzi s.
- pelvic congestion s.
- Pendred s.
- Pepper s.
- pericolic membrane s.
- periodic s.
- periodic somnolence s.
- persistent müllerian duct s.
- pertussis s.
- pertussis-like s.
- petrosphenoid s.
- Peutz-Jeghers s.
- Pfeiffer s.
- pharyngeal pouch s.
- PHC s.
- phobic anxiety-depersonalization s.
- pickwickian s.
- PIE s.
- Pierre Robin s.
- pigment dispersion s.
- pineal s.
- pituitary s.
- placental dysfunction s.
- placental hemangioma s.
- placental transfusion s.
- pleurideficiency s.

syndrome *(continued)*

- Plummer-Vinson s.
- pluriglandular s.
- Poland s.
- Polhemus-Schafer-Ivemark s.
- polyangiitis overlap s.
- polycystic ovary s.
- polyglandular s.
- polyposis coli s.
- poly-X s.
- pontine s.
- pontocerebellar angle s.
- popliteal entrapment s.
- popliteal pterygium s.
- popliteal web s.
- postcardiac injury s.
- postcardiotomy s.
- postcardiotomy psychosis s.
- postcholecystectomy s.
- postcommissurotomy s.
- postconcussional s.
- posterior cerebral artery s.
- posterior column s.
- posterior cord s.
- posterior cranial fossa s.
- posterior inferior cerebellar artery s.
- posterior lacertocondylar s.
- posterolateral s.
- postgastrectomy s.
- postgonococcal urethritis s.
- postinfarction s.
- postirradiation s.
- post–lumbar puncture s.
- postmaturity s.
- post–myocardial infarction s.
- postpartum panhypopituitary s.
- postpartum pituitary necrosis s.
- postperfusion s.
- postpericardiotomy s.
- postphlebitic s.
- postpump s. (PPS)
- post-thrombotic s.
- post-transfusion s.
- post-traumatic brain s.
- post-traumatic cervical s.
- postvalvulotomy s.
- Potter s.
- P pulmonale s.
- Prader-Willi s.
- preexcitation s.
- premature senility s.
- premenstrual s. (PMS)

syndrome *(continued)*
   premotor s.
   primary fibromyalgia s.
   prisoner of war s.
   pronator s.
   prune-belly s.
   pseudo–Argyll Robertson s.
   pseudoclaudication s.
   pseudo–Cushing s.
   pseudo–Turner s.
   puffy hand s.
   pulmonary acid aspiration s.
   pulmonary dysmaturity s.
   pulmonary infiltration with
      eosinophilia (PIE) s.
   pulmonary-renal s.
   punch-drunk s.
   Putnam-Dana s.
   pyramidal and hypoglossal
      nerve s.
   QT s.
   radial s.
   radial aplasia-
      thrombocytopenia s.
   radiation s.
   radicular s.
   radiculoneuritic s.
   Raeder s.
   Raeder paratrigeminal s.
   Ramsay Hunt s.
   Raymond-Cestan s.
   red diaper s.
   Reifenstein s.
   Reiter s.
   release s.
   Rendu-Osler-Weber s.
   residual ovary s.
   respiratory distress s. (RDS)
   respiratory distress s. (RDS) of
      newborn
   restless legs s.
   retraction s.
   retrolenticular s.
   retrolenticular capsule s.
   s. of retroparotid space
   retrosubthalamic s.
   Rett s.
   Reye s.
   Rh-null s.
   rib tip s.
   Richards-Rundle s.
   Richner-Hanhart s.
   Richter s.
   Rieger s.

syndrome *(continued)*
   right ovarian vein s.
   Riley-Day s.
   Riley-Smith s.
   Robert s.
   Robin s.
   Robinow s.
   Rochan-Duvigneaud s.
   Rokitansky-Küster-Hauser s.
   rolandic vein s.
   Rollet s.
   Romano-Ward s.
   Rosenberg-Chutorian s.
   Rosenthal s.
   Rosenthal-Kloepfer s.
   Rosewater s.
   rotational shift s.
   Roth (Rot) s.
   Roth-Bernhardt
      (Rot-Bernhardt) s.
   Rothmann-Makai s.
   Rothmund-Thomson s.
   Rotor s.
   Roussy-Dejerine s.
   Roussy-Lévy s.
   Rovsing s.
   RSH s.
   rubella s.
   Rubinstein s.
   Rubinstein-Taybi s.
   rubrospinal cerebellar
      peduncle s.
   Rud s.
   rudimentary testis s.
   Rundles-Falls s.
   runting s.
   Russell s.
   Russell-Silver s.
   Rust s.
   Ruvalcaba s.
   Sabin-Feldman s.
   Saethre-Chotzen s.
   sagittal imbalance s.
   Sakati-Nyhan s.
   salt-depletion s.
   salt-losing s.
   Sandifer s.
   Sanfilippo s.
   scalded skin s.,
      nonstaphylococcal
   scalded skin s., staphylococcal
   scalenus s.
   scalenus anticus s.
   scapulocostal s.

S

syndrome *(continued)*
    Schäfer s.
    Schanz s.
    Schaumann s.
    Scheie s.
    Schirmer s.
    Schmidt s.
    Schönlein-Henoch
      (Schoenlein-Henoch) s.
    Schüller s.
    Schüller-Christian s.
    Schultz s.
    Schwachman s.
    Schwartz-Jampel s.
    scimitar s.
    sea-blue histiocytes s.
    Seabright bantam s.
    sebaceous nevus s.
    Seckel s.
    second impact s.
    segmentary s.
    Selye s.
    Senear-Usher s.
    s. of sensory dissociation with
      brachial amyotrophy
    Senter s.
    Sertoli-cell–only s.
    serum sickness–like s.
    Sézary s.
    shaken baby s.
    Sheehan s.
    short-bowel s.
    short-gut s.
    short PR s.
    shoulder girdle s.
    shoulder-hand s.
    shoulder-neck s.
    Shwachman s.
    Shwachman-Diamond s.
    Shy-Drager s.
    Sicard s.
    sicca s.
    sick sinus s. (SSS)
    sideropenic s.
    Silfverskiold s.
    Silver s.
    Silver-Russell s.
    Silvestrini-Corda s.
    Simmonds s.
    Sipple s.
    Sjögren s.
    Sjögren-Larsson s.
    sleep apnea s.
    SLE-like s.
    slick-gut s.

syndrome *(continued)*
    Sluder s.
    Sly s.
    small left colon s.
    small-meal s.
    Smith-Lemli-Opitz s.
    social breakdown s.
    Sohval-Soffer s.
    somnolence s.
    Sorsby s.
    Sotos s.
    Sotos s. of cerebral gigantism
    space adaptation s.
    Spens s.
    spherophakia-brachymorphia s.
    spinal block s.
    splenic flexure s.
    split brain s.
    Sprinz-Dubin s.
    Sprinz Nelson s.
    Spurway s.
    stagnant loop s.
    staphylococcal scalded skin s.
    stasis s.
    static cerebellar s.
    steal s.
    Steele-Richardson-Olszewski s.
    steely-hair s.
    Stein-Leventhal s.
    steroid withdrawal s.
    Stevens-Johnson s.
    Stewart-Treves s.
    Stickler s.
    stiff heart s.
    stiff man s.
    Stilling s.
    Stilling-Türk-Duane s.
    stippled epiphyses s.
    Stokes s.
    Stokes-Adams s.
    Stokvis-Talma s.
    Strachan s.
    Strachan-Scott s.
    straight back s.
    striatal s.
    striocortical s.
    striopallidal s.
    stroke s.
    Sturge s.
    Sturge-Kalischer-Weber s.
    Sturge-Weber s.
    subclavian steal s.
    subcoracoid–pectoralis
      minor s.
    substantia nigra s.

syndrome *(continued)*

   subthalamic s.

   sudden infant death s. (SIDS)

   sudden unexplained death s. (SUDS)

   Sudeck-Leriche s.

   Sulzberger-Garbe s.

   sump s.

   superior caval s.

   superior cerebellar artery s.

   superior mesenteric artery s.

   superior midbrain s.

   superior oblique tendon sheath s.

   superior orbital fissure s.

   superior pontine s.

   superior sulcus tumor s.

   superior vena cava s.

   supine hypotensive s.

   suprarenogenic s.

   supraspinatus s.

   supravalvular aortic stenosis s.

   surdocardiac s.

   survivor s.

   swallowed blood s.

   sweat retention s.

   sweaty feet s.

   Sweet s.

   Swyer s.

   Swyer-James s.

   sylvian s.

   syringomyelic s.

   Takayasu s.

   Tapia s.

   TAR s.

   tarsal tunnel s.

   Taussig-Bing s.

   tegmental s.

   telangiectasia–pigmentation cataract s.

   temporal pyramidal apex s.

   temporomandibular dysfunction s.

   temporomandibular joint (TMJ) s.

   Terry s.

   Terson s.

   testicular dysgenesis s.

   testicular feminization s.

   testicular feminizing s.

   tethered cord s.

   tetra-X s.

   thalamic s.

   thalidomide s.

   Thibierge-Weissenbach s.

syndrome *(continued)*

   Thiele s.

   Thiemann s.

   third and fourth pharyngeal arch s.

   third and fourth pharyngeal pouch s.

   thoracic outlet s.

   Thorn s.

   thrombocytopenia–absent radius (TAR) s.

   thromboembolic s.

   thrombopathic s.

   Tietze s.

   Tolosa-Hunt s.

   Tommaselli s.

   TORCH (toxoplasmosis, other agents, rubella, cytomegalovirus, herpes simplex) s.

   Torres s.

   Touraine-Solente-Golé s.

   Tourette s.

   toxic fat s.

   toxic shock s.

   transcortical s.

   transfusion s.

   translocation Down s.

   transplant lung s.

   traumatic vasospastic s.

   Treacher Collins s.

   Treacher Collins–Franceschetti s.

   triad s.

   trichorhinophalangeal s.

   triparanol s.

   triple-A s.

   trisomy 8 s.

   trisomy 13 s.

   trisomy 18 s.

   trisomy 21 s.

   trisomy 22 s.

   trisomy C s.

   trisomy D s.

   trisomy E s.

   Troisier s.

   tropical splenomegaly s.

   Trousseau s.

   tuberohypophysial (tuberohypophyseal) s.

   tuberoinfundibular s.

   tumor lysis s.

   Turcot s.

   Turner s.

   Turner s., male

S

syndrome *(continued)*
    Ullrich-Feichtiger s.
    Ullrich-Turner s.
    ulnar tunnel s.
    unilateral hyperlucent lung s.
    unilateral nevoid
      telangiectasia s.
    Unna-Thost s.
    upper brachial plexus s.
    urethral s.
    Usher s.
    uveoparotid s.
    vagoaccessory s.
    van Buchem s.
    van der Hoeve s.
    vanishing testes s.
    vascular s.
    vasculitis-hypersensitivity s.
    velopalatine myoclonic s.
    Verner-Morrison s.
    Vernet s.
    vertebrobasilar s.
    vertical retraction s.
    Villaret s.
    Vinson s.
    Vogt s.
    Vogt-Koyanagi s.
    Vogt-Koyanagi-Harada s.
    Vohwinkel s.
    Volkmann s.
    vulnerable child s.
    Waardenburg s.
    WAGR s.
    Wallenberg s.
    Ward-Romano s.
    wasting s.
    Waterhouse-Friderichsen s.
    Watson s.
    WDHA s.
    Weber s.
    Weber-Cockayne s.
    Weber-Gubler s.
    Weber-Leyden s.
    Wegener s.
    Weil s.
    Weill-Marchesani s.
    Weingarten s.
    Wermer s.
    Werner s.
    Wernicke-Korsakoff s.
    West s.
    Weyers oligodactyly s.
    whiplash shake s.
    whistling face–windmill vane
      hand s.

syndrome *(continued)*
    Widal s.
    Willebrand s.
    Williams s.
    Williams-Campbell s.
    Wilson-Mikity s.
    Winter s.
    Wiskott-Aldrich s.
    withdrawal s.
    Wolff-Parkinson-White s.
      (WPW)
    Wolfram s.
    WPW s.
    Wright s.
    s. X
    X-linked lymphoproliferative s.
    XXXY s.
    XXY s.
    yellow nail s.
    Young s.
    ZE s.
    Zellweger s.
    Zieve s.
    Zinsser-Cole-Engman s.
    Zollinger-Ellison s. (ZES)
syndromic
synechia (synechiae)
    annular s.
    anterior s.
    circular s.
    s. pericardii
    posterior s.
    ring s.
    total anterior s.
    total posterior s.
    s. vulvae
synechialysis
synechotome
synechotomy
synechtenterotomy
synecology
synencephalocele
synencephalus
synencephaly
syneresis
synergenesis
synergetic
synergic
synergism
synergist
synergistic
synergy
synesthesia algica
synesthesialgia
syngamous

syngamy
syngenesiograft
syngenesioplastic
syngenesiotransplantation
syngenesis
syngnathia
syngonic
syngraft
synhexyl
synhidrosis
synizesis pupillae
synkaryon
synkinesis
    brachiobranchial s.
    contralateral s.
    coordination s.
    crurocrural s.
    imitative s.
    mouth-and-hand s.
    reflex s.
    spasmodic s.
synkinetic
synnecrosis
synnematin
synneurosis
synocha
synochal
synonychia
synonymize
synophrys
synophthalmia
synophthalmus
synoptophore
synorchidism
synorchism
synoscheos
synosteology
synosteotic
synosteotomy
synostosis (synostoses)
    cranial s.
    radioulnar s.
    sagittal s.
    tarsal s.
    transphalangeal s.
    tribasilar s.
synotia
synotus
synovectomy
    radioisotope s.
synovia
synovial
    s. biopsy
    s. chondrosarcoma
    s. frost

synovial *(continued)*
    s. histopathology
    s. osteochondromatosis
    s. sarcoma
    s. stromal cells
synovialis
synovianalysis
synovin
synovioblast
synoviocyte
synovioma
    benign s.
    malignant s.
synoviorthesis
synoviorthosis
synoviosarcoma
synoviparous
synovitis
    bursal s.
    chronic purulent s.
    dendritic s.
    dry s.
    filiarial s.
    fungous s.
    s. hyperplastica
    localized nodular s.
    pigmented
      villonodular s.
    proliferative s.
    puerperal s.
    purulent s.
    scarlatinal s.
    serous s.
    s. sicca
    simple s.
    suppurative s.
    tendinous s.
    transient s.
    traumatic s.
    tuberculous s.
    vaginal s.
    vibration s.
    villonodular s.
synpneumonic
synreflexia
syntactic
syntasis
syntaxis
syntectic
syntenic
syntenosis
synteny
synteresis
synteretic
syntexis

S

synthase
  lanosterol s.
  pantothenate s.
synthermal
synthesis
  s. of continuity
  de novo s.
  distributive s.
  DNA s.
  inducible enzyme s.
  morphologic s.
  protein s.
  unscheduled DNA s.
synthesize
synthesizer
  speech s.
synthetase
  heme s.
synthetic
synthetism
synthorax
syntonic
syntonin
syntopie, syntopy
syntopy
syntripsis
syntrophism
syntrophoblast
syntropic
syntropy
  inverse s.
synulosis
synulotic
synxenic
Syphacia obvelata
syphilemia
syphilid
  acuminate papular s.
  annular s.
  ecthymatous s.
  erythematous s.
  follicular s.
  macular s.
  papulosquamous s.
  pemphigoid s.
  pigmentary s.
  pustular s.
  roseolar s.
  secondary s.
  serpiginous s.
syphilidophthalmia
syphilis
  acquired s.
  anorectal s.
  cardiovascular s.

syphilis *(continued)*
  cerebrospinal s.
  congenital s.
  s. of conjunctiva
  s. d'emblée
  early s.
  early latent s.
  endemic s.
  equine s.
  gummatous s.
  s. hereditaria tarda
  s. of iris
  late s.
  late benign s.
  late latent s.
  latent s.
  latent s., early
  latent s., late
  meningovascular s.
  noduloulcerative s.
  nonvenereal s.
  parenchymatous s.
  prenatal s.
  primary s.
  secondary s.
  serologic test for s. (STS)
  tertiary s.
syphilitic
syphiloma
syphilomania
syphilomatous
syphilonechia
  s. sicca
  s. ulcerans
syphilophobia
syphilopsychosis
syrigmophonia
syrigmus
syringadenoma
  papillary s.
syringadenosis
syringe
  air s.
  aural s.
  chip s.
  continuous-flow s.
  dental s.
  ear s.
  fountain s.
  hand air s.
  hypodermic s.
  irrigating s.
  Luer s.
  Luer-Lok s.
  probe s.

syringe *(continued)*
    Toomey s.
    two-way s.
    water s.
    wound s.
syringectomy
syringitis
syringoadenoma
syringobulbia
syringocarcinoma
syringocele
syringocoele
syringocystadenoma
    papillary s.
    s. papilliferum
syringoencephalia
syringoencephalomyelia
syringoid
syringoma
    chondroid s.
    eruptive s.
syringomeningocele
    traumatic s.
syringomyelia
    s. atrophica
    posttraumatic s.
    traumatic s.
syringomyelitis
syringomyelobulbia
syringomyelocele
syringomyelus
syringopontia
syringotome
syringotomy
syrinx
syrosingopine
syrup
syssarcosis
syssarcotic
syssomus
systaltic
systatic
system
    ABO blood group s.
    accessory portal s. of Sappey
    adipose s.
    adrenergic s.
    alimentary s.
    anesthesia-breathing s.
    arch-loop-whorl s.
    ascending reticular-activating s.
    association s.
    autonomic nervous s.
    balanced lethal s.
    s. of Batson

system *(continued)*
    biliary s.
    biological s.
    blood group s.
    blood-vascular s.
    boarding-out s.
    body exhaust s.
    Boorman gastric cancer
      typing s.
    brain cooling s.
    brain stem-activating s.
    breathing s.
    buffer s.
    bulbospiral s.
    cardiovascular s.
    case s.
    catenary s.
    centimeter-gram-second
      (CGS) s.
    central nervous s. (CNS)
    centrencephalic s.
    cerebellorubral s.
    cerebellorubrospinal s.
    cerebrospinal s.
    CGS
      (centimeter-gram-second) s.
    CGS electromagnetic s.
    chemoreceptor s.
    chromaffin s.
    circle absorption s.
    circulatory s.
    coherent s. of units
    colloid s.
    colloidal s.
    complement s.
    complete nonrebreathing s.
    conducting s. of heart
    conduction s. of heart
    coordinate s.
    corticobulbar s.
    corticopontine projection s.
    corticopontocerebellar s.
    corticostrionigral s.
    craniosacral autonomic
      nervous s.
    cutaneous s.
    dentatorubral s.
    dentinal s.
    dermal s.
    dermoid s.
    digestive s.
    dioptric s.
    disperse s.
    dispersion s.
    dopaminergic s.

S

system *(continued)*
- dosimetric s.
- dual-probe s.
- duplex scanning s.
- ecological s.
- Edmondson Grading S.
- endocrine s.
- endothelial s.
- endovestibular s.
- exteroceptive nervous s.
- extracorticospinal s.
- extrapyramidal s.
- flush s.
- fusimotor s.
- Galton s. of classification of fingerprints
- gamma efferent s.
- gamma motor s.
- genital s.
- genitourinary s.
- glandular s.
- Grosse and Kempf locking nail s.
- H-2 histocompatibility s.
- haversian s.
- hematopoietic s.
- hemolytic s.
- Henry s. of classification of fingerprints
- hepatic duct s.
- hepatic portal s.
- heterogeneous s.
- hexaxial reference s.
- His-Purkinje s.
- HLA histocompatibility s.
- homogeneous s.
- hormonopoietic s.
- humoral amplification s's
- hypophyseoportal s., hypophysioportal s.
- hypothalamohypophyseal s.
- hypothalamo-hypophysial (hypothalamo-hypophyseal) s.
- hypothalamohypophysial (hypothalamohypophyseal) portal s.
- hypothalamoneurohypophysial (hypothalamoneur-ohypophyseal) s.
- hypoxia warning s.
- immune s.
- inducible s.
- integumentary s.
- interfusal motor s.

system *(continued)*
- International 10-20 s.
- International S. of Units
- interoceptive nervous s.
- interofective s.
- interrenal s.
- interstitial s.
- involuntary nervous s.
- Jewett-Strong s.
- kallikrein s.
- kallikrein-kinin s.
- keratinizing s.
- kinesiodic s.
- kinety s.
- kinin s.
- labyrinthine s.
- limbic s.
- linear s.
- Luhr maxillofacial s.
- lymphatic s.
- lymphoid s.
- lymphoreticular s.
- macrophage s.
- malpighian s.
- mammillary s.
- Manchester s.
- masticatory s.
- mastigont s.
- McIntire aspiration-irrigation s.
- melanocyte s.
- metameric nervous s.
- metanephric excretory s.
- metanephric secretory s.
- meter-kilogram-second (MKS) s.
- metric s.
- Meyer s.
- microcirculatory s.
- MKS (meter-kilogram-second) s.
- mobile artery and vein imaging s. (MAVIS)
- mononuclear phagocyte s. (MPS)
- muscular s.
- musculoskeletal s.
- neokinetic s.
- nervous s.
- neuromuscular s.
- nonspecific s.
- oculomotor s.
- open s.
- pallidal s.
- palm-and-sole s. of identification
- parasympathetic nervous s.

system *(continued)*
- peripheral nervous s.
- periventricular s.
- phagocytic s.
- pigmentary s.
- Pinel s.
- pituitary portal s.
- plenum s.
- pneumatic s. of temporal bone
- portal s.
- pressoreceptor s.
- projection s.
- properdin s.
- proprioceptive nervous s.
- Purkinje s.
- pyramidal s.
- renin-angiotensin s. (RAS)
- renin-angiotensin-
  aldosterone s.
- reproductive s.
- resonating s.
- respiratory s.
- reticular-activating s. (RAS)
- reticuloendothelial s. (RES)
- rubrospinal s.
- schlieren s.
- self s.
- sensory storage s.
- SI (Système International
  d'Unités) s.
- sinospiral s.
- skeletal s.
- somatic nervous s.
- somesthetic s.
- stomatognathic s.
- supraopticohypophyseal s.
- sympathetic nervous s.
- T s.
- thoracicolumbar autonomic
  nervous s.
- three-compartment s.
- three-phase s.
- TNM (tumor, node, metastasis)
  staging s.
- to-and-fro absorption s.
- triad s.
- two-compartment s.
- urinary s.
- urinary s., uropoietic s.
- urogenital s.
- uropoietic s.
- vagal autonomic s.
- vascular s.
- vasomotor s.

system *(continued)*
- vegetative nervous s.
- vertebral-basilar s.
- vertebral-venous s.
- vestibular s.
- villa s.
- visceral nervous s.

systema
- s. articulare
- s. conducens cordis
- s. digestorium
- s. genitale femininum
- s. genitale masculinum
- s. lymphoideum
- s. musculare
- s. nervosum
- s. nervosum autonomicum
- s. nervosum centrale
- s. nervosum periphericum
- s. respiratorium
- s. skeletale
- s. urinarium

systematic
systematics
systematization
systematology
Système International d'Unités (SI)
système sécant
systemic
- s. lupus
  erythematosus (SLE)
- s. sclerosis
- s. vasculitis
systemoid
systole
- aborted s.
- arterial s.
- atrial s.
- auricular s.
- cataplectic s.
- end s.
- extra s.
- frustrate s.
- hemic s.
- premature s.
- ventricular s.
systolic
- s. anterior motion (SAM)
- s. apical impulse
- s. click-murmur syndrome
- s. current
- s. function
- s. motion
- s. murmur

S

systolic *(continued)*
    s. pressure-time index
    s. reserve
    s. time interval
systolometer
systremma
syzygial

syzygiology
syzygy
Sz—schizophrenia
Szabo test
Szent-Györgyi reaction
Szymanowski operation
Szymanowski-Kuhnt operation

T

τ—
    tau (Greek letter)
T—
    temperature
    tension (intraocular)
    time
    tumor
T.—
    Taenia
    Treponema
    Trichophyton
    Trypanosoma
T– (T minus); T⁻—decreased
  intraocular tension (T–1, T–2,
  etc.)
T+ (T plus); T⁺—increased
  intraocular tension (T+1, T+2, etc.)
$T_{1/2}$—
    half-life
    half-time
T1 through T12—thoracic
  vertebrae 1–12
T_1-weighted [T1-]
T_2-weighted [T2-]
T_3 [T3]—triiodothyronine (test)
T_3 RU (resin uptake) [T3]
T_4 [T4]—thyroxine (test)
TA—
    therapeutic abortion
    toxin-antitoxin
T&A—tonsillectomy and
  adenoidectomy
TA-Ab—teichoic acid antibody
TA-AIDS—transfusion-associated
  AIDS
tab.—tablet
tabacosis
tabacum
tabagism

tabanid fly
tabatière anatomique
Tabb
    curet
    flap knife
tabby cat
    t.c. heart
    t.c. striations
tabella (tabellae)
tabernanthine
tabes
    diabetic t.
    t. dorsalis
    t. ergotica
    Friedreich t.
    t. infantum
    t. mesenterica
    t. spinalis
tabescent
tabetic
    t. arthropathy
    t. bladder
    t. crisis
    t. cuirass
    t. dissociation
    d. foot
    t. gait
    t. mask
    t. neurosyphilis
    t. otalgia
tabetiform
tabification
tablature
table
    Aub-Dubois t.
    external t. of calvaria
    inner t. of frontal bone
    inner t. of skull
    internal t. of calvaria

table *(continued)*
  outer t. of frontal bone
  outer t. of skull
  periodic t. of elements
  tilt t.
  vitreous t.
tablespoon (tbs., tbsp.)
tablet
  buccal t.
  dispensing t.
  enteric-coated t.
  hypodermic t.
  sublingual t.
  t. triturate
taboo
taboparalysis
taboparesis
tabourka
  bruit de t.
tabula (tabulae)
  t. externa ossis cranii
  t. interna ossis cranii
tabular
tabun
Tacaribe
  T. complex
  T. virus
TACE—
  transarterial
    chemoembolization
  tumor necrosis factor–
    alpha-converting enzyme
tache
  t. blanche
  t. bleuâtre
  t. cérébrale
  t. méningéale
  t. motrice
  t. noire
  t's noire sclérotique
  t. spinale
tachistoscopy
tachogram
tachography
tachyalimentation
tachyarrhythmia
  early atrial t.
  implantable atrial t.
    monitor
  malignant polymorphic
    ventricular t.
  uncontrollable t.
  uncontrolled t.
  ventricular t.
tachyauxesis

tachycardia
  antidromic t.
  antidromic atrioventricular
    (AV) reciprocating t.
  atrial t.
  atrioventricular (AV) t.
  atrioventricular (AV)
    junctional t.
  atrioventricular (AV) nodal
    reentrant t.
  atrioventricular (AV)
    reciprocating t.
  benign ventricular t.
  bidirectional ventricular t.
  bradycardia-t. syndrome
  chaotic atrial t.
  circus movement t.
  t.-dependent aberrancy
  double t.
  ectopic t.
  endless loop t.
  fetal t.
  junctional t.
  monomorphic ventricular t.
  multifocal atrial t.
  nodal t.
  nonparoxysmal junctional t.
  nonsustained ventricular t.
  orthodromic atrioventricular
    (AV) reciprocating t.
  orthostatic t.
  pacemaker-mediated t.
  paroxysmal t.
  paroxysmal atrial t.
  paroxysmal nodal t.
  paroxysmal supraventricular t.
  permanent junctional
    reciprocating t.
  polymorphic ventricular t.
  reciprocating t.
  reentrant t.
  reflex t.
  sinus t. (ST)
  sinus reentrant t.
  supraventricular t.
  sustained ventricular t.
  ventricular t.
tachycardiac
tachycardic
tachydysrhythmia
tachygastria
tachygenesis
tachykinin
tachylalia
tachylogia

T

tachymeter
tachyphagia
tachyphasia
tachyphemia
tachyphrasia
tachyphylaxis
tachypnea
    influenza A–induced t.
    influenza-associated t.
    intermittent t.
    transient t. of the newborn
      (TTN)
    virus-induced t.
tachysterol
tachysystole
    atrial t.
    uterine t.
tachytrophism
tachyzoite
tack operation
tactic
tacticity
tactile
    t. agnosia
    t. amnesia
    t. anesthesia
    t. aphasia
    t. cell, Merkel t. cell
    t. corpuscle of Meissner
    t. disk
    t. elevations
    t. fremitus
    t. hallucination
    t. hyperesthesia
    t. hypoesthesia
    t. meniscus
    t. receptor
    t. sense
taction
tactoid
tactual
TADAC—therapeutic abortion,
   dilation, aspiration, curettage
taenia (taeniae)
    taeniae acusticae
    t. choroidea
    taeniae coli
    t. fornicis
    t. of fourth ventricle
    t. libera
    medullary t. of thalamus
    t. mesocolica
    t. omentalis
    t. pontis
    t. telae
    t. terminalis

taenia (taeniae) *(continued)*
    t. thalami
    t. of third ventricle
    t. tubae
    t. ventriculi quarti
Taenia
    T. africana
    T. bremneri
    T. confusa
    T. cucurbitina
    T. mediocanellata
    T. philippina
    T. saginata
    T. solium
taeniacide
taeniafugal
taeniafuge
taenial
taeniasis
taeniform
Taenzer disease
tag
    anal skin t.
    auricular t's
    cutaneous t.
    radioactive t.
    sentinel t.
    skin t.
tagatose
tagged
    t. atom
    harmonic phase–t. MRI
    His-t. proteins
    t. red blood cells
tagging
tagliacotian
    t. cross-arm flap
    t. operation
    t. rhinoplasty
Tagliacozzi
    flap
    nasal reconstruction
    rhinoplasty
TAH—total abdominal
   hysterectomy
TAHBSO—total abdominal
   hysterectomy with bilateral
   salpingo-oophorectomy
tail
    axillary t.
    axillary t. of breast
    t. of caudate nucleus
    t. of epididymis
    t. of helix
    occult t.
    t. of pancreas

tail *(continued)*
- polyadenylate t.
- t. of Spence
- t. of spermatozoon
- t. of spleen

tailbone

tailor's
- t's ankle
- t's bunion
- t's bunionette deformity
- t's thumb

Takahara disease

Takahashi
- forceps
- punch

Takayasu
- arteritis
- disease
- pulseless disease
- syndrome

take
- graft t.

takeoff
- acute-angled t.
- t. angle
- t. of artery
- t. of celiac trunk
- high t. of right ventricular branch
- t. of vein

TAL—tendo Achillis lengthening

talalgia

talar

talc
- cosmetic t.
- t.-dusted contraceptive diaphragm
- t. dust exposure
- industrial t.
- inhaled t.
- t. pneumoconiosis
- t. pleurodesis
- t. poudrage
- t. retinopathy
- t. slurry
- thoracoscopic t. pleurodesis

talcosis
- intestinal t.
- intravenous t.
- pulmonary t.

talcum powder

talectomy
- primary t.
- salvage t.
- total t.

tali (genitive and plural of talus)

taliped

talipedic

talipes
- t. calcaneocavus
- t. calcaneovalgus
- t. calcaneus
- t. cavovarus
- t. cavus
- t. equinovalgus
- t. equinovarus
- t. equinus
- t. hobble splint
- t. valgus
- t. varus

talipomanus

Talma disease

talocalcaneal
- t. coalition
- t. joint
- t. ligament

talocalcanean

talocalcaneonavicular joint

talocrural
- t. joint
- t. region

talofibular ligament

talonavicular
- t. coalition
- t. joint
- t. ligament

talon noir

taloscaphoid

talotibial ligament

talus (tali)
- fovea of t.
- head of t.
- neck of t.

TAM—
- toxin-antitoxoid mixture
- transient abnormal myelopoiesis

tambour
- bruit de t.

TAME—toluene-sulfo-trypsin arginine methyl ester

TAMI—Thrombolysis and Angioplasty in Myocardial Infarction

Tamiami virus

Tamm-Horsfall
- mucoprotein
- protein

tampon
- t. action
- t.-associated toxic shock syndrome

T

tampon *(continued)*
    t. gauze
    Gibson-Mikulicz t.
    gynecological t.
    Merocel t.
    Mikulicz t.
    nasal t.
    obstetric t.
    pH-balanced t.
    pH-buffering t.
    Rapid Rhino nasal t.
    retained t.
    Rhino Rocket nasal t.
    self-administered t. ThinPrep test
    Trendelenburg t.
    t. tube
    vaginal t.
    vertically split Merocel t.
tamponade
    balloon t.
    bladder t.
    cardiac t.
    chronic t.
    t. effect
    esophageal t.
    esophageal balloon t.
    esophagogastric t.
    gas t.
    heart t.
    intracervical Foley catheter t.
    intraocular t.
    nasal t.
    pericardial t.
    postnasal balloon t.
    Rose t.
    silicone oil (SO) t.
    sulfur hexafluoride–air t.
    uterine balloon t.
tamponage
tamponing
tandem
tangential
    t. aneurysmectomy
    t. asymmetry
    t. cut
    t. excision
    t. force
    t. line
    t. irradiation
    t. radiotherapy
    t. speech
    t. splitting
    t. stapler excision
    t. topography corneal map

tangential *(continued)*
    t. traction
    t. view
tangentiality
Tangier disease
tangle
    intraneural fibrillary t's
    neurofibrillary t's
tank
    fish t. granuloma
    flotation t. therapy
    Hubbard t.
    saline-filled t.
    think t.
    t. ventilator
tannase
tannate
tanned
    t. appearance
    glutaraldehyde t. human umbilical vein graft
    t. red cell agglutination assay
    t. red cells (TRCs)
    t. skin
    t. and thickened peritoneum
Tanner
    developmental scale
    operation
    procedure
    stages (I–V)
tannic acid
tannin
tanning
Tanret
    reaction
    reagent
    test
Tansini operation
Tansley operation
tantalum (Ta)
    t. 182
    t. bronchogram
    t. clip
    t. mesh
    t. plate
    t. ring
    t. sheet
    t. wire
    t. wire suture
tantrum
tanycyte
Tanzer
    auricle reconstruction
    classification
TAO—thromboangiitis obliterans

tap
  bloody t.
  front t.
  heel t.
  mitral t.
  patellar t.
  spinal t.
  subdural t.
  tendon t.
TAP—tension by applanation
tape
  adhesive t.
  dental t.
  Montgomery t.
  sterile adhesive t.
tapeinocephalic
tapeinocephaly
taper
tapered crown
tapetal light reflex
tapetochoroidal dystrophy
tapetoretinal degeneration
tapetum (tapeta)
  t. cellulosum
  t. choroideae
  t. corporis callosi
  t. fibrosum
  t. lucidum
tapeworm
  African t.
  armed t.
  beef t.
  broad t.
  fish t.
  hydatid t.
  measly t.
  pork t.
  unarmed t.
taphephobia
Tapia syndrome
tapioca
tapir mouth
tapiroid cervix
tapotement
TAPVD—total anomalous
  pulmonary venous drainage
tar
  coal t.
  gas t.
  juniper t.
  pine t.
Tar symptom
TAR—thrombocytopenia–absent
  radius [syndrome]
tarantism

tarantula
  American t.
  black t.
  European t.
Tardieu
  spots
  test
tardive
  t. akathisia
  t. dyskinesia (TD)
  t. dystonia
target
  t. cell
  cold t. inhibition assay
  t. detection assay
  enriched t.
  t. erythrocyte
  t. gene
  t. lesion
  molecular t.
  t. organ
  t. protein
  t.-skin distance
  therapeutic t.
  t. tissue
targeting
  gene t.
targetoid hemosiderotic
  hemangioma
tarichatoxin
Tarin
  band
  fascia
  foramen
  fossa
  plate
  recess
  space
  taenia
Tarinus
  valve
  velum
Tarlov cyst
Tarnier
  forceps
  sign
Tarrant position
tarsadenitis
tarsal
tarsalgia
tarsalia
tarsalis
tarsectomy
tarsectopia
tarsi (plural of tarsus)

T

tarsitis
tarsocheiloplasty
tarsoclasis
tarsomalacia
tarsomegaly
tarsometatarsal
tarso-orbital
tarsophalangeal
tarsoplasty
tarsoptosis
tarsorrhaphy
tarsotarsal
tarsotibial
tarsotomy
tarsus (tarsi)
    bony t.
    t. inferior palpebrae
    t. osseus
    sinus tarsi
    t. superior palpebrae
tartar
    borated t.
    cream of t.
    t. emetic
tartarated
tartaric acid
tartarized
tartrate
    acid t.
    ammonium t.
    normal t.
    pyrantel t.
tartrated
task
    dichotic learning t's
    t. force
    t. oriented
    t.-specific activity
    t.-specific processing
tastant
TA-55 stapler
taste
    t. buds
    t. cells
    color t.
    t. corpuscle
    t. disorder
    t. dysfunction
    franklinic t.
    t. hairs
    impaired t.
    metallic t.
    t. pore
    t. receiving area
    t. ridges

taste-blindness
taster
TAT—
    tetanus antitoxin
    thematic apperception test
    thromboplastin activation test
    total antitryptic activity
    toxin-antitoxin
    turn-around time
    tyrosine aminotransferase
tattoo
    amalgam t.
    t.-associated endocarditis
    cosmetic t.
    dirt t.
    t. granuloma
    granuloma annulare–like t.
      reaction
    henna t.
    t.-induced vasculitis
    t. inks
    laser-assisted t. removal
    Monsel t.
    t. pigment
    Q-switched laser t. removal
    traumatic t.
tattooing
    accidental t.
    asphalt t.
    colonoscopic t.
    t. of cornea
    cosmetic t.
    temporary t.
Tatum clamp
tau
    Greek letter (τ; alphabetized
      as t)
    Kendall t.
Tauber spatula
taurine test
taurochenodeoxycholate
taurochenodeoxycholic acid
taurocholate
    tellurite t. gelatin agar
taurocholemia
taurocholic acid
taurocyamine
taurodontism
Taussig-Bing
    disease
    malformation
    syndrome
taut
    t. band of skeletal muscle
    t. foot

taut *(continued)*
    fully t. ligament
    myofascial t. bands
    t. skin
    t. tendon
tautomenial
tautomer
tautomeral cells
tautomerase
tautomeric
tautomerism
    keto-enol t.
    proton t.
    ring-chain t.
Tawara node
taxanes
taxine
taxis
taxon (taxa, taxons)
taxonomic
taxonomist
taxonomy
Tay
    choroiditis
    disease
    sign
    spot
Taylor
    apparatus
    brace
    position
    retractor
    scissors
    splint
    suture
Tay-Sachs disease
tazettine
TB—
    toluidine blue
    total base
    tracheobronchitis
    tubercle bacillus
    tuberculin
    tuberculosis
TBA—testosterone-binding affinity
T bandage
TBD—to be determined
TBE—tuberculin bacillin emulsion
TBF—total body fat
TBG—thyroxine-binding globulin
TBGP—total blood granulocyte pool
TBII—thyrotropin-binding
  inhibitory immunoglobulin
TBM—tuberculous meningitis
TBP—thyroxine-binding protein

TBPA—thyroxine-binding
  prealbumin
TB-RD—tuberculosis-respiratory
  disease
tbs., tbsp.—tablespoon
TBS—triethanolamine-buffered
  saline
TBSA—total body surface area
TBT—
    tolbutamide test
    tracheobronchial toilet
TBV—total blood volume
Tc—technetium
TC—
    tissue culture
    total capacity
    total cholesterol
    transhepatic cholangiography
TCA—
    tricarboxylic acid
    trichloroacetate
    trichloroacetic acid
TCE—trichloroethylene
T cell
T-cell
    T-c. activation
    adult T-c. leukemia
    T-c. anergy
    T-c. antibody labeling
    T-c. antigen receptor
    antigen-specific T-c. helper
      factor
    antigen-specific T-c.
      suppressor factor
    T-c. count
    cutaneous T-c. lymphoma
      (CTCL)
    T-c. dysfunction
    T-c. exhaustion
    T-c. function
    T-c. growth factor
    human T-c. leukemia virus
      (HTLV-1)
    human T-c. lymphotropic virus
      (types I–III)
    T-c. hybridoma
    T-c. infiltration
    T-c. infusion
    T-c. immunity
    T-c. lines
    T-c. lymphoma
    T-c. marker(s)
    T-c.–mediated hypersensitivity
    T-c.–mediated hypersensitivity
      reaction

T

T-cell *(continued)*
  T-c.–mediated immune reaction
  pan–T-c. antigen
  T-c. phenotype
  T-c. production
  T-c. proliferation
  T-c. proliferative response
  T-c. receptor
  T-c. response
TCGF—T-cell growth factor
TCH—total circulating hemoglobin
TCi—tetracurie(s)
TCI—transient cerebral ischemia
TCID—tissue culture infective dose
TCIE—transient cerebral ischemic episode
TCM—tissue culture medium
TCMI—T-cell–mediated immunity
TcR; TCR—T-cell receptor
TCT—
  thrombin-clotting time
  thyrocalcitonin
Td—tetanus-diphtheria
  [vaccine—adult booster dose]
TD—
  tardive dyskinesia
  tetanus-diphtheria [vaccine—pediatric initial dose]
  therapy discontinued
  thoracic duct
  threshold of discomfort
  thymus-dependent
  tic douloureux
  tone decay
  torsion dystonia
  total disability
  transverse diameter
  treatment discontinued
TDA—TSH-displacing antibody
TDE—tetrachlorodiphenylethane
TDF—thoracic duct fistula
TDI—
  toluene-diisocyanate
  total-dose infusion
TDP—thoracic duct pressure
TdT—terminal deoxynucleotidyl transferase
TDT—tone decay test
Te—tetanus
TE—
  echo time
  threshold energy
  tissue-equivalent
  tooth extracted

TE— *(continued)*
  total estrogen
  tracheoesophageal
Teale
  amputation
  forceps
  gorget
  operation
team
  surgical t.
tear
  annular t.
  bucket-handle t.
  cemental t.
  cementum t.
  Descemet membrane t.
  dural t.
  fishmouth t.
  full-thickness t.
  horseshoe t.
  labral t.
  Mallory-Weiss t.
  massive t.
  medial meniscus t.
  meniscal t.
  partial-thickness t.
  parenchymal t.
  perineal t.
  posterosuperior labral t.
  retinal t.
  retinal pigment epithelial (RPE) t.
  reverse horseshoe t.
  rotator cuff t.
  sphincter t.
  superficial t.
  tendinous t.
  vaginal t.
  wear and t. pigment
tear
  artificial t's
  t. break-up time
  crocodile t's
  t. deficiency
  t. drainage
  dry t's
  t. ducts
  t. film
  t. fluid concentration
  t. gas
  lower t. meniscus
  t. menisci
  preservative-free t. substitute
  t. sac
  Schirmer t. function test

tear *(continued)*
    total t. protein profile
    upper t. meniscus
    t. viscosity
    t. volume
Teare sling
tease, teased
teaspoon (tsp.)
TeBG; TEBG—testosterone-
  estradiol–binding globulin
TECA—technetium albumin
technetium (Tc)
    t. Tc 99m
    t. Tc 99m aggregated
      albumin kit
    t. Tc 99m albumin
    t. Tc 99m albumin aggregated
    t. Tc 99m albumin
      microspheres
    t. Tc 99m bicisate
    t. Tc 99m blood pool study
    t. Tc 99m colloid
    t. Tc 99m diphosphonate
    t. Tc 99m disofenin
    t. Tc 99m DTPA
    t. Tc 99m exametazime
    t. Tc 99m fanolesomab
    t. Tc 99m gluceptate
    t. Tc 99m HAM (human
      albumin microspheres)
      perfusion scan
    t. Tc 99m human serum
      albumin
    t. Tc 99m iminodiacetic acid
    t. Tc 99m-labeled
      macroaggregated human
      albumin
    t. Tc 99m lidofenin
    t. Tc 99m macroaggregates
    t. Tc 99m MDP
      (methylenediphosphonate,
      medronate)
    t. Tc 99m mebrofenin
    t. Tc 99m medronate
    t. Tc 99m mertiatide
    t. Tc 99m
      methylenediphosphonate
      (MDP, medronate)
    t. Tc 99m microspheres
    t. Tc 99m oxidronate
    t. Tc 99m pentetate (DTPA)
    t. Tc 99m pyrophosphate
    t. Tc 99m radiopharmaceutical
    t. Tc 99m red blood cell kit
    t. Tc 99m serum albumin kit

technetium (Tc) *(continued)*
    t. Tc 99m sestamibi
    t. Tc 99m sodium
      pertechnetate generator
    t. Tc 99m succimer
    t. Tc 99m sulfur colloid
    t. Tc 99m tetrofosmin
technical
technician
    audiologic t.
    dental t.
    emergency medical t. (EMT)
    laboratory t.
    lithotripter t.
    ophthalmic t.
    pharmacy t.
    radiologic t.
    sleep t.
    x-ray t.
technique
    abrasion t.
    absorption-elution t.
    absorption-inhibition t.
    Alexander t.
    Amplatz t.
    angle bisection t.
    aseptic t.
    Atkinson t.
    atrial-wall t.
    autoradiographic t.
    Baermann funnel t.
    Begg light-wire differential
      force t.
    bisection t.
    Bowen t.
    Brackin t.
    Brandt t.
    Bricker t.
    Brock t.
    Brown-Roberts-Wells t.
    Burhenne t.
    Buie t.
    cerebral flow image t.
    chromatographic-fluorometric t.
    clamp t.
    clonogenic t. for growing
      tumor cells in vitro
    Coffey t.
    Cohen t.
    competitive binding t.
    Conway t.
    Corbin t.
    Creech t.
    cross-fire t.
    Cutler-Beard t.

T

technique *(continued)*
>Denis Browne t.
>dilution-filtration t.
>dip slide t.
>direct fluorescent antibody t.
>DNA amplification t.
>Dotter-Judkins t.
>double antibody t.
>double-layer fluorescent
>>antibody t.
>drip infusion t.
>dye diffusion t.
>enzyme-multiplied
>>immunoassay t. (EMIT)
>Farr t.
>Fernandez t.
>Ferris Smith t.
>Ficoll-Hypaque t.
>fingerprinting t.
>fluorescent antibody t.
>flush t.
>Fones t.
>funicular suture t. in nerves
>George Lewis t.
>Gil-Vernet t.
>Glenn t.
>Glenn-Anderson t.
>Gruentzig (Grüntzig) t.
>guillotine t.
>hanging-drop t.
>helium dilution t.
>hemolytic plaque t.
>Heyman t.
>hybridoma t.
>immunoferritin t.
>immunoperoxidase t.
>indicator dilution t.
>indirect fluorescent antibody t.
>inhibition t.
>intermediate gel t.
>inversion-recovery t.
>Irving t.
>isolation-perfusion t.
>Jerne plaque t.
>Judkins t.
>Kleinschmidt t.
>Kristeller t.
>Krönig (Kroenig) t.
>La Roque t.
>Lash t.
>Laurell t.
>Leboyer t.
>LeDuc t.
>Leksell t.
>Lich t.

technique *(continued)*
>Lich-Gregoir t.
>Lotheissen-McVay t.
>Madden t.
>Maquet t.
>McGoon t.
>membrane filter t.
>Merendino t.
>microtiter t.
>Millen t.
>Mohs t.
>multiple pressure t.
>needle-through-needle t.
>Nars-Hunter t.
>Oakley-Fulthorpe t.
>open-drop t.
>opsonic t.
>Orr t.
>Orr-Loygue t.
>Ouchterlony t.
>Oudin t.
>Paquin t.
>parallel t.
>Paris t.
>peroxidase-antiperoxidase
>>(PAP) t.
>plaque t.
>play t.
>Politano-Leadbetter t.
>Pomeroy t.
>Ponka t.
>projective t.
>pulse echo t.
>push-back t.
>Q t.
>radioxenon t.
>Ravitch t.
>Rebuck skin window t.
>Regaud and Lacassagne t.
>renal micropuncture t.
>Richardson t.
>Riechert-Mundinger t.
>right-angle t.
>RNA amplification t.
>rosette t.
>sandwich t.
>saturation recovery t.
>Schultz-Dale t.
>Schuster t.
>scintillation counting t.
>Seldinger t.
>Sheehan-Dodge t.
>shoelace t.
>single layer
>>immunofluorescence t.

technique *(continued)*
    skin window t.
    Sones t.
    Southern blot t.
    squash t.
    stereotactic t.
    sterile t.
    Stockholm t.
    supervoltage t.
    Takatsy t.
    thermal expansion t.
    thermodilution t.
    time diffusion t.
    Todd-Wells t.
    transfusion t.
    Trueta t.
    Uchida t.
    ultrasound dilution t.
    van Lint t.
    vest-over-pants t.
    Warburg t.
    wax expansion t.
    Weigert-Pal t.
    Western blot t.
    Yasargil t.
    Ziehl-Neelsen t.
    zinc sulfate
technocausis
technologist
    certified nuclear medicine t.
    laboratory t.
    medical t.
    radiation therapy
      (radiotherapy) t.
    radiologic t.
    registered vascular t. (RVT)
    sleep t.
    x-ray t.
technology
    assisted reproductive t.
    gene t.
    recombinant DNA t.
tectal
tectobulbar tract
tectocephalic
tectocephaly
tectocerebellar tract
tectonic keratoplasty
tectorial membrane
tectorium (tectoria)
tectospinal
    t. decussation
    t. tract
tectum
    t. mesencephali

tectum *(continued)*
    t. of mesencephalon
    t. of midbrain
TED—
    threshold erythema dose
    thromboembolic disease
TED, T.E.D. (thromboembolic
  disease)
    hose
    stockings
TEE—transesophageal
  echocardiography
teeth (plural of tooth)
    accessional t.
    anatomic t.
    anterior t.
    auditory t.
    baby t.
    bicuspid t.
    buccal t.
    cheek t.
    cross-bite t.
    cross-pin t.
    deciduous t.
    diatoric t.
    Fournier t.
    fused t.
    Horner t.
    Hutchinson t.
    ISO System for T.
    labial t.
    t. ligation
    malacotic t.
    mandibular t.
    maxillary t.
    molar t.
    Moon t.
    morsal t.
    mottled t.
    nonanatomic t.
    permanent t.
    pinless t.
    posterior t.
    premature t.
    premolar t.
    primary t.
    rake t.
    rootless t.
    sclerotic t.
    screwdriver t.
    straight-pin t.
    succedaneous t.
    superior t.
    supernumerary t.
    temporary t.

T

teeth (plural of tooth) *(continued)*
  tube t.
  vital t.
  zero-degree t.
teething
TEF—tracheoesophageal fistula
Teflon
  catheter
  felt pledgets
  felt strips
  graft
  implant
  membrane
  mesh
  patch
  platinum-ribbon piston
  pledgeted sutures
  prosthesis
  septum
  sheath
  tape
  tube
teflurane anesthetic
tegmen (tegmina)
  t. mastoideotympanicum
  t. mastoideum
  t. tympani
  t. ventriculi quarti
tegmental
  anterior t. decussation
  t. cells
  t. decussations
  dorsal t. decussation
  t. field
  t. mesencephalic paralysis
  t. nuclei
  t. pontine reticular nucleus
  posterior t. decussation
  t. radiation
  t. syndrome
  t. tract
  ventral t. decussation
  t. wall of tympanic cavity
tegmentospinal tract
tegmentum (tegmenta)
  hypothalamic t.
  t. mesencephali
  t. of mesencephalon
  t. pontis
  t. rhombencephali
tegmina (plural of tegmen)
tegument
tegumental
tegumentary
Teichholz ejection fraction

Teichmann
  crystals
  test
teichoic acid
teichopsia
tela (telae)
  t. choroidea of fourth ventricle
  t. choroidea of third ventricle
  t. choroidea of lateral ventricle
  t. choroidea ventriculi lateralis
  t. choroidea ventriculi quarti
  t. choroidea ventriculi tertii
  t. subcutanea
  t. subcutanea abdominis
  t. subcutanea penis
  t. subcutanea perinei
  t. submucosa
  t. submucosa bronchiorum
  t. submucosa esophagi
  t. submucosa gastris
  t. submucosa intestini crassi
  t. submucosa intestini tenuis
  t. submucosa oesophagi
  t. submucosa pharyngis
  t. submucosa recti
  t. submucosa tracheae
  t. submucosa tubae uterinae
  t. submucosa ventriculi
  t. submucosa vesicae urinariae
  t. subserosa
  t. subserosa crassi
  t. subserosa gastris
  t. subserosa hepatis
  t. subserosa intestini tenuis
  t. subserosa peritonei
  t. subserosa tubae uterinae
  t. subserosa uteri
  t. subserosa ventriculi
  t. subserosa vesicae biliaris
  t. subserosa vesicae felleae
  t. subserosa vesicae urinariae
telalgia
telangiectasia
  ataxia-t. syndrome
  generalized essential t.
  hemorrhagic t.
  hereditary hemorrhagic t.
  t. macularis eruptiva
    perstans
  spider t.
  unilateral nevoid t.
telangiectasis (telangiectases)
  spider t.
  stellate t.
  t. syndrome

telangiectatic
    t. fibroma
    t. lipoma
    t. osteosarcoma
    t. sarcoma
    t. wart
telangiectodes
telangiitis
telangion
telangiosis
telar
telebinocular
telecanthus
telecardiogram
telecardiography
telecardiophone
teleceptive
teleceptor
telecobalt
telecord
telediagnosis
telefluoroscopy
telegraphic speech
telekinesis
telekinetic
telelectrocardiogram
telelectrocardiograph
telemedicine
telemetering capsule
telemetry
    cardiac t.
    continuous t. monitoring
    t. unit
telemnemonike
telencephalic
telencephalization
telencephalon
teleneurite
teleneuron
teleopsia
telepathy
telephone scatologia
teleradiography
teleradiotherapy
teleradium
telereceptor
teleroentgenography
telescope
    30-degree 4 mm rigid t.
    external t.
    Hopkins t.
    implantable miniature t.
      prosthesis
    intraocular t.
    intraocular Galilean t.

telescope *(continued)*
    right-angle t.
    rigid t.
telescopic denture
telestethoscope
telesthesia
teletherapy
telethermometer
television microscopy
Telfa dressing
TeLinde operation
tellurite taurocholate gelatin agar
tellurium (Te)
Tellyesniczky
    fluid
    mixture
telobranchial bodies
telocentric chromosome
telodendron (telodendra)
telogen
    t. defluvium
    t. effluvium
    t. phase
teloglia
telognosis
telolemma
telomerase
telomere
telomeric
    t. heterochromatin
    t. staining
telopeptide
telophase
telophragma
teloreceptor
telotism
TEM—transmission electron
  microscopy
temperament
    choleric t.
    epileptic t.
    melancholic t.
    phlegmatic t.
    sanguine t.
temperature (T, temp)
    absolute t.
    basal body t.
    body t.
    core t.
    critical t.
    t. curve
    maximum t.
    minimum t.
    normal t.
    optimum t.

T

temperature (T, temp) *(continued)*
  permissive t.
  restrictive t.
  room t.
  t. scale
  t. spots
  standard t. and pressure
    (STP, stp.)
  subnormal t.
temperature-sensitive mutation
temperate
  t. bacteriophage
  t. virus
template
  custom t.
  t. method
  stainless steel t.
  t. strand
  surgical t.
  wax t.
temple
Temple procedure
Templeton and Zim carpal tunnel
  projection
tempolabile
temporal
  t. aponeurosis
  t. arcade
  t. arteries
  t. arterioles of retina
  t. arteritis
  t. bone
  t. crescent
  t. crest of frontal bone
  t. diameter
  t. dispersion
  t. fascia
  t. fossa
  t. gyri
  t. hemianopia
  t. horn of lateral ventricle
  t. incision
  t. incisure
  t. line
  t. lobe
  t. lobectomy
  t. lobe epilepsy
  t. loop
  t. margin of parietal bone
  mesial t. sclerosis
  t. muscle
  t. nerves
  t. operculum
  t. pallor
  t. plane

temporal *(continued)*
  t. plexus
  t. pole of cerebral
    hemisphere
  t. process of mandible
  t. region
  t. squama
  t. sulcus
  t. sulci
  t. surface
  t. suture
  t. veins
  t. venule of retina
  t. wing of sphenoid bone
temporalis
  squama t.
temporoauricular
temporofacial
temporofrontal
temporohyoid
temporomalar
  t. foramen
  t. suture
temporomandibular
  t. articular veins
  t. dysfunction syndrome
  internal derangement of the
    t. joint
  t. joint (TMJ)
  t. joint ankylosis
  t. joint arthritis
  t. joint disease
  t. joint disorder
  t. joint pain
  t. joint reconstruction
  t. joint sounds
  t. joint syndrome
  t. ligament
temporomaxillary
temporo-occipital
temporoparietal muscle
temporoparietalis
temporopontile
temporopontine
  t. fibers
  t. tract
temporospatial
temporosphenoid
temporozygomatic suture
tempostabile
TEN—toxic epidermal
  necrolysis
tenable
tenacious
tenacity

tenaculum
  Adair t.
  Barrett t.
  Braun t.
  Cottle t.
  DeLee t.
  Duplay t.
  t. forceps
  Jackson t.
  Jacobs t.
  Kahn t.
  Lahey t.
  Marlex atraumatic t.
  Ritchie t.
  Schroeder t.
  sharp-toothed t.
  straight t.
  t. tendinum
Tenckhoff peritoneal
  catheter
tendency
  primary reaction t's
tender
  t. point
  retromandibular t. point
tenderness
  pencil t.
  rebound t.
tendines (plural of tendo)
tendineus
  arcus t.
  hiatus t.
tendinitis
  bicipital t.
  calcific t.
  t. ossificans traumatica
  t. stenosans
  stenosing t.
tendinoplasty
tendinosuture
tendinotrochanteric ligament
tendinous
  t. arch
  common t. ring
  Döllinger t. ring
  t. inscriptions
  t. intersection
  t. junctions
  t. membrane
  t. opening
  plantar t. sheath
  t. quittor
  t. sheaths
  t. synovitis
  t. zones of heart

tendo (tendines)
  t. Achillis
  t. calcaneus
  t. conjunctivus
  t. cordiformis
  t. cricooesophageus
  t. infundibuli
  t. oculi
tendolysis
tendomucin
tendon
  Achilles t.
  Achilles t. reflex time
  anterior patellar t.
  bowed t.
  calcaneal t.
  t. cartilage
  t. cells
  central t. of diaphragm
  central t. of perineum
  common t.
  common annular t.
  conjoined t.
  t. of conus
  cordiform t. of diaphragm
  coronary t
  t. corpuscles
  cricoesophageal t.
  fibrous s. of tendon
  giant cell tumor of t. sheath
  Golgi t. organ
  t. graft
  hamstring t.
  t. of Hector
  heel t.
  inferior patellar t.
  t. of infundibulum
  intermediate t. of diaphragm
  t. jerk
  membranaceous t.
  mucous sheath of t's
  t. organ
  palmaris longus t.
  patellar t.
  pulled t.
  t. reaction
  t. reflex
  t. release
  riders' t.
  t. sheath
  slipped t.
  snapping t.
  t. spindle
  stapedius t.
  superior oblique t.

T

tendon *(continued)*
    t. suture
    synovial sheath of t.
    Todaro t.
    t. transfer
    t. transplantation
    trefoil t.
    t. of Zinn
tendon tucker
    Bishop t.t.
    Bishop-Black t.t.
    Bishop-Peter t.t.
    Burch-Greenwood t.t.
    Fink t.t.
tendoplasty
tendosynovitis
tendotome
tendotomy
tendovaginal
tendovaginitis
tendril fibers
tenebric vertigo
tenectomy
Tenericutes
tenesmic
tenesmus
    rectal t.
    vesical t.
tenioid
teniotoxin
Tennison operation
Tennison-Randall operation
tenodesis
    t. orthosis
    t. splint
tenodynia
tenolysis
tenomyoplasty
tenomyotomy
Tenon
    capsule
    fascia
    membrane
    space
tenonectomy
tenonitis
tenonostosis
tenontagra
tenontodynia
tenontography
tenontolemmitis
tenontomyotomy
tenontophyma
tenontoplasty
tenontothecitis

tenontotomy
tenophyte
tenoplastic
tenoplasty
tenoreceptor
tenorrhaphy
tenosuspension
tenosynovectomy
tenosynovial chondrometaplasia
tenosynovioma
tenosynovitis
    t. acuta purulenta
    adhesive t.
    t. crepitans
    de Quervain t.
    gonococcic t.
    granulomatous t.
    t. granulosa
    t. hypertrophica
    infectious t.
    nodular t.
    t. serosa chronica
    t. stenosans
    stenosing t.
    tuberculous t.
    villonodular t.
    villous t.
tenotomized
tenotomy
    central slip t.
    curb t.
    fenestrated t.
    graduated t.
    intrasheath t.
    open t.
    partial t.
    percutaneous t.
    stapedial t.
    Z t.
tenovaginitis
TENS—
    transcutaneous electrical
        nerve stimulation
    transcutaneous electrical
        nerve stimulator
tense
Tensilon test
tensio-active
    t-a. molecules
    t-a. properties
tension
    arterial t.
    carbon dioxide t.
    t. cavities
    chronic t. headache

tension *(continued)*
    t. curves
    electric t.
    episodic t. headache
    t.-free hernioplasty
    t. headache
    high-t. pulse
    t. hydrocephalus
    interfacial surface t.
    intraocular t.
    intravenous t.
    t. lines
    lines of minimal t.
    low-t. glaucoma
    low-t. pulse
    muscular t.
    oxygen t.
    t. pneumothorax
    premenstrual t.
    relaxed skin t. lines
    surface t.
    t. suture
    tissue t.
    wall t.
tensor
    t. muscle of fascia lata
    t. tympani
    t. tympani muscle
    t. veli palatini
    t. veli palatini muscle
tent
    air flow t.
    Laminaria t.
    oxygen t.
    sponge t.
    steam t.
tentacle
tenting
    apical t. of mitral leaflets
    t. of hemidiaphragm
    mitral valve t.
    t. phenomenon
    t. of skin
    tricuspid valve t.
tentorial
tentorium (tentoria)
    t. cerebelli
    t. of cerebellum
    t. of hypophysis
tenuous
    t. airway
    t. balance
    t. blood supply
    t. cord
    t. course

tenuous *(continued)*
    t. flap
    t. hemodynamic status
    t. situation
TEP—thromboendophlebectomy
TEPP—tetraethyl pyrophosphate
teracurie (TCi)
teratic
teratism
teratoblastoma
teratocarcinogenesis
teratocarcinoma
teratogen
teratogenesis
teratogenetic
teratogenic
teratogenicity
teratogenous
teratoid
    t. parasite
    t. tumor
teratologic, teratological
teratologist
teratoma (teratomas, teratomata)
    benign cystic t.
    cystic t.
    differentiated t.
    immature t.
    malignant t.
    mature t.
    monodermal t.
    sacrococcygeal t.
    solid t.
    trophoblastic t.
    undifferentiated t.
teratomatous
teratospermia
terbium (Tb)
terebenthene
terebinthinate
terebinthinism
terebrant pain
terebrating
terebration
teres
    ligamentum t.
    t. major muscle
    t. minor muscle
    pronator t. muscle
tergal
term
    at t.
    t. infant
    ontogenetic t's
Terman test

terminad
terminaison
    t's en grappe
    t. en ligne
    t's en panier
    t. en plaque
terminal
    t. abutment
    t. addition enzyme
    t. artery
    axion t.
    t. bars
    bouton t.
    t. branch of deep peroneal
      nerve
    t. bronchiole
    t. bulb of Krause
    t. button
    C t.
    central t. of Wilson
    t. cisterns
    t. colic lymph nodes
    Deiters t. frame
    t. deletion
    t. deoxynucleotidyl transferase
      (TdT)
    t. device
    t. disinfection
    t. duct adenocarcinoma
    t. duct carcinoma
    t. edema
    en plaque t.
    t. enteritis
    t. filament
    t. fossa
    grapelike t's
    t. hair
    t. hinge position
    t. ileum
    t. insomnia
    Kühne t. plates
    t. latency
    t. leukocytosis
    t. ligature
    t. line of pelvis
    long t. repeats
    N t.
    t. nerve
    nerve t's
    t. nerve corpuscle
    NH2 t.
    t. notch of auricle
    t. nucleus
    t. occlusion
    t. plate

terminal *(continued)*
    t. pneumonia
    t. respiratory unit
    t. sac
    t. saccular period
    t. saccular phase
    t. saccules
    t. sinus
    subendocardial t. plexus
    t. sulcus of heart
    t. sulcus of tongue
    t. vein
    t. ventricle of spinal cord
    t. vertebra
    t. web
    Wilson central t.
terminale
    filum t.
    ganglion t.
terminalization
terminatio (terminationes)
termination
terminator
    DNA-chain t.
Terminologia Anatomica (TA)
terminology
terminoterminal anastomosis
terminus (termini)
termolecular
ternary
ternitrate
terpene
terpenism
terra silicea purificata
Terrien
    marginal corneal degeneration
    ulcer
territoriality
territory
    lymph t.
    vascular t.
    watershed t.
terror
    day t's
    night t's
Terry
    line
    syndrome
Terson operation
tertian
    double t.
    malignant t.
tertiary
    t. granule
    t. structure

tertigravida
tertipara
tesla (T)
tessellated
Tessier
    craniofacial cleft
    operation
test
    ABLB (alternate binaural
      loudness balance) t.
    Abrams t.
    absorption elution t.
    acetic acid t.
    acetic acid and potassium
      ferrocyanide t.
    acetoacetic acid t.
    acetone t.
    achievement t.
    acid clearance t.
    acid elution t.
    acidified serum t.
    acidity reduction t.
    acid-lability t.
    acidosis t.
    acid perfusion t.
    acid phosphatase t.
    acid reflux t.
    acoustic reflex t.
    ACTH stimulation t.
    active rosette t.
    acute toxicity t.
    Adamkiewicz t.
    adaptation t. of Rademaker
      and Garcin
    Addis t.
    Adler t.
    adrenaline t.
    adrenocortical inhibition t.
    Adson t.
    afterimage t.
    agglutination t.
    agglutination inhibition t.
    A/G ratio t.
    air-conduction t.
    AL t.
    Albarran t.
    albumin t.
    aldosterone t.
    aldosterone suppression t.
    alizarin t.
    alkali denaturation t.
    alkaline phosphatase t.
    alkali tolerance t.
    alkaloid t.
    allelism t.

test *(continued)*
    Allen t.
    Allen-Doisy t.
    Almén t.
    alpha t.
    alpha amino nitrogen t.
    alpha-fetoprotein (AFP) t.
    alternate binaural loudness
      balance (ABLB) t.
    alternate cover t.
    alternate loudness balance t.
    amebocyte lysate t.
    Ames t.
    amino acid t.
    aminopyrine breath t.
    Ammons Full-Range Picture
      Vocabulary t.
    amylase t.
    Anderson and Goldberger t.
    anesthetic t.
    angular deviation t.
    anterior drawer t.
    antibiotic sensitivity t.
    antibiotic susceptibility t.
    antibody absorption t.
    antibody screening t.
    anti–double-stranded DNA t.
    anti-DNA t.
    antiglobulin t. (AGT)
    antiglobulin consumption t.
    antiglobulin inhibition t.
    antihuman globulin (AHG) t.
    antihuman serum t.
    antimicrobial sensitivity t.
    antimicrobial susceptibility t.
    antimony trichloride t.
    anti-Rho-D titer t.
    antistreptolysin O (ASO) t.
    antistreptozyme t.
    antithrombin t.
    Apgar t.
    Apley compression t.
    apprehension t.
    Apt t.
    aptitude t.
    arginine stimulation t.
    arginine tolerance t. (ATT)
    Argo corn starch t.
    arm ergometry exercise t.
    arylsulfatase t.
    Aschner t.
    Aschner-Danini t.
    Ascoli t.
    ascorbate cyanide t.
    ascorbic acid t.

T

test *(continued)*

ASO (antistreptolysin O) t.
aspirin tolerance t.
association t.
atrial pacing t.
auditory acuity t.
augmented histamine t.
autohemolysis t.
automated reagin t. (ART)
Ayer t.
Ayer-Tobey t.
Babinski t.
Babinski-Weil t.
Bachman t.
bacteriolytic t.
bacteriophage neutralization t.
Baermann t.
balance t.
Balke-Ware t.
Bárány caloric t.
Bárány pointing t.
bar-reading t.
basophil degranulation t.
Bass-Watkins t.
battery of t's
bcr/abl protein t.
Becker t.
BEI (butanol extractable
   iodine) t.
Bekhterev (Bechterew) t.
Bence Jones protein t.
Bender Gestalt t.
Bender Visual-Motor Gestalt t.
Benedict t.
Bennet and Cash t.
bentiromide t.
bentonite flocculation t.
Benton t. for visual retention
benzidine t.
Berens 3-character t.
Bernard t.
Bernstein t.
beta t.
beta-hCG t.
BG (Bordet-Gengou) t.
β-galactosidase t. [beta-]
Bial t.
bicycle ergometer exercise t.
Bielschowsky head-tilting t.
bile acid breath t.
bile acid tolerance t.
bile esculin t.
bile pigment t.
bile solubility t.
biliary drainage t.

test *(continued)*

bilirubin t., direct
bilirubin t., indirect
bilirubin tolerance t.
binaural distorted speech t's
Binet t.
Binet-Simon t.
Bing t.
Biocept-G t.
Bischoff t.
bithermal caloric t.
biuret t.
Blackberg and Wanger t.
bleeding time t.
blocking t.
Block-Steiger t.
blood cholesterol t.
blood urea nitrogen (BUN) t.
Bloor t.
blot t.
Blumenau t.
Boas t.
Bodal t.
Bonanno t.
bone-conduction t.
Bonney t.
Bordet-Gengou (BG) t.
Boyden t.
bracelet t.
breath t.
breath-holding t.
breath hydrogen t.
Brenner t.
Brieger t.
Broadbent t.
bromphenol t.
bromsulfophthalein (BSP) t.
bronchial challenge t.
Bruck t.
BSP (bromsulfophthalein) t.
buccal smear t.
Burchard-Liebermann t.
butanol extractable iodine
   (BIE) t.
butyric acid t.
caffeine breath t.
Caille t.
calcium infusion t.
Callaway t.
Calmette t.
caloric t.
CAMP t.
capillary fragility t.
capillary resistance t.
captopril t.

test *(continued)*

carbohydrate t.
carbohydrate tolerance t.
carbohydrate utilization t.
carbon clearance t.
carbon dioxide combining
  power t.
carbon monoxide t.
carbon 13 breath t.
carbon 14 breath t.
cardiolipin t.
Carnot t.
carotid sinus t.
Carr-Price t.
Casoni intradermal t.
Castellani t.
catalase t.
catecholamine t.
catoptric t.
CCK (cholecystokinin) t.
CEA (carcinoembryonic
  antigen) t.
cellobiose-mannitol t.
cellophane tape t.
cephalin-cholesterol
  flocculation t.
cephalin flocculation t.
cervical posture t.
cetylpyridium chloride t.
challenge t.
Chediak t.
chemiluminescence t.
Chick-Martin t.
Chiene t.
Children's Apperception t.
  (CAT)
Chimani-Moos t.
chlormerodrin accumulation t.
chlorpromazine stimulation t.
cholecystokinin (CCK) t.
cholesterol t.
cholesterol-lecithin
  flocculation t.
cholinesterase t.
Chopra antimony t.
chorionic gonadotropin t.
Chrobak t.
chromatin t.
chromogenic cephalosporin t.
chronic toxicity t.
Chvostek t.
cis-trans t.
citrate t.
Clark t.
Clauberg t.

test *(continued)*

clivogram t.
clomiphene citrate
  challenge t.
clonidine suppression t.
coagulase t.
coagulation t.
cocaine t.
coccidioidin skin t.
Cohn t.
coin t.
colchicine t.
cold agglutinin t.
cold pressor t.
coliform t.
collateral circulation t.
Collin t.
colloidal gold t.
color perception t.
color vision t.
combined anterior pituitary t.
complement fixation (CF) t.
concentrating ability t.
concentration t.
concentration-dilution t.
confrontation field t.
conglutinating complement
  absorption t. (CCAT)
Congo red t.
conjunctival t.
Conn t.
consumption t.
contact t.
contraction stress t. (CST)
contralateral straight leg
  raising t.
contrast t.
controlled association t.
Coombs t., direct
Coombs t., indirect
copper t.
coproporphyrin t.
corneal t.
Corner-Allen t.
cortisone-glucose tolerance t.
cotton-tip applicator t.
cover t.
cover-uncover t.
Crafts t.
Craig t.
Crampton t.
C-reactive protein t.
creatine kinase (CK) t.
creatine phosphokinase
  (CPK) t.

T

test *(continued)*
- creatinine t.
- creatinine clearance t.
- cross agglutination t.
- crossed acoustic reflex t.
- cross-matching t.
- cuff t.
- Cuignet t.
- curare t.
- cyanide-nitroprusside t.
- Cybex t.
- cycle ergometer t.
- cysteine t.
- cystine t.
- cytosine t.
- cytotoxicity t.
- dark-adaptation t.
- darkroom t.
- Davidsohn differential absorption t.
- D-dimer t.
- decarboxylase t.
- Dehio t.
- dehydration t's
- dehydrocholate t.
- delayed auditory feedback t.
- Denes-Naunton t.
- Denver Developmental Screening T.
- deoxyribonuclease (DNase) t.
- deoxyuridine suppression t.
- dexamethasone suppression t.
- dextrose t.
- DFA (direct fluorescent antibody) t.
- DFA-TP (direct fluorescent antibody–*Treponema pallidum*) t.
- diabetes t.
- diacetyl t.
- Diagnex blue t.
- Dick t.
- Dienst t.
- differential t. for infectious mononucleosis
- diffusion t.
- dilution t.
- dimethylglyoxime t.
- dinitrophenylhydrazine t.
- diphtheria t.
- direct antiglobulin t.
- direct bilirubin t.
- direct Coombs t.
- direct fluorescent antibody (DFA) t.

test *(continued)*
- direct fluorescent antibody– *Treponema pallidum* (DFA-TP) t.
- direct immunofluorescence t.
- disk diffusion t.
- distribution-free t.
- dithionite t.
- Dix-Hallpike t.
- DNase (deoxyribonuclease) t.
- Doerfler-Stewart t.
- doll's eye t.
- Dolman t.
- Donath-Landsteiner t.
- Donders t.
- L-dopa response t.
- Dorn-Sugarman t.
- double-blind t.
- double-diffusion t.
- double-glucagon t.
- Draize t.
- draw-a-bicycle t.
- draw-a-family t.
- draw-a-person t.
- drawer t.
- Dreyer t.
- drinking t.
- Duane t.
- duck waddle t.
- duction t.
- Dugas t.
- Duke bleeding time t.
- duochrome t.
- dye exclusion t.
- dynamic t.
- E t.
- early pregnancy t.
- Ebbinghaus t.
- ECG stress t.
- echinococcus skin t.
- edrophonium chloride t.
- effort tolerance t.
- Ehrlich t.
- Einhorn string t.
- electrophoresis t.
- electrotransfer t.
- Elek t.
- ELISA (enzyme-linked immunosorbent assay) t.
- Ellsworth-Howard t.
- Ely t.
- EP (erythrocyte protoporphyrin) t.
- epithyroid iodine uptake t.

test *(continued)*

Epstein-Barr nuclear antigen t. (EBNA)
ergonovine t.
Erhard t.
Erichsen t.
E rosette t.
erythrocyte adherence t.
erythrocyte fragility t.
erythrocyte protoporphyrin (EP) t.
erythrocyte sedimentation rate (ESR) t.
Escherich t.
esophageal acid perfusion t.
estrogen receptor assay (ERA) t.
estrogen stimulation t.
estrogen suppression t.
euglobulin lysis t.
exercise t's
exercise stress t.
exercise tolerance t.
FAB (fluorescent antibody) t.
fabere (flexion, abduction, external rotation, extension) t.
face-hand t.
facial nerve function t.
Fahraeus t.
Fajersztajn t.
FANA (fluorescent antinuclear antibody) t.
Fantus t.
Farber t.
Farr t.
Farris t.
fat absorption t.
fecal fat t.
Fehling t.
femoral nerve stretch t.
FE_{Na} t. [FeNa] t.
fermentation t.
fern t.
ferric chloride t.
fetal acoustic stimulation t.
fetal electrocardiogram t.
Feulgen t.
fibrinogen t.
FIGLU excretion t.
Finckh t.
finger-to-finger t.
finger-nose t., finger-to-nose t.
fingerprint sweat t.
Finkelstein t.
Finn chamber t.

test *(continued)*

Fishberg concentration t.
Fishman-Doubilet t.
fistula t.
fixation t.
Flack t.
flicker t.
flocculation t.
fluctuation t.
Fluhmann t.
fluorescein dilaurate t.
fluorescein dye disappearance t.
fluorescent antibody (FAB) t.
fluorescent antinuclear antibody (FANA) t.
fluorescent treponemal antibody (FTA) t.
fluorescent treponemal antibody absorption (FTA-ABS) t.
foam stability t.
Folin and Wu t.
food challenge t.
forced duction t.
formaldehyde t.
formol-gel t.
40 millimeter t.
Foshay t.
Fouchet t.
four diopter base-out prism t.
Fournier t.
four-prism-diopter t.
Fowler t.
fragility t.
Francis t.
Fränkel t.
free association t.
free urinary cortisol t.
Frei t.
Friberg t.
Friderichsen t.
Friedman t.
Friedman-Lapham t.
friend t.
Frostig Developmental T. of Visual Perception
fructosamine t.
fructose tolerance t.
FTA (fluorescent treponemal antibody) t.
FTA-ABS (fluorescent treponemal antibody absorption) t.
fundus reflex t.
Funkenstein t.
furfurol t.

T

test *(continued)*

Gaenslen t.
galactose breath t.
galactose tolerance t.
β-galactosidase t. [beta-]
gallbladder function t.
Galli-Mainini t.
galvanic t.
gastric function t.
gastrointestinal blood loss t.
gastrointestinal protein loss t.
Gault t.
gaze t. for ocular and
    vestibular functioning
gelatin agglutination t.
gel diffusion t.
Gellé t.
Gerhardt t.
germ tube t. for *Candida
    albicans*
Gerrard t.
Gesell t.
Gibbon and Landis t.
Gies biuret t.
globulin t.
glucagon response t.
glucagon stimulation t.
glucose t.
glucose absorption t.
glucose oxidase paper strip t.
glucose suppression t.
glucose tolerance t. (GTT)
Gluzinski t.
glycerol t.
glycerophosphate t.
glycogen storage t.
glycosylated hemoglobin t.
glycuronates t.
glycyltryptophan t.
glyoxylic acid t.
Gmelin t.
Goetsch t.
Gofman t.
gold number t.
gold-sol t.
gonadotropin-releasing
    hormone stimulation t.
Goodenough Draw-a-Man t.
Goodenough Draw-a-Person t.
Goodenough-Harris
    Draw-a-Person t.
goodness-of-fit t.
Gordon biological t.
Göthlin (Goethlin) t.

test *(continued)*

graded exercise t. (GXT)
Graefe t.
Graham t.
Gravindex t.
Gregerson and Boas t.
Griess t.
Grigg t.
Gross t.
group t.
Gruber-Widal t.
guaiac t.
Guerreiro-Machado t.
Gunning t.
Gunning-Lieben t.
Günzberg t.
Guthrie t.
Gutzeit t.
Haagensen t.
HAI (hemagglutination
    inhibition) t.
Haines t.
Hallion t.
Hallpike t.
Halstead-Reitan t.
Ham t.
Hamburger t.
Hamel t.
Hamilton t.
Hammarsten t.
Hammerschlag t.
Hamolsky t.
Hanfmann-Kasanin t.
Hanger t.
Hanger-Rose skin t.
hanging-drop t.
Hanke and Koessler t.
hapten inhibition t.
Harding and Ruttan t.
harmonic acceleration t.
Harris and Ray t.
Harrison spot t.
Hart t.
hatching t.
Hay t.
head-tilt t.
Heaf t.
heat stability t.
heel-knee t., heel-to-knee t.
heel-shin t., heel-to-shin t.
heel-tap t.
Heinz body t.
Heller t.
hemadsorption t.

test *(continued)*

hemadsorption inhibition t.
hemagglutination t.
hemagglutination inhibition
   (HI, HAI) t.
hematein t.
hematin t.
heme t.
Hemoccult t.
hemoglobin t.
hemolytic plaque t.
hemosiderin t.
Hench-Aldrich t.
Hendler screening t.
Henle-Coenen t.
Hennebert t.
Henshaw t.
hepatic function t.
Hering t.
Herter t.
Herzberg t.
Hess capillary t.
heterophile antibody t.
HI (hemagglutination
   inhibition) t.
Hickey-Hare t.
Hildebrandt t.
Hines and Brown t.
Hinton t.
hippuric acid t.
Hirschberg t. for strabismus
Histalog t.
histamine flare t.
histamine stimulation t.
histidine loading t.
histoplasmin skin t.
Hitzenberg t.
Hitzig t.
HIVAGEN t.
Hoesch t.
Hoffmann t.
Hofmeister t.
Hogben t.
Hollander t.
Holmgren t.
homogentisic acid oxidase t.
Hopkins-Cole t.
Hopkins thiophene t.
Hoppe-Seyler t.
hormone t.
horse cell t.
house-tree-person (HTP) t.
Howard t.
Howell t.

test *(continued)*

HTP (house-tree-person) t.
Huddleson t.
Huhner t.
Huppert t.
Huppert-Cole t.
Hurtley t.
hydrochloric acid t.
hydrogen breath t.
hydrogen peroxide t.
hydrostatic t.
hydroxyaromatic acid t.
17-hydroxycorticosteroid t.
5-hydroxyindoleacetic acid t.
hydroxylamine t.
hyperemia t.
hyperventilation t.
hypochlorite-orcinol t.
hypo-osmotic swelling t. for
   sperm viability
hypoxanthine t.
icterus index t.
IFA (indirect fluorescent
   antibody) t.
Ilimow t.
Ilosvay t.
imidazole t.
immobilization t.
immunodiffusion t.
immunofluorescence t.
immunologic t.
immunologic pregnancy t.
impedance audiometry t.
IMViC t.
incomplete sentences t.
indican t.
indigo-carmine t.
indigo red t.
indirect antiglobulin t.
indirect bilirubin t.
indirect Coombs t.
indirect fluorescent antibody
   (IFA) t.
indirect hemagglutination t.
indirect immunofluorescence t.
indocyanine green t.
indole t.
indophenol t.
induced hypercalciuria t.
induced hypoglycemia t.
induced phosphaturia t.
inhalation challenge t.
inhibition t.
inkblot t.

T

test *(continued)*

inoculation t.
inositol t.
insulin clearance t.
insulin sensitivity t.
insulin tolerance t.
intelligence t. (IQ)
interference t.
intracutaneous t.
intradermal t.
intradermal tuberculin t.
intravenous secretin t.
inulin clearance t.
in vitro t.
iodide-perchlorate discharge t.
iodine t. for starch
iodine I 131 uptake t.
iodoform t.
[131]I-oleic acid t. [I 131-]
Iowa pressure articulation t.
iron-binding capacity t.
irresistible impulse t.
irrigation t.
ischemic forearm t.
Ishihara t.
Isojima sperm immobilization t.
isopropanol precipitation t.
[131]I uptake t. [I 131-]
Ivy bleeding time t.
Jacoby t.
Jacquemin t.
Jadassohn t.
Jadassohn-Bloch t.
Jaeger t.
Jaffé t.
Jaksch t.
Janet t.
Jansen t.
Javorski (Jaworski) t.
Jenning t.
jerk t.
Johnson t.
Jolles t.
Jones t.
Jones-Cantarow t.
Jorissen t.
Kahn t.
Kantor and Gies t.
Kapeller-Adler t.
Kaplan t.
Kapsinow t.
Kashiwado t.
Kastle t.
Kastle-Meyer t.
Katayama t.

test *(continued)*

Kathrein t.
Kato t.
Keller ultraviolet t.
Kelling t.
Kentmann t.
Kerner t.
17-ketogenic steroid t.
ketone body t.
17-ketosteroid t.
Kibrick gelatin agglutination t.
kidney function t.
Killian t.
Kinberg t.
King-Devick test for
   evaluation of saccade
Kjeldahl t.
Kleihauer t.
Kleihauer-Betke t.
Klimow t.
Kline flocculation t.
Knapp t.
knee dropping t.
Knott t.
Kober t.
Kolmer t.
Kolmogorov-Smirnov t.
Kondo t.
Korotkoff t.
Kossel t.
Kowarsky t.
Kremer t.
Krokiewicz t.
Kuhlmann t.
Külz t.
Kunkel t.
Kupperman t.
Kurzrok-Miller t.
Kveim t.
Kveim-Siltzbach t.
t. of labor
labyrinthine t.
Lachman anterior drawer t.
lactate dehydrogenase t.
lactic acid t.
lactose t.
lactose tolerance t.
Ladendorff t.
Lancaster red-green t.
Lancefield precipitation t.
Landau t.
Lang t. for taurine
Lange t. for acetone in urine
Lange colloidal gold t.
lantern t.

test *(continued)*

LAP (leucine aminopeptidase) t.
laryngeal mirror t.
Lasègue t.
lateral pivot shift t.
latex agglutination t.
latex fixation t.
latex particle agglutination t.
latex slide agglutination t.
Laurell rocket t.
Lautier t.
LE (lupus erythematosus) t.
Leach t.
Lebbin t.
Lechini t.
Lee t.
Legal t.
leishmanin t.
Le Nobel t.
Leo t.
lepromin t.
Lesser t.
leucine t.
leucine aminopeptidase
  (LAP) t.
leucine tolerance t.
leukocyte adherence inhibition t.
leukocyte bactericidal t.
leukocyte migration t.
Levinson t.
levulose t.
levulose tolerance t.
Lewis and Pickering t.
Lezak malingering t.
Lichtheim t.
Lieben t.
Lieben-Ralfe t.
Liebermann t.
Liebermann-Burchard t.
Liebig t.
Ligat t.
Lignières (Lignieres) t.
limulus t.
limulus lysate t.
Lindemann t.
Linder t.
Linzenmeier t.
lipase t.
lipid t.
Lipps t.
litmus milk t.
liver function t. (LFT)
Livierato t.
Lombard t.
long-term toxicity t.

test *(continued)*

Löwenthal (Lowenthal) t.
Lücke t. for hippuric acid
Luebert t.
Luenbach-Koeppe t.
Lundh t.
lupus band t.
lupus erythematosus (LE)
  cell t.
Lyle and Curtman t.
lymphocyte proliferation t.
lymphocyte transfer t.
Machado t.
Machado-Guerreiro t.
Machover Human Figure t.
MacMunn t.
macrophage migration t.
MacWilliam t.
magnesionitric t.
magnesium t.
Magpie t.
maintenance of wakefulness t.
malaria film t.
mallein t.
malonate t.
Malot t.
maltose t.
Maly t.
Mancini t.
Mann-Whitney t.
Mann-Whitney U t.
Mann-Whitney-Wilcoxon t.
manometric t.
Mantoux skin t.
manual muscle t.
Manzullo t.
Marchetti t.
Maréchal t.
Maréchal-Rosin t.
Marlow t.
Marquis t.
Marshall t.
Marshall-Marchetti t.
Maschke t.
Masset t.
mast cell degranulation t.
Master two-step exercise t.
mastic t.
Matas t.
match t.
Mátéfy t.
Mathews t.
Matzker t.
Maumené t.
Mauthner t.

T

test *(continued)*

- maximal exercise t.
- Mayer t.
- Mayerhofer t.
- Mazzotti t.
- McMurray t.
- McNemar t.
- mecalil provocation t.
- mecholyl t.
- MEGX (monoethylglycinexylidide) t.
- Méhu t.
- Meigs t.
- melanin t.
- Meltzer-Lyon t.
- Mendel t.
- Mendelsohn t.
- meningitis t.
- mercaptoethanol agglutination inhibition t.
- mercury t.
- Mester t.
- metabisulfate t.
- methacetin breath t.
- methylene blue t.
- methylphenylhydrazine t.
- methyl red t.
- metoclopramide stimulation t.
- Metopirone t.
- metyrapone t.
- Michailow t.
- microhemagglutination t. for *Treponema pallidum* (MHA-TP)
- microimmunofluorescence t.
- microprecipitation t.
- Middlebrook-Dubos hemagglutination t.
- MIF (migration inhibitory factor) t.
- migration inhibitory factor t. (MIF t.)
- Millard t.
- Miller-Kurzrok t.
- Millon t.
- Mills t.
- Mingazzini t.
- minimal caloric t.
- Minnesota Multiphasic Personality Inventory (MMPI) t.
- mirror t.
- Mitscherlich t.
- Mitsuda t.
- Mittelmeyer t.

test *(continued)*

- mixed agglutination t.
- mixed leukocyte culture t.
- mixed lymphocyte culture t.
- mixed triglyceride breath t.
- MLB (monaural loudness balance) t.
- mobility t.
- modified Rinne t.
- Moerner-Sjöqvist t.
- Mohr t.
- Molisch t.
- Moloney t.
- Moloney-Underwood t.
- monaural distorted speech t's
- monaural loudness balance (MLB) t.
- monocyte function t.
- monoethylglycinexylidide (MEGX) t. for liver function
- mononucleosis spot t.
- Monospot t.
- Mono-Vac t.
- Montenegro t.
- Montigne t.
- Morelli t.
- Moretti t.
- Moritz t.
- Mörner t.
- Moro t.
- morphine t.
- Morton t.
- Moschcowitz t.
- Mosenthal t.
- motility t.
- Moynihan t.
- mucin clot t.
- mucoprotein t.
- Mulder t.
- Müller t.
- multiple-puncture t.
- multiple sleep latency t.
- mumps sensitivity t.
- mumps skin t.
- murexide t.
- Murphy t.
- mycobiologic t.
- mycologic t.
- Myers and Fine t.
- Mylius t.
- Naffziger t.
- Nagel t. for color vision
- Nagler t. for *Clostridium perfringens*
- Nakayama t.

test *(continued)*

Nardi t.
Nathan t.
NBT (nitroblue tetrazolium) t.
Nencki t.
neostigmine t.
Nessler t.
Neubauer and Fischer t.
Neufeld t.
neuraminidase inhibition t.
neutralization t.
niacin t.
Nickerson-Kveim t.
nicotine t.
Ninhydrin t.
Nippe t.
nitrate reduction t.
nitrate utilization t.
Nitrazine t.
nitric acid t.
nitric acid–magnesium
  sulfate t.
nitrite t.
nitroblue tetrazolium (NBT) t.
nitrogenous compounds t.
nitrogen partition t.
nitrogen retention t.
nitrogen washout t.
nitroprusside t.
nitroso-indole-nitrate t.
N-MID osteocalcin ELISA t.
Nobel t.
nocturnal penile tumescence
  (NPT) t.
Noguchi t.
Nonne t.
Nonne-Apelt t.
nonparametric t.
nonprotein nitrogen t.
nonstress t. (NST)
nontreponemal antigen t.
nonverbal intelligence t.
norethindrone t.
norethynodrel t.
NPT (nocturnal penile
  tumescence) t.
nucleic acid t.
nucleic acid amplification t.
nystagmus t.
Oakley-Fulthorpe t.
Ober t.
Obermayer t.
Obermüller (Obermueller) t.
obturator t.
occult blood t.

test *(continued)*

octanoic acid breath t.
Octopus perimetry t.
olfactory nerve t.
Oliver t.
one-stage prothrombin time t.
ONPG t.
optokinetic drum t.
Optochin t.
oral lactose tolerance t.
orcinol t.
organic acid t.
orientation t.
orthotoluidine t.
Ortolani t.
osazone t.
Osgood-Haskins t.
osmotic fragility t.
Osterberg t.
Ott t.
Ouchterlony t.
Oudin t.
ovarian hyperemia t.
ox cell hemolysin t.
oxidase t.
oxyphenylsulfonic acid t.
oxytocin challenge t. (OCT)
oxytocin sensitivity t.
p24 antigen t.
Pachon t. for collateral
  circulation
Paget t.
PAM (postauricular myogenic)
  reflex t.
pancreatic function t.
pancreozymin-secretin t.
Pandy t.
Pap (Papanicolaou) t.
PAP (prostatic acid
  phosphatase) t.
parallel swing t.
parentage t.
Parnum t.
partial thromboplastin time
  (PTT) t.
PAS (periodic acid–Schiff) t.
passive agglutination t.
passive cutaneous
  anaphylaxis t.
passive protection t.
passive transfer t.
patch t.
paternity t.
Patrick t.
Patterson t.

T

test *(continued)*

patting t.
Paul t.
Paul-Bunnell t.
Paul-Bunnell-Barrett t.
Paul-Bunnell-Davidsohn t.
Pavy t.
PCA (passive cutaneous anaphylaxis) t.
Pélouse-Moore t.
pendular eye-tracking t. (PETT)
pendulousness of legs t.
pentagastrin stimulation t. for gastric function
pentose t.
Penzoldt t.
Penzoldt-Fischer t.
pepsin t.
peptide t.
peptone t.
perchlorate discharge t.
perchloride t.
performance t.
Peria t.
periodic acid–Schiff (PAS) t.
peritoneal equilibration t.
Perls t. for hemosiderin
permanganate t.
peroxidase t.
Perthes t.
Petri t.
Pettenkofer t.
Petzetaki t.
pH t.
phage neutralization t.
Phalen t.
phenacetin t.
phenol t.
phenolphthalein t.
phenolsulfonphthalein t.
phentolamine t.
phenylalanine deaminase t.
phenylhydrazine t.
phenylketonuria t.
phlorizin t.
phosphatase t.
phospholipid t.
phosphoric acid t.
photopatch t.
photostress t.
phthalein t.
Piazza t.
picrotoxin t.
pinch t.
Pincus t.

test *(continued)*

pineapple t.
pine wood t. for indole
Piotrowski t.
Piria t. for tyrosine
pivot-shift t.
P-K (Prausnitz-Küstner) t.
plantar ischemia t.
plasma ACTH t.
plasma cortisol t.
plasma hemoglobin t.
platelet aggregation t.
pneumatic t.
Pohl t.
pointing t.
Politzer t.
Pollacci t.
polystyrene latex t.
Porges-Meier t.
Porges-Salomon t.
porphobilinogen t.
porphyrin t.
Porter t.
Porter-Silber chromogens t.
Porteus maze t.
positive washout t.
Posner t.
postauricular myogenic (PAM) reflex t.
postcoital t.
posterior drawer t.
potassium t.
potassium cyanide t.
potassium iodide t.
P and P (prothrombin and proconvertin) t.
PPD (purified protein derivative) t.
Prausnitz-Küstner (P-K) t.
precipitation t.
precipitin t.
Pregl t.
pregnancy t.
Prendergast t.
Preyer t.
prism adaption t.
Proetz t.
progesterone withdrawal t.
projective t.
projective human figure drawing t.
prolactin t.
prolonged toxicity t.
pronation-supination t.

test *(continued)*

prostatic acid phosphatase (PAP) t.
protection t.
protein t.
protein truncation t.
proteinuria t.
proteose t.
prothrombin t. (PT)
prothrombin consumption t.
prothrombin-proconvertin (P and P) t.
proverbs t.
provocative t.
psoas t.
psychological t.
psychomotor t.
pulmonary function t. (PFT)
pulp t.
Purdy t.
purine bodies t.
pus t.
Pyramidon t.
Q-tip t.
quadriceps t.
qualitative fecal fat t.
quantitation t.
quantitative gel diffusion t.
Queckenstedt t.
Queckenstedt-Stookey t.
quellung t.
Quick t. (for liver function)
Quick tourniquet t. (for prothrombin time)
Quinlan t.
Raabe t.
Rabuteau t.
Race-Coombs t.
radial diffusion t.
radioactive fibrinogen uptake t.
radioactive iodine (RAI) uptake t.
radioallergosorbent t. (RAST)
radioimmunoprecipitation t.
radioimmunosorbent t. (RIST)
radioiodine t.
radioisotope renal excretion t.
radioisotope renogram t.
RAI (radioactive iodine) t.
RA latex fixation t.
Ralfe t.
Ramon flocculation t.
Randolph t.
Rantzman t.
rapid plasma reagin (RPR) t's

test *(continued)*

rapid plasma reagin (RPR) circle card t.
rapid serum amylase t.
Raygat t.
Rebuck t.
recruitment t.
red t.
red cell adherence t.
red glass t.
Rees t.
Rehberg t.
Rehfuss t.
Reichl t.
Reinsch t.
Reitan-Indiana aphasic screening t.
Remont t.
renal function t. (RFT)
renin stimulation t.
renin suppression t.
resorcinol t.
resorcinol–hydrochloric acid t.
Reuss t.
Reynold t.
rheumatoid arthritis (RA) t.
rheumatoid factor (RF) t.
RhoGAM t.
rhubarb t.
Rideal-Walker t.
RIF t.
ring t.
Rinne t.
Rivalta t.
Roberts t.
Robinson-Kepler t.
Robinson-Kepler-Power water t.
Rocher drawer t.
rollover t.
Romberg t.
Ronchese t.
Roos t.
Rorschach inkblot t.
Rose t.
rose bengal t.
Rosenbach-Gmelin t.
Rosenheim-Drummond t.
Rosenthal t.
Rosenzweig picture frustration t.
Rose-Waaler t.
Rosin t.
Ross-Jones t.
rotation t.
Rotazyme t.

T

test *(continued)*

Rothera t.
Rotter t.
Rous t.
Roussin t.
Rowntree and Geraghty t.
RPR (rapid plasma reagin) t.
Rubin t.
Rubino t.
Rubner t.
Ruhemann t.
ruler t.
Rumpel-Leede t.
Russell viper venom t.
Russo t.
Ruttan and Hardisty t.
Saathoff t.
Sabin-Feldman dye t.
saccharimeter t.
saccharin t.
Sakaguchi t.
salicylic acid t.
saline fragility t.
saline suppression t.
Salkowski t.
Salkowski-Ludwig t.
Salkowski and Schipper t.
Salomon t.
sand t.
Sandrock t.
Sanford t.
santonin t.
Saundby t.
scarification t.
Schaffer t.
Schalfijew t.
Schalm t.
Scherer t.
Schick t.
Schiff t.
Schiller t. for cervical cancer
Schilling t. for GI absorption
   of B12
Schirmer t.
Schlesinger t.
Schlichter t.
Schober t.
Schönbein (Schoenbein) t.
Schroeder t.
Schulte t. for proteins
Schultze t. for cellulose
Schumm t.
Schwabach t.
sciatic stretch t.
Scivoletto t.

test *(continued)*

scleroscope t.
SCMC t. for cervical factor
   infertility
scratch t.
screening t.
Seashore t.
secretin t.
secretin-cholecystokinin t.
secretin injection t.
secretin-pancreozymin t.
secretin stimulation t.
sedimentation t.
SeHCAT (selenium Se
   75–labeled homocholic acid)
   t. for absorption of bile salts
Seidel t.
Seidlitz powder t.
Selivanoff (Seliwanow) t.
semen analysis t.
senna t.
sensitized sheep cell
   agglutination t.
sentence completion t.
Sereny t.
serologic t.
serologic t. for syphilis (STS)
serology t.
serum alkaline phosphatase t.
serum bactericidal activity t.
serum bilirubin t.
serum calcium t.
serum creatine kinase (CK) t.
serum creatinine t.
serum enzyme t.
serum gastrin t.
serum globulin t.
serum neutralization t.
serum phosphorus t.
sex chromatin t.
shadow t.
sham feeding t.
Shear t.
sheep cell agglutination t.
short increment sensitivity
   index (SISI) t.
short-term toxicity t.
shuttle walking t.
Sia water t. for
   macroglobulinemia
Sibley-Lehninger t.
Sicard-Cantelouble t.
sickle cell t.
sickling t.
Siebold and Bradbury t.

test *(continued)*

   silver t.
   silver nitroprusside t.
   Simonelli t.
   Sims t.
   Sims-Huhner t.
   single-breath nitrogen
     washout t.
   single-breath oxygen t.
   single diffusion t.
   single radial diffusion t.
   single radial hemolysis t.
   single-tail t.
   SISI (short increment
     sensitivity index) t.
   skatole t.
   skin t.
   skin-puncture t.
   skin window t.
   slide agglutination t.
   slide flocculation t.
   Slocum t.
   small increment sensitivity
     index (SISI) t.
   SMA profile t. (SMA-12, SMA-
     21, etc.)
   smear t.
   Smith t.
   Snellen t.
   Snider match t.
   sniff t.
   Snyder t.
   sodium t.
   Soldaini t.
   Solera t.
   solubility t.
   Sonnenschein t.
   sorting t.
   soy bean t. (for urease)
   specific gravity t.
   specific red cell adherence t.
   spectroscopic t.
   sperm agglutination t.
   sperm–cervical mucus contact t.
   sperm immobilization t.
   sphenopalatine t.
   Spiegler t.
   Spiro t.
   split renal function t.
   sponge t.
   Spurling t.
   squatting t.
   STA (standard tube
     agglutination) t.
   Stamey t.

test *(continued)*

   standing plasma t.
   Stanford-Binet t.
   starch t.
   starch hydrolysis t.
   station t.
   Staub-Traugott t.
   Stein t.
   Stenger t.
   stereognostic t.
   Sterneedle tuberculin t.
   stiff wrist t.
   stimulation t.
   Stock t.
   Stokvis t.
   Stoll t.
   stool guaiac t.
   Storck t.
   straight leg raising t.
     (SLRT)
   Strassburg t.
   Straus biological t.
   streptolysin O t.
   streptozyme t.
   stress t.
   string t.
   Struve t.
   strychnine t.
   Stypven time t.
   subchronic toxicity t.
   submaximal exercise t.
   sucrose hemolysis t.
   sucrose lysis t.
   sucrose tolerance t.
   sulfobromophthalein excretion
     t. for liver function
   sulfosalicylic acid t.
   sulfur t.
   Sulkowitch t.
   Sullivan t.
   suppression t.
   susceptibility t.
   sweat t.
   sweating t.
   swinging flashlight t.
   syphilis t.
   Szabo t.
   Szondi t.
   T_3 resin uptake t. [T3]
   T_3 suppression t. [T3]
   T_3 uptake t. [T3]
   T_4 RIA t. [T4]
   Takata-Ara t.
   tanned red cell (TRC) t.
   tannic acid t.

T

test *(continued)*

 Tanret t.
 Tardieu t.
 taurine t.
 Taylor t.
 Teichmann t.
 tellurite t.
 Tensilon t.
 Terman t.
 tetrazolium t.
 thalleioquin t.
 thallium stress t.
 Thayer-Martin t.
 thematic apperception t. (TAT)
 thermal t.
 thiamine t.
 thin layer rapid use
  epicutaneous (TRUE) t.
 thiochrome t.
 thiocyanate t.
 Thomas t.
 Thormählen t. for melanin in
  urine
 Thorn t.
 threshold tone decay t.
 thromboplastin generation t.
  (TGT)
 Thudichum t. for creatinine
 thumbnail t.
 thymol turbidity t.
 thyroid antibody t.
 thyroid function t. (TFT)
 thyroid-stimulating hormone
  (TSH) t.
 thyroid-stimulating hormone
  stimulation t.
 thyroid suppression t.
 thyrotropin-releasing
  hormone t.
 thyrotropin-releasing hormone
  stimulation t.
 thyroxine-binding index t.
 Tidy t.
 tilt table t.
 tine t.
 Tinel t.
 tine tuberculin t. (Rosenthal)
 Tizzoni t.
 Tobey-Ayer t.
 tolbutamide tolerance t.
 tolerance t.
 Tollens, Neuberg, and
  Schwket t.
 tone decay t.
 tongue t.

test *(continued)*

 Töpfer (Toepfer) t.
 Torquay t.
 torsion t.
 tourniquet t.
 toxigenicity t.
 Toynbee t. for patency of
  auditory t.
 TPHA (*Treponema pallidum*
  hemagglutination) t.
 TPI (*Treponema pallidum*
  immobilization) t.
 traction t.
 Trambusti t.
 transcriptase reverse t.
 transillumination t.
 trapeze t.
 tray agglutination t.
 TRC (tanned red cells) t.
 treadmill exercise t. (TET)
 treadmill stress t. (TST)
 Trendelenburg t.
 treponemal antigen t. (TAT)
 treponemal hemagglutination
  (TPHA) t.
 Treponema pallidum
  complement fixation t's
 Treponema pallidum
  hemagglutination (TPHA) t.
 Treponema pallidum
  immobilization (TPI) t.
 Tretop t.
 TRH t., TRH-stimulation t.
 Triboulet t.
 trichophytin t.
 tricresol peroxidase t.
 triiodothyronine (T_3 [T3]) red
  cell uptake t.
 triiodothyronine (T_3 [T3])
  resin uptake t.
 triiodothyronine (T_3 [T3])
  uptake t.
 triketohydrindene hydrate t.
 triolein breath t.
 triple t.
 Trommer t.
 Trousseau t.
 TRUE t.
 trypsin t.
 tryptophan load t.
 TSH t., TSH-stimulation t.
 t. tube
 tuberculin t.
 tuberculin patch t.
 tuberculin t., Sterneedle

test *(continued)*
    tuberculin titer t.
    tube-slide agglutination t.
    tubular reabsorption of
        phosphate t.
    Tuffier t.
    tuning fork t.
    T water fructose intolerance t.
    two-glass t.
    two-stage prothrombin time t.
    two-step exercise t.
    typhoid fever t.
    tyrosine t.
    Tyson t.
    Tzanck t.
    Udránszky t.
    Uffelmann t.
    Ulrich t.
    ultrasound t.
    Ultzmann t.
    Umber t.
    unheated serum reagin
        (USR) t.
    Unterberger t.
    uracil t.
    urea t.
    urea breath t.
    urea clearance t.
    urea concentration t.
    urea nitrogen t.
    urease t.
    Urecholine supersensitivity t.
    uric acid t.
    urine acetone t.
    urine chloride t.
    urine concentration t.
    urobilin t.
    urobilinogen t.
    urochromogen t.
    urorrhodin t.
    USR (unheated serum reagin) t.
    vaginal cornification t.
    Valenta t.
    Valsalva t.
    van den Bergh t.
    van den Velden t.
    vanillylmandelic acid (VMA) t.
    Van Slyke t.
    Van Slyke and Cullen t.
    Vaughan and Novy t.
    VDRL t.
    ventilation t.
    virulence t.
    virus neutralization t.
    Visscher-Bowman t.

test *(continued)*
    visual field t.
    visual-motor gestalt t.
    Vitali t.
    vitality t.
    vitamin t.
    vitamin A absorption t.
    vitamin K t.
    VMA (vanillylmandelic
        acid) t.
    Voelcker and Joseph t.
    Vogel and Lee t.
    Voges-Proskauer t.
    Volhard t.
    Vollmer t.
    von Aldor t.
    von Jaksch t.
    von Maschke t.
    von Recklinghausen t.
    von Zeynek and Mencki t.
    W4D (Worth four-dot) t.
    Waaler-Rose t.
    Wada t.
    Wagner t.
    WAIS (Wechsler Adult
        Intelligence Scale) t.
    Waldenström t.
    walking t.
    Walter bromide t.
    Wampole t.
    Wang t.
    Warren t.
    washout t.
    Wassermann t.
    Wassermann-fast t.
    Wassermann reaction t.
    watch t.
    water deprivation t.
    water-gurgle t.
    water provocative t.
    Watson-Schwartz t.
    Weber t.
    Wechsler Adult Intelligence
        Scale (WAIS) t.
    Wechsler Intelligence Scale for
        Children (WISC) t.
    Weichbrodt t.
    Weidel t.
    Weigl-Goldstein-Scheerer t.
    Weil-Felix t.
    Weinberg t.
    Weiss t.
    Weiss permanganate t.
    Weisz t.
    Welland t.

T

test *(continued)*

Well-Cogen latex
   agglutination t.
Wenzell t.
Weppen t.
Werner t.
Wernicke t.
Westergren sedimentation
   rate t.
Western blot t.
Western blot electrotransfer t.
Wetzel t.
Weyl t.
Wheeler and Johnson t.
whiff t
whisper t.
whistle t.
Whitaker t. for resistance of
   ureters
Whiteside t.
Widal serum t.
Wilkinson and Peter t.
Williamson blood t.
Wilson t.
Winckler t.
wipe t.
wire loop t.
Wishart t.
Witz t.
Woldman t.
Wolff-Eisner t.
Wolff-Junghans t.
Woodbury t.
word association t.
Wormley t.
Worm-Müller t.
worsted t.
Worth four-dot (W4D) t.
Wright t.
Wurster t.
xanthine t.
X-chromatin t.
Xenopus t., *X. laevis* t.
xylidine t.
D-xylose absorption t.
D-xylose breath t.
xylose concentration test
D-xylose tolerance t.
Y-chromatin t.
Yergason t.
Yerkes-Bridges t.
Young t.
Zaleski t.
Zangemeister t.
Zappacosta t.

test *(continued)*

Zeisel t.
Zeller t.
Ziehen t.
zinc flocculation t.
zinc fluorescence t.
zinc turbidity t.
Zondek-Aschheim t.
Zouchlos t.
Zung depression scale t.
Zwenger t.
testa (testae)
testaceous
testalgia
Tes-Tape
test card
   stigmometric t.c.
testectomy
testes (plural of testis)
testicle
   atrophic t.
   ectopic t.
   hidden t.
   high intra-abdominal t.
   nonpalpable t.
   palpable t.
   retained t.
   retractile t.
   Sertoli cell tumor of the t.
   t. torsion
   undescended t.
testicular
   t. appendage
   t. artery
   t. compression reflex
   t. duct
   embryonic t. regression
      syndrome
   t. enlargement
   t. feminization syndrome
   t. fine-needle aspiration
   t. hormone
   incomplete t. feminization
   t. microlithiasis
   percutaneous t. sperm
      aspiration
   Pick t. adenoma
   t. shock
   t. sperm extraction
   t. tumor
   t. vein
testiculoma ovarii
testiculus (testiculi)
testimony
   expert t.

testing
- histocompatibility t.
- nondestructive t.
- reality t.
- visual field t.

testis (testes)
- abdominal t.
- adenocarcinoma of infantile t.
- ascending t.
- blood-t. barrier
- canalicular t.
- Cooper irritable t.
- t. cords
- cryptorchid t.
- ectopic t.
- femoral t.
- gliding t.
- inguinal t.
- intra-abdominal t.
- inverted t.
- mesothelioma of t.
- obstructed t.
- peeping t.
- perineal t.
- pulpy t.
- t. redux
- retained t.
- retractile t.
- rudimentary t. syndrome
- undescended t.
- vanishing t.

testitis

test meal
- barium t.m.
- fatty t.m.
- Lundh t.m.
- standard t.m.
- U-13 C palmitate t.m.

testoid

testopathy

testosterone
- t.-estradiol–binding globulin
- ethinyl t.
- methyl t.
- t. 17β-dehydrogenase [17-beta-]

test type
- Jaeger t.t.
- Landolt t.t.
- Snellen t.t.

tetanic
- t. contraction
- t. convulsion
- t. spasm

tetaniform

tetanization

tetanize

tetanocannabin

tetanode

tetanoid paraplegia

tetanolysin

tetanospasmin

tetanus
- t. antitoxin
- t. bacillus
- cephalic t.
- cerebral t.
- cryptogenic t.
- diphtheria and t. toxoids
- generalized t.
- t. immune globulin
- localized t.
- neonatal t.
- t. neonatorum
- t. toxin
- t. toxoid

tetany
- t. of alkalosis
- duration t.
- gastric t.
- hyperventilation t.
- hypoparathyroid t.
- infantile t.
- latent t.
- neonatal t.
- t. of newborn
- parathyroid t.
- parathyroprival t.
- phosphate t.
- physiological t.
- postoperative t.
- postsurgical t.
- rheumatic t.
- thyroprival t.

tetartanope

tetartanopia

tetartanopic

tetartanopsia

tethered
- t. cord syndrome
- t. nerves

tetraboric acid

tetrabrachius

tetrachirus

tetrachloride
- carbon t.

tetrachloroethane poisoning

tetrachloroethylene

tetrachromic

tetracosanoic acid

tetracrotic
tetracyclic antidepressant
tetrad
    Fallot t.
    narcoleptic t.
tetradactylous
tetradactyly
tetraethyl pyrophosphate
tetragonum lumbale
tetragonus
tetrahedron chest
tetrahydric
tetrahydrobiopterin deficiency
tetrahydrocannabinol (THC)
tetrahydrofolate (THF)
tetrahydrofolic acid
tetraiodophenolphthalein
tetralogy
    t. of Eisenmenger
    t. of Fallot
tetramethylammonium hydroxide
tetramine
tetranopsia
Tetranychus
    T. montensis
    T. telarius
tetraodon poisoning
tetraodontoxin
tetraodontoxism
tetraotus
tetraparesis
tetrapeptide
tetraplegia
tetraploid
tetraploidy
tetrapus
tetrasaccharide
tetrascelus
tetrasomic
tetrasomy 12p
tetrastichiasis
tetrathionate broth
tetratomic molecule
tetrodonic acid
tetrodotoxin
tetrodotoxism
tetroxide
    nitrogen t.
    osmium t.
tetryl
Teutleben ligament
Tevdek suture
Texas catheter
text blindness
textiform

textoblastic
Textor operation
textural
texture
textus (textus)
TF—
    tactile fremitus
    tetralogy of Fallot
    thymol flocculation
    tissue-damaging factor
    total flow
    transfer factor
    tuberculin filtrate
TFA—total fatty acid(s)
TFCC—triangular fibrocartilage
    complex
TFE—tetrafluoroethylene
TG—
    thioguanine
    thyroglobulin
    toxic goiter
    triglyceride
TGA—
    transient global amnesia
    transposition of the great
      arteries
TGAR—total graft area rejected
TGC—time gain compensation
TGF—
    T-cell growth factor
    transforming growth factor
TG-globulin
TGT—thromboplastin generation
    test
TGV—transposition of the great
    vessels
θ—theta (Greek letter)
THA—total hip arthroplasty
thalamectomy
thalamencephalic
thalamencephalon
thalami (genitive and plural of
    thalamus)
thalamic
    t. fasciculus
    t. hyperesthetic anesthesia
    t. nuclei
    t. peduncles
    t. radiations
    t. syndrome
    t. tubercle
thalamocortical
    t. fibers
    t. projections
thalamogeniculate artery

thalamolenticular
thalamomammillary
    t. bundle
    t. fasciculus
thalamoparietal fibers
thalamoperforating artery
thalamostriate
    t. arteries
    t. radiation
    t. veins
thalamotegmental
thalamotemporal radiation
thalamotomy
    anterior t.
    dorsomedial t.
    parafascicular t. (PFT)
thalamotuberal artery
thalamus (thalami)
    dorsal t.
    optic t.
    radiations of t.
    stalks of t.
    ventral t.
thalassemia
    α-t. [alpha-]
    β-t. [beta-]
    δ-t. [delta-]
    δ-β-t. [delta beta-]
    hemoglobin C–t.
    hemoglobin C–β-t. [C–beta-]
    hemoglobin E–t.
    hemoglobin E–α-t. [E-alpha-]
    hemoglobin E–β-t. [E-beta-]
    hemoglobin Lepore–β-t. [-beta-]
    hemoglobin S-t.
    hemoglobin S–α-t. [S-alpha-]
    hemoglobin S–β-t. [S-beta-]
    heterozygous β-t. [beta-]
    homozygous β-t. [beta-]
    t. intermedia
    t. major
    t. minor
    sickle cell–t.
thalassin
thalleioquin test
thallitoxicosis
thallium (Tl)
    t. 201 imaging
    t. myocardial scan
    t. perfusion scintigraphy
    t. stress testing
thallous chloride Tl 201
thalposis
thalpotic
thanatobiologic

thanatognomonic
thanatoid
thanatophidia
thanatophidial
thanatophobia
thanatophoric
    t. dwarf
    t. dysplasia
thanatopsis
thanatosis
Thayer-Martin culture medium
Thaysen disease
THC—tetrahydrocannabinol
theaism
thebaic
thebaine
thebesian
    t. circulation
    t. foramina
    t. valve
    t. veins
theca (thecae)
    t. cells
    t. cell tumor
    t. externa
    t. of follicle of von Baer
    t. folliculi
    t. interna
    t.-lutein cyst
    t. medullare spinalis
    t. vertebralis
thecal
    t. abscess
    t. cyst
    t. puncture
    t. whitlow
thecitis
thecoma
thecomatosis
thecosis
thecostegnosis
Theden bandage
Theile
    canal
    glands
Theiler
    disease
    virus
Theis retractor
thelalgia
thelarche
    exaggerated t.
    fluctuating t.
    precocious t.
    premature t.

T

theleplasty
thelerethism
theliolymphocyte
thelitis
thelium (thelia)
thelorrhagia
thenad
thenal
thenar eminence
Theobald probe
theobroma oil
theotherapy
theque
therapeutic
    t. agent
    t. benefit
    t. concentration
    t. drugs
    t. effect
    t. guidelines
    t. iridectomy
    t. milieu
    t. options
    t. regimen
    t. target
therapeutics
    cellular t.
    rational t.
    specific t.
therapist
    certified craniosacral t.
    corrective t.
    family t.
    low-vision t.
    music t.
    occupational t.
    physical t.
    radiation t.
    rehabilitation t.
    respiratory t.
    sex t.
    speech t.
therapy
    ablation t.
    active t.
    adjuvant t.
    aerosol t.
    alkali t.
    analytic t.
    androgen ablation t.
    anticoagulant t.
    anticonvulsant t.
    antiplatelet t.
    art t.
    autolymphocyte t.

therapy *(continued)*
    autoserum t.
    aversion t.
    beam t.
    behavior t.
    behavioral marital t.
    bilateral electroconvulsive t.
    bile acid t.
    biological t.
    blunderbuss t.
    buffer t.
    carbon dioxide t.
    cardiac resynchronization t.
    Chaoul t.
    chelation t.
    client-centered t.
    cognitive t.
    collapse t.
    color t.
    combined t.
    combined-modality t.
    compression t.
    conditioning t.
    conjoint t.
    contact t.
    continuous sleep t.
    convulsive t.
    corrective t.
    couples t.
    craniosacral t.
    dance t.
    deleading t.
    diathermic t.
    diet t.
    drug t.
    electric convulsive t.
    electric shock t.
    electroconvulsive t. (ECT)
    electrodermal activity t.
    electromagnetic field t.
    electron beam t.
    electroshock t. (EST)
    emotionally focused t.
    endocrine t.
    endocrine ablative t.
    enzyme t.
    estrogen replacement t. (ERT)
    external beam t.
    family t.
    fango t.
    fever t.
    fibrinolytic t.
    first line t.
    gene t.
    gestalt t. (also: Gestalt)

therapy *(continued)*
    Goeckerman t.
    gold t.
    grenz ray t.
    grid t.
    group t.
    heat t.
    highly active antiretroviral t.
      (HAART)
    hormonal t.
    hormone replacement t. (HRT)
    humidification t.
    hyperbaric oxygen (HBO) t.
    hypoglycemic t.
    immunization t.
    immunosuppressive t.
    induction t.
    inhalation t.
    insulin coma t.
    interstitial radiation t.
    intradiscal electrothermal t.
    intraosseous t.
    intrathecal t.
    intravenous t.
    larval t.
    light t.
    lithium t.
    locoregional t.
    maggot t.
    magnetic field t.
    maintenance t.
    manipulative t.
    marital t.
    massage t.
    milieu t.
    Morita t.
    movement t.
    multimodality t.
    multiple t.
    music t.
    myofunctional t.
    neoadjuvant t.
    nondirective t.
    nonspecific t.
    nutritional t.
    occupational t.
    oral rehydration t. (ORT)
    orthomolecular t.
    osteopathic manipulative t.
      (OMT)
    oxygen t.
    pancreatic enzyme t.
    paraspecific t.
    parenteral t.
    photodynamic t.

therapy *(continued)*
    physical t.
    plasma t.
    play t.
    poetry t.
    polarity t.
    preoperative t.
    presurgical t.
    primal t.
    protective t.
    proton beam t.
    psychoanalytic t.
    pulp canal t.
    pulse t.
    PUVA (psoralens and
      ultraviolet A light) t.
    radiation t.
    radiofrequency t.
    radionuclide t.
    radium t.
    rational t.
    recreational t.
    reflex t.
    relaxation t.
    renal replacement t.
    replacement t.
    respiratory t.
    root canal t.
    rotation t.
    salvage t.
    sclerosing t.
    serum t.
    sex t.
    shock t.
    short-wave t.
    sleep t.
    social t.
    solar t.
    somatic cell gene t.
    sparing t.
    specific t.
    speech t.
    spinal manipulative t. (SMT)
    strategic t.
    subcoma insulin t.
    substitution t.
    substitutive t.
    suggestion t.
    supportive t.
    telecobalt t.
    thrombolytic t.
    thyroid replacement t.
    thyroxine replacement t.
    Trager t.
    ultrasonic t.

T

therapy *(continued)*
    unilateral electroconvulsive t.
    vaccine t.
    virus-directed enzyme
      prodrug t.
    x-ray t.
    zone t.
thermacogenesis
thermal
    t. anesthesia
    t. ataxia
    t. biofeedback
    British t. unit (BTU)
    t. burn
    t. capacity
    t. cataract
    t. conductivity
    t. diffusion
    t. dilution curve
    t. dilution method
    t. dilution technique
    t. expansion
    t. neutron
    t. receptor
    t. relaxation time
    t. sweating
thermalgesia
thermalgia
thermanalgesia
thermanesthesia
thermesthesia
thermhyperesthesia
thermhypesthesia
thermic
    t. effect
    t. fever
    t. inversion
thermionic
    t. emission
    t. rectifier
thermionics
Thermoactinomyces vulgaris
thermocauterectomy
thermocautery
thermochemistry
thermochroic
thermochroism
thermochrosis
thermocoagulation
    radiofrequency t.
thermocurrent
thermodiffusion
thermodilution
    t. catheter
    t. technique

thermoduric
thermodynamics
thermoexcitory
Thermo-flex suture
thermogenesis
    dietary induced t.
    nonshivering t.
    shivering t.
thermogenetic
thermogenic anhidrosis
thermogenics
thermogenous
thermogram
    liquid crystal t.
thermograph
    continuous scan t.
thermographic
thermography
    infrared tympanic t.
    liquid crystal t. (LCT)
thermohyperalgesia
thermohyperesthesia
thermohypesthesia
thermoinactivation
thermoinhibitory
thermojunction
thermolabile
thermolamp
thermoluminescence
thermoluminescent
thermolysis
thermolytic
thermomassage
thermometer
    alcohol t.
    axilla t.
    Celsius t.
    centigrade t.
    clinical t.
    Fahrenheit t.
    fever t.
    infrared tympanic t.
    mercury t.
    oral t.
    rectal t.
    resistance t.
    self-registering t.
    surface t.
    tympanic t.
thermonuclear
thermopalpation
thermopenetration
thermophilic
thermoplastic
thermoplegia

thermoprecipitation
thermoradiotherapy
thermoregulation
thermoregulator
thermoresistance
thermoresistant
thermostabile
thermostasis
thermostat
   hypothalamic t.
thermosteresis
thermotactic
thermotaxis
thermotherapy
   diode laser t.
   endometrial laser intrauterine
     t. (ELITT)
   laser interstitial t. (LITT)
   transpupillary t.
   transurethral microwave t.
     (TUMT)
   water-induced t.
thermotolerant
thermotonometer
thermotoxin
theta—Greek letter
  (θ; alphabetized as th)
theta antigen
THFA—tetrahydrofolic acid
thiaminase (I and II)
thiamine
   t. hydrochloride
   t. mononitrate
   t. pyrophosphate (TPP)
thiazide
   t. diabetes
   t. diuretics
thiazine-eosinate stain
Thibierge-Weissenbach
  syndrome
thick-layer autoradiography
thickness
   deep partial-t. burn
   full-t. burn
   full-t. graft
   half-value t.
   partial-t. burn
   split-t. skin graft
   superficial partial-t. burn
   triceps skinfold (TSF) t.
Thiele syndrome
Thiemann disease
Thiersch
   graft
   knife

Thiersch *(continued)*
   operation
   suture
Thiersch-Duplay
   operation
   urethroplasty
thigh
   t. bone
   cricket t.
   drivers' t.
   Heilbronner t.
thigh-lift
thigmesthesia
thigmotactic
thigmotaxis
thigmotropic
thigmotropism
thimble-shaped nail shedding
thimerosal
thinking
   abstract t.
   autistic t.
   concrete t.
   critical t.
   delusional t.
   dereistic t.
   disordered t.
   disorganized t.
   irrational t.
   magical t.
   negative t.
   preoperational t.
   pressured t.
   primary process t.
   rational t.
   secondary process t.
thin-layer chromatography
  (TLC)
   instant t.l.c. (ITLC)
thioalcohol
thioarsenite
thiobarbiturate
thiobarbituric acid
thiocarbamide
thiochrome
thioctic acid
thiocyanate
   t. space
   t. test
thiocyanic acid
thiodotherapy
thioester
thioether
thioethylamine
thioflavine

T

thiogalactoside
  isopropyl t.
thioglucose
thioglycolate (THIO) broth
thioglycolic acid
thiolase
thiolate
thiolhistidine
thiomersalate
thioneine
thionin
thionine
thionyl
thiopanic acid
thiopectic
thioredoxin
thioredoxin reductase
thiosemicarbazone
thiostrepton
thiosulfate sulfurtransferase
thiosulfuric acid
thioxanthene
thiozine
third-spacing
third ventriculostomy
thirst
  insensible t.
  real t.
  subliminal t.
  true t.
  twilight t.
Thiry fistula
Thiry-Vella fistula
thlipsencephalus
Thoma
  ampulla
  fluid
Thomas
  collar
  curet
  operation
  pessary
  sign
  splint
  test
Thomas-Warren incision
Thoma-Zeiss
  cell
  counting chamber
Thompson
  catheter
  dermatoplasty
  lithotrite
  operation
  prosthesis

Thompson *(continued)*
  resectoscope
  syndrome
Thoms
  forceps
  method
  pelvimeter
  test
Thoms-Allis forceps
Thomsen
  antibody
  disease
Thomsen-Friedenreich antigen
Thoms-Gaylor forceps
Thomson
  clamp
  disease
  poikiloderma congenitale
  scattering
  sign
thoracalgia
thoracectomy
thoracentesis
thoraces (plural of thorax)
thoracic
  t. aorta
  t. aortofemoral bypass
  t. aortography
  t. aperture
  t. arteries
  asphyxiating t. dystrophy
  t. axis
  t. bones
  t. cavity
  t. column
  t. constriction of esophagus
  t. curvature
  t. diaphragm
  t. duct
  t. empyema
  t. esophagus
  t. fascia
  first t. ganglion
  t. fistula
  Fourmentin t. index
  t. index
  inferior t. opening
  t. inlet
  t. insufficiency syndrome
  t. joint
  t. kidney
  t. kyphosis
  t. laminectomy
  t. limb
  t. nerves

thoracic *(continued)*
  t. opening
  t. outlet
  t. outlet syndrome
  t. plane
  t. respiration
  t. skeleton
  t. spine
  t. stomach
  superior t. aperture
    syndrome
  superior t. opening
  t. synovial joints
  t. veins
thoracicoabdominal
thoracicoacromial artery
thoracicohumeral
thoracicolumbar division
thoracispinal
thoracoabdominal
  incision
thoracoacromial
thoracoceloschisis
thoracocentesis
thoracocyllosis
thoracocyrtosis
thoracodelphus
thoracodidymus
thoracodorsal
thoracodynia
thoracogastrodidymus
thoracogastropagus
thoracogastroschisis
thoracolaparotomy
thoracolumbar
thoracolysis
thoracomelus parasiticus
thoracometry
thoracomyodynia
thoracoomphalopagus
thoracopagus
  t. epigastricus
  t. parasiticus
thoracoparacephalus
thoracopathy
thoracoplasty
  costoversion t.
  lateral t.
thoracoschisis
thoracoscope
thoracoscopy
thoracostenosis
thoracostomy tube
thoracotomy incision
Thoraeus filter

thorax (thoraces)
  amazon t.
  barrel-shaped t.
  cholesterol t.
  Peyrot t.
  pyriform t.
Thorek
  aspirator
  scissors
Thorek-Feldman scissors
Thorek-Mixter forceps
Thorel bundle
thorium (Th)
  t. dioxide
  radioactive t.
  sodium t. tartrate
Thorn maneuver
Thorn salt-depletion syndrome
Thornton
  nail
  plate
  screw
  sign
Thornwald perforator
Thorpe
  calipers
  forceps
  plastic lens
  scissors
Thorpe-Castroviejo scissors
Thorpe-Westcott scissors
thought
  audible t.
  t. broadcasting
  t. insertion
  t. withdrawal
thread
  mucous t's
  Simonart t.
thread-elastic ligature
threadworm
three-bottle drainage system
three-chambered heart
three-dimensional
  t-d. computed tomography
  t-d. echocardiography
  t-d. images
  t-d. imaging technique
  t-d. model
  t-d. optical coherence
    tomography
  t-d. ultrasonography (3D-US)
three-phase system
three-pillow orthopnea
threonine (Thr., T) dehydratase

T

threonyl
threose
threpsis
threshold
    absolute t.
    achromatic t.
    alpha t.
    anaerobic t.
    audiometric t.
    auditory t.
    chromatic t.
    colorless visual t.
    t. of consciousness
    convulsant t.
    defibrillation t.
    differential t.
    differential light t.
    differential sensory t.
    t. of discomfort
    displacement t.
    t. dose
    double-point t.
    epileptic t.
    erythema t.
    t. erythema dose
    excretion t.
    fibrillation t.
    flicker fusion t.
    t. for two-point discrimination
    galvanic t.
    Geiger t.
    light t.
    myoclonic t.
    neuron t.
    t. of nose
    olfactory t.
    pacing t.
    pain t.
    t. percussion
    t. potential
    relational t.
    renal t.
    renal t. for glucose
    resolution t.
    sensing t.
    sensitivity t.
    speech reception t. (SRT)
    stimulus t.
    t. stimulus
    stretch t.
    swallowing t.
    thrombotic t. velocity
    t. of visual sensation
thrill
    aneurysmal t.
    aortic t.

thrill *(continued)*
    arterial t.
    arteriovenous t.
    diastolic t.
    fat t.
    hydatid t.
    presystolic t.
    purring t.
    systolic t.
thrix annulata
throat
    septic sore t.
    sore t.
    streptococcal sore t.
    trench t.
    ulcerated sore t.
    ulceromembranous
      sore t.
throb, throbbing
Throckmorton
    reflex
    sign
throe, throes
thrombase
thrombasthenia
    Glanzmann t.
thrombectomy
thrombi (plural of thrombus)
thrombin
    t. time
    topical t.
thrombinogen
thromboagglutinin
thromboangiitis obliterans
thromboaortopathy
    occlusive t.
thromboarteritis purulenta
thromboclasis
thromboclastic
thrombocyst
thrombocytapheresis
thrombocytasthenia
thrombocyte
thrombocythemia
    essential t.
    hemorrhagic t.
    idiopathic t.
    primary t.
thrombocytic
thrombocytin
thrombocytocrit
thrombocytolysis
thrombocytopathia
thrombocytopathic
thrombocytopathy
    constitutional t.

thrombocytopenia
    t. with absence of radius
    essential t.
    HIV-associated t.
    idiopathic t.
    immune t.
    malignant t.
    secondary t.
    thrombotic t.
thrombocytopenic purpura (TP)
thrombocytopoiesis
thrombocytopoietic
thrombocytosis
thromboelastogram
thromboelastography
thromboembolectomy
thromboembolic
thromboembolism
thromboendarterectomy
    coronary t.
thromboendarteritis
thrombogenesis
thrombogenic
thromboid
thrombokinase
thrombokinesis
thrombokinetics
thrombolymphangitis
thrombolysis
thrombolytic
thrombomodulin
thrombon
thrombopathy
thrombophilia
thrombophlebitis
    iliofemoral t.
    intracranial t.
    t. migrans
    postpartum t.
    postpartum iliofemoral t.
    t. purulenta
    t. saltans
    septic t.
    spinal t.
    suppurative t.
thromboplastic
thromboplastin
    extrinsic t.
    intrinsic t.
    tissue t.
thromboplastinogen
thrombopoiesis
thrombopoietic
thrombopoietin
thrombose, thrombosed
thrombosinusitis

thrombosis
    agonal t.
    arterial t.
    atrophic t.
    ball-valve t.
    calcarine t.
    cardiac t.
    catheter-induced t.
    cavernous sinus t.
    cerebellar t.
    cerebral t.
    coronary t.
    creeping t.
    deep venous t. (DVT)
    dilatation t.
    effort t.
    iliofemoral t.
    infective t.
    intracardiac t.
    intraventricular t.
    jumping t.
    marantic t.
    marasmic t.
    mesenteric t.
    mesenteric arterial t.
    migrating t.
    mural t.
    placental t.
    plate t.
    platelet t.
    propagating t.
    puerperal t.
    renal vein t.
    Ribbert t.
    sinus t.
    suppurative venous t.
    traumatic t.
    venous t.
thrombostasis
thrombosthenin
thrombotic
thrombotonin
thromboxane
thrombus (thrombi)
    agglutinative t.
    agonal t.
    agony t.
    annular t.
    antemortem t.
    ball t.
    ball-valve t.
    bile t.
    blood platelet t.
    calcified t.
    canalized t.
    coral t.

T

thrombus (thrombi) *(continued)*
    coronary t.
    currant jelly t.
    fibrin t.
    hyaline t.
    infective t.
    laminated t.
    lateral t.
    marantic t.
    marasmic t.
    milk t.
    mixed t.
    mural t.
    obstructive t.
    occluding t.
    occlusive t.
    organized t.
    pale t.
    parasitic t.
    parietal t.
    phagocytic t.
    pigmentary t.
    plate t.
    platelet t.
    postmortem t.
    primary t.
    propagated t.
    red t.
    saddle t.
    septic t.
    stratified t.
    t. stripper
    traumatic t.
    valvular t.
    white t.
through-and-through
  suture
throwback
thrush
    t. breast, t. breast
      heart
    Candida albicans t.
    oral t.
    vaginal t.
thrust
    extensor t.
    paraspinal t.
    spinal t.
    tongue t.
thrypsis
Thudichum
    speculum
    test
thulium (Tm)
    t. thumb-printing

thumb
    bifid t.
    cortical t.
    tennis t.
    trigger t.
thumbprinting
thumbsucking
thumps
thunderclap headache
Thygeson keratitis
thymectomize
thymectomy
    neonatal t.
      syndrome
thymelcosis
thymic
    t. hypoplasia
    t. peptide
    t. transplantation
thymicolymphatic
thymidine
    t. diphosphoric acid
    t. kinase
    t. triphosphoric acid
thymidylate
thymidylate synthase
thymidylic acid
thymidylyl
thymin
thymine dimer
thyminic acid
thymitis
    autoimmune t.
thymocyte
thymohydroquinone
thymokesis
thymokinetic
thymol
thymoleptic
thymolize
thymolphthalein
thymolsulfonphthalein
thymolysis
thymolytic
thymoma
thymometastasis
thymopathic
thymopathy
thymopentin
thymopoietin
thymoprivous
thymosin
thymotoxic
thymotoxin
thymotrophic

thymus
    accessory t.
    t. persistens hyperplastica
    persistent t.
thymus-dependent
thymusectomy
thymus-independent
thyroactive
thyroadenitis
thyroaplasia
thyroarytenoid
thyrocalcitonin
thyrocardiac
thyrocarditis
thyrocele
thyrochondrotomy
thyrocolloid
thyrocricotomy
thyroepiglottic
thyrofissure
thyrogenous
thyroglobulin
thyroglossal
thyrohyal
thyrohyoid laryngotomy
thyroid
    aberrant t.
    accessory t.
    t. cartilage
    t. crisis
    t. deficiency
    ectopic t.
    t. gland
    intrathoracic t.
    lingual t.
    t. lobectomy
    t. nodule
    t. peroxidase
    retrosternal t.
    t.-stimulating hormone (TSH)
    t. storm
    substernal t.
thyroidal lymph node scintigraphy
thyroidea
    t. accessoria
    t. ima
thyroidectomize
thyroidectomy
    medical t.
thyroidism
thyroiditis
    acute t.
    acute nonsuppurative t.
    acute suppurative t.
    autoimmune t.

thyroiditis *(continued)*
    chronic t.
    chronic atrophic t.
    chronic fibrous t.
    chronic lymphadenoid t.
    chronic lymphocytic t.
    de Quervain t.
    experimental allergic t.
    focal lymphocytic t.
    giant cell t.
    giant follicular t.
    granulomatous t.
    Hashimoto t.
    invasive t.
    ligneous t.
    lymphocytic t.
    lymphoid t.
    painless t.
    parasitic t.
    postpartum t.
    pseudotuberculous t.
    pyogenic t.
    Riedel t.
    silent t.
    subacute t.
    subacute diffuse t.
    subacute granulomatous t.
    subacute lymphocytic t.
    woody t.
thyroidization
    de Quervain t.
thyroidotomy
thyroidotoxin
thyrointoxication
thyrolaryngeal
thyrolingual
thyrolytic
thyromegaly
thyromimetic
thyronine
thyroparathyroidectomy
thyroparathyroprivic
thyropathy
thyropenia
thyropharyngeal
thyroprival
thyroprivia
thyroprivic
thyroprivous
thyroptosis
thyrotherapy
thyrotome
thyrotomy
thyrotoxemia
thyrotoxic

thyrotoxic heart disease
thyrotoxicosis factitia
thyrotroph
thyrotropic
thyrotropin
    human chorionic t.
thyroxine
    levo t.
    radioactive t.
    t. radioisotope assay (T4 [T4] RIA)
thyroxinic
Ti—titanium
TI—
    time interval
    transverse inlet
    tricuspid incompetence
    tricuspid insufficiency
TIA—transient ischemic attack
TIBC—total iron-binding capacity
tibia
    saber t.
    saber-scabbard t.
    saber-shaped t.
    t. valga
    t. vara
tibiad
tibial plateau
tibiale
    t. externum
    t. posticum
tibialgia
tibialis
tibiocalcanean
tibiofemoral
tibiofibular
tibionavicular
tibioperoneal
tibioscaphoid
tibiotarsal
tibolone
tibric acid
tic
    blinking t.
    bowing t.
    compulsive t.
    convulsive t.
    degenerative t.
    t. de Guinon
    t. de pensée
    t. de sommeil
    diaphragmatic t.
    t. douloureux
    facial t.
    gesticulatory t.

tic *(continued)*
    habit t.
    laryngeal t.
    local t.
    mimic t.
    motor t.
    t. nondouloureux
    progressive choreic t.
    respiratory t.
    rocking t.
    rotatory t.
    saltatory t.
    spasmodic t.
    wide-eyed t.
    winking t.
TIC—trypsin-inhibitory capacity
tick
    deer t.
    t. paralysis
    seed t.
tickle
tickling
tick-tack sounds
t.i.d.—three times a day (L. ter in die)
TID—titrated initial dose
tidal drainage system
tidal volume (TV)
tide
    acid t.
    alkaline t.
    fat t.
    red t.
tie
    stick t.
TIE—transient ischemic episode
Tiemann catheter
Thiersch graft
Tietze
    disease
    syndrome
TIG—tetanus immunoglobulin
tiger
    t. gut suture
    t. heart
    t. lily heart
tiglic acid
tigroid
Tillaux disease
tilmus
tilt
    angle of t.
    head t.
    pelvic t.
    t. table
    t. table test

tilting-disk prosthesis
Timberlake obturator
timbre
    t. métallique
time (T)
    Achilles tendon reflex t.
    acquisition t.
    action t.
    activated coagulation t.
    activated clotting t. (ACT)
    activated partial
      thromboplastin t.
      (APTT, aPTT)
    adaptation t.
    A-H conduction t.
    apex t.
    acquisition t.
    arm-lung t.
    association t.
    biologic t.
    bleeding t.
    blocking t.
    chromoscopy t.
    circulation t.
    clot retraction t.
    clotting t.
    coagulation t.
    colonic transit t.
    conduction t.
    counter resolving t.
    dead t.
    decimal reduction t. (D)
    deep tendon reflex relaxation t.
    delay t.
    dextrinizing t.
    doubling t.
    echo t. (TE)
    ejection t.
    euglobulin clot lysis t.
    expiratory pause t.
    fading t.
    filter bleeding t.
    t. of flight
    forced expiratory t. (FET)
    forced expiratory t. in seconds
      (FETS)
    gastric emptying t.
    generation t.
    H-R conduction t.
    H-V conduction t.
    inertia t.
    insensitive t.
    inspiratory pause t.
    interpulse t.
    intra-atrial conduction t.

time (T) *(continued)*
    inversion t.
    isovolumic relaxation t. (IVRT)
    Ivy bleeding t.
    lead t.
    left ventricular ejection t.
      (LVET)
    longitudinal relaxation t.
    mean circulating t.
    mean generation t.
    median survival t.
    occlusion t. (OT)
    one-stage prothrombin t.
    P-A conduction t.
    partial thromboplastin t. (PTT)
    perception t.
    P-H conduction t.
    plasma clot t.
    prothrombin t. (PT)
    pulmonary circulation t.
    reaction t.
    real-t.
    recalcification t.
    recognition t.
    recovery t.
    relaxation t.
    repetition t. (TR)
    reptilase t.
    resolving t.
    response t.
    retention t.
    retinocortical t.
    rise t.
    Russell viper venom t.
    secondary bleeding t.
    sedimentation t.
    serum prothrombin t.
    sinoatrial conduction t.
      (SACT)
    sinoatrial recovery t. (SART)
    spin-lattice relaxation t.
    spin-spin relaxation t.
    stimulus-response t.
    Stypven t.
    survival t.
    synaptic transmission t.
    systolic ejection t. (SET)
    T_1 relaxation t. [T1]
    T_2 relaxation t. [T2]
    template bleeding t.
    thermal death t.
    thermal relaxation t.
    thrombin t. (TT)
    thrombin clotting t.
    tincture of t.

T

time (T) *(continued)*
>   transit t.
>   transverse relaxation t.
>   treadmill walking t.
>   turn-around time (TAT)
>   ventricular activation t.

time-activity curve

TIMI—Thrombolysis in Myocardial Infarction (classification)

tin (Sn)
>   t. chloride
>   t. with indium 113m
>   t. oxide

tinctable

tinction

tinctorial

tincturation

tincture
>   belladonna t.
>   benzethonium chloride t.
>   camphorated opium t.
>   compound benzoin t.
>   deodorized t. of opium
>   iodine t.
>   mother t.
>   opium t.
>   strong iodine t.
>   t. of time

tinea
>   t. amiantacea
>   asbestoslike t.
>   t. axillaris
>   t. barbae
>   t. capitis
>   t. ciliorum
>   t. circinata
>   t. corporis
>   t. cruris
>   t. decalvans
>   t. faciale
>   t. faciei
>   t. favosa
>   t. furfuracea
>   t. galli
>   t. glabrosa
>   t. imbricata
>   t. inguinalis
>   t. interdigitalis
>   t. kerion
>   t. manus
>   t. manuum
>   t. nigra
>   t. nigra palmaris
>   t. nodosa
>   t. pedis

tinea *(continued)*
>   t. profunda
>   t. sycosis
>   t. tarsi
>   t. tondens
>   t. tonsurans
>   t. unguium
>   t. versicolor

Tinel
>   sign
>   test

tine test

tingibility

tingible

tingle

tingling
>   distal t. on percussion

tinkle
>   high-pitched t's
>   peristaltic t's
>   rushes, gurgles, and t's

tinkling sounds

tinnitus
>   t. aurium
>   bilateral t.
>   central t.
>   chronic t.
>   clicking t.
>   cochlear t.
>   debilitating t.
>   decompensated t.
>   intermittent
>   ipsilateral t.
>   Leudet t.
>   metallic t.
>   nonpulsatile
>   nonvibratory t.
>   objective t.
>   pulsatile t.
>   sensorineural t.
>   subjective t.
>   tonal t.
>   unilateral t.
>   vibratory t.

tip
>   t. of nose
>   pinched nasal t.
>   policeman's t.
>   root t.
>   t. of sacral bone
>   t. of tongue
>   Woolner t.

tipping

TIPS—transjugular intrahepatic portosystemic shunt

tiqueur
tiring
TIS—tumor in situ
Tischler forceps
Tissot spirometer
tissue
    accidental t.
    adenoid t.
    adipose t.
    adipose t., white
    adipose t., yellow
    adrenogenic t.
    analogous t.
    aponeurotic t.
    areolar t.
    areolar connective t.
    basement t.
    bony t.
    brown adipose t.
    bursa-equivalent t.
    bursal equivalent t.
    cancellous t.
    cartilaginous t.
    cavernous t.
    cellular t.
    chondroid t.
    chordal t.
    chromaffin t.
    cicatricial t.
    compact t.
    connective t.
    cribriform t.
    critical t.
    dartoid t.
    dense fibrous connective t.
    elastic t.
    elastic t., yellow
    embryonal connective t.
    endometrial t.
    endothelial t.
    episcleral t.
    epithelial t.
    epivaginal connective t.
    erectile t.
    erectile t. of penis
    t. expander
    extracellular t.
    extraperitoneal t.
    t. factor
    fatty t.
    fibroareolar t.
    fibrocellular t.
    fibroelastic t.
    fibrohyaline t.
    fibrous t.

tissue *(continued)*
    fibrous t., white
    t. forceps
    Gamgee t.
    gelatinous t.
    glandular t.
    granulation t.
    gut-associated lymphoid t.
      (GALT)
    hematopoietic t.
    heterologous t.
    heterotopic t.
    His-Purkinje t.
    homologous t.
    hyperplastic t.
    indifferent t.
    inflammatory t.
    interrenal t.
    interstitial t.
    junctional t.
    keratinized t.
    Kuhnt intermediary t.
    laminated t.
    lardaceous t.
    loose connective t.
    lymphadenoid t.
    lymphatic t.
    lymphoid t.
    mesenchymal t.
    metanephrogenic t.
    mucoid t.
    mucous t.
    multilocular adipose t.
    muscular t.
    myeloid t.
    nephrogenic t.
    nerve t.
    nervous t.
    nodal t.
    osseous t.
    osteogenic t.
    osteoid t.
    parenchymatous t.
    periapical t.
    periodontal t.
    periosteal t.
    pigmented connective t.
    t. plasminogen activator
      (t-PA, tPA, TPA)
    protochondral t.
    pseudoerectile t.
    reticular t.
    reticulated t.
    retroperitoneal t.
    rubber t.

T

tissue *(continued)*
    scar t.
    scleral t.
    sclerous t's
    shock t.
    skeletal t.
    splenic t.
    subcutaneous t.
    subcutaneous fatty t.
    sustentacular t.
    symplastic t.
    target t.
    tendinous t.
    tuberculosis granulation t.
    tuberculous granulation t.
    vesicular supporting t.
tissue-active
tissue-borne
tissular
TIT—triiodothyronine
titanate
    lead zirconate t.
titanium (Ti)
    t. dioxide
    t. dioxide pneumoconiosis
titer
    agglutination t.
    antihyaluronidase t.
    anti-Rh_0-D t.
    antistreptolysin O t. (ASO t.)
    anti-teichoic acid t.
    CF antibody t.
    HI (hemagglutination
      inhibition) t.
    rubella t.
    TORCH t.
    whole complement t.
titillation
titrant
titrate
titration
    colorimetric t.
    complexometric t.
    coulometric t.
    Dean and Webb t.
    formol t.
    potentiometric t.
titrimetric
titrimetry
Titterington position
titubant
titubation
    lingual t.
TIVC—thoracic inferior vena cava
Tivnen forceps

TK—thymidine kinase
TKA—transketolase activity
Tl—thallium
TL—
    temporal lobe
    thymus leukemia (antigen)
    time lapse
    time-limited
    total lipids
    tubal ligation
TLA—translumbar aortogram
TLC—
    tender loving care
    thin-layer chromatography
    total lung capacity
TLD—
    transcutaneous lumbar
      diskectomy
    tumor lethal dose
TLE—thin-layer electrophoresis
TLSO—thoracolumbosacral
    orthosis
TLV—threshold limit value
TM—transport maximum
T_m—melting temperature
TM—
    temporomandibular
    time motion
    trademark
    transmetatarsal
    tympanic membrane
TMAb—thyroid microsomal
    antibody
TMAS—Taylor Manifest Anxiety
    Scale
TMI—
    threatened myocardial
      infarction
    transmandibular implant
    transmural infarction
TMIF—tumor-cell migration–
    inhibition factor
TMJ—temporomandibular joint
TMJ syndrome
TMV—tobacco mosaic virus
Tn—normal intraocular tension
TND—term normal delivery
TNF—tumor necrosis factor
TNI—total nodal irradiation
TNM—tumor, nodes, metastases
TNM staging system
TNS—transcutaneous nerve
    stimulation
TNT—trinitrotoluene
TNTC—too numerous to count

TO—telephone order
TOA—tubo-ovarian abscess
toadskin
toadstool
tobacco
tobaccoism
Tobey rongeur
Tobey-Ayer test
Tobold
    forceps
    knife
Tobruk splint
tocodynamometer
tocography
tocolysis
tocolytic
tocopherol
    α-t. [alpha-]
    α-t. acetate
    α-t. acid succinate
    alpha-t. equivalent
tocophobia
TOCP—triorthocresyl
  phosphate
Todaro tendon
Todd
    bodies
    cirrhosis
    gouge
    palsy
    paralysis
    process
toddler
toe
    claw t.
    t. drop brace
    great t.
    hammer t.
    little t.
    mallet t.
    Morton t.
    pigeon t.
    seedy t.
    stiff t.
    tennis t.
    up-going t.
toeing-in
toeing-out
toenail
    ingrowing t.
Toennis scissors
toewalking
togavirus
toilet
    pulmonary t.

Toison
    fluid
    solution
Tokelau ringworm
Toldt
    ligament
    membrane
    white line
tolerance
    acoustic t.
    acquired t.
    acquired drug t.
    adaptation t.
    adoptive t.
    alkali t.
    crossed t.
    drug t.
    G t.
    glucose t.
    high-dose t.
    high-zone t.
    immune t.
    immunologic t.
    impaired glucose t. (IGT)
    low-dose t.
    low-zone t.
    self t.
    species t.
    split t.
tolerant
toleration
tolerogen
tolerogenic
Tollens test
Tolosa-Hunt syndrome
toluene diisocyanate (TDI)
toluidine blue O
toluylene red
tomatine
tomentum cerebri
Tomes
    fiber
    fibril
    layer
    process
Tom Jones
    closure
    suture
Tommaselli
    disease
    syndrome
tomogram
tomography
    axial transverse t.
    circular t.

T

tomography *(continued)*
  computed t. (CT)
  computerized axial t. (CAT)
  contrast-enhanced computed
    t. (CECT)
  cranial computed t. (CCT)
  dynamic computed t.
  electron beam computed t.
  emission t.
  emission computed t. (ECT)
  emission computerized axial t.
    (ECAT)
  focal plane t.
  high-resolution computerized t.
  hypocycloidal t.
  linear t.
  longitudinal section t.
  metrizamide-assisted
    computed t.
  nuclear magnetic resonance t.
  panoramic t.
  pluridirectional t.
  positron emission t. (PET)
  positron emission transaxial
    t. (PETT)
  quantitative computed t.
  radionuclide emission t.
  rotational t.
  simultaneous multifilm t.
  single photon emission
    computed t. (SPECT)
  skip t.
  ultrasonic t.
  wide-angle t.
tonaphasia
tone
  arterial t.
  feeling t.
  heart t's
  muscle t.
  myogenic t.
  nervous t.
  neurogenic t.
  peripheral vasomotor t.
  plastic t.
  Traube double t.
  Williams tracheal t.
tongs
  Barton t.
  Barton-Cone t.
  Cherry t.
  Crutchfield t.
  Crutchfield-Raney t.
  Raney-Crutchfield t.
  skull t.

tongue
  adherent t.
  amyloid t.
  antibiotic t.
  baked t.
  bald t.
  beefy t.
  bifid t.
  burning t.
  cardinal t.
  cerebriform t.
  choreic t.
  cleft t.
  coated t.
  cobble-stone t.
  crocodile t.
  dotted t.
  double t.
  earthy t.
  encrusted t.
  fern leaf t.
  filmy t.
  fissured t.
  flat t.
  furred t.
  furrowed t.
  geographic t.
  grooved t.
  hairy t.
  lobulated t.
  magenta t.
  mappy t.
  parrot t.
  plicated t.
  raspberry t.
  raw-beef t.
  Sandwith bald t.
  scrotal t.
  smokers' t.
  smooth t.
  t. of sphenoid bone
  split t.
  stippled t.
  strawberry t.
  strawberry t., red
  strawberry t., white
  t.-tie, t.-tied
  trombone t. sign
  white t.
  wrinkled t.
tongue-and-groove suture
tonic
  bitter t.
  cardiac t.
  digestive t.

tonic *(continued)*
    general t.
    intestinal t.
    stomachic t.
    vascular t.
tonic-clonic
tonicity
tonicize
tonics
toning
    gold t.
tonka bean
tonofibril
tonofilament
tonogram
tonography
    carotid compression t.
tonometer
    air-puff t.
    applanation t.
    Draeger t.
    electronic t.
    Gärtner t.
    Goldmann applanation t.
    impression t.
    indentation t.
    MacKay-Marg electronic t.
    Musken t.
    Perkins t.
    pneumatic t.
    Recklinghausen t.
    Schiotz t.
    Sklar-Schiotz t.
tonometry
    applanation t.
    digital t.
    impression t.
    indentation t.
tonoplast
tonoscope
tonsil
    adenoid t.
    buried t.
    t. of cerebellum
    eustachian t.
    faucial t.
    Gerlach t.
    hypertrophied t.
    intestinal t.
    lingual t.
    Luschka t.
    nasopharyngeal t.
    palatine t.
    pharyngeal t.
    t. snare

tonsil *(continued)*
    submerged t.
    third t.
    t. of torus tubarius
    tubal t's
tonsilla (tonsillae)
    t. cerebelli
    t. of cerebellum
    t. lingualis
    t. palatina
    t. pharyngealis
    t. tubaria
tonsillar
    t. artery
    t. calculus
    t. capsule
    t. crypts
    t. hernia
    t. herniation
    t. nerves
    t. pits
    t. plexus
    t. sinus
    t. snare
tonsillectome
    Ballenger-Sluder t.
    Beck-Mueller t.
    Beck-Schenck t.
    Brown t.
    Daniels t.
    LaForce t.
    Mack t.
    Myles t.
    Sauer t.
    Sauer-Sluder t.
    Searcy t.
    Sluder t.
    Sluder-Demarest t.
    Sluder-Sauer t.
    Tydings t.
    Whiting t.
tonsillectomy
    t. and adenoidectomy (T&A)
    dissection t.
    guillotine t.
tonsillitic
tonsillitis
    acute t.
    caseous t.
    chronic t.
    follicular t.
    herpetic t.
    lacunar t.
    lingual t.
    mycotic t.

T

tonsillitis *(continued)*
    streptococcal t.
    suppurative t.
tonsilloadenoidectomy
tonsillohemisporosis
tonsillolith
tonsillomycosis
tonsillopathy
tonsillopharyngitis
tonsillotome
tonsillotomy
tonsillotyphoid
tonus
    acerebral t.
    chemical t.
    myogenic t.
    neurogenic t.
Tooke knife
Toomey
    evacuator
    syringe
tooth (teeth)
    abutment t.
    accessional teeth
    accessory t.
    acrylic resin t.
    anatomic t., anatomical t.
    anchor t.
    ankylosed t.
    anterior teeth
    artificial t.
    t. atrophy
    auditory teeth
    auditory teeth of Huschke
    t. of axis
    baby teeth
    back t.
    t. banding
    bicuspid t.
    buccal teeth
    buck t.
    canine t.
    carnassial t.
    cheek teeth
    cog t. of malleus
    conical t.
    connate t.
    corner t.
    cross-bite teeth, crossbite
      teeth
    cross-pin teeth
    cuspid t.
    cuspidate t.
    cuspless t.
    cutting t.
    dead t.

tooth (teeth) *(continued)*
    deciduous teeth
    devitalized t.
    diatoric teeth
    drifting t.
    embedded t.
    t. of epistropheus
    extruded t.
    eye t.
    Fournier teeth
    fused teeth
    geminate t., geminated t.
    ghost t.
    Goslee t.
    hag teeth
    Horner teeth
    Huschke auditory teeth
    Hutchinson teeth
    hutchinsonian t.
    impacted t.
    incisor t.
    labial teeth
    malacotic teeth
    malposed t.
    mandibular teeth
    maxillary teeth
    metal insert t.
    migrating t.
    milk t.
    molar teeth
    Moon teeth
    morsal teeth
    mottled teeth
    mulberry t.
    multicuspid t.
    natal t.
    neonatal t.
    nonanatomic teeth
    nonvital t.
    notched t.
    peg t., pegged t.
    peg-shaped t.
    permanent teeth
    pink t. of Mummery
    pinless teeth
    posterior teeth
    predeciduous t.
    premature teeth
    premolar teeth
    primary teeth
    protruding t.
    pulpless t.
    rake teeth
    rootless teeth
    rotated t.
    sclerotic teeth

tooth (teeth) *(continued)*
    screwdriver teeth
    second t.
    shell t.
    snaggle t.
    spaced t.
    stomach t.
    straight-pin teeth
    submerged t.
    succedaneous teeth
    successional teeth
    superior teeth
    supernumerary teeth
    supplemental teeth
    temporary teeth
    third molar t.
    tube teeth
    Turner t.
    unerupted t.
    vital teeth
    wandering t.
    wisdom t.
    zero-degree teeth
Tooth [eponym]
    atrophy
    disease
    type
toothache
tooth-borne
toothbrushing
toothed
toothpick
    balsa wood t.
top
    spinning t.
topagnosia
topagnosis
topalgia
topectomy
topesthesia
tophaceous
topholipoma
tophus (tophi)
    auricular t.
    dental t.
    gouty tophi
    t. of pinna
    t. syphiliticus
topical
Topinard
    angle
    line
topognosis
topographic
    t. anatomy
    t. percussion

topographical
topography
topoisomerase (type I and II)
topoisomerase inhibitor
toposcopic catheter
TOPS—Take Off Pounds Sensibly
TOPV—trivalent oral poliovirus
    vaccine
TORCH—toxoplasmosis, other
    agents, rubella, cytomegalovirus,
    herpes simplex
TORCH
    infection
    syndrome
    titer
torcular Herophili
Torek operation
tori (plural of torus)
toric lens
Torkildsen
    operation
    shunt
Tornwaldt (Thornwaldt)
    abscess
    bursa
    bursitis
    cyst
    disease
    syndrome
torose
torous
TORP—total ossicular replacement
    prosthesis
torpent
torpid
torpidity
Torpin operation
torpor
    t. retinae
    summer t.
    winter t.
torque
torquing
Torre syndrome
torrefaction
torrefy
torricellian vacuum
torr unit
torsades de pointes
torsion
    lateral t.
    negative t.
    positive t.
torsive
torsiversion
torso

T

torticollar
torticollis
    acute t.
    congenital t.
    dermatogenic t.
    fixed t.
    hysteric t., hysterical t.
    infantile t.
    intermittent t.
    labyrinthine t.
    mental t.
    myogenic t.
    nasopharyngeal t.
    neurogenic t.
    ocular t.
    paralytic t.
    reflex t.
    rheumatoid t.
    spasmodic t.
    spastic t.
    spurious t.
    symptomatic t.
tortipelvis
tortua facies
tortuous
    t. aorta
    t. bowel
    t. ureter
    t. veins
tortured expression
toruloid
Torulopsis glabrata
torulosis
torulus (toruli)
    toruli tactiles
torus (tori)
    t. aorticus
    t. fracture
    t. frontalis
    t. levatorius
    t. mandibularis
    t. occipitalis
    palatine t.
    t. palatinus
    t. tubarius
    t. uretericus
total
    t. abdominal hysterectomy
      (TAH)
    t. hip arthroplasty
    t. hysterectomy
    t. knee arthroplasty
    t. laryngectomy
    t. mastectomy
    t. maxillary osteotomy

total *(continued)*
    t. rhinectomy
    t. vaginal hysterectomy (TVH)
Toti operation
Toti-Mosher operation
totipotency
totipotential
totipotentiality
touch
    abdominal t.
    double t.
    rectal t.
    royal t.
    therapeutic t. (TT)
    vaginal t.
    vesical t.
Touraine
    aphthosis
    syndrome (III)
Touraine-Solente-Golé syndrome
Tourette (Gilles de la Tourette)
    disease
    syndrome
tourniquet
    automatic rotating t.
    Bethune lung t.
    Esmarch t.
    forceps t.
    garrote t.
    Lynn Thomas t.
    t. paralysis
    pneumatic t.
    Rumel t.
    scalp t.
    Shenstone t.
    Spanish t.
    torcular t.
    windlass t.
Touton giant cell
towel
    Backhaus t. clamp
    t. clip
Towne
    position
    projection radiograph
    view
Townley prosthesis
toxanemia
toxaphene
toxemia
    eclamptic t.
    eclamptogenic t.
    hydatid t.
    preeclamptic t.
    t. of pregnancy

toxemic
toxic
toxicant
toxication
toxicide
toxicity
    antibiotic t.
    bismuth t.
    cadmium t.
    digitalis t.
    iron dextran t.
    mercury t.
    O_2 t.
    osmotic diuretic t.
    oxygen t.
    phenacetin t.
    salicylate t.
    sulfonamide t.
toxicogenic
toxicoid
toxicologist
toxicology
    forensic t.
    predictive t.
    prospective t.
    retrospective t.
toxicopathy
toxicopectic
toxicopexis
toxicophidia
toxicophobia
toxicosis
    exogenic t.
    gestational t.
    hemorrhagic capillary t.
    proteinogenous t.
    retention t.
    T_3 t.
    T3 [T3] t.
toxic shock
    t.s. syndrome (TSS)
toxiferous
toxigenic
    t. bacterium
    t. diarrhea
toxigenicity test
toxignomic
toximetry
toxin
    A-B t's
    Amanita t.
    animal t.
    anthrax t.
    antitetanus t.
    bacterial t's

toxin *(continued)*
    botulinal t.
    botulinum t.
    botulinus t.
    cholera t.
    clostridial t.
    dermonecrotic t.
    Dick t.
    dinoflagellate t.
    diphtheria t.
    diphtheria t. for Schick test
    dysentery t.
    epidermolytic t.
    erythrogenic t.
    extracellular t.
    fatigue t.
    fugu t.
    fusarial t.
    gas gangrene t.
    inactivated diagnostic
      diphtheria t.
    intracellular t.
    labile t. (LT)
    necrotizing t.
    perfringens alpha t.
    perfringens theta t.
    plague t.
    plant t.
    pseudomonal t.
    Shiga t.
    Shiga-like t.
    soluble t.
    stable t. (ST)
    staphylococcal t.
    streptococcal t.
    T-2 t.
    tetanus t.
toxin-antitoxin (TA)
toxinemia
toxinosis
toxisterol
Toxocara
    T. canis
    T. cati
toxocaral
toxocariasis
toxogen
toxoglobulin
toxoid
    adsorbed t.
    bacterial t.
    Clostridium perfringens t.
    diphtheria t.
    diphtheria and tetanus t's
    formol t.

T

toxoid *(continued)*
    tetanus t.
    tetanus and diphtheria t's
toxoid-antitoxin floccule
toxoid-antitoxoid
toxoneme
toxonosis
toxopexic
toxophil
toxophilic
Toxoplasma gondii
toxoplasmic
    t. chorioretinitis
    t. encephalitis
    t. encephalomyelitis
    t. meningoencephalitis
    t. retinochoroiditis
    t. uveitis
toxoplasmosis
    acquired t.
    congenital t.
    ocular t.
    pulmonary t.
toxoprotein
Toynbee
    corpuscles
    experiment
    law
    ligament
    otoscope
    speculum
TP—
    temperature and pressure
    threshold potential
    thrombocytopenic purpura
    total protein
t-PA, tPA, TPA—tissue
  plasminogen activator
TPA—*Treponema pallidum*
  agglutination
TPBF—total pulmonary blood flow
TPC—thromboplastic plasma
  component
TPCF—*Treponema pallidum*
  complement fixation
TPG—transplacental gradient
TPH—transplacental hemorrhage
TPHA—*Treponema pallidum*
  hemagglutination assay
TPI—
    Treponema pallidum
      immobilization (test)
    triose phosphate isomerase
TPI cardiolipin test
T-piece

TPN—total parenteral nutrition
TPPN—total peripheral parenteral
  nutrition
TPR—
    temperature, pulse,
      respiration
    total pulmonary resistance
TPS—tumor polysaccharide
  substance
TPT—typhoid-paratyphoid
TPT vaccine
TPVR—total pulmonary vascular
  resistance
TQ—tourniquet
tr—trace
TR—tricuspid regurgitation
trabecula (trabeculae)
    arachnoid trabeculae
    trabeculae arachnoideae
    trabeculae of bone
    trabeculae carneae cordis
    trabeculae cordis
    trabeculae corporis spongiosi
      penis
    trabeculae corporum
      cavernosorum penis
    trabeculae of corpus
      spongiosum of penis
    t. cranii
    fleshy trabeculae of heart
    trabeculae lienis
    trabeculae nodi lymphatici
    trabeculae nodi lymphoidei
    Rathke trabeculae
    septomarginal t.
    t. septomarginalis
    trabeculae of spleen
    trabeculae splenicae
trabecular
    t. adenoma
    t. carcinoma of the skin
    t. meshwork
    t. osteoma
    t. region
    t. substance of bone
    t. veins
trabecularism
trabecular-tubular adenoma
trabeculate
trabeculated bladder
trabeculation of bladder dome
trabeculectomy
trabeculoplasty
    argon laser t.
    laser t.

trace
- contact t's
- t. elements
- memory t.
- t. mineral

tracer
- arrow-point t.
- Gothic arch t.
- needle-point t.
- radioactive t.
- stylus t.

trachea (tracheae)
- cervical t.
- scabbard t.

tracheaectasy

tracheal
- t. atresia
- t. cannula
- t. length
- t. mucus
- t. mucus velocity
- t. stenosis
- t. tube
- t. tug

trachealgia

tracheitis sicca

trachelectomy

trachelism

trachelismus

trachelitis

trachelocystitis

trachelodynia

trachelomastoid muscle

trachelopexy

tracheloplasty

trachelorrhaphy

tracheloschisis

trachelotomy

tracheobronchial
- t. lymph nodes
- t. tree
- t. tuberculosis

tracheobronchitis

tracheobronchomegaly

tracheobronchoscopy

tracheocele

tracheocutaneous fistula

tracheoesophageal
- t. fistula
- t. folds
- t. puncture
- t. spasm

tracheofistulization

tracheogenic

tracheolaryngeal

tracheole

tracheomalacia

tracheopathia osteoplastica

tracheopharyngeal

tracheophony

tracheoplasty
- slide t.

tracheorrhagia

tracheorrhaphy

tracheoscope

tracheoscopic

tracheoscopy
- percervical t.
- peroral t.

tracheostenosis

tracheostoma

tracheostomize

tracheostomy
- Bose t. hook
- t. hook
- t. mask
- Moore t. button
- post-t. stenosis
- t. tube

tracheotome
- Sierra-Sheldon t.

tracheotomize

tracheotomy
- inferior t.
- superior t.
- t. tube

trachoma (trachomata)
- Arlt t.
- brawny t.
- Türck t.
- t. of vocal bands

trachomata

trachomatous

trachychromatic

trachyonychia

trachyphonia

tracing
- arrow-point t.
- cephalometric t.
- contact t.
- extraoral t.
- flat t.
- Gothic arch t.
- intraoral t.
- needle-point t.
- pantographic t.
- stylus t.

track
- bear t's
- germ t.

T

track *(continued)*
- ionization t.
- needle t's

tracking

tract
- afferent t.
- alimentary t.
- anterior cerebrospinal t.
- anterior corticospinal t.
- anterior intersegmental t's of spinal cord
- anterior pyramidal t.
- anterior reticulospinal t.
- anterior spinocerebellar t.
- anterior spinothalamic t.
- arcuatofloccular t.
- ascending t.
- ascending and descending association t's of cord
- ascending t's of spinal cord
- association t.
- atrio-His t.
- atriohisian t.
- Bekhterev (Bechterew) t.
- biliary t.
- Bruce t.
- t of Bruce and Muir
- bulbar t.
- bulboreticulospinal t.
- Burdach t.
- central tegmental t.
- central t. of acoustic nerve
- central t. of auditory nerve
- central t. of cochlear nerve
- central t. of cranial nerves
- central t. of tegmental t.
- central t. of thymus
- central t. of trigeminal nerve
- cerebellorubral t.
- cerebellorubrospinal t.
- cerebellospinal t.
- cerebellotegmental t's of bulb
- cerebellothalamic t.
- cerebellovestibular t.
- Collier t.
- comma t. of Schultze
- commissurospinal t.
- conariohypophyseal t.
- cornucommissural t.
- corticobulbar t.
- corticocerebellar t.
- corticohypothalamic t's
- corticonuclear t.
- corticopontine t.
- corticopontocerebellar t's

tract *(continued)*
- corticorubral t.
- corticospinal t.
- corticospinal t., anterior
- corticospinal t., crossed
- corticospinal t., direct
- corticospinal t., lateral
- corticospinal t. of medulla oblongata
- corticospinal t's of spinal cord
- corticotectal t.
- corticothalamic t.
- crossed corticospinal t.
- crossed marginal t.
- crossed pyramidal t.
- dead t.
- Deiters t.
- dentatothalamic t.
- descending t.
- descending t's of spinal cord
- descending vestibular t.
- digestive t.
- direct cerebellar t. of Flechsig
- direct corticospinal t.
- direct pyramidal t.
- direct vestibulocerebellar t.
- dopaminergic t.
- dorsal intersegmental t's of spinal cord
- dorsolateral t.
- efferent t.
- extracorticospinal t.
- extrapyramidal t.
- fastigiobulbar t's
- fiber t's of spinal cord
- Flechsig t.
- flow t. of the heart
- Foville t.
- fronto-occipital t.
- frontopontine t.
- gastrointestinal (GI) t.
- generative t.
- geniculocalcarine t.
- geniculostriate t.
- geniculotemporal t.
- genital t.
- genitourinary (GU) t.
- Goll t.
- Gowers t.
- Gudden t.
- habenular t.
- habenulointerpeduncular t.
- habenulopeduncular t.
- Helweg t.
- Hoche t.

tract *(continued)*

hypothalamohypophyseal (hypothalamohypophysial) t.
iliopubic t.
iliotibial t.
intermediolateral t.
internuncial t.
intersegmental t's of spinal cord
intersegmental t's of spinal cord, anterior
intersegmental t's of spinal cord, dorsal
intersegmental t's of spinal cord, lateral
intersegmental t's of spinal cord, posterior
intersegmental t's of spinal cord, ventral
interstitiospinal t.
intestinal t.
lateral intersegmental t's of spinal cord
lateral t. of isthmus
lateral olfactory t.
lateral pyramidal t.
lenticulothalamic t.
Lissauer t.
Löwenthal (Lowenthal) t.
lower respiratory t.
Maissiat t.
mammillopeduncular t.
mammillotegmental t.
mammillothalamic t.
Marchi t.
marginal t's
marginal t., crossed
mesencephalic t. of trigeminal nerve
Meynert t.
Monakow t.
motor t.
nigrostriatal t.
occipitopontile t.
occipitopontine t.
olfactory t.
olivocerebellar t.
olivospinal t.
optic t.
pallidoreticular t.
pallidosubthalamic t.
pallidotegmental t.
pallidothalamic t.
parietopontine t.
peduncular t., transverse

tract *(continued)*

periependymal t.
periventricular t.
t. of Philippe-Gombault t.
pontocerebellar t.
portal t.
posterior intersegmental t's of spinal cord
prepyramidal t.
projection t.
pyramidal t.
pyramidal t., anterior
pyramidal t., crossed
pyramidal t., direct
pyramidal t., lateral
pyramidal t., pyramidal t. of medulla oblongata
pyramidal t's of spinal cord
respiratory t.
reticulo-olivary t.
reticulospinal t.
rubrobulbar t.
rubro-olivary t.
rubroreticular t.
rubrospinal t.
rubrothalamic t.
t. of Schütz t.
semilunar t.
seminal t.
sensory t.
septomarginal t.
solitary t. of medulla oblongata
spinal t. of trigeminal nerve
spinal vestibular t.
spinocerebellar t.
spinocerebellar t., anterior
spinocerebellar t., direct
spinocerebellar t., dorsal
spinocerebellar t., posterior
spinocervical t.
spinocervicothalamic t.
spino-olivary t.
spinotectal t.
spinothalamic t.
spinothalamic t., anterior
Spitzka-Lissauer t.
Spitzka marginal t.
strionigral t.
striothalamic t.
sulcomarginal t.
supraopticohypophyseal (supraopticohypophysial) t.
sympathetic t.
tectobulbar t.

T

tract *(continued)*
    tectocerebellar t.
    tectospinal t.
    tegmental t.
    tegmentospinal t.
    temporopontile t.
    temporopontine t.
    thalamocortical t.
    thalamo-occipital t.
    thalamo-olivary t.
    tracheobronchial t.
    transverse peduncular t.
    triangular t.
    triangular t. of Philippe-
        Gombault
    trigeminothalamic t.
    tuberohypophysial
        (tuberohypophyseal) t.
    tuberoinfundibular t.
    Türck t.
    upper respiratory t.
    urinary t.
    urogenital t.
    uveal t.
    ventral corticospinal t.
    ventral intersegmental t's of
        spinal cord
    ventral pyramidal t.
    ventral reticulospinal t.
    ventral spinocerebellar t.
    ventral spinothalamic t.
    vestibulocerebellar t.
    vestibulo-ocular t.
    vestibulo-ovular t.
    vestibulospinal t.
    t. of Vicq d'Azyr t.
    vocal t.
    Waldeyer t.
tractellum (tractella)
traction
    axis t.
    Bryant t.
    Buck t.
    cervical t.
    Crutchfield skeletal t.
    elastic t.
    elastic finger t.
    external t.
    halo t.
    halo-pelvic t.
    halter t.
    intermaxillary t.
    internal t.
    intramaxillary t.
    intraoral elastic t.

traction *(continued)*
    isometric t.
    lumbar t.
    maxillomandibular t.
    Russell t.
    skeletal t.
    skin t.
    t. suture
    tongue t.
    vertebral t.
    vitreous t.
    weight t.
    windlass t.
traction handle
    Barton t.h.
    Bill t.h.
    Luikart-Bill t.h.
tractology
tractor
    Lowsley t.
    prostatic t.
    Syms t.
    urethral t.
    Young t.
tractotomy
    descending root t.
    intramedullary t.
    mesencephalic t.
    pyramidal t.
    Sjöqvist t.
    spinothalamic t.
    trigeminal t.
tractus (tractus)
    t. bulboreticulospinalis
    t. centralis thymi
    t. corticopontinus
    t. corticospinalis anterior
    t. corticospinalis lateralis
    t. corticospinalis ventralis
    t. dorsolateralis
    t. frontopontinus
    t. habenulo-interpeduncularis
    t. hypothalamohypophysealis
        (hypothalamohypophysialis)
    t. iliopubicus
    t. iliotibialis
    t. mesencephalicus nervi
        trigemini
    t. olfactorius
    t. olivocerebellaris
    t. olivocochlearis
    t. opticus
    t. pontoreticulospinalis
    t. pyramidalis
    t. pyramidalis anterior

tractus (tractus) *(continued)*
    t. pyramidalis lateralis
    t. reticulospinalis anterior
    t. reticulospinalis ventralis
    t. rubrospinalis
    t. solitarius medullae
      oblongatae
    t. spinalis nervi trigeminalis
    t. spinalis nervi trigemini
    t. spinocerebellaris anterior
    t. spinocerebellaris dorsalis
    t. spinocerebellaris posterior
    t. spinocerebellaris ventralis
    t. spino-olivaris
    t. spinoreticularis
    t. spinotectalis
    t. spinothalamicus anterior
    t. spinothalamicus lateralis
    t. spinothalamicus ventralis
    t. spiralis foraminosus
    t. tectobulbaris
    t. tectospinalis
    t. tegmentalis centralis
    t. trigeminothalamicus
    t. vestibulospinalis
    t. vestibulospinalis lateralis
tragacanth
    gum t.
    Indian t.
    t. mucilage
tragal
tragedy
Trager
    approach
    therapy
tragi (plural of tragus)
tragion
tragophonia
tragophony
tragopodia
tragus (tragi)
    accessory t.
TRAIDS—transfusion-related
  AIDS
train
    t. of four
    t. of pulses
trainable
training
    assertiveness t.
    auditory t.
    bladder t.
    bowel t.
    expressive t.
    habit t.

training *(continued)*
    sensitivity t.
    toilet t.
Trainor-Nida operation
trait
    dominant t.
    Hageman t.
    recessive t.
    secretor t.
    sickle cell t.
    single gene t.
    thalassemia t.
trajector
TRAM—
    transverse rectus abdominis
      myocutaneous (flap)
    Treatment Rating Assessment
      Matrix
    Treatment Response
      Assessment Method
Trambusti
    reaction
    test
trance
    alcoholic t.
    hypnotic t.
    induced t.
    somnambulistic t.
tranexamic acid
tranquilizer
    major t.
    minor t.
transabdominal cholangiography
transacetylase
transacetylation
transacylase
transacylation
transaldolase
transamidation
transamidinase
transaminase
transamination
transanimation
transantral ethmoidectomy
transaortic endarterectomy
transatrial
transaudient
transaxial
transaxonal
transbasal
transcalent
transcalvarial
transcarbamoylase
transcarboxylase
transcatheter

T

transcavitary
transcervical
transclomiphene
transcondylar
transcondyloid
transcorneal
transcortical
transcortin
transcricothyroid
transcript
    primary t.
transcriptase
    reverse t.
transcription
    complementary t.
    reverse t.
    symmetric t.
transcutaneous
transdermal
transdermic
transdetermination
transdiaphragmatic
transducer
    acoustic t.
    bone-conduction t.
    electrochemical t.
    neuroendocrine t.
    piezoelectric t.
    pressure t.
    quarter-wave t.
    rotating t.
    sector t.
    ultrasound t.
transducin
transductant
transduction
    abortive t.
    vestibular t.
transduodenal
transdural
transect
transection
    t. incision
    spinal t.
transepidermal
transethmoidal
transfaunation
transfection
transfectoma
transfer
    adoptive t.
    Bunnell tendon t.
    egg t.
    embryo t.
    group t.

transfer *(continued)*
    linear energy t. (LET)
    nuclear t.
    passive t.
    phosphate-group t.
    placental t.
    temporalis t.
    tendon t.
transferase
transference
    counter t., countertransference
    institutional t.
transferrin
transfix
transfixing suture
transfixion suture
transformation
    antigenic t.
    asbestos t.
    bacterial t.
    blast t.
    Bliss t.
    fast Fourier f.
    globular-fibrous t.
    lymphocyte t.
    membranous t.
transformer
    filament t.
    high-voltage t.
    ratio t.
    resonance t.
    step-down t.
    step-up t.
transformiminase
transfructosylase
transfuse
transfusion
    arterial t.
    autologous t.
    bone marrow t.
    cell saver t.
    direct t.
    drip t.
    exchange t.
    exsanguination t.
    fetomaternal t.
    granulocyte t.
    immediate t.
    indirect t.
    intra-arterial t.
    intraperitoneal t.
    intrauterine t.
    leukocyte t.
    mediate t.
    placental t.

transfusion *(continued)*
   replacement t.
   sternal t.
   substitution t.
transfusional
transgenic
transglucosylase
transglutaminase
transglycosidation
transglycosylase
transhemophilin
transhepatic
   t. cholangiography (TC)
   direct percutaneous t.
     cholangiography
   fine-needle t. cholangiography
     (FNTC)
   percutaneous t. biliary
     drainage (PTBD)
   percutaneous t.
     cholangiography (PTC)
   percutaneous t. portography
transhiatal
transhydrogenase
transhyoid pharyngotomy
transient
   t. ischemia
   t. obscuration
transiliac
transilient
transillumination
transilluminator
transinsular
transischiac
transisthmian
transistor
   field-effect t.
transition
   cervicothoracic t.
   forbidden t.
   isomeric t.
transitional
transketolase
translateral
translation
   nick t.
translingual pharyngotomy
translocase
translocation
   balanced t.
   t. Down syndrome
   group t.
   insertional t.
   nonreciprocal t.
   reciprocal t.

translocation *(continued)*
   robertsonian t.
   unbalanced t.
translucent
translumbar aortography
transluminal
   percutaneous t. angioplasty
     (PTA)
   percutaneous t. atrial
     valvuloplasty (PTAV)
   percutaneous t. coronary
     angioplasty (PTCA)
   percutaneous t. mitral
     valvuloplasty (PTMV)
   percutaneous t. renal
     angioplasty (PTRA)
transmeatal
   t. atticotomy
   t. incision
   t. tympanotomy
transmethylase
transmethylation
transmigration
   external t.
   internal t.
transmissibility
transmissible
transmission
   cochlear t.
   cyclical t.
   direct t.
   duplex t.
   horizontal t.
   humoral t.
   insect t.
   neurochemical t.
   neurohumoral t.
   neuromuscular t.
   placental t.
   synaptic t.
   vertical t.
transmission electron microscopy
   (TEM)
transmittance
transmitter
transmural
transmutation
transnasal
transocular
transonance
transonic
transorbital
   t. leukotomy
   t. lobotomy
transovarial

T

transpalatal
transparent
transparietal
transpeptidation
transperineal
transperitoneal
transphosphorylase
transphosphorylation
transpiration
    pulmonary t.
transpire
transplacental
transplant
    autogenous t.
    cadaveric t.
    corneal t.
    Gallie t.
    homogenous t.
    living donor t.
    living related-donor t.
transplantar
transplantation
    allogeneic t.
    allogeneic marrow t.
    bone marrow t.
    corneal t.
    heart t.
    heterotopic t.
    homotopic t.
    kidney t.
    liver t.
    lung t.
    orthotopic t.
    orthotopic liver t.
    pancreatic t.
    pancreaticoduodenal t.
    renal t.
    syngeneic t.
    syngenesioplastic t.
    tendon t.
    tooth t.
transpleural
transport
    active t.
    active renal tubular t.
    bulk t.
    competitive t.
    competitive renal
      tubular t.
    membrane t.
    ovum t.
    passive t.
    tubal t.
transposase
transpose

transposition
    t. of affect
    t. of aorta
    t. of appendix
    t. of arterial stems
    t. of arterial trunk
    t. of colon
    congenitally corrected t.
    corrected t. of great vessels
    t. of the great arteries (TGA)
    t. of great vessels
    t. of intestine
    partial t. of great vessels
    t. of pulmonary veins
    t. of stomach
transposon
transpubic
transpulmonary
transrectal
transrectus incision
transsacral
transscleral
transsection
transsegmental
transseptal
    t. alveolectomy
    t. catheterization
transsexual
transsexualism
transsphenoidal hypophysectomy
transsternal
transsuccinylase
transsynaptic
transtadial
transtemporal
transtentorial
transthalamic
transthermia
transthoracic nephrectomy
transthyretin
transthyroid pharyngotomy
transtracheal
    percutaneous t.
      bronchography
transtrochanteric osteotomy
transtympanic labyrinthectomy
transudate
    pleural t.
transudation
transuranic
transuranium
transureteroureterostomy
transurethral
    t. prostatectomy
    t. resection (TUR)

transurethral *(continued)*
  t. resection of bladder (TURB)
  t. resection of prostate (TURP)
transvaginal
transvaterian
transvector
transvenous
transventricular
  t. closed valvotomy
  t. pulmonary valvotomy
transversalis
transverse
  axial t. tomography
  t. colon
  t. incision
  t. magnetization
  t. palatine suture
  t. pharyngotomy
  t. suture of Krause
transversectomy
transversion
transversocostal
transversotomy
transversourethralis
transversus abdominis muscle
transvesical
  suprapubic t. prostatectomy
transvestism
transvestite
Trantas
  dots
  operation
trap
  Luken t.
trap-door incision
trapezial
trapeziform
trapeziometacarpal
trapezium
trapezoid
Trapp
  coefficient
  formula
Traube
  curves
  dyspnea
  gallop rhythm
  heart
  heart murmur
  murmur
  sign
  space
Traube-Hering
  curves
  waves

trauma (traumas, traumata)
  acoustic t.
  birth t.
  occlusal t.
  perinatal t.
  periodontal t.
  potential t.
  primary occlusal t.
  psychic t.
  secondary occlusal t.
traumasthenia
traumata
traumatherapy
traumatic
traumatism
  occlusal t.
  periodontal t.
traumatize
traumatogenic
traumatologist
traumatology
traumatopathy
traumatophilia
traumatopnea
traumatropism
Trautmann triangle
Travel operation
Travenol needle
tray
  acrylic resin t.
  impression t.
TRBF—total renal blood flow
TRC—
  tanned red cells (test)
  total ridge-count
Treacher Collins syndrome
Treacher Collins-Franceschetti
  syndrome
treadmill
  t. exercise test (TET)
  t. stress test (TST)
treatment
  active t.
  ambulatory insulin t.
  Ascoli t.
  Beard t.
  Bell t.
  Bergonié t.
  Bier t.
  Bird t.
  Bouchardat t.
  Brandt t.
  Brehmer t.
  Brown-Séquard t.
  Calot t.

T

treatment *(continued)*
  carbon dioxide t.
  Carrel t.
  Carrel-Dakin t.
  Castellani t.
  causal t.
  Chervin t.
  choline t.
  closed t. of burns
  Coffey-Humber t.
  conservative t.
  continuous sleep t.
  Cox t.
  cross-fire t.
  curative t.
  Dancel t.
  dietetic t.
  drip t.
  drug t.
  electric shock t.
  electroconvulsive t.
  electroshock t.
  Elliott t.
  empiric t.
  eventration t.
  expectant t.
  fever t.
  Fichera t.
  Fitz Gerald t.
  Forlanini t.
  fractionated t.
  Fränkel t.
  Frenkel t.
  Gennerich t.
  Girard t.
  Goeckerman t.
  Guinard t.
  Hartel t.
  high-frequency t.
  hygienic t.
  hyperbaric oxygen t.
  hypoglycemic shock t.
  isoserum t.
  Jacquet biokinetic t.
  Karell t.
  Keating-Hart t.
  Kenny t.
  Killgren t.
  Klapp creeping t.
  Koga t.
  Lambotte t.
  Lerich t.
  light t.
  maintenance t.
  Matas t.

treatment *(continued)*
  McPheeters t.
  medical t.
  medicinal t.
  Murphy t.
  Noorden t.
  Nordach t.
  oatmeal t.
  Ochsner t.
  Oertel t.
  open t. of burns
  organ t.
  Orr t.
  palliative t.
  Pasteur t.
  Paul t.
  Plummer t.
  Politzer t.
  Potter t.
  preventive t.
  Proetz t.
  prolonged sleep t.
  prophylactic t.
  protracted t.
  radical t.
  rational t.
  Roeder t.
  Rollier t.
  root canal t.
  Rotunda t.
  Schlösser (Schloesser) t.
  sewage t.
  shock t.
  slush t.
  solar t.
  specific t.
  Stoker t.
  Stroganoff (Stroganov) t.
  subcoma insulin t.
  supporting t.
  supportive t.
  surgical t.
  symptomatic t.
  Tallerman t.
  teleradium t.
  thyroid t.
  total-push t.
  Trueta t.
  underwater t.
  venous heart t.
  Yeo t.
tree
  arterial t.
  bronchial t.
  laryngotracheobronchial t.

tree *(continued)*
    tracheobronchial t.
    vascular t.
    venous t.
trehalose
Treitz
    arch
    fossa
    hernia
    ligament
    muscle
trematode
trematodiasis
trematoid
trembles
tremelloid
tremellose
tremens
    delirium t.
tremogram
tremor
    action t.
    alternating t.
    arsenic t.
    benign familial t.
    bread-crumbling t.
    coarse t.
    coin-counting t.
    congenital t. syndrome
    continuous t.
    effort t.
    enhanced physiologic t.
    essential t.
    familial t.
    fine t.
    flapping t.
    hereditary essential t.
    heredofamilial t.
    intention t.
    intermittent t.
    kinetic t.
    t. linguae
    t. mercurialis
    metallic t.
    motor t.
    muscular t.
    orthostatic t.
    parkinsonian t.
    passive t.
    persistent t.
    physiologic t.
    pill-rolling t.
    postural t.
    purring t.
    rest t., resting t.

tremor *(continued)*
    senile t.
    static t.
    striocerebellar t.
    toxic t.
    trombone t. of tongue
    volitional t.
tremulous
    t. arousals
    benign t. parkinsonism
    t. hand movements
    t. iris
    t. movements
    t. myoclonus
Trendelenburg
    gait
    operation
    position
    symptom
    test
Trendelenburg-Crafoord
    clamp
trepanation
trephination
    corneoscleral t.
    dental t.
trephine
    Arruga t.
    Barraquer t.
    Castroviejo t.
    DeVilbiss t.
    Elliot t.
    Grieshaber t.
    Michel t.
    Paufique t.
    Turkel t.
trephinement
trephiner
trephining
trepidant
trepidatio cordis
trepidation
Treponema
    T. carateum
    T. denticola
    T. mucosum
    T. pallidum
    T. pertenue
    T. vincentii
treponemal
treponematosis
treponeme
treponemiasis
treponemicidal
trepopnea

T

treppe
Treves operation
Trevor disease
TRF—thyrotropin-releasing factor
TRH—thyrotropin-releasing
  hormone
triacetate
    glyceryl t.
triacid
    Ehrlich t. stain
triacylglycerol lipase
triad
    acute compression t.
    adrenomedullary t.
    AGR t.
    anal t.
    Andersen t.
    Beck t.
    Charcot t.
    Dieulafoy t.
    Falta t.
    Gougerot t.
    Grancher t.
    hepatic t's
    Hutchinson t.
    Kartagener t.
    t. of Luciani
    Marburg t.
    meningitic t.
    Merseburg t.
    Oppenheim t.
    Osler t.
    portal t's
    t. of retinal cone
    Saint t.
    t. of Schultz
    t. of skeletal muscle
    Whipple t.
triaditis
    portal t.
triage
trial
    Bernoulli t's
    blind t.
    clinical t.
    crossover t.
    double-blind t.
    t. of labor
    phase I t.
    phase II t.
    phase III t.
    preventive t.
    randomized controlled t.
triallylamine
triamelia

triamine
triamylose
triangle
    Alsberg t.
    anal t.
    anterior t. of neck
    aortic t.
    Assézat t.
    auditory t.
    auricular t.
    t. of auscultation
    axillary t.
    Béclard t.
    Bolton t.
    Bonwill t.
    brachial t.
    Bryant t.
    t. of Budde
    Burger scalene t.
    Burow t.
    Calot t.
    cardiohepatic t.
    carotid t.
    carotid t., inferior
    carotid t., superior
    cephalic t.
    cervical t.
    clavipectoral t.
    Codman t.
    color t.
    crural t.
    cystohepatic t.
    digastric t.
    Dunham t's
    Einthoven t.
    Elaut t.
    t. of elbow
    t. of election
    extravesical t.
    facial t.
    Farabeuf t.
    femoral t.
    fetal t.
    frontal t.
    Garland t.
    Gerhardt t.
    Gombault-Philippe t.
    Grocco t.
    Grynfeltt t.
    t. of Grynfeltt and
      Lesgaft
    Henke t.
    Hesselbach t.
    hypoglossal t.
    hypoglossohyoid t.

triangle *(continued)*
    iliofemoral t.
    infraclavicular t.
    inguinal t.
    Jackson safety t.
    Kanavel t.
    Korányi-Grocco t.
    Langenbeck t.
    Lesshaft t.
    Lieutaud t.
    Livingston t.
    lumbar t.
    lumbocostoabdominal t.
    lymphoid t.
    Macewen t.
    Malgaigne t.
    mesenteric t.
    Minor t.
    Mohrenheim t.
    muscular t.
    t. of necessity
    t's of neck
    nodal t.
    occipital t.
    occipital t., inferior
    omoclavicular t.
    omotracheal t.
    palatal t.
    paravertebral t.
    Pawlik t.
    Petit t.
    Petit lumbar t.
    Pinaud t.
    Pirogoff t.
    popliteal t. of femur
    posterior t. of neck
    pubourethral t.
    Rauchfuss t.
    reactive t.
    rectal t.
    Reil t.
    retromandibular t.
    retromolar t.
    sacral t.
    t. of safety
    Scarpa t.
    Sherren t.
    sternocostal t.
    subclavian t.
    subinguinal t.
    submandibular t.
    submaxillary t.
    submental t.
    suboccipital t.
    superior lumbar t.

triangle *(continued)*
    suprameatal t.
    surgical t.
    surgical lumbar t.
    tracheal t.
    Trautmann t.
    Tweed t.
    umbilicomammillary t.
    urogenital t.
    vaginal t.
    vesical t.
    von Weber t.
    Ward t.
    Weber t.
    Wernicke t.
triangular
triangularis
triangulation
triantebrachia
triatomic molecule
triatrial heart
triatriatum
    cor t.
triazenes
tribasic
tribenoside
tribology
triboluminescence
tribrachia
tribrachius
tribulosis
tributyrinase
TRIC—trachoma-inclusion
    conjunctivitis
tricarboxylic acid
tricellular
tricephalus
triceps surae
triceptor
tricheiria
trichiasis
trichilemmoma
Trichinella spiralis
trichiniferous
trichinization
trichinoscope
trichinosed
trichinosis
trichinotic
trichinous
trichion (trichia)
trichite
trichlorfon
trichloride
trichloroacetaldehyde

T

trichloroacetic acid
trichloroethylene
trichloromethane
trichloromethylchloroformate
trichloromonofluoromethane
trichlorophenol
2,4,5-trichlorophenoxyacetic acid
trichlorotrivinylarsine
trichlorphon
trichoadenoma
trichobacteria
trichobezoar
Trichobilharzia ocellata
trichoblastoma
trichocardia
trichocephaliasis
trichocephalosis
trichoclasia
trichoclasis
trichocyst
trichodiscoma
trichodysplasia
trichodystrophy
trichoepithelioma
    desmoplastic t.
    multiple t.
    solitary t.
trichoesthesia
trichofolliculoma
trichoglossia
trichohyalin
trichoid
tricholemmoma
tricholeukocyte
tricholith
trichology
trichomalacia
trichome
trichomegaly
trichomonacidal
trichomonacide
trichomonad
trichomonal
Trichomonas
    T. buccalis
    T. tenax
    T. vaginalis
trichomoniasis
    urogenital t.
    vaginal t.
trichomycosis
    t. axillaris
    t. nodosa
    t. nodularis
    pubic t.

trichonodosis
trichopathic
trichopathy
trichophagia
trichophytic
    granuloma
trichophytid
trichophytin test
trichophytobezoar
Trichophyton
    T. concentricum
    T. mentagrophytes
    T. rubrum
    T. tonsurans
    T. verrucosum
    T. violaceum
trichophytosis
trichopoliodystrophy
Trichoptera
trichoptilosis
trichorhinophalangeal
    syndrome
trichorrhexis
    t. invaginata
    t. nodosa
trichoschisis
trichosiderin
trichosis carunculae
Trichosporon
    T. beigelii
    T. cutaneum
trichosporonosis
trichosporosis
trichostasis spinulosa
trichostrongyliasis
trichostrongylosis
Trichostrongylus
    T. probolurus
    T. vitrinus
trichothecenes
Trichothecium roseum
trichothiodystrophy
trichotillomania
trichotomous
trichotoxin
trichroic
trichroism
trichromacy
    anomalous t.
trichromat
trichromatic
    anomalous t. vision
    t. vision
trichromatism
trichromatopsia

trichrome
    Gomori t. stain
    Milligan t. stain
    t. stain
    t. vitiligo
trichromic
trichterbrust
trichuriasis
Trichuris trichiura
tricipital
tricornute
tricresol
tricresyl phosphate (TCP)
tricrotic
tricrotism
tricuspid
    t. annular plane systolic
      excursion
    t. annular velocity
    t. annulus
    t. annulus systolic
      displacement
    t. annulus systolic velocity
    t. aortic valve
    t. atresia
    t. inflow
    t. insufficiency
    t. jet velocity
    t. opening snap
    t. regurgitant jet velocity
    t. regurgitant velocity
    t. regurgitation
    t. stenosis
    t. valve
tricyclic
tridactylism
tridactylous
tridentate
trident hand
tridermic tumor
tridermogenesis
tridermoma
triencephalus
triethylamine
trifacial
trifid
Tri-Flow incentive spirometry
trifocal
trifurcate
trifurcation
    t. aneurysm
    de novo t. lesion
    t. graft
    internal carotid artery t.
    t. lesion

trifurcation *(continued)*
    left main coronary artery t.
    middle cerebral artery t.
    popliteal t.
    portal vein t.
    t. vessel imaging
trigastric
trigeminal
    t. neuralgia
    t. rhizotomy
    t. tractotomy
trigeminus
trigeminy
trigger
    t. point
    t. thumb
triglycerides
trigona
trigonal
    deep t. muscle
    t. muscles
    superficial t. muscle
trigone
    bladder t.
    carotid t.
    cerebral t.
    collateral t. of fourth ventricle
    collateral t. of lateral ventricle.
    fibrous t. of heart
    Henke t.
    hypoglossal t.
    iliopectineal t.
    interpeduncular t.
    t. of lateral lemniscus
    olfactory t.
    omoclavicular t.
    pontocerebellar t.
    retromolar t.
    t. of urinary bladder
    urogenital t.
    vagal t.
    vesical t.
trigonelline
trigonid
trigonitis
trigonocephalic
trigonocephalus
trigonocephaly
trigonum (trigona)
    t. auscultationis
    t. caroticum
    t. cervicale
    t. cervicale anterius
    t. cervicale posterius
    t. clavipectorale

T

trigonum (trigona) *(continued)*
    t. collaterale ventriculi
      lateralis
    t. colli anterius
    t. colli laterale
    t. coracoacromiale
    t. cystohepaticum
    t. deltoideopectorale
    t. deltopectorale
    t. femorale
    t. fibrosum dextrum cordis
    t. fibrosum sinistrum cordis
    t. habenulae
    t. hypoglossale
    t. inguinale
    t. lemnisci lateralis
    t. lumbale inferius
    t. lumbale superius
    t. lumbare
    t. lumbocostale
    t. musculare
    t. nervi hypoglossi
    t. nervi vagi
    t. olfactorium
    t. omoclaviculare
    t. omotracheale
    t. pontocerebellare
    t. sternocostale
    t. submandibulare
    t. submentale
    t. urogenitale
    t. vagale
    t. vesicae urinariae
trihydrate
trihydric alcohol
trihydrol
trihydroxide
triiniodymus
triiodide
triiodoethionic acid
triiodomethane
triiodothyronine (T_3, [T3])
    free t. index
    t. resin uptake
    t. resin uptake test
    reverse t. (rT_3, [rT3])
    total t.
trilabe
trilaminar
trilateral
trilaurin
trileaflet
    t. aortic prosthesis
    t. aortic valve prolapse
    t. heart valve

trilinolein
trilobate
trilobed
trilocular heart
trilogy of Fallot
trimagnesium phosphate
trimalleolar fracture
trimellitic anhydride (TMA)
    t. flu
    t. pneumonitis
trimensual
trimer
trimercuric
trimeric
trimester
trimethylxanthine
trimorphous
trinegative
trinitrate
    glyceryl t.
trinitrocellulose
trinitroglycerin
trinitroglycerol
trinitrotoluene poisoning
trinocular microscope
trinomial
trinucleate
trinucleotide repeat
triocephalus
Triodontophorus diminutus
triolein breath test
triopathy
triophthalmos
triopodymus
triorchid
triorchidism
triose
    t. kinase
    t. phosphate
    t. phosphate isomerase
triotus
trioxide
trioxypurine
tripalmitate
    glyceryl t.
tripalmitin
tripara
triparanol syndrome
tripartite
tripeptide
tripeptidyl-peptidase
triphalangeal
triphalangism
trip-hammer pulse
triphasic

triphenylmethane
triphosphate
    adenosine t.
    cytidine t.
    deoxyadenosine t.
    deoxycytidine t.
    deoxyguanosine t.
    deoxythymidine t.
    deoxyuridine t.
    guanosine t.
    inosine t.
    inositol 1,4,5-t.
    uridine t.
triphosphopyridine nucleotide
Tripier
    amputation
    operation
triplane fracture
triple
    t.-angle
    t. arthrodesis
    t.-A syndrome
    t. blind
    t. discharge
    t.-lumen drain
    Mallory t. stain
    t. mask
    t. phosphate
    t. phosphate calculus
    t. point
    t. response
    t. rhythm
    t. staining
    t. sugar iron (TSI) agar
    t. sulfa
    t. syndactyly
    t. test
    t. vision
    t.-voiding cystography
    t.-X chromosomal aberration
triplegia
triplet
    t. code
    t. repeat disorders
    t. state
triplex
triploblastic
triploid
triploidy
triplokoria
triplopia
tripod
    t. cane
    Haller t.
    t. of life

tripod *(continued)*
    t. position
    vital t.
tripodia
tripoding
tripoli
tripositive
triprosopus
tripus
triquetral
triquetrous
triquetrum
triradial
triradiate
triradiation
triradius
trisaccharide
Tri-screen
trismic
trismoid
trismus
trisomic
trisomy
    t. 8 syndrome
    t. 9, 9p
    t. 11q syndrome
    t. 13 syndrome
    t. 13-15
    t. 13-15 D
    t. 16-18
    t. 18 E
    t. 18 syndrome
    t. 21 syndrome
    t. 22 syndrome
    t. C syndrome
    t. D syndrome
    t. E syndrome
trisplanchnic
trisporic acids
tristearin
tristichia
tristimania
trisubstituted
trisulcate
trisulfate
trisulfide
tritan
tritanomal
tritanomalous
tritanomaly
tritanope
tritanopia
tritanopic
tritanopsia
tritiate

T

triticeous
triticeum
tritium
tritocone
tritoconid
triton
tritubercular
triturable
triturate
    tablet t.
trituration
triturator
trivalence
trivalent
trivalve
trizonal
TRMC—tetramethylrhodamino-
  isothiocyanate
tRNA—transfer RNA
TRNG—tetracycline-resistant
  Neisseria gonorrhoeae
trocar
    Allen t.
    Barnes t.
    Beardsley cecostomy t.
    Campbell t.
    t. catheter
    Coakley t.
    Duke t.
    Durham t.
    Hurwitz t.
    Ingram t. catheter
    Lichtwicz t.
    Ochsner t.
    Patterson t.
    piloting t.
    Potain t.
    rectal t.
    Southey t.
trochanter
    greater t.
    lesser t.
    t. major
    t. minor
    rudimentary t.
    small t.
    t. tertius
    third t.
trochanteric
trochanteritis
trochanterplasty
trochantinian
troche
trochinian
trochiscation
trochiscus (trochisci)

trochiter
trochiterian
trochlea (trochleae)
    t. fibularis calcanei
    t. humeri
    t. of humerus
    muscular t.
    t. muscularis
    t. musculi obliqui superioris
      bulbi
    peroneal t. of calcaneus
    t. peronealis calcanei
    t. phalangis manus
    t. phalangis pedis
    t. of superior oblique muscle
    t. tali
    t. of talus
trochlear
trochleariform
trochlearis
trochocephaly
trochoid
trochoides
Troisier
    ganglion
    node
    sign
    syndrome
Troisier-Hanot-Chauffard
    syndrome
troland
Trolard
    net
    plexus
    vein
Tröltsch (Troeltsch)
    corpuscles
    recesses
    spaces
    speculum
Trombicula
    T. muscae domesticae
    T. muscarum
trombiculiasis
tromophonia
tropaeolin
    t. D
    t. G
tropate
tropeine
tropeinism
trophectoderm
trophedema
    congenital t.
    hereditary t.
trophic

trophicity
trophism
trophoblast
trophoblastic
trophoblastoma
trophocyte
trophoderm
trophodermatoneurosis
trophodynamics
tropholecithal
tropholecithus
trophology
trophoneurosis
    disseminated t.
    facial t.
    lingual t.
    muscular t.
    t. of Romberg
trophoneurotic
trophonosis
trophont
trophonucleus
trophopathy
trophoplast
trophospongium
  (trophospongia)
trophotaxis
trophotherapy
trophotropic
trophotropism
trophozoite
tropia
tropic acid
tropical
tropidine
tropin
tropine
tropism
tropochrome
tropocollagen
tropoelastin
tropometer
tropomyosin A
troponin
    t. C
    t. I
    t. T
trough
    gingival t.
    Langmuir t.
    peak and t. level
    synaptic t's
    vestibular t.
trousers
    MAST (military [or medical]
      antishock treatment) t.

Trousseau
    bougie
    dilator
    phenomenon
    sign
    spot
    syndrome
    twitching
Trousseau-Jackson dilator
Trousseau-Lallemand bodies
Troutman
    chisel
    gouge
    implant
    operation
TRP—tubular reabsorption of
  phosphate
TRPT—theoretical renal
  phosphorus threshold
TRU—turbidity-reducing unit
Truc operation
true suture
Trueta
    method
    technique
    treatment
truly
truncal
    t. obesity
    t. vagotomy
truncate
truncoconal
truncus (trunci)
    t. arteriosus
    t. arteriosus, persistent
    t. brachiocephalicus
    t. bronchomediastinalis
    t. coeliacus
    t. corporis callosi
    t. costocervicalis
    t. encephali
    t. encephalicus
    t. fasciculi atrioventricularis
    t. inferior plexus brachialis
    trunci intestinales
    t. jugularis
    t. linguofacialis
    t. lumbalis
    t. lumbaris
    t. lumbosacralis
    trunci lymphatici
    t. medius plexus brachialis
    t. nervi accessorii
    t. nervi spinalis
    trunci plexus brachialis
    t. pulmonalis

T

truncus (trunci) *(continued)*
    t. subclavius
    t. superior plexus brachialis
    t. sympatheticus
    t. sympathicus
    t. thyreocervicalis
    t. vagalis anterior
    t. vagalis posterior
trunk
    anterior gastric t.
    t. of atrioventricular
      bundle
    basilar t.
    t's of brachial plexus
    brachiocephalic t.
    bronchomediastinal t.
    t. of bundle of His
    celiac t.
    t. of corpus callosum
    costocervical t.
    inferior t. of brachial plexus
    intestinal t's
    intestinal lymphatic t's
    jugular t.
    left bronchomediastinal t.
    linguofacial t.
    lumbar t.
    lumbosacral t.
    lymphatic t's
    middle t. of brachial plexus
    nerve t.
    posterior gastric t.
    pulmonary t.
    right bronchomediastinal t.
    subclavian t.
    superior t. of brachial
      plexus
    sympathetic t.
    sympathetic ganglionated t.
    thyrocervical t.
    vagal t. anterior
    vagal t. posterior
TRUS—transrectal
  ultrasonography
trusion
truss
    carotid t.
    t. mattress
    nasal t.
    yarn t.
try-in
trypan blue
trypanid
trypanocidal
trypanolysis

trypanolytic
Trypanosoma
    T. cruzi
    T. neotomae
    T. nigeriense
    T. rangeli
    T. theileri
trypanosomal
trypanosomatic
trypanosomatid
trypanosomatotropic
trypanosome
trypanosomiasis
    acute t.
    African t.
    American t.
    Brazilian t.
    chronic t.
    Congo t.
    Cruz t.
    t. cruzi
    East African t.
    Gambian t.
    Rhodesian t.
    South American t.
    West African t.
trypanosomic
trypanosomicidal
trypanosomicide
trypanosomid
trypanosomosis
trypan red
tryparosan
tryparsamide
trypesis
trypochetes
trypomastigote
tryponarsyl
trypotan
trypsin
    crystallized t.
    t. inhibitor
trypsinize
tryptamine
tryptase
tryptic
tryptone
L-tryptophan
tryptophan 2,3-dioxygenase
tryptophanase
tryptophanuria
tryptophyl
TS—
    test solution
    thoracic surgery

TS— *(continued)*
    tricuspid stenosis
    triple strength
    tropical sprue
TSA—tumor-specific antigen
T₄SA—thyroxine-specific activity
TSB—trypticase soy broth
TSC—technetium sulfur colloid
TSD—
    target skin distance
    Tay-Sachs disease
TSE—trisodium edetate
tsetse fly
TSF—
    tissue-coding factor
    triceps skinfold
TSH—thyroid-stimulating hormone
T-shaped incision
TSH-RF—thyroid-stimulating hormone–releasing factor
TSI—thyroid-stimulating immunoglobulins
tsp.—teaspoon(s), teaspoonful
TSP—total serum protein
TSPAP—total serum prostatic acid phosphatase
TSR—thyroid-to-serum ratio
TST—tumor skin test
TSTA—tumor-specific transplantation antigen
T-strain mycoplasma
tsutsugamushi disease
TSY—trypticase soy yeast
TT—
    therapeutic touch
    thrombin time
    total thyroxine
    total time
    transit time
    transthoracic
TTD—tissue tolerance dose
TTH—thyrotropic hormone
TTP—thrombotic thrombocytopenic purpura
TTS—temporary threshold shift
TTT—tolbutamide tolerance test
T tube
T-tube
    T-t. cholangiogram
    T-t. cholangiography
TU—
    thiouracil
    toxic unit
    tuberculin unit

tuba (tubae)
    t. acustica
    t. auditiva
    t. auditoria
    t. uterina
tubal
    t. ligation
    t. occlusion
    t. pregnancy
    t. sterilization
tubatorsion
Tubbs dilator
tube
    Abbott-Miller t.
    Abbott-Rawson t.
    Aberdeen t.
    Adson suction t.
    air t.
    Alder Hey t.
    Andrews-Pynchon suction t.
    Anthony t.
    Argyle chest t.
    Argyle endotracheal t.
    Atkins-Cannard tracheotomy t.
    auditory t.
    auscultation t.
    Ayre t.
    Baker jejunostomy t.
    Baker self-sumping t.
    Beardsley empyema t.
    Bellocq t.
    Blakemore esophageal t.
    Blakemore nasogastric t.
    Blakemore-Sengstaken t.
    Bouchut laryngeal t.
    Bowman t's
    breathing t.
    bronchial t.
    Broyles t.
    buccal t.
    Buie rectal suction t.
    Cantor t.
    capillary t.
    Carabelli endobronchial t.
    cardiac t.
    Carlens t.
    Carman rectal t.
    Carrel t.
    Castelli t.
    cathode-ray t. (CRT)
    Cattell t.
    Celestin t.
    t. cell
    cerebromedullary t.
    Chaffin-Pratt t.

T

tube *(continued)*
- Chaoul t.
- chest t.
- Chevalier Jackson t.
- collecting t's
- Coolidge x-ray t.
- corneal t's
- Craigie t.
- Crookes t.
- cuffed t.
- Debove t.
- Diamond t.
- digestive t.
- discharge t.
- Dobbhoff feeding t.
- Donaldson t.
- Dotter t.
- drainage t.
- drawing t.
- duodenal t.
- Durham t.
- electron multiplier t.
- embryonic fallopian t.
- empyema t.
- end t.
- endobronchial t.
- endocardial t.
- endotracheal t.
- Esmarch t.
- esophageal t.
- eustachian t.
- Ewald t.
- fallopian t.
- t. feeding
- fermentation t.
- Ferrein t's
- fiberoptic t.
- Frazier suction t.
- Fuller t.
- fusion t's
- Gabriel Tucker t.
- Geiger-Müller t.
- glow modular t.
- Greiling t.
- grenz ray t.
- Guisez t.
- Harris t.
- Holinger t.
- horizontal t.
- hot-cathode t.
- House t.
- image intensifier t.
- Immergut t.
- intestinal t.
- intratracheal t. (IT)

tube *(continued)*
- intubation t.
- Jackson t.
- Jackson-Pratt t.
- Johnson t.
- Jutte t.
- KCH t.
- Kelly t.
- Killian t.
- Kistner t.
- Kobelt t's
- Kuhn t.
- Lanz t.
- LaRocca t.
- laryngostomy t.
- Lennarson t.
- Lepley-Ernst t.
- Levin t.
- Lewis t.
- Lindeman-Silverstein t.
- Linton t.
- lobster-tail t.
- Lore-Lawrence t.
- Luer t.
- MacKenty t.
- Martin t.
- medullary t.
- Mett (Mette) test t.
- Miller-Abbott (MA) t.
- Millin t.
- Minnesota t.
- Montgomery T t.
- Morch t.
- Mosher t.
- Mueller-Frazier t.
- Mueller-Pool t.
- Mueller-Pynchon t.
- Mueller-Yankauer t.
- Nachlas t.
- nasogastric t.
- nasopharyngeal t.
- nasotracheal t.
- Negus t.
- nephrostomy t.
- neural t.
- New t.
- O'Beirne t.
- observation t.
- Ochsner t.
- Olshevsky t.
- orotracheal t.
- otopharyngeal t.
- ovarian t's
- Paparella t.
- Parker t.

tube *(continued)*
>   Paul-Mixter t.
>   Per-Lee t.
>   Pflüger t's
>   pharyngotympanic t.
>   photomultiplier t. (PMT)
>   Pilling t.
>   Polisar-Lyons t.
>   Pool t.
>   Pudenz t.
>   pus t.
>   Pynchon t.
>   rectal t.
>   Rehfuss t.
>   Reuter t.
>   Robertshaw t.
>   Roida t.
>   roll t.
>   Rosen t.
>   rotating anode t.
>   Rubin t.
>   Ruysch t.
>   Ryle t.
>   Sachs suction t.
>   Schachowa spiral t's
>   Schall t.
>   sediment t.
>   sedimentation t.
>   Sengstaken t.
>   Sengstaken-Blakemore t.
>   Shea t.
>   Sheehy t.
>   Shepard t.
>   Shiley t.
>   Shiner t.
>   Southey-Leech t.
>   Souttar t.
>   speaking t.
>   sputum t.
>   stomach t.
>   suction t.
>   sump t.
>   T t.
>   tampon t.
>   Teflon t.
>   test t.
>   thoracostomy t.
>   Thunberg t.
>   tracheal t.
>   tracheostomy t.
>   Tucker t.
>   tympanostomy t.
>   U t.
>   uterine t.
>   vacuum t.

tube *(continued)*
>   Valentine t.
>   valve t.
>   Veillon t.
>   ventilation t.
>   Venturi myringotomy t.
>   vertical t.
>   Voltolini t.
>   Wangensteen t.
>   Welch-Allyn t.
>   Wintrobe t.
>   x-ray t.
>   Yankauer t.

tubectomy

tuber (tubers, tubera)
>   t. angle
>   t. calcanei
>   t. cinereum
>   t. cochleae
>   eustachian t.
>   external t. of Henle
>   frontal t.
>   t. frontale
>   iliopubic t.
>   t. ischiadicum
>   t. maxillae
>   maxillary t.
>   mental t.
>   omental t. of body of pancreas
>   t. omentale corporis pancreatis
>   t. omentale hepatis
>   omental t. of liver
>   papillary t.
>   parietal t.
>   t. parietale
>   t. radii
>   t. of radius
>   sciatic t.
>   t. vermis
>   t. zygomaticum

tubercle
>   accessory t.
>   acoustic t.
>   adductor t. of femur
>   amygdaloid t. of Schwalbe
>   anal t.
>   anatomical t.
>   anterior t. of atlas
>   anterior t. of calcaneus
>   anterior t. of cervical
>   vertebrae
>   anterior t. of humerus
>   anterior obturator t.
>   t. of anterior scalene muscle
>   anterior t. of thalamus

tubercle *(continued)*

articular t. of temporal bone
t. of atlas, anterior
t. of atlas, posterior
auditory t.
auricular t.
Babès t's
brachial t. of humerus
calcaneal t.
Carabelli t.
carotid t.
caseous t.
caudal t. of liver
cervical t's
t. of cervical vertebrae, anterior
t. of cervical vertebrae, posterior
Chassaignac t.
condyloid t.
conglomerate t.
conoid t.
corniculate t.
costal t.
crude t.
t. of cuneate nucleus
cuneiform t.
t. of Czermak
Darwin t.
darwinian t.
deltoid t.
dental t.
dissection t.
dorsal t. of radius
ear t.
epiglottic t.
external t. of humerus
external mental t.
Farre t's
t. of femur
fibrous t.
t. of fibula, posterior
genital t.
Gerdy t.
Ghon t.
gracile t.
gray t.
greater t. of calcaneus
greater t. of humerus
t. of greater multangular bone
hard t.
hepatic t.
hippocampal t.
His t.
t. of humerus

tubercle *(continued)*

t. of humerus, anterior, of Meckel
t. of humerus, anterior, of Weber
t. of humerus, external
t. of humerus, greater
t. of humerus, internal
t. of humerus, lesser
t. of humerus, posterior
iliac t.
t. of iliac crest
iliopectineal t.
iliopubic t.
inferior genial t.
inferior t. of Humphrey
inferior thyroid t.
infraglenoid t.
intercolumnar t.
intercondylar t., lateral
intercondylar t., medial
internal t. of humerus
intravascular t.
jugular t. of occipital bone
labial t.
lacrimal t.
lateral intercondylar t.
lateral orbital t.
lateral palpebral t.
lateral t. of posterior process of talus
lesser t. of calcaneus
lesser t. of humerus
Lisfranc t.
Lister t.
Lower t.
Luschka t.
lymphoid t.
mammillary t's
mammillary t. of hypothalamus
marginal t. of zygomatic bone
medial intercondylar t.
medial t. of posterior process of talus
mental t., external
mental t. of mandible
miliary t.
Montgomery t's
Morgagni t.
Müller t.
müllerian t.
muscular t. of atlas
naked t.
t. of navicular bone

tubercle *(continued)*

    nuchal t.
    t. of nucleus cuneatus
    t. of nucleus gracilis
    obturator t., anterior
    obturator t., posterior
    olfactory t.
    orbital t.
    palpebral t.
    papillary t.
    paramolar t.
    peroneal t.
    peroneal t. of calcaneus
    pharyngeal t.
    t. of philtrum
    plantar t.
    posterior t. of atlas
    posterior t. of cervical
      vertebrae
    posterior t. of fibula
    posterior t. of humerus
    posterior obturator t.
    t. of posterior process of talus,
      lateral
    t. of posterior process of talus,
      medial
    posterior t. of sixth cervical
      vertebra
    posterior t. of thalamus
    postglenoid t.
    postmortem t.
    pterygoid t.
    pubic t.
    t. of pubic bone
    t. of rib
    t. of Rolando
    t. of root of zygoma
    t. of Santorini
    scalene t.
    t. of scaphoid bone
    sebaceous t.
    t. of sella turcica
    t. for serratus anterior
      muscle
    t. of sixth cervical vertebra,
      anterior
    t. of sixth cervical vertebra,
      carotid
    t. of sixth cervical vertebra,
      posterior
    spinous t.
    superior t. of Henle
    superior t. of Humphrey
    superior thyroid t.
    supraglenoid t.

tubercle *(continued)*

    supratragic t.
    t. of thalamus, anterior
    t. of thalamus, posterior
    thyroid t., inferior
    thyroid t., superior
    t. of tibia
    transverse t. of fourth tarsal
      bone
    t. of trapezium
    trochanteric t.
    trochlear t.
    t. of ulna
    t. of upper lip
    t's of vertebra
    Whitnall t.
    Wrisberg t.
    yellow t.
    t. of zygoma
    zygomatic t.

tubercula (plural of tuberculum)
tubercular
tuberculase
tuberculate, tuberculated
tuberculation
tuberculid

    micronodular t.
    papular t.
    papulonecrotic t.
    rosacea-like t.

tuberculin

    Koch t.
    Old t. (OT)
    purified protein derivative
      (PPD) t.
    Seibert t.

tuberculinization
tuberculitis
tuberculization
tuberculocele
tuberculocidal
tuberculocide
tuberculoderm
tuberculoderma
tuberculofibroid
tuberculoid
tuberculoidin
tuberculoma en plaque
tuberculosis (TB)

    abdominal t.
    active t.
    acute miliary t.
    adrenal t.
    adult t.
    aerogenic t.

T

tuberculosis (TB) *(continued)*
  anthracotic t.
  attenuated t.
  atypical t.
  basal t.
  t. of bone
  t. of bones and joints
  bronchogenic t.
  bronchopneumonic t.
  caseous t.
  cerebral t.
  cestodic t.
  childhood t.
  chronic fibroid t.
  chronic ulcerative t.
  cutaneous t.
  cystic t. of bones
  disseminated t.
  endogenous t.
  endothelial t.
  esophageal t.
  extrapulmonary t.
  extrathoracic t.
  exudative t.
  fibrocaseous t.
  fibrosing t.
  gastrointestinal t.
  genital t.
  genitourinary t.
  glandular t.
  hematogenous t.
  hilar t.
  hilus t.
  ileocecal t.
  inhalation t.
  intestinal t.
  t. of intestines
  intrathoracic t.
  t. of kidney and bladder
  laryngeal t.
  t. of larynx
  latent t.
  t. of lungs
  t. of lymph nodes
  lymphogenous t.
  lymphoid t.
  meningeal t.
  miliary t.
  minimal t.
  moderately advanced t.
  open t.
  oral t.
  orificial t.
  papulonecrotic t.
  postprimary t.

tuberculosis (TB) *(continued)*
  primary t.
  primary inoculation t.
  productive t.
  pulmonary t.
  quiescent t.
  reinfection t.
  renal t.
  t. of serous membranes
  skeletal t.
  t. of skin
  spinal t.
  t. of spine
  surgical t.
  tracheobronchial t.
  warty t.
tuberculostatic
tuberculotic
tuberculotoxin
tuberculous
  t. dactylitis
  t. keratoconjunctivitis
  t. meningitis
  t. peritonitis
  t. spondylitis
tuberculum (tubercula)
  t. adductorium femoris
  t. anterius atlantis
  t. anterius thalami
  t. arthriticum
  t. articulare ossis temporalis
  t. auriculae
  t. auriculae (Darwini)
  t. calcanei
  t. caroticum
  t. cinereum
  t. conoideum
  t. corniculatum
  t. coronae
  t. costae
  t. cuneatum
  t. cuneiforme
  t. dentale
  t. dentis
  t. dolorosum
  t. dorsale radii
  t. epiglotticum
  t. gracile
  t. iliacum
  t. impar
  t. infraglenoidale
  t. intercondylare laterale
  t. intercondylare mediale
  t. intercondyloideum
  t. intercondyloideum laterale

tuberculum (tubercula) *(continued)*
t. intercondyloideum mediale
t. intervenosum
t. jugulare ossis occipitalis
t. labii superioris
t. laterale processus
  posterioris tali
t. majus humeri
t. marginale ossis zygomatici
t. mediale
t. mediale processus
  posterioris tali
t. mentale mandibulae
t. minus humeri
t. musculi scaleni anterioris
t. obturatorium anterius
t. obturatorium posterius
t. ossis multanguli majoris
t. ossis navicularis
t. ossis scaphoidei
t. ossis trapezii
t. pharyngeum
t. posterius atlantis
t. posterius vertebrae
  cervicalis
t. pubicum
t. sellae turcicae
t. septi
t. supraglenoidale
t. supratragicum
t. thyroideum inferius
t. thyroideum superius
t. trigeminale
tuberosis
tuberositas (tuberositates)
t. coracoidea
t. costae II
t. costalis claviculae
t. deltoidea humeri
t. femoris externa
t. femoris interna
t. glutea femoris
t. iliaca
t. infraglenoidalis
t. masseterica
t. musculi serrati anterioris
t. ossis cuboidei
t. ossis metatarsalis primi
t. ossis metatarsalis quinti
t. ossis navicularis
t. patellaris
t. phalangis distalis manus
t. phalangis distalis pedis
t. pterygoidea mandibulae
t. radii

tuberositas (tuberositates)
(continued)
t. sacralis
t. supraglenoidalis scapulae
t. tibiae
t. tibiae externa
t. tibiae interna
t. ulnae
t. unguicularis manus
t. unguicularis pedis
tuberosity
t. for anterior serratus muscle
bicipital t.
t. of calcaneus
t. of carpal bone
t. of clavicle
coracoid t.
costal t. of clavicle
t. of cuboid bone
deltoid t. of humerus
distal t. of finger
distal t. of toe
t. of femur, internal
t. of femur, lateral
t. of femur, medial
t. of fifth metatarsal
t. of first carpal bone
t. of first metatarsal
t. of fourth tarsal bone
frontal t.
gluteal t. of femur
t. of greater multangular bone
greater t. of humerus
t's of humerus (greater, lesser)
iliac t.
infraglenoid t.
ischial t.
t. of ischium
lesser t. of humerus
malar t.
masseteric t.
t. of maxilla
maxillary t.
t. of metatarsal bone
t. of navicular bone
omental t.
omental t. of liver
omental t. of pancreas
parietal t.
patellar t.
pterygoid t. of mandible
t. of pubic bone
pyramidal t. of palatine bone
radial t.
t. of radius

T

tuberosity *(continued)*
    sacral t.
    t. of scaphoid bone
    scapular t. of Henle
    t. of second rib
    t. for serratus anterior muscle
    supraglenoid t.
    t. of tarsal bone
    t. of tibia, external
    t. of tibia, internal
    tibial t.
    t. of trapezium
    t. of ulna
    ungual t.
    unguicular t.
tuberous sclerosis
tubi (plural of tubus)
tubiferous
tuboabdominal pregnancy
tuboadnexopexy
tubocurarine
    t. chloride
    dimethyl t. iodide
tubogastrostomy
tuboligamentous
tubo-ovarian
tubo-ovariectomy
tubo-ovariotomy
tubo-ovaritis
tuboperitoneal
tuboplasty
    balloon t.
    eustachian t.
tuborrhea
tubotorsion
tubotympanal
tubotympanic recess
tubotympanum
tubouterine
tubovaginal
tubular
    t. necrosis
    t. proteinuria
    t. stenosis
tubule
    Albarran t.
    Bellini t's
    biliferous t.
    caroticotympanic t's
    collecting t's
    collecting t's of mesonephros
    connecting t's
    convoluted t's
    convoluted t., distal
    convoluted t., proximal

tubule *(continued)*
    convoluted renal t's
    convoluted seminiferous t's
    dental t's
    dentinal t's
    discharging t's
    distal convoluted t.
    t's of the epoöphoron
    Ferrein t's
    galactophorous t's
    Henle t's
    Kobelt t's
    lactiferous t's
    malpighian t.
    mesonephric t's
    metanephric t's
    Miescher t.
    outer t's of the parovarium
    paraurethral t's
    pronephric t's
    proximal convoluted t.
    Rainey t.
    renal t's
    renal t's, convoluted
    renal t's, straight
    segmental t's
    seminiferous t's
    seminiferous t's,
      convoluted
    seminiferous t's, straight
    Skene t's
    spiral t's
    straight t's
    straight renal t's
    straight seminiferous t's
    subtracheal t.
    testicular t.
    tracheal t.
    transverse t.
    T t's
    urine-collecting t.
    uriniferous t.
    uriniparous t.
    vertical t's
tubuli (plural of tubulus)
tubuliform
tubulin
tubulitis
tubulization
tubuloacinar
tubuloacinous
tubulocyst
tubulointerstitial
tubulopathy
tubuloracemose

tubulorrhexis
  ischemic t.
tubulosaccular
tubulous
tubulovesicle
tubulovesicular
tubulovillous
tubulus (tubuli)
  t. attenuatus
  t. colligens rectus
  t. contortus distalis
  t. contortus proximalis
  t. rectus distalis
  t. rectus proximalis
  t. renalis arcuatus
  t. renalis colligens
  tubuli seminiferi
    contorti
  tubuli seminiferi recti
tubus (tubi)
tuck
tucker
  Bishop tendon t.
  Bishop-Black tendon t.
  Bishop-Peter tendon t.
  Burch-Greenwood
    tendon t.
  Fink tendon t.
Tucker
  bronchoscope
  dilator
  esophagoscope
  laryngoscope
  tube
Tucker-McLane forceps
tucking
Tudor-Edwards costotome
Tuffier
  method
  operation
  retractor
  rib spreader
  test
Tuffier-Raney retractor
tuft
  enamel t's
  hair t's
  malpighian t.
  renal t.
  synovial t's
  ungual t.
tufting
TUG—total urinary gonadotropin
tug, tugging
  tracheal t.

tularemia
  gastrointestinal t.
  glandular t.
  oculoglandular t.
  oropharyngeal t.
  pneumonic t.
  pulmonary t.
  pulmonic t.
  typhoidal t.
  ulceroglandular t.
tularine
tulle gras
  t.g. dressing
  t.g. gauze
Tullio phenomenon
Tulpius valve
tumefacient
tumefaction
tumefy
tumentia
  vasomotor t.
tumescence
  nocturnal penile t. (NPT)
  penile t.
tumescent
tumor
  Abrikosov (Abrikossoff) t.
  Ackerman t.
  acoustic t.
  acoustic nerve t.
  acute splenic t.
  adenoid t.
  adenomatoid t.
  adenomatoid odontogenic t.
  adipose t.
  adrenal rest t.
  t. albus
  alpha cell t.
  alveolar t.
  alveolar cell t.
  ameloblastic adenomatoid t.
  amyloid t.
  aneurysmal giant cell t.
  angiomatoid t.
  angle t.
  aniline t.
  aortic body t.
  argentaffin carcinoid t.
  ascites t.
  benign t.
  benign mixed t.
  benign triton t.
  t. blush
  Brenner t.
  Brodie t.

T

tumor *(continued)*

    Brooke t.
    brown t.
    brown fat t.
    Brown-Pearce t.
    Burkitt t.
    Burkitt-like t.
    Buschke-Löwenstein
      (Buschke-Loewenstein) t.
    butyroid t.
    calcifying epithelial
      odontogenic t.
    carcinoid t. of bronchus
    carotid body t.
    cartilaginous t.
    cavernous t.
    cellular t.
    cerebellopontine angle t.
    chemoreceptor t.
    chromaffin cell t.
    chromophil t.
    clear cell odontogenic t.
    Cock t.
    Codman t.
    t. colli
    collision t.
    colloid t.
    colloid ovarian t.
    connective tissue t.
    corticoadrenal t.
    craniopharyngeal duct t.
    Cushing t.
    cystic t.
    dermoid t.
    desmoid t.
    dumb-bell t.
    dysontogenetic t.
    Ehrlich t.
    eighth-nerve t.
    eiloid t.
    embryonal t.
    embryoplastic t.
    encysted t.
    endodermal sinus t.
    eosinophilic t.
    eosinophilic t. of the pituitary
    epidermoid t.
    epithelial t.
    erectile t.
    Ewing t.
    extramedullary t.
    extramedullary
      hematopoietic t.
    false t.
    fatty t.

tumor *(continued)*

    fecal t.
    fibrocellular t.
    fibroid t.
    fibroplastic t.
    fibrous t.
    fungating t.
    Furth pituitary t.
    ganglion nodosum t.
    G-cell t.
    gelatinous t.
    germ cell t.
    germ cell testicular t.
    germinal t.
    giant cell t.
    giant cell t. of bone
    giant cell t. of tendon sheath
    glomus t.
    glomus jugulare t.
    gonadal-stromal t.
    granular cell t.
    granulation t.
    granulosa t.
    granulosa cell t.
    granulosa-theca cell t.
    Grawitz t.
    Gubler t.
    gummy t.
    heterologous t.
    heterotypic t.
    hilar cell t.
    hilus cell t.
    histioid t.
    homoiotypic t.
    homologous t.
    Hortega cell t.
    hourglass t.
    Hürthle cell t.
    hypernephroid t.
    hypopharyngeal t.
    t. immunity
    infiltrating t.
    innocent t.
    interstitial cell t.
    intramedullary t.
    iron-hard t.
    islet cell t.
    ivory-like t.
    Jensen t.
    juxtaglomerular t.
    Koenen t.
    Krompecher t.
    Krukenberg t.
    lacteal t.
    Leydig cell t.

tumor *(continued)*
  t. lienis
  lipoid cell t.
  lipoid cell t. of ovary
  luteinized granulosa-theca
    cell t.
  Malherbe t.
  malignant t.
  malignant mixed mesodermal t.
  malignant triton t.
  march t.
  margaroid t.
  mast cell t.
  melanotic neuroectodermal t.
  Merkel cell t.
  mesenchymal t.
  mesodermal mixed t.
  metastatic t.
  migrated t.
  migratory t.
  mixed t.
  mixed t. of salivary glands
  mixed t. of skin
  mixed-tissue t.
  mucinous t.
  mucoepidermoid t.
  mucous t.
  müllerian mixed t.
  muscular t.
  t. necrosis factor
  Nélaton t.
  neuroectodermal t.
  neuroepithelial t.
  neurogenic t.
  nonencapsulated sclerosing t.
  nonresponsive t.
  oat cell t.
  odontogenic t.
  oozing t.
  organoid t.
  oxyphil cell t.
  pacinian t.
  Pancoast t.
  papillary t.
  paraffin t.
  parasagittal t.
  parasellar t.
  paravertebral t.
  parvilocular pseudomucinous t.
  pearl t.
  pearly t.
  Perlmann t.
  phantom t.
  phyllodes t.
  Pindborg t.

tumor *(continued)*
  pineal t.
  plasma cell t.
  t. plop
  polypoid t.
  pontine t.
  pontine angle t.
  potato t.
  Pott puffy t.
  pregnancy t.
  premalignant fibroepithelial t.
  pseudointraligamentous t.
  pulmonary sulcus t.
  radiocurable t.
  radioresistant t.
  radiosensitive t.
  ranine t.
  Rathke pouch t.
  Recklinghausen t.
  recurring digital fibrous t's of
    childhood
  responsive t.
  retinal anlage t.
  rhabdoid t.
  Ringertz t.
  sacrococcygeal t.
  salivary mixed cutaneous t.
  sand t.
  Schiller t.
  Schmincke t.
  Schwann cell t.
  Scully t.
  sellar t.
  sentinel t.
  serous t.
  Sertoli cell t.
  Sertoli-Leydig cell t.
  sheath t.
  solid t.
  t.-specific antigen
  Spiegler t's
  stercoral t.
  sulcus t.
  superior sulcus t.
  supratentorial t.
  teratoid t.
  theca cell t.
  thoracic inlet t.
  thrombus t.
  thymic t.
  transition t.
  tridermic t.
  true t.
  turban t.
  varicose t.

T

tumor *(continued)*
    vascular t.
    villous t.
    vitelline t.
    Warthin t.
    white t.
    Wilms t.
    xanthomatous giant cell t. of
      tendon sheath
    Yoshida t.
    Zollinger-Ellison (ZE) t.
tumorectomy
tumoricidal
tumorigenesis
tumorigenic
tumorlet
tumorous
TUNA—transurethral needle
  ablation
tungsten (W)
tunic
    Bichat t.
    Brücke t.
    fibrous t. of eyeball
    fibrous t. of liver
    mucous t.
    muscular t.
    pharyngeal t.
    pharyngobasilar t.
    proper t.
    Ruysch t.
    t's of spermatic cord
tunica (tunicae)
    t. abdominalis
    t. adventitia
    t. adventitia ductus
      deferentis
    t. adventitia esophagi
    t. adventitia oesophagi
    t. adventitia tubae uterinae
    t. adventitia ureteris
    t. adventitia vasorum
    t. adventitia vesiculae
      seminalis
    t. albuginea corporis
      spongiosi
    t. albuginea corporum
      cavernosorum
    t. albuginea ovarii
    t. albuginea testis
    t. conjunctiva
    t. conjunctiva bulbi
    t. conjunctiva palpebrarum
    t. dartos
    t. decidua
    t. externa thecae folliculi

tunica (tunicae) *(continued)*
    t. externa vasorum
      (adventitia)
    t. fibrosa
    t. fibrosa bulbi
    t. fibrosa hepatis
    t. fibrosa oculi
    t. fibrosa renis
    t. fibrosa splenica
    tunicae funiculi spermatici
    t. interna bulbi
    t. interna thecae folliculi
    t. intima vasorum
    t. media vasorum
    t. mucosa
    t. mucosa bronchiorum
    t. mucosa cavitatis
      tympanicae
    t. mucosa ductus deferentis
    t. mucosa esophagi
    t. mucosa gastris
    t. mucosa intestini crassi
    t. mucosa intestini tenuis
    t. mucosa laryngis
    t. mucosa linguae
    t. mucosa nasi
    t. mucosa oesophagi
    t. mucosa oris
    t. mucosa pharyngis
    t. mucosa recti
    t. mucosa tracheae
    t. mucosa tubae auditivae
    t. mucosa tubae uterinae
    t. mucosa tympanica
    t. mucosa ureteris
    t. mucosa urethrae femininae
    t. mucosa uteri
    t. mucosa vaginae
    t. mucosa ventriculi
    t. mucosa vesicae biliaris
    t. mucosa vesicae felleae
    t. mucosa vesiculae seminalis
    t. muscularis
    t. muscularis bronchiorum
    t. muscularis coli
    t. muscularis ductus
      deferentis
    t. muscularis esophagi
    t. muscularis gastris
    t. muscularis intestini tenuis
    t. muscularis oesophagi
    t. muscularis pharyngis
    t. muscularis recti
    t. muscularis tracheae
    t. muscularis tubae uterinae
    t. muscularis ureteris

tunica (tunicae) *(continued)*
  t. muscularis urethrae
    femininae
  t. muscularis uteri
  t. muscularis vaginae
  t. muscularis ventriculi
  t. muscularis vesicae biliaris
  t. muscularis vesicae felleae
  t. muscularis vesicae
    urinariae
  t. muscularis vesiculae
    seminalis
  t. nervea of Brücke
  t. propria
  t. ruyschiana
  t. sensoria bulbi
  t. serosa
  t. serosa gastris
  t. serosa hepatis
  t. serosa intestini tenuis
  t. serosa lienis
  t. serosa peritonei
  t. serosa splenis
  t. serosa testis
  t. serosa tubae uterinae
  t. serosa uteri
  t. serosa ventriculi
  t. serosa vesicae biliaris
  t. serosa vesicae felleae
  t. serosa vesicae urinariae
  t. spongiosa urethrae
    femininae
  t. spongiosa vaginae
  tunicae testis
  t. uvea
  t. vaginalis testis
  t. vasculosa
  t. vasculosa bulbi
  t. vasculosa lentis
  t. vasculosa oculi
  t. vasculosa testis
tunicary
tunicate
tunicin
tuning fork
  Hartmann t.f.
tunnel
  aortico-left ventricular t.
  carpal t.
  cervical t's
  t. of Corti
  cubital t.
  flexor t.
  inner t.
  outer t.
  tarsal t.

tunnel *(continued)*
  t. view
  Witzel t.
tunneled bougie
tunneler
  Crawford-Cooley t.
  DeBakey t.
tunnel vision
Tuohy needle
TUR—transurethral resection
turanose
TURB—transurethral resection of
  bladder
turbid
turbidimetric
turbidimetry
turbidity
turbinal
turbinate
  ethmoid t.
  inferior t.
  middle nasal t.
  nasal t.
  t. of Santorini
  sphenoid t.
  superior nasal t.
  t. of Zuckerkandl
turbinated
turbinectomy
turbinotome
turbinotomy
Türck
  bundle
  cell
  column
  degeneration
  fasciculus
  trachoma
  zone
Turcot syndrome
turgescence
turgescent
turgid
turgidization
turgor vitalis
Türk
  cell
  irradiation leukocyte
  irritation leukocyte
Turkel
  needle
  punch
  trephine
turmeric
turmschädel
  (turmschaedel)

T

twitching
  fascicular t.
  fibrillar t.
  Trousseau t.
TWL—transepidermal water loss
two-bottle drainage system
two-dimensional
  t.-d. chromatography
  t.-d. echocardiography (TDE)
two-emulsion autoradiography
two-flight dyspnea
two-pillow orthopnea
Twort-d'Herelle phenomenon
Tx—
  traction
  treatment
TXA$_2$—thromboxane A$_2$
TXB$_2$—thromboxane B$_2$
Tydings
  forceps
  knife
  snare
  tonsillectome
Tydings-Lakeside forceps
tylectomy
tylion
tyloma
tylosis
tylotic
tympanal
tympanectomy
tympania
tympanic
  t. neurectomy
  t. plethysmography
tympanichord
tympanicity
tympanism
tympanites
  false t.
  uterine t.
tympanitic
tympanitis
tympanocentesis
tympanoeustachian
tympanogenic
tympanogram
tympanohyal
tympanolabyrinthopexy
tympanomalleal
tympanomandibular
tympanomastoiditis
tympanomastoid suture
tympanomeatal
tympanometric

tympanometry
tympano-ossicular system
tympanoplastic
tympanoplasty
  combined approach t.
  intact canal-wall t.
  t., types 2–5
tympanosclerosis
tympanosclerotic
tympanosis
tympanosquamosal
tympanostapedial
tympanostomy tube
tympanosympathectomy
tympanotemporal
tympanotomy
  posterior t.
  transmeatal t.
tympanous
tympanum
tympany
  bell t.
  Skoda t.
  skodaic t.
  t. of the stomach
Tyndall
  light
  phenomenon
tyndallization
type
  amyostatic-kinetic t.
  asthenic t.
  athletic t.
  Aztec t.
  basic personality t.
  blood t.
  body t.
  buffalo t.
  Charcot-Marie t.
  Charcot-Marie-Tooth t.
  constitutional t.
  cycloid t.
  Dejerine t.
  Dejerine-Landouzy t.
  Duchenne t.
  Duchenne-Aran t.
  Duchenne-Landouzy t.
  Duchenne-t. muscular
    dystrophy
  Duffy blood antibody t.
  dysplastic t.
  Erb-Zimmerlin t.
  Fazio-Londe t.
  Hutchison t.
  Kell blood antibody t.

T

type *(continued)*
    Kidd blood antibody t.
    Kretschmer t's
    Landouzy t.
    Landouzy-Dejerine t.
    leg t.
    Leichtenstern t.
    Levi-Lorain t.
    Leyden-Möbius t.
    Lorain t.
    mating t.
    Nothnagel t.
    personality t.
    phage t.
    Putnam t.
    pyknic t.
    Raymond t. of apoplexy
    Remak t.
    Runeberg t.
    scapulohumeral t.
    schizoid t.
    Schultze t.
    Simmerlin t.
    Strümpell t.
    sympatheticotonic t.
    test t.
    Tooth t.
    Werdnig-Hoffmann t.
    Wernicke-Mann t.
    wild t.
    Zimmerlin t.
type-specific
typhemia
typhinia
typhlectasis
typhlectomy
typhloappendicitis
typhlodicliditis
typhlolexia
typhlology
typhlomegaly
typhlopexy
typhlosis
typhlostomy
typhlotomy
typhloureterostomy
typhobacterin
typhoid
    ambulatory t.
    latent t.
    provocation t.
typhoidal
typhoid-paratyphoid (TPT) vaccine
typhomania
Typhonium trilobatum

typhous
typhus
    Australian tick t.
    benign t.
    canine t.
    chigger-borne t.
    classic t.
    collapsing t.
    endemic t.
    epidemic t.
    epidemic louse-borne t.
    European t.
    exanthematous t.
    flea-borne t.
    Gubler-Robin t.
    Hildenbrand t.
    Indian tick t.
    Kenya tick t.
    latent t.
    louse-borne t.
    Mexican t.
    mite-borne t.
    murine t.
    North Asian tick t.
    North Queensland
      tick t.
    petechial t.
    Queensland tick t.
    rat t.
    recrudescent t.
    rural t.
    São Paulo t.
    scrub t.
    shop t.
    Siberian tick t.
    sporadic t.
    tick t.
    tick-borne t.
    Toulon t.
    tropical t.
    urban t.
typical
typing
    ABO t.
    ABO-Rh t.
    t. of blood
    colicin t.
    HLA t.
    phage t.
    primed lymphocyte
      t. (PLT)
    tissue t.
tyramine oxidase
tyrannism
tyresin

tyrogenous
tyroid
tyromatosis
Tyrophagus
    T. castellani
    T. farinae
    T. longior
tyrosamine
tyrosinase
tyrosine aminotransferase
    t.a. deficiency
    neonatal t.a.
tyrosinemia
    hepatorenal t.
    hereditary t.
    neonatal t.
    type I t.
    type II t.
tyrosinosis
tyrosinuria

tyrosis
tyrosyl
tyrosyluria
tyrothricin
tyrotoxicon
tyrotoxicosis
tyrotoxism
Tyrrell
    fascia
    hook
Tyson
    crypts
    glands
tysonian
tysonitis
tyvelose
Tzanck
    cell
    smear
    test

U

υ—upsilon (Greek letter)
μ—mu (Greek letter; alphabetized as m)
U—
    international unit
    unknown
    upper
    urology
    unit
UA—
    uric acid
    urinalysis
    uterine aspiration
UAP—uterine arterial pressure
uarthritis
UBBC—unsaturated vitamin B_{12}-binding capacity
uberous
uberty
UBF—uterine blood flow
UBI—ultraviolet blood irradiation
ubiquinol
ubiquinol-cytochrome c reductase
ubiquinol dehydrogenase
ubiquinone
ubiquitin

ubiquitous
UC—
    urea clearance
    urethral catheterization
    uterine contraction
U&C—usual and customary
UCD, UChD—usual childhood diseases
UCG—urinary chorionic gonadotropin
Uchida
    operation
    technique
UCP—urinary coproporphyrin
UCS—unconditioned stimulus
UCTS—undifferentiated connective tissue syndrome
UD—urethral discharge
UDCA—ursodeoxycholic acid
UDP—
    uridine diphosphate
    urine drug panel
UDPG—uridine diphosphate-glucose
UDPGA—uridine diphosphoglucuronic acid

UDP-galactose
UDP-galactose 4-epimerase
UDP-glucose
UDP-glucose 6-dehydrogenase
UDP-glucose 4-epimerase
UDP-glucose-hexose-1-phosphate
   uridylyltransferase
UDP-glucose
   pyrophosphorylase
UDP-glucuronate
UDP-glucuronate decarboxylase
UDP-hexose
UDP-iduronate
UDP-*N*-acetylgalactosamine
UDP-*N*-acetylglucosamine
UDP-*N*-acetylglucosamine
   4-epimerase
UDP-*N*-acetylglucosamine-
   lysosomal-enzyme *N*-acetyl
   glucosaminephosphotransferase
UDP-*N*-acetylglucosamine
   pyrophosphorylase
UDP-xylose
Udránszky test
UDS—urine drug screen
UE—upper extremity
UFA—unesterified fatty acid(s)
Uffelmann
   reagent
   test
UG—urogenital
UGI—upper gastrointestinal
UGI
   endoscopy
   series
   study
   tract
UH—upper half
Uhl anomaly
UI—uroporphyrin isomerase
UIBC—unsaturated iron-binding
   capacity
UIF—undegraded insulin factor
UIQ—upper inner quadrant
UK—
   unknown
   urokinase
UL—upper lobe
U&L—upper and lower
ulaganactesis
ulalgia
ulatrophy
   afunctional u.
   atrophic u.
   calcic u.

ulatrophy *(continued)*
   ischemic u.
   traumatic u.
ulcer
   acute vulvar u.
   Aden u.
   Allingham u.
   amebic u.
   amputating u.
   anastomotic u.
   aphthous u.
   arterial u.
   arteriosclerotic u.
   atheromatous u.
   atonic u.
   Bahia u.
   Bairnsdale u.
   Barrett u.
   Bazin u.
   Bouveret-Duguet u.
   burrowing phagedenic u.
   Buruli u.
   Cameron u.
   catarrhal corneal u.
   chancroid u.
   chicle u.
   chiclero u.
   chrome u.
   cold u.
   concealed u.
   contact u.
   contact u. of larynx
   corneal u.
   corneal marginal u.
   creeping u.
   Cruveilhier u.
   Curling u.
   Cushing u.
   Cushing-Rokitansky u.
   cutaneous u.
   decubital u.
   decubitus u.
   dendriform u.
   dendritic u.
   diabetic u.
   Dieulafoy u.
   diphtheritic u.
   duodenal u.
   elusive u.
   endemic u.
   eosinophilic u.
   esophageal u.
   exuberant u.
   factitial u.
   Fenwick-Hunner u.

ulcer *(continued)*
    fissured u.
    fistulous u.
    flask u.
    follicular u.
    frenal u.
    fungous u.
    gastric u.
    gastroduodenal u.
    gastrojejunal u.
    giant peptic u.
    girdle u.
    gouty u.
    gravitational u.
    groin u.
    gummatous u.
    herpetic u.
    Hunner u.
    hyperkeratotic u.
    hypertensive ischemic u.
    hypopyon u.
    hypostatic u.
    indolent u.
    Jacob u.
    jejunal u.
    kissing u's
    Kocher dilatation u.
    Kurunegala u.
    Lipschütz (Lipschuetz) u.
    lupoid u.
    Malabar u.
    Mann-Williamson u.
    marginal u.
    marginal corneal u.
    Marjolin u.
    Meleney chronic
      undermining u.
    Mooren u.
    mycobacterial u.
    mycotic u.
    neurogenic u.
    neurotrophic u.
    NSAID u.
    Parrot u.
    penetrating u.
    penetrating u. of foot
    peptic u.
    perambulating u.
    perforating u.
    perforating u. of foot
    phagedenic u.
    plantar u.
    plantar neurotrophic u.
    pneumococcus u.
    postbulbar u.

ulcer *(continued)*
    post-thrombotic u.
    pressure u.
    pudendal u.
    radiation u.
    ring u.
    rodent u.
    Rokitansky-Cushing u.
    round u.
    Saemisch u.
    scorbutic u.
    sea anemone u.
    secondary jejunal u.
    serpiginous u.
    serpiginous corneal u.
    simple u.
    sloughing u.
    soft u.
    stasis u.
    stercoraceous u.
    stercoral u.
    stoma u.
    stomal u.
    stress u.
    sublingual u.
    submucous u.
    symptomatic u.
    syphilitic u.
    tanner's u.
    Terrien u.
    transparent u. of cornea
    trophic u.
    trophoneurotic u.
    tropical u.
    tropical phagedenic u.
    undermining
      burrowing u.
    varicose u.
    venereal u.
    venous u.
    venous stasis u.
    warty u.
    Yemen u.
    Zambezi u.
ulcera (plural of ulcus)
ulcerate
ulcerated sore throat
ulcerating
    u. adenocarcinoma
    u. atherosclerotic lesion
    u. blister
    congenital u. hemangioma
    u. cutaneous mass
    u. dermatosis
    u. dermonecrosis

U

ulcerating *(continued)*
>   intractable u. enterocolitis of infancy
>   u. leg varicosities
>   u. lesion
>   u. mass
>   u. plaques
>   u. tumor

ulceration
>   aggressive Mooren u.
>   central u.
>   chronic u.
>   colonic u.
>   u. of Daguet
>   ischemic u.
>   ischemic duodenal u.
>   radiation-induced u.
>   tracheal u.
>   venous u.
>   widespread u.

ulcerative
>   acute necrotizing u. gingivitis
>   u. cellulitis
>   u. colitis
>   u. dermatosis
>   u. endocarditis
>   u. inflammation
>   u. keratitis
>   u. lichen planus
>   u. lymphangitis
>   u. mutilating acropathy
>   necrotizing u. gingivoperiodontitis
>   necrotizing u. gingivostomatitis
>   u. nodular lesion
>   nonhealing u. nodule
>   u. pharyngitis
>   u. process
>   u. proctitis
>   u. stomatitis
>   u. vulvitis
>   u. wound

ulcerocavernous
ulcerogangrenous
ulcerogenic
ulceroglandular
ulcerogranuloma
ulceromembranous
ulcerous

ulcus (ulcera)
>   u. ambulans
>   u. corneae serpens
>   u. interdigitale

ulcus (ulcera) *(continued)*
>   u. serpens corneae
>   u. vulvae acutum

ulectomy
ulegyria
ulerythema ophryogenes
uliginous
Ullmann line
Ulloa operation
Ullrich
>   retractor
>   syndrome

Ullrich-Feichtiger syndrome
Ullrich-Turner syndrome
ULN—upper limit of normal
ulna
ulnad
ulnar
>   u. artery
>   u. bone
>   u. canal
>   u. clubhand
>   u. collateral artery
>   u. condyle of humerus
>   u. crest
>   u. deviation
>   u. deviation splint
>   u. drift
>   u. drift deformity
>   u. eminence of wrist
>   u. fossa
>   u. groove
>   u. hemimelia
>   u. ligament
>   u. malleolus
>   u. nerve
>   u. notch
>   u. palsy
>   u. reflex
>   u. ridge of wrist
>   u. tunnel syndrome
>   u. veins

ulnare
ulnaris
ulnen
ulnocarpal
ulnoradial
ulotomy
ulotripsis
ULQ—upper left quadrant
ultimate
ultimisternal
ultimobranchial
ultimum moriens
ultrabrachycephalic

ultracentrifugation
ultracentrifuge
ultradian
ultradolichocephalic
ultrafilter
ultrafiltrate
ultrafiltration
    sequential u.-hemodialysis
ultraligation
ultramicrochemistry
ultramicropipet
ultramicroscope
ultramicroscopic
ultramicroscopy
ultramicrotome
ultrapasteurization
ultrasonic
    u. cardiography
    u. labyrinthectomy
    u. microscope
    u. tomography
ultrasonics
ultrasonogram
    B scan u.
    renal u.
ultrasonograph
ultrasonographic
ultrasonography
    A-mode u.
    B-mode u.
    continuous wave Doppler u.
    Doppler u.
    duplex u.
    endorectal u.
    endoscopic u.
    gray-scale u.
    intravascular u.
    pulsed-wave Doppler u.
    real-time u.
    transcranial Doppler u.
    transrectal u.
ultrasonometry
ultrasound
    u. diathermy
    u. dilution technique
    Doppler u.
    u. Doppler flowmeter
    real-time u.
    u. transducer
ultrastructure
UltraTag RBC
ultraviolet
    u. A (UVA)
    u. B (UVB)
    u. C (UVC)

ultraviolet *(continued)*
    far u.
    u. microscope
    near u.
ultravisible
Ultravist
ultromotivity
Ultzmann test
ululation
UM—uracil mustard
umbauzonen
umbelliferone
umbelliferous
umber
Umber test
umbilical
    u. artery
    u. canal
    u. catheter
    u. circulation
    u. cord
    u. cyst
    u. diphtheria
    u. duct
    u. eventration
    u. fascia
    u. fissure
    u. fistula
    u. fold
    u. fossa of liver
    u. granuloma
    u. hernia
    u. ligament
    u. notch
    u. plane
    u. portography
    u. region
    u. ring
    u. scissors
    u. souffle
    u. vein
    u. vein graft
    u. vesicle
umbilicate
umbilicated
umbilication
umbilicoplasty
umbilicus
    amniotic u.
    decidual u.
    posterior u.
umbo (umbones)
    u. membranae tympani
    u. membranae tympanicae
    u. of tympanic membrane

U

umbonate
umbones
umbra
umbrascopy
umbrella
    Mobin-Uddin u.
UMP—uridine monophosphate
UMP synthase deficiency
UN—urea nitrogen
unabsorbable, nonabsorbable
    n. surgical suture
unarousable
unazotized
unbalance
unbeknownst
uncal
uncarthrosis
unci (genitive and plural of uncus)
unciform
unciforme
uncinal
uncinate
    u. epilepsy
    u. gyrus
    u. process
    u. seizure
uncinatum
uncipressure
uncompensated
uncomplemented
unconditioned
unconscious
unconsciousness
unco-ossified
uncotomy
uncoupling
uncovertebral
uncrossed
unction
unctuous
uncus (unci)
    u. corporis vertebrae cervicalis
    u. gyri fornicati
    u. gyri hippocampi
    u. gyri parahippocampalis
    u. of hamate bone
undecenoic acid
undecylenic acid
underachiever
underbite
undercut
underdrive
underhorn
underlay myringoplasty
undernutrition

undersensing
understain
undertoe
underwater seal drainage
    system
underweight
Underwood disease
undescended testis
undifferentiated
    acute u. leukemia
    u. carcinoma of the thyroid
      gland
    u. cell leukemia
    u. lymphoma
    u. schizophrenia
    u. somatoform disorder
undifferentiation
undine
undinism
undoing
Undritz anomaly
undulant fever
undulate
undulating membrane
undulation
    jugular u.
    respiratory u.
unengaged
ungual
    u. phalanx
    u. process
    u. tuberosity
unguent
unguenti (genitive of unguentum)
unguentum (unguenta)
unguiculate
unguiculus
unguis (ungues)
    u. incarnatus
    u. ventriculi lateralis
      cerebri
ungula
ungulate
unguligrade
uniarticular
uniarticulate
uniaural
uniaxial
unibasal
unicalyceal
unicameral
unicellular
unicentral
uniceps
unicollis

unicornous
unicornuate
unicuspid
unicuspidate
unidirectional
unifascicular
unifocal
uniforate
Uniform Anatomical Gift Act
unigeminal
unigerminal
uniglandular
unigravida
unilaminar
unilateral
    u. anesthesia
    u. emphysema
    u. gliosis
    u. hemianopia
    u. hermaphroditism
    u. hyperhidrosis
    u. hypertrophy
    u. neglect
    u. nevoid telangiectasia
      syndrome
    u. nystagmus
    u. partial denture
    u. strabismus
unilobar
unilocular
unimodal
uninephrectomy
uninephric
uninhibited neurogenic bladder
uninterrupted suture
uninuclear
uninucleated
uniocular
union
    faulty u.
    immediate u.
    primary u.
    syngamic nuclear u.
    vicious u.
uniovular
unipara
uniparental
uniparous
unipennate
unipolar
    augmented u. limb lead
    u. depression
    u. disorder
    u. lead
    u. limb lead

unipolar *(continued)*
    u. neuron
    u. pacemaker
    u. pacing
    u. precordial leads
    u. spongioblastoma
uniport
uniporter
unipotency
unipotent
unipotential
unirritable
uniseptate
unisexual
unit
    absolute u.
    alcohol and drug dependency
      u. (ADDU)
    Allen-Doisy u.
    amboceptor u.
    American Drug Manufacturers
      Association u.
    androgen u.
    Angström u.
    Ansbacher u.
    antigen u.
    antitoxic u.
    antivenene u.
    atomic mass u. (amu.)
    atomic weight u.
    base u.
    Bethesda u.
    Bodansky u.
    Bovie u.
    British thermal u. (BTU)
    burn u.
    cardiac care u. (CCU)
    cardiology intensive care u.
      (CICU)
    C. G. S. (centimeter-gram-
      second) u.
    CH_{50} [CH50] u.
    clinical u.
    cobalt 60 beam therapy u.
    coherent u.
    coincidence u.
    Collip u.
    colony-forming u. (CFU)
    colony-forming u.–culture
      (CFU-C)
    colony-forming u.–erythroid
      (CFU-E)
    colony-forming u.–
      granulocyte-macrophage
      (CFU-GM)

U

unit *(continued)*

- colony-forming u.–spleen (CFU-S)
- complement u.
- u. of convergence
- Corner-Allen u.
- coronary care u. (CCU)
- coronary intensive care u. (CICU)
- corpus luteum hormone u.
- critical care u. (CCU)
- crossover u.
- dental u.
- derived u.
- detoxification (detox) u.
- digitalis u.
- electromagnetic u's
- u. of energy
- enzyme u.
- estrone u.
- Felton u.
- flotation u.
- u. of force
- Gutman u.
- Hampson u.
- u. of heat
- hemolytic u.
- Hertz (Hz) u.
- Hounsfield (H) u.
- insulin u.
- intensive care u. (ICU)
- intensive coronary care u. (ICCU)
- u. of intermedin
- international u. (IU)
- international androgen u.
- international u. of enzyme activity
- international u. of estrogenic activity
- international estrone u.
- international u. of gonadotrophic activity
- international u. of immunological activity
- international insulin u.
- international u. of luteinizing activity
- international u. of male hormone
- international u. of penicillin
- international u. of progestational activity
- international progesterone u.
- international prolactin u.

unit *(continued)*

- international u. of vitamin A
- international u. of vitamin D
- Karmen u.
- Kienböck u. (X)
- King u.
- King-Armstrong u.
- Lf (limes flocculating) u. (LfU)
- lung u.
- Mache u.
- map u.
- medical intensive care u. (MICU)
- minimal hemolytic u.
- Mira u.
- Montevideo u's
- morgan u. (M)
- motor u.
- mouse u.
- muscle u.
- neonatal intensive care u. (NICU)
- nerve u.
- neurological intensive care u. (NICU)
- Noon pollen u.
- u. of oxytocin
- parathyroid u.
- u. of penicillin
- pepsin u.
- peripheral resistance u. (PRU)
- pilosebaceous u.
- plaque-forming u.
- postanesthesia care u (PACU)
- progesterone u.
- prolactin u.
- psychiatric u.
- pulmonary intensive care u. (PICU)
- quantum u.
- rat u.
- respiratory care u. (RCU)
- Russell u.
- sensation u.
- Shinowara-Jones-Reinhard u.
- SI (Système International) u.
- Siegbahn u.
- skin test u.
- slow-motor u.
- Somogyi u.
- special care u. (SCU)
- specific smell u.
- Steenbock u. of vitamin D
- sudanophobic u.
- supplementary u.

unit *(continued)*
    surgical intensive care u.
      (SICU)
    Svedberg flotation u.
    terminal airway u.
    terminal respiratory u.
    Thayer-Doisy u.
    u. of thyrotrophic activity
    Todd u.
    toxic u.
    toxin u.
    tuberculin u. (TU)
    turbidity-reducing u. (TRU)
    unified atomic mass u.
    USP (United States
      Pharmacopeia) u.
    u. of vasopressin
    vitamin A u.
    u. of vitamin B_1 [B1]
    vitamin D u.
    Voegtlin u.
    Wohlegemuth u.
    u. of work
    x-ray u.
unitage
unitary
United States Adopted Names
  (USAN) Council
United States Pharmacopeia
  (USP)
uniterminal
unitless
univalence
univalent
univariate
univitelline
unmedullated
unmyelinated
Unna
    alkaline methylene blue
    boot
    cell
    dermatosis
    disease
    extractor
    nevus
    paste
    paste boot
    syndrome
Unna-Pappenheim stain
Unna-Thost
    disease
    syndrome
unnecessary
unofficial

unorganized
unphysiologic
unprimed
unresponsive
unrest
    peristaltic u.
unsaturated compounds
Unschuld sign
unstriated
untenable
untoward effects
Unverricht
    disease
    myoclonia
    syndrome
Unverricht-Lundborg type of
  epilepsy
unvoiced
UOQ—upper outer quadrant
UP—
    upright posture
    ureteropelvic
U/P—urine-plasma ratio
UPG—uroporphyrinogen
up-gaze
UPI—uteroplacental
  insufficiency
UPJ—ureteropelvic junction
UPOR—usual place of residence
UPP—urethral pressure profile
UPP, UPPP—
  uvulopalatopharyngoplasty
upper GI series
upregulation
uprighting
upsiloid
upsilon—Greek letter
  (υ; alphabetized as u)
upstream
uptake
    absolute iodine u. (AIU)
    iodine-131 u.
    radioactive iodine u.
    RAI (radioactive iodine) u.
    resin u.
UR—
    unconditioned response
    upper respiratory
    utilization review
urachal
    u. adenocarcinoma
    u. cyst
    u. diverticulum
    u. fistula
    u. fold

U

urachal *(continued)*
    u. fossa
    u. sinus
urachovesical
urachus
    patent u.
uracrasia
uracratia
uraniscus
uranium (U)
uranoplastic
uranoplasty
uranoplegia
uranorrhaphy
uranoschisis
uranostaphyloplasty
uranostaphylorrhaphy
uranostaphyloschisis
uranyl
urarthritis
urate
uratemia
urate oxidase
uratic
uratohistechia
uratoma
uratosis
uraturia
Urbach-Oppenheim disease
Urbach-Wiethe disease
urceiform
urceolate
URD—upper respiratory disease
urea
    blood u. nitrogen (BUN)
    u. nitrogen (UN)
    plasma u.
    sterile u.
    u. stibamine
ureagenetic
ureal
ureaplasma
Ureaplasma
    U. parvum
    U. urealyticum
ureapoiesis
urease
urechitin
urechitoxin
uredema
ureic
ureide
uremia
    azotemic u.
    extrarenal u.

uremia *(continued)*
    prerenal u.
    puerperal u.
    retention u.
uremic medullary cystic disease
uremigenic
ureolysis
ureolytic
ureotelic
uresis
ureter
    aberrant u.
    circumcaval u.
    double u.
    ectopic u.
    postcaval u.
    retrocaval u.
    retroiliac u.
ureteral
    u. catheter
    u. colic
    u. duplication
    u. electromyography
    u. jet
    u. meatoscopy
    u. meatus
    u. neocystostomy
    u. neuromuscular dysplasia
    u. reduplication
    u. reflux
    u. reimplantation
    u. stent
    u. valve
ureteralgia
ureterectasia
ureterectasis
ureterectomy
ureteric ridge
ureteritis
    u. cystica
    u. glandularis
ureteroarterial
ureterocele
    ectopic u.
ureterocelectomy
ureterocervical
ureterocolonic
ureterocolostomy
ureterocutaneostomy
ureterocutaneous
ureterocystanastomosis
ureterocystoneostomy
ureterocystoscope
ureterocystostomy
ureteroduodenal

ureteroenteric
ureteroenteroanastomosis
ureteroenterostomy
ureterogram
ureterography
ureterohydronephrosis
ureteroileal neocystostomy
ureteroileostomy
ureterointestinal
ureterolith
ureterolithiasis
ureterolithotomy
ureterolysis
ureteromeatotomy
ureteroneocystostomy
ureteroneopyelostomy
ureteronephrectomy
ureteronephroscopy
ureteropathy
ureteropelvic
ureteropelvioneostomy
ureteropelvioplasty
    Culp u.
    Culp-DeWeerd u.
    Foley u.
    Foley Y-type u.
    Foley Y-V u.
    Scardino u.
    Scardino-Prince u.
ureteroplasty
ureteroproctostomy
ureteropyelitis
ureteropyelography
ureteropyeloneostomy
ureteropyelonephrostomy
ureteropyeloplasty
ureteropyelostomy
ureteropyosis
ureterorectal
ureterorectoneostomy
ureterorectostomy
ureterorenoscope
ureterorenoscopy
ureterorrhagia
ureterorrhaphy
ureteroscope
ureteroscopy
ureterosigmoidostomy
ureterostenosis
ureterostoma
ureterostomy
    cutaneous u.
ureterotomy
ureteroureteral
ureteroureterostomy

ureterouterine
ureterovaginal
ureterovascular
ureterovesical
ureterovesicoplasty
    Leadbetter-Politano u.
ureterovesicostomy
urethra
    anterior u.
    cavernous u.
    double u.
    female u.
    u. feminina
    imperforate u.
    male u.
    u. masculina
    membranous u.
    u. muliebris
    penile u.
    posterior u.
    primary u.
    prostatic u.
    spongy u.
    u. virilis
urethral
    u. artery
    u. atresia
    u. calculus
    u. caruncle
    u. catheter
    u. crest
    u. diverticulum
    u. duplication
    u. fever
    u. folds
    u. glands
    u. groove
    u. hematuria
    u. lacunae
    u. meatus
    u. plate
    u. pressure
    u. pressure profilometry
    prostatic u. polyps
    u. ridge
    u. sound
    u. speculum
    u. sphincter
    u. syndrome
    u. valve
urethralgia
urethratresia
urethrectomy
urethremphraxis
urethrism

U

urethritis
   atrophic u.
   u. cystica
   u. glandularis
   gonococcal u.
   gonorrheal u.
   gouty u.
   u. granulosa
   nongonococcal u.
   nonspecific u.
   u. orificii externi
   u. petrificans
   polypoid u.
   prophylactic u.
   senile u.
   simple u.
   specific u.
   u. venerea
urethroanal
urethrobulbar
urethrocele
urethrocystitis
urethrocystocele
urethrocystogram
urethrocystography
urethrocystometry
urethrocystopexy
urethrocystoscopy
urethrodynia
urethrogram
   excretory u.
urethrograph
urethrography
urethroileal
urethrometer
urethrometry
urethropenile
urethroperineal
urethroperineoscrotal
urethropexy
   Lapides u.
urethroplasty
   Thiersch-Duplay u.
   Turner-Warwick u.
urethroprostatic
urethrorectal
urethrorrhagia
urethrorrhaphy
urethrorrhea
urethroscope
urethroscopic
urethroscopy
urethroscrotal
urethrospasm
urethrostaxis

urethrostenosis
urethrostomy
urethrotome
   dilating u.
   Maisonneuve u.
   Otis u.
urethrotomy
   external u.
   internal u.
urethrotrigonitis
urethrovaginal
urethrovesical
   u. angle
   u. suspension
uretic
URF—unidentified reading frame
urgency
urhidrosis crystallina
URI—upper respiratory infection
urian
uric acid
uricacidemia
uricaciduria
uricase
uricemia
uricocholia
uricolysis
uricolytic
uricometer
   Ruhemann u.
uricopoiesis
uricosuria
uricosuric
uricotelic
uricotelism
Uricult
uridine
   u. diphosphate
   acetylgalactosamine
   u. diphosphate
   acetylglucosamine
   u. diphosphate galactose
   u. diphosphate glucose
   u. diphosphate (UDP)
   u. diphosphogalactose-4-
   epimerase
   u. diphosphoglucose
   u. diphosphoglucose
   dehydrogenase
   u. diphosphoglucuronate
   u. monophosphate (UMP)
   u. 5´-phosphate
   u. triphosphate (UTP)
uridrosis
uridylate

uridylic acid
uridyl transferase
uridylyl
urinacidometer
urinal
    condom u.
urinalysis
urinary
    u. abscess
    u. anion gap
    u. bladder
    u. calculus
    u. cast
    u. continence
    continent u. diversion
    continent u. reservoir
    u. cylinder
    u. cyst
    u. diversion
    u. fistula
    u. frequency
    u. incontinence
    internal u. meatus
    u. lithiasis
    u. meatus
    u. output
    u. reflex
    u. retention
    u. schistosomiasis
    u. sediment
    u. siderosis
    u. sodium
    u. space
    u. sphincter
    u. stasis
    u. stuttering
    u. tract
    u. tract infection
    u. urgency
    u. voiding
urinate
urination
    precipitant u.
    stuttering u.
urine
    Bence Jones u.
    black u.
    chylous u.
    clean-catch u. specimen
    cloudy u.
    crude u.
    u. cytology
    diabetic u.
    u. drug panel (UDP)
    u. drug screen (UDS)

urine *(continued)*
    febrile u.
    gouty u.
    milky u.
    nebulous u.
    residual u.
    straw-colored u.
    voided u.
urine urea nitrogen (UUN)
urinidrosis
uriniferous
urinocryoscopy
urinogenital
urinogenous
urinoglucosometer
urinoma
urinometry
urinophilous
urinosexual
urinothorax
urinous
uriposia
urishiol
uroacidimeter
uroammoniac
uroanthelone
urobenzoic acid
urobilin
urobilinemia
urobilinogen
urobilinogenemia
urobilinogenuria
urobilinoid
urobilinuria
urocanase deficiency
urocanate hydratase
urocanic acid
urocele
urochezia
urochordate
urochrome
urochromogen
uroclepsia
urocystitis
urodialysis
urodilatin
urodynamic
urodynamics
urodynia
urodysfunction
uroedema
uroenterone
uroerythrin
uroflavin
urofollitropin

U

urofuscin
urofuscohematin
urogenital
    u. diaphragm
    u. ridge
    u. sinus
    u. trigone
urogenous
urogram
urography
    ascending u.
    cystoscopic u.
    descending u.
    drip infusion u.
    excretion u.
    excretory u.
    intravenous u. (IVU)
    magnetic resonance u.
    oral u.
    percutaneous
      antegrade u.
    retrograde u.
urogravimeter
urogynecology
urohematin
urohematoporphyrin
urokinase
urolagnia
urolith
urolithiasis
urolithic
urolithotomy
urologic, urological
urologist
urology
uromancy
uromelanin
uromelus
urometric
urometry
uronate
uronephrosis
uronic acid
uropathogen
uropathy
    obstructive u.
uropepsinogen
urophanic
urophein
urophilia
urophobia
urophosphometer
uropod
uropoiesis
uropoietic

uroporphyria
    erythropoietic u.
uroporphyrin
uroporphyrinogen
    u. decarboxylase
    u. I synthase
    u. III synthase
uroprotection
uroprotective
uropsammus
uropterin
uroradiology
urosaccharometry
uroschesis
uroscopic
uroscopy
urosemiology
urosepsis
uroseptic
urospectrin
urostalagmometry
urothelial
urothelium
urotoxic
urotoxicity
urotoxin
uroxin
URQ—upper right quadrant
ursodeoxycholate
ursodeoxycholic acid
ursodeoxycholylglycine
ursodeoxycholyltaurine
ursodiol
URTI—upper respiratory tract
    infection
Urtica dioica
urticant
urticaria
    acute u.
    aquagenic u.
    u. bullosa
    bullous u.
    cholinergic u.
    chronic u.
    cold u.
    contact u.
    endemic u.
    u. endemica
    u. epidemica
    u. factitia
    factitious u.
    u. febrilis
    giant u.
    u. gigantea
    heat u.

urticaria *(continued)*
    hemorrhagic u.
    u. hemorrhagica
    heredofamilial u.
    light u.
    u. maritima
    u. medicamentosa
    Milton u.
    u. multiformis endemica
    papular u.
    u. papulosa
    u. perstans
    u. petechialis
    u. photogenica
    physical u.
    u. pigmentosa
    pressure u.
    solar u.
    u. solaris
    u. subcutanea
    subcutaneous u.
urticarial
urticariogenic
urticarious
urticate
urtication
urushiol
US—
    ultrasonic
    ultrasonography
    ultrasound
USAN—United States Adopted
  Names
USDA—United States Department
  of Agriculture
U-shaped incision
Usher
    disease
    syndrome
USN—ultrasonic nebulizer
usnein
usnic acid
USO—unilateral salpingo-
  oophorectomy
USP—United States Pharmacopeia
USPHS—United States Public
  Health Service
USR—unheated serum reagin
ustilaginism
Ustilago
    U. maydis
    U. zeae
ustion
ustulation
uta

UTBG—unbound
  thyroxine–binding globulin
uteralgia
uteri (plural of uterus)
uterine
    u. appendages
    u. artery
    u. calculus
    u. canal
    u. cavity
    u. colic
    u. contractions
    u. corpus carcinoma
    u. cycle
    u. dehiscence
    dysfunctional u. bleeding
      (DUB)
    u. dysmenorrhea
    u. forceps
    u. glands
    u. hernia
    u. insufficiency
    u. leiomyoma
    u. luteolysin
    u. milk
    u. myoma
    u. myomectomy
    u. neck
    u. orifice of uterine tube
    u. peristalsis
    u. placenta
    u. plexus
    u. probe
    u. prolapse
    u. segment
    u. sinuses
    u. souffle
    u. sound
    u. stimulant
    u. tube
    u. tympanites
    u. veins
    u. venography
    u. venous plexus
uteroabdominal
uterocervical
uterodynia
uterofixation
uterogenic
uterogestation
uteroglobulin
uterography
uterolith
uterometer
uterometry

U

utero-ovarian
uteropelvic
uteropelvioplasty
    Scardino u.
uteropexy
uteroplacental
    u. insufficiency
    u. ischemia
uteroplasty
uterorectal
uterosacral
    u. block
    u. ligaments
uterosalpingogram
uterosalpingography
uterosclerosis
uteroscope
uterothermometry
uterotomy
uterotonic
uterotropic
uterotubal
uterovaginal
uteroventral
uterovesical
uterus (uteri)
    arcuate u.
    u. arcuatus
    u. bicornis
    u. bicornis bicollis
    u. bicornis unicollis
    bicornuate u.
    bifid u.
    u. biforis
    u. bilocularis
    bipartite u.
    u. bipartitus
    boggy u.
    bosselated u.
    capped u.
    cochleate u.
    u. cordiformis
    Couvelaire u.
    u. didelphys
    double-mouthed u.
    duplex u., u. duplex
    embryonic u.
    fetal u.
    fibroid u.
    fibromyomata uteri
    gravid u.
    u. incudiformis
    infantile u.
    masculine u.
    u. masculinus

uterus (uteri) *(continued)*
    ovoid u.
    u. parvicollis
    Piskacek u.
    u. planifundalis
    pubescent u.
    ribbon u.
    u. rudimentarius
    sacculated u.
    saddle-shaped u.
    scarred u.
    septate u.
    u. septus
    u. simplex
    subseptate u.
    u. subseptus
    u. triangularis
    u. unicornis
    unicornuate u.
    unscarred u.
UTI—urinary tract infection
utilization
    red cell u. (RCU)
    u. review (UR)
UTP—uridine triphosphate
UTP–glucose-1-phosphate
   uridylyltransferase
UTP–hexose-1-phosphate
   uridylyltransferase
utricle
    prostatic u.
    urethral u.
utricular
utriculitis
utriculosaccular
utriculus (utriculi)
    u. masculinus
    u. prostaticus
    u. vestibuli
utriform
utrophin
U-tube
UU—urine urobilinogen
UUN—urine urea nitrogen
UV—
    ultraviolet
    umbilical vein
    ureterovesical
    urethrovesical
    urine volume
uva (uvae)
    u. ursi
UVA—
    ultraviolet A
    urethrovesical angle

UVB—ultraviolet B
UVC—ultraviolet C
uvea
uveal
uveitic
uveitis
    anterior u.
    Förster u.
    granulomatous u.
    heterochromic u.
    lens-induced u.
    nongranulomatous u.
    phacoanaphylactic u.
    phacoantigenic u.
    phacotoxic u.
    posterior u.
    sympathetic u.
    toxoplasmic u.
    tuberculous u.
uveomeningitis
uveoparotid
uveoscleritis
uviform
U virus—Uppsala virus
UVJ—
    ureterovesical junction
    urethrovesical junction

UVL—ultraviolet light
UVP—uterine venous pressure
uvula (uvulae)
    bifid u.
    u. of bladder
    u. cerebelli
    u. of cerebellum
    cleft u.
    u. fissura
    forked u.
    Lieutaud u.
    u. palatina
    palatine u.
    split u.
    u. vermis
    u. vesicae
    u. vesicae urinariae
uvular
uvularis
uvulectomy
uvulitis
uvulopalatopharyngoplasty
    (UPPP)
uvulopalatoplasty (UPP)
uvuloptosis
uvulotome
uvulotomy

V

v—nu (Greek letter;
    alphabetized as n)
v.—vein (L. vena)
V—
    vein
    velocity
    vision
    visual acuity
    volt(s)
    volume
V.—Vibrio
Va—visual acuity
V_a—arterial ventilation
V_A—alveolar
    ventilation
VA—
    vacuum aspiration
    ventriculoatrial
    vertebral artery

VA, V.A.—
    Veterans Administration
    Veterans Affairs
vaccenic acid
vaccinal
vaccinate
vaccination
    booster v.
    smallpox v.
vaccinator
vaccinatum
    eczema v.
vaccine
    acellular v.
    adjuvant v.
    adsorbed diphtheria and
      tetanus toxoids and
      pertussis v.
    anthrax v. adsorbed

vaccine *(continued)*
- anthrax spore v.
- antirabies v.
- attenuated v.
- attenuated live v.
- attenuated viral v.
- attenuated virus v.
- autogenous v.
- bacterial v.
- BCG (bacille Calmette-Guérin) v.
- Calmette v.
- cholera v.
- conjugate v.
- diphtheria and tetanus toxoids and pertussis vaccine adsorbed and Haemophilus b conjugate v.
- DTaP (diphtheria and tetanus toxoids and acellular pertussis) v.
- DPT (diphtheria, pertussis and tetanus toxoids) v.
- DTP (diphtheria, tetanus toxoids and pertussis) v.
- *Haemophilus* b (HIB) conjugate v.
- *Haemophilus* b (HIB) polysaccharide v.
- hepatitis A v. inactivated
- hepatitis B v. inactivated
- hepatitis B v. (recombinant)
- heptavalent pneumococcal conjugate v.
- heterologous v.
- heterotypic v.
- human diploid cell v.
- influenza virus v.
- Japanese encephalitis virus v.
- live v.
- Lyme disease v. (recombinant OspA)
- measles, mumps, rubella and varicella virus v. live
- measles, mumps, and rubella virus (MMR) v. live
- measles and rubella virus v. live
- measles virus v. live
- meningococcal conjugate v.
- meningococcal polysaccharide v.
- mixed v.
- MMR (measles, mumps, and rubella) v.

vaccine *(continued)*
- modified live viral v.
- modified live virus v.
- monovalent v.
- multivalent v.
- mumps virus v. live
- PCEC (purified chick embryo cell) v.
- pertussis v.
- pertussis v., acellular
- plague v.
- pneumococcal heptavalent conjugate v.
- pneumococcal v. polyvalent
- poliomyelitis v.
- poliovirus v. inactivated (IPV)
- poliovirus v. live oral (OPV)
- poliovirus v. live oral trivalent (TOPV)
- polyvalent v.
- purified chick embryo cell (PCEC) v.
- quadrivalent human papillomavirus (HPV) recombinant v.
- rabies v.
- rabies v. adsorbed
- replicative v.
- rotavirus v. live oral
- rubella and mumps virus v. live
- rubella virus v. live
- Sabin v.
- Salk v.
- 7-valent pneumococcal conjugate v.
- smallpox v.
- split-virus v.
- streptococcus v.
- streptococcus group E v.
- subunit v.
- subvirion v.
- Tdap (diphtheria and reduced tetanus toxoids and acellular pertussis) v.
- tetanus v.
- triple v.
- trivalent v.
- tuberculosis v.
- tularemia v.
- typhoid v.
- typhoid v. live oral
- typhoid Vi polysaccharide v.
- varicella virus v. live
- whooping cough v.
- yellow fever v.

vaccinia
  fetal v.
  generalized v.
  v. immune globulin
  v. necrosum
  progressive v.
vaccinial
vacciniform
vaccinogen
vaccinogenous
vaccinostyle
vaccinotherapy
vacillate
VACTERL (vertebral, anal, cardiac, tracheal, esophageal, renal, and limb) association
vacuolar
  v. membrane
  v. myelopathy
vacuolate
vacuolated
vacuolation
vacuole
  autophagic v.
  condensing v's
  contractile v.
  digestive v.
  food v.
vacuome
vacuum
  v. drainage system
  v. extraction operation
  high v.
  torricellian v.
  v. tube
vacuuming
VAD—ventricular assist device
vadum
vagabond's disease
vagal
vagectomy
vagi (plural of vagus)
vagina (vaginae)
  v. bulbi
  v. carotica fasciae cervicalis
  v. communis musculorum flexorum
  v. communis tendinum musculorum fibularium
  v. communis tendinum musculorum peroneorum
  v. externa nervi optici
  v. femoris
  v. fibrosa

vagina (vaginae) *(continued)*
  vaginae fibrosae digitorum manus
  vaginae fibrosae digitorum pedis
  v. fibrosa tendinis
  v. interna nervi optici
  v. masculina
  v. mucosa
  v. mucosa tendinis
  v. musculi recti abdominis
  vaginae nervi optici
  v. oculi
  v. plantaris tendinis musculi fibularis longi
  v. plantaris tendinis musculi peronei longi
  v. processus styloidei
  vaginae synoviales digitorum manus
  vaginae synoviales digitorum pedis
  vaginae synoviales tendinum digitorum manus
  vaginae synoviales tendinum digitorum pedis
  v. synovialis
  v. synovialis communis musculorum flexorum
  v. synovialis intertubercularis
  v. synovialis musculi obliqui superioris
  v. synovialis musculorum peroneorum communis
  v. synovialis tendinis
  v. synovialis tendinis musculi flexoris carpi radialis
  v. synovialis tendinis musculi flexoris hallucis longi
  v. synovialis tendinis musculi tibialis posterioris
  v. tendinis
  v. tendinis musculi extensoris carpi ulnaris
  v. tendinis musculi extensoris digiti minimi
  v. tendinis musculi extensoris hallucis longi
  v. tendinis musculi extensoris pollicis longi
  v. tendinis musculi fibularis longi plantaris
  v. tendinis musculi flexoris carpi radialis

V

vagina (vaginae) *(continued)*
v. tendinis musculi flexoris hallucis longi
v. tendinis musculi flexoris pollicis longi
v. tendinis musculi obliqui superioris
v. tendinis musculi tibialis anterioris
v. tendinis musculi tibialis posterioris
vaginae tendinum digitorum manus
vaginae tendinum digitorum pedis
v. tendinum musculorum abductoris longi et extensoris brevis pollicis
v. tendinum musculorum extensoris digitorum communis et extensoris indicis
v. tendinum musculorum extensoris digitorum et extensoris indicis
v. tendinum musculorum extensorum carpi radialium
v. vasorum
vaginal
v. artery
v. bulb
v. candidiasis
v. celiotomy
v. coat of testis
v. columns
v. cuff
v. delivery
v. diaphragm
Doyen v. hysterectomy
v. folds
v. gland
Heaney v. hysterectomy
v. hernia
v. hysterectomy (VH)
v. hysterotomy
v. intraepithelial neoplasia (VIN)
v. introitus
laparoscopic-assisted v. hysteroscopy (LAVH)
v. laparotomy
v. ligaments of fingers
v. ligaments of toes
v. lithotomy

vaginal *(continued)*
Mayo-Ward v. hysterectomy
v. myomectomy
v. nerves
v. orifice
v. ovariotomy
v. plate
v. plexus
v. plug
posterior v. hernia
v. prolapse
Schauta-Amreich v. hysterectomy
Schauta radical v. hysterectomy
v. septum
v. speculum
v. synovitis
total v. hysterectomy (TVH)
v. trichomoniasis
v. vault
v. wall sling
vaginalis
processus v.
Trichomonas v.
vaginalitis
plastic v.
vaginapexy
vaginate
vaginectomy
vaginiperineotomy
vaginismus
perineal v.
posterior v.
superficial v.
vulvar v.
vaginitis
v. adhaesiva
adhesive v.
atrophic v.
Candida v.
candidal v.
desquamative inflammatory v.
v. emphysematosa
emphysematous v.
granular v.
monilial v.
senile v.
v. testis
Trichomonas v.
vaginoabdominal
vaginocele
vaginocervical
vaginocutaneous

vaginodynia
vaginofixation
vaginogram
vaginography
vaginolabial
vaginomycosis
vaginopathy
vaginoperineal
vaginoperineoplasty
vaginoperineorrhaphy
vaginoperineotomy
vaginoperitoneal
vaginopexy
vaginoplasty
vaginoscope
vaginoscopy
vaginosis
    bacterial v.
vaginotomy
vaginovesical
vaginovulvar
vagitus
    v. uterinus
    v. vaginalis
vagoaccessorius
vagoglossopharyngeal
vagogram
vagolysis
vagolytic
vagomimetic
vagosplanchnic
vagosympathetic
vagotomy
    bilateral v.
    hemigastrectomy and v.
      (H&V)
    highly selective v.
    medical v.
    parietal cell v.
    posterior truncal v.
    pyloroplasty and v. (P&V)
    selective v.
    surgical v.
    truncal v.
vagotonia
vagotonic
vagotony
vagotropic
vagovagal
vagrant
vagus
Vail neuralgia
VALE—visual acuity, left eye
valence
valency

Valentin
    corpuscles
    ganglion
    nerve
    pseudoganglion
Valentine
    position
    splint
    tube
valerian
valeric acid
valetudinarian
valetudinarianism
valgus
    v. correction
    cubitus v.
    v. deformity
    v. extension overload
      syndrome
    v. femoral osteotomy
    hallux abducto v.
    hallux v. angle
    hallux v. deformity
    hallux v. et rigidus
    high tibial v. osteotomy
    v. knee
    v. laxity
    v. load
    v. osteotomy
    v. positioning
    v. rotation
    v. torque
    v. stress
    v. stress test
    varus-v. motion
validation
    consensual v.
validity
    face v.
valinemia
valine transaminase
vallate
vallecula (valleculae)
    v. cerebelli
    v. of cerebellum
    epiglottic v.
    v. epiglottica
    v. sylvii
vallecular
Valleix
    points
    sign
valley of cerebellum
vallicepobufagin
Valli-Ritter law

V

vallum (valla)
    v. unguis
valnoctamide
valproic acid
Valsalva
    experiment
    ligaments
    maneuver
    method
    procedure
    sinus
    test
    zone
value
    normal v's
    reference v's
    survival v.
valva (valvae)
    v. aortae
    v. atrioventricularis dextra
    v. atrioventricularis sinistra
    v. ilealis
    v. ileocaecalis
    v. mitralis
    v. pulmonaria
    v. tricuspidalis
    v. trunci pulmonalis
valval
valvar
valvate
valve
    anal v's
    anterior urethral v's
    v. of aorta
    aortic v.
    artificial v.
    atrioventricular v.
    atrioventricular v., left
    atrioventricular v., right
    Ball v's
    ball-type v.
    Bauhin v.
    Béraud v.
    Bianchi v.
    bicuspid v.
    bicuspid aortic v.
    bicuspid pulmonary v.
    bileaflet v.
    bioprosthetic v.
    Björk-Shiley v.
    Blom-Singer v.
    Bochdalek v.
    caged-ball v.
    cardiac v's
    cardiac v., artificial

valve *(continued)*
    Carpentier-Edwards v.
    caval v.
    v. of colon
    congenital ureteric v's
    congenital urethral v.
    Cooley-Cutter v.
    coronary v.
    v. of coronary sinus
    directional v.
    Dua antireflux v.
    duckbill v.
    Duromedics v.
    escape v.
    eustachian v.
    expiratory v.
    fallopian v.
    femoral v.
    flail mitral v.
    flair v.
    floppy mitral v.
    flow-control v.
    Foltz v.
    v. of foramen ovale
    Gerlach v.
    glutaraldehyde-tanned porcine
      heart v.
    Guérin v.
    Hancock v.
    Hasner v.
    heart v's
    heart v., artificial
    Heimlich v.
    Heister v.
    Heyer v.
    Hoboken v.
    homograft v.
    Houston v's
    Huschke v.
    hymenal v. of male urethra
    ileal v.
    ileocecal v.
    ileocolic v.
    v. of inferior vena cava
    inspiratory v.
    Ionescu v.
    Ionescu-Shiley v.
    Kerckring (Kerkring) v's
    Kohlrausch v's
    Krause v.
    left atrioventricular v.
    LeVeen peritoneal v.
    Lillehei-Kaster v.
    lymphatic v.
    v. of Macalister

valve *(continued)*
- Medtronic-Hall v.
- Mercier v.
- mitral v.
- monocuspid aortic v.
- Morgagni v's
- nasal v.
- v. of navicular fossa
- nonrebreathing v.
- O'Beirne v.
- Omnicarbon v.
- Omniscience v.
- oxygen flush v.
- parachute mitral v.
- pop-off v.
- porcine v.
- posterior urethral v's
- pressure-limiting v.
- prosthetic cardiac v.
- prosthetic heart v.
- Pudenz v.
- Pudenz-Heyer v.
- pulmonary v.
- v. of pulmonary trunk
- pyloric v.
- quadricuspid v.
- quadricuspid aortic v.
- quadricuspid pulmonary v.
- relief v.
- right atrioventricular v.
- Rosenmüller v.
- St. Jude Medical v.
- semilunar v.
- semilunar v's of colon
- semilunar v's of
  Morgagni
- semilunar v's of rectum
- sigmoid v's of colon
- sinoatrial v., sinuatrial v.
- v. of sinus venosus
- speaking v.
- spiral v. of cystic duct
- spiral v. of Heister
- Spitz-Holter v.
- Starr-Edwards v.
- v. of Sylvius
- Taillefer v.
- Tarinus v.
- Terrier v.
- thebesian v.
- thermionic v.
- tilting-disk v.
- tissue v.
- tracheostoma v.
- tricuspid v.

valve *(continued)*
- v. tube
- v. of Tulpius
- unidirectional v.
- ureteral v.
- urethral v's
- v. of Varolius
- v's of veins
- venous v.
- v. of vermiform appendix
- v. of Vieussens
- Willis v.

valvectomy

valved

valviform

valvoplasty

valvotome

valvotomy
- mitral v.
- pulmonary v.
- rectal v.
- transventricular closed v.
- transventricular pulmonary v.

valvula (valvulae)
- Amussat v.
- valvulae anales
- valvulae conniventes
- v. foraminis ovalis
- v. fossae navicularis
- Gerlach v.
- v. ileocaecalis
- v. ileocolica
- v. lymphaticum
- v. semilunaris
- v. semilunaris anterior valvae trunci pulmonalis
- v. semilunaris dextra valvae aortae
- v. semilunaris dextra valvae trunci pulmonalis
- v. semilunaris posterior valvae aortae
- v. semilunaris valvae sinistra aortae
- v. semilunaris sinistra valvae trunci pulmonalis
- v. sinus coronarii
- v. spiralis
- v. venae cavae inferioris
- v. venosa
- v. vestibuli

valvular
- v. aortic stenosis
- v. stenosis

valvulate

V

valvule
    v. of Béraud
    v. of Bochdalek
    v. of Foltz
    v. of Guérin
valvulectomy
valvulitis
    rheumatic v.
    uricemic v.
valvuloplasty
    aortic v.
    balloon v.
    catheter balloon v. (CBV)
    mitral v.
    percutaneous transluminal
      atrial v. (PTAV)
    percutaneous transluminal
      mitral v. (PTMV)
valvulotome
    Himmelstein v.
valvulotomy
VAMP—
    vinblastine, doxorubicin,
      methotrexate, and
      prednisone
    vincristine, actinomycin,
      methotrexate, prednisone
    vincristine, Adriamycin,
      methylprednisolone
vampire bat
vanadate
vanadic acid
vanadium (V)
vanadiumism
van Bogaert
    encephalitis
    sclerosing leukoencephalitis
van Bogaert-Bertrand disease
van Bogaert-Divry syndrome
van Bogaert-Nyssen-Peiffer disease
van Bogaert-Scherer-Epstein
  syndrome
van Buchem
    disease
    syndrome
van Buren
    dilator
    disease
    forceps
    operation
    sound
Van de Graaff generator
van den Bergh
    disease
    test
Vanderbilt forceps

van der Hoeve
    syndrome
van der Hoeve-de Kleyn
  syndrome
van der Waals radius
Van Doren forceps
van Gehuchten
    cells
    method
Vanghetti prosthesis
van Gieson stain
van Gorder operation
van Hook operation
van Hoorne (van Hoorn, van
  Horne) canal
vanilla
vanillal
vanillic acid diethylamide
vanillin
    ethyl v.
vanillism
vanillylmandelic acid (VMA)
van Lint
    akinesia
    block
    technique
van Millingen
    graft
    operation
Vannas scissors
Van Slyke
    formula
    method
    tests
Van Slyke-Cullen
    method
    test
Van Slyke-Fitz method
Van Slyke and Neill method
Vanzetti sign
vapocauterization
vapo-coolant
vapor (vapores, vapors)
vaporarium
vaporization
vaporize
vaporizer
    anesthetic v.
    Copper Kettle v.
    Fluotec v.
    Vernitrol v.
vapotherapy
Vaquez disease
Vaquez-Osler disease
VARE—visual acuity, right eye
variability

variable
    acoustic v.
    confounding v.
    continuous v.
    dependent v.
    discrete v.
    dummy v.
    explanatory v.
    independent v.
    intervening v.
    predictor v.
    random v.
variance
    environmental v.
    genetic v.
variant
    alpha v.
    v. angina
    Haenel v.
    L-phase v.
    petit mal v.
variate
    binary v.
    continuous v.
    discrete v.
variation
    allotypic v.
    antigenic v.
    continuous v.
    discontinuous v.
    diurnal v.
    genetic v.
    genotypic v.
    idiotypic v.
    impressed v.
    inborn v.
    isotypic v.
    meristic v.
    microbial v.
    phase v.
    phenotypic v.
    quasicontinuous v.
    saltatory v.
    sampling v.
    smooth-rough (S-R) v.
varicated
varication
variceal
varicectomy
varicella
    v. gangrenosa
    v. pneumonia
    v. virus vaccine live
    v.-zoster immune globulin
        (VZIG)
    v.-zoster virus

varicellation
varicelliform
    Kaposi v. eruption
varicelloid
varices (plural of varix)
variciform
varicoblepharon
varicocele
    v. embolization
    idiopathic v.
    ovarian v.
    palpable v.
    pelvic v.
    utero-ovarian v.
varicocelectomy
varicography
varicoid
varicomphalus
varicophlebitis
varicose vein
varicosis
varicosity
varicotomy
varicula
variety
variola
    v. caprina
    v. haemorrhagica
    v. major
    v. ovina
    v. sine eruptione
variolar
variolate
variolation
varioliform
varioloid
variolous
varix (varices)
    anastomotic v.
    aneurysmal v.
    aneurysmoid v.
    arterial v.
    cirsoid v.
    esophageal varices
    lymph v.
    v. lymphaticus
varnish
    cavity v.
varolian
Varolius
    bridge
    valve
varus
    v. alignment
    v. angulation
    v. collapse

V

varus *(continued)*
  cubitus v.
  v. deformity
  v. displacement
  elbow v. torque
  hallux v.
  v. knee
  v. laxity
  metatarsus primus v.
  v. position, v. positioning
  v. rotation
  v. stress
  v. thrust
  v.-valgus motion
vas (vasa)
  v. aberrans
  v. aberrans of Roth
  vasa aberrantis hepatis
  v. afferens glomeruli
  vasa afferentia
    lymphoglandulae
  vasa afferentia nodi
    lymphatici
  v. anastomoticum
  vasa auris internae
  vasa brevia
  v. capillare
  v. collaterale
  v. deferens
  v. efferens glomeruli
  vasa efferentia
    lymphoglandulae
  vasa efferentia nodi lymphatici
  vasa lymphatica
  v. lymphaticum profundum
  v. lymphaticum superficiale
  v. lymphocapillare
  vasa nervorum
  vasa praevia
  v. prominens ductus cochlearis
  vasa recta renis
  vasa sanguinea auris internae
  vasa sanguinea retinae
  v. sinusoideum
  v. spirale
  vasa vasorum
  vasa vorticosa
vasalgia
vasalium
VASC—Verbal Auditory Screen for
  Children
vascular
  articular v. network
  v. atrophy
  v. bed

vascular *(continued)*
  v. birthmark
  v. bud
  v. cecal fold
  v. circle
  v. coat
  v. compartment
  v. deafness
  v. dementia
  Dieulafoy v.
    malformation
  v. ejection sound
  encephalotrigeminal v.
    syndrome
  v. endothelial growth factor
  v. endothelium
  v. foot plate
  v. funnel
  gastric antral v. ectasia
  v. gland
  v. goiter
  v. groove
  v. hamartoma
  v. headache
  v. hemophilia
  v. hypertension
  v. hypotension
  v. impedance
  v. insufficiency
  v. keratitis
  knitted v. prosthesis
  v. lacuna
  v. lamina of choroid
  v. layer of eyeball
  v. leak syndrome
  v. leiomyoma
  v. malformation
  v. membrane
  v. murmur
  v. myxoma
  v. nephritis
  v. nerves
  v. nevus
  v. osteitis
  v. parabiosis
  peripheral v. resistance
  v. plexus
  v. poison
  v. pole of renal corpuscle
  pulmonary v. resistance
  v. reflex
  v. resistance
  v. ring
  v. rosacea
  v. sclerosis

vascular *(continued)*
    v. sedative
    v. sensation
    v. spider
    v. stenosis
    v. stimulus
    v. styptic
    v. syndrome
    v. system
    v. tumor
    v. tunic of eyeball
    visceral v. space
    v. zone
vascularity
vascularization
vascularize
vasculature
vasculi
vasculitic
vasculitis
    allergic v.
    consecutive v.
    epineurial v.
    granulomatous v.
    hypersensitivity v.
    leukocytoclastic v.
    livedo v.
    livedoid v.
    lymphomatoid v.
    necrotizing v.
    nodular v.
    overlap v.
    retinal v.
    segmented
      hyalinizing v.
    septic v.
    urticarial v.
vasculocardiac
vasculogenesis
vasculogenic
vasculolymphatic
vasculopathy
vasculotoxic
vasculum (vascula)
    v. aberrans
vasectomized
vasectomy
    crossover v.
Vaseline gauze
    dressing
vasifaction
vasifactive
vasiform
vasitis nodosa
vasoactive amines

vasoconstriction
    active v.
    passive v.
vasoconstrictive
vasoconstrictor
vasocorona
vasodepression
vasodepressor
vasodilatation
    active v.
    passive v.
vasodilation
    reflex v.
vasodilative
vasodilator
vasoepididymography
vasoepididymostomy
vasofactive
vasoformative
vasoganglion
vasography
vasohypertonic
vasohypotonic
vasoinert
vasoinhibitor
vasoinhibitory
vasolabile
vasoligation
vasoligature
vasomotion
vasomotor
vasomotorial
vasomotoricity
vasomotorium
vasomotory
vasoneuropathy
vasoneurosis
vasoparalysis
vasoparesis
vasopermeability
vasopressin
    arginine v. (AVP)
    v. 8-lysine
    v. tannate
vasopressinase
vasopressor
vasopuncture
vasoreflex
vasorelaxation
vasoresection
vasorrhaphy
vasosection
vasosensory
vasospasm
    refractory ergonovine-induced v.

V

vasospasmolytic
vasospastic
vasostimulant
vasostomy
vasotocin
    arginine v.
vasotomy
vasotonia
vasotonic
vasotribe
vasotripsy
vasotrophic
vasotropic
vasovagal
vasovasostomy
vasovesiculectomy
vasovesiculitis
vastus lateralis
Vater
    ampulla (ampulla of Vater)
    corpuscles
    duct
    papilla
Vater-Pacini corpuscles
vault
    cartilaginous v.
    cranial v.
    v. of pharynx
    vaginal v.
VB—viable birth
VC—
    acuity of color vision
    vena cava
    ventilatory capacity
    vital capacity
VCE—vagina, (ecto)cervix, and
    endocervix (smear)
VCG—vectorcardiogram
VCU, VCUG—voiding
    cystourethrogram
VD—venereal disease
–V.D.—negative vertical divergence
+V.D.—positive vertical divergence
VDA—visual discriminatory acuity
VDG—venereal disease–gonorrhea
VDH—vascular disease of the
    heart
VDP—vincristine, daunorubicin,
    prednisone
VDRL—Venereal Disease Research
    Laboratories
VDS—venereal disease–syphilis
VE—
    visual efficiency
    volumic ejection

Veau
    elevator
    operation
Veau-Axhausen operation
vection
vector
    biological v.
    cardiac v.
    cloning v.
    expression v.
    instantaneous v.
    macroscopic magnetization v.
    manifest v.
    mechanical v.
    P v.
    recombinant v.
    spatial v.
    T v.
vector-borne
vectorcardiogram (VCG)
vectorcardiograph
vectorcardiography (VCG)
    spatial v.
vectorial
vectorscope
Vedder
    agar
    culture medium
VEE—
    vagina, ectocervix, and
      endocervix (smear)
    Venezuelan equine
      encephalomyelitis (virus)
Veenema retractor
Veenema-Gusberg needle
VEE smear
vegan
veganism
vegetable
vegetal
vegetality
vegetarian
vegetarianism
vegetation
    adenoid v.
    aortic valve v's
    bacterial v's
    candidal v.
    cardiac valve v's
    dendritic v.
    mitral valve leaflet v's
    pacemaker lead v.
    septic v.
    verrucous v's
vegetative

vehicle
    motor vehicle accident (MVA)
veil
    v. cells
    Fick v.
    Hottentot v.
    Jackson v.
    Sattler v.
    vitreous v's
Veillon tube
Veillonella parvula
vein
    accompanying v.
    accompanying v. of hypoglossal
      nerve
    anastomotic v., inferior
    anastomotic v., superior
    angular v.
    antebrachial cephalic v.
    antebrachial v., median
    anticlinal v.
    appendicular v.
    v. of aqueduct of cochlea
    v. of aqueduct of vestibule
    arciform v's
    arcuate v.
    arcuate v's of kidney
    arterial v.
    arterial v. of Soemmering
    ascending v's of Rosenthal
    atrial v., lateral
    atrial v., medial
    atrioventricular v's of heart
    auditory v's, internal
    auricular v's, anterior
    auricular v., posterior
    axillary v.
    azygos v.
    azygos v., left
    azygos v., lesser superior
    basal v.
    basilic v.
    basilic v., median
    brachial v's
    Braune v.
    v. of bulb of penis
    v. of bulb of vestibule
    Burow v.
    v. of canaliculus of cochlea
    capillary v.
    capsular v.
    cardiac v's, anterior
    cardiac v., great
    cardiac v., middle
    cardiac v., small

vein *(continued)*
    cardiac v's, smallest
    carotid v., external
    cavernous v's of penis
    central v.
    central v. of retina
    central v. of suprarenal gland
    cephalic v.
    cephalic v., accessory
    cephalic v., median
    cerebellar v's, inferior
    cerebellar v's, superior
    cerebral v's, anterior
    cerebral v's, deep
    cerebral v., deep middle
    cerebral v., great
    cerebral v's, inferior
    cerebral v's, internal
    cerebral v's, superficial
    cerebral v's, superficial middle
    cerebral v's, superior
    cervical v., deep
    cervical v's, transverse
    choroid v., inferior
    choroid v., superior
    ciliary v's, anterior
    ciliary v's, posterior
    cilioretinal v.
    circumflex femoral v's, lateral
    circumflex femoral v's, medial
    circumflex iliac v., deep
    circumflex iliac v., superficial
    v. of cochlear canaliculus
    colic v., left
    colic v., middle
    colic v., right
    companion v.
    coronary v., left
    v. of corpus callosum, dorsal
    v. of corpus callosum, posterior
    cubital v., median
    cutaneous v.
    cutaneous v., ulnar
    cystic v.
    deep v.
    deep v. of thigh
    deep v. of tongue
    digital v's of foot, common
    digital v's of foot, dorsal
    digital v's, palmar
    digital v's, plantar
    diploic v., anterior temporal
    diploic v., frontal
    diploic v., occipital
    diploic v., posterior temporal

V

vein *(continued)*

    dorsal v. of clitoris, deep
    dorsal v's of clitoris, superficial
    dorsal v. of penis, deep
    dorsal v's of penis, superficial
    dorsal v's of tongue
    emissary v.
    emissary v., condylar
    emissary v., mastoid
    emissary v., occipital
    emissary v., parietal
    emulgent v.
    epigastric v., inferior
    epigastric v., superficial
    epigastric v's, superior
    epiploic v., left
    epiploic v., right
    facial v.
    facial v., anterior
    facial v., common
    facial v., deep
    facial v., posterior
    facial v., transverse
    femoral v.
    femoral v., deep
    femoropopliteal v.
    Galen v.
    gastric v., left
    gastric v., right
    gastric v's, short
    gastroepiploic v., left
    gastroepiploic v., right
    gastro-omental v., left
    gastro-omental v., right
    gluteal v's, inferior
    gluteal v's, superior
    gonadal v's
    hemiazygos v.
    hemiazygos v., accessory
    hemorrhoidal v's, inferior
    hemorrhoidal v's, middle
    hemorrhoidal v., superior
    hepatic v. catheterization
    hepatic v., intermediate
    hepatic v., middle
    hypogastric v.
    hypophysioportal v's
    ileocolic v.
    iliac v., common
    iliac v., external
    iliac v., internal
    iliolumbar v.
    infralobar v.
    infrasegmental v.
    innominate v's

vein *(continued)*

    intercalated v.
    intercapitular v's of foot
    intercapitular v's of hand
    intercostal v's, anterior
    intercostal v., highest
    intercostal v., left superior
    intercostal v's, posterior
    intercostal v., right superior
    interlobar v.
    interlobular v's of kidney
    interlobular v's of liver
    intermediate v.
    intermediate colic v.
    interosseous v's of foot, dorsal
    interosseous metacarpal v's,
      dorsal
    intersegmental v.
    intervertebral v.
    intrasegmental v.
    jugular v., anterior
    jugular v., anterior horizontal
    jugular v., external
    jugular v., internal
    Krukenberg v's
    Kuhnt postcentral v.
    labial v's, anterior
    labial v's, inferior
    labial v's, posterior
    labial v., superior
    labyrinthine v's
    lacrimal v.
    laryngeal v., inferior
    laryngeal v., superior
    Latarjet v.
    v. of lateral recess of fourth
      ventricle
    v. of lateral ventricle, lateral
    v. of lateral ventricle, medial
    levoatriocardinal v.
    lingual v.
    lingual v., deep
    lingual v's, dorsal
    lumbar v., ascending
    mammary v's, external
    mammary v., internal
    Mayo v.
    median v. of elbow
    median v. of forearm
    median v. of neck
    meningeal v's, middle
    mesenteric v., inferior
    mesenteric v., superior
    metacarpal v's, dorsal
    metacarpal v's, palmar

vein *(continued)*

nasal v's, external
nasofrontal v.
oblique v. of left atrium
occipital v's
v. of olfactory gyrus
ophthalmic v., inferior
ophthalmic v., superior
ophthalmomeningeal v.
ovarian v.
ovarian v., left
ovarian v., right
palatine v.
palatine v., external
palpebral v's, inferior
palpebral v's, superior
parietal v. of Santorini
parotid v's, anterior
parotid v's, posterior
petrosal v.
phrenic v's, inferior
phrenic v's, superior
pontomesencephalic v., anterior
popliteal v.
portal v.
portal v. of liver
posterior conjunctival v.
posterior v. of left ventricle
precentral v. of cerebellum
prepyloric v.
v. of pterygoid canal
pudendal v's, external
pudendal v., internal
pulmonary v's
pulmonary v., left inferior
pulmonary v., left superior
pulmonary v., right inferior
pulmonary v., right superior
pyloric v.
radial v., external, of Soemmering
ranine v.
rectal v's, inferior
rectal v's, middle
rectal v., superior
retinal v.
retromandibular v.
retroperitoneal v.
Retzius v's
revehent v.
Rosenthal v.
Ruysch v's
sacral v's, lateral
sacral v., middle

vein *(continued)*

saphenous v.
saphenous v., accessory
saphenous v., great
saphenous v., small
scrotal v's, anterior
scrotal v's, posterior
v. of septum pellucidum, anterior
v. of septum pellucidum, posterior
small v. of heart
spermatic v.
sphenopalatine v.
spinal v's, anterior and posterior
spiral v. of modiolus
splenic v.
stellate v's of kidney
Stensen v's
sternocleidomastoid v.
stylomastoid v.
subclavian v.
subcostal v.
sublingual v.
submental v.
superficial v.
supraorbital v.
suprarenal v., left
suprarenal v., right
suprascapular v.
sylvian v.
v. of sylvian fossa
systemic v.
temporal v's, deep
temporal v., middle
temporal v's, superficial
terminal v.
testicular v., left
testicular v., right
thalamostriate v's, inferior
thalamostriate v., superior
thebesian v's
v's of Thebesius
thoracic v's, internal
thoracic v., lateral
thoracoacromial v.
thymic v's
thyroid v., inferior
thyroid v's, middle
thyroid v., superior
tibial v's, anterior
tibial v's, posterior
tonsillar v.
transverse v. of face

V

vein *(continued)*
 transverse v's of neck
 Trolard v.
 ulnar v's
 umbilical v.
 umbilical v., left
 v. of uncus
 varicose v.
 ventricular v's of heart, right
 ventricular v., inferior
 v. of vermis, inferior
 v. of vermis, superior
 vertebral v.
 vertebral v., accessory
 vertebral v., anterior
 vertebral v's, superficial
 vesalian v.
veinlet
vela
velamen (velamina)
 v. vulvae
velamentous
velamentum (velamenta)
 velamenta cerebri
velar
Velcro
 binder
 dressing
 rales
vellosine
vellus
 v. hair
 v. olivae
velocimetry
 laser-Doppler v. (LDV)
velocity
 conduction v.
 high-v. particles
 limiting v.
 maximum v.
 nerve conduction v.
 propagation v.
 PSA (prostate-specific antigen) v.
 sedimentation v.
 sensory conduction v.
 thrombotic threshold v.
velopharyngeal
velopharynx
veloplasty
velour
Velpeau
 axillary view
 bandage
 deformity
 hernia

velum (vela)
 anterior medullary v.
 artificial v.
 Baker v.
 caudal medullary v.
 inferior medullary v.
 v. interpositum cerebri
 v. medullare anterius
 v. medullare caudale
 v. medullare inferius
 v. medullare posterius
 v. medullare rostralis
 v. medullare superius
 medullary v., anterior
 medullary v., cranial
 medullary v., inferior
 medullary v., posterior
 medullary v., rostral
 medullary v., superior
 nursing v.
 palatine v.
 v. palatinum
 pharyngeal v.
 posterior medullary v.
 rostral medullary v.
 superior medullary v.
 v. of Tarinus
 v. transversum
VEM—vasoexcitor material
vena (venae)
 venae advehentes
 v. anastomotica inferior
 v. anastomotica superior
 v. angularis
 venae anteriores cerebri
 v. anterior septi pellucidi
 v. appendicularis
 v. aqueductus cochleae
 v. aqueductus vestibuli
 venae arcuatae renis
 venae articulares
 venae atriales dextrae
 venae atriales sinistrae
 venae auriculares
  anteriores
 v. auricularis posterior
 v. axillaris
 v. azygos
 v. basalis
 v. basilica
 venae basivertebrales
 venae brachiales
 v. brachiocephalica
 venae bronchiales
 v. bulbi penis

vena (venae) *(continued)*
- v. bulbi vestibuli
- v. canalis pterygoidei
- venae cardiacae anteriores
- v. cardiaca magna
- v. cardiaca media
- v. cardiaca parva
- v. cava, venae cavae
- v. cava inferior
- v. cava superior
- venae cavernosae penis
- v. centralis glandulae
  suprarenalis
- venae centralis hepatis
- venae centralis retinae
- v. cephalica
- v. cephalica accessoria
- venae cerebelli
- venae cerebri
- v. cervicalis profunda
- v. choroidea inferior
- v. choroidea superior
- venae ciliares
- venae circumflexae femoris
  laterales
- venae circumflexae femoris
  mediales
- v. circumflexa ilium profunda
- v. circumflexa ilium
  superficialis
- v. colica dextra
- v. colica media
- v. colica sinistra
- venae columnae vertebralis
- v. comitans
- v. comitans nervi hypoglossi
- venae conjunctivales
- venae cordis
- venae cordis anteriores
- v. cordis magna
- v. cordis media
- venae cordis minimae
- v. cordis parva
- venae costoaxillares
- v. cutanea
- v. cystica
- venae digitales communes
  pedis
- venae digitales dorsales pedis
- venae digitales palmares
- venae digitales plantares
- venae diploicae
- v. diploica frontalis
- v. diploica occipitalis
- v. diploica temporalis anterior

vena (venae) *(continued)*
- v. diploica temporalis posterior
- venae directae laterales
- venae dorsales linguae
- v. dorsalis profunda clitoridis
- v. dorsalis profunda penis
- v. emissaria
- v. emissaria condylaris
- v. emissaria mastoidea
- v. emissaria occipitalis
- v. emissaria parietalis
- v. encephali
- v. epigastrica inferior
- v. epigastrica superficialis
- venae episclerales
- venae esophageales
- venae ethmoidales
- v. facialis
- v. femoralis
- venae fibulares
- venae frontales
- v. gastrica dextra
- venae gastricae breves
- v. gastrica sinistra
- v. gastroepiploica dextra
- v. gastroepiploica sinistra
- v. gastroomentalis dextra
- v. gastroomentalis sinistra
- venae geniculares
- venae genus
- venae gluteae inferiores
- venae gluteae superiores
- v. gyri olfactorii
- v. hemiazygos
- v. hemiazygos accessoria
- v. hepatica dextra
- venae hepaticae
- v. hepatica intermedia
- v. hepatica media
- v. hepatica sinistra
- venae ileales
- v. ileocolica
- v. iliaca communis
- v. iliaca externa
- v. iliaca interna
- v. iliolumbalis
- inferior v. cava
- venae inferiores cerebelli
- venae inferiores cerebri
- v. inferior vermis
- venae insulares
- venae intercapitulares manus
- venae intercapitulares pedis
- venae intercostales anteriores
- venae intercostales posteriores

vena (venae) *(continued)*

v. intercostalis superior dextra
v. intercostalis superior sinistra
v. intercostalis suprema
venae interlobares renis
venae interlobulares hepatis
venae interlobulares renis
venae internae cerebri
v. intervertebralis
venae jejunales
v. jugularis anterior
v. jugularis externa
v. jugularis interna
venae labiales anteriores
venae labiales inferiores
venae labiales posteriores
v. labialis superior
venae labyrinthi
venae labyrinthinae
v. lacrimalis
v. laryngea inferior
v. laryngea superior
v. lateralis atrii
v. lateralis ventriculi lateralis
v. lienalis
v. lingualis
v. lingularis
venae lumbales
v. lumbalis ascendens
v. magna cerebri
venae maxillares
v. medialis ventriculi lateralis
v. mediana antebrachii
v. mediana cubiti
venae mediastinales
vena media superficialis cerebri
venae medullae oblongatae
venae meningeae
venae meningeae mediae
v. mesenterica inferior
v. mesenterica superior
venae metacarpales dorsales
venae metacarpales palmares
venae metatarsales dorsales
venae metatarsales plantares
venae musculophrenicae
venae nasales externae
v. nasofrontalis
venae nuclei caudati
v. obliqua atrii sinistri
venae obturatoriae
venae occipitales
v. occipitalis

vena (venae) *(continued)*

venae oesophageales
v. ophthalmica inferior
v. ophthalmica superior
v. ovarica dextra
v. ovarica sinistra
v. palatina externa
venae palpebrales
venae palpebrales inferiores
venae palpebrales superiores
venae pancreaticae
venae pancreaticoduodenales
venae paraumbilicales
venae parietales
venae parotideae
venae pectorales
venae pedunculares
venae perforantes
venae pericardiacae
venae pericardiacophrenicae
venae peroneae
persistent left superior v. cava
v. petrosa
venae pharyngeae
venae phrenicae inferiores
venae phrenicae superiores
venae pontis
v. pontomesencephalica anterior
v. poplitea
v. portae hepatis
v. posterior corporis callosi
v. posterior septi pellucidi
v. precentralis cerebelli
venae prefrontales
v. prepylorica
v. profunda
venae profundae cerebri
venae profundae clitoridis
v. profunda faciei
v. profunda femoris
v. profunda linguae
venae pudendae externae
v. pudenda interna
venae pulmonales
v. pulmonalis dextra inferior
v. pulmonalis dextra superior
v. pulmonalis sinistra inferior
v. pulmonalis sinistra superior
venae radiales
v. recessus lateralis ventriculi quarti
venae rectales inferiores
venae rectales mediae
v. rectalis superior

vena (venae) *(continued)*
- venae renales
- venae renis
- v. retromandibularis
- venae revehentes
- venae sacrales laterales
- v. sacralis mediana
- v. saphena accessoria
- v. saphena magna
- v. saphena parva
- v. scapularis dorsalis
- venae sclerales
- venae scrotales anteriores
- venae scrotales posteriores
- venae sigmoideae
- venae spinales anteriores
- venae spinales posteriores
- v. splenica
- venae stellatae renis
- v. sternocleidomastoidea
- v. stylomastoidea
- v. subclavia
- v. subcostalis
- venae subcutaneae abdominis
- v. sublingualis
- v. submentalis
- venae superficiales cerebri
- venae superficiales membri inferioris
- venae superficiales membri superioris
- v. superficialis
- superior v. cava
- venae superiores cerebelli
- venae superiores cerebri
- v. superior vermis
- v. supraorbitalis
- venae suprarenales
- v. suprarenalis dextra
- v. suprarenalis sinistra
- v. suprascapularis
- venae supratrochleares
- venae surales
- venae temporales profundae
- venae temporales superficiales
- v. temporalis media
- v. terminalis
- v. testicularis dextra
- v. testicularis sinistra
- venae thalamostriatae inferiores
- v. thalamostriata superior
- venae thoracicae internae
- v. thoracica lateralis
- v. thoracoacromialis

vena (venae) *(continued)*
- venae thoracoepigastricae
- venae thymicae
- v. thyroidea ima
- v. thyroidea inferioris
- v. thyroidea mediae
- v. thyroidea superior
- venae tibiales anteriores
- venae tibiales posteriores
- venae tracheales
- venae transversae cervicis
- venae transversae colli
- v. transversa facialis
- v. transversa faciei
- venae trunci encephalici
- venae tympanicae
- venae ulnares
- v. umbilicalis
- v. uncalis
- venae uterinae
- venae vasorum
- venae ventriculares dextrae
- venae ventriculares sinistrae
- v. ventricularis inferior
- v. ventriculi dextri anteriores
- v. ventriculi sinistri posterior
- v. vertebralis
- v. vertebralis accessoria
- v. vertebralis anterior
- venae vesicales
- venae vestibulares
- venae vorticosae

Venable-Stuck nail
vena cava (venae cavae)
- inferior v.c. (IVC)
- superior v.c. (SVC)
venacavogram
venacavography
- inferior v. (IVCV)
venae cavae (plural of vena cava)
venation
venectasia
venectomy
veneer
- full v.
venenation
venene
veneniferous
venenific
venenosity
venereal disease (VD)
venereologist
venipuncture
venisection
venisuture

venoatrial
venoauricular
venoclysis
venofibrosis
venogram
    computed tomography (CT) v.
    contrast v.
    coronary sinus v.
    levophase coronary v.
    renal v.
venography
    ascending v.
    descending v.
    extradural v.
    impedance v.
    intraosseous v.
    limb v.
    peripheral v.
    portal v.
    radionuclide v.
    selective v.
    splenic v.
    splenoportal v.
    subtraction v.
    uterine v.
    vertebral v.
venom
    bee v.
    cobra v.
    kokoi v.
    moccasin v.
    rattlesnake v.
    Russell viper v.
    snake v.
    spider v.
    toad v.
    viper v.
venomization
venomosalivary
venomotor
venomous
veno-occlusive
venoperitoneostomy
venopressor
venorrhaphy
    lateral v.
venosclerosis
venose
venosinal
venosity
venostasis
venotomy
venous
    v. angiocardiography
    v. aortography

venous (continued)
    v. cannula
    dynamic v. plethysmography
    v. hum
    v. occlusion plethysmography
    v. pressure
    v. pulse
    v. resistance
    v. return curve
    v. smooth muscle
    v. thromboembolism
    v. thrombosis
venovenostomy
vent
    pulmonic alveolar v's
Ventaire
venter (ventres)
    v. anterior musculi digastrici
    v. frontalis musculi
        occipitofrontalis
    v. ilii
    v. imus
    v. inferior musculi omohyoidei
    v. medius
    v. musculi
    v. occipitalis musculi
        occipitofrontalis
    v. posterior musculi digastrici
    v. propendens
    v. scapulae
    v. superior musculi omohyoidei
    v. supremus
ventilate
ventilation
    alveolar v.
    arterial v.
    artificial v.
    assist/control mode v.
    assisted v.
    v. bronchoscope
    constant positive-pressure v.
    control-mode v.
    dead space v.
    downward v.
    exhausting v.
    expired air v.
    intermittent demand v.
    intermittent mandatory v.
        (IMV)
    intermittent mandatory v.,
        synchronized
    intermittent positive-pressure
        v. (IPPV)
    maximum voluntary v. (MVV)
    mechanical v.

ventilation (*continued*)
  middle ear v.
  minute v.
  natural v.
  negative-pressure v.
  v.-perfusion (V/Q) ratio
  v.-perfusion (V/Q) scan
  plenum v.
  v. scintigraphy
  synchronized intermittent
    mandatory v.
  v. threshold
  total v.
  v. tube
  upward v.
  vacuum v.
  walking v.
ventilator
  mechanical v.
  pressure-cycled v.
  tank v.
  time-cycled v.
  volume-cycled v.
ventilatory
ventilometer
ventilometry
Ventimask
ventplant
ventrad
ventral celiotomy
ventralis
ventricle
  aortic v. of heart
  v. of Arantius
  auxiliary v.
  v's of the brain
  cerebral v.
  v. of cerebrum
  v. of cord
  double-inlet v.
  double-outlet right v.
  Duncan v.
  fifth v.
  first v. of brain
  first v. of cerebrum
  fourth v. of brain
  fourth v. of cerebrum
  v's of the heart
  Krause v.
  v. of larynx
  lateral v. of brain
  lateral v. of cerebrum
  left v. of heart
  Morgagni v.
  optic v.

ventricle (*continued*)
  pineal v.
  primitive v.
  right v. of heart
  second v. of brain
  second v. of cerebrum
  single v.
  sixth v.
  v. of spinal cord
  v. of Sylvius terminal
  terminal v. of spinal cord
  third v. of brain
  third v. of cerebrum
  third v. of spinal cord
  Verga v.
  Vieussens v.
ventricornu
ventricornual
ventricose
ventricular
  v. arrhythmia
  v. assist device
  Berlin Heart v. assist
    device
  v. cannula
  v. catheter
  v. contour
  v. dilatation
  v. ectopy
  v. end-diastolic volume
  v. end-systolic pressure
  v. fibrillation
  v. filling
  v. flutter
  v. function
  v. fusion
  v. gradient
  v. hypertrophy
  v. interdependence
  v. mapping
  v. pacing
  v. performance
  v. premature beat
  v. premature contractions
  v. pressure-volume loop
  v. reentry
  v. relaxation
  v. rhythm
  v. septal defect (VSD)
  v. septum
  v. systole
  v. tachyarrhythmia
  v. tachycardia
  v. wall motion
  v. wall shortening

V

ventriculi (plural of ventriculus)
ventriculitis
ventriculoarterial coupling
ventriculoatriostomy
ventriculocisternostomy
ventriculocordectomy
ventriculofiberscope
ventriculofiberscopic
ventriculogram
ventriculography
    bubble v.
    cardiac v.
    cerebral v.
    contrast v.
    isotope v.
    radionuclide v.
ventriculomegaly
ventriculometry
ventriculomyotomy
ventriculonector
ventriculoperitoneal
ventriculophasic
ventriculoplasty
ventriculopuncture
ventriculoscope
ventriculoscopy
ventriculostium
ventriculostomy
ventriculosubarachnoid
ventriculovenostomy
ventriculus (ventriculi)
    v. cordis
    v. cordis dexter
    v. cordis sinister
    v. dexter cerebri
    v. laryngis
    v. lateralis cerebri
    v. medius
    v. quartus cerebri
    v. quintus
    v. sinister cerebri
    v. terminalis medullae spinalis
    tertius cerebri
ventricumbent
ventriduct
ventriduction
ventriflexion
ventrimesal
ventrimeson
ventrocystorrhaphy
ventrodorsad
ventrodorsal
ventrofixation
ventrohysteropexy
ventroinguinal

ventrolateral
ventromedial
ventromedian
ventroposterior
ventroptosia
ventroptosis
ventroscopy
ventrose
ventrosuspension
ventrotomy
ventrovesicofixation
Venturi
    effect
    mask
    meter spirometer
    myringotomy tube
    principle
    tube
venturimeter
venula (venulae)
    v. macularis inferior
    v. macularis superior
    v. medialis retinae
    v. nasalis retinae inferior
    v. nasalis retinae superior
    v. postcapillaris
    venulae rectae renis
    v. retinae medialis
    venulae stellatae renis
    v. temporalis retinae inferior
    v. temporalis retinae
      superior
venular
venule
    high endothelial v's
    inferior macular v.
    inferior nasal v. of retina
    inferior temporal v. of retina
    medial v. of retina
    nasal v. of retina, inferior and
      superior
    postcapillary v's
    stellate v's of kidney
    straight v's of kidney
    superior macular v.
    superior nasal v. of retina
    superior temporal v. of retina
    temporal v. of retina, inferior
      and superior
venulitis
    cutaneous necrotizing v.
Venus
    collar of V.
VEP—visual evoked potential
VER—visual evoked response

Veraguth fold
verbal
Verbiest syndrome
verbigeration
verbomania
Verbrugge clamp
verdohemin
verdohemochromogen
verdohemoglobin
verdoperoxidase
Veress needle
Verga
    lacrimal groove
    ventricle
verge
    anal v.
vergence
Verhoeff
    forceps
    operation
    scissors
    stain
    suture
vermes
vermetoid
vermian
vermicidal
vermicide
vermicular
vermiculation
vermicule
    traveling v.
vermiculous
vermiform
vermifugal
vermifuge
vermifuges
vermilion border
vermilionectomy
vermin
verminal
vermination
verminotic
verminous
vermis
    v. cerebelli
    inferior v.
    superior v.
vermix
vermography
vernal
    v. catarrh
    v. conjunctivitis
Verner-Morrison
  syndrome

Vernet
    paralysis (paralyses)
    syndrome
Verneuil
    canals
    disease
    neuroma
    operation
vernier
Vernier [eponym]
  acuity
vernix caseosa
Vernon-David
    operation
    proctoscope
    sigmoidoscope
    speculum
Vernonia anthelmintica
Verocay bodies
verruca (verrucae)
    v. acuminata, verrucae
      acuminatae
    v. digitata
    v. filiformis
    v. glabra
    v. mollusciformis
    v. necrogenica
    v. peruana
    v. peruviana
    v. plana
    v. plana juvenilis
    v. plantaris
    v. seborrheica
    v. senilis
    v. simplex
    v. tuberculosa
    v. vulgaris
verruciform
verrucose
verrucosis
    lymphostatic v.
verrucosity
verrucous
verruga peruana
versicolor
    tinea v.
version
    abdominal v.
    bimanual v.
    bipolar v.
    Braxton-Hicks v.
    cephalic v.
    combined v.
    Denman spontaneous v.
    external v.

version *(continued)*
  Hicks v.
  internal v.
  pelvic v.
  podalic v.
  Potter v.
  spontaneous v.
  Wigand v.
  Wright v.
Verstraeten bruit
vertebra (vertebrae)
  abdominal vertebrae
  basilar v.
  butterfly v.
  caudal vertebrae
  caudate vertebrae
  cervical vertebrae (C1–C7)
  vertebrae cervicales
  cleft v.
  vertebrae coccygeae
  coccygeal vertebrae
  codfish v.
  vertebrae colli
  cranial v.
  v. dentata
  false vertebrae
  hourglass v.
  H-shaped v.
  ivory v.
  vertebrae lumbales
  lumbar vertebrae (L1–L5)
  v. magna
  movable v.
  odontoid v.
  picture frame v.
  v. plana
  primitive v.
  v. prominens
  prominent v.
  sacral vertebrae (S1–S5)
  vertebrae sacrales
  vertebrae spuriae
  sternal v.
  tail v.
  terminal v., great
  vertebrae thoracales
  thoracic vertebrae (T1–T12)
  vertebrae thoracicae
  toothed v.
  tricuspid v.
  true vertebrae
  v. vera
vertebral
  v. angiography
  v. arteriography

vertebral *(continued)*
  v. artery
  v. compression fracture
  v. osteomyelitis
  v. venography
vertebrarium
vertebrarterial
vertebrate
vertebrate collagenase
vertebrated
vertebrectomy
vertebrobasilar
vertebrochondral
vertebrocostal
vertebrodidymus
vertebrofemoral
vertebrogenic
vertebroiliac
vertebromammary
vertebrosacral
vertebrosternal
vertex (vertices)
  v. of bony cranium
  v. cordis
  v. of cornea
  v. corneae
  v. cranii
  v. cranii ossei
  v. of urinary bladder
  v. vesicae urinariae
vertical
  Eckhout v. gastroplasty
  v. hemilaryngectomy
  v. incision
  v. mattress suture
  v. tube
verticalis
verticillate
Verticillium graphii
verticomental
vertiginous
vertigo
  v. ab stomacho laeso
  alternobaric v.
  angiopathic v.
  apoplectic v.
  arteriosclerotic v.
  auditory v.
  aural v.
  benign paroxysmal positional v.
  benign paroxysmal postural v.
  cardiac v.
  cardiovascular v.
  central v.
  cerebral v.

vertigo *(continued)*
  disabling positional v.
  disorientation v.
  encephalic v.
  endemic paralytic v.
  epidemic v.
  epileptic v.
  essential v.
  galvanic v.
  gastric v.
  height v.
  horizontal v.
  hysterical v.
  labyrinthine v.
  laryngeal v.
  lateral v.
  lithemic v.
  mechanical v.
  neurasthenic v.
  nocturnal v.
  objective v.
  ocular v.
  organic v.
  paralytic v.
  paralyzing v.
  paroxysmal
    positional v.
  peripheral v.
  positional v.
  post-traumatic v.
  postural v.
  pressure v.
  primary v.
  residual v.
  rider's v.
  rotary v.
  rotatory v.
  sham-movement v.
  special sense v.
  stomachal v.
  subjective v.
  systematic v.
  systemic v.
  tenebric v.
  toxemic v.
  toxic v.
  vertical v.
  vestibular v.
  voltaic v.
vertigraphy
verumontanitis
verumontanum
Verwey operation
vesalian
vesalianum

Vesalius
  foramen
  ligament
vesica (vesicae)
  v. biliaris
  v. fellea
  v. prostatica
  v. urinaria
vesical
  v. compliance
  v. diverticulectomy
  v. exstrophy
  v. external sphincter
    dyssynergia (VSD)
  v. fibrosis
  v. fistula
  v. neck
vesicant
vesicants
vesicate
vesication
vesicatory
vesicle
  acoustic v.
  acrosomal v.
  air v's
  allantoic v.
  amniocardiac v's
  anhidrotic v.
  archoplasmic v.
  auditory v.
  Baer v.
  blastodermic v.
  brain v's
  brain v's, primary
  brain v's, secondary
  cephalic v's
  cerebral v's
  v's of cerebral hemispheres
  cervical v.
  chorionic v.
  coated v.
  compound v.
  concentrating v's
  encephalic v's
  endocytic v's
  germinal v.
  graafian v's
  intermediate v's
  lens v.
  lung v's
  Malpighi v's
  matrix v's
  medullary coccygeal v.
  micropinocytotic v.

V

vesicle *(continued)*
- midbrain v.
- multilocular v.
- Naboth v's
- ocular v.
- olfactory v.
- ophthalmic v.
- optic v.
- otic v.
- phagocytotic v.
- pinocytotic v.
- pituitary v.
- plasmalemmal v.
- primitive brain v.
- prostatic v.
- pulmonary v's
- Purkinje v.
- secondary cerebral v's
- secretory v's
- seminal v.
- sense v.
- spermatic v.
- spermatic v., false
- synaptic v's
- telencephalic v's
- transfer v's
- transitional v's
- transport v's
- umbilical v.
- Unna v.
- water expulsion v.

vesicoabdominal
vesicobullous
vesicocavernous
vesicocele
vesicocervical
vesicoclysis
vesicocolonic
vesicoenteric
vesicofixation
vesicointestinal
vesicoperineal
vesicoprostatic
vesicopubic
vesicopustule
vesicorectal
vesicorectostomy
vesicorenal
vesicosigmoid
vesicosigmoidostomy
vesicospinal
vesicostomy
- cutaneous v.

vesicotomy
vesicoumbilical

vesicourachal
vesicoureteral
- v. reflux (VUR)
- v. regurgitation

vesicoureteric
vesicourethral
vesicouterine
vesicouterovaginal
vesicovaginal lithotomy
vesicovaginorectal
vesicula (vesiculae)
- v. bilis
- v. fellea
- v. germinativa
- vesiculae graafianae
- vesiculae nabothi
- v. ophthalmica
- v. prostatica
- v. seminalis
- v. serosa

vesicular
- v. bullous pemphigoid
- v. dermatophytid
- v. ringworm
- v. stomatitis

vesiculate
vesiculated
vesiculation
vesiculectomy
vesiculiform
vesiculitis
- seminal v.

vesiculobronchial
vesiculobullous
vesiculocavernous
vesiculogram
- seminal v.

vesiculography
vesiculopapular
vesiculoprostatitis
vesiculopustular
vesiculotomy
- seminal v.

vesiculotubular
vesiculotympanic
Veslingius line
vesperal
vessel
- absorbent v's
- afferent v. of glomerulus
- afferent v's of lymph node
- anastomotic v.
- arterioluminal v's
- arteriosinusoidal v's
- bile v.

vessel *(continued)*
    blood v.
    chyliferous v's
    circumflex v.
    collateral v.
    efferent v. of glomerulus
    efferent v's of lymph node
    external pudic v.
    ghost v.
    great v's
    hemorrhoidal v's
    hypogastric v.
    iliac v.
    internal spermatic v.
    Jungbluth v's
    lacteal v's
    lymphatic v.
    lymphatic v., deep
    lymphatic v., superficial
    lymphocapillary v.
    nutrient v's
    pudendal v.
    pudic v.
    sinusoidal v.
    Warburg v.
Vest telescope
vestibula (plural of vestibulum)
vestibular
    v. bulb
    v. nerve
    v. neuronitis
    v. reflex
    v. system
vestibule
    v. of aorta
    buccal v.
    v. of ear
    Gibson v.
    labial v.
    laryngeal v.
    v. of larynx
    v. of mouth
    nasal v.
    v. of nose
    v. of omental bursa
    v. of oral cavity
    v. of pharynx
    Sibson v.
    urogenital v.
    v. of vagina
    v. of vulva
vestibulectomy
vestibulocerebellar
vestibulocerebellum
vestibulocochlear

vestibulogenic
vestibulo-ocular reflex
vestibulopathy
vestibuloplasty
vestibulospinal
vestibulotomy
vestibulourethral
vestibulum (vestibula)
    v. auris
    v. bursae omentalis
    v. glottidis
    v. laryngis
    v. nasale
    v. nasi
    v. oris
    v. vaginae
vestige
    caudal medullary v.
    coccygeal v.
    v. of vaginal process
    wolffian v's
vestigial
vestigium (vestigia)
    v. processus vaginalis
vest-over-pants
    technique
vesuvine
veterinarian
veterinary
v.f.—field of vision
VF—
        left leg electrode
        ventricular fluid
        visual field
        ventricular fibrillation
        vocal fremitus
VFib—ventricular fibrillation
VFP—ventricular fluid
    pressure
VG—ventricular gallop
VH—
        vaginal hysterectomy
        venous hematocrit
        ventricular hypertrophy
        viral hepatitis
        vitreous hemorrhage
VHD—
        valvular heart disease
        viral hematodepressive
            disease
VHF—visual half-field
via (viae)
    v. naturales
VIA—virus-inactivating agent
viability

V

viable
  v. alternative
  v. birth
  v. fetus
vial
vibesate
vibex (vibices)
vibration
  bone-conduction v.
  chest wall v.
vibrative
vibratode
vibrator
vibratory angioedema
vibrio (vibrios, vibriones)
  Celebes v.
  cholera v.
  El Tor v.
  v. group EF-6, v. group F
  NAG (nonagglutinating) v's
  noncholera v's
  paracholera v's
Vibrio
  V. alginolyticus
  V. cholerae
  V. cholerae biovar *El Tor*
  V. cincinnatiensis
  V. fluvialis
  V. furnissii
  V. hollisae
  V. leonardii
  V. massauah
  V. metschnikovii
  V. mimicus
  V. parahaemolyticus
  V. vulnificus
vibriocidal
vibriolysis
vibriosis
vibrissa (vibrissae)
vibroacoustic
vibrocardiogram
vibrocardiography
vibrolode
vibromassage
vicarious
vicinal
vicine
vicious
Vicq d'Azyr
  band
  body
  bundle
  fasciculus
  foramen

Vicq d'Azyr *(continued)*
  operation
  stripe
  tract
Vicryl suture
Victoreen dosimeter
Vidal operation
videodensitometric
videodensitometry
videognosis
videomicroscopy
vidian
  v. artery
  v. canal
  v. nerve
Vi-drape
Vienna speculum
Vieth-Muller horopter
Vieussens
  annulus
  ansa
  foramen
  limbus
  valve
  vein
  ventricle
view
  apical lordotic v.
  Arcelin v's
  ball catcher's v.
  Chausse v.
  comparison v.
  coned-down v.
  decubitus v.
  dorsal v.
  frog-leg v.
  Hampton v.
  kyphotic v.
  lateral v.
  lateral decubitus v.
  Law v.
  lordotic v.
  Mayer v.
  normal anteroposterior v.
  oblique v.
  overcouch v.
  Owen v.
  panoramic v.
  pantomographic v.
  parasternal long axis v.
  plantar v.
  posterior v.
  profile ray v.
  recumbent v.
  Schüller v.

view *(continued)*
>> scottie dog v.
>> scout v.
>> skyline v.
>> Stenvers v.
>> stereoscopic v.
>> stress v.
>> submentovertical v.
>> superoinferior v.
>> swimmer's v.
>> tangential v.
>> Towne v.
>> tunnel v.
>> Velpeau axillary v.
>> Waters v.

VIG—vaccinia-immune globulin
vigilambulism
vigilance
vigintinormal
Vignal cells
vigor
>> hybrid v.

Villaret syndrome
villi (plural of villus)
villiferous
villikinin
villitis
villoglandular
villoma
villonodular
villose, villous
>> v. adenoma
>> v. arthritis
>> v. duct cancer
>> v. papillae of tongue
>> v. papilloma
>> v. placenta
>> v. tenosynovitis
>> v. tumor

villositis
villosity
villus (villi)
>> amniotic v.
>> anchoring v.
>> arachnoid villi
>> chorionic v.
>> v. of choroid plexus
>> colonic villi
>> floating v.
>> free v.
>> intestinal villi
>> villi intestinales
>> jejunal villi
>> labial v.
>> lingual villi

villus (villi) *(continued)*
>> pericardial v.
>> pleural villi
>> villi pleurales
>> primary v.
>> secondary v.
>> villi of small intestine
>> synovial villi
>> villi synoviales
>> tertiary v.
>> zonary v.

villusectomy
vimentin
Vim-Silverman needle
vinca
vincaleukoblastine
vincamine
Vincent
>> angina
>> gingivitis
>> infection
>> spirillum
>> stomatitis
>> tonsillitis

vincofos
vinculum (vincula)
>> v. breve
>> v. breve digitorum manus
>> v. linguae
>> vincula lingulae cerebelli
>> v. longum
>> v. longum digitorum manus
>> vincula tendinum digitorum manus
>> vincula tendinum digitorum pedis
>> vincula of tendons of fingers
>> vincula of tendons of toes

Vineberg operation
vinegar
vinegaroon
Vinson syndrome
vinyl
>> v. acetate
>> v. chloride
>> v. ether

viocid
Vioform dressing
violacein
violaceous
violation
violescent
violet
>> amethyst v.
>> ammonium oxalate crystal v.

V

violet *(continued)*
- aniline gentian v.
- bismuth v.
- bismuth crystal v.
- v. 7 B or C
- cresyl v.
- cresylecht v.
- crystal v.
- v. G
- gentian v.
- hexamethyl v.
- Hofmann v.
- iodine v.
- iris v.
- Lauth v.
- methyl v.
- methylene v.
- neutral v.
- Paris v.
- pentamethyl v.
- visual v.

viosterol

VIP—
- vasoactive intestinal polypeptide
- very important patient
- voluntary interruption of pregnancy

viper
- European v.
- Gaboon v.
- nose-horned v.
- palm v.
- pit v.
- rhinoceros v.
- Russell v.
- sand v.
- true v.

viperine

vipoma

viraginity

viral
- v. arthritis
- attenuated v. vaccine
- v. bronchitis
- v. bronchopneumonia
- v. cirrhosis
- v. cystitis
- v. dysentery
- v. encephalomyelitis
- v. esophagitis
- v. gastroenteritis
- v. hemagglutination
- v. hemorrhagic fevers
- v. hepatitis

viral *(continued)*
- v. keratoconjunctivitis
- v. load
- v. meningitis
- modified live v. vaccine
- v. myelitis
- v. myocarditis
- v. neutralization
- v. oncogene
- v. papular dermatitis
- v. parotitis
- v. particle
- v. pericarditis
- v. pneumonia

Virchow
- angle
- cell
- corpuscle
- crystal
- degeneration
- granulation
- knife
- line
- node

Virchow-Hassall body

Virchow-Robin spaces

viremia

virgin

virginal

virginity

viricidal

viridin

viridobufagin

virile

virilescence

virilia

virilism
- adrenal v.

virility

virilization

virilize

virilizing

virion

viripotent

virocyte

virogene

virogenetic

viroid

virolactia

virologist

virology

viromicrosome

viropexis

viroplasm

virose
virosis (viroses)
virostatic
Viro-Tec suture
Virtus forceps
virucidal
virucide
virulence
virulent
virulicidal
viruliferous
viruria
virus
    Abelson murine leukemia v.
    acute
      laryngotracheobronchitis v.
    adeno-associated v. (AAV)
    Amapari v.
    animal v's
    Apeú v.
    Apoi v.
    arbor v's (arbovirus)
    Argentine hemorrhagic fever v.
    arthropod-borne v.
    attenuated v.
    Australian X disease v.
    B v.
    bacterial v.
    Bangui v.
    Banzi v.
    Batai v.
    bat salivary gland v.
    Bhanja v.
    Bittner v.
    Bolivian hemorrhagic fever v.
    Brunhilde v.
    Bunyamwera v.
    Bussuquara v.
    Bwamba fever v.
    CA v.
    Cache valley v.
    California v.
    California encephalitis v.
    California myxoma v.
    Calovo v.
    cancer-inducing v.
    Candiru v.
    Carparu v.
    Catu v.
    CCA (chimpanzee coryza
      agent) v.
    CELO (chicken-embryo-
      lethalorphan) v.
    central European tick-borne
      encephalitis v.

virus *(continued)*
    Chagres v.
    Chandipura v.
    Changuinola v.
    Chenuda v.
    Chikungunya v.
    Coe v.
    Colorado tick fever (CTF) v.
    Columbia SK v.
    common cold v's
    Congo v.
    contagious pustular
      dermatitis v.
    coryza v.
    cowpox v.
    Coxsackie v. [now:
      coxsackievirus]
    Crimean-Congo hemorrhagic
      fever v.
    Crimean hemorrhagic fever v.
    croup-associated (CA) v.
    CTF (Colorado tick fever) v.
    C-type v.
    cytomegalic inclusion disease v.
    defective v.
    dengue v.
    DNA v's
    Dugbe v.
    Duvenhage v.
    eastern equine
      encephalomyelitis v.
    EB (Epstein-Barr) v.
    Ebola v.
    EEE (eastern equine
      encephalomyelitis) v.
    EMC (encephalomyocarditis) v.
    encephalomyocarditis
      (EMC) v.
    enteric v.
    enteric cytopathogenic bovine
      orphan (ECBO) v.
      [now: ecbovirus]
    enteric cytopathogenic dog
      orphan (ECDO) v.
      [now: ecdovirus]
    enteric cytopathogenic human
      orphan (ECHO) v.
      [now: echovirus]
    enteric cytopathogenic
      monkey orphan
      (ECMO) v. [now: ecmovirus]
    enteric cytopathogenic swine
      orphan (ECSO) v.
      [now: ecsovirus]
    enteric orphan v's

virus *(continued)*

    epidemic keratoconjunctivitis v.
    epidemic pleurodynia v.
    Epstein-Barr v., (EB v., EBV)
    equine encephalomyelitis v.
    equine influenza v.
    Everglades v.
    exanthematous disease v.
    FA v.
    filamentous bacterial v.
    filterable v.
    filtrable v.
    v. fixé
    fixed v.
    foamy v.
    Friend v.
    Ganjam v.
    German measles v.
    Germisten v.
    Graffi v.
    granulosis v.
    Gross v.
    Guama v.
    Guaroa v.
    Hantaan v.
    Hazara v.
    helper v.
    hemadsorption v., type 1
      (HA1)
    hemadsorption v., type 2
      (HA2)
    hemagglutinating v. of Japan
    hemorrhagic fever v.
    hepadna v.
    hepatitis v.
    hepatitis A v. (HAV)
    hepatitis B v. (HBV)
    hepatitis C v. (HCV)
    hepatitis D v. (HDV)
    hepatitis delta v.
    hepatitis E v.
    hepatitis G v. (HGV)
    hepatitis GB v. (HGBV, HGBV-
      A, HGBV-B, HGBV-C)
    herpangina v.
    herpes B v.
    herpes simplex v. (HSV)
    herpes zoster v.
    human immunodeficiency v.
      (HIV)
    human papilloma v. (HPV)
    human T-lymphotropic v. 1
      (HTLV-1)
    human T-lymphotropic v. 2
      (HTLV-2)

virus *(continued)*

    human wart v.
    Ilesha v.
    Ilheus v.
    immunodeficiency v.
    inclusion v.
    inclusion conjunctivitis v.
    infectious porcine
      encephalomyelitis v.
    infectious wart v.
    influenza v.
    Ingwavuma v.
    iridescent v.
    Itaqui v.
    Japanese B encephalitis v.
    JC v.
    JH (Johns Hopkins) v.
    Junin v.
    K v.
    Karimabad v.
    Kemerovo v.
    Keystone v.
    Korean hemorrhagic fever v.
    Kumba v.
    Kyasanur Forest disease v.
    lactic dehydrogenase v.
    Langat v.
    Lansing v.
    Lassa v.
    Lassa fever v.
    latent v.
    latent rat v.
    Latino v.
    LCM (lymphocytic
      choriomeningitis) v.
    Lenny v.
    Leon v.
    leukemia v.
    leukemia-sarcoma v.
    Lokern v.
    louping ill v.
    Lumbo v.
    Lunyo v.
    lymphadenopathy-associated
      v. (LAV)
    lymphocytic choriomeningitis
      v. (LCM)
    lymphogranuloma venereum v.
    lysogenic v.
    lytic v.
    M-25 v.
    Machupo v.
    Madrid v.
    maedi v.
    Makonde v.

virus *(continued)*
- mammary tumor v.
- Marburg v.
- Marcy v.
- Marituba v.
- masked v.
- Mayaro v.
- McKrae herpes v.
- measles v.
- Mengo v.
- milker's node v.
- MM v.
- Modoc v.
- molluscum contagiosum v.
- Moloney v.
- monkeypox v.
- Mossuril v.
- mouse mammary tumor v.
- Mucambo v.
- mumps v.
- murine leukemia v.
- Murray Valley encephalitis v.
- Murutucu v.
- myxoma v.
- myxomatosis v.
- Nakiwogo v.
- Negishi v.
- Nepuyo v.
- neurotrophic v.
- neurotropic v.
- v. neutralization test
- newborn pneumonitis v.
- Newcastle disease v.
- non-A, non B-hepatitis v.
- nononcogenic v.
- Norwalk v.
- Ntaya v.
- Nyando v.
- Omsk hemorrhagic fever v.
- oncogenic v.
- O'nyong-nyong v.
- orf v.
- Oriboca v.
- ornithosis v.
- Oropouche v.
- orphan v's
- Ossa v.
- pantropic v.
- papilloma v.
- pappataci fever v.
- parainfluenza v.
- Parana v.
- paravaccinia v.
- parrot v.
- pharyngoconjunctival fever v.

virus *(continued)*
- phlebotomus fever v.
- Pichinde v.
- Piry v.
- pneumonitis v.
- poliomyelitis v.
- polyoma v.
- Pongola v.
- Powassan v.
- pox v. (poxvirus)
- pseudocowpox v.
- psittacosis v.
- Punta Toro v.
- Quaranfil v.
- rabies v.
- Rauscher v.
- respiratory syncytial v. (RSV)
- Restan v.
- Rift Valley fever v.
- Riley v.
- RNA v's
- Ross River v.
- Rous-associated v. (RAV)
- Rous sarcoma v. (RSV)
- RS (respiratory syncytial) v.
- rubella v.
- Russian autumn encephalitis v.
- Russian spring-summer encephalitis v.
- SA v.
- St. Louis encephalitis v.
- salivary gland v.
- satellite v.
- Schwartz leukemia v.
- Semliki Forest v.
- Semunya v.
- Sendai v.
- Shope papilloma v.
- sigma v.
- Simbu v.
- simian v. (SV)
- simian v. 40 (SV40)
- Sindbis v.
- slow v.
- smallpox v.
- Spondweni v.
- street v.
- Tacaribe v.
- Tahyna v.
- Tamiami v.
- Tataguine v.
- temperate v.
- Tensaw v.
- Teschen v.
- Theiler v.

V

virus *(continued)*
    Thogoto v.
    tick-borne v's
    tobacco mosaic v. (TMV)
    trachoma v.
    trivittatus v.
    tumor v.
    Turlock v.
    2060 v.
    type C v.
    U (Uppsala) v.
    Uganda S v.
    unorganized v.
    Uppsala (U) v.
    Uruma v.
    vaccinia v.
    vacuolating v.
    varicella-zoster v.
    variola v.
    Venezuelan equine
      encephalomyelitis
      (VEE) v.
    vesicular stomatitis v.
    wart v.
    WEE (western equine
      encephalomyelitis) v.
    Wesselsbron v.
    western equine
      encephalomyelitis
      (WEE) v.
    West Nile v.
    Wyeomyia v.
    Yaba v.
    yabalike disease v.
    Yale SK v.
    yellow fever v.
    Zika v.
    Zimmermann v.
virustatic
vis (vires)
    v. a fronte
    v. a tergo
    v. conservatrix
    v. formativa
    v. in situ
    v. medicatrix naturae
    v. vitae
    v. vitalis
VIS—vaginal irrigation
  smear
vis-á-vis
VISC—vitreous infusion suction
  cutter
viscera (plural of viscus)
viscerad

visceral
    v. angiography
    v. aortography
    v. arteriography
    v. larva migrans
    v. leishmaniasis
    v. schistosomiasis
    selective v. aortography
    v. syphilis
visceralgia
visceralism
viscerimotor
viscerocranium
viscerogenic
viscerography
visceroinhibitory
visceromegaly
visceromotor
visceroparietal
visceroperitoneal
visceropleural
visceroptosis
viscerosensory
visceroskeletal
visceroskeleton
viscerosomatic
viscerotome
viscerotomy
viscerotonia
viscerotrophic
viscerotropic
viscid
viscidity
viscoelasticity
viscogel
viscose
viscosimeter
    monolayer v.
    Ostwald v.
    Stormer v.
viscosimetry
viscosity
    absolute v.
    dynamic v.
    kinematic v.
viscous
viscus (viscera)
visile
vision
    achromatic v.
    binocular v.
    central v.
    chromatic v.
    color v.
    day v.

vision *(continued)*
 dichromatic v.
 direct v.
 double v.
 epileptic panoramic v.
 facial v.
 foveal v.
 gun-barrel v.
 half v.
 halo v.
 haploscopic v.
 indirect v.
 iridescent v.
 low v.
 monocular v.
 multiple v.
 night v.
 v. null
 v. obscure
 oscillating v.
 peripheral v.
 photopic v.
 Pick v.
 pseudoscopic v.
 rainbow v.
 rod v.
 scotopic v.
 shaft v.
 solid v.
 stereoscopic v.
 triple v.
 tubular v.
 tunnel v.
 twilight v.
 violet v.
 word v.
 yellow v.
Visipaque
visor
 v. osteotomy
 v./sandwich osteotomy
Visscher-Bowman test
visual
 v. acuity
 v. axis
 v. cliff
 v. cortex
 v. evoked potential (VEP)
 v. field examination
 v. purple
visualization
 double-contrast v.
 laryngoscopic v.
visualize
visuoauditory

visuognosis
visuopsychic
visuosensory
visus
 v. decoloratus
 v. diminutus
 v. diurnus
 v. nocturnus
 v. senilis
 v. triplex
visuscope
vita glass
vitagonist
vital
vitalism
vitality
 pulp v.
Vitallium
 drill
 implant
 mesh
 prosthesis
 screw
vitamer
vitamin
 v. A
 v. A_1 [A1]
 v. A_2 [A2]
 v. A acid
 v. A esters
 anticanitic v.
 antihemorrhagic v.
 anti-infection v.
 antineuritic v.
 antipellagra v.
 antirachitic v.
 antiscorbutic v.
 antisterility v.
 antixerophthalmic v.
 v. B
 v. B_1 [B1]
 v. B_2 [B2]
 v. B_2 phosphate
 v. B_6 [B6]
 v. B_{12} [B12]
 v. B_{12b} [B12b]
 v. B_{17} [B17]
 v. B_c [Bc]
 v. B_c [Bc] conjugate
 v. B complex
 v. B_t [Bt]
 v. C
 v. D
 v. D_2 [D2]
 v. D_3 [D3]

V

vitamin *(continued)*
    v. D_4 [D4]
    v. E
    fat-soluble v's
    v. G
    v. H
    v. K
    v. K_1 [K1]
    v. K_2 [K2]
    v. K_3 [K3]
    v. L
    v. M
    v. P
    permeability v.
    therapeutic v's
    water-soluble v's
vitaminogenic
vitaminoid
vitaminology
vitanition
vitellarium
vitellary
vitellicle
vitellin
vitelline
vitellogenesis
vitellolutein
vitellomesenteric
vitellorubin
vitellose
vitellus ovi
vitiate
vitiatin
vitiation
vitiliginous
vitiligo (vitiligines)
    v. capitis
    Cazenave v.
    Celsus v.
    circumscribed v.
    v. iridis
    perinevic v.
vitium
    v. conformationis
    v. cordis
    v. primae formationis
vitodynamics
Vitrasert
vitrectomy
    open sky v.
    pars plana v.
vitrector
    Kaufman v.
vitreocapsulitis
vitreoretinal

vitreoretinopathy
    familial exudative v.
vitreous
    anterior v.
    v. base
    v. body
    v. bulge
    detached v.
    v. floater
    v. hemorrhage
    v. humor
    v. opacity
    persistent hyperplastic
      primary v.
    primary v.
    primary persistent
      hyperplastic v.
    secondary v.
    v. tap
    tertiary v.
    v. touch
vitreum
vitrina
vitriol
    blue v.
vitritis
vitropressure
vividialysis
vividiffusion
viviparity
viviparous
vivipation
vivisection
vivisectionist
Vladimiroff operation
Vladimiroff-Mikulicz amputation
VLBW—very low birth weight
VLDL—very-low-density
    lipoprotein
V leads: V_1–V_6 [V1–V6]
VMA—vanillylmandelic acid
    (test)
V_{max} [V-max]—maximum velocity of
    an enzyme-catalyzed reaction
VMD—Doctor of Veterinary
    Medicine (L. Veterinariae
    Medicinae Doctor)
VMR—vasomotor rhinitis
VN—virus-neutralizing
VNS—villonodular synovitis
VO—verbal order
vocal
vocalization
    epileptic v.
    iterative v.

voces (plural of vox)
vocis (genitive of vox)
Voegtlin unit
Vogel
     curet
     operation
Voges-Proskauer
     broth
     reaction
     test
Vogt
     angle
     cataract
     cornea
     degeneration
     disease
     girdle
     point
     syndrome
Vogt-Hueter point
Vogt-Koyanagi syndrome
Vogt-Koyanagi-Harada syndrome
Vogt-Spielmeyer disease
Vohwinkel syndrome
voice
     amphoric v.
     bronchial v.
     cavernous v.
     double v.
     eunuchoid v.
     myxedema v.
     whispered v.
voiceprint
void
voiding
     v. cystourethrography (VCUG)
     isotope v. cystourethrography
        (IVCU)
     radionuclide v.
        cystourethrography
Voigt
     boundary lines
     line
Voillemier point
Voit nucleus
voix de Polichinelle
vola (volae)
     v. manus
     v. pedis
volar
volardorsal
volaris
volatile
volatilization
volatilize

volatilizer
volenti non fit injuria
Volhard
     nephritis
     test
Volhard and Fahr method
volition
volitional
Volkmann
     canal
     contracture
     curet
     deformity
     disease
     membrane
     operation
     paralysis
     retractor
     splint
     spoon
     subluxation
volley
     antidromic v.
Vollmer test
volt (V)
     electron v. (eV; ev)
voltage
     effective v.
     inverse v.
     peak v.
     pulsating v.
     ripple v.
voltaic
voltaism
voltammeter
voltampere
voltmeter
     electrostatic v.
     sphere gap v.
Voltolini
     disease
     tube
volume
     alveolar v.
     alveolar dead-space v.
     atomic v.
     blood v.
     circulation v.
     v. of circulation
     v. content
     v. of distribution
     end-diastolic v. (EDV)
     end-systolic v. (ESV)
     expiratory reserve v. (ERV)
     forced expiratory v. (FEV)

V

volume *(continued)*
    gram-molecular v.
    v. imaging
    inspiratory reserve v. (IRV)
    inspiratory triggering v.
    maximal expiratory v.
    mean corpuscular v. (MCV)
    minute v.
    molar v.
    normal v.
    packed-cell v. (PCV)
    v. of packed red cells (VPRC)
    partial v.
    plasma v.
    red cell v.
    residual v. (RV)
    standard v.
    stroke v. (SV)
    target v.
    tidal v.
volumetric
volumette
volumometer
voluntary
voluntomotory
volute
volutin granules
volvulate
volvulosis
volvulus
    v. of colon
    gastric v.
    v. neonatorum
vomer
vomerine
vomerobasilar
vomeronasal
vomica
    nux v.
vomit
    Barcoo v.
    bilious v.
    black v.
    coffee-grounds v.
vomiting
    cerebral v.
    cyclic v.
    dry v.
    explosive v.
    fecal v.
    hysterical v.
    morning v.
    periodic v.
    pernicious v.
    v. of pregnancy

vomiting *(continued)*
    projectile v.
    recurrent v.
    stercoraceous v.
vomitive
vomito negro
vomitory
vomiturition
vomitus
    coffee-grounds v.
    v. cruentus
    v. gravidarum
    v. matutinus
von Bergmann hernia
von Burow operation
von Economo
    disease
    encephalitis
von Fernwald sign
von Gies joint
von Haberer-Finney
    gastroenterostomy
von Hippel (Hippel)
    disease
    keratoplasty
    operation
    trephine
von Hippel-Lindau
    disease
    syndrome
von Kossa stain
von Petz clamp
von Poehl test
von Saal pin
von Sonnenberg sump drain
    catheter
von Willebrand (Willebrand)
    disease
    factor
    factor deficiency
    syndrome
Voorhees
    bag
    needle
Voronoff operation
vortex (vortices)
    coccygeal v.
    v. coccygeus
    v. cordis
    v. dystrophy
    Fleischer v.
    v. of heart
    v. lentis
    vortices pilorum
vorticose

VOS—vision, left eye
(L. visio oculus sinister)
Vossius lenticular ring
Vossius ring
voussure
vox (voces)
  v. cholerica
voxel (*vol*ume *el*ement)
voyeur
voyeurism
VP—
    variegate porphyria
    vasopressin
    venipuncture
    venous pressure
    volume pressure
    vulnerable period
V&P—vagotomy and pyloroplasty
VPB—ventricular premature beat
VPC—
    ventricular premature
      complex
    ventricular premature
      contraction
    volume of packed cells
    volume per cent
VPD—ventricular premature
depolarization
VPF—vascular permeability factor
V-plasty
VPRC—volume of packed red cells
V/Q
    distribution
    imbalance
    nonuniformity
    ratio
    scan
V/Q—ventilation-perfusion
VR—
    valve replacement
    vascular resistance
    venous return
    ventilation ratio
    vocal resonance
    vocational rehabilitation
VR&E—vocational rehabilitation
and education
VRI—viral respiratory infection
Vrolik disease
vs—vibration seconds
vs.—against (L. versus)
VS—
    vaccination scar
    venisection
    ventricular septum

VS— *(continued)*
    verbal scale (IQ)
    vital signs
    volumetric solution
    without glasses
VSD—ventricular septal
defect
VSG—variable surface
glycoprotein
V-shaped incision
VSS—vital signs stable
VSV—vesicular stomatitis
virus
VSW—ventricular stroke
work
VT—
    tidal volume
    vacuum tuberculin
    ventricular tachycardia
V&T—volume and tension
vuerometer
vulcanite
vulcanize
vulgaris
    acne v.
    verruca v.
vulgarobufotoxin
vulnera (plural of vulnus)
vulnerability
vulnerable
vulnerant
vulnerary
vulnerate
vulnus (vulnera)
vulsella, vulsellum
    v. forceps
vulva
    v. clausa
    fused v.
vulvae
    kraurosis v.
    noma v.
vulval
vulvar
vulvectomy
vulvismus
vulvitis
    adhesive v.
    creamy v.
    diabetic v.
    diphtheritic v.
    eczematiform v.
    erosive v.
    follicular v.
    intertriginous v.

V

vulvitis *(continued)*
 irritative leukoplakic v.
 leukoplakic v.
 monilial v.
 phlegmonous v.
 plasma cell v.
 v. plasmocellularis
 pseudoleukoplakic v.
 ulcerative v.
vulvocrural
vulvopathy
vulvorectal
vulvouterine
vulvovaginal

vulvovaginitis
 infectious pustular v.
 mycotic v.
 senile v.
v/v—volume (of solute) per volume
 (of solvent)
VV—viper venom
VW—vessel wall
V-Y operation
V-Y plasty
VZ—varicella-zoster
VZIG—varicella-zoster immune
 globulin
VZV—varicella-zoster virus

ω—omega (Greek letter;
 alphabetized as o)
W—
 watt(s)
 Weber (test)
 weight
 widowed
 wife
W+—weakly positive
Waaler-Rose
 reaction
 test
Waardenburg
 disease
 syndrome
Wachendorf membrane
Wada
 prosthesis
 test
wadding
 appearance of shotgun w. on
 CT
 shot-retaining w.
Wadsworth-Todd cautery
wafer
 acrylic w.
 arthroscopic w.
 procedure
 bite impression w.
 carmustine polymer w.
 cartilage-retaining w. resection
 osteotomy

wafer *(continued)*
 dental impression w.
 Feldon open w. procedure
 Gliadel w.
 occlusal w. splint
 silicon w.
 ulna-shortening open w.
 procedure
 wax bite w.
Wagener retinitis
Wagner
 corpuscles
 disease
 hammer
 line
 punch
 spot
 syndrome
 theory
Wagner-Jauregg treatment
Wagstaffe fracture
WAIS—Wechsler Adult Intelligence
 Scale
waist
wakefulness
Waksman
Walcher position
Waldeau forceps
Waldenström
 disease
 macroglobulinemia
 syndrome

Waldeyer
    colon
    fluid
    fossa
    gland
    layer
    ring
    sulcus
Wales dilator
walk
    shuttle w. test
    6-minute walk t.
walker
    rigid w.
    rolling w.
Walker
    appliance
    carcinoma
    dissector
    lid everter
    lissencephaly
    pin
    retractor
    scissors
Walker-Warburg syndrome
walking
    w. aid
    chromosome w.
    heel w.
    reflex w.
    sleep w.
    w. stick
    w. test
wall
    anterior abdominal w.
      syndrome
    anterior gastric w.
    anterior w. of stomach
    anterior w. of tympanic cavity
    anterior w. of vagina
    axial w.
    bladder w.
    canal w. down mastoidectomy
    canal w. down
      tympanomastoidectomy
    canal w. up mastoidectomy
    canal w. up
      tympanomastoidectomy
    capillary w. of glomerulus
    carotid w. of tympanic cavity
    cavity w.
    cell w.
    chest w.
    external w. of cochlear duct
    gastric w.

wall *(continued)*
    germ w.
    gingival w.
    hollow w.
    inferior w. of orbit
    inferior w. of tympanic cavity
    inner w. of glomerular capsule
    intact canal w. mastoidectomy
    intact canal w.
      tympanomastoidectomy
    jugular w. of tympanic cavity
    labyrinthine w. of middle ear
    lateral w. of nasal cavity
    lateral w. of orbit
    lateral w. of tympanic cavity
    mastoid w. of tympanic cavity
    medial w. of middle ear
    medial w. of nasal cavity
    medial w. of orbit
    medial w. of tympanic cavity
    membranous w. of trachea
    membranous w. of tympanic
      cavity
    nail w.
    outer w. of glomerular capsule
    parietal w. of glomerular
      capsule
    party w.
    periotic w.
    posterior gastric w.
    posterior w. of stomach
    posterior w. of tympanic
      cavity
    posterior w. of vagina
    pulpal w.
    splanchnic w.
    subpulpal w.
    superior w. of orbit
    tegmental w. of middle ear
    tympanic w. of cochlear duct
    vestibular w. of cochlear duct
    visceral w.
Walldius prosthesis
Wallenberg syndrome
wallerian
    degeneration
    law
walleye
Wallgren aseptic meningitis
Wallhauser-Whitehead
    method
Walsh
    curet
    pressure ring
Walsham forceps

Walter
- bromide test
- forceps
- spud

Walter-Deaver retractor

Walthard
- cell
- cell rests
- inclusions
- islets

Walther
- clamp
- dilator
- ducts
- forceps
- oblique ligament
- sound

Walther-Crenshaw clamp

Walton
- forceps
- punch

Walton-Schubert
- forceps

Wampole test

wandering
- w. abscess
- w. atrial pacemaker
- w. cell
- dementia-related w.
- w. gallbladder
- w. goiter
- w. histiocyte
- w. kidney
- w. liver
- multiple, chaotically w.
  - electrical wavelets
- w. pacemaker lead
- w. pain
- pathologic tooth w.
- w. pneumonia
- w. rash
- w. spleen
- w. tooth

wanderlust

Wangensteen
- apparatus
- awl
- carrier
- clamp
- colostomy
- dissector
- drainage
- dressing
- forceps
- operation

Wangensteen *(continued)*
- suction
- tube

Wappler cystoscope

warbles
- cutaneous w.

Warburg
- apparatus
- technique
- theory
- vessel

Ward-French needle

Wardill
- method
- palatoplasty

Wardill-Kilner operation

Ward-Mayo vaginal hysterectomy

Ward triangle

warfare
- biological w.
- chemical w.

Waring
- method
- system

warm-blooded

Warren
- incision
- operation
- shunt

wart
- acuminate w.
- anatomical w.
- butcher's w.
- cadaver w.
- common w.
- digitate w.
- filiform w.
- flat w.
- fugitive w.
- genital w.
- Hassall-Henle w's
- juvenile w.
- juvenile plane w.
- moist w.
- mosaic w.
- necrogenic w.
- periungual w.
- Peruvian w.
- pitch w.
- plane w.
- plantar w.
- pointed w.
- postmortem w.
- prosector's w.
- seborrheic w.

wart *(continued)*
    seed w.
    soft w.
    telangiectatic w.
    tuberculous w.
    venereal w.
Wartenberg
    disease
    neuralgia
    phenomenon
    sign
    symptom
Warthin tumor
Warthin-Finkeldey cell
Warthin-Starry silver stain
warty
    w.-basaloid vulvar
       intraepithelial neoplasia
       (VIN)
    w. carcinoma
    w. changes
    w. dyskeratoma
    w. excrescences
    w. growths
    w. lesions
    w. tuberculosis
    vulvar intraepithelial
       neoplasia (VIN) of w. type
WAS—Wiskott-Aldrich syndrome
wash
    w. bottle
    eye w.
    jet w.
    mouth w.
washed
    w. clot
    w. sperm
washing
    bronchial w's
    sperm w.
washout
    w. cannula
    nitrogen w. test, single-breath
    w. pyelography
wasp
wasserhelle cell
Wassermann
    fast test
    reaction
Wassermann-fast
Wassilieff disease
wastage
    birth w.
    pregnancy w.
    reproductive w.

waste
    nitrogenous w.
    phonetic w. of the breath
wasting
    w. disease
    w. syndrome
water
    w. of adhesion
    ammonia w.
    ammonia w., stronger
    aniline w.
    aromatic w.
    bacteriostatic w. for injection
    bag of w's
    body w.
    bound w.
    w. brash
    capillary w.
    chlorine w.
    cinnamon w.
    w. of combustion
    concentrated anise w.
    concentrated camphor w.
    concentrated caraway w.
    w. of crystallization
    deionized w.
    distilled w.
    egg w.
    false w's
    w. for injection
    w. for injection, bacteriostatic
    w. for injection, sterile
    free w.
    Goulard w.
    ground w.
    hamamelis w.
    hard w.
    heavy w.
    w. of hydration
    lead w.
    lime w.
    metabolic w.
    mineral w.
    orange flower w.
    peppermint w.
    peptone w.
    potable w.
    purified w.
    rose w.
    rose w., stronger
    saline w.
    soft w.
    spearmint w.
    sterile w. for injection
    stronger ammonia w.

water *(continued)*
    stronger rose w.
    witch-hazel w.
water-borne
    w. infection
    w. transmission
Waterhouse-Friderichsen syndrome
Waterman bronchoscope
Waters
    cesarean section
    operation
    projection
    view
water-seal drainage system
watershed
    abdominal w's
    w. areas of frontal lobes
    w. basins
    w. event
    w. infarction
    parasagittal w. territory
        infarct
    w. sign
Waterston
    operation
    shunt
Watkins
    transposition operation for
        uterine prolapse
    uterine prolapse
Watkins-Wertheim operation
Watson
    method
    operation
Watson-Alagille syndrome
Watsonius watsoni
Watson-Jones
    incision
    operation
Watson-Schwartz test
Watson-Williams
    forceps
    punch
watt (W)
    w. per kilogram (W/kg)
    w. per square meter (W/m² [W/m2])
    w. per steradian (W/sr)
wattage
watt-hour
wattmeter
Watts clamp
Watzke
    forceps
    sleeve

Waugh operation
wave
    A w.
    activation w.
    afterpotential w.
    alpha w.
    anacrotic w.
    anadicrotic w.
    arterial w.
    beta w.
    brain w.
    C w.
    cannon w.
    catacrotic w.
    catadicrotic w.
    complex w's
    continuous w. (CW)
    contraction w.
    cove-plane T w.
    delta w's
    dicrotic w.
    electroencephalographic
        w's
    electromagnetic w's
    Erb w's
    excitation w.
    F w.
    ff w's
    fibrillary w's
    fibrillation w's
    flat-top w's
    fluid w.
    flutter w.
    gamma w.
    glottal w.
    H w.
    kappa w's
    lambda w's
    Liesegang w's
    light w's
    longitudinal w.
    microelectric w.
    monomorphic w.
    monorhythmic w's
    Osborne w.
    oscillation w.
    overflow w.
    P w.
    papillary w.
    percussion w.
    peridicrotic w.
    peristaltic w.
    in phase w's
    phrenic w.
    plateau w.

wave *(continued)*
    P mitrale w.
    polymorphic w's
    polyrhythmic w's
    postextrasystolic T w.
    P pulmonale w.
    predicrotic w.
    pre-excitation w.
    pulse w.
    Q w.
    QRS w.
    QS w.
    R w.
    radio w's
    random w.
    recoil w.
    respiratory w.
    S w.
    sharp w.
    shear w.
    short w.
    sine w.
    slow occipital w's
    slow posterior w's
    sonic w's
    standing w's
    Stephenson w.
    stimulus w.
    supersonic w's
    T w.
    theta w's
    tidal w.
    transverse w.
    Traube-Hering w's
    traveling w.
    tricrotic w.
    U w.
    ultrashort w.
    ultrasonic w's
    v w.
    V_1 [V1] w.
    V_2 [V2] w.
    vasomotor w.
    ventricular w.
    x w.
    y w.
waveform
wavelength
    Compton w.
    effective w.
    equivalent w.
    minimum w.
waveshape
wave-speed
  mechanism

wax
    baseplate w.
    blockout w.
    bone w.
    boxing w.
    candelilla w.
    carding w.
    carnauba w.
    casting w.
    cetyl esters w.
    w. D
    dental w.
    dental inlay casting w.
    ear w.
    emulsifying w.
    grave w.
    Horsley w.
    inlay casting w.
    inlay pattern w.
    mycobacteria w. D
    palm w.
    paraffin w.
    set-up w.
    sticky w.
    try-in w.
    tubercle bacillus w.
    utility w.
    vegetable w.
    white w.
    yellow w.
waxed and waned
    fever w.a.w.
    symptoms w.a.w.
waxing
waxing up
wax-tipped bougie
Wb—weber(s)
WB—
    weightbearing
      (weight-bearing)
    whole blood
    Willowbrook (virus)
WBC—
    white blood cell
    white blood count
WBC/hpf—white blood cell(s) per
  high-power field
WBF—whole-blood folate
WBH—whole-blood
  hematocrit
WBR—whole-body
  radiation
WC—
    whooping cough
    work capacity

W

WD—
- wallerian degeneration
- well-developed
- well-differentiated

W4D—Worth four-dot (test)

WDLL—well-differentiated lymphocytic lymphoma

WDWN—well-developed, well-nourished

wean

weaning

wear
- interproximal w.
- occlusal w.

Weavenit
- patch graft
- prosthesis

web
- antral w.
- w. of duodenum
- esophageal w.
- interdigital w.
- laryngeal w.
- pyloric w.
- subsynaptic w.
- terminal w.

Webb
- bolt
- stripper

webbed
- w. fingers
- w. neck
- w. penis
- w. toes

webbing
- congenital w. of neck
- skin w.

weber (Wb)

Weber
- catheter
- corpuscle
- disease
- glands
- insufflator
- knife
- law
- organ
- paradox
- paralysis
- point
- sign
- symptom
- syndrome
- test

Weber (continued)
- triangle
- zone

Weber-Christian
- disease
- panniculitis
- syndrome

Weber-Cockayne syndrome

Weber-Fechner law

Weber-Fergusson incision

Webster
- line
- operation
- retractor
- test

Wechsler
- Adult Intelligence Scale (WAIS)
- Intelligence Scale for Children (WISC)

Weck clip

Weck-cel sponge

wedge
- w. angiogram
- w. compression fracture
- dental w.
- w. elevator
- w. incision
- w. pressure
- pulmonary artery w. pressure (PAWP)
- w. resection
- step w.

wedge-and-groove joint

WEE—western equine encephalomyelitis

weed
- jimson w.

Weeks
- bacillus
- needle
- operation
- speculum

weep

weepiness

weeping
- w. cerebrospinal fluid (CSF) leak
- w. eruption
- w. infection
- w. lesion
- w. lymphedema
- w. nodule
- w. willow–shaped pattern
- w. sinew

weeping *(continued)*
   w. sore
   w. wound
Wegener
   granulomatosis
   syndrome
Wegner rebound effect
Weichbrodt
   reaction
   test
Weichselbaum diplococcus
Weigert
   law
   method
   stain
Weigert-Pal
   method
   technique
weight
   apothecaries' w.
   atomic w. (at. wt.)
   avoirdupois w.
   birth w., birthweight
   combining w.
   equivalent w.
   gram-atomic w.
   gram-molecular w.
   molecular w. (mol. wt.)
   troy w.
weightbearing, weight-bearing
   w. activity
   asymmetry on w.
   w. brace
   w. exercises
   w. flexion
   full w.
   limited w.
   w. position
   w. radiographs
   w. total contact cast
   w. view
   w. x-rays
weighted speculum
Weigl-Goldstein-Scheerer test
Weil
   basal layer
   disease
   forceps
   stain
   syndrome
   zone
Weil-Felix
   reaction
   test
Weill sign

Weill-Marchesani syndrome
Weill-Reys syndrome
Weill-Reys-Adie syndrome
Weinberg
   retractor
   test
Weingarten syndrome
Weinstein syndrome
Weir Mitchell
   disease
   treatment
Weisman
   curet
   forceps
Weisman-Graves speculum
Weiss
   reflex
   sign
   test
Weitbrecht
   cord
   foramen
   ligament
Weitlaner retractor
Welch bacillus
Welch-Allyn
   anoscope
   forceps
   hook
   laryngoscope
   otoscope
   probe
   proctoscope
   sigmoidoscope
   speculum
   tube
Welcker
   angle
   method
welder's lung
Welland test
well baby checkup
well-being
   sense of w.
wellness
   overall w.
   w. program
Wells syndrome
welt
wen
Wenckebach
   cycle
   disease
   heart block
   period

Wenckebach *(continued)*
    phenomenon
    sign
Werdnig-Hoffmann
    atrophy
    disease
    paralysis
    syndrome
    type
Werlhof disease
Wermer syndrome
Werner
    disease
    syndrome
    test
Werner-His disease
Wernicke
    aphasia
    area
    campus
    disease
    encephalopathy
    reaction
    sign
    syndrome
Wernicke-Korsakoff
    psychosis
    syndrome
Wernicke-Mann
    hemiplegia
    type
Wertheim
    clamp
    forceps
    operation
    radical hysterectomy
    splint
Wertheim-Cullen
    clamp
    forceps
Wertheim-Reverdin clamp
Wertheim-Schauta operation
Wesolowski prosthesis
Wesson retractor
West
    operation
    skull
    spasm
    syndrome
Westcott scissors
Wester
    clamp
    scissors
Westergren method
Westermark sign

Western
    blot electrotransfer
     test
    blot test
    blotting
western equine encephalomyelitis
    (WEE)
West Nile
    encephalitis
    fever
    virus
Westphal
    nucleus
    phenomenon
    pupillary reflex
    sign
    symptom
    zone
Westphal-Piltz
    phenomenon
    reflex
Westphal-Strümpell
    disease
    pseudosclerosis
wet mount
wet-nurse
wet prep
wet-to-dry dressing
Wetzel
    grid
    test
Weve
    electrode
    operation
Wever-Bray
    effect
    phenomenon
WF—
    Weil-Felix (reaction)
    white female
WFR—Weil-Felix
    reaction
WH—well-healed
Wharton
    duct
    gelatin
    jelly
    operation
wheal
wheat bran
wheel
    Burlew w.
    Carborundum w.
    lathe w.
    rag w.

Wheeler
    cystotome
    implant
    knife
    operation
    spatula
wheeze
    asthmatoid w.
wheezing
whelk poison
whelk poisoning
whereupon
wherewithal
W hernia
whey
whiff test
whip catheter
Whipple
    disease
    incision
    operation
    syndrome
    test
    triad
whipstitch suture
whipworm
whirlpool
    w. bath
    w. folliculitis
whisper test
whispered
    w. bronchophony
    w. pectoriloquy
    w. speech
    w. voice
    w. resonance
whispering
    postictal w. voice
Whisperjet nebulizer
whistle
    w. bougie
    w. deformity
    glottal w.
    high-pitched w. tinnitus
    inspiratory w.
    notch and w. deformity
    w. notch deformity
    peak flow w.
    slide w. breath sounds
    W. Watch device
    w. wheeze
whistle-cut aperture
whistle-tip
    w.-t. catheter
    w.-t. drain

Whitacre operation
white
    w. braided suture
    w. line of Toldt
    w. silk suture
    visual w.
White
    classification
    disease
    forceps
    operation
Whitehead operation
whiteleg
White-Lillie forceps
white matter disease
White-Oslay forceps
White-Proud retractor
Whitfield ointment
Whiting
    curet
    rongeur
    tonsillectome
whitlow
    herpetic w.
    melanotic w.
    painless w.
    perionychial w.
    thecal w.
Whitman
    frame
    operation
Whitmore
    bacillus
    disease
    fever
    melioidosis
Whitnall tubercle
WHO—World Health Organization
whole-body counting
whoop
whooping cough
WHO periodontal probe
whorl
    bone w.
    coccygeal w.
    concentric perivascular w's
    hair w's
    intravascular w's of spindle
      cells
    lens w.
    loops and w's
    w's of nerve fibers
    w. patterns
    spindle cells in w.-like fashion
    w's and streaks

whorled
  w. bundles
  w. configuration of spindle
    cells
  w. hypermelanosis
  w. hyperpigmentation
  w. nevoid hypermelanosis
  w. pattern
  w. stripes
Whytt disease
WIA—wounded in action
WIC—Women, Infants and
  Children
Wicherkiewicz operation
wick
  antibiotic-soaked w.
  cotton w.
  cotton w. soaked in mitomycin C
  ear w.
  endocervical w. sampling
  w.-in-needle method
  iris w.
  medicated w.
  mydriatic-soaked w.
  w. specimen
wicked away
Wickersheimer
  fluid
  medium
Wickham striae
Widal
  reaction
  serum test
  syndrome
  test
Widal-Abrami disease
wide-angle tomography
Widmark conjunctivitis
width
  line w.
  pulse w.
  window w.
Wiedemann syndrome
Wiener
  hook
  operation
  speculum
Wiener-Pierce rasp
Wies operation
Wigand
  maneuver
  version
Wigby-Taylor position
Wilbur-Addis test
Wild operating microscope

Wilde
  forceps
  incision
  punch
Wilde-Bruening snare
Wilder
  diet
  scoop
  sign
Wildervanck syndrome
Wilkins disease
Wilks
  disease
  symptom complex
  syndrome
will
  living w.
Willett
  clamp
  forceps
William pelvimeter
Williams
  clamp
  exercise
  forceps
  operation
  probe
  sign
  speculum
  syndrome
  tracheal tone
Williams-Campbell syndrome
Williamson
  blood test
  sign
Williams-Richardson operation
Willis
  antrum
  circle
  cords
  disease
  nerve
  pancreas
  paracusis
Wills anemia
Wilman clamp
Wilmer
  operation
  scissors
Wilms
  operation
  tumor
Wilson
  awl
  block

Wilson *(continued)*
    bolt
    chamber
    clamp
    degeneration
    disease
    leads
    lichen
    muscle
    plate
    pronator sign
    rib spreader
    stripper
    syndrome
    test
    wrench
Wilson-McKeever operation
Wilson-Mikity syndrome
Wiltberger spreader
Wimshurst machine
wind
    electric w.
windburn
windchill
windigo
windlass
    Spanish w.
window
    acoustic w.
    aortic w.
    aorticopulmonary w.
    beryllium w.
    cochlear w.
    energy w.
    found w.
    oval w.
    Rebuck skin w.
    round w.
    skin w.
    vestibular w.
windowing
windpipe
wind-sucking
Winer catheter
wing
    ash-like w.
    external white w.
    great w. of sphenoid bone
    greater w. of sphenoid bone
    w. of ilium
    w. of Ingrassia
    internal white w.
    lateral w. of sacrum
    lateral w. of sphenoid bone
    lesser w. of sphenoid bone

wing *(continued)*
    Maddox w.
    major w. of sphenoid bone
    minor w. of sphenoid bone
    w. of nose
    orbital w. of sphenoid bone
    small w. of sphenoid bone
    sphenoid w.
    w's of sphenoid bone
    superior w. of sphenoid bone
    temporal w. of sphenoid bone
    w. of vomer
Winiwarter operation
wink
    anal w.
    w. incision
    smile-w. phenomenon
Winkelman
    disease
    paralysis
winking
    w. coronary sinus
    eye-w. tics
    jaw w.
    jaw w. phenomenon
    jaw w. ptosis
    jaw w. syndrome
    Marcus Gunn jaw w. synkinesis
    opticofacial w. reflex
    w. spasm
Winkler disease
Winslow
    foramen
    ligament
    pancreas
    star
Winter arch bar
wintergreen
Wintrobe
    hematocrit
    method
    tube
Wintrobe and Landsberg method
wipe-out syndrome
wire
    alignment w.
    alveolar w.
    arch w.
    arch w., ideal
    w. bivalve speculum
    cable w. suture
    continuous loop w.
    diagnostic w.
    Gigli w. saw
    guide w., guidewire

wire *(continued)*
- interdental w.
- intraoral w.
- Ivy w.
- Johnston twin w. appliance
- K w., Kirschner w.
- Kirschner w. splint
- ligature w.
- w.-loop lesion
- measuring w.
- Medrafil w. suture
- w. mesh
- olive w.
- orthodontic w.
- over-the-w. technique
- pigtail-shaped w. tip catheter
- pull-out w. suture
- Risdon w.
- separating w.
- silver w. suture
- w. speculum
- straight-w. Alexander technique
- w. suture
- tantalum w.
- tantalum w. suture
- twin w.

wiring
- aortic aneurysm w.
- cerclage w.
- circumferential w.
- continuous loop w.
- craniofacial suspension w.
- eyelet w.
- figure-of-eight w. fixation
- figure-of-eight w. technique
- Gilmer w.
- interdental w.
- intravascular
  - ultrasound-guided w.
- Ivy w.
- Ivy loop w.
- multiple loop w.
- perialveolar w.
- piriform aperture w.
- single loop w.
- silver w.
- Stout w.
- sublaminar w.
- tension-band w.

Wirsung
- canal
- duct

wiry pulse

WISC—Wechsler Intelligence Scale for Children

Wise operation

Wishard catheter
Wishart test
Wis-Hipple laryngoscope
Wiskott-Aldrich syndrome
Wissler-Fanconi syndrome
witch hazel
withdrawal
- w. reflex
- w. symptoms
- w. syndrome
- thought w.

witigo
witkop
Witkop disease
Witkop-Von Sallman disease
Wittner forceps
Witts anemia
Witzel
- enterostomy
- gastrostomy
- operation
witzelsucht
wizened appearance
wk.—week
WL—
- waiting list
- wavelength
- work load

WM—white male
WMF—white middle-aged female
WMM—white middle-aged male
WMR—work metabolic rate
WN—well-nourished
WNF—well-nourished female
WNL—within normal limits
WNM—well-nourished male
w/o, wo—without
WO—water in oil
wobble trajectory
Wolf
- laparoscope
- method
- peritoneoscope
- syndrome

Wolfe
- graft
- operation

Wolfe-Krause graft
Wolfenden position
Wolff
- corpus
- duct
- law

Wolff-Eisner
- reaction
- test

wolffian
    w. body
    w. cyst
    w. duct
    w. vestiges
Wolff-Parkinson-White
  syndrome
Wölfler (Woelfler)
    gastroenterostomy
    sign
    suture
Wolfram syndrome
Wolfring glands
wolfsbane
Wolf-Schindler gastroscope
Wolfson
    clamp
    retractor
Wolman disease
womb
wood
    w. alcohol
    w. creosote
    Panama w.
    w. tick
Wood
    filter
    glass
    lamp
    light
    needle
    operation
    sign
wooden
    w. resonance
    w. tongue
Woodman operation
Woodson
    elevator
    spatula
woody thyroiditis
Wookey
    neck flap
    pharyngoesophageal
      reconstruction
wool
    collodion w.
    cotton w.
    lumpy w.
    w. worker's pneumonia
wooly hair disease
word salad
Woringer-Kolopp disease
working through
work-up
World Health Organization (WHO)

worm
    bilharzia w.
    bladder w.
    case w.
    w. of cerebellum
    eye w.
    flat w.
    fluke w.
    pork w.
    screw w., screwworm
    trichina w.
wormian
    w. bone
    w. ossicles
Worth
    four-dot test
    operation
wound
    aseptic w.
    avulsion w.
    blowing w.
    contused w.
    crease w. of head
    defense w's
    entrance w.
    exit w.
    hesitation w's
    incised w.
    lacerated w.
    nonpenetrating w.
    open w.
    penetrating w.
    perforating w.
    puncture w.
    septic w.
    seton w.
    stab w.
    subcutaneous w.
    sucking w.
    summer w's
    tangential w.
    tetanus-prone w.
woven
    w. bone
    w. loop stone dislodger
    w. vascular prosthesis
WP—
    weakly positive
    working point
W-plasty
W-plasty revision
WPW—Wolff-Parkinson-White
  (syndrome)
WR—
    Wassermann reaction
    weakly reactive

wraparound artifact
wrapping
    fundic w.
    vein w.
WRCs—washed red cells
WRE—whole ragweed extract
wreath
    w. cell
    daughter w.
    hippocratic w.
    w.-like arrangement
    w.-like distribution
    w.-like nuclei
    w.-like spots
    w. pattern corneal infiltrates
    w.-shaped nuclei
Wreden sign
wrench
    Wilson w.
Wright
    operation
    plate
    respirometer-spirometer
    snare
    stain
    syndrome
    version
wrinkle
    coarse w's
    fine w's
wrinkled surface
Wrisberg
    cartilage
    ganglion

Wrisberg *(continued)*
    ligament
    line
    nerve
    tubercle
wrist
    tennis w.
wristdrop
writhing in pain
writing
    mirror w.
    specular w.
wryneck
ws—watts-second
W-shaped incision
wt.—weight
Wuchereria bancrofti
wuchereriasis
Wullstein
    bur
    forceps
    knife
    operation
    retractor
Wullstein-House forceps
Wützer operation
WV—whispered voice
Wylie
    dilator
    operation
    pessary
    stripper
Wynn method
W-Y operation

Ξ—xi (Greek letter)
χ—chi (Greek letter; alphabetized
    as ch)
x—
    homeopathic symbol for the
        decimal scale of potencies
        $(1/10^x)$
    times
X—
    Kienböck unit of x-ray
        dosage
    magnification

X— *(continued)*
    start of anesthesia
    symbol for an unknown
xanchromatic
xanthan gum solution
xanthelasma
    generalized x.
    x. palpebrarum
xanthelasmatosis
xanthematin
xanthene
xanthic calculus

xanthin
xanthine
    x. bases
    x. dehydrogenase
    x. oxidase
    x. test
    tyrosine x. agar
xanthinuria
xanthinuric
xanthism
xanthochromatic
xanthochromia
    x. striata palmaris
xanthochromic
xanthocyanopsia
xanthocyte
xanthoderma
xanthoerythrodermia perstans
xanthofibroma
xanthogranuloma
    juvenile x.
    necrobiotic x.
xanthogranulomatosis
xanthogranulomatous
    x. cholecystitis
    x. pyelonephritis
xanthokyanopy
xanthoma (xanthomas,
   xanthomata)
    x. cell
    disseminated x.
    x. disseminatum
    eruptive x.
    fibrous x.
    generalized plane x.
    x. multiplex
    x. palpebrarum
    planar x.
    plane x.
    x. striatum palmare
    x. tendinosum
    tendinous x.
    x. tuberosum
    tuberous x.
    verruciform x.
xanthomatosis
    biliary hypercholesterolemic x.
    x. bulbi
    cerebrotendinous x.
    chronic idiopathic x.
    x. corneae
    x. generalisata ossium
    hypercholesterolemic x.
    x. iridis
    primary familial x.

xanthomatosis *(continued)*
    verruciform x.
    Wolman x.
xanthomatous granuloma
xanthone
xanthophore
xanthophyll
xanthopia
xanthoproteic acid
xanthoprotein
xanthopsia
xanthopsin
xanthopsis
xanthopterin
xanthosarcoma
xanthosine
    x. monophosphate (XMP)
xanthosis
xanthotoxin
xanthous albinism
xanthurenic acid
xanthuria
xanthydrol reaction
xanthyl
xanthylic acid
X axis
X-bite
X-body
XC—excretory cystogram
X chromatin
Xe—xenon
xenoantigen
xenobiotic
xenocytophilic
xenodiagnosis
xenodiagnostic
xenogeneic
    x. antigen
    x. graft
    x. transplantation
xenogenous
xenograft
    bovine valved x. conduit
    Carpentier-Edwards porcine x.
    concordant x.
    Contegra x.
    discordant x.
    Hancock porcine x.
    x. hyperacute rejection
    Ionescu-Shiley pericardial x.
    orthotopic x.
    porcine x.
    porcine dermal x.
    x. rejection
    stentless aortic root x.

xenograft *(continued)*
   x. survival
   Zimmer patch x.
xenology
xenon (Xe)
   x. arc lamp
   x. Xe 127
   x. Xe 133
xenoparasite
xenophobia
xenophonia
xenophthalmia
Xenopus laevis test
xenotransplantation
xenotropic
xenyl
xenylamine
xerocollyrium
xerocyte
xerocytosis
   hereditary x.
xeroderma pigmentosum
xerodermia
xerodermoid
   pigmented x.
Xeroform gauze
  dressing
xerogel
xerography
xeroma
xeromammography
xeromenia
xeromycteria
xerophthalmia
xerophthalmus
xeroradiography
xerosialography
xerosis
   x. conjunctivae
   conjunctival x.
   x. corneae
   corneal x.
   Corynebacterium x.
   x. cutis
   generalized x.
   x. parenchymatosa
   x. superficialis
xerostomia
xerotic keratitis
xerotomography
xerotripsis
Xg blood group
X histiocytosis
xi—Greek letter
  (Ξ; alphabetized as x)

xiphicostal ligaments of
  Macalister
xiphisternal
   x. crunching sound
   x. joint
xiphisternum
xiphocostal
xiphodidymus
xiphodymus
xiphodynia
xiphoid
   x. angles
   x. appendix
   x. bone
   x. cartilage
   x. process
xiphoiditis
xiphoomphaloischiopagus
xiphopagus
XIST gene
XLA—X-linked
  agammaglobulinemia
X-linked
   X. cutis laxa
   X. hypogammaglobulinemia
   X. ichthyosis
   X. recessive
    inheritance
XM—crossmatch
XMP—xanthosine
  monophosphate
XO—one X chromosome
XOAN—X-linked ocular
  albinism
X-Prep
x-radiation
x-ray
   hard x-r.
   x-r. microscope
   projection x-r.
    microscope
   soft x-r.
   spark x-r's
   x-r. tube
XS—xiphisternum
XT—exotropia
Xu—x-unit
XU—excretory urogram
XXY syndrome
xylan
xylene
xylidine
xylitol
  dehydrogenase
Xylocaine

xylol
xylopyranose
xylose
 D-x.
  x.-lysine-deoxycholate (XLD)
   agar
  x.-lysine-Tergitol 4 (XLTR) agar
xyloside

xylulose
 x. 5-phosphate
 x. reductase
xylyl
xysma
xyster
XYZ leads
X-zone

Y

γ—gamma (Greek letter;
  alphabetized as g)
ψ—psi (Greek letter;
  alphabetized as ps)
y—ordinate
y.—year(s)
YAG—yttrium-aluminum-garnet
YAG laser therapy
Yale SK virus
yang
Yankauer
  bronchoscope
  catheter
  curet
  esophagoscope
  forceps
  laryngoscope
  operation
  probe
  punch
  speculum
  tube
Yankauer-Little
  forceps
yarrow
Yasargil
  clip
  retractor
Yates correction
yaw
  guinea corn y.
  mother y.
  ringworm y.
yawn
yawning
  contagious y.
  disabling y.
  drug-induced y.

yawning *(continued)*
  excessive y.
  pathological y.
yaws
  crab y.
  foot y.
  forest y.
Y axis
Yb—ytterbium
Y chromatin
yd.—yard(s)
yeast
  bakers' y.
  brewers' y.
  dried y.
  y. extract
  y. extract agar
  false y.
  imperfect y.
  perfect y.
  sporogenous y.
  true y.
Yellen clamp
yellow
  acid y.
  alizarin y.
  y. atrophy
  y. blindness
  y. body of ovary
  brilliant y.
  butter y.
  canary y.
  y. cartilage
  corallin y., y. corallin
  y. cross
  y. enzymes
  fast y.
  y. fat disease

yellow *(continued)*
  y. fever
  y. fever vaccine
  y. fever virus
  y. fibrocartilage
  y. hepatization
  imperial y.
  y. jacket
  y. ligaments
  Manchester y.
  y. marrow
  Martius y.
  metanil y.
  metaniline y. (extra)
  y. mutant oculocutaneous
    albinism
  y. nail syndrome
  naphthol y.
  naphthol y. S
  y. ointment
  Philadelphia y.
  y. phosphorus
  rhubarb y.
  y. soft paraffin
  y. spot
  y. vision
  visual y.
  y. wax
Yeoman
  forceps
  proctoscope
  sigmoidoscope
Yeo treatment
yerba santa
Yergason test
Yerkes-Bridges test
Yerkes discrimination box
Yersinia
  Y. enterocolitica
  Y. frederiksenii
  Y. intermedia
  Y. kristensenii
  Y. pestis
  Y. pseudotuberculosis
yersiniosis
yew tree
YF—yellow fever
yield strength
yin
yin/yang principle
Y incision, Y-type incision
y/o, Y/O—
  year-old
  years old
YOB—year of birth

yoga
  ashtanga y.
  hatha y.
  Iyengar y.
  kundalini y.
yogurt
yohimbi bark
yohimbine
yoke
  alveolar y's of mandible
  alveolar y's of maxilla
  sphenoidal y.
yoked muscles
yolk
  accessory y.
  y. cavity
  y. duct
  egg y.
  formative y.
  y. membrane
  y. nucleus
  nutritive y.
  y. plug
  y. space
  y. stalk
yolk sac
  y.s. carcinoma
  y.s. endoderm
  y-s. placenta
  y.s. tumor
Yorke-Mason incision
Young
  clamp
  dilator
  enucleator
  forceps
  needle holder
  operation
  retractor
  rule
  syndrome
  test
  tractor
Young-Dees-Leadbetter
  procedure
Young-Helmholtz theory
Young-Millin needle holder
Yount operation
yo-yo dieting
yperite
Y-plasty
  Foley Y-p.
  Schweizer-Foley Y-p.
ypsiliform
ypsiloid

YS—
  yellow spot (of the
    retina)
  yolk sac
YST—yolk sac tumor
Y suture

Yt blood group
ytterbium (Yb) pentetate sodium
yttrium Y 90 ibritumomab
  tiuxetan
Y-type incision
Yuzpe method

Z

Z—zeta (Greek letter)
Zachary-Cope-DeMartel
  clamp
Zahn
  infarct
  lines
  ribs
Zahorsky disease
Zaleski test
Zancolli operation
Zander
  apparatus
  cells
Zappert chamber
Zaufal sign
Z/D—zero defects
ZE, Z-E—Zollinger-Ellison
  (tumor, syndrome)
zearalenone
zeatin
zebra body
zedoary
zed reaction
Zeeman effect
zein
zeiosis
Zeis glands
Zeisel test
zeisian
  z. gland
  z. stye
zeism
zeismus
Zeiss
  counting cell
  microscope
  photocoagulator
zeitgeber
Zellweger
  syndrome

Zenker
  crystals
  degeneration
  diverticulum
  fixative
  fluid
  forceps
  leiomyoma
  necrosis
  paralysis
  pouch
  solution
zenkerism
zenkerize
zeolite
zeoscope
zeranol
zero
  absolute z.
  audiometric z.
  z. balance
  z. degree teeth
  limes z.
  physiologic z.
  z. potential
Zero Balancing
zeta
  Greek letter (Z; alphabetized
    as z)
  z. potential
  z. sedimentation ratio
zetacrit
Zetafuge
zeugopodium
Z-flap incision
Zickel nail fixation
Ziegler
  cautery
  forceps
  knife

Ziegler *(continued)*
>   operation
>   probe
Ziehen test
Ziehen-Oppenheim disease
Ziehl carbolfuchsin stain
Ziehl-Neelsen
>   carbolfuchsin
>   carbolfuchsin solution
>   staining method
Zielke instrumentation
Zieman operation
Ziemssen motor point
Zierdt-Garavelli disease
Zieve syndrome
ZIFT—zygote intrafallopian transfer
zigzag
>   z. incision
>   z. laceration
zigzagplasty
Zimaloy prosthesis
Zimany bilobed flap
Zimmer
>   method
>   pin
>   prosthesis
>   screw
>   splint
Zimmerlin
>   atrophy
>   type
Zimmermann
>   corpuscle
>   pericyte
Zimmermann-Laband syndrome
zinc (Zn)
>   z. acetate
>   z. carbonate
>   z. chloride
>   z. colic
>   z. finger
>   z. finger protein
>   z. fume fever
>   z. gelatin
>   z. gelatin-impregnated gauze
>   z. gluconate
>   z. oxide
>   z. oxide-eugenol cement
>   z. oxide gauze
>   z. oxide and salicylic acid paste
>   z. phosphate cement
>   z. phosphide
>   z. poisoning

zinc (Zn) *(continued)*
>   z. protoporphyrin
>   z. stearate
>   z. sulfate
>   z. undecylenate
>   white z.
zincalism
zinciferous
zincoid
Zinn
>   annulus
>   artery
>   cap
>   circlet
>   circulus
>   corona
>   fibra
>   ligament
>   membrane
>   ring
>   tendon
>   zonule
Zinsser-Cole-Engman syndrome
Zinsser-Engman-Cole syndrome
zipper
Zipser clamp
zirconium (Zr)
>   z. granuloma
>   z. with niobium 95
Z lines
zoanthropic
zoanthropy
zoic
zoite
Zollinger forceps
Zollinger-Ellison (ZE)
>   syndrome
>   tumor
Zöllner
>   figures
>   lines
zona (zonae)
>   z. arcuata
>   z. cartilaginea
>   z. ciliaris
>   z. denticulata
>   z. dermatica
>   z. epithelioserosa
>   z. externa medullae renalis
>   z. fasciculata
>   z. glomerulosa
>   z. granulosa
>   z. hemorrhoidalis
>   z. incerta
>   z. interna medullae renalis

zona (zonae) *(continued)*
 z. ophthalmica
 z. orbicularis articulationis
  coxae
 z. pectinata
 z. pellucida
 z. perforata
 z. radiata
 z. reticularis
 z. striata
 z. tecta
 z. transitionalis analis
 z. vasculosa
zonal
 zonal aberration
 z. gastritis
 z. layer of cerebral cortex
 z. layer of superior colliculus
 z. layer of thalamus
 z. ligament of thigh
zonary placenta
zonate
Zondek-Aschheim test
zone
 abdominal z's
 active z.
 z. of adhesion
 adoral z. of membranelles
 algogenic z.
 analgesic z.
 anal transitional z.
 androgenic z.
 anelectrotonic z.
 z. of antemortem wound
 z. of antibody excess
 z. of antigen excess
 apical z.
 arcuate z.
 Barnes z.
 biokinetic z.
 border z.
 cell-free z.
 cell-poor z.
 cell-rich z.
 central z.
 cervical z.
 chemoreceptor trigger z.
 chondrogenic z.
 ciliary z.
 z. of coagulation
 comfort z.
 contact area z.
 cornuradicular z.
 coronal z.
 Cozzolino z.

zone *(continued)*
 Daseler z.
 dead z.
 definitive z. of adrenal cortex
 dendritic z.
 denticulate z.
 dentofacial z.
 z's of discontinuity
 dolorogenic z.
 dorsal z. of His
 ectopic z.
 ectopic z. of Schulte
 z. electrophoresis
 entry z.
 ependymal z.
 epigastric z.
 epileptogenic z.
 epileptogenous z.
 z. of equivalence
 ergotropic z.
 erogenous z.
 erotogenic z.
 z. of exclusion
 extravisual z's
 far z.
 fascicular z.
 fetal z. of adrenal cortex
 Flechsig primordial z's
 focal z.
 Fraunhofer z.
 Fresnel z.
 glomerular z.
 Golgi z.
 grenz z.
 H z.
 Head z's
 hemorrhoidal z.
 Hess z.
 His z's
 z's of hyperalgesia
 z. of hyperemia
 hyperesthetic z.
 hypnogenic z.
 hypogastric z.
 hysterogenic z.
 hysterogenous z.
 inhibition z.
 inner z. of renal medulla
 intermediate z. of spinal cord
 interpalpebral z.
 Kambin triangular working z.
 keratogenous z.
 language z.
 lateral z. of hypothalamus
 Lissauer marginal z.

Z

zone *(continued)*

Looser transformation z's
mantle z.
marginal z.
maturation z.
medial z. of hypothalamus
median root z.
medullary z.
mesogastric z.
motor z.
multiplication z.
near z.
nephrogenic z.
neutral z.
neutral z. of His
Nitabuch z.
notogenetic z.
nuclear z.
occlusal z.
z. of optimal proportions
orbicular z. of hip joint
organizer z.
outer z. of renal medulla
z. of oval nuclei
papillary z.
z. of partial preservation
pectinate z.
pellucid z.
perifollicular z.
peripheral z.
peripolar z.
periurethral z.
periventricular z.
placental z.
z. of plateaus and furrows
polar z.
pupillary z.
z. of rarefaction
reticular z.
Rolando z.
root z.
z. of round nuclei
rugae z.
z's of Schreger
sclerotic z.
segmental z.
Spitzka marginal z.
z. of stasis
subcostal z.
sudanophobic z.
tendinous z's of heart
thymus-dependent z.
thymus-independent z.
transformation z.
transition z., transitional z.

zone *(continued)*

transitional and
respiratory z.
triangular working z.
trigger z.
trophotropic z. of Hess
Türck z.
umbau z's
Valsalva z.
vascular z.
ventral z. of His
vermilion z.
vermilion transitional z.
visual z.
Weber z.
Weil basal z.
Wernicke z.
Westphal z.
X z.
z. of Zinn
zone plate
Fresnel z.p.
zonesthesia
zonifugal
zoning
zonipetal
zonography
stereoscopic z.
zonoskeleton
zonula (zonulae)
z. adherens
z. ciliaris
z. occludens
zonular
z. band
z. cataract
z. fibers
z. keratitis
z. spaces
zonule
ciliary z.
lens z.
z. of Zinn
zonulitis
zonulolysis
enzymatic z.
zonulotomy
zoo blot
zoochemistry
zooerastia
zoogenous
zoograft
zoografting
zooid
zoolagnia

zoology
    experimental z.
Zoon
    balanitis
    erythroplasia
zoonosis (zoonoses)
zoonotic
zoophilia
zoophilic
zoophilism
    erotic z.
zoophilous
zoophobia
zooplasty
zooprecipitin
zooprophylaxis
zoopsia
zoosadism
zoospermia
zoosporangium (zoosporangia)
zootoxin
zoster
    dermatomal z.
    disseminated z.
    herpes z.
    z. immune globulin (ZIG)
    ophthalmic z.
    z. ophthalmicus
    z. oticus
    z. sine eruptione
    z. sine herpete
    varicella z.
zosteriform
zosteroid
Zovickian flap
Z-plasty
    incision
    operation
    revision
Z-shaped incision
Zsigmondy
    gold number method
    test
ZSR—zeta sedimentation ratio
Z suture
zuckerguss
zuckergussdarm
zuckergussleber
Zuckerkandl
    bodies
    convolution
    dehiscence
    fascia
    gland
    organs

Zumbusch (von Zumbusch) psoriasis
Zung depression scale
Zwanck pessary
Zweifel-DeLee cranioclast
zwitterion
zygal fissure
zygapophyseal joints
zygapophysis (zygapophyses)
    z. inferior
    z. superior
zygia
zygion
zygodactyly
zygoma
zygomatic
    z. arch
    z. bone
    z. crest
    z. foramen of Arnold
    z. foramen of Meckel
    z. foramina
    z. fossa
    z. head
    z. margin
    z. muscle
    z. nerve
    z. process of frontal bone
    z. process of maxilla
    z. process of temporal bone
    z. region
    z. tubercle
zygomaticoauricular index
zygomaticofacial
    z. branch of zygomatic nerve
    z. foramen
    z. nerve
zygomaticofrontal suture
zygomaticomaxillary suture
zygomaticoorbital
    z. artery
    z. foramen
zygomaticosphenoid
zygomaticotemporal
    z. branch of zygomatic nerve
    z. canal
    z. foramen
    z. nerve
    z. suture
zygomaticus
    z. major muscle
    z. minor muscle
zygomaxillare
zygomaxillary
zygomycosis
zygon

Z

zygonema
zygopodium
zygosis
zygosity
zygosperm
zygosphere
zygostyle
zygote
    duplex z.
    z. intrafallopian transfer
    z. nucleus

zygotene
zygotic
zymochemistry
zymogen
    z. cell of stomach
    z. granules
    lab z.
zymogenic
zymogenous
zymosan
zymosterol